O9-AIC-725

LIPPINCOTT'S REVIEW FOR

NCLEX-RN

LIPPINCOTT'S REVIEW FOR

NCLEX-RN

SEVENTH EDITION

Diane M. Billings, RN, EdD, FAAN

Professor of Nursing and Associate Dean for Teaching
Learning and Information Resources
Center for Teaching and Lifelong Learning
Indiana University
School of Nursing
Indianapolis, Indiana

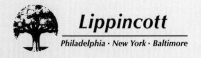

Lippincott
Philadelphia · New York · Baltimore

Acquisitions Editor: Margaret Zuccarini
Managing Editor: Barclay Cunningham
Senior Project Editor: Sandra Cherrey Scheinin
Senior Production Manager: Helen Ewan
Production Coordinator: Nannette Winski
Art Director: Carolyn O'Brien
Senior Manufacturing Manager: William Alberti
Printer: Courier/Kendallville

Edition 7

Copyright © 2002 by Lippincott Williams & Wilkins.
Copyright © 1998 by Lippincott-Raven Publishers. All rights reserved. This book is protected by copyright. No part of it may be reproduced, stored in a retrieval system, or transmitted in any form or by any means — electronic, mechanical, photocopy, recording, or otherwise — without prior written permission of the publisher, except for brief quotations embodied in critical articles and reviews and testing and evaluation materials provided by publisher to instructors whose schools have adopted its accompanying textbook. Printed in the United States of America. For information write Lippincott Williams & Wilkins, 530 Walnut Street, Philadelphia, PA 19106.

Materials appearing in this book prepared by individuals as part of their official duties as U.S. Government employees are not covered by the above-mentioned copyright.

9   8   7   6   5   4   3   2

Library of Congress Cataloging-in-Publication Data

Billings, Diane McGovern.
   Lippincott's review for NCLEX-RN.—7th ed. / Diane M. Billings.
     p. ; cm.
   Includes bibliographical references.
   ISBN 0-7817-3069-4 (alk. paper)
     1. Nursing—Examinations, questions, etc. I. Title: Review for NCLEX-RN. II. Title.
   [DNLM: 1. Nursing—Examination Questions. WY 18.2 B598L 2002]
   RT55 .B55 2002
   610.73'076—dc21   2001029913

Care has been taken to confirm the accuracy of the information presented and to describe generally accepted practices. However, the authors, editors, and publisher are not responsible for errors or omissions or for any consequences from application of the information in this book and make no warranty, express or implied, with respect to the content of the publication.

The authors, editors, and publisher have exerted every effort to ensure that drug selection and dosage set forth in this text are in accordance with the current recommendations and practice at the time of publication. However, in view of ongoing research, changes in government regulations, and the constant flow of information relating to drug therapy and drug reactions, the reader is urged to check the package insert for each drug for any change in indications and dosage and for added warnings and precautions. This is particularly important when the recommended agent is a new or infrequently employed drug.

Some drugs and medical devices presented in this publication have Food and Drug Administration (FDA) clearance for limited use in restricted research settings. It is the responsibility of the health care provider to ascertain the FDA status of each drug or device planned for use in his or her clinical practice.

Contributors

Karen Bawel, *RN, PhD*
Assistant Professor
University of Southern Indiana School of Nursing
and Health Professions
Evansville, IN

Carol Bostrom, *RN, MSN, CS*
Clinical Assistant Professor
Indiana University School of Nursing
Indianapolis, IN

Karen Cobb, *RN, EdD*
Associate Professor of Nursing
Indiana University School of Nursing
Indianapolis, IN

Linda Evinger, *MSN*
Instructor
University of Southern Indiana School
of Nursing and Health Professions
Evansville, IN

Judith A. Halstead, *RN, DNS*
Associate Professor of Nursing
Director of Instructional Services and Resources
University of Southern Indiana School
of Nursing and Health Professions
Evansville, IN

W. Gale Hoehn, *RN, MSN*
Instructor
University of Southern Indiana School
of Nursing and Health Professions
Evansville, IN

Julie L. McCullough, *PhD,RD*
Assistant Professor of Nutrition
University of Southern Indiana School of Nursing
and Health Professions
Evansville, IN

Virginia Richardson, *RN, DNS, CPNP*
Associate Professor of Nursing
Indiana University School of Nursing
Indianapolis, IN

Gayle Roux, *PhD, RN, CNS, NP-C*
Assistant Professor of Nursing
University of Southern Indiana School of Nursing
and Health Professions
Evansville, IN

Lee Schwecke, *EdD, MSN*
Associate Professor of Psychiatric Mental Health
Nursing
Indiana University School of Nursing
Indianapolis, IN

Mary Ann Wehmer, *RN, MSN, CNOR*
Instructor
University of Southern Indiana School
of Nursing and Health Professions
Evansville, IN

Contributors to Previous Editions

Susan Bennett, *RN, DNS*
Associate Professor of Nursing
Indiana University School of Nursing
Indianapolis, IN

Patricia Henry, *RN, MSN*
Lecturer
Indiana University School of Nursing
South Bend, IN

Reviewers

Coreen Arioto, MSNC, RN
School Nurse, Pasadena Unified School District
Pasadena, CA
Former Emergency Advice Manager, Kaiser
  Permanente
Los Angeles, CA

Marilyn Bratt, RN, MS
Adjunct Faculty
Marquette University, Concordia University, and
  University of Wisconsin—Milwaukee
Departments of Nursing
Mequon, WI

Donna Bumpus, MSN
Assistant Professor
Lamar University
Department of Nursing
Beaumont, TX

Patricia Clark
Associate Professor of Nursing
Abraham Baldwin College
Division of Nursing
Tifton, GA

Patricia Dumphy, MSN, RNC
Perinatal Clinical Nurse Specialist/Lecturer
University of Pennsylvania
School of Nursing
Philadelphia, PA

Linda Ferguson, RN, MN
Professor
University of Saskatchewan
Department of Nursing
Saskatoon, Saskatchewan

Regina Grazel, RNC, MSN, CNSC
Clinical Nurse Specialist—Perinatal
Our Lady of Lourdes Medical Center
Camden, NJ
Clinical Instructor Maternal–Child Nursing
Villanova University
Villanova, PA

Janet Gysi, MA, ARNP-C
Associate Professor of Nursing
Abraham Baldwin College
Division of Nursing
Tifton, GA

Dorothy Herron, RN, CS, PhD
Assistant Professor
University of Maryland
Adult Health Department
Baltimore, MD

Mary Ellen Howell, MN, RNC
Instructor
Medical University of South Carolina
  at Francis Marion College of Nursing
Florence, SC

Marty Hucks, MN, FNP
Nursing Instructor
Medical University of South Carolina
  at Francis Marion College of Nursing
Florence, SC

Elizabeth Jerabeck, RN, BSN
Senior Nurse Counselor, Viahealth Link
  Call Center
Rochester, NY

Jodi MacLennan, RN, CAN, QMRP
Director of Health and Human Resources
Partnerships for Minnesota Futures, Inc.
St. Paul, MN

Dorothy Obester, PhD, MSN, BSN

Professor of Nursing
Saint Francis College of Nursing
Loretto, PA

Karen Koozer Olson, PhD, FNP-CS

Professor and Outreach Coordinator
Texas A&M University—Corpus Christi
School of Nursing and Health Sciences
Corpus Christi, TX

Kathy Roberts, RN, MSN

Assistant Professor
Lamar University
Department of Nursing
Beaumont, TX

Pamela Stetina, RN, MN

Assistant Professor of Nursing
Texas A&M University—Corpus Christi
School of Nursing and Health Sciences
Corpus Christi, TX

Patricia Stockert, RN, MS

Associate Professor
St. Francis Medical Center
College of Nursing
Peoria, IL

Donna Wilsker, RN, MSN

Assistant Professor
Lamar University
Department of Nursing
Beaumont, TX

Preface

This book and the accompanying CD-ROM are written for students and nurses who are preparing to take the NCLEX-RN licensing exam. Students also find this book helpful for review when preparing for course exams, final exams, or competency exams.

This book includes:

- Approximately 4,000 practice test questions
- Questions written for all clinical areas of nursing (child-bearing family and their neonate; nursing care of infants, children, and adolescents; nursing care of adults with medical and surgical health problems; and nursing care of clients with psychiatric disorders and mental health problems)
- Questions organized by health problems to facilitate review for course-specific exams
- Questions with teaching feedback and rationale for both correct and incorrect answers
- Questions using figures, diagrams, and illustrations to test analysis and critical thinking
- Questions to provide practice for calculating drug dosage and intravenous drip rates
- Questions in a special section at the end of each unit on general client needs to emphasize important NCLEX-RN test plan categories of growth and development, pharmacologic and parenteral therapies, and management of care
- Questions emphasizing current nursing practice in the areas of home care, health promotion, cancer nursing, end-of-life care, perioperative care and community health
- Questions organized in five comprehensive tests designed to resemble the format of the NCLEX-RN

- A CD-ROM with more than 1,000 questions. The CD-ROM simulates NCLEX questions by using questions formatted for a computer screen, a mouse interface, and a pulldown calculator. The CD-ROM can be used to customize tests for specific review and practice.
- A description of the current NCLEX-RN test plan of the National Council of State Boards of Nursing, Inc.
- A tear-out study plan and checklist to guide systematic preparation for the licensing examination
- Information about developing study skills, taking multiple choice examinations, and managing test anxiety
- Tips for studying from students who have successfully passed the NCLEX-RN exam
- Address and telephone number of the National Council of State Boards of Nursing. Inc., and for each state board of nursing

I would like to acknowledge the item writers for this edition—Karen Bawel, Carol Bostrom, Karen Cobb, Linda Evinger, Judith Halstead, Gale Hoehn, Julie McCollough, Virginia Richardson, Gayle Roux, Lee Schwecke, Mary Ann Wehmer—nationally recognized content experts, creative test-item writers, and valued colleagues. Thanks go to Lisa Gillen, Resarach Assistant. Thanks also to Jennifer Brogan, Acquisitions Editor; Barclay Cunningham, Managing Editor; and Hilarie Surrena, Editorial Assistant—the Lippincott Williams & Wilkins team who brought this book to life.

This edition of the book is dedicated to Karen Cobb, consummate item writer, valued colleague.

Diane M. Billings, EdD, RN, FAAN

Contents

Introduction

OVERVIEW OF THIS BOOK AND CD-ROM

This review book and CD-ROM have been developed to help you prepare for the National Council of State Boards of Nursing Licensing Examination for Registered Nurses (NCLEX-RN) and other nursing exams you will encounter while you are in nursing school and beyond. The test items in the book are organized around major clinical areas of nursing: obstetric nursing, pediatric nursing, medical-surgical nursing, and psychiatric nursing. Each test presents a variety of situations commonly encountered in nursing practice.

The first section of the book is organized according to the four major areas of clinical nursing practice. Within these areas, tests are grouped according to health problems. The final test at the end of each clinical section provides additional practice in the areas of growth and development, pharmacologic and parenteral therapies, and management of care. The second section of the book contains five comprehensive exams written to simulate the NCLEX-RN by placing test items in random order.

This book also has a CD-ROM with more than 1,000 questions. You may take a test in the four content areas, arrange a test to present questions in random order, or select questions for particular review and practice. You will be able to print out test results to gauge your progress. The CD-ROM is designed to simulate the actual NCLEX-RN exam by formatting questions on a computer screen and using the keyboard and mouse to answer the questions. (For more information, see the Website for the National Council of State Boards of Nursing, Inc. at http://www.ncsbn.org) It also features a pull-down calculator for use in answering questions that require you to calculate drug doses and drip rates for intravenous infusions.

HOW TO USE THIS BOOK AND CD-ROM

We suggest that you begin your review by using the practice exams in the book to identify areas of strength and areas needing further study. Each exam contains specific case-study questions written in the style of the NCLEX-RN. Answers include rationales and are coded according to the NCLEX-RN test plan, including step of the nursing process and client needs categories. You may wish to score the results of each practice test and identify areas that need further review. Pay particular attention to the last test in each clinical section, called General Client Needs. The questions in this section have been designed to provide additional practice in the areas that have presented difficulty for test applicants. To evaluate your results after completing each exam, divide the number of your correct responses by the total number of questions in the test and multiply by 100. For example, if you answered 72 of 90 items correctly, you would divide 72 by 90 and multiply by 100, for a result of 80%. If you answered more than 75% of the items in an area correctly, you are most likely prepared to answer questions in that area on the NCLEX-RN. If you answered fewer than 75% of the questions correctly, you need to determine why. Did you answer incorrectly because of lack of content knowledge or because you did not read carefully? Use this information to guide your study.

After reviewing the specific content areas in the practice exams, take the comprehensive exams. These exams more realistically reflect the NCLEX-RN because each test presents a variety of situations commonly encountered in nursing practice and across all clinical disciplines. Underlying knowledge, skills, and abilities related to the basic physiopsychosocial sciences, fundamentals of nursing, pharmacology and other therapeutic measures, communicable diseases, legal and ethical considerations, and nutrition are included in items as needed to plan nursing care for individual clients or groups of clients.

Finally, use the CD-ROM to simulate taking computerized adaptive tests. Note how the questions are presented on the computer screen, and practice answering questions without using a pencil. Use the diagnostic features of the CD-ROM to identify areas for further study and develop your own customized test for focused review.

INFORMATION ABOUT THE LICENSING EXAMINATION

The NCLEX-RN is administered to graduates of nursing schools to test the knowledge, abilities, and skills necessary for entry-level safe and effective nursing practice. The examination is developed by the National Council of State Boards of Nursing, Inc., an organization with representation from all state boards of nursing.[1] The same examination is used in all 50 states, the District of Columbia, and United States possessions. Students who have graduated from baccalaureate, diploma, and associate-degree programs in nursing must pass this examination to meet licensing requirements in the United States.

THE TEST PLAN

The National Council of State Boards of Nursing, Inc. prepares the test plan used to develop the licensing examination. The test plan, or framework of the examination, is based on the results of a job analysis conducted every 3 years of the entry-level performance of newly licensed registered nurses, and on expert judgement provided by members of the National Council's Examination Committee and a Job Analysis Panel of Experts.[1] The questions are written by nurse clinicians and nurse educators nominated by the Council of State Boards of Nursing to serve as item writers, and they reflect nursing practice in all parts of the country.

The questions for the test are formulated on health care situations that registered nurses commonly encounter, addressing two components: (1) client needs categories and (2) integrated concepts and process such as the nursing process, caring, communication and documentation, cultural awareness, self-care, and teaching/learning (Table 1). Representative items test knowledge of these components as they relate to specific health care situations in all of the four major areas of client needs. The questions developed for the test plan were written to test knowledge, comprehension, application, and analysis of nursing knowledge at these levels of the cognitive domain; most of the questions on the NCLEX-RN test at the level of application and analysis. The following sections explain how the nursing process, client needs and related subcategories, and cognitive levels are used to formulate test questions.

The Nursing Process

The five phases of the nursing process are: (1) assessment, (2) analysis, (3) planning, (4) implementation, and (5) evaluation. The NCLEX-RN test plan includes questions from all steps of the nursing process.

Assessment. Assessment involves establishing a data base. The nurse gathers objective and subjective information about the client, then verifies the data and communicates information gained from the assessment.

Analysis. Analysis involves identifying actual or potential health care needs or problems based on assessment data. The nurse interprets the data, collects additional data as indicated, and identifies and communicates the client's nursing diagnoses. The

TABLE 1.
TEST PLAN STRUCTURE

The framework of *Client Needs* was selected for the NCLEX-RN examination because it provides a universal structure for defining nursing actions and competencies across all settings for all clients.

Client Needs

Four major categories of *Client Needs* organize the content of the *NCLEX-RN®* Test Plan. These client needs are further divided into subcategories that define the content contained within each of the four major *Client Needs* categories. These categories and subcategories are:

A. Safe, Effective Care Environment
    1. Management of Care
    2. Safety and Infection Control
B. Health Promotion and Maintenance
    3. Growth and Development Through the Life Span
    4. Prevention and Early Detection of Disease
C. Psychosocial Integrity
    5. Coping and Adaptation
    6. Psychosocial Adaptation
D. Physiologic Integrity
    7. Basic Care and Comfort
    8. Pharmacologic and Parental Therapies
    9. Reduction of Risk Potential
    10. Physiologic Adaptation

Integrated Concepts and Processes

The following concepts and processes fundamental to the practice of nursing are integrated throughout the four major categories of *Client Needs*:

- Nursing Process
- Caring
- Communication and Documentation
- Cultural Awareness
- Self-care
- Teaching/Learning

Used by permission of the National Council of State Boards of Nursing, Inc., Chicago, IL

nurse also determines the congruency between the client's needs and the ability of the health care team members to meet those needs.

Planning. Planning involves setting goals for meeting the client's needs and designing strategies to attain those goals. The nurse determines the goals of care, develops and modifies the plan, collaborates with other health team members for delivery of the client's care, and formulates expected outcomes of nursing interventions.

Implementation. Implementation involves initiating and completing actions necessary to accomplish the defined goals. The nurse organizes and manages the client's care; performs or assists the client in performing activities of daily living; counsels and teaches the client, significant others, and health care team members; and provides care to attain the established client goals. The nurse also provides care to optimize the achievement of the client's health care goals; supervises, coordinates, and evaluates delivery of the client's care as provided by nursing staff; and records and exchanges information.

Evaluation. Evaluation determines goal achievement. The nurse compares actual with expected outcomes of therapy, evaluates compliance with prescribed or proscribed therapy, and records and describes the client's response to therapy or care. The nurse also modifies the plan, as indicated, and reorders priorities.

The five phases of the nursing process are equally important. Therefore, each is represented by an equal number of items on the NCLEX-RN, and integrated throughout the exam.

Client Needs Categories

The health needs of clients are grouped under four broad categories: (1) safe, effective care environment; (2) health promotion and maintenance; (3) psychosocial integrity; and (4) physiologic integrity. Each category of needs includes subcategories of related and specified needs (Table 2). The percentage of test items in each subcategory on the NCLEX-RN examination is shown in Table 3.

Cognitive Level of Questions

Each test item is written to test a variety of levels of the cognitive domain. The cognitive level of questions refers to the type of mental activity required to answer the question as defined in a taxonomy of the cognitive domain.[2] The lowest level of the taxonomy is the *knowledge* level, the ability to recall facts about principles, concepts, theories, terms, or procedures. Questions at this level ask you to define, identify, or select. *Comprehension* requires understanding data; questions ask you to interpret, explain, distinguish, or predict. *Application* involves using information in new situations. At this level, you are expected to solve problems, modify plans, manipulate data, and demonstrate appropriate use of information. *Analysis* requires recognizing relationships between parts. Questions at this level ask you to analyze, evaluate, select, differentiate, or interpret data from a variety of sources, and to think critically and set priorities. The highest level of the cognitive domain is *synthesis*. Here you must put data together in new and meaningful ways. Test questions can be written to test at all levels of the

cognitive domain, but those questions that are written for the NCLEX-RN are generally written at knowledge, comprehension, application, and analysis levels, with the majority of the questions testing at the levels of application and analysis.

The Test Items

Each test item of the NLCEX-RN has been developed as a performance-based multiple choice question.[3] The *background (situation)* is a client-based scenario that gives information about the client that is needed to answer the question. The question that follows is based on the information given in the situation. As you answer the question, relate the answer to the background information. Pay particular attention to information about the client's age, family status, health status, ethnicity, or point in the care plan (eg, early admission versus preparation for discharge).

The *stem (question)* poses the problem to solve. The stem may be written as a direct questions, such as "what should the nurse do first?" or as an incomplete sentence such as "The nurse should..."

The answers (options) are possible responses to the stem. Each stem has one correct option and three incorrect options. The options may be written as complete sentences or may complete the sentence stated as a question.

The test questions also use figures, diagrams, and tables to frame the question and answers.[4] For example, the candidate may be asked to look at an ECG strip and analyze the data or determine nursing priorities. The test questions will also use figures and diagrams to ask the candidate to identify parts of a figure (eg, to identify the location for the site of an intramuscular injection).

EXAM FORMAT

Computer Adaptive Testing

The NCLEX-RN is administered using computer adaptive testing (CAT) procedures. CAT uses a computer to randomly generate questions from an item pool in order to administer individually tailored examinations. CAT has several advantages. For example, an exam can be given in less time because there are potentially fewer questions for each candidate. CAT exams also can be administered frequently, allowing a graduate of a nursing program to take the exam close to graduation, receive the results quickly, and enter the work force as a registered nurse in less time than is possible with paper and pencil exams. Study results also show that because CAT is self-paced, there is less stress on the candidate.

CAT uses the memory and speed of the computer to administer a test for each candidate. The test is generated from a large pool of questions (a test item bank) based on

TABLE 2.
CATEGORIES AND SUBCATEGORIES OF CLIENT NEEDS

A. Safe, Effective Care Environment

1. *Management of Care*—providing integrated, cost-effective care to clients by coordinating, supervising, and/or collaborating with members of the multidisciplinary health care team.

   Related content includes but is **not limited** to:

   - Advance Directives
   - Advocacy
   - Case Management
   - Client Rights
   - Concepts of Management
   - Confidentiality
   - Consultation with Members of the Health Care Team
   - Continuity of Care
   - Continuous Quality Improvement
   - Delegation
   - Establishing Priorities
   - Ethical Practice
   - Incident/Irregular Occurrence/Variance Reports
   - Informed Consent
   - Legal Responsibilities
   - Organ Donation
   - Referrals
   - Resource Management
   - Supervision

2. *Safety and Infection Control*—protecting clients and health care personnel from environmental hazards.

   Related content includes but is **not limited** to:

   - Accident Prevention
   - Disaster Planning
   - Error Prevention
   - Handling Hazardous and Infectious Materials
   - Medical and Surgical Asepsis
   - Standard (Universal) and Other Precautions
   - Use of Restraints

B. Health Promotion and Maintenance

3. *Growth and Development Through the Life Span*—assisting the client and significant others through the normal expected stages of growth and development, from conception through advanced old age.

   Related content includes but is **not limited** to:

   - Aging Process
   - Ante/Intra/Postpartum and Newborn
   - Developmental Stages and Transitions
   - Expected Body Image Changes
   - Family Planning
   - Family Systems
   - Human Sexuality

4. *Prevention and/or Early Detection of Health Problems*—assisting clients to recognize alterations in health and to develop health practices that promote and support wellness.

   Related content includes but is **not limited** to:

   - Disease Prevention
   - Health and Wellness
   - Health Promotion Programs
   - Health Screening
   - Immunizations
   - Lifestyle Choices
   - Techniques of Physical Assessment

C. Psychosocial Integrity

5. *Coping and Adaptation*—promoting the client's and/or significant others' ability to cope, adapt, and/or problem solve situations related to illnesses, disabilities, or stressful events.

   Related content includes but is **not limited** to:

   - Coping Mechanisms
   - End of Life
   - Grief and Loss
   - Mental Health Concepts
   - Religious and Spiritual Influences on Health
   - Sensory/Perceptual Alterations
   - Situational Role Changes
   - Stress Management
   - Support Systems
   - Therapeutic Interactions
   - Unexpected Body Image Changes

(continues)

TABLE 2.
CATEGORIES AND SUBCATEGORIES OF CLIENT NEEDS *(Continued)*

6. *Psychosocial Adaptation*—managing and providing care for clients with acute or chronic mental illnesses, as well as maladaptive behaviors.

Related content includes but is **not limited** to:

- Behavioral Interventions
- Chemical Dependency
- Child Abuse/Neglect
- Crisis Intervention
- Domestic Violence
- Elder Abuse/Neglect
- Psychopathology
- Sexual Abuse
- Therapeutic Milieu

D. Physiologic Integrity

The nurse promotes physical health and well-being by providing care and comfort, reducing client risk potential, and managing the client's health alterations.

7. *Basic Care and Comfort*—providing comfort and assistance in the performance of activities of daily living.

Related content includes but is **not limited** to:

- Assistive Devices
- Elimination
- Mobility/Immobility
- Nonpharmacologic Comfort Interventions
- Nutrition and Oral Hydration
- Palliative/Comfort Care
- Personal Hygiene
- Rest and Sleep

8. *Pharmacologic and Parenteral Therapies*—managing and providing care related to the administration of medications and parenteral therapies.

Related content includes but is **not limited** to:

- Adverse Effects/Contraindications
- Blood and Blood Products
- Central Venous Access Devices
- Chemotherapy
- Expected Effects
- Intravenous Therapy
- Medication Administration
- Parenteral Fluids
- Pharmacologic Actions
- Pharmacologic Agents
- Pharmacologic Interactions
- Pharmacologic Pain Management
- Side Effects
- Total Parenteral Nutrition

9. *Reduction of Risk Potential*—reducing the likelihood that clients will develop complications or health problems related to existing conditions, treatments, or procedures.

Related content includes but is **not limited** to:

- Diagnostic Tests
- Laboratory Values
- Pathophysiology
- Potential for Alterations in Body Systems
- Potential for Complications of Diagnostic Tests, Procedures, Surgery, and Health Alterations
- Therapeutic Procedures

10. *Physiologic Adaptation*—managing and providing care for clients with acute, chronic, or life-threatening physical health conditions.

Related content includes but is **not limited** to:

- Alterations in Body Systems
- Fluid and Electrolyte Imbalances
- Hemodynamics
- Infectious Diseases
- Medical Emergencies
- Pathophysiology
- Radiation Therapy
- Respiratory Care
- Unexpected Response to Therapies

Used by permission of the National Council of State Boards of Nursing, Inc., Chicago, IL

TABLE 3.
TEST PLAN AND DISTRIBUTION OF CONTENT

Categories	Percentage of Test Questions
A. Safe, Effective Care Environment	
1. Management of Care	7–13%
2. Safety and Infection Control	5–11%
B. Health Promotion and Maintenance	
3. Growth and Development Through the Life Span	7–13%
4. Prevention and Early Detection of Disease	5–11%
C. Psychosocial Integrity	
5. Coping and Adaptation	5–11%
6. Psychosocial Adaptation	5–11%
D. Physiologic Integrity	
7. Basic Care and Comfort	7–13%
8. Pharmacologic and Parenteral Therapies	5–11%
9. Reduction of Risk Potential	12–18%
10. Physiologic Adaptation	12–18%

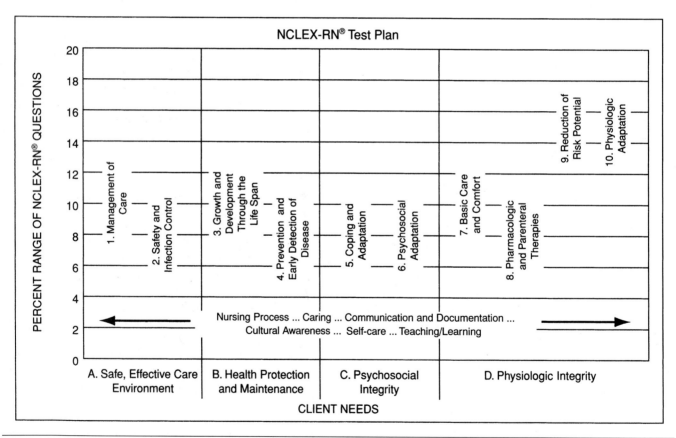

Used by permission of the National Council of State Boards of Nursing, Inc., Chicago, IL

the NCLEX-RN test plan. The examination begins as the computer randomly selects a question of medium difficulty for each candidate. The next question is based on the response to the previous question. If the question is answered correctly, an item of similar or greater difficulty is generated; if it is answered incorrectly, a less-difficult item is selected. Thus, the test is adapted for each candidate. Once competence has been determined, the exam is completed at a passing level.

The exams for all candidates are derived from the same large pool of test items. They contain comparable questions for each component of the test plan. Although the questions are not exactly the same, they test the same knowledge, skills, and abilities from the test plan. All candidates must meet the requirements of the test plan and achieve the same passing score. Each candidate, therefore, has the same opportunity to demonstrate competence. Although one candidate may answer fewer questions, all candidates have the opportunity to answer a sufficient number of questions to demonstrate competence until the stability of passing or failing is established or the time limit expires.

Exam Locations

The Council of State Boards of Nursing contracts with vendors in each state to serve as exam sites. Your school of nursing can inform you of the location nearest you. You can also contact your state board of nursing for information. (See the Appendix for the address.) You can also find updated information from the National Council of State Boards of Nursing, Inc. at its Website (*http://www.nscbn.org*).

The National Council of State Boards of Nursing, Inc. contracts with testing centers who offer the NCLEX-RN exam. Generally, each center has several computer stations equipped with adequate lighting and scratch paper for candidates' use. The computers have surge-protection devices to prevent data loss. Secured storage areas outside of the testing room are provided for storage of personal articles. Each testing center maintains comprehensive security, using audio and video camera monitoring.

The exam site is designed so that candidates can take breaks. There is a mandatory 10-minute break after 2 hours and an optional break 1.5 hours after that.

Scheduling the Examination

The first step is to apply to the state board of nursing in the state in which you plan to take the examination. Within about 30 days, you will receive an authorization to test card with information about testing centers and additional procedures. Testing centers are open Monday through Saturday, about 15 hours each day.

Computer Use and Screen Design

Test questions are presented on the computer screen (monitor); you select your answer and use the keyboard or a mouse to enter your answer. The CD-ROM included with this book provides you with an opportunity to simulate taking computer-generated examinations. At every testing site, written directions are provided at each computer exam station. There are also tutorials and practice questions on the computer that you can complete to be sure you understand how to use the computer before you begin the exam.

For further information about the NCLEX-RN, the test plan, test questions, or exam format, visit the Council's Website at *http://www.ncsbn.org*, or write to the National Council of State Boards of Nursing, Inc. For information about the dates, requirements, and specifics of writing the examination in your state, contact your state board of nursing. The addresses and telephone numbers of the National Council of State Boards of Nursing, Inc. and each state board of nursing are provided in the Appendix.

PREPARING FOR THE EXAM

Studying for the NCLEX-RN or other similar exam, requires careful planning and preparation. You can make the best use of your time by developing a systematic approach to study that includes assessing your strengths and weaknesses, developing a study plan, and evaluating progress on a regular basis. Use the Personal Study Plan in Box 1 to help develop your own study plan.

Assessing Study Needs

The first step in developing a study plan is to determine which content areas you know well and which areas you need to review further. Follow these steps to assess your knowledge, skills, and abilities:

1. **Review your success in nursing school.** Review your record of achievement in courses in the nursing curriculum. Subjects in which you received high grades, that you found easy to learn, or in which you have had additional clinical practice or work experience are likely areas of strength. On the other hand, subjects you found difficult to learn or did not achieve high grades in should be areas for concentrated review. Also consider content areas that you have not studied for a while. Recent course work will be the most familiar and, therefore, may require the least amount of study. You also can use the practice exams in this book to identify areas needing further study. Begin with the subjects you find most difficult or in which you have the least confidence.

BOX 1. PERSONAL STUDY PLAN

Assess Study Needs

1. Review your success in nursing school.

   - I did best in these courses: _____
   - I needed to study harder in these courses:_____
   - I took these courses near the beginning of the curriculum: _____
   - I scored best on these practice exams in this book: _____
   - I am not satisfied with my scores on these practice exams in this book: _____
   - I need further study in these content areas:_____
   - I need further study in these areas of the nursing process: _____
   - I need further study in these areas of client needs: _____

2. Review your test-taking skills.

   - I can identify the components of a test question.
   - I read questions carefully before answering.
   - I can make reasonable guesses if I am not certain of the correct answer.

3. Review your test-anxiety management skills.

   - I can do relaxation and deep-breathing exercises.
   - I can visualize success.
   - I can give myself positive feedback.
   - I can concentrate for extended periods of time.

4. Review your computer skills.

   - I am able to use a computer to read and answer test questions.
   - I have used the practice disk accompanying this book.

Develop a Study Plan

- I will study in this location: _____
- I will study at these times and dates: _____
- I have assembled all of the materials I need to study: _____
- I will study with a study group: _____

Evaluate Progress

- I have completed the practice tests in this book:_____
- I have completed the comprehensive tests in this book: _____
- I need to improve my scores in these areas:_____
- I am prepared to take the NCLEX-RN examination: _____

(continues)

BOX 1. PERSONAL STUDY PLAN (*Continued*)

Strategies for Taking Tests

- Read the question carefully.

- Anticipate the correct answer.

- Read for key words.

- Base answers on nursing knowledge.

- Identify the components of the test item.

Strategies for Managing Test Anxiety

- Mental rehearsal

- Relaxation

- Deep breathing

- Positive self-talk

- Distraction

- Concentration

---

2. **Assess your test-taking skills.** Using effective test-taking skills contributes to exam success. What have you done in the past to make you confident about taking a test? How do you feel when you are in the exam situation? What has worked in the past to help you be successful? Review these strategies to build on past successes and work on problem areas. Consider additional strategies suggested in the following section, Test-Taking Strategies. You can practice these skills by simulating the testing situation using the practice tests and comprehensive exams in this review book.

3. **Assess your skills for taking computer-administered exams.** Although previous computer experience is not necessary to take the NCLEX-RN, you may wish to familiarize yourself with the differences between taking a paper-and-pencil exam and taking exams administered by the computer. Use Table 4, "Differences Between Paper-and-Pencil and Computer-Administered Exams," to review these differences. If you have not used a computer before, find a learning resource center at your college, university, library, or hospital where you can become familiar with basic computer keyboard skills. Use the CD-ROM accompanying this review book to simulate the experience of taking questions using a computer. Practice reading questions from the computer screen. If you are accustomed to underlining key words or making notes in the margins of paper and pencil tests, adapt these strategies to reading and answering the questions on the computer screen.

Developing a Study Plan

Once you have identified areas of strength and areas needing further study, develop a specific plan and begin to study regularly. Students who study a small amount of content over a longer period of time tend to have higher success rates than students who wait until the last few weeks before the exam and then "cram." Consider these suggestions:

1. **Identify a place for study.** The area should be quiet and have room for your books and papers. This area might be in your home, at your nursing school, or in a library. Be sure your friends and family understand the importance of not interrupting you when you are studying.

2. **Establish regular study times.** Make appointments with yourself to ensure a commitment to study. Frequent, short study periods (1–2 hours) are preferable to sporadic, extended study periods. Plan to finish your studying 1 week before the NCLEX-RN; last-minute cramming tends to increase anxiety.

3. **Obtain all necessary resources.** As you begin to study, it is helpful to have easy access to textbooks, notes,

TABLE 4.
DIFFERENCES BETWEEN PAPER-AND-PENCIL AND COMPUTER-ADMINISTERED EXAMS

Exam Feature	Paper-and-Pencil Exams	Computer-Administered Exams
Question layout	Linear	Blocked, with stem of the question or the case study on the left, options on the right
Question design	Case study with several related questions following the case study	All information related to the question is presented in the stem
Ability to read questions randomly	Yes	No, one question presented at a time
Ability to skip question if not sure of answer	Yes	No, must answer each question before receiving the next one
Ability to underline or circle key words; make margin notes	Yes	No
Scratch paper available	Yes	Yes
Proctor	Rotates among tables	Can observe all candidates simultaneously; video monitors used
Ergonomics	Sit at desk	Sit at computer
Breaks	Yes	Yes

and study guides. Suggested readings are included at the end of each unit in this book.

4. **Make the best use of your time.** Make review cards that you can carry with you to study during free moments throughout the day. Some students tape record review notes and listen to the tapes while driving or exercising.

5. **Develop effective study skills.** Study skills enable you to acquire, organize, remember, and use the information you need to take the NCLEX-RN. These skills include outlining, summarizing, reviewing, and practicing test-taking. Some students prefer to study alone, while others benefit from study groups; know which approach works best for you, and develop your study plan accordingly. You can use this book to learn, refine, and practice your study skills. Study skill suggestions include the following:

- Use study skills with which you are familiar and that have worked well for you in the past. Recall effective study behaviors that you used in nursing school, such as reviewing highlighted text, outlines, or content maps. What are your learning style preferences? Do you study best in a quiet room, or do you prefer music in the background? Are you most alert in the morning or evening? Do you like to eat while you study? Does it help you to concentrate and learn if you make notes as you study? Learn what works best for you, and use it to optimize your study plan.

- Study to learn, not to memorize. The NCLEX-RN tests application of knowledge. When reviewing content, continually ask yourself, "How is this information used in client care?"

- Anticipate questions. As you study, formulate questions around the content. Practice giving a rationale for your answer to these questions. If you work in a study group, have each member contribute questions.

- Study common, not unique, nursing care situations. The NCLEX-RN tests minimum competence for nursing practice; therefore, focus on common health problems and client needs.

- Simulate test-taking. The comprehensive tests in Section Two of this book are designed to simulate the random order in which questions appear in the NCLEX-RN. Use these tests to focus on areas of common concern in nursing care rather than on the traditional content delineations of adult, pediatric, psychiatric, and childbearing clients. Make additional copies of answer sheets, and retake the exams on which you had low scores.

- Give yourself positive feedback. Use positive self-talk strategies to build your confidence. Reward yourself as you study. Engage in a favorite activity after a successful study session.

Evaluating Your Progress

Periodically determine if you are on schedule with your study plan. Note if your scores on the practice and comprehensive tests improve. Do not spend time on content you have mastered, on areas in which you obtained high scores on the practice exam, or on areas with which you feel confident. Set priorities for study on areas needing additional review.

TEST-TAKING STRATEGIES

Knowing how to take a test is as important as knowing the content being tested. Strategies for taking tests can be learned and used to improve test scores. Here are some suggestions for building a repertoire of effective test-taking strategies:

1. Understand the components of the test item. Typically, test items consist of a situation or background information, a question, and four possible answers (Fig. 1).
2. Understand which step of the nursing process is being tested. For example, as you read the question, determine whether the question is asking you to set priorities (planning) or judge outcomes (evaluation).
3. Understand client needs. As you read the question, consider the question in the context of client needs. Be sure to understand if the question is asking you to determine what to do "first" or to select the nursing action that is "best."
4. Read the question carefully. This is one of the most important aspects of effective test taking. Do not rush. Ask yourself, "What is this question asking?" and "What is the expected response?" If necessary, rephrase the question in your own words. Do not read meaning into a question that is not intended, and do not make a question more difficult than it is. If you do not understand the question, try to figure it out. If, for example, the question is asking about the fluid balance needs of a client with pheochro-

mocytoma and you do not remember what pheochromocytoma is, then try to answer the question based on your knowledge of principles of fluid balance. The exam questions reflect national nursing practice standards and are not written to test knowledge of procedures or practices at specific health care agencies. Thus, it is important to answer the question from the framework of best nursing practice, not unique practices.

5. Look for key words that provide clues to the correct answer. For instance, words such as *except, not,* or *but* can change the meaning of a question; words such as *first, next,* and *most* ask you to establish a priority or use an order or sequence of steps.
6. Be certain you understand the meaning of all words in the question. If you see a word you do not know, try to figure out its meaning from a familiar base of the word or from the context of the question.
7. Attempt to answer the question before you see the answers, then look for the answer that is similar to the one you generated.
8. Base answers on nursing knowledge. Remember that the NCLEX-RN is used to test for safe practice and that you have learned the information needed to answer the question.
9. If you do not know the answer, make a reasonable guess. Hunches and intuition are often correct. If you do not know the answer, do not waste time and energy; give yourself permission to not know every question, and move on to the next one. In CAT, you must answer each question before the next item is administered, and because the level of difficulty will be adjusted as you answer each question, it is likely that you will know the answer to one of the next questions.

STRATEGIES FOR MANAGING TEST ANXIETY

All test takers experience some anxiety. A certain amount of anxiety is motivating, but be prepared to control unwanted anxiety. Develop the following anxiety management strategies, practice them while you are taking the comprehensive examinations in this book, and use them during the exam as needed.

- **Mental rehearsal.** Mental rehearsal involves reviewing the events and environment during the examination. Anticipate how you will feel, what the setting will be like, how you will take the exam, what the computer screen will look like, and how you will talk to yourself during the exam. Visualize your success. Rehearse what you will do if you have test anxiety.

Background ⇩	⇩ Stem
SITUATION: The parents of children attending an elementary school and a high school invite the school nurse to attend some of their Parent-Teacher Association meetings to discuss common health problems related to their youngsters.	**QUESTION 1:** One parent asks about head lice (pediculosis capitis). The nurse discusses the symptoms with the parents. Which of the following symptoms is *most* common when a child has been infected with head lice? 1. Itching of the scalp. 2. Scaling of the scalp. 3. Serous weeping on the scalp surface. 4. Pinpoint hemorrhagic spots on the scalp surface.

⇧ Answers

Figure 1. Sample text item, computer adaptive testing format: background (situation), stem (question), and answers (options).

- **Relaxation exercises.** Relaxation exercises involve tensing and relaxing various muscle groups to relieve the physical effects of anxiety. Practice systematically contracting and relaxing muscle groups from your toes to your neck to release energy for concentration. You can do these exercises during the exam to promote relaxation.

- **Deep breathing.** Taking deep breaths by inhaling slowly while counting to 5 and then exhaling slowly while counting to 10 increases oxygen flow to the lungs and brain. Deep breathing also decreases tension and helps manage anxiety by focusing your thoughts on the breathing and away from worries.

- **Positive self-talk.** Talking to yourself in a positive way serves to correct negative thoughts (eg, "I can't pass this test" and "I don't know the answers to any of these questions") and reinforces a positive self-concept. Replace negative thoughts with positive ones, telling yourself, "I can do this" and "I studied well and am prepared."

- **Distraction.** Thinking about something else can clear your mind of negative or unwanted thoughts. Think of something fun, something you enjoy. Plan now what you will think about to distract yourself during the exam.

- **Concentration**. During the exam, be prepared to concentrate. Have tunnel vision. Do not worry if others finish the test before you. Remember that everyone has his or her own speed for taking tests and that each test is individualized. Do not rush; you will have plenty of time. Focus; do not let noises from the keyboard next to you divert your attention. Do not become overwhelmed by the testing environment. Use positive self-talk as you begin the exam.

TIPS FROM STUDENTS WHO HAVE PASSED THE NCLEX-RN

Students who have successfully passed the NCLEX-RN offer these tips for preparing for and taking this exam.

- Study regularly several months before taking the exam. Be sure you are well prepared.

- Use practice questions until you can score at least 75% on the exam. Use practice exams with at least 2,000 questions so you test yourself with a wide range of content and style of questions.

- Make sure you know the date, time, and place the exam will be given; how to get to the exam site; how long it takes to drive there; and where you can park. It may be helpful to visit the exam site and see the room where the exam will be given.

- Visualize yourself in the room, taking the test. Use mental rehearsal to practice anxiety managing strategies.

- Organize the information you will need to bring to the testing center the night before the exam. You will need to present your authorization to test. You will also need to provide two forms of identification, one of which must be photo identification (eg, driver's license or passport).

- Make sure you are physically prepared. Get enough rest before the examination; fatigue can impair concentration. If you are working, it may be advisable not to work the day before the exam; if you are working on a shift that is different from the time of the exam, adjust your work schedule several days ahead of time.

- Avoid planning time-consuming activities (eg, weddings, vacation trips) immediately before the exam.

- Do not use any drugs you usually do not use (including caffeine and nicotine), and do not use alcohol for 2 days before the exam.

- Eat regular meals before the exam. Remember that high-carbohydrate foods provide energy, but excessive sugar and caffeine can cause hyperactivity.

- Dress comfortably, in layers that can be added or removed according to your comfort level.

The authors of this review book and CD-ROM offer you our best wishes for success on any of the exams you will be taking throughout your academic career. We are confident that your review and preparation has given you a good foundation for a positive testing experience!

REFERENCES

1. National Council of State Boards of Nursing. (2000). *Test plan for the National Council Licensure Examination for Registered Nurses.* Chicago: Author.
2. Bloom, B.S. (1956). *Taxonomy of educational objectives. Handbook I: Cognitive domain.* New York: David McKay.
3. Chornick, N.L. and Wendt, A.L. (1997). NCLEX-RN: From job analysis study to examination. *Journal of Nursing Education, 36*(8), 378–382.
4. Wendt, A. & Brown, P. (2000). The NCLEX examination: Preparing for future nursing practice. *Nurse Educator, 25*(6), 297–300.

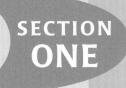

PRACTICE TESTS

PART

I

The Nursing Care of the Childbearing Family and Their Neonate

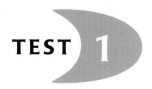

TEST 1

Antepartum Care

▶ **The Preconception Client**

▶ **The Pregnant Client Receiving Prenatal Care**

▶ **The Pregnant Client in Childbirth Preparation Classes**

▶ **The Pregnant Client With Risk Factors**

▶ **Correct Answers and Rationale**

Select the best answer and indicate your choice by filling in the circle in front of the option.

The Preconception Client

1. After the nurse instructs a 20-year-old nulligravid client on how to perform a breast self-examination, which of the following client statements indicates that the teaching has been successful?
   - ○ 1. "I should perform breast self-examination on the day my menstrual flow begins."
   - ○ 2. "It's important that I perform breast self-examination on the same day each month."
   - ○ 3. "If I notice that one of my breasts is much smaller than the other, I shouldn't worry."
   - ○ 4. "If there is some discharge from my nipples, I should avoid squeezing them."

2. Assessment of a 16-year-old nulligravid client who visits the clinic and asks for information on contraceptives reveals a menstrual cycle of 28 days. The nurse formulates a nursing diagnosis of Deficient Knowledge related to ovulation and fertility management. Which of the following would be important to include in the teaching plan for the client?
   - ○ 1. The ovum survives for 96 hours after ovulation, making conception possible during this time.
   - ○ 2. The basal body temperature falls at least 0.2°F after ovulation has occurred.
   - ○ 3. Ovulation usually occurs on day 14, plus or minus 2 days, before the onset of the next menstrual cycle.
   - ○ 4. Most women can tell they have ovulated because of severe pain and thick, scant cervical mucus.

3. Which of the following instructions about activities during menstruation would the nurse include when counseling an adolescent who has just begun to menstruate?
   - ○ 1. Take a mild analgesic for the menstrual pain.
   - ○ 2. Avoid cold foods if menstrual pain persists.
   - ○ 3. Stop exercise while menstruating.
   - ○ 4. Avoid sexual intercourse during menstruation.

4. After conducting a class for female adolescents about human reproduction, which of the following statements indicates that the school nurse's teaching has been effective?
   - ○ 1. "Under ideal conditions, sperm can reach the ovum in 15 to 30 minutes, resulting in pregnancy."
   - ○ 2. "I won't become pregnant if I abstain from intercourse during the last 14 days of my menstrual cycle."
   - ○ 3. "Sperm from a healthy male usually remain viable in the female reproductive tract for 96 hours."
   - ○ 4. "After an ovum is fertilized by a sperm, the ovum then contains 21 pairs of chromosomes."

5. A 20-year-old nulligravid client expresses a desire to learn more about the symptothermal method of family planning. Which of the following would the nurse include in the teaching plan?
   - ○ 1. This method has a 50% failure rate during the first year of use.
   - ○ 2. Couples must abstain from coitus for 5 days after the menses.
   - ○ 3. Cervical mucus is carefully monitored for changes.
   - ○ 4. The male partner uses condoms for significant effectiveness.

6. Before advising a 24-year-old client desiring oral contraceptives for family planning, the nurse would assess the client for signs and symptoms of which of the following?
   - ○ 1. Anemia.
   - ○ 2. Hypertension.
   - ○ 3. Dysmenorrhea.
   - ○ 4. Acne vulgaris.

7. After instructing a 20-year-old nulligravid client about side effects of oral contraceptives, the nurse determines that the she needs further instruction when the client states which of the following as a side effect?

5

○ 1. Weight gain.
○ 2. Nausea.
○ 3. Headache.
○ 4. Ovarian cancer.

8. While discussing reproductive health with a group of female adolescents, one of the adolescents asks the nurse, "Where is the ovum fertilized?" The nurse responds by stating that fertilization normally occurs at which of the following sites?
○ 1. Uterus.
○ 2. Vagina.
○ 3. Fallopian tube.
○ 4. Cervix.

9. A 22-year-old nulligravid client tells the nurse that she and her husband have been considering using condoms for family planning. Which of the following instructions would the nurse include about the use of condoms as a method for family planning?
○ 1. Using a spermicide with the condom offers added protection against pregnancy.
○ 2. Natural skin condoms protect against sexually transmitted diseases.
○ 3. The typical failure rate for couples using condoms is about 25%.
○ 4. Condom users frequently report penile gland sensitivity.

10. Which of the following would the nurse include in the teaching plan for a 32-year-old female client requesting information about using a diaphragm for family planning?
○ 1. Douching with an acidic solution after intercourse is recommended.
○ 2. Diaphragms should not be used if the client develops acute cervicitis.
○ 3. The diaphragm should be washed in a weak solution of bleach and water.
○ 4. The diaphragm should be left in place for 2 hours after intercourse.

11. After being examined and fitted for a diaphragm, a 24-year-old client receives instructions about its use. Which of the following client statements indicates a need for *further* teaching?
○ 1. "I can continue to use the diaphragm for about 2 to 3 years if I keep it protected in the case."
○ 2. "If I get pregnant, I will have to be refitted for another diaphragm after the delivery."
○ 3. "Before inserting the diaphragm I should coat the rim with contraceptive jelly."
○ 4. "If I gain or lose 20 pounds, I can still use the same diaphragm."

12. A 22-year-old client tells the nurse that she and her husband are trying to conceive a baby. When teaching the client about reducing the incidence of neural tube defects in newborns, the nurse would empha-

size the need for intake of which of the following nutrients?
○ 1. Iron.
○ 2. Folic acid.
○ 3. Calcium.
○ 4. Magnesium.

13. When describing a vasectomy to a couple inquiring about this procedure, the nurse would explain that which of the following is clamped or excised?
○ 1. Ejaculatory duct.
○ 2. Seminiferous tubules.
○ 3. Seminal vesicles.
○ 4. Vas deferens.

14. A 39-year-old multigravid client asks the nurse for information about female sterilization with a tubal ligation. Which of the following client statements indicates effective teaching?
○ 1. "My fallopian tubes will be tied off through a small abdominal incision."
○ 2. "Reversal of a tubal ligation is easily done, with a pregnancy success rate of 80%."
○ 3. "After this procedure, I must abstain from intercourse for at least 3 weeks."
○ 4. "Both of my ovaries will be removed during the tubal ligation procedure."

15. When discussing sexual arousal and orgasm with a 25-year-old nulliparous client, which of the following would the nurse include as the *primary* anatomic female structure involved?
○ 1. Vaginal wall.
○ 2. Clitoris.
○ 3. Mons pubis.
○ 4. Vulvovaginal glands.

16. A 20-year-old woman desiring to use a cervical cap for family planning is instructed on its use. Which of the following client statements would indicate to the nurse that the client needs *further* instruction?
○ 1. "Cervical caps can be left in place longer than a diaphragm."
○ 2. "Using a cervical cap may increase the risk of irritation."
○ 3. "Cervical caps usually fit better than a diaphragm."
○ 4. "Many women are unable to use cervical caps."

17. A 23-year-old nullipara visiting the clinic for a routine examination tells the nurse that she desires to use the basal body temperature method for family planning. The nurse should instruct the client to do which of the following?
○ 1. Check the cervical mucus to see if it is thick and sparse.
○ 2. Take her temperature at the same time every morning.
○ 3. Document ovulation when the temperature decreases at least 1°F.

○ 4. Avoid coitus for 10 days after a slight rise in temperature.

18. A couple visiting the infertility clinic for the first time ask the nurse, "What causes infertility in a woman?" Which of the following would the nurse include in the response as one of the most common factors?
   ○ 1. Absence of an ovary.
   ○ 2. Overproduction of prolactin.
   ○ 3. Anovulation.
   ○ 4. Immunologic factors.

19. A couple visiting the infertility clinic for the first time state that they have been trying to conceive for the past 2 years without success. After a history and physical examination of both partners, the nurse determines that an appropriate goal for the couple would be to accomplish which of the following by the end of this visit?
   ○ 1. Choose an appropriate infertility treatment method.
   ○ 2. Acknowledge that only 50% of infertile couples achieve a pregnancy.
   ○ 3. Discuss alternative methods of having a family, such as adoption.
   ○ 4. Describe each of the potential causes and possible treatment modalities.

20. A client is scheduled to have in vitro fertilization (IVF) as an infertility treatment. Which of the following client statements about IVF indicates that the client understands this procedure?
   ○ 1. "IVF requires supplemental estrogen to enhance the implantation process."
   ○ 2. "The pregnancy rate with IVF is higher than with gamete intrafallopian transfer (GIFT)."
   ○ 3. "IVF involves bypassing the blocked or absent fallopian tubes."
   ○ 4. "Both ova and sperm are instilled into the open end of a fallopian tube."

21. A 20-year-old nulligravid client tells the nurse that her mother had a friend who died from hemorrhage about 10 years ago during a vaginal delivery. Which of the following responses would be *most* helpful?
   ○ 1. "Today's modern technology has resulted in a low maternal mortality rate."
   ○ 2. "Don't concern yourself with things that happened in the past."
   ○ 3. "In the United States, mothers seldom die in childbirth."
   ○ 4. "What is it that concerns you about pregnancy, labor, and delivery?"

22. A 19-year-old nulligravid client visiting the clinic for a routine examination asks the nurse about cervical mucus changes that occur during the menstrual cycle. Which of the following statements would the nurse expect to include in the client's teaching plan?

○ 1. About midway through the menstrual cycle, cervical mucus is thick and sticky.
○ 2. During ovulation, the cervix remains dry without any mucus production.
○ 3. As ovulation approaches, cervical mucus is abundant and clear.
○ 4. Cervical mucus disappears immediately after ovulation, resuming with menses.

23. When instructing a client about the proper use of condoms for pregnancy prevention, which of the following instructions would be included to ensure maximum effectiveness?
   ○ 1. Place the condom over the erect penis before coitus.
   ○ 2. Withdraw the condom after coitus when the penis is flaccid.
   ○ 3. Ensure that the condom is pulled tightly over the penis before coitus.
   ○ 4. Obtain a prescription for a condom with nonoxynol 9.

24. A multigravid client will be using medroxyprogesterone acetate (Depo-Provera) as a family planning method. After the nurse instructs the client about this method, which of the following client statements indicates effective teaching?
   ○ 1. "This method of family planning requires monthly injections."
   ○ 2. "I should have my first injection during my menstrual cycle."
   ○ 3. "One possible side effect is absence of a menstrual period."
   ○ 4. "This drug will be given by subcutaneous injections."

25. Which of the following would the nurse expect to include in the teaching plan for a 30-year-old multiparous client who will be using an intrauterine device (IUD) for family planning?
   ○ 1. Amenorrhea is a common side effect of IUDs.
   ○ 2. The client needs to use additional protection for conception.
   ○ 3. IUDs are more costly than other forms of contraception.
   ○ 4. Severe cramping may occur when the IUD is inserted.

26. After counseling a 35-year-old client about breast self-examination and mammography, the nurse determines that the client has understood the instructions when the client states which of the following?
   ○ 1. "I should have a mammogram every year once I'm 40."
   ○ 2. "I should schedule a mammography examination during my menstrual period."
   ○ 3. "Mammography screening is inexpensive."
   ○ 4. "Mammography is an extremely painful procedure."

27. After instructing a 40-year-old woman about osteoporosis after menopause, the nurse determines that the client needs *further* instruction when the client states which of the following?
    ○ 1. "One cup of yogurt is the equivalent of one glass of milk."
    ○ 2. "Women who do not eat dairy products should consider calcium supplements."
    ○ 3. "African American women are at the greatest risk for osteoporosis."
    ○ 4. "Estrogen therapy at menopause can reduce the risk of osteoporosis."

28. When developing a teaching plan about sexually transmitted diseases for an 18-year-old female client, which of the following treatments would the nurse need to keep in mind?
    ○ 1. Acyclovir (Zovirax) can be used to cure herpes genitalis.
    ○ 2. *Chlamydia trachomatis* infections are usually treated with penicillin.
    ○ 3. Ceftriaxone sodium (Rocephin) may be used to treat *Neisseria gonorrhoeae* infections.
    ○ 4. Metronidazole (Flagyl) is used to treat condylomata acuminata.

29. The physician prescribes raloxifene hydrochloride (Evista) for a 60-year-old woman. The nurse should instruct the client that this drug is useful in preventing which of the following?
    ○ 1. Hot flashes.
    ○ 2. Osteoporosis.
    ○ 3. Hyperglycemia.
    ○ 4. Migraine headaches.

30. A couple is visiting the clinic because they have been unable to conceive a baby after 3 years of frequent coitus. After discussing the various causes of male infertility, the nurse determines that the male partner needs *further* instruction when he states which of the following as a cause?
    ○ 1. Seminal fluid with an alkaline pH.
    ○ 2. Frequent exposure to heat sources.
    ○ 3. Abnormal hormonal stimulation.
    ○ 4. Immunologic factors.

31. A 24-year-old woman is being assessed for a malformation of the uterus. Figure 1 indicates which of the following uterine malformations?
    ○ 1. Septate uterus.
    ○ 2. Bicornate uterus.
    ○ 3. Double uterus.
    ○ 4. Uterus didelphys.

The Pregnant Client Receiving Prenatal Care

32. When preparing a 20-year-old client who reports missing one menstrual period and suspects that she

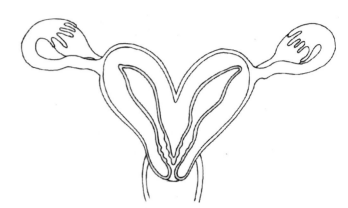

Figure 1.

is pregnant for a radioimmunoassay pregnancy test, which of the following would the nurse need to keep in mind about this test?
    ○ 1. It has a high degree of accuracy within 1 week after ovulation.
    ○ 2. It is identical in nature to an over-the-counter home pregnancy test.
    ○ 3. A positive result is considered a presumptive sign of pregnancy.
    ○ 4. A urine sample is needed to obtain quicker results.

33. After instructing a female client about the radioimmunoassay pregnancy test, the nurse determines that the client understands the instructions when the client states that which of the following hormones is evaluated by this test?
    ○ 1. Prolactin.
    ○ 2. Follicle-stimulating hormone.
    ○ 3. Luteinizing hormone.
    ○ 4. Human chorionic gonadotrophin (hCG).

34. Using Nägele's rule for a client whose last normal menstrual period began on May 10, the nurse determines that the client's estimated date of delivery would be which of the following?
    ○ 1. January 13.
    ○ 2. January 17.
    ○ 3. February 13.
    ○ 4. February 17.

35. After instructing a primigravid client about the functions of the placenta, the nurse determines that the client needs additional teaching when she says that which of the following hormones is produced by the placenta?
    ○ 1. Estrogen.
    ○ 2. Progesterone.
    ○ 3. Human chorionic gonadotrophin.
    ○ 4. Testosterone.

36. A client, about 8 weeks pregnant, asks the nurse when she will be able to hear the fetal heartbeat. The nurse would respond by telling the client that the

fetal heartbeat can be heard with a Doppler ultrasound device when the gestation is as early as which of the following?
- ○ 1. 4 weeks.
- ○ 2. 8 weeks.
- ○ 3. 15 weeks.
- ○ 4. 18 weeks.

37. A 20-year-old married client with a positive pregnancy test states, "Is it really true? I can't believe I'm going to have a baby!" Which of the following responses by the nurse would be *most* appropriate at this time?
- ○ 1. "Would you like some booklets on the pregnancy experience?"
- ○ 2. "Yes it is true. How does that make you feel?"
- ○ 3. "You should be delighted that you are pregnant."
- ○ 4. "Weren't you and your husband trying to have a baby?"

38. A newly diagnosed pregnant client tells the nurse, "If I'm going to have all of these discomforts, I'm not sure I want to be pregnant!" The nurse interprets the client's statement as an indication of which of the following?
- ○ 1. Fear of pregnancy outcome.
- ○ 2. Rejection of the pregnancy.
- ○ 3. Normal ambivalence.
- ○ 4. Inability to care for the newborn.

39. When caring for a newly diagnosed primigravid client at 10 weeks' gestation who is experiencing breast tenderness, amenorrhea, nausea and vomiting, and urinary frequency, which of the following would the nurse identify as a *priority* nursing diagnosis?
- ○ 1. Readiness for Enhanced Family Coping related to pregnancy confirmation.
- ○ 2. Ineffective Sexuality Patterns related to fear of spontaneous abortion.
- ○ 3. Compromised Family Coping related to the discomforts of pregnancy.
- ○ 4. Imbalanced Nutrition: Less than Body Requirements related to increased demands of pregnancy.

40. A client, approximately 11 weeks pregnant, and her husband are seen in the antepartal clinic. The client's husband tells the nurse that he has been experiencing nausea and vomiting and fatigue along with his wife. The nurse interprets these findings as suggesting that the client's husband is experiencing which of the following?
- ○ 1. Ptyalism.
- ○ 2. Mittelschmerz.
- ○ 3. Couvade syndrome.
- ○ 4. Pica.

41. A primigravid client asks the nurse if she can continue to have a glass of wine with dinner during her pregnancy. Which of the following would be the nurse's *best* response?
- ○ 1. "The effects of alcohol on a fetus during pregnancy are unknown."
- ○ 2. "You should limit your consumption to beer and wine."
- ○ 3. "You should abstain from drinking alcoholic beverages."
- ○ 4. "You may have 1 drink or 2 ounces of alcohol per day."

42. Examination of a primigravid client complaining of increased vaginal secretions since becoming pregnant reveals clear, highly acidic vaginal secretions. The client denies any perineal itching or burning. The nurse interprets these findings as a response related to which of the following?
- ○ 1. A decrease in vaginal glycogen stores.
- ○ 2. Development of a sexually transmitted disease.
- ○ 3. Prevention of expulsion of the cervical mucus plug.
- ○ 4. Control of the growth of pathologic bacteria.

43. When measuring the fundal height of a primigravid client at 20 weeks' gestation, the nurse would anticipate locating the fundal height at which of the following points?
- ○ 1. Halfway between the client's symphysis pubis and umbilicus.
- ○ 2. At about the level of the client's umbilicus.
- ○ 3. Between the client's umbilicus and xyphoid process.
- ○ 4. Near the client's xyphoid process and compressing the diaphragm.

44. A primigravid client visiting the antepartal clinic at 8 weeks' gestation tells the nurse that she wants an amniocentesis because there is a history of hemophilia A in her family. The nurse instructs the client that newer techniques now allow amniocentesis to be performed as early as which of the following?
- ○ 1. 8 weeks' gestation.
- ○ 2. 10 weeks' gestation.
- ○ 3. 12 weeks' gestation.
- ○ 4. 14 weeks' gestation.

45. After instructing a primigravida about desired weight gain during pregnancy, the nurse determines that the teaching has been successful when the client states which of the following?
- ○ 1. "A total weight gain of approximately 20 pounds (9 kg) is recommended."
- ○ 2. "A weight gain of 6.6 pounds (3 kg) in the second and third trimesters is considered normal."
- ○ 3. "A weight gain of about 12 pounds (5.5 kg) every trimester is recommended."
- ○ 4. "Although it varies, a gain of 25 to 35 pounds (11.4 to 14.5 kg) is about average."

46. When developing a teaching plan for a client who is 8 weeks pregnant, which of the following foods would the nurse suggest to meet the client's need for increased folic acid?
    ○ 1. Spinach.
    ○ 2. Bananas.
    ○ 3. Seafood.
    ○ 4. Yogurt.

47. The nurse instructs a primigravida about the importance of sufficient vitamin A in her diet. The nurse knows that the instructions have been effective when the client indicates that she should include which of the following in her diet?
    ○ 1. Buttermilk and cheese.
    ○ 2. Strawberries and cantaloupe.
    ○ 3. Egg yolks and squash.
    ○ 4. Oranges and tomatoes.

48. When developing a meal-planning guide about foods rich in riboflavin for a primigravid client, the nurse would expect to instruct the client to include at least two daily servings of which of the following foods?
    ○ 1. Fresh fruit.
    ○ 2. Prunes.
    ○ 3. Potatoes.
    ○ 4. Enriched cereals.

49. The nurse instructs a primigravida to increase her intake of foods high in magnesium because of its role with which of the following?
    ○ 1. Prevention of demineralization of the mother's bones.
    ○ 2. Synthesis of proteins, nucleic acids, and fats.
    ○ 3. Amino acid metabolism.
    ○ 4. Synthesis of neural pathways in the fetus.

50. When caring for a primigravid client at 9 weeks' gestation who immigrated to the United States from Vietnam 1 year ago, the nurse would assess the client's diet for a deficiency of which of the following?
    ○ 1. Calcium.
    ○ 2. Vitamin E.
    ○ 3. Vitamin C.
    ○ 4. Iodine.

51. Which of the following statements by a primigravid client scheduled for chorionic villi sampling indicates effective teaching about the procedure?
    ○ 1. "A fiberoptic fetoscope will be inserted through a small incision into my uterus."
    ○ 2. "I can't have anything to eat or drink after midnight on the day of the procedure."
    ○ 3. "The procedure involves the insertion of a thin catheter into my uterus."
    ○ 4. "I need to drink 32 to 40 ounces of fluid 1 to 2 hours before the procedure."

52. A 34-year-old multigravid client at 16 weeks' gestation who received regular prenatal care for all of her previous pregnancies tells the nurse that she has already felt the baby move. The nurse interprets this as which of the following?
    ○ 1. The possibility that the client is carrying twins.
    ○ 2. Unusual because most multiparous clients do not experience quickening until 30 weeks' gestation.
    ○ 3. Evidence that the client's estimated date of delivery is probably off by a few weeks.
    ○ 4. Normal because multiparous clients can experience quickening between 14 and 20 weeks' gestation.

53. A desire for which of the following diagnostic tests would be *most* important to ascertain for a primigravid client in the second trimester of her pregnancy?
    ○ 1. Culdocentesis to detect abnormalities.
    ○ 2. Chorionic villus sampling.
    ○ 3. Ultrasound testing.
    ○ 4. α-Fetoprotein (AFP) testing.

54. When performing Leopold's maneuvers, which of the following would the nurse ask the client to do to ensure optimal comfort and accuracy?
    ○ 1. Breathe deeply for 1 minute.
    ○ 2. Empty her bladder.
    ○ 3. Drink a full glass of water.
    ○ 4. Lie on her left side.

55. The nurse is assessing fetal position for a 32-year-old client in her eighth month of pregnancy. From Figure 2, the fetal position can be described as which of the following?
    ○ 1. Left occipital transverse.
    ○ 2. Left occipital anterior.
    ○ 3. Right occipital transverse.
    ○ 4. Right occipital anterior.

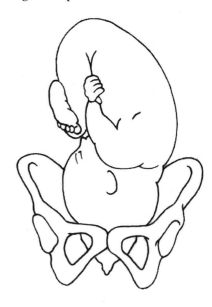

Figure 2.

56. Which of the following statements by the nurse would be *most* appropriate when responding to a primigravid client who asks, "What should I do about this brown discoloration across my nose and cheeks?"
    ○ 1. "This usually disappears after delivery."
    ○ 2. "It is a sign of skin melanoma."
    ○ 3. "The discoloration is due to dilated capillaries."
    ○ 4. "It will fade if you use a prescribed cream."

57. A 36-year-old primigravid client at 22 weeks' gestation without any complications to date is being seen in the clinic for a routine visit. The nurse expects to assess the client's fundal height for which of the following reasons?
    ○ 1. Determine the level of uterine activity.
    ○ 2. Identify the need for increased weight gain.
    ○ 3. Assess the location of the placenta.
    ○ 4. Estimate the fetal gestational age.

58. After reviewing the physician's explanation of amniocentesis with a multigravid client, which of the following, if reported by the client as a *primary* risk of the procedure, would indicate successful teaching?
    ○ 1. Premature rupture of the membranes.
    ○ 2. Possible premature labor.
    ○ 3. Fetal limb malformations.
    ○ 4. Fetal organ malformations.

59. A primigravida at 28 weeks' gestation tells the nurse that she and her husband wish to drive to visit relatives who live several hundred miles away. Which of the following recommendations by the nurse would be *best*?
    ○ 1. "Try to avoid traveling anywhere in the car during your third trimester."
    ○ 2. "Limit the time you spend in the car to a maximum of 4 to 5 hours."
    ○ 3. "Taking the trip is okay if you stop every 1 to 2 hours and walk."
    ○ 4. "Avoid wearing your seat belt in the car to prevent injury to the fetus."

60. Which of the following recommendations would be *most* helpful to suggest to a primigravid client at 37 weeks' gestation who is complaining of leg cramps?
    ○ 1. Change positions frequently throughout the day.
    ○ 2. Alternately flex and extend the legs.
    ○ 3. Straighten the knee and push upward on the toes.
    ○ 4. Lie prone in bed with the legs elevated.

61. Which of the following recommendations would be the *most* appropriate preventative measure to suggest to a primigravid client at 30 weeks' gestation who is experiencing occasional heartburn?
    ○ 1. Eat smaller and more frequent meals during the day.

○ 2. Take a pinch of baking soda with water before meals.
○ 3. Decrease fluid intake to four glasses daily.
○ 4. Drink several cups of regular tea throughout the day.

62. When performing Leopold's maneuvers on a primigravid client at 22 weeks' gestation, the nurse performs the first maneuver to do which of the following?
    ○ 1. Locate the fetal back and spine.
    ○ 2. Determine what is in the fundus.
    ○ 3. Determine whether the fetal head is at the pelvic inlet.
    ○ 4. Identify the degree of fetal descent and flexion.

63. A primigravid adolescent client at approximately 15 weeks' gestation who is visiting the prenatal clinic with her mother is to undergo AFP screening. When developing the teaching plan for this client, the nurse would include information about which of the following?
    ○ 1. Ultrasonography usually accompanies AFP testing.
    ○ 2. Results are usually very accurate until 20 weeks' gestation.
    ○ 3. A clean-catch midstream urine specimen is needed.
    ○ 4. Increased levels of AFP are associated with neural tube defects.

64. Which of the following statements *best* identifies the rationale for why the nurse reinforces the need for continued prenatal care throughout the pregnancy with an adolescent primigravid client?
    ○ 1. Pregnant adolescents are at high risk for pregnancy-induced hypertension.
    ○ 2. Gestational diabetes during pregnancy often develops in adolescents.
    ○ 3. Adolescents need additional instruction related to common discomforts.
    ○ 4. The father of the baby is rarely involved in the pregnancy.

65. An adolescent primigravid client at 20 weeks' gestation weighs 120 pounds, having gained only 5 pounds since becoming pregnant. She states, "I haven't had any appetite." Which of the following would be the *most* appropriate nursing diagnosis for this client?
    ○ 1. Knowledge Deficit about fetal development as evidenced by lack of sufficient weight gain.
    ○ 2. Noncompliance with diet related to fear of body image changes.
    ○ 3. Imbalanced Nutrition: Less Than Body Requirements related to lack of appetite.
    ○ 4. Chronic Low Self-esteem related to poor appetite and decreased weight gain.

66. Which of the following would be included in the teaching plan about pregnancy-related breast changes for a primigravid client?
    ○ 1. Growth of the milk ducts is greatest during the first 8 weeks of gestation.
    ○ 2. Enlargement of the breasts indicates adequate levels of progesterone.
    ○ 3. Colostrum is usually secreted by about the 16th week of gestation.
    ○ 4. Darkening of the areola occurs during the last month of pregnancy.

67. When the nurse is planning a class for primigravid clients about the common discomforts of pregnancy, which of the following physiologic changes of pregnancy would the nurse need to keep in mind?
    ○ 1. The temperature decreases slightly early in pregnancy.
    ○ 2. Cardiac output increases by 25% to 50% during pregnancy.
    ○ 3. The circulating fibrinogen level decreases as much as 50% during pregnancy.
    ○ 4. The anterior pituitary gland secretes oxytocin late in pregnancy.

68. When teaching a primigravida at 24 weeks' gestation about the diagnostic tests to determine fetal well-being, which of the following would the nurse include?
    ○ 1. A fetal biophysical profile involves assessments of breathing movements, body movements, tone, amniotic fluid volume, and fetal heart rate reactivity.
    ○ 2. A reactive nonstress test is an ominous sign and requires further evaluation with fetal echocardiography.
    ○ 3. Contraction stress testing, performed on most pregnant women, can be initiated as early as 16 weeks' gestation.
    ○ 4. Percutaneous umbilical blood sampling uses a needle inserted through the vagina to obtain a sample.

69. When teaching a primigravid client how to do Kegel exercises several times a day, the nurse explains that the primary purpose of these exercises is to accomplish which of the following?
    ○ 1. Prevent vaginal swelling.
    ○ 2. Alleviate lower back discomfort.
    ○ 3. Strengthen the perineal muscles.
    ○ 4. Strengthen the abdominal muscles.

70. During a routine clinic visit, a 25-year-old multigravid client who initiated prenatal care at 10 weeks' gestation and is now in her third trimester states, "I've been having strange dreams about the baby. Last week I dreamed he was covered with hair." Which of the following would be the nurse's *best* response?

○ 1. "Dreams like the ones that you describe are very unusual. Please tell me more about them."
○ 2. "Often when a mother has these dreams, she is trying to cope with becoming a parent."
○ 3. "Dreams about the baby late in pregnancy usually mean that labor is about to begin soon."
○ 4. "It's not uncommon to have dreams about the baby, particularly in the third trimester."

71. A primigravida at 36 weeks' gestation tells the nurse that she has been experiencing insomnia for the past 2 weeks. Which of the following suggestions would be *most* helpful?
    ○ 1. Practice relaxation techniques before bedtime.
    ○ 2. Drink a cup of hot chocolate before bedtime.
    ○ 3. Drink a small glass of wine with dinner.
    ○ 4. Exercise for 30 minutes just before bedtime.

72. Which of the following client statements indicates a need for additional teaching about self-care during pregnancy?
    ○ 1. "I should use nonskid pads when I take a shower or bath."
    ○ 2. "I should avoid using soap on my nipples to prevent drying."
    ○ 3. "I should sit in a hot tub for 20 minutes to relax after working."
    ○ 4. "I should avoid douching even if my vaginal secretions increase."

73. To obtain the obstetric conjugate measurement, the nurse practitioner would do which of the following?
    ○ 1. Add 1.5 cm to the transverse diameter.
    ○ 2. First measure the angle of the pubic arch.
    ○ 3. Subtract 1.5 to 2 cm from the diagonal conjugate.
    ○ 4. Measure the diameter of the pelvic inlet.

74. After discussing the pelvic changes that occur during pregnancy with a group of student nurses, the instructor determines that the students understand the instruction when they state that the uterus receives its blood supply directly from the uterine artery and which of the following?
    ○ 1. Ovarian artery.
    ○ 2. Iliac artery.
    ○ 3. Hypogastric artery.
    ○ 4. Pulmonary artery.

The Pregnant Client in Childbirth Preparation Classes

75. When preparing a series of Preparation for Parenting classes for primigravidas and their partners about endocrine changes that normally occur during pregnancy, which of the following would be included?
    ○ 1. Human placental lactogen maintains the corpus luteum.

○ 2. Progesterone is responsible for hyperpigmentation and vascular skin changes.

○ 3. Estrogen relaxes smooth muscle in the respiratory tract.

○ 4. The thyroid enlarges with an increase in basal metabolic rate.

76. When developing a series of parent classes on fetal development, which of the following would the nurse include as being developed by the end of the third month (9 to 12 weeks)?

○ 1. External genitalia.

○ 2. Myelinization of nerves.

○ 3. Brown fat stores.

○ 4. Air ducts and alveoli.

77. A primigravid client attending parenthood classes tells the nurse that there is a history of twins in her family. On which of the following would the nurse base the response to the client?

○ 1. Monozygotic twins result from fertilization of two ova by different sperm.

○ 2. Monozygotic twins occur by chance regardless of race or heredity.

○ 3. Dizygotic twins are usually of the same sex.

○ 4. Dizygotic twins occur more often in primigravid than in multigravid clients.

78. During a 2-hour childbirth preparation class focusing on the labor and delivery process for primigravidas, the nurse describes the first maneuver that the fetus goes through during the labor process when the head is the presenting part as which of the following?

○ 1. Engagement.

○ 2. Flexion.

○ 3. Descent.

○ 4. Internal rotation.

79. A primigravida in a Preparation for Parenting class asks how much blood is lost during an uncomplicated delivery. Which of the following would be the nurse's best response?

○ 1. "The maximum blood loss considered within normal limits is 500 mL."

○ 2. "The minimum blood loss considered within normal limits is 1000 mL."

○ 3. "Blood loss during a delivery is rarely estimated unless there is a hemorrhage."

○ 4. "It would be very unusual if you lost more than 100 mL of blood during the delivery."

80. Which of the following statements by a primigravid client about the amniotic fluid and sac indicates the need for *further* teaching?

○ 1. "The amniotic fluid helps to dilate the cervix once labor begins."

○ 2. "Fetal nutrients are provided by the amniotic fluid."

○ 3. "Amniotic fluid provides a cushion against impact of the maternal abdomen."

○ 4. "The fetus is kept at a stable temperature by the amniotic fluid and sac."

81. During a childbirth preparation class, a primigravid client at 36 weeks' gestation tells the nurse, "My lower back has really been bothering me lately." Which of the following exercises suggested by the nurse would be *most* helpful?

○ 1. Pelvic rocking.

○ 2. Deep breathing.

○ 3. Tailor sitting.

○ 4. Squatting.

82. When developing a teaching plan for a childbirth education class for a group of primigravid clients about pain during labor and delivery, which of the following would the nurse expect to discuss as the *primary* cause of pain in the first stage of labor?

○ 1. Dilation of the uterine blood vessels.

○ 2. Hypoxia to the uterine muscle fibers.

○ 3. Distention of the upper uterine segment.

○ 4. Status of the amniotic membranes.

83. During a "Preparation for Parenting" class, one of the participants asks the nurse, "How will I know if I am really in labor?" Which of the following statements about true labor contractions would be the nurse's *best* response?

○ 1. "Walking around helps to decrease true contractions."

○ 2. "True labor contractions may disappear with ambulation, rest, or sleep."

○ 3. "The duration and frequency of true labor contractions remain the same."

○ 4. "True labor contractions are felt first in the lower back, then the abdomen."

84. After instructing participants in a childbirth education class about methods to cope with discomforts of the first stage of labor, the nurse determines that one of the pregnant clients needs *further* instruction when she says that she has been practicing which of the following?

○ 1. Biofeedback.

○ 2. Effleurage.

○ 3. Guided imagery.

○ 4. Pelvic tilt exercises.

85. After a "Preparation for Parenting" class session, a pregnant client tells the nurse that she has had some yellow-gray frothy vaginal discharge and local itching. The nurse's *best* action is to advise the client to do which of the following?

○ 1. Use an over-the-counter cream for yeast infections.

○ 2. Schedule an appointment at the clinic for an examination.

○ 3. Administer a vinegar douche under low pressure.

○ 4. Prepare for preterm labor and delivery.

86. During childbirth preparation classes for a group of adolescent primigravidas, one of the clients asks, "How does the baby breathe inside of me?" The nurse responds by explaining fetal circulation, stating that circulation of oxygenated blood from the placenta begins with which of the following?
    ○ 1. Umbilical artery.
    ○ 2. Foramen ovale.
    ○ 3. Ductus arteriosus.
    ○ 4. Umbilical vein.

87. Which of the following instructions would the nurse expect to include in the teaching plan for a group of primigravid clients attending a parenting class about the placenta and the umbilical cord?
    ○ 1. The highest oxygen content is found in the umbilical artery.
    ○ 2. About 10% of umbilical cords have only two vessels.
    ○ 3. The cord normally inserts in the center of the placenta.
    ○ 4. A nuchal cord usually occurs when the cord is abnormally short.

88. The topic of physiologic changes that occur during pregnancy is to be included in a parenting class for primigravid clients who are in their first half of pregnancy. Which of the following would be important for the nurse to include in the teaching plan?
    ○ 1. Decreased plasma volume.
    ○ 2. Increased risk for urinary tract infections.
    ○ 3. Increased peripheral vascular resistance.
    ○ 4. Increased hemoglobin levels.

89. While preparing a childbirth education class for a group of nursing students, the nurse expects to emphasize the need for continued prenatal care and postpartum well-baby care for all clients. Which of the following should be included in the teaching plan?
    ○ 1. The maternal mortality rate has been steadily increasing in the United States during the past 20 years.
    ○ 2. The infant mortality rate is defined as the number of infant deaths before the age of 1 year per 1000 live births.
    ○ 3. The perinatal mortality rate is the number of deaths among infants younger than 12 months of age per 1000 live births.
    ○ 4. The neonatal mortality rate is the number of infant deaths before the age of 12 months per 1000 live births.

90. When developing a teaching plan for a group of nursing students about the role of the placenta, which of the following would the nurse expect to incorporate?
    ○ 1. The placenta is formed by the fusion of chorionic villi and the decidua basalis.

○ 2. Viruses generally do not cross the placental barrier.
○ 3. The total weight of a term placenta is 1000 to 1500 g.
○ 4. In the male fetus, human placental lactogen promotes synthesis of testosterone.

The Pregnant Client With Risk Factors

91. After conducting a presentation to a group of adolescent parents on the topic of adolescent pregnancy, the nurse determines that one of the parents needs *further* instruction when the parent says that adolescents are at greater risk for which of the following?
    ○ 1. Denial of the pregnancy.
    ○ 2. Low-birth-weight infant.
    ○ 3. Cephalopelvic disproportion.
    ○ 4. Congenital anomalies.

92. A dilation and curettage (D&C) is scheduled for a primigravid client admitted to the hospital at 10 weeks' gestation with abdominal cramping, bright red vaginal spotting, and passage of some of the products of conception. The nurse anticipates that the client will most likely express which of the following feelings?
    ○ 1. Ambivalence.
    ○ 2. Anxiety.
    ○ 3. Fear.
    ○ 4. Guilt.

93. When providing care to the client who has undergone a D&C after a spontaneous abortion, the nurse administers hydroxyzine (Vistaril) as ordered, primarily for which of the following reasons?
    ○ 1. To counteract nausea.
    ○ 2. To reduce pain discomfort.
    ○ 3. To decrease uterine cramping.
    ○ 4. To promote uterine contractility.

94. On entering the room of a client who has undergone a D&C for a spontaneous abortion, the nurse finds the client crying. Which of the following comments by the nurse would be *most* appropriate?
    ○ 1. "Are you having a great deal of uterine pain?"
    ○ 2. "Often spontaneous abortion means a defective embryo."
    ○ 3. "I'm truly sorry you lost your baby."
    ○ 4. "You should try to get pregnant again as soon as possible."

95. Rho(D) immune globulin (RhoGAM) is ordered for a client before she is discharged after a spontaneous abortion. The nurse understands that the rationale for administration is to prevent which of the following?
    ○ 1. Development of a future Rh-positive fetus.
    ○ 2. An antibody response to Rh-negative blood.

○ 3. A future pregnancy resulting in abortion.

○ 4. Development of Rh-positive antibodies.

96. A multigravid client who stands for long periods while working in a factory visits the prenatal clinic at 35 weeks' gestation, stating, "The varicose veins in my legs have really been bothering me lately." Which of the following instructions would be *most* helpful?

○ 1. Perform slow contraction and relaxation of the feet and ankles twice daily.

○ 2. Take frequent rest periods with the legs elevated above the hips.

○ 3. Avoid support hose that reach above the leg varicosities.

○ 4. Take a leave of absence from your job to avoid prolonged standing.

97. A multigravid client at 36 weeks' gestation has been diagnosed with condylomata acuminata. Which of the following would the nurse include when teaching the client about the disorder and current therapies?

○ 1. Cryotherapy may be used to remove the warts.

○ 2. Podophyllin solution may be used to decrease the size of the warts.

○ 3. A 25% trichloroacetic acid solution can eradicate the disorder.

○ 4. Condolymata acuminata has been associated with ovarian cancer.

98. A primigravid client at 8 weeks' gestation tells the nurse that since having had sexual relations with a new partner 2 weeks ago, she has noticed flu-like symptoms, enlarged lymph nodes, and clusters of vesicles on her vagina. The nurse refers the client to a physician because the nurse suspects which of the following sexually transmitted diseases?

○ 1. Gonorrhea.

○ 2. *Chlamydia trachomatis* infection.

○ 3. Syphilis.

○ 4. Herpes genitalis.

99. While caring for a 24-year-old primigravid client scheduled for emergency surgery because of a probable ectopic pregnancy, the nurse would expect to do which of the following?

○ 1. Witness an informed consent for surgery.

○ 2. Assess the client for massive external bleeding.

○ 3. Explain that the fallopian tube can be salvaged.

○ 4. Monitor the client for uterine contractions.

100. A 30-year-old gravida IV, para III client at 30 weeks' gestation is admitted to the hospital for evaluation. The client has experienced two neonatal deaths becaue of hemolytic disease of the newborn. An amniocentesis is to be performed to evaluate bilirubin density. The nurse would obtain a specimen container that is which of the following?

○ 1. Dark.

○ 2. Clear.

○ 3. Green.

○ 4. Amber.

101. A multigravid client at 32 weeks' gestation has experienced hemolytic disease of the newborn in a previous pregnancy. The nurse would prepare the client for frequent antibody titer evaluations obtained from which of the following?

○ 1. Placental blood.

○ 2. Amniotic fluid.

○ 3. Fetal blood.

○ 4. Maternal blood.

Correct Answers and Rationale

The letters in parentheses following the rationale identify the step of the nursing process (A, D, P, I, E) and client needs (1, 2, 3, 4, 5, 6, 7, 8, 9, 10). See the inside front cover for the key.

The Preconception Client

1. 4. The nurse determines that the client has understood the instructions when the client says that she should not squeeze her nipples if there is a discharge present. If the client notices a discharge or bleeding, she should notify her physician or health care provider, because this may be symptomatic of underlying disease. Ideally, breast self-examination should be performed about 1 week after the onset of menses because hormonal influences on breast tissue are at a low ebb at this time. The client should perform breast self-examination on the same day each month only if she has stopped menstruating (eg, menopause). The client's breasts should mirror each other. If one breast is significantly larger than the other, or if there is "pitting" disease, a tumor may be present. (E, 9)

2. 3. For a client with a menstrual cycle of 28 days, ovulation usually occurs on day 14, plus or minus 2 days, before the onset of the next menstrual cycle. Stated another way, the menstrual period begins about 2 weeks after ovulation has occurred. Ovulation does not usually occur during the menses component of the cycle when the uterine lining is being shed. In most women, the ovum survives for about 12 to 24 hours after ovulation, during which time conception is possible. The basal body temperature rises 0.5° to 1.0°F when ovulation occurs. Although some women experience some pelvic discomfort during ovulation (mittelschmerz), severe or unusual pain is rare. After ovulation, the cervical mucus is thin and copious. (P, 3)

3. 1. The nurse should instruct the client to take a mild analgesic, such as ibuprofen, if menstrual pain or "cramps" are present. The client should also eat foods rich in iron and should continue moderate exercise during menstruation, which increases abdominal tone. Avoiding cold foods will not decrease dysmenorrhea. Sexual intercourse is not prohibited during menstruation, but the male partner should wear a condom to prevent exposure to blood. (I, 3)

4. 1. Under ideal conditions, sperm can reach the ovum in 15 to 30 minutes. This is an important point to make with adolescents who may be sexually active. Many people believe that the time interval is much longer and that they can wait to take steps to prevent conception until after intercourse. Without protection, pregnancy and sexually transmitted diseases can occur. When using the abstinence or calendar method, the couple should abstain from intercourse on the days of the menstrual cycle when the woman is most likely to conceive. Using a 28-day cycle as an example, a couple should abstain from coitus 3 to 4 days before ovulation (days 10 through 14) and 3 to 4 days after ovulation (days 15 through 18). Sperm from a healthy male can remain viable for 24 to 72 hours in the female reproductive tract. If the female client ovulates after coitus, there is a possibility that fertilization can occur. Before fertilization, the ovum and sperm each contain 23 chromosomes. After fertilization, the conceptus contains 46 chromosomes unless there is a chromosomal abnormality. (E, 3)

5. 3. The symptothermal method is a natural method of fertility management that depends on knowing when ovulation has occurred. Because regular menstrual cycles can vary by 1 to 2 days in either direction, the symptothermal method requires daily basal body temperature assessments plus close monitoring of cervical mucus changes. The method relies on abstinence during the period of ovulation, which occurs approximately 14 days before the beginning of the next cycle. Abstinence from coitus for 5 days after menses is unnecessary because it is unlikely that ovulation will occur during this time period (days 1 through 10). Typically, the failure rate for this method is between 10% and 20%. Although a condom may increase the effectiveness of this method, most clients who choose natural methods are not interested in chemical or barrier types of family planning. (P, 3)

6. 2. Before advising a client about oral contraceptives, the nurse needs to assess for signs and symptoms of hypertension. Clients who have hypertension, thrombophlebitis, obesity, or a family history of cerebral or cardiovascular accident are poor candidates for oral contraceptives. In addition, women who smoke, are older than 40 years of age, or have a history of pulmonary disease should be advised to use a different method. Iron-deficiency anemia, dysmenorrhea, and acne are not contraindications for the use of oral contraceptives. Iron-deficiency anemia is a common disorder in young women. Oral contraceptives decrease the amount of menstrual flow and thus decrease the amount of iron lost through menses, thereby providing a beneficial effect when used by clients with anemia.

Low-dose oral contraceptives to prevent ovulation may be effective in decreasing the severity of dysmenorrhea (painful menstruation). Dysmenorrhea is thought to be caused by the release of prostaglandins in response to tissue destruction during the ischemic phase of the menstrual cycle. Use of oral contraceptives often improves facial acne. (A, 9)

7. 4. The nurse determines that the client needs further instruction when the client says that one of the side effects of oral contraceptive use is ovarian cancer. Some studies suggest that ovarian and endometrial cancer are reduced in women using oral contraceptives. Other side effects of oral contraceptives include weight gain, nausea, headache, breakthrough bleeding, and monilial infections. The most serious side effect is thrombophlebitis. (E, 8)

8. 3. Fertilization normally occurs in the outer third of the fallopian tube. Although there have been reports of fertilization outside the fallopian tube, this is not a normal occurrence. (I, 3)

9. 1. The typical failure rate of a condom is approximately 12% to 14%. Adding a spermicide can decrease this potential failure rate because it offers additional protection against pregnancy. Natural skin condoms do not offer the same protection against sexually transmitted diseases caused by viruses as latex condoms do. Unlike latex condoms, natural skin (membrane) condoms do not prevent the passage of viruses. Most condom users report decreased penile gland sensitivity. However, some users do report an increased sensitivity or allergic reaction (such as a rash) to latex, necessitating the use of another method of family planning or a switch to a natural skin condom. (I, 3)

10. 2. The teaching plan should include a caution that diaphragms should not be used if the client develops acute cervicitis, possibly aggravated by contact with the rubber of the diaphragm. Some studies have also associated diaphragm use with increased incidence of urinary tract infections. Douching after use of a diaphragm and intercourse is not recommended because pregnancy could occur. The diaphragm should be inspected and washed with mild soap and water after each use. A diaphragm should be left in place for at least 6 hours but no longer than 24 hours after intercourse. More spermicidal jelly or cream should be used if intercourse is repeated during this period. (P, 9)

11. 4. A client would need additional instructions when she says that she can still use the same diaphragm if she gains or loses 20 pounds. Gaining or losing more than 15 pounds can change the pelvic and vaginal contours to such a degree that the diaphragm will no longer protect the client against pregnancy. The diaphragm can be used for 2 to 3 years if it is cared for and well protected

in its case. The client should be refitted for another diaphragm after pregnancy and delivery of a newborn because weight changes and physiologic changes of pregnancy can alter the pelvic and vaginal contours, thus affecting the effectiveness of the diaphragm. The client should use a spermicidal jelly or cream before inserting the diaphragm. (E, 9)

12. 2. Folic acid (folate) can reduce the incidence of neural tube defects in newborns. Adequate intake of folic acid is especially important just before conception and during the first 6 weeks after conception. Folic acid supplements may be prescribed, especially after conception occurs. Foods that are rich in folic acid include fruits and green leafy vegetables. Iron, calcium, and magnesium are not associated with reducing the risk for neural tube defects. Iron is necessary to maintain iron stores during pregnancy and postpartum. Calcium is important for bone density of the mother and bone formation in the developing fetus. Magnesium aids in the synthesis of proteins and fats in the mother. It also is important in promoting cell growth in the fetus. Magnesium can be found in dark green leafy vegetables. (I, 9)

13. 4. In vasectomy, a common procedure for male sterilization, the vas deferens (ductus deferens) is cut and tied. Coagulation may also be used to create an obstruction in the vas deferens and block the passage of sperm. (I, 3)

14. 1. Tubal ligation, a female sterilization procedure, involves ligation (tying off) or cauterization of the fallopian tubes through a small abdominal incision (laparotomy). Reversal of a tubal ligation is not easily done, and the pregnancy success rate after reversal is about 30%. After a tubal ligation, the client may engage in intercourse 2 to 3 days after the procedure. The ovaries are not generally removed during a tubal ligation. An oophorectomy involves removal of one or both ovaries. (E, 3)

15. 2. Although the vaginal wall and cervix may be sensitive structures, the primary anatomic female structure involved in sexual arousal is the clitoris. Composed of erectile tissue with a plentiful arterial blood supply, the clitoris is especially sensitive to foreplay, temperature, and movements of the shaft of the penis against its surface. The mons pubis—the round, fleshy prominence over the symphysis pubis—forms the anterior border of the external reproductive organs. Covered with varying amounts of pubic hair, the mons pubis is not associated with sexual arousal. The vulvovaginal glands include the Skene and Bartholin glands with ducts that lie within the vestibule. These glands provide lubrication for the urethra and vaginal introitus. They are not the primary anatomic organ associated with sexual arousal because they do not contain the highly sensitive erectile tissues of the clitoris. (I, 3)

16. 3. The client needs further instruction when she says that cervical caps fit better than the diaphragm. Many women are unable to use cervical caps because their cervix is too short for the cap to fit the cervix properly. A cervical cap may remain in place for up to 48 hours after intercourse, whereas it is recommended that a diaphragm be left in place for only 24 hours. The cervical cap is associated with cervical irritation. (E, 9)

17. 2. The basal body temperature method requires that the client take her temperature each morning before arising, preferably at the same time each day before eating or any other activity. Just before the day of ovulation, the temperature falls by 0.5°F. At the time of ovulation, the temperature rises 0.4° to 0.8°F because of increased progesterone secretion in response to the luteinizing hormone. The temperature remains higher for the rest of the menstrual cycle. The client should keep a diary of about 6 months of menstrual cycles to calculate "safe" days. There is no mucus for the first 3 or 4 days after menses, and then thick, sticky mucus begins to appear. As estrogen increases, the mucus changes to clear, slippery, and stretchy. This condition, termed *spinnbarkeit*, is present during ovulation. After ovulation, the mucus decreases in amount and becomes thick and sticky again until menses. Because the ovum typically survives about 24 hours and sperm can survive up to 72 hours, couples must avoid coitus when the cervical mucus is copious and for about 3 to 4 days before and after ovulation to avoid a pregnancy. (I, 3)

18. 3. The most common factor in female infertility is ovarian dysfunction, particularly anovulation. Other common factors include blocked fallopian tubes and cervical factors such as infection and inflammation. The causes of infertility can be determined in about 80% to 90% of couples investigated, but in about 10% to 20% of the cases no cause can be found. Less frequent causes include endometriosis, vaginitis, polycystic ovaries, overproduction of prolactin, immunologic factors, inadequate secretion of progesterone, and stenosis of the cervical os (possibly preventing sperm transport). Immunologic factors do play a role in female infertility; however, they are less common than anovulation. Overproduction of prolactin is also a less frequent cause of infertility in women. Absence of an ovary is an extremely rare cause of infertility. (I, 3)

19. 4. By the end of the first visit, the couple should be able to identify potential causes and treatment modalities for infertility. If their evaluation shows that a treatment or procedure may help them to conceive, the couple must then decide how to proceed, considering all of the various treatments before selecting one. Treatments can be difficult, painful, or risky. The first visit is not the appropriate time to decide on a treatment plan because the couple need time to adjust to the diagnosis of infertility, a crisis for most couples. Although the couple may be in a hurry for definitive therapy, a thorough assessment of both partners is necessary before a treatment plan can be initiated. The success rate for achieving a pregnancy depends on both the cause and the effectiveness of the treatment, and in some cases it may be only as high as 30%. The couple may desire information about alternatives to treatment, but insufficient data are available to suggest that a specific treatment modality may not be successful. Suggesting that the couple consider adoption at this time may inappropriately imply that the couple has no other choice. If a specific therapy may result in a pregnancy, the couple should have time to consider these options. After a thorough evaluation, adoption may be considered by the couple as an alternative to the costly, time-consuming, and sometimes painful treatments for infertility. (P, 3)

20. 3. The client's understanding of the procedure is demonstrated by the statement describing IVF as a technique that involves bypassing the blocked or absent fallopian tubes. The physician removes the ova by laparoscope- or ultrasound-guided transvaginal retrieval and mixes them with prepared sperm from the woman's partner or a donor. Two days later, up to four embryos are returned to the uterus to increase the likelihood of a successful pregnancy. Supplemental progesterone, not estrogen, is given to enhance the implantation process. Both GIFT and tubal embryo transfer have a higher pregnancy rate than IVF. However, these procedures cannot be used for clients who have blocked or absent fallopian tubes because the fertilized ova are placed into the fallopian tubes, subsequently entering the uterus naturally for implantation. In IVF, fertilization of the ova by the sperm occurs outside the client's body. In GIFT, both ova and sperm are implanted into the fallopian tubes and allowed to fertilize within the woman's body. (E, 9)

21. 4. The client is verbalizing concerns about death during childbirth, thus providing the nurse with an opportunity to gather additional data. Asking the client about these concerns would be most helpful to determine the client's knowledge base and to provide the nurse with the opportunity to answer any questions and clarify any misconceptions. Although the maternal mortality rate is low in the United States, maternal deaths do occur, even with modern technology. Leading causes of maternal mortality in the United States include embolism, pregnancy-induced hypertension, hemorrhage, ectopic pregnancy, and infection. Telling

the client not to concern herself about what has happened in the past is not useful. It only serves to discount the client's concerns and block further therapeutic communication. Also, postponing or ignoring the client's need for a discussion about complications of pregnancy may further increase the client's anxiety. (I, 3)

22. 3. As ovulation approaches, cervical mucus is abundant and clear, resembling raw egg white. Ovulation generally occurs 14 days (plus or minus 2 days) before the beginning of menses. During the luteal phase of the cycle, which occurs after ovulation, the cervical mucus is thick and sticky, making it difficult for sperm to pass. Changes in the cervical mucus are related to the influences of estrogen and progesterone. Cervical mucus is always present. (P, 3)

23. 1. To ensure maximum effectiveness, the condom should always be placed over the erect penis before coitus. Some couples find condom use objectional because foreplay may have to be interrupted to apply the condom. The penis, covered by the condom, should be withdrawn before the penis becomes flaccid. Otherwise sperm may escape from the condom, providing an opportunity for possible fertilization. Rather than having the condom pulled tightly over the penis before coitus, space should be left at the tip of the penis to allow the condom to hold the sperm. The client does not need a prescription for a condom with nonoxynol 9 because these are sold over the counter. (I, 9)

24. 3. With medroxyprogesterone acetate, irregular menstrual cycles and amenorrhea are common side effects. Other side effects include weight gain, breakthrough bleeding, headaches, and depression. This method requires deep intramuscular injections every 3 months. The first injection should occur within 5 days after menses. (E, 9)

25. 4. Severe cramping and pain may occur as the device is passed through the internal cervical os. The insertion of the device is generally done when the client is having her menses, because it is unlikely that she is pregnant at that time. Common side effects of IUDs are heavy menstrual bleeding and subsequent anemia, not amenorrhea. Uterine infection or ectopic pregnancy may occur. The IUD has an effectiveness rate of 98%. Therefore, additional protection is not necessary to prevent pregnancy. IUDs generally are less costly than other forms of contraception because they do not require additional expense. Only one insertion is necessary, in comparison to daily doses of oral contraceptives or the need for spermicides in conjunction with diaphragm use. (I, 9)

26. 1. The American Cancer Society recommends an annual mammography screening examination for all women after the age of 40. Some high-risk women may begin annual screening at an earlier age. Some women have never had a mammogram because of fear or misconceptions. Mammography should be scheduled after the client's menses to reduce complaints of breast tenderness. Mammography screening is considered expensive, especially by low-income women. Although some discomfort is common because the breast is placed between two plates during the screening process, the procedure should not be considered extremely painful. (E, 4)

27. 3. Small-boned, fair-skinned women of northern European descent are at the greatest risk for osteoporosis, not African American women. One cup of yogurt or 1.5 ounces of hard cheese is the equivalent of one glass of milk. Women who do not eat dairy products, such as women who are lactose intolerant, should consider using calcium supplements. Inadequate lifetime intake of calcium is a major risk factor for osteoporosis. Estrogen therapy, or some of the newer medications that are non–estrogen based, can greatly reduce the incidence of osteoporosis. (E, 9)

28. 3. Ceftriaxone sodium (Rocephin) may be used to treat *Neisseria gonorrhoeae* infections and is often combined with doxycycline. Both the client and her partner should be treated if gonorrhea is present. Acyclovir (Zovirax) can be used to treat herpes genitalis; however, the drug does not cure the disease. *Chlamydia trachomatis* infections are usually treated with antibiotics such as doxycycline hyclate (Vivox, Vibramycin) or azithromycin (Zithromax). Metronidazole (Flagyl) is used to treat trichomoniasis vaginalis, not condylomata acuminata (genital warts). (P, 8)

29. 2. Raloxifene hydrochloride (Evista), an estrogen receptor modulator, increases bone mineral density without stimulating the endometrium. The drug is useful in preventing osteoporosis in postmenopausal women. This drug is contraindicated for women who smoke cigarettes or who have a history of venous thrombosis. Raloxifene does not prevent hot flashes, hyperglycemia, or migraine headaches. One of its side effects is increased headaches. (I, 9)

30. 1. The client needs further instruction when he says that one cause of male infertility is decreased sperm count due to seminal fluid that has an alkaline pH. A slightly alkaline pH is necessary to protect the sperm from the acidic secretions of the vagina and is a normal finding. An alkaline pH is not associated with decreased sperm count. However, seminal fluid that is abnormal in amount, consistency, or chemical composition suggests obstruction, inflammation, or infection, which can decrease sperm production. The typical number of sperm produced during ejaculation is 400 million. Frequent exposure to heat sources, such as

saunas and hot tubs, can decrease sperm production, as can abnormal hormonal stimulation. Immunologic factors produced by the man against his own sperm (autoantibodies) or by the woman can cause the sperm to clump or be unable to penetrate the ovum, thus contributing to infertility. (E, 3)

31. 2. A bicornate uterus has a "Y" shape and appears to be a double uterus but in fact has only one cervix. A septate uterus contains a septum that extends from the fetus to the cervix, thus dividing the uterus into two separate compartments. A double uterus has two uteri, each of which has a cervix. A uterus didelphys occurs when both uteri of a double uterus are fully formed. (A, 10)

The Pregnant Client Receiving Prenatal Care

32. 1. The radioimmunoassay pregnancy test, which uses an antiserum with specificity for the β-subunit of human chorionic gonadotrophin (hCG) in blood plasma, is highly accurate within 1 week after ovulation. The test is performed in a laboratory. Over-the-counter or home pregnancy tests are performed on urine and use the hemagglutination inhibition method. Radioimmuno-assay tests usually use blood serum. A positive pregnancy test is considered a probable sign of pregnancy. Certain conditions other than pregnancy, such as choriocarcinoma, can cause increased hCG levels. The radioimmunoassay pregnancy test can be use with blood or urine specimens. However, urine specimens are rarely used today in the health care setting because serum results can be obtained earlier. (I, 9)

33. 4. The hormone analyzed in most pregnancy tests is hCG. In the pregnant woman, trace amounts of hCG appear in the serum as early as 24 to 48 hours after implantation owing to the trophoblast production of this hormone. Prolactin, follicle-stimulating hormone, and luteinizing hormone are not used to detect pregnancy. Prolactin is the hormone secreted by the pituitary gland to prepare the breasts for lactation. Follicle-stimulating hormone is involved in follicle maturation during the menstrual cycle. Luteinizing hormone is responsible for stimulating ovulation. (E, 9)

34. 4. When using Nägele's rule to determine the estimated date of delivery, the nurse would count back 3 calendar months from the first day of the last menstrual period and add 7 days. This means the client's estimated date of delivery is February 17. (A, 3)

35. 4. The placenta does not produce testosterone. Human placental lactogen, hCG, estrogen, and progesterone are hormones produced by the placenta during pregnancy. The hormone hCG stimulates the synthesis of estrogen and progesterone early in the pregnancy until the placenta can assume this role. Estrogen results in uterine and breast enlargement. Progesterone aids in maintaining the endometrium, inhibiting uterine contractility, and developing the breasts for lactation. The placenta also produces some nutrients for the embryo and exchanges oxygen, nutrients, and waste products through the chorionic villi. (E, 3)

36. 2. With a Doppler ultrasound device, the fetal heartbeat can be heard as early as 8 weeks' gestation. With a fetoscope, the fetal heartbeat can be heard between 17 and 20 weeks' gestation. (I, 3)

37. 2. This client is expressing a feeling of surprise about having a baby. Therefore, the nurse's best response would be to confirm the pregnancy, which is something that the client already suspects, and then ascertain how the client is feeling now that the suspicion is confirmed. Studies have shown that a common reaction to pregnancy is summarized as ambivalence or "someday, but not now." Such feelings are normal and are experienced by many women early in pregnancy. Offering a pamphlet on pregnancy does not respond to the client's feelings. Telling the client that she should be delighted ignores, rather than addresses, the client's feelings. Also, doing so imposes the nurse's opinion on the client. Ambivalence is a common reaction to pregnancy. Telling the client that she should be delighted may lead to feelings of guilt. Asking the client if she and her husband were trying to have a baby is a "yes–no" question and is not helpful. In addition, it ignores the client's underlying feelings. (I, 5)

38. 3. Women normally experience ambivalence when pregnancy is confirmed, even if the pregnancy was planned. Although the client's culture may play a role in openly accepting the pregnancy, most new mothers who have been ambivalent initially accept the reality by the end of the first trimester. Ambivalence also may be expressed throughout the pregnancy; this is believed to be related to the amount of physical discomfort. The nurse should become concerned and perhaps contact a social worker if the client expresses ambivalence in the third trimester. The client's statement reflects ambivalence, not fear. There is no evidence to suggest or imply that the client is rejecting the fetus. The client's statement reflects ambivalence about the pregnancy, not her ability to care to the newborn. (D, 5)

39. 4. The priority nursing diagnosis at this time relates to nutrition, and the necessary health teaching involves a definite need for appropriate nutrition to meet the needs of the growing fetus. Pregnancy places additional demands on the body, and adequate nutrition is important for fetal well-being throughout pregnancy. Readiness for Enhanced Family Coping related to pregnancy confirmation is not a priority at this time. The developing fetus is the priority; the fetus requires adequate nutrition throughout the pregnancy. Insufficient information is provided in the scenario to support a nursing diagnosis of Ineffective Sexuality Patterns or Compromised Family Coping. (D, 9)

40. 3. Couvade syndrome refers to the situation in which the expectant father experiences some of the discomforts of pregnancy along with the pregnant woman as a means of identifying with the pregnancy. Ptyalism is the term for excessive salivation. Mittelschmerz is the lower abdominal discomfort felt by some women during ovulation. Pica refers to an oral craving for substances such as clay or starch that some pregnant clients experience. (D, 5)

41. 3. Maternal alcohol use may result in fetal alcohol syndrome, marked by mild to moderate mental retardation, physical growth retardation, central nervous system disorders, and feeding difficulties. Because there is no definitive answer as to how much alcohol can be safely consumed by a pregnant woman, it is recommended that pregnant clients be taught to abstain from drinking alcohol during pregnancy. Smoking and other medications also may affect the fetus. (I, 9)

42. 4. An increase in clear, highly acidic vaginal secretions is a normal finding during pregnancy that aids in controlling the growth of pathologic bacteria. Vaginal secretions increase because of the influence of estrogen secretion and increased vaginal and cervical vascularity. The highly acidic nature of the vaginal secretions is caused by the action of *Lactobacillus acidophilus*, which increases the lactic acid content of the secretions. The increased acidity helps to make the vagina resistant to bacterial growth. During pregnancy, estrogen secretion fosters a glycogen-rich environment. Unfortunately, this glycogen-rich, acidic environment fosters the development of yeast (*Candida albicans*) infection, manifested by itching, burning, and a cheese-like vaginal discharge. If the client had a sexually transmitted disease, most likely she would complain of additional symptoms, such as lesions in the genital area or changes in color, consistency, or odor of the vaginal secretions. An increase in vaginal secretions does not help prevent expulsion of the mucus plug. The mucus plug is held in the place by the cervix until the cervix becomes ripe. (D, 3)

43. 2. Measurement of the client's fundal height is a gross estimate of fetal gestational age. At 20 weeks' gestation, the fundal height should be at about the level of the client's umbilicus. The fundus typically is over the symphysis pubis at 12 weeks. A fundal height measurement between these two areas would suggest a fetus with a gestational age between 12 and 20 weeks. The fundal height increases approximately 1 cm/week

after 20 weeks' gestation. The fundus typically reaches the xiphoid process at approximately 36 weeks' gestation. A fundal height between the umbilicus and the xiphoid process would suggest a fetus with a gestational age between 20 and 36 weeks. The fundus then often returns to about 4 cm below the xiphoid owing to lightening at 40 weeks. Additionally, pressure on the diaphragm occurs late in pregnancy. Therefore, a fundal height measurement near the xiphoid process with diaphragmatic compression suggests a fetus near the gestational age of 36 weeks or older. (A, 3)

44. 3. Previously it was believed that amniocentesis should not be performed until 14 to 16 weeks' gestation because of risk to the fetus and also to allow for a generous amount of amniotic fluid to form. However, with the newer techniques of amniocentesis analysis, only 1 mL of fluid is required and the test can be performed as early as 12 weeks' gestation, which is especially useful for identifying genetic disorders. Gestation of 8 or 10 weeks is too early for amniocentesis because the procedure can result in premature labor and subsequent abortion. (I, 4)

45. 4. The National Academy of Sciences Institute of Medicine recommends that women gain between 25 and 35 pounds during pregnancy. These guidelines were developed to decrease the risk of intrauterine growth retardation. It is believed that the pattern of weight gain is as important as the total amount of weight gained. Underweight women and women carrying twins should have a greater weight gain. Typically, women should gain 3.5 pounds during the first trimester and then 1 pound/week during the remainder of the pregnancy (24 weeks) for a total of about 27 to 28 pounds. A weight gain of only 6.6 pounds in the second and third trimesters is not considered normal because the client should be gaining about 1 pound/week, or 12 pounds during the second and third trimesters. Gaining 12 pounds during each trimester would total 36 pounds, which is slightly more than the recommended weight gain. In addition, nausea and vomiting during the first trimester can contribute to a lack of appetite and smaller weight gain during this trimester. (E, 3)

46. 1. Green leafy vegetables, such as asparagus, spinach, brussels sprouts, and broccoli, are rich sources of folic acid. The pregnant woman needs to eat foods high in folic acid to prevent folic acid deficits, which may result in neural tube defects in the newborn. A well-balanced diet must include whole grains, dairy products, and fresh fruits; however, bananas are rich in potassium, seafood is rich in iodine, and yogurt is rich in calcium, not folic acid. (P, 9)

47. 3. Egg yolks and squash and other yellow vegetables are rich sources of vitamin A. Pregnant women should avoid megadoses of vitamin A because fetal malformations may occur. Buttermilk and cheese are good sources of calcium. Strawberries, cantaloupe, citrus fruits (eg, oranges), and tomatoes are good sources of vitamin C, not vitamin A. (E, 7)

48. 4. Riboflavin forms coenzymes needed to release energy. Enriched grain products (eg, cereals, breads), deep green leafy vegetables, milk, veal, beef, and cheddar cheese are rich sources of riboflavin. Fresh fruit is rich in vitamin C and fiber. Prunes are rich in iron, fiber, and vitamin C. Potatoes are a source of vitamin C and carbohydrates. (P, 7)

49. 2. Magnesium aids in the synthesis of protein, nucleic acids, proteins, and fats. It is important for cell growth and neuromuscular function. Magnesium also activates the enzymes for metabolism of protein and energy. Calcium prevents demineralization of the mother's bones. Vitamin B$_6$ is important for amino acid metabolism. Folic acid assists in the development of neural pathways in the fetus. (I, 7)

50. 1. The diet for Vietnamese Americans typically consists of small portions of meat and ample amounts of rice. Fresh milk may not have been readily available in Vietnam, and many Asian clients are lactose intolerant. Therefore, the nurse would need to assess the client's diet for deficiencies of calcium and possibly iron. Traditionally, Southeast Asian diets have an abundance of dark green leafy vegetables, such as mustard greens and bok choy, which contain adequate amounts of vitamin E and vitamin C. Seafood, which contains iodine, is usually adequate in the diets of Southeast Asian women. (A, 9)

51. 3. Chorionic villi sampling, which can be performed between 8 and 10 weeks' gestation, involves the insertion of a thin catheter into the vagina and uterus to obtain a sample of the chorionic cells. It is a useful diagnostic test to determine trisomy 13, translocations, fragile X syndrome, and trisomy 18. Fetoscopy is performed with a small fiberoptic fetoscope inserted through a small incision into the client's uterus to inspect the fetus for gross abnormalities. There are no food or fluid restrictions necessary before chorionic villi sampling. Ideally, the client should empty the bladder before this procedure. A full bladder would be needed if the client were scheduled to have an ultrasound examination. (E, 9)

52. 4. Although most multiparous women experience quickening at about 17.5 weeks' gestation, some women may perceive it between 14 and 20 weeks' gestation because they have been pregnant before and know what to expect. This does not suggest a twin pregnancy. If the multiparous client does not experience quickening by 20 weeks gestation, further investi-

gation is warranted, because the fetus may have died, or perhaps a hydatidiform mole, rather than a fetus, is present. There is no evidence that the client's expected date of delivery is erroneous. (D, 3)

53. 4. AFP testing is usually performed between the 15th and 18th weeks of gestation. Abnormally high levels found in maternal serum may be indicative of neural tube defects such as anencephaly and spina bifida. Low levels may indicate trisomy 21 (Down syndrome). Culdocentesis is used to confirm a tubal pregnancy. Chorionic villus sampling is done as early as 10 weeks' gestation to detect anomalies. Ultrasound testing may be done in the first trimester to determine fetal viability and in the third trimester to determine pelvic adequacy and fetal or placental position. (A, 9)

54. 2. Leopold's maneuvers involve abdominal palpation. The client should empty her bladder before the nurse palpates the abdomen. Doing so increases the client's comfort and makes palpation more accurate. Although breathing deeply may help to relax the client, it has no effect on the accuracy of the results of Leopold's maneuvers. The client does not need to drink a full glass of water before the examination. The client should be lying in a supine position with the head slightly elevated for greater comfort and with the knees drawn up slightly. (I, 4)

55. 1. In left occipital transverse lie, the occiput faces the woman's left hip. In left occipital anterior lie, the occiput faces the left anterior segment of the woman's pelvis. In right occipital transverse lie, the occiput faces the woman's right hip. In right occipital anterior lie, the occiput faces the right anterior segment of the woman's pelvis. (D, 10)

56. 1. Discoloration on the face that commonly appears during pregnancy, called *chloasma* (mask of pregnancy), usually fades postpartum and is of no clinical significance. The client who is bothered by her appearance may be able to decrease its prominence with ordinary makeup. No treatment is necessary for this condition. Chloasma is not a sign of skin melanoma. It is not caused by dilated capillaries. Rather, it results from increased secretion of melanocyte-stimulating hormones caused by estrogen and progesterone secretion. (I, 3)

57. 4. Assessment of fundal height is a gross estimate of gestational age. By 20 weeks' gestation, the height of the fundus should be at the level of the umbilicus, after which it should increase 1 cm for each week of gestation until approximately 36 weeks' gestation. Fundal height that is significantly different from that implied by the estimated gestational age warrants further evaluation (eg, ultrasound examination), because it possibly indicates multiple pregnancy or fetal growth retar-

dation. Fundal height estimation will not determine uterine activity or a need for increased weight gain. Ultrasound examination, not fundal height estimation, will locate the placenta. (P, 3)

58. 2. One of the primary risks of amniocentesis is stimulation of the uterus and subsequent preterm labor. Other risks include hemorrhage from penetration of the placenta, infection of the amniotic fluid, and puncture of the fetus. There is little risk for rupture of the membranes, fetal organ malformations, or fetal limb malformations if a practitioner skilled in using ultrasound performs the procedure. Fetal limb malformations have been associated with percutaneous umbilical blood sampling. (E, 9)

59. 3. Automobile travel is not contraindicated during pregnancy unless the client develops complications. There is no set maximum number of hours allowed. The client traveling by automobile should be advised to take intermittent breaks of 10 to 15 minutes, including walking, every 1 to 2 hours to stimulate the circulation, which becomes sluggish during long periods of sitting. The pregnant client should always wear a seat belt when traveling by automobile. The client should be aware of the nearest health care facility in the city to which she is traveling. (I, 9)

60. 3. Leg cramps are thought to result from excessive amounts of phosphorus absorbed from milk products. Straightening the knee and pushing upward on the toes is an effective measure to relieve leg cramps. Also, decreasing milk intake and supplementing with calcium lactate may help to reduce the cramping. Keeping the legs warm and elevating them are good preventive measures. Changing positions frequently aids venous return but is not helpful in relieving leg cramps. Alternately flexing and extending the legs will not help to relieve the leg cramp. Lying prone in the bed is a difficult position for a client at 37 weeks' gestation to achieve and maintain because of the increase in abdominal size and therefore is not considered helpful. (I, 7)

61. 1. Eating smaller and more frequent meals may help prevent heartburn because acid production is decreased and stomach displacement is reduced. Heartburn can occur at any time during pregnancy. Contributing factors include stress, tension, worry, fatigue, caffeine, and smoking. Certain spicy foods (eg, tacos) may trigger heartburn in the pregnant client. The client should be advised to avoid sodium bicarbonate antacids (eg, Alka-Seltzer), baking soda, Bicitra or sodium citrate, and fatty foods, which are high in sodium and can contribute to fluid retention. Increasing, not decreasing, fluid intake may help to relieve heartburn by diluting gastric juices. Caffeinated prod-

ucts such as coffee or tea can stimulate acid formation in the stomach, further contributing to heartburn. (I, 7)

62. 2. In the first maneuver, which is done with the nurse facing the client's head, both hands are used to palpate and determine which fetal body part (eg, the head or buttocks) is in the fundus. This first maneuver helps to determine the presenting part of the fetus. In the second maneuver, also done with the nurse facing the client's head, the palms of both hands are used to palpate the sides of the uterus and determine the location of the fetal back and spine. In the third maneuver, one hand gently grasps the lower portion of the abdomen just above the symphysis pubis to determine whether the fetal head is at the pelvic inlet. The fourth maneuver, done with the nurse facing the client's feet, determines the degree of fetal descent and flexion into the pelvis. (I, 3)

63. 4. Increased AFP levels are associated with neural tube defects, such as spina bifida, anencephaly, and encephalocele. Ultrasonography is used to confirm a neural tube defect only when AFP levels are increased. Because AFP levels are usually highest at 15 to 18 weeks' gestation, this is the optimum time for testing. Performing the test after this time leads to inaccurate results. The client's blood, not urine, is used for the sample. (P, 9)

64. 1. Prenatal care is often the most critical factor influencing pregnancy outcome. This is especially true for adolescents, because the most significant medical complication in pregnant adolescents is pregnancy-induced hypertension. Continued prenatal care helps to allow for early detection and prompt intervention should the complication arise. Other risks for adolescents include low-birth-weight infant, preterm labor, iron-deficiency anemia, and cephalopelvic disproportion. Gestational diabetes can occur with any pregnancy regardless of the age of the mother. Generally, all first-time mothers need instruction related to discomforts. Adolescent mothers have better nutrition when they attend group classes and are subject to peer pressure. No evidence demonstrates that most adolescents lack support systems. Fathers may abandon mothers at any time during the pregnancy; other fathers, regardless of age, are supportive throughout the pregnancy. (D, 3)

65. 3. The most appropriate nursing diagnosis for this client is Impaired Nutrition: Less Than Body Requirements related to lack of appetite. The evidence of gaining only 5 pounds since the beginning of pregnancy supports this diagnosis. Additional supportive evidence is the client's statement that she has no appetite. The nurse needs to gather additional data to determine the reason for the client's poor appetite, such as a physiologic or psychological problem. More information is needed to support a nursing diagnosis of Knowledge Deficit, Noncompliance, or Chronic Low Self-esteem. These nursing diagnoses may be appropriate after the reason for the client s poor appetite is determined. (D, 9)

66. 3. Colostrum is usually secreted by about the 16th week of gestation in preparation for breast-feeding. Growth of the milk ducts is greatest in the last trimester, not in the first 8 weeks of gestation. Enlargement of the breasts is usually caused by estrogen, not progesterone. Darkening of the areola can occur as early as the sixth week of gestation. (I, 3)

67. 2. During pregnancy, the circulatory system undergoes tremendous changes. Cardiac output increases by 25% to 50%, and circulatory blood volume increases by about 30%. The client may experience transient hypotension and dizziness with sudden position changes. Early in pregnancy there is a slight increase in the temperature, and clients may attribute this to a sinus infection or a cold. The client may feel warm, but this sensation is transient. The level of circulating fibrinogen increases as much as 50% during pregnancy, probably because of increased estrogen. Any calf tenderness should be reported, because it may indicate a clot. Late in pregnancy, the posterior pituitary gland secretes oxytocin. The client may experience painful Braxton Hicks contractions or early labor symptoms. (P, 3)

68. 1. The fetal biophysical profile includes fetal breathing movements, fetal body movements, tone, amniotic fluid volume, and fetal heart rate reactivity. A reactive nonstress test is a sign of fetal well-being and does not require further evaluation. A nonreactive nonstress test requires further evaluation. A contraction stress test or oxytocin challenge test should be performed only on women who are at risk for fetal distress during labor. The contraction stress test is rarely performed before 28 weeks gestation because of the possibility of initiating labor. Percutaneous umbilical cord sampling requires the insertion of a needle through the abdomen to obtain a fetal blood sample. (I, 9)

69. 3. The purpose of Kegel exercises is to strengthen the perineal muscles in preparation for the labor process. These movements strengthen the pubococcygeal muscle, which surrounds the urinary meatus and vagina. No evidence is available to support the idea that these exercises prevent vulvar edema, alleviate lower back discomfort, or strengthen the abdominal muscles. (I, 7)

70. 4. During the third trimester, it is not uncommon for clients to have dreams or fantasies about the baby. Sometimes the dreams are about infants who are malformed or, in this example, covered with hair. There is no evidence to suggest that the client is trying to cope

with becoming a parent. Having dreams about the baby does not mean that labor will begin soon. (I, 5)

71. 1. Insomnia in the later part of pregnancy is not uncommon because the client has difficulty getting into a position of comfort. This is further compounded by frequent nocturia. The best suggestion would be to advise the client to practice relaxation techniques before bedtime. The client should avoid caffeine products such as chocolate and coffee before going to bed because caffeine is a stimulant. Alcohol consumption, regardless of the type or amount, should be avoided. Exercise is advised during the day, but it should be avoided before bedtime because exercise can stimulate the client and decrease the client s ability to fall asleep. (I, 7)

72. 3. The client needs further instruction when she says it is permissible to sit in a hot tub for 20 minutes to relax after working. Hot tubs and saunas should be avoided, particularly in the first trimester, because their use can lead to maternal hyperthermia, which is associated with fetal anomalies such as central nervous system defects. The client should use nonskid pads in the shower or bath to avoid slipping because the client s center of gravity has shifted and she may fall. The client should avoid using soap on the nipples to prevent removal of the natural protective oils. Douching is not recommended for pregnant women because it can destroy the normal flora and increase the client s risk for infection. (E, 3)

73. 3. The obstetric conjugate can be estimated by subtracting 1.5 to 2 cm from the diagonal conjugate, which can be measured during a pelvic examination. (I, 3)

74. 1. The uterus receives its blood supply from the uterine and ovarian arteries. The ovarian artery is a branch of the abdominal aorta. It enters the broad ligament and supplies the ovary with blood. Its main stem makes its way to the upper margin of the uterus. The ovarian blood supply drains into two ovarian veins. (E, 3)

The Pregnant Client in Childbirth Preparation Classes

75. 4. Thyroid enlargement and increased basal body metabolism are common occurrences during pregnancy. Human placental lactogen does not maintain the corpus luteum. Rather, it enhances milk production. Estrogen, not progesterone, is responsible for hyperpigmentation and vascular skin changes. Progesterone, not estrogen, relaxes smooth muscle in the respiratory tract. (P, 3)

76. 1. Although sex is not easily identified at 9 to 12 weeks, external genitalia are developed at this period of fetal

development. Myelinization of the nerves begins at about 20 weeks' gestation. Brown fat stores develop at approximately 21 to 24 weeks. Air ducts and alveoli develop later in the gestational period, at approximately 25 to 28 weeks. (P, 3)

77. 2. Monozygotic twinning is independent of race, age, parity, or heredity. Monozygotic twins result from the fertilization of one ovum by two different sperm. Dizygotic twinning occurs with the fertilization of more than one ovum during conception. Dizygotic twins may be of the same sex or different sexes. Dizygotic twinning is correlated with increased parity, becoming pregnant within 1 month after stopping oral contraception, and infertility treatments. African Americans have a higher rate of dizygotic twins than Caucasian Americans do. (I, 3)

78. 3. If the head is the presenting part, the normal maneuvers during labor and delivery are descent, flexion, internal rotation, extension, external rotation, and expulsion. These maneuvers are called the cardinal movements. They maneuvers occur as the fetal head passes through the maternal pelvis during the normal labor process. Engagement refers to the fetus' entering the true pelvis. (I, 3)

79. 1. In a normal delivery and for the first 24 hours postpartum, a total blood loss not exceeding 500 mL is considered normal. Blood loss during delivery is almost always estimated because it provides a valuable indicator for possible hemorrhage. A blood loss of 1000 mL is considered hemorrhage. (I, 3)

80. 2. Although the amniotic fluid promotes normal prenatal development by allowing symmetric development, it does not provide the fetus with nutrients. Rather, nutrients are provided by the placenta. The amniotic fluid does help dilate the cervix once labor begins by pressure and gravity forces. The amniotic fluid helps to protect the fetus from injury by cushioning against impact of the maternal abdomen and allows room and buoyancy for fetal movement. The amniotic fluid and sac keep the fetus at a stable temperature by maintaining a neutral thermal environment. (E, 3)

81. 1. Pelvic rocking helps to relieve backache during pregnancy and early labor by making the spine more flexible. Deep breathing exercises assist with relaxation and pain relief during labor. Tailor sitting and squatting help stretch the perineal muscles in preparation for labor. (I, 3)

82. 2. Pain during the first stage of labor is primarily caused by hypoxia of the uterine and cervical muscle cells during contraction, stretching of the lower uterine segment, dilation of the cervix and perineum, and pressure on adjacent structures. A client's perceptions of pain, her cultural background, fear, and anxiety can influence pain. (I, 3)

83. 4. With true labor, the contractions are felt first in the lower back and then the abdomen. They gradually increase in frequency and duration and do not disappear with ambulation, rest, or sleep. In true labor, the cervix dilates and effaces. Walking tends to increase true contractions. False labor contractions disappear with ambulation, rest, or sleep. False labor contractions often remain the same in duration and frequency. Clients who are experiencing false labor may have pain, even though the contractions are not very effective. (I, 3)

84. 4. Pelvic tilt exercises are useful to alleviate backache during pregnancy and labor but are not useful for the pain from contractions. Biofeedback (a conscious effort to control the response to pain), effleurage (light uterine massage), and guided imagery (focusing on a pleasant scene) are appropriate pain relief techniques to practice before labor begins. Various breathing exercises also can help to alleviate the discomfort from contraction pain. (E, 3)

85. 2. Increased vaginal discharge is normal during pregnancy, but yellow-gray frothy discharge with local itching is associated with infection (eg, *Trichomonas vaginalis*). The client's symptoms must be further assessed by a health professional because the client needs treatment for this condition. *T. vaginalis* infection is commonly treated with metronidazole (Flagyl). However, this drug is not used in the first trimester. In the first trimester, the typical treatment is topical clotrimazole. Although a yeast infection is associated with vaginal itching, the vaginal discharge is cheese-like. Furthermore, because the client may have a serious vaginal infection, over-the-counter medications are not advised until the client has been evaluated. Douching is not recommended during pregnancy because it would predispose the client to an ascending infection. The client is not exhibiting signs and symptoms of preterm labor, such as contractions or leaking fluid. And although the client's complaints are suggestive of a trichomonas infection, which can lead to preterm labor and premature rupture of the membranes, further evaluation is needed to confirm the cause of the infection. (I, 3)

86. 4. The umbilical cord normally consists of two arteries and one vein. Oxygen and other nutrients are carried to the fetal circulation by the umbilical vein. The umbilical arteries carry oxygen-poor blood back to the placenta. The foramen ovale is a shunt that allows blood returning from the lungs to mix. The ductus arteriosus allows oxygenated blood via the umbilical vein to be carried to the inferior vena cava. (I, 3)

87. 3. The umbilical cord normally inserts in the center of the placenta. A velamentous cord does not insert centrally into the placenta, and cord vessels branch out, which can lead to fetal hemorrhage. The highest oxygen content is found in the umbilical vein. Oxygenated blood flows through the umbilical vein to the fetus. Blood leaving the fetus to return to the placenta flows through the two umbilical arteries. About 1% of umbilical cords have only one artery. A nuchal cord occurs when the cord is wrapped around the fetus' neck, often because the cord is longer than normal. (P, 3)

88. 2. During pregnancy, urinary tract infections are more common because of urinary stasis. Clients need instructions about increasing fluid volume intake. Plasma volume increases during pregnancy. The increase in plasma volume is more pronounced and occurs earlier than the increase in red blood cell mass, possibly resulting in physiologic anemia. Peripheral vascular resistance decreases during pregnancy, providing a relatively stable blood pressure. Hemoglobin levels decrease during pregnancy even though there is an increase in blood volume. (P, 3)

89. 2. Infant mortality rate is defined as the number of deaths of infants younger than 1 year of age per 1000 live births. Maternal mortality in the United States has been steadily decreasing; however, African American infants have a higher mortality rate than caucasian infants. The perinatal mortality rate includes all stillborn infants with a gestational age of 28 weeks or more plus all neonatal deaths before 7 days of age per 1000 of this population. The neonatal mortality rate is the number of deaths of infants younger than 28 days of age per 1000 live births. (P, 3)

90. 1. The placenta is formed by fusion of the chorionic villi and the decidua basalis. Many viruses, such as rubella, chickenpox, mumps, measles, and cytomegalovirus, as well as the bacterium *Treponema pallidum*, can cross the placenta and infect the fetus. Larger molecules have more difficulty, with the exception of immunoglobulin G. The weight of a term placenta is 400 to 600 g, or about one sixth of the weight of the newborn. Human placental lactogen promotes normal nutrition and growth of the fetus and maternal breast development for lactation. Human placental lactogen does not affect testosterone production. (P, 3)

The Pregnant Client With Risk Factors

91. 4. Additional teaching is needed when the parent says that adolescents are at greater risk for congenital anomalies. Although adolescents are at greater risk for denial of the pregnancy, lack of prenatal care, low-birth-weight infant, cephalopelvic disproportion, anemia, and nutritional deficits and have a higher maternal mortality rate, studies reveal that congenital anomalies are not more frequent in adolescent pregnancies. (E, 3)

92. 4. With a spontaneous abortion, many clients and their partners feel an acute sense of loss. Their grieving often includes feelings of guilt, which may be expressed as wondering whether the woman could have done something to prevent the loss. Anger, sadness, and disappointment are also common emotions after a pregnancy loss. Ambivalence, anxiety, and fear are not common emotions after a spontaneous abortion. (P, 5)

93. 1. Hydroxyzine (Vistaril) has a tranquilizing effect and also decreases nausea and vomiting. It does not decrease fluid retention, reduce pain, decrease uterine cramping, or promote uterine contractility. One of the side effects of the medication is sleepiness. Ibuprofen may decrease pain from uterine cramping. Oxytocin may be used to increase uterine contractility. (I, 8)

94. 3. The death of a fetus at any time during pregnancy is a tragedy for most parents. After a spontaneous abortion, the client and family members can be expected to suffer from grief for several months or longer. When offering support, a simple statement such as "I'm truly sorry you lost your baby" is most appropriate. Therapeutic communication techniques help the client and family understand the meaning of the loss, move less stressfully through the grief process, and share feelings. Asking the client whether she is experiencing a great deal of uterine pain is inappropriate because this is a "yes–no" question and doesn't allow the client to express her feelings. Saying that the embryo was defective is inappropriate because this may lead the client to think that she contributed to the fetus' demise. This is not the appropriate time to discuss embryonic or fetal malformations. However, the nurse should explain to the client that this situation was not her fault. Telling the client that she should get pregnant again as soon as possible is not therapeutic and discounts the feelings of expectant mothers who have already begun to bond with the fetus. (I, 5)

95. 4. Rh sensitization can be prevented by Rho(D) immune globulin, which clears the maternal circulation of Rh-positive cells before sensitization can occur, thereby blocking maternal antibody production to Rh-positive cells. Administration of this drug will not prevent future Rh-positive fetuses, nor will it prevent future abortions. Rh-negative mothers do not develop sensitivities if the fetus is also Rh negative. (I, 8)

96. 2. The client with leg varicosities should take frequent rest periods with the legs elevated above the hips to promote venous circulation. The client should avoid constrictive clothing, but support hose that reach above the varicosities may help alleviate the pain. Contracting and relaxing the feet and ankles twice daily is not helpful because it does not promote circulation. Taking a leave of absence from work may not be possible because of economic reasons. The client should try to rest with her legs elevated or walk around for a few minutes every 2 hours while on the job. (I, 9)

97. 1. Cryotherapy, electrocautery, or laser therapy may be used to remove the genital warts. Podophyllin solution should not be used to decrease their size while the client is pregnant, because fetal malformations may result. A 25% trichloroacetic acid solution can decrease the size of the warts, but because this disease is caused by a virus, the disorder may recur. Condolymata acuminata has been associated with cervical cancer, and the client should have semiannual or annual Pap smears to detect cervical dysplasia. (I, 8)

98. 4. The client is reporting symptoms typically associated with herpes genitalis. Some women have no symptoms of gonorrhea. Others may experience vaginal itching and a thick, purulent vaginal discharge. *C. trachomatis* infection in women is often asymptomatic, but symptoms may include a yellowish discharge and painful urination. The first symptom of syphilis is a painless chancre. (A, 10)

99. 1. The client may need surgery to remove a ruptured fallopian tube where the pregnancy has occurred, and the nurse is usually responsible for witnessing the signature on the informed consent. Usually, if bleeding is occurring, it is internal. Typically there is only scant vaginal bleeding with no discoloration. The nurse cannot determine whether the fallopian tube can be salvaged; this can be accomplished only during surgery. If the tube has ruptured, it must be removed. If the tube has not ruptured, a linear salpingostomy may be done to salvage the tube for future pregnancies. With an ectopic pregnancy, although the client is experiencing abdominal pain, she is not having uterine contractions. (P, 10)

100. 1. The optical density of the amniotic fluid is evaluated for bilirubin level with a spectrophotometer. The higher the optical density, the more bilirubin is present in the fluid, indicating that fetal red blood cells are being destroyed. From these findings, the severity of the disease can be estimated. Because light destroys bilirubin, specimens should be kept in a dark container until the analysis is complete. A clear, green, or amber container would allow light to enter, thus destroying bilirubin. (I, 9)

101. 4. For the Rh-negative client who may be pregnant with an Rh-positive fetus, an indirect Coombs test measures antibodies in the maternal blood. Titers should be performed monthly during the first and second trimesters and biweekly during the third trimester and the week before the due date. (I, 3)

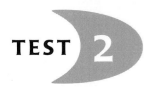

TEST 2

Complications of Pregnancy

Select the one best answer, and indicate your choice by filling in the circle in front of the option.

The Client With Preeclampsia/Eclampsia

1. At 32 weeks' gestation, a 15-year-old primigravid client who is 5 feet, 2 inches tall has gained a total of 20 pounds, with a 1-pound gain in the last 2 weeks. Urinalysis reveals negative glucose and a trace of protein. The nurse determines that which of the following factors increases this client risk for preeclampsia?
   ○ 1. Total weight gain.
   ○ 2. Short stature.
   ○ 3. Adolescent age group.
   ○ 4. Proteinuria.

2. A primigravid client's baseline blood pressure at her initial visit at 12 weeks' gestation was 110/70 mm Hg. During an assessment at 38 weeks' gestation, which of the following data would indicate mild preeclampsia?
   ○ 1. Blood pressure of 160/110 mm Hg on two separate occasions.
   ○ 2. Proteinuria, more than 5 g in 24 hours.
   ○ 3. Serum creatinine concentration of 1.4 mL/dL.
   ○ 4. Weight gain of 2 pounds in the last week.

3. When making a home visit to a 19-year-old primigravid client at 38 weeks' gestation diagnosed with mild preeclampsia and mild peripheral edema requiring bed rest at home for the past 2 weeks, which of the following would the nurse identify as the client's priority nursing diagnosis?
   ○ 1. Noncompliance related to poor nutrition and lack of exercise during pregnancy.
   ○ 2. Delayed Growth and Development related to required bed rest and subsequent immobility.
   ○ 3. Deficient Fluid Volume related to fluid shift from intravascular to extravascular space.
   ○ 4. Situational Low Self-Esteem related to prolonged bed rest and pregnancy complications.

4. During a home visit to a 16-year-old client at 34 weeks' gestation diagnosed with mild preeclampsia, assessment reveals that the client has gained 2 pounds in the past week and her current blood pressure is 130/86 mm Hg. Which of the following assessment findings would provide further evidence to support the client's diagnosis?
   ○ 1. Pounding headache after reading.
   ○ 2. History of urinary tract infection.
   ○ 3. Frequent voiding in large amounts.
   ○ 4. Mild edema in hands and face.

5. When developing the teaching plan for a primigravid client at 30 weeks' gestation diagnosed with mild preeclampsia who is being treated at home, which of the following would the nurse identify as the *most* appropriate client-centered goal?
   ○ 1. Return visit to the prenatal clinic in approximately 4 weeks.
   ○ 2. Decreased edema after 1 week of a low-protein, low-fiber diet.
   ○ 3. Bed rest on the left side during the day, with bathroom privileges.
   ○ 4. Immediate reporting of adverse reactions to magnesium sulfate therapy.

6. After instructing a primigravid client at 38 weeks' gestation about how preeclampsia can affect both the client and the growing fetus, the nurse realizes that the client needs additional instruction when she

says that preeclampsia can lead to which of the following?

○ 1. Hydrocephalic infant.

○ 2. Abruptio placenta.

○ 3. Intrauterine growth retardation.

○ 4. Poor placental perfusion.

7. After instructing a multigravid client diagnosed with mild preeclampsia how to keep a record of fetal movement patterns at home, the nurse determines that the teaching has been effective when the client says that she will count the number of times the baby moves during which of the following time spans?

○ 1. 30-minute period three times a day.

○ 2. 45-minute period after lunch each day.

○ 3. 1-hour period each day.

○ 4. 12-hour period each week.

8. When teaching a multigravid client diagnosed with mild preeclampsia about nutritional needs, which of the following types of diet would the nurse discuss?

○ 1. High-residue diet.

○ 2. Low-sodium diet.

○ 3. Regular diet.

○ 4. High-protein diet.

9. In response to a question from a 40-year-old multigravid client diagnosed with mild preeclampsia about the causes of this problem, the nurse teaches the client about the various theories surrounding the conditions associated with preeclampsia. Which of the following, if stated by the client as an associated condition, would indicate the need for additional teaching?

○ 1. Multifetal pregnancy.

○ 2. Diabetes mellitus.

○ 3. Age older than 35 years.

○ 4. Iron deficiency.

10. A 17-year-old client at 33 weeks' gestation diagnosed with mild preeclampsia is prescribed bed rest at home. The nurse instructs the client to contact the health care provider immediately if she experiences which of the following?

○ 1. Blurred vision.

○ 2. Ankle edema.

○ 3. Increased energy levels.

○ 4. Mild backache.

11. One week after her prenatal visit, a primigravid client at 38 weeks' gestation diagnosed with mild preeclampsia calls the clinic nurse complaining of a continuous headache for the past 2 days accompanied by nausea. The client does not want to take aspirin. Which of the following responses by the nurse would be *most* appropriate?

○ 1. "Take two acetaminophen tablets. They aren't as likely to upset your stomach."

○ 2. "I think the doctor should see you today. Can you come to the clinic this morning?"

○ 3. "You need to lie down and rest. Have you tried placing a cool compress over your head?"

○ 4. "I'll ask the doctor to call in a prescription for aspirin with codeine. What's your pharmacy's number?"

12. When reviewing the prenatal records of a 16-year-old primigravid client at 37 weeks' gestation diagnosed with severe preeclampsia, the nurse would interpret which of the following as *most* indicative of the client's diagnosis?

○ 1. Blood pressure of 138/94 mm Hg.

○ 2. Severe blurring of vision.

○ 3. Less than 2 g protein in a 24-hour sample.

○ 4. Weight gain of 0.5 pound in 1 week.

13. When preparing the room for admission of a multigravid client at 36 weeks' gestation diagnosed with severe preeclampsia, which of the following would the nurse obtain?

○ 1. Oxytocin infusion solution.

○ 2. Disposable tongue blades.

○ 3. Portable ultrasound machine.

○ 4. Padding for the side rails.

14. The physician orders intravenous magnesium sulfate for a primigravid client at 38 weeks' gestation diagnosed with severe preeclampsia. Which of the following medications would the nurse have readily available at the client's bedside?

○ 1. Diazepam (Valium).

○ 2. Hydralazine (Apresoline).

○ 3. Calcium gluconate.

○ 4. Phenytoin (Dilantin).

15. For the client who is receiving intravenous magnesium sulfate for severe preeclampsia, which of the following assessment findings would alert the nurse to suspect hypermagnesemia?

○ 1. Decreased deep tendon reflexes.

○ 2. Cool skin temperature.

○ 3. Rapid pulse rate.

○ 4. Tingling in the toes.

16. A 28-year-old multigravida at 37 weeks' gestation arrives at the emergency department via ambulance with a blood pressure of 160/104 mm Hg and +3 reflexes without clonus. The client, who is diagnosed with severe preeclampsia, asks the nurse, "What is the cure for my high blood pressure?" Which of the following would the nurse identify as the primary cure?

○ 1. Administration of glucocorticoids (Betamethasone).

○ 2. Vaginal or cesarean delivery of the fetus.

○ 3. Sedation with phenytoin (Dilantin).

○ 4. Reduction of fluid retention with thiazide diuretics.

17. Which of the following would the nurse identify as the priority to achieve when developing the plan of

care for a primigravid client at 38 weeks' gestation who is hospitalized with severe preeclampsia and receiving intravenous magnesium sulfate?

○ 1. Decreased generalized edema within 8 hours.

○ 2. Decreased urinary output during the first 24 hours.

○ 3. Sedation and decreased reflex excitability within 48 hours.

○ 4. Absence of any seizure activity during the first 48 hours.

18. When administering intravenous magnesium sulfate as ordered for a client at 34 weeks' gestation with severe preeclampsia, the nurse would explain to the client and her family that this drug acts as which of the following?

○ 1. Peripheral vasodilator.

○ 2. Antihypertensive.

○ 3. Central nervous system depressant.

○ 4. Sedative/hypnotic.

19. Soon after admission of a primigravida at 38 weeks' gestation with severe preeclampsia, the physician orders a continuous intravenous infusion of 5% dextrose in Ringer's solution and 4 g of magnesium sulfate. While the medication is being administered, which of the following signs should the nurse report immediately?

○ 1. Respiratory rate of 12 breaths/minute.

○ 2. Patellar reflex of +2.

○ 3. Blood pressure of 160/88 mm Hg.

○ 4. Urinary output exceeding intake.

20. Which of the following would be the most appropriate nursing diagnosis for a primigravid client at 38 weeks' gestation who was just admitted for eclampsia after experiencing a seizure in her home?

○ 1. Risk for Injury related to possibility of further convulsions.

○ 2. Deficient Knowledge related to symptoms of preeclampsia.

○ 3. Hypertensive Crisis related to severe preeclampsia.

○ 4. Situational Low Self-Esteem related to hospitalization and sedation.

21. As the nurse enters the room of a newly admitted primigravid client diagnosed with severe preeclampsia, the client begins to experience a seizure. Which of the following should the nurse do *first*?

○ 1. Insert an airway to improve oxygenation.

○ 2. Note the time when the seizure begins and ends.

○ 3. Call for immediate assistance.

○ 4. Turn the client to her left side.

22. After administering hydralazine (Apresoline) 5 mg intravenously as ordered for a primigravid client with severe preeclampsia at 39 weeks' gestation, the nurse would be alert for which of the following?

○ 1. Tachycardia.

○ 2. Bradypnea.

○ 3. Polyuria.

○ 4. Dysphagia.

23. A primigravid client with severe preeclampsia exhibits hyperactive, very brisk patellar reflexes with ankle clonus present and two movements after the reflex. The nurse documents these findings as which of the following?

○ 1. 1+.

○ 2. 2+.

○ 3. 3+.

○ 4. 4+.

24. A 16-year-old unmarried primigravid client at 37 weeks' gestation with severe preeclampsia is in early active labor. Her mother is at the bedside. The client's blood pressure is 164/110 mm Hg. Which of the following would alert the nurse that the client may be about to experience a seizure?

○ 1. Decreased contraction intensity.

○ 2. Decreased temperature.

○ 3. Epigastric pain.

○ 4. Hyporeflexia.

25. Fifteen minutes after a client experiences an eclamptic seizure, the nurse assesses the client for which of the following?

○ 1. Polyuria.

○ 2. Facial flushing.

○ 3. Hypotension.

○ 4. Uterine contractions.

26. If a client at 36 weeks' gestation with eclampsia begins to exhibit signs of labor after an eclamptic seizure, for which of the following would the nurse assess?

○ 1. Abruptio placenta.

○ 2. Transverse lie.

○ 3. Placenta accreta.

○ 4. Uterine atony.

27. For a multigravid client at 39 weeks' gestation with suspected HELLP syndrome, the nurse would immediately notify the physician for which of the following laboratory test results?

○ 1. Hyperfibrinogenemia.

○ 2. Decreased liver enzymes.

○ 3. Thrombocytopenia.

○ 4. Hypernatremia.

The Pregnant Client With a Chronic Hypertensive Disorder

28. An obese 36-year-old multigravida at 12 weeks' gestation has a history of chronic hypertension. She was treated with methyldopa (Aldomet) before becoming pregnant. When counseling the client

about diet during pregnancy, the nurse realizes that the client needs additional instruction when she states which of the following?
- ○ 1. "I need to reduce my caloric intake to 1200 calories a day."
- ○ 2. "A regular diet is recommended during pregnancy."
- ○ 3. "I should eat more frequent meals if I get heartburn."
- ○ 4. "I need to consume more fluids and fiber each day."

29. After instructing a multigravid client at 10 weeks' gestation diagnosed with chronic hypertension about the need for frequent prenatal visits, the nurse determines that the instructions have been successful when the client states which of the following?
- ○ 1. "I may develop hyperthyroidism because of my high blood pressure."
- ○ 2. "I need close monitoring because I may have a small-for-gestational-age infant."
- ○ 3. "It's possible that I will have excess amniotic fluid and may need a cesarean section."
- ○ 4. "I may develop placenta accreta, so I need to keep my clinic appointments."

The Pregnant Client With Third-Trimester Bleeding

30. A 24-year-old client, gravida III, para I, at 32 weeks' gestation, is admitted to the hospital because of vaginal bleeding. After reviewing the client's history, which of the following factors might lead the nurse to suspect abruptio placenta?
- ○ 1. Several hypotensive episodes.
- ○ 2. Previous low transverse cesarean delivery.
- ○ 3. One induced abortion.
- ○ 4. History of cocaine use.

31. When caring for a multigravid client admitted to the hospital with vaginal bleeding at 38 weeks' gestation, which of the following would the nurse anticipate administering intravenously if the client develops disseminated intravascular coagulation (DIC)?
- ○ 1. Ringer's lactate solution.
- ○ 2. Fresh frozen platelets.
- ○ 3. 5% dextrose solution.
- ○ 4. Warfarin sodium (Coumadin).

32. When assessing a 34-year-old multigravid client at 34 weeks' gestation experiencing moderate vaginal bleeding, which of the following would *most* likely alert the nurse that placenta previa is present?
- ○ 1. Painless vaginal bleeding.
- ○ 2. Uterine tetany.
- ○ 3. Intermittent pain with spotting.
- ○ 4. Dull lower back pain.

33. After giving instruction about the cause of the vaginal bleeding to a multigravid client at 36 weeks' gestation diagnosed with placenta previa, the nurse determines that the teaching has been effective when the client says that the bleeding results from which of the following?
- ○ 1. Diminished clotting factors.
- ○ 2. Exposure of maternal blood sinuses.
- ○ 3. Increased platelet levels.
- ○ 4. A large-for-gestational-age fetus.

34. During an interview, a multigravid client at 35 weeks' gestation who was admitted to the hospital with placenta previa and ordered to strict bed rest states, "My last baby was born 6 weeks early and had to stay in a special care nursery." Which of the following would the nurse formulate as the priority nursing diagnosis?
- ○ 1. Risk for Constipation related to bed rest.
- ○ 2. Interrupted Family Processes related to hospitalization.
- ○ 3. Anxiety related to unknown outcome of client/fetus.
- ○ 4. Impaired Physical Mobility related to vaginal bleeding.

35. The physician orders whole blood replacement for a multigravid client with abruptio placenta. Before administering the intravenous blood product, which of the following should the nurse do *first*?
- ○ 1. Validate client information and the blood product with another nurse.
- ○ 2. Check the vital signs before transfusing over 5 to 6 hours.
- ○ 3. Ask the client if she has ever had any allergies.
- ○ 4. Administer 100 mL of 5% dextrose solution intravenously.

36. Following a cesarean delivery for abruptio placenta, a multigravid client tells the nurse, "I feel like such a failure. None of my other deliveries were like this." The nurse's response to the client is based on the understanding of which of the following?
- ○ 1. The client will most likely have postpartum blues.
- ○ 2. Maternal–infant bonding is likely to be difficult.
- ○ 3. The client's feeling of grief is a normal reaction.
- ○ 4. This type of delivery was necessary to save the client's life.

37. Which of the following actions would the nurse anticipate as the *highest* priority when preparing for the admission of a multigravid client at 36 weeks' gestation with a probable diagnosis of abruptio placenta?
- ○ 1. Preparing the client for a vaginal examination.
- ○ 2. Obtaining a brief history from the client.
- ○ 3. Inserting a large-gauge intravenous catheter.
- ○ 4. Preparing the client for an ultrasound scan.

The Pregnant Client With Preterm Labor

38. A 31-year-old client, gravida III, para 0, at 32 weeks' gestation, is admitted to the hospital with contractions of moderate intensity occurring every 3 to 4 minutes. The client, who has previously delivered two nonviable fetuses at 30 weeks' gestation, is crying on admission. The client asks, "What causes preterm labor?" After giving instruction about various risks for preterm labor, the nurse determines that additional explanation is needed when the client says that preterm labor is often associated with which of the following?
    ○ 1. Age older than 30 years.
    ○ 2. Polyhydramnios.
    ○ 3. Chronic hypertension.
    ○ 4. Multifetal gestation.

39. A multigravid client at 34 weeks' gestation who is leaking amniotic fluid has just been hospitalized with a diagnosis of preterm labor. The client's contractions are 20 minutes apart, lasting 20 to 30 seconds. Her cervix is dilated at 2 cm. The client tells the nurse, "Why is God punishing me? I go to church every Sunday. What did I do wrong to cause this?" Which of the following would be the *priority* nursing diagnosis?
    ○ 1. Risk for Impaired Parenting related to hospitalization.
    ○ 2. Spiritual Distress related to feelings of guilt and preterm labor.
    ○ 3. Risk for Infection related to possible chorioamnionitis.
    ○ 4. Disturbed Body Image related to pregnancy and hospitalization.

40. A multigravida at 34 weeks' gestation is being treated with indomethacin (Indocin) to halt preterm labor. If the client should deliver a preterm infant, the nurse would notify the nursery personnel about this therapy because of the possibility for which of the following?
    ○ 1. Pulmonary hypertension.
    ○ 2. Respiratory distress syndrome (RDS).
    ○ 3. Hyperbilirubinemia.
    ○ 4. Cardiomyopathy.

41. The nurse is preparing to administer terbutaline (Brethine) to a multigravid client in preterm labor. Before administering this drug intravenously, the nurse should assess which of the following?
    ○ 1. Hematocrit level.
    ○ 2. Weight gain.
    ○ 3. Urinary output.
    ○ 4. Heart rate.

42. In which of the following maternal locations would the nurse place the ultrasound transducer of the external electronic fetal heart rate monitor if a fetus at 34 weeks' gestation is in the left occipitoanterior (LOA) position?
    ○ 1. Near the symphysis pubis.
    ○ 2. Two inches above the umbilicus.
    ○ 3. Below the umbilicus on the side of the fundus.
    ○ 4. At the level of the umbilicus.

43. The physician orders betamethasone (Celestone) for a 34-year-old multigravid client at 32 weeks' gestation who is experiencing preterm labor. Previously, the client has experienced one infant death due to preterm birth at 28 weeks' gestation. The nurse explains that this drug is given for which of the following reasons?
    ○ 1. To enhance fetal lung maturity.
    ○ 2. To counter the effects of tocolytic therapy.
    ○ 3. To treat chorioamnionitis.
    ○ 4. To decrease neonatal production of surfactant.

44. The nurse is caring for a multigravid client at 34 weeks' gestation diagnosed with preterm labor. The client has delivered two stillborn infants at 30 weeks' gestation. The client is scheduled for a sonogram before an amniocentesis. Which of the following would be a *priority* nursing diagnosis for the client?
    ○ 1. Acute Pain related to abnormal uterine contractions.
    ○ 2. Anxiety related to diagnostic tests for fetal well-being.
    ○ 3. Ineffective Coping related to hospitalization.
    ○ 4. Deficient Knowledge related to consequences of preterm birth.

45. When preparing a multigravid client at 34 weeks' gestation experiencing preterm labor for the shake test performed on amniotic fluid, the nurse would instruct the client that this test is done to evaluate the maturity of which of the following fetal systems?
    ○ 1. Urinary.
    ○ 2. Gastrointestinal.
    ○ 3. Cardiovascular.
    ○ 4. Pulmonary.

The Pregnant Client With Premature Rupture of the Membranes

46. The nurse is planning care for a multigravid client hospitalized at 36 weeks' gestation with confirmed rupture of membranes and no evidence of labor. Which of the following would the nurse expect the physician to order?
    ○ 1. Frequent assessments of cervical dilation.
    ○ 2. Intravenous oxytocin administration.
    ○ 3. Vaginal culture for *Neisseria gonorrhoeae*.
    ○ 4. Sonogram for amniotic fluid volume index.

47. A multigravida at 34 weeks' gestation visits the hospital because she suspects that her water has broken. After testing the leaking fluid with nitrazine paper, the nurse confirms that the client's membranes have ruptured when the paper turns which of the following colors?
   ○ 1. Yellow.
   ○ 2. Green.
   ○ 3. Blue.
   ○ 4. Red.

48. A primigravid client at 30 weeks' gestation has been admitted to the hospital with premature rupture of the membranes without contractions. Her cervix is 2 cm dilated and 50% effaced. Which of the following would be a priority assessment for this client?
   ○ 1. Red blood cell count.
   ○ 2. Degree of discomfort.
   ○ 3. Urinary output.
   ○ 4. Temperature.

49. A multigravida at 34 weeks' gestation with premature rupture of the membranes tests positive for streptococcus B. The client is having contractions every 4 to 6 minutes. Her vital signs are as follows: blood pressure, 120/80 mm Hg; temperature, 100°F (37.8°C); pulse, 100 bpm; respirations, 18 breaths/minute. Which of the following would the nurse expect the physician to order?
   ○ 1. Intravenous ampicillin sulfate (Polycillin-N).
   ○ 2. Intravenous gentamicin sulfate (Garamycin).
   ○ 3. Intramuscular betamethasone (Celestone).
   ○ 4. Intramuscular cefaclor (Ceclor).

50. A primigravida at 36 weeks' gestation with premature rupture of the membranes is to be discharged home on bed rest with follow-up by the home health nurse. After instruction about care while at home, which of the following client statements indicates effective teaching?
   ○ 1. "It is permissible to douche if the fluid irritates my vaginal area."
   ○ 2. "I can take either a tub bath or a shower when I feel like it."
   ○ 3. "I should limit my fluid intake to less than 1 quart daily."
   ○ 4. "I should contact the doctor if my temperature is 100.4°F or higher."

51. A primigravid client at 34 weeks' gestation is experiencing contractions every 3 to 4 minutes lasting for 35 seconds. Her cervix is 2 cm dilated and 50% effaced. While the nurse is assessing the client's vital signs, the client says, "I think my bag of water just broke." Which of the following would the nurse do *first*?
   ○ 1. Check the status of the fetal heart rate.
   ○ 2. Turn the client to her right side.
   ○ 3. Test the leaking fluid with nitrazine paper.
   ○ 4. Perform a sterile vaginal examination.

The Pregnant Client With Diabetes Mellitus

52. A 27-year-old primigravid client with insulin-dependent diabetes at 34 weeks' gestation undergoes a nonstress test, the results of which are documented as reactive. The nurse tells the client that the test results indicate which of the following?
   ○ 1. A contraction stress test is necessary.
   ○ 2. The nonstress test should be repeated.
   ○ 3. Chorionic villus sampling is necessary.
   ○ 4. There is evidence of fetal well-being.

53. A primigravida with insulin-dependent diabetes tells the nurse that the contraction stress test performed earlier in the day was suspicious. The nurse interprets this test result as indicating that the fetal heart rate pattern showed which of the following?
   ○ 1. Frequent late decelerations.
   ○ 2. Decreased fetal movement.
   ○ 3. Inconsistent late decelerations.
   ○ 4. Lack of fetal movement.

54. Which of the following statements about a fetal biophysical profile would be incorporated into the teaching plan for a primigravid client with insulin-dependent diabetes?
   ○ 1. Determines fetal lung maturity.
   ○ 2. Is noninvasive using real-time ultrasound.
   ○ 3. Will correlate with the newborn's Apgar score.
   ○ 4. Requires the client to have an empty bladder.

55. A 30-year-old multigravid client at 8 weeks' gestation has a history of insulin-dependent diabetes since age 20 years. When explaining about the importance of blood glucose control during pregnancy, which of the following would the nurse expect to occur with respect to the client's insulin needs during the first trimester?
   ○ 1. They will increase.
   ○ 2. They will decrease.
   ○ 3. They will remain constant.
   ○ 4. They will be unpredictable.

56. The nurse explains the complications of pregnancy that occur with diabetes to a primigravid client at 10 weeks' gestation who has a 5-year history of insulin-dependent diabetes. Which of the following, if stated by the client as a complication, indicates the need for additional teaching?
   ○ 1. *Candida albicans* infection.
   ○ 2. Twin-to-twin transfer.
   ○ 3. Polyhydramnios.
   ○ 4. Preeclampsia.

57. When developing a teaching plan for a primigravid client with insulin-dependent diabetes about monitoring blood glucose control and insulin dosages at home, which of the following would the nurse expect to include as a desired target range for blood glucose levels?

○ 1. 40 to 60 mg/dL between 2 and 4 PM.

○ 2. 60 to 100 mg/dL before meals and bedtime snacks.

○ 3. 110 to 140 mg/dL before meals and bedtime snacks.

○ 4. 140 to 160 mg/dL 1 hour after meals.

58. When teaching a primigravid client with diabetes about common causes of hyperglycemia during pregnancy, which of the following would the nurse include?

○ 1. Fetal macrosomia.

○ 2. Obesity before conception.

○ 3. Maternal infection.

○ 4. Pregnancy-induced hypertension.

59. After teaching a diabetic primigravida about symptoms of hyperglycemia and hypoglycemia, the nurse determines that the client understands the instruction when she says that hyperglycemia may be manifested by which of the following?

○ 1. Dehydration.

○ 2. Pallor.

○ 3. Sweating.

○ 4. Nervousness.

60. At 38 weeks' gestation, a primigravid client with poorly controlled diabetes and severe preeclampsia is admitted for a cesarean delivery. The nurse explains to the client that delivery helps to prevent which of the following?

○ 1. Neonatal hyperbilirubinemia.

○ 2. Congenital anomalies.

○ 3. Perinatal asphyxia.

○ 4. Stillbirth.

61. A primigravid client with diabetes at 39 weeks' gestation is seen in the high-risk clinic. The physician estimates that the fetus weighs at least 4500 g (10 pounds). The client asks, "What causes the baby to be so large?" The nurse's response is based on the understanding that fetal macrosomia is usually related to which of the following?

○ 1. Family history of large infants.

○ 2. Fetal anomalies.

○ 3. Maternal hyperglycemia.

○ 4. Maternal hypertension.

62. With plans to breast-feed her neonate, a pregnant client with insulin-dependent diabetes asks the nurse about insulin needs during the postpartum period. Which of the following statements about postpartal insulin requirements for breast-feeding mothers would the nurse include in the explanation?

○ 1. They fall significantly in the immediate postpartum period.

○ 2. They remain the same as during the labor process.

○ 3. They usually increase in the immediate postpartum period.

○ 4. They need constant adjustment during the first 24 hours.

The Pregnant Client With Heart Disease

63. After instruction of a primigravid client at 8 weeks' gestation diagnosed with class I heart disease about self-care during pregnancy, which of the following client statements would indicate the need for additional teaching?

○ 1. "I should avoid being near people who have a cold."

○ 2. "I may be given antibiotics during my pregnancy."

○ 3. "I should reduce my intake of protein in my diet."

○ 4. "I should limit my salt intake at meals."

64. While caring for a primigravid client with class II heart disease at 28 weeks' gestation, the nurse would instruct the client to contact her physician immediately if the client experiences which of the following?

○ 1. Mild ankle edema.

○ 2. Emotional stress on the job.

○ 3. Weight gain of 1 pound in 1 week.

○ 4. Increased dyspnea at rest.

65. When developing the collaborative plan of care for a multigravid client at 10 weeks' gestation with a history of cardiac disease who was being treated with digitalis therapy before this pregnancy, which of the following would the nurse anticipate happening with the client's drug therapy regimen?

○ 1. Need for an increased dosage.

○ 2. Continuation of the same dosage.

○ 3. Switching to a different medication.

○ 4. Addition of a diuretic to the regimen.

66. Which of the following anticoagulants would the nurse expect to administer when caring for a primigravid client at 12 weeks' gestation who has class II cardiac disease due to mitral valve stenosis?

○ 1. Heparin.

○ 2. Warfarin (Coumadin).

○ 3. Enoxaparin (Lovenox).

○ 4. Ardeparin (Normiflo).

67. A primigravida with class II heart disease who is visiting the clinic at 8 weeks' gestation tells the nurse that she has been maintaining a low-sodium, 1800-calorie diet. Which of the following instructions should the nurse give the client?

○ 1. Avoid folic acid supplements to prevent megaloblastic anemia.

○ 2. Severely restrict sodium intake throughout the pregnancy.

○ 3. Take iron supplements with milk to enhance absorption.

○ 4. Increase caloric intake to 2200 calories daily to promote fetal growth.

The Client With an Ectopic Pregnancy

68. On arrival at the emergency department, a client tells the nurse that she suspects that she may be pregnant but has been having a small amount of bleeding and has severe pain in the lower abdomen. The client's blood pressure is 70/50 mm Hg and her pulse rate is 120 bpm. The nurse notifies the physician immediately because which of the following is suspected?
    - ○ 1. Ectopic pregnancy.
    - ○ 2. Abruptio placenta.
    - ○ 3. Gestational trophoblastic disease.
    - ○ 4. Complete abortion.

69. A multigravid client seen in the emergency department complaining of sharp abdominal pain and vaginal spotting is diagnosed with an ectopic pregnancy. When explaining to the client and family members about an ectopic pregnancy, which of the following would the nurse include as the most common site of implantation?
    - ○ 1. Fallopian tube.
    - ○ 2. Intestine.
    - ○ 3. Interstitial lining.
    - ○ 4. Ovary.

70. A multigravid client at 8 weeks' gestation is admitted with a diagnosis of "probable ectopic pregnancy." Which of the following would be the *most* appropriate nursing diagnosis for this client?
    - ○ 1. Fear related to the outcome of possible surgery.
    - ○ 2. Ineffective Coping related to ectopic pregnancy.
    - ○ 3. Disturbed Body Image related to surgical scarring.
    - ○ 4. Anticipatory Grieving related to the loss of the pregnancy.

71. Before surgery to remove an ectopic pregnancy and the fallopian tube, which of the following would alert the nurse to the possibility of tubal rupture?
    - ○ 1. Amount of vaginal bleeding and discharge.
    - ○ 2. Falling hematocrit and hemoglobin levels.
    - ○ 3. Slow, bounding pulse rate of 80 bpm.
    - ○ 4. Marked abdominal edema.

72. A multigravid client diagnosed with a probable ruptured ectopic pregnancy is scheduled for emergency surgery. In addition to monitoring the client's blood pressure before surgery, which of the following would the nurse assess?
    - ○ 1. Uterine cramping.
    - ○ 2. Abdominal distention.
    - ○ 3. Hemoglobin and hematocrit.
    - ○ 4. Pulse rate.

73. A 36-year-old multigravid client is admitted to the hospital with possible ruptured ectopic pregnancy. When obtaining the client's history, which of the following would be *most* important to identify as a predisposing factor?
    - ○ 1. Urinary tract infection.
    - ○ 2. Marijuana use during pregnancy.
    - ○ 3. Episodes of pelvic inflammatory disease.
    - ○ 4. Use of estrogen-progestin contraceptives.

74. After surgery to remove a ruptured fallopian tube, a multigravid client receives discharge instructions about potential complications to report to her physician. Which of the following, if stated by the client as a complication, indicates a need for additional teaching?
    - ○ 1. Pain.
    - ○ 2. Headache.
    - ○ 3. Fever.
    - ○ 4. Bleeding.

75. A multigravid client is admitted to the hospital with a diagnosis of ectopic pregnancy. The nurse anticipates that, because the client's fallopian tube has not yet ruptured, which of the following may be ordered?
    - ○ 1. Progestin contraceptives (Prodox).
    - ○ 2. Medroxyprogesterone (Depo-Provera).
    - ○ 3. Methotrexate.
    - ○ 4. Dyphylline (Dilor).

The Client With Hyperemesis Gravidarum

76. After instruction of a primigravid client at 8 weeks' gestation about measures to overcome early morning nausea and vomiting, which of the following client statements indicates the need for additional teaching?
    - ○ 1. "I'll eat dry crackers or toast before arising in the morning."
    - ○ 2. "I'll drink adequate fluids separate from my meals or snacks."
    - ○ 3. "I'll eat two large meals daily with frequent protein snacks."
    - ○ 4. "I'll snack on a small amount of carbohydrates throughout the day."

77. A multigravid client thought to be at 14 weeks' gestation reports that she is experiencing such severe morning sickness that "she has not been able to keep anything down for a week." The nurse should assess for signs and symptoms of which of the following?
    - ○ 1. Hypercalcemia.
    - ○ 2. Hypobilirubinemia.
    - ○ 3. Hypokalemia.
    - ○ 4. Hyperglycemia.

78. A multigravid client is admitted at 16 weeks' gestation with a diagnosis of hyperemesis gravidarum. The nurse should explain to the client that hyper-

emesis gravidarum is thought to be related to high levels of which of the following hormones?

○ 1. Progesterone.
○ 2. Estrogen.
○ 3. Somatotropin.
○ 4. Aldosterone.

79. The physician orders 1000 mL of Ringer's lactate intravenously over an 8-hour period for a 29-year-old primigravid client at 16 weeks' gestation with hyperemesis gravidarum. The nurse would administer the intravenous infusion at which of the following rates?

○ 1. 60 mL per hour.
○ 2. 100 mL per hour.
○ 3. 125 mL per hour.
○ 4. 150 mL per hour.

80. A primigravid client admitted to the hospital with a diagnosis of hyperemesis gravidarum will be placed on NPO status and receive intravenous therapy. Which of the following would the nurse *most* likely include when explaining to the client about oral intake of food and fluids?

○ 1. Withholding them indefinitely until acidosis is corrected.
○ 2. Giving them in small quantities whenever the client desires.
○ 3. Providing them as clear liquids after 24 hours if vomiting subsides.
○ 4. Withholding them until total parenteral nutrition replaces lost electrolytes.

The Pregnant Client With a Hydatidiform Mole

81. A 38-year-old client at about 14 weeks' gestation is admitted to the hospital with a diagnosis of com-

plete hydatidiform mole. Soon after admission, the nurse would assess the client for signs and symptoms of which of the following?

○ 1. Pregnancy-induced hypertension.
○ 2. Gestational diabetes.
○ 3. Hypothyroidism.
○ 4. Polycythemia.

82. After a dilation and curettage to evacuate a molar pregnancy, assessing the client for signs and symptoms of which of the following would be *most* important?

○ 1. Urinary tract infection.
○ 2. Hemorrhage.
○ 3. Abdominal distention.
○ 4. Chorioamnionitis.

83. When preparing a multigravid client who has undergone evacuation of a hydatidiform mole for discharge, the nurse explains the need for follow-up care. The nurse determines that the client understands the instruction when she says that she is at risk for developing which of the following?

○ 1. Ectopic pregnancy.
○ 2. Choriocarcinoma.
○ 3. Multifetal pregnancies.
○ 4. Infertility.

84. After suction and evacuation of a complete hydatidiform mole, the 28-year-old multigravid client asks the nurse when she can become pregnant again. The nurse would advise the client not to become pregnant again for at least which of the following time spans?

○ 1. 6 months.
○ 2. 12 months.
○ 3. 18 months.
○ 4. 24 months.

Correct Answers and Rationale

The letters in parentheses following the rationale identify the step of the nursing process (A, D, P, I, E) and client needs (1, 2, 3, 4, 5, 6, 7, 8, 9, 10). See the inside front cover for the key.

The Client With Preeclampsia/Eclampsia

1. 3. Clients with increased risk for preeclampsia include primigravid clients younger than 20 years or older than 40 years of age, clients with five or more pregnancies, women of color, women with multifetal pregnancies, women with diabetes or heart disease, and women with hydramnios. A total weight gain of 20 pounds at 32 weeks' gestation with a 1-pound weight gain in the last 2 weeks is within normal limits. Short stature is not associated with the development of preeclampsia. A trace amount of protein in the urine is common during pregnancy. However, protein amounts of 1+ or more may be a symptom of pregnancy-induced hypertension. (A, 9)

2. 4. A weight gain of 2 pounds in the last week during the third trimester and mild peripheral edema are associated with mild preeclampsia. With severe preeclampsia, peripheral edema is extensive. Blood pressure readings of 160 mm Hg systolic and 100 mm Hg diastolic on two separate occasions and oliguria (urine output less than 400 mL in 24 hours) are signs of severe preeclampsia. Proteinuria, 3+ to 4+ or more than 5 g in a 24-hour sample, also indicates severe preeclampsia. Normal serum creatinine levels range from 0.5 to 1.1 mL/dL. A serum creatinine concentration of 1.4 ml/dL is greatly elevated, indicating severe preeclampsia. (D, 10)

3. 3. Because the client has peripheral edema with preeclampsia, the most appropriate nursing diagnosis is Deficient Fluid Volume related to fluid shift from intravascular to extravascular space. The scenario supplies no data to suggest Noncompliance. If the client refused to remain on bed rest, then Noncompliance would be the priority diagnosis. The scenario also supplies no data to suggest Delayed Growth and Development. If the client exhibited regression to an immature stage or child-like behaviors such as thumb-sucking, then Delayed Growth and Development would be an appropriate diagnosis. The client may be experiencing Social Isolation related to the prolonged bed rest, but there is no evidence of Situational Low Self-Esteem. Evidence of low self-esteem would include a disheveled appearance or statements by the client such as "I look so awful" or "I'm really fat." (D, 10)

4. 4. The diagnosis of mild preeclampsia is further confirmed if the client exhibits mild edema in the hands, fingers, and/or face resulting from fluid retention. A pounding headache after reading may indicate that a more severe form of preeclampsia is developing. A history of a urinary tract infection is not related to preeclampsia unless the client develops diabetes with renal impairment. Frequent voiding in large amounts is not related to preeclampsia. Women in the third trimester of pregnancy often void frequently in large amounts because of increased fluid intake and pressure of the uterus on the bladder. Diabetes, age younger than 20 years or older than 40 years, and multifetal pregnancy (eg, twins) are associated with preeclampsia. (A, 10)

5. 3. The client with mild preeclampsia is often treated at home with activity restriction. Bed rest for most of the day with the client lying in the left lateral recumbent position is recommended. This position helps to decrease pressure on the vena cava, thus increasing venous return, circulatory volume, and renal and placental perfusion. A decrease in angiotensin II improves renal blood flow, lowers blood pressure, and increases diuresis. Typically, the client is monitored with home visits twice a week. The client usually returns to the clinic every 2 weeks until 36 weeks' gestation. After that time, clinic visits occur at least every week or more often, if needed. The client's diet needs to be well balanced, with ample protein intake. Fiber intake may need to be increased to prevent complications from prolonged bed rest, such as constipation. If magnesium sulfate is necessary, as in severe preeclampsia, the drug is usually administered intravenously, and the client is carefully monitored in the hospital setting because of the possible risk for seizure activity. (P, 10)

6. 1. Congenital anomalies such as hydrocephalus are not associated with preeclampsia. Conditions such as stillbirth, prematurity, intrauterine growth retardation, abruptio placenta, and poor placental perfusion are associated with preeclampsia. Abruptio placenta occurs because of severe vasoconstriction. Intrauterine growth retardation is possible owing to poor placental perfusion. Poor placental perfusion results from increased vasoconstriction. (E, 10)

7. 3. Numerous methods have been proposed to record the maternal perceptions of fetal movement or "kick counts." A commonly used method is the Cardiff count-to-10 method. The client begins counting fetal movements at a specified time (eg, 8 AM) and notes the time when the 10th movement is felt. If the client does not feel at least 6 movements in a 1-hour period, she

should notify the health care provider. The fetus typically moves an average of 1 to 2 times every 10 minutes or 10 to 12 times per hour. A 30- or 45-minute period is not enough time to evaluate fetal movement accurately. The client should monitor fetal movements more frequently than 1 time per week. One hour of monitoring each day is adequate. (E, 9)

8. 3. For clients with mild preeclampsia, a regular diet with ample protein and calories is recommended. Sodium and fluid intake should not be restricted or increased. A high-residue diet is not necessary. If the client experiences constipation, she should increase the fiber in her diet, such as by eating raw fruits and vegetables, and increase fluid intake. A high-protein diet is unnecessary. (P, 7)

9. 4. Iron deficiency can lead to anemia, but this has not been linked to preeclampsia. Although the exact cause of preeclampsia is not yet known, several theories have been proposed. Conditions that make a client more susceptible to preeclampsia include multifetal pregnancy, impaired vascular invasion of the uterine lining, genetic predisposition, age older than 35 years, hydramnios, low socioeconomic status, and diabetes mellitus. Calcium deficiency also has been implicated by some researchers. Multifetal pregnancy (eg, twins) is associated with preeclampsia. This is related to an increased incidence of hydramnios, which is common in multifetal pregnancies. Diabetes mellitus is associated with preeclampsia; this is related to increased vasoconstriction, which is common in diabetes. Preeclampsia occurs more frequently in clients who are older than 35 years; this is thought by some researchers to be related to underlying hypertension. (E, 10)

10. 1. Severe headache, visual disturbances such as blurred vision, and epigastric pain are associated with the development of severe preeclampsia and possibly eclampsia. These danger signs and symptoms must be reported immediately. Severe headache and visual disturbances are related to severe vasoconstriction and a severe increase in blood pressure. Epigastric pain is related to hepatic dysfunction. Ankle edema is common during the third trimester. However, facial edema is associated with increased fluid retention and the progression from mild to severe preeclampsia. Increased energy levels are not associated with a progression of the client's preeclampsia or the development of complications. In fact, some women report an "energy spurt" before the onset of labor. Mild backache is a common discomfort of pregnancy, unrelated to a progression of the client's preeclampsia. It also may be associated with bed rest when the mattress is not firm. Some multiparous women have reported a mild backache as a sign of impending labor. (I, 9)

11. 2. A client with preeclampsia complaining of a continuous headache for 2 days should be seen by a health care provider immediately. Continuous headache, drowsiness, and mental confusion indicate poor cerebral perfusion and are symptoms of severe preeclampsia. Immediate care is recommended because these symptoms may lead to eclampsia or seizures if left untreated. Advising the client to take two acetaminophen tablets would be inappropriate and may lead to further complications if the client is not evaluated and treated. Although the application of cool compresses may ease the pain temporarily, this would delay treatment. Aspirin with codeine may temporarily relieve the client's headache. However, this delays immediate treatment, which is crucial. Additionally, pregnant women are advised not to take aspirin at this time because it may cause clotting problems in the neonate. Codeine generally is not prescribed. (I, 9)

12. 2. Signs of severe preeclampsia include blood pressure of 160/110 mm Hg or greater measured at two different times at least 6 hours apart, severe blurring of vision or seeing spots in front of the eyes, oliguria, proteinuria of 5 g or greater in a 24-hour specimen, a serum creatinine concentration of 1.2 mL/dL, and a urine specific gravity of 1.04 or greater. A blood pressure of 138/94 mm Hg would suggest mild preeclampsia, as would proteinuria of less than 2 g in a 24-hour urine specimen. A weight gain of 1 pound per week in the third trimester is normal. However, a weight gain of 2 pounds or more suggests severe preeclampsia. (D, 10)

13. 4. The client with severe preeclampsia may develop eclampsia, which is characterized by seizures. The client needs a darkened, quiet room and side rails with thick padding. This helps decrease the potential for injury should a seizure occur. Airways, a suction machine, and oxygen also should be available. If the client is to undergo induction of labor, oxytocin infusion solution can be obtained at a later time. Tongue blades are not necessary. However, the emergency cart should be placed nearby in case the client experiences a seizure. In many hospitals, the client with severe preeclampsia is admitted to the labor area, where she and the fetus can be closely monitored. The safety of the client and her fetus is the priority. (P, 10)

14. 3. The client receiving magnesium sulfate intravenously is at risk for possible toxicity. The antidote for magnesium sulfate toxicity is calcium gluconate, which should be readily available at the client's bedside. Diazepam (Valium), used to treat anxiety, usually is not given to pregnant women. Hydralazine (Apresoline) would be used to treat hypertension, and phenytoin (Dilantin) would be used to treat seizures. (I, 8)

15. 1. Typical signs of hypermagnesemia include decreased deep tendon reflexes, sweating or a flushing of

the skin, oliguria, impaired respirations, and lethargy progressing to coma as the toxicity increases. The nurse should check the client's patellar, biceps, and radial reflexes regularly during magnesium sulfate therapy. A rapid pulse rate commonly occurs in hypomagnesemia. Tingling in the toes may suggest hypocalcemia, not hypermagnesemia. (A, 8)

16. 2. The only known cure for severe preeclampsia is delivery of the fetus. In severe cases, labor induction is initiated or a cesarean section is performed. However, some women remain hypertensive even after delivery. Early diagnosis and careful management are used to control the disease. Medical treatment for severe preeclampsia includes bed rest in a quiet, darkened room; a regular diet; restoration of fluid and electrolyte balance; sedation; and antihypertensive medications. Glucocorticoids such as betamethasone are used to enhance fetal lung maturity. Phenytoin may be used to control seizures in eclampsia; however, it is not a first-line drug, and it exerts no curative effect on the client's hypertension. Additionally, the drug usually is not prescribed for pregnant women because of the significant risk for fetal malformations. Although reduction of fluid retention may make the client more comfortable, thiazide diuretics can result in serious sodium and potassium depletion, hemorrhagic pancreatitis, and neonatal thrombocytopenia. (I, 10)

17. 4. The highest priority for a client with severe preeclampsia is to prevent seizures, thereby minimizing the possibility of adverse effects on the mother and fetus, and then to deliver the infant safely. Efforts to decrease edema, reduce blood pressure, increase urine output, limit kidney damage, and maintain sedation are desirable but are not as important as preventing seizures. It would take several days or weeks for the edema to be decreased. Sedation and decreased reflex excitability can occur with the administration of intravenous magnesium sulfate, which peaks in 30 minutes. However, sedation and reflex excitability would occur much sooner than 48 hours. (P, 10)

18. 3. Magnesium sulfate, an anticonvulsant, acts as a central nervous system depressant by blocking peripheral neuromuscular transmissions and decreasing the amount of acetylcholine liberated. Although the drug relaxes smooth muscle and reduces vasoconstriction, it does not act as a peripheral vasodilator or a sedative/hypnotic. Other drugs, such as hydralazine (Apresoline), labetalol (Normodyne), or nifedipine (Procardia), may be used to control blood pressure in a client with severe preeclampsia. (I, 8)

19. 1. A respiratory rate of 12 breaths/minute suggests potential respiratory depression, an adverse effect of magnesium sulfate therapy. The medication must be stopped and the physician should be notified immediately. A patellar reflex of +2 is normal. Absence of a patellar reflex suggests magnesium toxicity. A blood pressure reading of 160/88 mm Hg would be a common finding in a client with severe preeclampsia. Urinary output exceeding intake is not likely in a client receiving intravenous magnesium sulfate. Oliguria is more common. (A, 8)

20. 1. The most appropriate nursing diagnosis at this time is Risk for Injury related to possibility of further seizure activity. Unless the client's blood pressure can be brought under control, the risk of another seizure is high. The scenario provides no information to suggest Deficient Knowledge or Situational Low Self-Esteem. Questions about the causes or treatment would suggest a knowledge deficit. Client statements about her appearance or feeling depressed would suggest a self-esteem disturbance. Hypertensive Crisis is a medical diagnosis, not a nursing diagnosis. (D, 9)

21. 3. If a client begins to have a seizure, the first action by the nurse is to remain with the client and call for immediate assistance. The nurse needs to have some assistance in managing this client. After the seizure, the client needs intensive monitoring. An airway can be inserted, if appropriate, after the seizure ends. Noting the time the seizure begins and ends, and turning the client to her left side, should be done after assistance is obtained (I, 9)

22. 1. One of the most common side effects of the drug hydralazine (Apresoline) is tachycardia. Therefore, the nurse should assess the client's heart rate and pulse. Hydralazine acts to lower blood pressure by peripheral dilation without interfering with placental circulation. Bradypnea and polyuria are usually not associated with hydralazine use. Polyuria is not usually associated with hydralazine use. Dysphagia is not a typical side effect of hydralazine. (A, 8)

23. 4. These findings would be documented as 4+ with clonus. 1+ indicates a diminished response; 2+ indicates a normal response; 3+ indicates a response that is brisker than average but not abnormal. Mild clonus is said to be present when there are two movements. (A, 10)

24. 3. Epigastric pain or acute right upper quadrant pain is associated with the development of eclampsia and an impending seizure; this is thought to be related to liver ischemia. Decreased contraction intensity is unrelated to the severity of the preeclampsia. Typically, the client's temperature increases because of increased cerebral pressure. A decrease in temperature is unrelated to an impending seizure. Hyporeflexia is not associated with an impending seizure. Typically, the client would exhibit hyperreflexia. (A, 10)

25. 4. After an eclamptic seizure, the client often falls into a deep sleep or coma. The nurse must continually monitor the client for signs of impending labor, because the client will not be able to verbalize that contractions are occurring. Oliguria is more common than polyuria after an eclamptic seizure. Facial flushing is not common unless it is caused by a reaction to a medication. Typically, the client remains hypertensive unless medications such as magnesium sulfate are administered. (A, 10)

26. 1. After an eclamptic seizure, the client is at risk for abruptio placenta due to severe vasoconstriction resulting in hemorrhage into the decidua basalis. Abruptio placenta is manifested by a board-like abdomen and nonreassuring fetal heart rate tracing. Transverse lie or shoulder presentation, placenta accreta, and uterine atony are not related to eclampsia. Causes of a transverse lie may include relaxation of the abdominal wall secondary to grand multiparity, preterm fetus, placenta previa, abnormal uterus, contracted pelvis, and excessive amniotic fluid. Placenta accreta, a rare phenomenon, refers to a condition in which the placenta abnormally adheres to the uterine lining. Uterine atony, or relaxed uterus, may occur after delivery, leading to postpartum hemorrhage. (A, 10)

27. 3. HELLP syndrome refers to a form of severe preeclampsia involving *h*emolysis, *e*levated *l*iver enzymes, and *l*ow *p*latelet count, also termed thrombocytopenia. This syndrome occurs in 4% to 12% of clients with severe preeclampsia. It is a serious syndrome with a maternal mortality rate as high as 24%. Hypofibrinogenemia is associated with HELLP syndrome because of vascular damage resulting from vasospasm. The increase in liver enzymes in HELLP is a result of obstruction of the hepatic blood flow by fibrin deposits. Hyponatremia may be a complication of HELLP, but it is not one of the underlying problems associated with this condition. (I, 9)

The Pregnant Client With a Chronic Hypertensive Disorder

28. 1. Pregnancy is not the time for clients to begin a diet. Clients with chronic hypertension need to consume adequate calories to support fetal growth and development. They also need an adequate protein intake. Meat and beans are good sources of protein. Most pregnant women report that eating more frequent, smaller meals decreases heartburn resulting from the reflux of acidic secretions into the lower esophagus. Pregnant women need adequate hydration (fluids) and fiber to prevent constipation. (E, 7)

29. 2. Women with chronic hypertension during pregnancy are at risk for complications such as preeclampsia (about 25%), abruptio placenta, and intrauterine growth retardation, resulting in a small-for-gestational-age infant. There is no association between chronic hypertension and hyperthyroidism. Pregnant women with chronic hypertension are not at an increased risk for hydramnios (polyhydramnios), abnormally large amount of amniotic fluid. Clients with diabetes and multiple gestations are at risk for this condition. Placenta accreta, a rare placental abnormality, refers to a condition in which the placenta abnormally adheres to the uterine lining. It is not associated with chronic hypertension. (E, 9)

The Pregnant Client With Third-Trimester Bleeding

30. 4. Although the exact cause of abruptio placenta is unknown, possible contributing factors include excessive intrauterine pressure caused by hydramnios or multiple pregnancy, cocaine use, cigarette smoking, alcohol ingestion, trauma, increased maternal age and parity, and amniotomy. A history of hypertension is associated with an increased risk for abruptio placenta. A previous low transverse cesarean section delivery and a history of one induced abortion are associated with increased risk of placenta previa, not abruptio placenta. (D, 10)

31. 2. Treatment of DIC includes treating the causative factor, replacing maternal coagulation factors, and supporting physiologic functions. Intravenous infusions of whole blood, fresh-frozen plasma, or platelets are used to replace depleted maternal coagulation factors. Although Ringer's lactate solution and 5% dextrose solution may be used as intravenous fluid replacement, the client needs blood component therapy. Therefore, normal saline must be used. Intravenous heparin, not warfarin sodium (Coumadin) may be administered to halt the clotting cascade. (P, 10)

32. 1. The most common assessment finding associated with placenta previa is painless vaginal bleeding. With placenta previa, the placenta is abnormally implanted, covering a portion or all of the cervical os. Uterine tetany, intermittent pain with spotting, and dull lower back pain are not associated with placenta previa. Uterine tetany is associated with oxytocin administration. Intermittent pain with spotting commonly is associated with a spontaneous abortion. Dull lower back pain is often associated with poor maternal posture or a urinary tract infection with renal involvement. (A, 10)

33. 2. Bleeding precipitated by placenta previa results from exposure of the maternal sinuses when placental villi are torn from the uterine wall as the lower uterine segment contracts and dilates in the later weeks of pregnancy. The bleeding is not initiated because of diminished clotting factors. Diminished clotting factors are associated with DIC. Increased platelet levels would suggest an increased risk for clotting. A large-

for-gestational-age fetus may be related to hereditary factors or diabetes. (E, 10)

34. 3. The client's statement reflects concern for her present fetus based on her previous experience. Therefore, the priority diagnosis is Anxiety. This is further supported by the fact that the client is at only 35 weeks' gestation, and delivery at this time most likely would result in a preterm neonate. The client needs a supportive nurse who will allow her to express her feelings. The client may be at risk for constipation after prolonged bed rest, but the priority at this time is the client's anxiety. There is no evidence presented to support a diagnosis of Interrupted Family Processes. Expression of concerns related to the family, such as "I'm worried about my other children," would suggest this diagnosis. A diagnosis of Impaired Physical Mobility is inappropriate because the client is still able to move about in bed. (D, 5)

35. 1. When administering blood replacement therapy, extreme caution is needed. Before administering any blood product, the nurse should validate the client information and the blood product with another nurse to prevent administration of the wrong blood transfusion. Although baseline vital signs are necessary, the infusion of blood should be initiated slowly for the first 10 to 15 minutes. Then if the client experiences evidence of a reaction, the rate of infusion is adjusted to ensure that the blood product is infused over 2 to 4 hours. The client can be asked if she has ever had a reaction to a blood product, but a general question about allergies may not elicit the most complete response about any reactions to blood product administration. Blood transfusions are typically given with intravenous normal saline solution, not dextrose solutions. (I, 8)

36. 3. Feelings of loss, grief, and guilt are normal after a cesarean section delivery, particularly if it was not planned. The nurse should support the client, listen with empathy, and allow the client time to grieve. The likelihood of the client's experiencing postpartum blues is not known, and no evidence is presented. Although maternal–infant bonding may be delayed owing to neonatal complications or maternal pain and subsequent medications, it should not be difficult. Although the nurse is aware that that this type of delivery was necessary to save the client's life, using this as the basis for the response does not acknowledge the mother's feelings. (P, 5)

37. 3. Abruptio placenta is a medical emergency because the degree of hypovolemic shock may be out of proportion to visible blood loss. On admission, the nurse should plan to first insert a large-gauge intravenous catheter for fluid replacement and oxygen by mask to decrease fetal anoxia. Vaginal examination usually is not performed on pregnant clients who are experienc-

ing third-trimester bleeding due to abruptio placenta because it can result in damage to the placenta and further fetal anoxia. The client's history can be obtained once the client has been admitted and the intravenous line has been started. The goal is to get the fetus delivered, usually by emergency cesarean delivery. The nurse should also plan to monitor the client's vital signs and the fetal heart rate. Ultrasound is of limited use in the diagnosis of abruptio placenta. (P, 9)

The Pregnant Client With Preterm Labor

38. 1. Although the exact cause of preterm labor has not been determined, various risk factors are associated with this condition. Age younger than 19 or older than 40 years has been associated with preterm labor. Other factors associated with preterm labor include polyhydramnios, poor pregnancy weight gain, multifetal gestation, prior preterm delivery, cervical incompetence, reproductive tract infection, urinary tract infection, renal disease, and chronic hypertension. (E, 9)

39. 2. The priority nursing diagnosis at this time is Spiritual Distress related to feelings of guilt. The client is visibly upset, asking why is God punishing her and what she did wrong to cause the preterm labor. The nurse needs to be supportive and allow the client to verbalize her feelings. The client may desire to speak to a member of the clergy. There is no evidence to suggest a risk for impaired parenting. Evidence such as statements about poor mothering abilities or lack of family support would suggest this nursing diagnosis. Although the client's amniotic fluid is leaking, this may cease with bed rest and other treatments for preterm labor. Risk for Infection may be a priority later in the client's care. No evidence is suggested to support a diagnosis of Disturbed Body Image. Statements about the client's appearance or body would suggest this diagnosis. (D, 3)

40. 1. Indomethacin (Indocin) has been successfully used to halt preterm labor. However, if the client should deliver a preterm infant, the nurse would notify the nursery personnel about the tocolytic therapy because this drug can lead to premature closure of the fetal ductus arteriosus, resulting in pulmonary hypertension. Prematurity is associated with RDS because of the immaturity of the fetal lungs. RDS is not a result of indomethacin. Hyperbilirubinemia, common in preterm infants, can result from oxytocin infusion. Use of indomethacin to halt preterm labor is not associated with cardiomyopathy in the infant. (I, 8)

41. 4. Tachycardia is a common side effect of terbutaline therapy. If the client's heart rate is 130 bpm or faster, the nurse should contact the physician before administering the medication. After the drug has been administered, the client should also be carefully monitored for dyspnea or other symptoms of pulmonary edema. Other side effects include premature ventricular contractions, increased stroke volume, increased systolic pressure with decreased diastolic pressure, palpitations, tremors, nausea and vomiting, and shortness of breath. Other adverse effects include hyperglycemia, metabolic acidosis, hypokalemia, and anemia. Terbutaline has no known effects on the client's hemoglobin or hematocrit levels, or on weight. However, the drug can cause nausea. Terbutaline may result in perspiration, but there are no known effects on urinary output. (A, 8)

42. 3. As the uterus contracts, the abdominal wall rises and, when external monitoring is used, presses against the transducer. This movement is transmitted into an electrical current, which is then recorded. With the fetus in the LOA position, the cardiotransducer should be placed below the umbilicus on the side of the fundus, where the fetal back is located and uterine displacement during contractions is greatest. If the fetal back is near the symphysis pubis, the fetus is presenting as a transverse lie. If the fetus is in a breech position, the fetal back may be at or above the umbilicus. (I, 9)

43. 1. Betamethasone therapy is indicated when the fetal lungs are immature. The fetus must be between 28 and 34 weeks' gestation and delivery must be delayed for 24 to 48 hours for the drug to achieve a therapeutic effect. Betamethasone is not an antagonist for tocolytic therapy. It increases, not decreases, the production of neonatal surfactant. Antibiotics would be used to treat chorioamnionitis. (I, 8)

44. 2. For this client, who has experienced two stillbirths, the most appropriate diagnosis is Anxiety related to diagnostic tests for fetal well-being. With most antepartal diagnostic tests, pain is absent or minimal. Information to support the diagnoses of Ineffective Coping or Deficient Knowledge is lacking. (D, 9)

45. 4. The shake test helps determine the maturity of the fetal pulmonary system. The test is based on the fact that surfactant foams when mixed with ethanol. The more stable the foam, the more mature the fetal pulmonary system. Although the shake test is inexpensive and provides rapid results, problems have been noted with its reliability. Therefore, the lecithin-sphingomyelin ratio is usually determined in conjunction with the shake test. (P, 9)

The Pregnant Client With Premature Rupture of the Membranes

46. 3. Because an intrauterine infection may occur when membranes have ruptured, vaginal cultures for *N. gon-*

orrhoeae, β-streptococci, and chlamydia are usually taken. Prophylactic antibiotics may be prescribed to reduce the risk of infection in the newborn. Frequent vaginal examinations should be avoided because they can further increase the client's risk for infection. Intravenous oxytocin to initiate labor may be used if an infection occurs. Bed rest can sometimes prolong the pregnancy and prevent a preterm birth. A sonogram may be used to validate rupture of the membranes with an amniotic fluid index. However, it is not needed if the physician has confirmed the rupture. (I, 9)

47. 3. If the client's membranes have ruptured, the nitrazine paper will turn blue, an alkaline reaction. A yellow color may indicate urine, an acidic reaction. Nitrazine paper does not turn green or red at any time. However, red may indicate blood cells on the paper. (A, 9)

48. 4. Premature rupture of the membranes is often associated with chorioamnionitis, or an infection. A priority assessment for the nurse to make is to document the client's temperature every 2 to 4 hours. Temperature elevation may indicate an infection. Lethargy and an elevated white blood cell count also indicate an infection. The red blood cell count would provide information related to anemia, not infection. The client is not in labor. Therefore, assessing the degree of discomfort is not a priority at this time. Urinary output is not a reliable indicator of an infection such as chorioamnionitis. (A, 9)

49. 1. Because streptococcus B is a gram-positive bacteria, the physician probably will order intravenous ampicillin to treat the mother's infection and prevent fetal infection. Gentamicin sulfate, which acts on gram-negative bacteria, would be inappropriate. Administering a corticosteroid, such as betamethasone, is inappropriate because the premature rupture of the membranes enhances fetal lung maturity. The lack of amniotic fluid causes early maturation of lung tissue. Cefaclor, which is available only in the oral form, is used for upper and lower respiratory tract infections and urinary tract infections by gram-negative staphylococci. (P, 8)

50. 4. Because of the client's increased risk for infection, successful teaching is indicated when the client states that she will contact the doctor if her temperature is 100.4°F (38°C) or greater. The client should be instructed to monitor her temperature twice daily. The client should refrain from coitus, tub bathing, and douching, which can increase the potential for infection. A fluid intake of at least 2 L daily is recommended to prevent potential urinary tract infection. (E, 9)

51. 1. The priority is to determine whether a prolapsed cord has occurred as a result of the spontaneous rupture of membranes. The nurse's first action should be to check the status of the fetal heart rate. Complications of premature rupture of the membranes include a prolapsed cord or increased pressure on the fetal umbilical cord inhibiting fetal nutrient supply. Variable decelerations or fetal bradycardia may be seen on the external fetal monitor. The cord also may be visible. Turning the client to her right side is not necessary. If the cord does prolapse, the client should be placed in a knee-to-chest or Trendelenburg position. Checking the fluid with nitrazine paper and vaginal examination are appropriate once the status of the fetus has been evaluated. (I, 9)

The Pregnant Client With Diabetes Mellitus

52. 4. The nonstress test is considered reactive when two or more fetal heart rate accelerations of at least 15 bpm occur (from a baseline fetal heart rate of 120 to 160 bpm), along with fetal movement, during a 10- to 20-minute period. A reactive nonstress test indicates fetal heart rate accelerations and well-being. There is no indication for further evaluation (eg, contraction stress test). However, contraction stress tests are often scheduled for pregnant clients with insulin-dependent diabetes in the latter part of pregnancy. Chorionic villus sampling is usually performed early in the pregnancy to detect fetal abnormalities. (I, 9)

53. 3. A contraction stress test is used to evaluate fetal well-being during a simulated labor. A suspicious contraction stress test indicates inconsistent late deceleration patterns requiring further evaluation. A negative contraction stress test indicates no fetal heart rate late decelerations and is considered normal. A positive contraction stress test indicates fetal compromise with frequent late decelerations. Fetal movements are one of the parameters of a biophysical profile and are detected with nonstress testing. Decreased fetal movements may indicate central nervous system dysfunction or prematurity. (D, 9)

54. 2. The fetal biophysical profile, a noninvasive test using real-time ultrasound, assesses five parameters: fetal heart rate reactivity, fetal breathing movements, gross fetal body movements, fetal tone, and amniotic fluid volume. Fetal heart rate reactivity is determined by a nonstress test; the other four parameters are determined by ultrasound scanning. The results are available as soon as the test is completed and interpreted. The lecithin-sphingomyelin ratio is used to determine fetal lung maturity. Although the fetal biophysical profile is useful in predicting which fetuses may be at greater risk for compromise, there is no correlation with the newborn's Apgar score. The biophysical score is sometimes referred to as the fetal Apgar score. A score of 8 to 10 indicates fetal well-being. Use of an ultrasound requires the mother to have a full bladder. (P, 8)

55. 2. During the first trimester, it is not unusual for insulin needs to decrease, often as a result of nausea and vomiting. Progressive insulin resistance is characteristic of pregnancy, particularly the second half of pregnancy. It is not unusual for insulin needs to increase by as much as four times the nonpregnant dose after about the 24th week of gestation. This resistance is caused by the production of human placental lactogen, also called human chorionic somatotropin, by the placenta and by other hormones such as estrogen and progesterone, which are insulin antagonists. (I, 8)

56. 2. Clients who are pregnant and have diabetes are not at greater risk for multifetal pregnancy and subsequent twin-to-twin transfer unless they have undergone fertility treatments. The pregnant diabetic client is at higher risk for complications such as infection, polyhydramnios, ketoacidosis, and preeclampsia, compared with the pregnant nondiabetic client. (E, 9)

57. 2. The goal is to maintain blood plasma glucose levels at 60 to 100 mg/dL before meals and bedtime snacks. A range of 40 to 60 mg/dL indicates hypoglycemia. A range of 110 to 140 mg/dL suggests hyperglycemia. A range of 140 to 160 mg/dL 1 hour after meals suggests hyperglycemia. The target range 1 hour after meals is 100 to 120 mg/dL. (P, 8)

58. 3. Maternal infection is the most common cause of maternal hyperglycemia and can lead to ketoacidosis, coma, and death. The client should notify the physician immediately if she experiences symptoms of an infection. Fetal macrosomia, obesity before conception, and pregnancy-induced hypertension are not associated with maternal hyperglycemia during pregnancy. (I, 10)

59. 1. Dehydration, polyuria, fatigue, flushed hot skin, dry mouth, fatigue, and drowsiness are manifestations of hyperglycemia. Hyperglycemia is a medical emergency and requires immediate action to prevent maternal and fetal mortality. Pallor, sweating, and nervousness are early signs of hypoglycemia, not hyperglycemia. (E, 9)

60. 4. Stillbirths caused by placental insufficiency occur with increased frequency in women with diabetes and severe preeclampsia. Clients with poorly controlled diabetes may experience unanticipated stillbirth as a result of premature aging of the placenta. Therefore, labor is frequently induced in these clients before term. If induction of labor fails, a cesarean delivery will be necessary. Induction and cesarean delivery do not prevent neonatal hyperbilirubinemia, congenital anomalies, or perinatal asphyxia. (I, 9)

61. 3. Maternal hyperglycemia and poor control of the mother's diabetes mellitus have been implicated in fetal macrosomia. When the mother is hyperglycemic, large amounts of amino acids, free fatty acids, and glu-

cose are transferred to the fetus. Although maternal insulin does not cross the placenta, the fetal pancreas responds by hypertrophy of the islet cells of the pancreas. The islet cells produce large amounts of insulin, which acts as a growth hormone. A family history of large infants usually is not the reason for large-for-gestational-age fetuses in diabetic mothers. Maternal hypertension is associated with small-for-gestational-age fetuses because of vasoconstriction of the maternal and placental blood vessels. (D, 10)

62. 1. Insulin needs fall significantly for the first 24 hours postpartum because the client has usually been NPO for a period of time during labor and the labor process has used maternal glycogen stores. If the client breastfeeds, lower blood glucose levels decrease the insulin requirements. With insulin resistance gone, often the client needs little or no insulin during the immediate postpartum period. Although the need for insulin decreases during the intrapartum period, the insulin requirements fall further during the first 24 hours postpartum. After the first 24 hours postpartum, insulin requirements may fluctuate markedly, needing constant adjustment during the next few days as the mother's body returns to a nonpregnant state. (I, 8)

The Pregnant Client With Heart Disease

63. 3. The client needs a diet that is adequate in protein and calories to prevent anemia, which can place additional strain on the cardiac system, further compromising the client's cardiac status. The client should avoid contact with people who have infections because of the increased risk for developing endocarditis. The client may need antibiotics during the pregnancy to prevent endocarditis. Limiting sodium intake can help to prevent excessive expansion of blood volume and decrease cardiac workload. (E, 9)

64. 4. Increased dyspnea at rest must be reported immediately because it may be indicative of increasing congestive heart failure. Mild ankle edema in the third trimester is a common finding. However, generalized or pitting edema, suggesting increasing congestive heart failure, must be reported immediately. Emotional stress on the job increases cardiac demand. However, it needs to be reported only if the client experiences symptoms, such as palpitations or irregular heart rate, indicating heart failure related to the increased stress. Weight gain of 1 pound per week is a normal finding during the third trimester. (I, 9)

65. 2. Unless the client has cardiac decompensation during the pregnancy, she will most likely be able to continue taking the same dose of medication. The client may be prescribed prophylactic antibiotics, particularly if she has had rheumatic fever. The medication would

be switched only if digitalis toxicity occurs. A diuretic is added only if congestive heart failure is not controlled by sodium and activity restrictions. (P, 1)

66. 1. Although there is no completely safe anticoagulant therapy during pregnancy, heparin is typically the drug of choice. Warfarin (Coumadin), a pregnancy category D drug, can cause fetal malformations. Enoxaprin (Lovenox) is not typically prescribed because it can result in thrombocytopenia. Ardeparin (Normiflo) also can cause fetal malformations. (I, 8)

67. 4. The client can continue a low-sodium diet but should increase the caloric intake to 2200 calories daily to provide adequate nutrients to support fetal growth and development. Folic acid supplements, a standard component of care, are used to prevent folic acid deficiency, which is associated with megaloblastic anemia during pregnancy. Severe restriction of sodium intake is not recommended because sodium is necessary to maintain fluid volume. Iron supplements should be taken with acidic foods and fluids (eg, citrus juices) for maximum absorption. Milk decreases the absorption of iron. (I, 9)

The Client With an Ectopic Pregnancy

68. 1. The client's signs and symptoms indicate a probable ectopic pregnancy, which can be confirmed by ultrasound examination or by culdocentesis. The physician is notified immediately because hypovolemic shock may develop without external bleeding. Once the fallopian tube ruptures, blood will enter the pelvic cavity, resulting in shock. Abruptio placenta would be manifested by a board-like uterus in the third trimester. Gestational trophoblastic disease would be suspected if the client exhibited no fetal heart rate and symptoms of pregnancy-induced hypertension before 20 weeks' gestation. A client with a complete abortion would exhibit a normal pulse and blood pressure with scant vaginal bleeding. (D, 10)

69. 1. An ectopic pregnancy is defined as any gestation located outside the uterus. About 95% of ectopic pregnancies occur in the fallopian tube. Ectopic pregnancies are the second most common cause of bleeding early in pregnancy; they are commonly associated with pelvic inflammatory disease and scars from tubal surgery. An intestinal implantation is extremely rare, occurring in fewer than 1% of ectopic pregnancies. Interstitial implantation occurs in fewer than 3% of ectopic pregnancies. Ovarian implantation is extremely rare, occurring in fewer than 1% of ectopic pregnancies. (I, 10)

70. 4. The most appropriate nursing diagnosis for this client is Anticipatory Grieving related to the loss of the pregnancy. Most women form an emotional attachment to the fetus during the first trimester of pregnancy. This is a crisis for the client, and she needs emotional support. More information, such as a client's expression of being afraid, is needed to support a nursing diagnosis of Fear related to surgery. Demonstration of inappropriate behaviors (eg, screaming or yelling) would be needed to support a nursing diagnosis of Ineffective Coping. A statement such as "I don't want any scars on my body" would be needed to support a nursing diagnosis of Disturbed Body Image. (D, 5)

71. 2. Falling hematocrit and hemoglobin levels are indicators of shock, which occurs if the tube ruptures. Other common symptoms of tubal rupture include severe knife-like lower quadrant abdominal pain and referred shoulder pain. The amount of vaginal bleeding that is evident is a poor estimate of actual blood loss. Slight vaginal bleeding, often described as spotting, is common. A rapid, thready pulse, a symptom of shock, is more common with tubal rupture than is a slow, bounding pulse. Abdominal edema is not associated with tubal rupture in ectopic pregnancy. (A, 9)

72. 4. Fallopian tube rupture is an emergency situation because of extensive bleeding into the peritoneal cavity. Shock soon develops if precautionary measures are not taken. The nurse readying a client for surgery should be especially careful to monitor blood pressure and pulse rate for signs of impending shock. The nurse should be prepared to administer fluids, blood, or plasma expanders as necessary through an intravenous line that should already be in place. Because the fertilized ovum has implanted outside the uterus, uterine cramping is unlikely. However, abdominal tenderness or knife-like pain may occur. Abdominal fullness may be present, but abdominal distention is rare unless peritonitis has developed. Although the hemoglobin and hematocrit may be checked routinely before surgery, the laboratory results may not truly reflect the presence or degree of acute hemorrhage. (A, 9)

73. 3. Anything that causes a narrowing or constriction in the fallopian tubes so that a fertilized ovum cannot be properly transported to the uterus for implantation predisposes to an ectopic pregnancy. Pelvic inflammatory disease is the most common cause of constricted or narrow tubes. Developmental defects are other possible causes. Ectopic pregnancy is not related to urinary tract infections. Use of marijuana during pregnancy is not associated with ectopic pregnancy, but its use can result in some intelligence reduction if the mother's use during pregnancy was extensive. Progestin-only contraceptives and intrauterine devices have been associated with ectopic pregnancy. (A, 10)

74. 2. The client should not experience a headache or dizziness. Symptoms that the client should report include pain (caused by stretching of the tube), bleeding (suggestive of possible hemorrhage), and temperature elevation (suggestive of infection). The client should also be instructed that infertility may occur as a result of the removal of one fallopian tube. (E, 9)

75. 3. Because the fallopian tube has not yet ruptured, methotrexate may be given, followed by leucovorin. This chemotherapeutic agent attacks the fast-growing zygote and trophoblast cells. RU-486 is also effective. A hysterosalpingogram is usually performed after chemotherapy to determine whether the tube is still patent. Progestin-only contraceptives and medroxyprogesterone are ineffective in clearing the fallopian tube. Dyphylline is a bronchodilator and is not used. (P, 8)

The Client With Hyperemesis Gravidarum

76. 3. The client needs further instructions when she says she should eat two meals a day with frequent protein snacks to decrease the nausea and vomiting. The client should eat more frequent, smaller meals, with frequent carbohydrate snacks to decrease the nausea and vomiting. Eating dry crackers or toast before arising, consuming fluids separately from meals, and avoiding greasy or spicy foods may also help to decrease the nausea and vomiting. (E, 7)

77. 3. Gastrointestinal secretion losses from excessive vomiting, diarrhea, and excessive perspiration can result in hypokalemia, hyponatremia, decreased chloride levels, metabolic alkalosis, and eventual acidosis if precautionary measures are not taken. Ketones may be present in the urine. Dehydration can lead to poor maternal and fetal outcomes. Persistent vomiting can lead to hypocalcemia, not hypercalcemia. Hyperbilirubinemia, not hypobilirubinemia, is typical in clients with hyperemesis. Persistent vomiting may affect liver function and subsequently the excretion of bilirubin from the body. Hypoglycemia, not hyperglycemia, may occur as a result of decreased intake of food and fluids, decreased metabolism of nutrients, and excessive vomiting. (A, 9)

78. 2. Although the cause of hyperemesis is still unclear, it is thought to be related to high estrogen levels or to trophoblastic activity or gonadotrophin production. Hyperemesis is also associated with infectious conditions, such as hepatitis or encephalitis, intestinal obstruction, peptic ulcer, and hydatidiform mole. (I, 10)

79. 3. 1000 mL divided by 8 hours equals 125 mL per hour. (I, 8)

80. 3. Usually the client remains NPO for at least 24 hours with intravenous therapy. Total parenteral nutrition is started only if other measures fail. If the client is not vomiting after 24 hours, she may be offered clear liquids. If she tolerates liquids, then dry

toast, crackers, or cereal may be given every 2 to 3 hours. The client should be given a choice of foods. The temperature of the foods and fluids should be appropriate (ie, hot foods served hot and cold foods served cold). (I, 10)

The Pregnant Client With a Hydatidiform Mole

81. 1. Hydatidiform mole is suspected when the following are present: pregnancy-induced hypertension before the 24th week of gestation, brownish or prune-colored vaginal bleeding, anemia, absence of fetal heart tones, passage of hydropic vessels, uterine enlargement greater than expected for gestational age, and increased human chorionic gonadotrophin (hCG) levels. Gestational diabetes is related to an increased risk for preeclampsia and urinary tract infections, but it is not associated with hydatidiform mole. Hyperthyroidism, not hypothyroidism, occurs occasionally with hydatidiform mole. If it does occur, it can be a serious complication, possibly life-threatening to the mother and fetus from cardiac problems. Polycythemia is not associated with hydatidiform mole. Rather, anemia from blood loss is associated with molar pregnancies. (A, 9)

82. 2. After dilation and curettage to evacuate a molar pregnancy, the nurse should assess the client's vital signs and monitor for signs of hemorrhage, because the surgical procedure may have traumatized the uterine lining, leading to hemorrhage. Urinary tract infections, not common after evacuation of a molar pregnancy, are most commonly related to urinary catheterization. Typically, urinary catheters are not used during evacuation of a molar pregnancy. The client should not experience abdominal distention, because the contents of the uterus have been removed. Chorioamnionitis is an inflammation of the amniotic fluid membranes. With complete mole, no embryonic or fetal tissue or membranes are present. (A, 9)

83. 2. A client who has had a hydatidiform mole removed should have regular checkups to rule out the presence of choriocarcinoma, which may complicate the client's clinical picture. The client's hCG levels are monitored for 1 year. During this time, she should be advised not to become pregnant because this would be reflected in rising hCG levels. (E, 9)

84. 2. A client who has experienced a molar pregnancy is at risk for development of choriocarcinoma and requires close monitoring of hCG levels. Pregnancy would interfere with monitoring these levels. High hCG titers are common for up to 7 weeks after the evacuation of the mole, but then these levels gradually begin to decline. Clients should have a pelvic examination and a blood test for hCG titers every month for 6 months and then every 2 months for 1 year. Gradually declining hCG levels suggest no complications. Increasing levels are indicative of a malignancy and should be treated with methotrexate. If after 1 year the hCG levels are negative, the client is theoretically free of the risk of a malignancy developing and could plan another pregnancy. (I, 9)

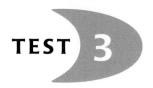
The Birth Experience

▶ **The Primigravid Client in Labor**

▶ **The Multigravid Client in Labor**

▶ **The Intrapartal Client With Risk Factors**

▶ **Correct Answers and Rationale**

Select the best answer and indicate your choice by filling in the circle in front of the option.

The Primigravid Client in Labor

1. The physician orders intermittent fetal heart rate monitoring for a 20-year-old obese primigravid client at 40 weeks' gestation who is admitted to the birthing center in the first stage of labor. The nurse would monitor the client's fetal heart rate pattern at which of the following intervals?
   ○ 1. Every 15 minutes during the latent phase.
   ○ 2. Every 30 minutes during the active phase.
   ○ 3. Every 60 minutes during the initial phase.
   ○ 4. Every 2 hours during the transition phase.

2. Assessment reveals that the fetus of a primigravid client is at +1 station. The nurse interprets this finding as indicating that the fetal presenting part is positioned at which of the following?
   ○ 1. 1 cm above the ischial spines.
   ○ 2. 1 cm below the ischial spines.
   ○ 3. 1 cm above the ischial tuberosities.
   ○ 4. 1 cm below the sacral promontory.

3. Assessment of a primigravid client in active labor who has had no analgesia or anesthesia reveals complete cervical effacement, dilation of 7 cm, and the fetus at 0 station. Which of the following behaviors would the nurse anticipate that the client will exhibit during this phase of labor?
   ○ 1. Excitement.
   ○ 2. Loss of control.
   ○ 3. Numbness of the legs.
   ○ 4. Feelings of relief.

4. While caring for a moderately obese primigravida in active labor at term, the nurse would expect to monitor the client for signs of which of the following?
   ○ 1. Hypotonic reflexes.
   ○ 2. Increased uterine resting tone.
   ○ 3. Soft tissue dystocia.
   ○ 4. Increased fear and anxiety.

5. The nurse is caring for a primigravid client in active labor at 42 weeks' gestation. The client has had no analgesia or anesthesia and has been in the second stage of labor for 2¹/₂ hours. The nurse determines that the client may be exhibiting symptoms of which of the following?
   ○ 1. Shoulder dystocia.
   ○ 2. Twin gestation.
   ○ 3. Anencephaly.
   ○ 4. Breech presentation.

6. The physician has ordered prostaglandin gel to be administered vaginally to a newly admitted primigravid client. Which of the following would indicate to the nurse that the client has had a therapeutic response to the medication?
   ○ 1. Resting period of 2 minutes between contractions.
   ○ 2. Normal patellar and elbow reflexes for the past 2 hours.
   ○ 3. Softening of the cervix and beginning effacement.
   ○ 4. Leaking of clear amniotic fluid in small amounts.

7. A primigravid client is admitted as an outpatient for an external cephalic version. For which of the following would the nurse assess the client as a possible contraindication for the procedure?
   ○ 1. Multiple gestation.
   ○ 2. Breech presentation.
   ○ 3. Maternal Rh-negative blood type.
   ○ 4. History of gestational diabetes.

8. A primigravida is admitted to the labor suite with ruptured membranes and contractions occurring every 2 to 3 minutes and lasting 45 seconds. After 6 hours of labor, the client's contractions are now every 7 to 10 minutes, lasting 30 seconds. Which of the following would the nurse anticipate that the physician will order?
   ○ 1. Morphine sulfate.
   ○ 2. Oxytocin (Pitocin).
   ○ 3. Nalbuphine (Nubain).
   ○ 4. Ampicillin.

9. A primigravid client in the second stage of labor feels the urge to push. The client has had no analgesia or anesthesia. Anatomically, which of the following would be the *best* position for the client to assume?
   ○ 1. Dorsal recumbent.
   ○ 2. Lithotomy.
   ○ 3. Hands and knees.
   ○ 4. Squatting.

10. A 21-year-old primigravid client at 40 weeks' gestation is admitted to the hospital in active labor. The client's cervix is 7 cm and completely effaced at 0 station. During the transition phase of labor, which of the following would the nurse identify as a *priority* nursing diagnosis?
    ○ 1. Impaired Urinary Elimination related to NPO status.
    ○ 2. Risk for Injury related to hyperventilation and dizziness.
    ○ 3. Ineffective Coping related to lack of confidence.
    ○ 4. Pain related to increasing frequency and intensity of uterine contractions.

11. A 24-year-old primigravid client who delivers a viable term neonate is ordered to receive oxytocin intravenously after delivery of the placenta. Which of the following signs would indicate to the nurse that the placenta is about to be delivered?
    ○ 1. The cord lengthens outside the vagina.
    ○ 2. There is decreased vaginal bleeding.
    ○ 3. The uterus cannot be palpated.
    ○ 4. Uterus changes to discoid shape.

12. A primiparous client, who has just delivered a healthy term neonate after 12 hours of labor, holds and looks at her neonate and begins to cry. The nurse correctly interprets this behavior as a sign of which of the following?
    ○ 1. Disappointment in the baby's gender.
    ○ 2. Grief over the ending of the pregnancy.
    ○ 3. A normal response to the birth.
    ○ 4. Indication of postpartum "blues."

13. The cervix of a 15-year-old primigravida admitted to the labor area is 2 cm dilated and 50% effaced. Her membranes are intact, and contractions are occurring every 5 to 6 minutes. Which of the following would the nurse recommend after the client is admitted?
    ○ 1. Resting in the right lateral recumbent position.
    ○ 2. Lying in the left lateral recumbent position.
    ○ 3. Walking around in the hallway until she gets tired.
    ○ 4. Sitting in a comfortable chair for a period of time.

14. Which of the following would the nurse include in the teaching plan for a 16-year-old primigravid client in early labor concerning active relaxation techniques to help her cope with pain?
    ○ 1. Relaxing uninvolved body muscles during uterine contractions.
    ○ 2. Practicing being in a deep, meditative, sleep-like state.
    ○ 3. Focusing on an object in the room during the contractions.
    ○ 4. Breathing rapidly and deeply between contractions.

15. A primigravid client in early labor asks the nurse what *effleurage* means. The nurse explains that effleurage is a type of massage involving which of the following?
    ○ 1. Deep kneading of superficial muscles.
    ○ 2. Secure grasping of muscular tissues.
    ○ 3. Light stroking of the skin surface.
    ○ 4. Prolonged pressure on specific sites.

16. A 24-year-old primigravid client in active labor requests use of the jet hydrotherapy tub to aid in pain relief. The nurse bases the response on the understanding that this therapy is often contraindicated for clients with which of the following?
    ○ 1. Ruptured membranes.
    ○ 2. Multifetal gestation.
    ○ 3. Diabetes mellitus.
    ○ 4. Hypotonic labor patterns.

17. A primigravid client admitted to the labor area in early labor tells the nurse that her brother was born with cystic fibrosis. When teaching the client about this disorder, the nurse understands that this disorder is considered as which of the following?
    ○ 1. X-linked recessive.
    ○ 2. X-linked dominant.
    ○ 3. Autosomal recessive.
    ○ 4. Autosomal dominant.

18. The physician orders an amniocentesis for a primigravid client at 37 weeks' gestation in early labor to determine fetal lung maturity. The nurse expects the fluid sample to be tested for which of the following?
    ○ 1. Amount of bilirubin present.
    ○ 2. Presence of red blood cells.
    ○ 3. Barr body determination.
    ○ 4. Lecithin-sphingomyelin (L/S) ratio.

19. Assessment of a 15-year-old primigravid client at term in active labor reveals cervical dilation at 7 cm with complete effacement. Because the client is only 15 years old, which of the following would the nurse assess the client for during labor?
    ○ 1. Uterine inversion.
    ○ 2. Cephalopelvic disproportion (CPD).
    ○ 3. Rapid third stage of labor.
    ○ 4. Decreased ability to push.

20. The nurse is working on a busy labor and delivery unit with other nurses and a licensed practical

nurse. Which of the following labor clients would the nurse assign to the licensed practical nurse?
- ○ 1. A gravida IV, para III client with a history of gestational diabetes.
- ○ 2. A gravida III, para I, Ab I client at 35 weeks' gestation.
- ○ 3. A gravida I, para 0 client with leaking green amniotic fluid.
- ○ 4. A gravida II, para I client with a history of hyperemesis gravidarum.

21. A 19-year-old primigravid client at 38 weeks' gestation is admitted to the hospital in active labor that began 8 hours ago. When the client's cervix is 7 cm dilated and the presenting part is at +1 station, the client tells the nurse, "I need to push!" Which of the following would the nurse do *next*?
- ○ 1. Use the McDonald procedure to widen the pelvic opening.
- ○ 2. Increase the rate of oxygen and intravenous fluids.
- ○ 3. Instruct the client to use a pant-blow pattern of breathing.
- ○ 4. Tell the client to push only when absolutely necessary.

22. Which of the following would be the priority when caring for a primigravid client whose cervix is dilated at 8 cm when the fetus is at 1+ station and the client has had no analgesia or anesthesia?
- ○ 1. Giving frequent sips of water.
- ○ 2. Applying extra blankets for warmth.
- ○ 3. Providing frequent perineal cleansing.
- ○ 4. Offering encouragement and support.

23. To determine whether a primigravid client in labor with a fetus in the left occipitoanterior (LOA) position is completely dilated, the nurse performs a vaginal examination. During the examination the nurse would expect to palpate which of the following cranial sutures?
- ○ 1. Sagittal.
- ○ 2. Lambdoidal.
- ○ 3. Coronal.
- ○ 4. Frontal.

24. After a lengthy labor process, a primigravid client delivers a healthy newborn boy with a moderate amount of skull molding. Which of the following would the nurse include when explaining to the parents about this condition?
- ○ 1. It is typically seen with breech deliveries.
- ○ 2. It usually lasts a day or two before resolving.
- ○ 3. It is unusual when the brow is the presenting part.
- ○ 4. Surgical intervention may be necessary to alleviate pressure.

25. After delivery of a viable neonate, a 20-year-old primiparous client comments to her mother and the nurse about the baby. Which of the following comments would the nurse interpret as a possible sign of potential maternal–infant bonding problems?
- ○ 1. "He's got my funny-looking ears!"
- ○ 2. "I think my mother should give him the first feeding."
- ○ 3. "He's a lot bigger than I expected him to be."
- ○ 4. "I want to buy him a blue outfit to wear when we get home."

26. Assessment of a 23-year-old primigravid client at term who is admitted to the birthing unit in active labor reveals that her cervix is 4 cm dilated and 100% effaced. Contractions are occurring every 4 minutes. When developing the teaching plan, which of the following statements about the gate-control theory of pain would the nurse expect to include?
- ○ 1. Input from the large sensory fibers opens the gate.
- ○ 2. Labor pain is a matter of individual perception.
- ○ 3. Slow abdominal breathing can open the gate.
- ○ 4. The gating mechanism is in the spinal cord.

27. The nurse explains to a newly admitted primigravid client in active labor that, according to the gate-control theory of pain, a closed gate means that the client should experience which of the following?
- ○ 1. No pain.
- ○ 2. Sharp pain.
- ○ 3. Light pain.
- ○ 4. Moderate pain.

28. The cervix of a primigravid client in active labor who received epidural anesthesia 4 hours ago is now completely dilated, and the client is ready to begin pushing. Before the client begins to push, which of the following would the nurse assess?
- ○ 1. Fetal heart rate variability.
- ○ 2. Cervical dilation again.
- ○ 3. Vital signs.
- ○ 4. Bladder status.

29. For the past 8 hours, a 20-year-old primigravid client in active labor with intact membranes has been experiencing regular contractions. Fetal heart rate is 136 bpm with good variability. After determining that the client is still in the latent phase of labor, for which of the following would the nurse expect to observe the client closely?
- ○ 1. Exhaustion.
- ○ 2. Chills and fever.
- ○ 3. Fluid overload.
- ○ 4. Meconium-stained fluid.

30. A primigravid client whose cervix is 7 cm dilated with the fetus at 0 station and in a left occipitoposterior (LOP) position requests pain relief for severe back pain. In developing the plan of care for this client, the nurse would anticipate which of the following?

○ 1. Providing firm pressure to the client's sacral area.

○ 2. Preparing the client for a cesarean delivery.

○ 3. Preparing the client for a precipitate delivery.

○ 4. Maintaining the client in a left side-lying position.

31. A primigravida in active labor has had no anesthesia. The client's cervix is 7 cm dilated, and she is starting to feel considerable discomfort during contractions. The nurse suggests that the client change from slow chest breathing to which of the following?

○ 1. Rapid, shallow chest breathing.

○ 2. Deep chest breathing.

○ 3. Rapid pant-blow breathing.

○ 4. Slow abdominal breathing.

32. A 16-year-old primigravida, with a history of attending one prenatal visit, is admitted to the hospital in active labor at 37 weeks' gestation. Her cervix is 7 cm dilated with the presenting part at 0 station. She enters the labor unit appearing anxious and hyperventilating. Because of the hyperventilation, the nurse would assess the client for symptoms of which of the following?

○ 1. Metabolic alkalosis.

○ 2. Metabolic acidosis.

○ 3. Respiratory alkalosis.

○ 4. Respiratory acidosis.

33. The physician orders scalp stimulation of the fetal head for a primigravid client in active labor. When explaining to the client about this procedure, which of the following would the nurse include as the purpose?

○ 1. Assessment of the fetal hematocrit level.

○ 2. Increase in the strength of the contractions.

○ 3. Increase in the fetal heart rate and variability.

○ 4. Assessment of fetal position.

34. The nurse is caring for a primigravid client in active labor who has had two fetal blood samplings to check for fetal hypoxia. The nurse determines that the fetus is showing signs of acidosis when the scalp blood pH is below which of the following?

○ 1. 7.5.

○ 2. 7.4.

○ 3. 7.3.

○ 4. 7.2.

35. Assessment of a primigravid client reveals cervical dilation at 8 cm and complete effacement. The client complains of severe back pain during this phase of labor. The nurse explains that the client's severe back pain is most likely caused by the fetal occiput's being in a position that is identified as which of the following?

○ 1. Breech.

○ 2. Transverse.

○ 3. Posterior.

○ 4. Anterior.

36. When performing Leopold's maneuvers on a primigravid client, the nurse is palpating the uterus as shown in Figure 1. Which of the following maneuvers is the nurse performing?

○ 1. First maneuver.

○ 2. Second maneuver.

○ 3. Third maneuver.

○ 4. Fourth maneuver.

37. Before placing the fetal monitoring device on a primigravid client's fundus, the nurse performs Leopold's maneuvers. When performing the third maneuver, the nurse explains that this maneuver is done for which of the following reasons?

○ 1. To determine whether the fetal presenting part is engaged.

○ 2. To locate the fetal cephalic prominence.

○ 3. To distinguish between a breech and a cephalic presentation.

○ 4. To locate the position of the fetal arms and legs.

38. A primigravid client in active labor with a fetus in LOP position complains of severe back pressure. Which of the following would be the priority nursing diagnosis for this client?

○ 1. Anxiety related to fear of maternal–fetal outcomes.

○ 2. Ineffective Coping related to lack of experience in labor.

○ 3. Urinary Retention related to prolonged labor process.

○ 4. Pain related to occipitoposterior position and prolonged fetal descent.

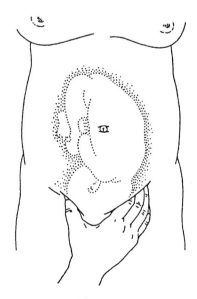

Figure 1.

39. One-half hour after vaginal delivery of a term neonate, the nurse palpates the fundus of a primigravid client, noting several large clots and a small trickle of bright red vaginal bleeding. The client's blood pressure is 136/92 mm Hg. Which of the following would the nurse do *next*?
○ 1. Continue to monitor the client's fundus every 15 minutes.
○ 2. Ask the physician for an order for methylergonovine (Methergine).
○ 3. Immediately notify the physician of the client's symptoms.
○ 4. Change the client's perineal pads every 15 minutes.

The Multigravid Client in Labor

40. A 31-year-old multigravid client at 39 weeks' gestation admitted to the hospital in active labor is receiving intravenous lactated Ringer's solution and a continuous epidural anesthetic. During the first hour after administration of the anesthetic, the nurse would monitor the client for which of the following?
○ 1. Hypotension.
○ 2. Diaphoresis.
○ 3. Headache.
○ 4. Tremors.

41. The nurse, while shopping in a local department store, hears a multiparous woman say loudly, "I think the baby's coming." After asking someone to call 911, the nurse assists the client to deliver a term neonate. While waiting for the ambulance, the nurse suggests that the mother initiate breast-feeding, primarily for which of the following reasons?
○ 1. To begin the parental–infant bonding process.
○ 2. To prevent neonatal hypothermia.
○ 3. To provide glucose to the neonate.
○ 4. To contract the mother's uterus.

42. Approximately 15 minutes after delivery of a viable term neonate, a multiparous client complains of a chill. Which of the following would the nurse do *next*?
○ 1. Assess the client's pulse rate.
○ 2. Decrease the rate of intravenous fluids.
○ 3. Provide the client with a warm blanket.
○ 4. Assess the amount of blood loss.

43. The physician plans to perform an amniotomy on a multiparous client admitted to the labor area at 41 weeks' gestation for labor induction. After the amniotomy, which of the following would the nurse expect do *first*?
○ 1. Monitor the client's contraction pattern.
○ 2. Assess the fetal heart rate for 1 full minute.

○ 3. Assess the client's temperature and pulse.
○ 4. Document the color of the amniotic fluid.

44. Which of the following nursing diagnoses would the nurse identify as the priority after delivery for a multiparous client who received an epidural anesthetic?
○ 1. Pain related to episiotomy and exhaustive pushing efforts.
○ 2. Anxiety related to inability to move legs and toes.
○ 3. Risk for Injury related to epidural anesthesia.
○ 4. Excess Fluid Volume overload related to labor process and intravenous fluids.

45. Which of the following would the nurse expect as a common finding for a multiparous client delivering a viable neonate at 41 weeks' gestation with the aid of a vacuum extractor?
○ 1. Neonatal scalp edema.
○ 2. Uterine separation.
○ 3. Maternal lacerations.
○ 4. Neonatal intracranial hemorrhage.

46. The nurse is assessing fetal presentation in a multiparous client. Figure 2 indicates which of the following types of presentation?
○ 1. Frank breech.
○ 2. Complete breech.
○ 3. Footling breech.
○ 4. Vertex.

47. Two hours ago, a multigravid client was admitted in active labor with her cervix dilated at 5 cm and completely effaced and the fetus at 0 station. Currently, the client is experiencing nausea and vomiting, a slight chill with perspiration beads on her lip, and extreme irritability. Which of the following actions would be *most* appropriate at this time?

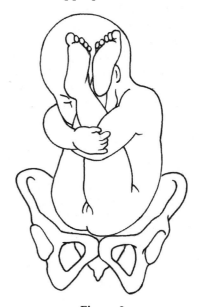

Figure 2.

○ 1. Warm the temperature of the room by a few degrees.

○ 2. Increase the rate of intravenous fluid administration.

○ 3. Obtain an order for an intramuscular antiemetic medication.

○ 4. Assess the client's cervical dilation and station.

48. When assessing the frequency of contractions of a multiparous client in active labor admitted to the birthing area, the nurse should assess the interval between which of the following?

○ 1. Acme of one contraction to the beginning of the next contraction.

○ 2. Beginning of one contraction to the end of the next contraction.

○ 3. End of one contraction to the end of the next contraction.

○ 4. Beginning of one contraction to the beginning of the next contraction.

49. While the nurse is caring for a multiparous client in active labor at 36 weeks' gestation, the client tells the nurse, "I think my water just broke." Which of the following would the nurse do *first*?

○ 1. Turn the client to the right side.

○ 2. Assess the color, amount, and odor of the fluid.

○ 3. Assess the fetal heart rate pattern.

○ 4. Check the client's cervical dilation.

50. A multigravid client admitted to the labor area is scheduled for a cesarean delivery under spinal anesthesia. After instructions by the anesthesiologist, the nurse determines that the client has understood the instructions when she says which of the following?

○ 1. "The medication will be administered while I am in a side-lying position."

○ 2. "The anesthetic may cause a severe headache which is treatable."

○ 3. "My blood pressure may increase if I lie down too soon after the injection."

○ 4. "I can expect immediate anesthesia that can be reversed very easily."

51. When developing the plan of care for a multiparous client in active labor who receives an epidural anesthetic, which of the following would the nurse anticipate that the physician will order if the client develops moderate hypotension?

○ 1. Ephedrine sulfate.

○ 2. Epinephrine (Adrenalin chloride).

○ 3. Methylergonovine (Methergine).

○ 4. Atropine sulfate.

52. The physician determines that the fetus of a multipara in active labor is in distress, necessitating a cesarean delivery with general anesthesia. Before the cesarean delivery, the anesthesiologist orders cimetidine 300 mg PO (Tagamet). The nurse prepares to administer this drug based on the understanding that it reduces which of the following?

○ 1. Incidence of bronchospasm.

○ 2. Oral and respiratory secretions.

○ 3. Acid level of the stomach contents.

○ 4. Incidence of postoperative gastric ulcer.

53. The nurse prepares a 26-year-old multiparous client at 40 weeks' gestation admitted to the hospital's labor unit for induction of labor for lumbar epidural anesthesia. Before anesthesia administration, the nurse instructs the client to assume which of the following positions?

○ 1. Lithotomy.

○ 2. Side-lying.

○ 3. Knee-to-chest.

○ 4. Prone.

54. The nurse is assessing the perineal changes of a multigravida in the second stage of labor. Figure 3 represents which of the following perineal changes?

○ 1. Anterior–posterior slit.

○ 2. Oval opening.

○ 3. Circular shape.

○ 4. Crowning.

55. After suctioning to clear the airway of a term neonate who appears in good condition after spontaneous vaginal delivery, which of the following would the nurse do *next*?

○ 1. Place the infant in a radiant warmer.

○ 2. Instill erythromycin in the eyes.

○ 3. Obtain the neonate's weight.

○ 4. Put identification bracelets on each wrist.

The Intrapartal Client With Risk Factors

56. A multigravid client is in active labor with twins at 38 weeks' gestation. The nurse would monitor the client closely for symptoms of which of the following?

○ 1. Pregnancy-induced hypertension.

○ 2. Urinary tract infection.

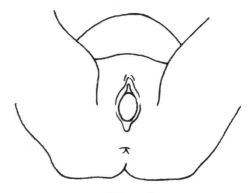

Figure 3.

○ 3. Chorioamnionitis.

○ 4. Precipitous delivery.

57. A 39-year-old multigravid client at 39 weeks' gestation admitted to the hospital in active labor has been diagnosed with class II heart disease. To ensure cardiac emptying and adequate oxygenation during labor, the nurse plans to encourage the client to do which of the following?

○ 1. Breathe slowly after each contraction.

○ 2. Avoid the use of analgesics for the labor pain.

○ 3. Remain in a side-lying position with the head elevated.

○ 4. Request local anesthesia for vaginal delivery.

58. When developing the plan of care for a multigravid client with class III heart disease, which of the following areas would the nurse expect to assess frequently?

○ 1. Dehydration.

○ 2. Nausea and vomiting.

○ 3. Iron-deficiency anemia.

○ 4. Tachycardia.

59. A multigravida in active labor has been diagnosed with class II heart disease and a prosthetic valve replacement. When developing the plan of care for this client, the nurse would anticipate that the physician most likely will order which of the following medications?

○ 1. Anticoagulants.

○ 2. Antibiotics.

○ 3. Diuretics.

○ 4. Folic acid supplements.

60. A 22-year-old primigravid client at 39 weeks' gestation with class B, pregestational insulin-dependent diabetes is admitted to the hospital for induction of labor. The fetus is in a cephalic position, and the client's cervix is dilated 2 cm. The physician has ordered prostaglandin E_2 gel (Dinoprostone) for the client. Before administering prostaglandin E_2 gel to the client, which of the following would the nurse do *first*?

○ 1. Assess the frequency of uterine contractions.

○ 2. Place the client in a side-lying position.

○ 3. Determine whether the membranes have ruptured.

○ 4. Prepare the client for an amniotomy.

61. A multigravid client at 39 weeks' gestation diagnosed with insulin-dependent diabetes is admitted for induction of labor with oxytocin (Pitocin). Which of the following would the nurse include in the teaching plan as a possible disadvantage of this procedure?

○ 1. Urinary frequency.

○ 2. Maternal hypoglycemia.

○ 3. Preterm birth.

○ 4. Neonatal jaundice.

62. Which of the following nursing diagnoses would be the priority for a multigravid diabetic client at 38 weeks' gestation who is scheduled for labor induction with oxytocin (Pitocin)?

○ 1. Risk for Deficient Fluid Volume related to oxytocin infusion.

○ 2. Pain related to prolonged labor and uterine ischemia.

○ 3. Fear related to possible need for cesarean delivery.

○ 4. Risk for Injury, maternal or fetal, related to potential uterine hyperstimulation.

63. A multigravid client is receiving oxytocin (Pitocin) augmentation. When the client's cervix is dilated to 6 cm, her membranes rupture spontaneously with meconium-stained amniotic fluid. Which of the following would the nurse do *next*?

○ 1. Increase the rate of the oxytocin infusion.

○ 2. Turn the client to a knee-to-chest position.

○ 3. Assess cervical dilation and effacement.

○ 4. Monitor the fetal heart rate continuously.

64. A multigravid client in active labor at 39 weeks' gestation has a history of smoking one to two packs of cigarettes daily. For which of the following would the nurse be alert when assessing the client's neonate?

○ 1. Hyperirritability.

○ 2. Hyperbilirubinemia.

○ 3. Low birth weight.

○ 4. Hypocalcemia.

65. A primigravid client who has had a prolonged labor but now is completely dilated has received epidural anesthesia. Which of the following would the nurse expect to include in the teaching plan about pushing?

○ 1. The client needs to push for at least 1 to 3 minutes.

○ 2. Pushing is most effective when the client holds her breath.

○ 3. The client should be urged to push with an open glottis.

○ 4. Pushing is limited to times when she feels the urge.

66. The physician determines that outlet forceps are needed to assist in the delivery of a primigravid client in active labor with a large-for-gestational-size fetus. The nurse reinforces the physician's explanation for using forceps based on the understanding about which of the following concerning the location of the fetal skull?

○ 1. It is engaged past the inlet.

○ 2. It is at +1 station.

○ 3. It is visible at the perineal floor.

○ 4. It has reached the level of the ischial spines.

67. The physician orders an amnioinfusion for a primi-

gravid client at term who is diagnosed with oligo-hydramnios. Which of the following would the nurse include in the client's teaching plan about the purpose of this procedure?

○ 1. To decrease the frequency and severity of variable decelerations.

○ 2. To minimize the possibility of fetal metabolic alkalosis.

○ 3. To increase the fetal heart rate accelerations during a contraction.

○ 4. To raise the amniotic fluid index to more than 15 cm.

68. A primigravid client at 37 weeks' gestation who has been diagnosed with pregnancy-induced hypertension is to be admitted to the labor and delivery area. Which of the following client care rooms would the nurse determine to be *most* appropriate for this client?

○ 1. A brightly lit private room at the end of the hall from the nurse's station.

○ 2. A semiprivate room midway down the hall from the nurse's station.

○ 3. A private room with many windows that is near the operating room.

○ 4. A darkened private room as close to the nurse's station as possible.

69. A multigravid client is admitted to the labor area from the emergency room. At the time of admission, the fetal head is crowning, and the client yells "The baby's coming!" To help the client remain calm and cooperative during the imminent delivery, which of the following responses by the nurse would be *most* appropriate?

○ 1. "You're right, the baby is coming, so just relax."

○ 2. "Please don't push because you'll tear your cervix."

○ 3. "Your doctor will be here as soon as possible."

○ 4. "I'll explain what's happening to guide you as we go along."

70. The nurse is caring for a multigravid client who speaks little English. As the nurse enters the client's room, the nurse observes the client squatting in the bed and the fetal head crowning. After calling for assistance and checking for the umbilical cord around the fetal neck, which of the following would the nurse do *next*?

○ 1. Tell the client to push between contractions.

○ 2. Hold the neonate's head down to promote drainage of secretions.

○ 3. Apply gentle upward traction on the neonate's anterior shoulder.

○ 4. Massage the perineum to stretch the perineal tissues.

71. During the first hour after a precipitous delivery, the nurse would monitor a multiparous client for signs and symptoms of which of the following?

○ 1. Postpartum blues.

○ 2. Uterine atony.

○ 3. Intrauterine infection.

○ 4. Urinary tract infection.

72. A multigravid client in labor at 38 weeks' gestation has been diagnosed with Rh sensitization and probable fetal hydrops and anemia. When the nurse observes the fetal heart rate pattern on the monitor, which of the following patterns is *most* likely?

○ 1. Early deceleration pattern.

○ 2. Sinusoidal pattern.

○ 3. Variable deceleration pattern.

○ 4. Late deceleration pattern.

73. The physician orders oxytocin to be added to the intravenous fluids of a 30-year-old multigravid client at 37 weeks' gestation with twins after vaginal delivery. The nurse anticipates administering the oxytocin after delivery of which of the following?

○ 1. First placenta.

○ 2. First twin.

○ 3. Second placenta.

○ 4. Second twin.

74. The nurse in the labor and delivery area receives a telephone call from the emergency room announcing that a multigravid client in active labor is being transferred to the labor area. The client has had no prenatal care. When the client arrives by stretcher, she says, "I think the baby's coming . . . Help!" The fetal skull is crowning. Which of the following would be a priority assessment for the nurse to make?

○ 1. Estimated date of delivery.

○ 2. Amniotic fluid status.

○ 3. Gravida and parity.

○ 4. Prenatal history.

75. A multiparous client delivers dizygotic twins at 37 weeks' gestation. The twin neonates require additional hospitalization after the client is discharged. In planning the family's care, an appropriate goal for the nurse to formulate is that, while the twins are hospitalized, the parents will do which of the following?

○ 1. Discuss how they will cope with twin infants at home.

○ 2. Participate in care of the twins as much as possible.

○ 3. Take turns providing 24-hour observation of the twins.

○ 4. Identify complications that may occur as the twins develop.

76. A primigravida at 41 weeks' gestation is admitted to the hospital's labor and delivery unit in active labor. After 25 hours of labor with membranes ruptured for 24 hours, the client delivers a healthy neonate vaginally with a midline episiotomy. Which of the following would the nurse identify as a priority nursing diagnosis for the client?

○ 1. Activity Intolerance related to difficult labor process.

○ 2. Sleep Deprivation related to prolonged labor.

○ 3. Situational Low Self-Esteem related to lengthy labor process.

○ 4. Risk for Infection related to birth trauma and prolonged ruptured membranes.

77. The nurse is caring for a primiparous client and her neonate immediately after delivery. The neonate was born at 41 weeks' gestation and weighs 4082 g (9 pounds). Signs and symptoms of which of the following would be a priority assessment in the neonate?

○ 1. Anemia.

○ 2. Hypoglycemia.

○ 3. Delayed meconium.

○ 4. Elevated bilirubin.

78. A multigravid client in active labor at term is diagnosed with polyhydramnios. The physician has instructed the client about possible neonatal complications related to the polyhydramnios. The nurse determines that the client has understood the instructions when the client states that polyhydramnios is associated with which of the following in the fetus or neonate?

○ 1. Renal dysfunction.

○ 2. Intrauterine growth retardation.

○ 3. Pulmonary hypoplasia.

○ 4. Gastrointestinal disorders.

79. A primigravid client at 39 weeks' gestation is admitted to the hospital in active labor. On admission, the client's cervix is 6 cm dilated. After 2 hours of active labor, the client's cervix is still dilated at 6 cm with 100% effacement at −1 station. Contractions are 3 to 5 minutes apart, lasting 45 seconds, and of moderate intensity. The nurse determines that the client is most likely experiencing which of the following?

○ 1. Cephalopelvic disproportion.

○ 2. Prolonged latent phase.

○ 3. Prolonged transitional phase.

○ 4. Hypotonic contraction pattern.

80. The physician who elects to perform a cesarean delivery on a primigravid client for fetal distress has informed the client of possible risks during the procedure. When the nurse asks the client to sign the consent form, the client's husband says, "I'll sign it for her. She's too upset by what is happening to make this decision." Which of the following actions would be *most* appropriate?

○ 1. Ask the client if this is acceptable to her.

○ 2. Have the client and her husband both sign the consent form.

○ 3. Ask the client to sign the consent form.

○ 4. Ask the doctor to witness the consent form.

81. A multigravid client at term is admitted to the hospital for a trial labor and possible vaginal birth. She has a history of previous cesarean delivery because of fetal distress. When the client is 4 cm dilated, she receives nalbuphine (Nubain) intravenously. While monitoring the fetal heart rate, the nurse observes minimal variability and a rate of 120 bpm. The nurse should explain to the client that the decreased variability is most likely caused by which of the following?

○ 1. Maternal fatigue.

○ 2. Fetal malposition.

○ 3. Small-for-gestational-age fetus.

○ 4. Effects of analgesic medication.

82. The nurse is caring for a primipara in active labor when the fetus develops severe bradycardia with late decelerations, and an emergency cesarean delivery is performed with the client under general anesthesia. After the delivery, the client tells the nurse, "I feel terrible. This is exactly what I didn't want to happen!" Which of the following would be a priority nursing diagnosis for this client?

○ 1. Interrupted Family Processes related to cesarean delivery.

○ 2. Anxiety related to incisional scar and neonatal outcome.

○ 3. Pain related to surgical incision and uterine cramping.

○ 4. Situational Low Self-Esteem related to inability to deliver vaginally.

83. During a scheduled cesarean delivery of a primigravid client with a fetus at 39 weeks' gestation in a breech presentation, a neonatologist is present in the operating room. The nurse explains to the client that the neonatologist is present because neonates born by cesarean delivery tend to have an increased incidence of which of the following?

○ 1. Congenital anomalies.

○ 2. Pulmonary hypertension.

○ 3. Meconium aspiration syndrome.

○ 4. Respiratory distress syndrome.

84. A 28-year-old multigravid client at 28 weeks' gestation diagnosed with acute pyelonephritis is receiving intravenous fluids and antibiotics. After teaching the client about the rationale for the aggressive therapy, the nurse determines that the client needs *further* instruction when she says that acute pyelonephritis can lead to which of the following?

○ 1. Preterm labor.

○ 2. Maternal sepsis.

○ 3. Intrauterine growth retardation.

○ 4. Congenital fetal anomalies.

85. A primigravid client at 38 weeks' gestation is admitted to the labor suite in active labor. The client's physical assessment reveals a chlamydial infection.

The nurse explains that if the infection is left untreated, the neonate may develop which of the following?
○ 1. Conjunctivitis.
○ 2. Heart disease.
○ 3. Harlequin sign.
○ 4. Brain damage.

86. A 34-year-old primigravid client at 39 weeks' gestation admitted to the hospital in active labor has type B Rh-negative blood. The nurse would instruct the client that if the neonate is Rh positive, the client will receive an Rh immune globulin (RHIG) injection for which of the following reasons?
○ 1. To prevent Rh-positive sensitization with the next pregnancy.
○ 2. To provide active antibody protection for this pregnancy.
○ 3. To decrease the amount of Rh-minus sensitization for the next pregnancy.
○ 4. To destroy fetal Rh-positive cells during the next pregnancy.

87. A 16-year-old primigravid client admitted at 38 weeks' gestation with severe pregnancy-induced hypertension is given intravenous magnesium sulfate and lactated Ringer's solution. Which of the following would the nurse expect to assess?
○ 1. Urinary output every 8 hours.
○ 2. Deep tendon reflexes every 4 hours.
○ 3. Respiratory rate every hour.
○ 4. Blood pressure every 6 hours.

88. The labor and delivery room nurse has received a telephone call from the emergency room indicating that a multigravid client in early labor and diagnosed with probable placenta previa will be arriving soon. In preparation for the client's arrival, the nurse anticipates that the physician will order which of the following?
○ 1. Whole blood replacement.
○ 2. Continuous blood pressure monitoring.
○ 3. Internal fetal heart rate monitoring.
○ 4. An immediate cesarean delivery.

89. During admission, a multigravida in early active labor acts somewhat euphoric and tells the nurse that she smoked some crack cocaine before coming to the hospital. In addition to fetal heart rate assessment, the nurse should monitor the client for symptoms of which of the following?
○ 1. Placenta previa.
○ 2. Ruptured uterus.
○ 3. Maternal hypotension.
○ 4. Abruptio placenta.

90. A primigravid client in early labor tells the nurse that she was exposed to rubella at about 14 weeks' gestation. After delivery, the nurse should assess the neonate for which of the following?

○ 1. Hydrocephaly.
○ 2. Cardiac disorders.
○ 3. Renal disorders.
○ 4. Bulging fontanels.

91. A primigravid client in early labor with abruptio placenta develops disseminated intravascular coagulation (DIC). Which of the following would the nurse expect the physician to order?
○ 1. Magnesium sulfate.
○ 2. Warfarin sodium (Coumadin).
○ 3. Fresh-frozen platelets.
○ 4. Meperidine hydrochloride (Demerol).

92. A multigravid client diagnosed with chronic hypertension is now in early labor at 34 weeks' gestation. The physician has ordered intravenous terbutaline (Brethine) 5 μg/minute, with the dose increased every 10 minutes until a maximum dosage of 80 μg/minute is achieved. The nurse determines that the medication has had a therapeutic effect when which of the following is observed?
○ 1. Increase in fetal heart rate accelerations.
○ 2. Decrease in the frequency and number of contractions.
○ 3. Increased variability of the fetal heart rate.
○ 4. Decrease in the maternal pulse rate.

93. A primigravid client who was successfully treated for preterm labor at 30 weeks' gestation had a history of mild hyperthyroidism before becoming pregnant. The nurse should instruct the client to do which of the following?
○ 1. Continue taking low-dose oral propyl-thio-uracil (PTU) as ordered.
○ 2. Discontinue taking the methimazole (Tapazole) until after delivery.
○ 3. Consider breast-feeding the neonate after the delivery.
○ 4. Contact the physician if bradycardia occurs.

94. A primigravid client at 37 weeks' gestation has been hospitalized for several days with severe pregnancy-induced hypertension. While caring for the client, the nurse observes that the client is beginning to have a seizure. Which of the following would the nurse do *first*?
○ 1. Pad the side rails of the client's bed.
○ 2. Turn the client to the right side.
○ 3. Insert a padded tongue blade into the client's mouth.
○ 4. Call for immediate assistance in the client's room.

95. While assessing a primigravida client admitted at 36 weeks' gestation, the nurse observes multiple bruises on the client's face, neck, and abdomen. When asked about the bruises, the client admits that her boyfriend beats her now and then and says, "I want to leave him because I'm afraid he will hurt

the baby." Which of the following would be the nurse's *most* appropriate action?

○ 1. Tell the client to leave the boyfriend immediately.

○ 2. Ask the client when she last felt the baby move.

○ 3. Refer the client to a social worker for possible options.

○ 4. Report the incident to the unit nursing supervisor.

96. A multigravid client in active labor at term suddenly sits up and says, "I can't breathe! My chest hurts really bad!" The client's skin begins to turn a dusky gray color. After calling for assistance, which of the following would the nurse do *next*?

○ 1. Administer oxygen by face mask.

○ 2. Begin cardiopulmonary resuscitation.

○ 3. Administer intravenous oxytocin.

○ 4. Obtain an order for intravenous fibrinogen.

Correct Answers and Rationale

The letters in parentheses following the rationale identify the step of the nursing process (A, D, P, I, E) and client needs (1, 2, 3, 4, 5, 6, 7, 8, 9, 10). See the inside front cover for the key.

The Primigravid Client in Labor

1. 2. Labor is categorized into three phases: latent, active, and transition. During the active stage of labor, intermittent fetal monitoring is performed every 30 minutes to detect changes in fetal heart rate such as bradycardia, tachycardia, or decelerations. If complications develop, more frequent or continuous electronic fetal monitoring may be needed. During the latent phase intermittent monitoring is usually performed every 2 hours, because contractions during this time are usually less frequent. During the transition phase intermittent monitoring is performed every 5 to 15 minutes, because the client is getting closer to delivery of the baby. There is no initial phase of labor. (I, 9)

2. 2. The ischial spines are used as landmarks to determine the descent of the fetal presenting part. The station +1 means that the presenting part is 1 cm below the level of the ischial spines. The station −1 means that the presenting part is 1 cm above the level of the ischial spines. The ischial tuberosities and sacral promontory are not used to determine the fetal station. (D, 9)

3. 2. Assessment findings indicate that the client is in the transition phase of labor. During this phase, it is not unusual for clients to exhibit a loss of control or irritability. Leg tremors, nausea, vomiting, and an urge to bear down also are common. Excitement is associated with the latent phase of labor. Numbness of the legs may occur when epidural anesthesia has been given; however, it is rare when no anesthesia is given. Feelings of relief generally occur during the second stage, when the client begins bearing-down efforts. (P, 3)

4. 3. The obese pregnant client is more susceptible to soft tissue dystocia, which can impede the progress of labor. Symptoms of soft tissue dystocia would include an arrest of labor, prolonged labor, or an arrest of descent of the fetus. Hypotonic reflexes are associated with magnesium sulfate therapy, and increased uterine resting tone is associated with the transition phase or second stage of labor, not with obesity and pregnancy. Increased fear and anxiety are also not associated with obesity. However, they

may be associated with a primigravida who does not know what to expect during labor. (A, 9)

5. 1. Shoulder dystocia is most apt to occur in clients with diabetes, multiparity, or postdate pregnancies. A prolonged second stage and arrest of descent are signs of shoulder dystocia. Asking the client to flex her thighs sharply on her abdomen (McRobert's maneuver) may widen the pelvic outlet and allow the shoulder to deliver. Twin gestations are typically suspected by an oversized uterus and can be confirmed with ultrasound. Anencephaly would not contribute to a prolonged second stage. However, hydrocephaly can complicate delivery because the enlarged fetal skull can prevent descent. Breech presentation would be suspected by palpation of the buttocks or feet during a vaginal examination and can be confirmed by ultrasound visualization of the presenting part. (D, 9)

6. 3. Prostaglandin gel may be used for cervical ripening before the induction of labor with oxytocin. It is usually administered by catheter or suppository, or by vaginal insertion. Two to three doses are usually needed to begin the softening process. Common side effects include nausea, vomiting, and diarrhea. Continuous fetal heart rate monitoring and close monitoring of maternal vital signs are necessary to detect subtle changes or adverse effects. (E, 8)

7. 1. External cephalic version is the turning of the fetus from a breech position to the vertex position to prevent the need for a cesarean delivery. Gentle pressure is used to rotate the fetus in a forward direction to a cephalic lie. Contraindications to the procedure include multiple gestation because of the potential for fetal injury or uterine injury, severe oligohydramnios (decreased amniotic fluid), contraindications to a vaginal birth (eg, cephalopelvic disproportion), and unexplained third trimester bleeding. If the mother has Rh-negative blood type, the procedure can be performed and Rh immunoglobulin should be administered in case minimal bleeding occurs. A history of gestational diabetes is not a contraindication unless the fetus is large for gestational age and the client has cephalopelvic disproportion. (A, 9)

8. 2. Augmentation of labor with oxytocin (Pitocin) is needed when labor contractions begin spontaneously but then become so weak, irregular, or ineffective (hypotonic) that assistance is needed to strengthen them. Often this condition is the administration of analgesia or anesthesia early in the labor process. Morphine sulfate analgesia is administered to clients who

are experiencing hypertonic contractions, to allow the client to rest. Nubain is an analgesic and may result in further hypotonic contractions. Ampicillin is an antibiotic; there is no justification for administration of an antibiotic at this time. (D, 8)

9. 4. Anatomically, the best position for the client to assume is the squatting position because this enhances pelvic diameters and allows gravity to assist in the expulsion stage of labor. This position also provides for natural pressure anesthesia as the fetal presenting part presses on the stretched perineum. If the client is extremely fatigued from a lengthy labor process, she may prefer the dorsal recumbent position. However, this position is not considered the best position anatomically. The lithotomy position may be ineffective and uncomfortable for a client who is ready to push. The hands and knees position may help to alleviate some back pain. However, this position can cause discomfort to the arms and wrists and is tiring over a long period of time. (I, 3)

10. 4. During transition, contractions are increasing in frequency, duration, and intensity. The most appropriate nursing diagnosis is Pain related to strength and duration of the contractions. Insufficient information is provided in the scenario to support the other listed nursing diagnoses. Impaired Urinary Elimination would be appropriate if the client had a full bladder and was unable to void. Risk for Injury might apply if the client were completely out of control or thrashing around in the bed. Ineffective Coping might apply if the client said, "I can't do this" or something similar. (D, 3)

11. 1. The most reliable sign that the placenta has detached from the uterine wall is lengthening of the cord outside the vagina. Other signs include a change in the shape of the uterus from discoid to globular and a sudden gush of vaginal blood. Usually, when placenta detachment occurs, the uterus becomes more firm. This process takes about 5 minutes. If the placenta does not separate, manual removal may be necessary to prevent postpartum hemorrhage. (A, 3)

12. 3. Childbirth is a very emotional experience. An expression of happiness with tears is a normal reaction. Cultural factors, exhaustion, and anxieties over the new role can all affect maternal responses, so the nurse must be sensitive to the client's emotional expressions. There is no evidence to suggest that the mother is disappointed in the baby's gender, grieving over the end of the pregnancy, or a candidate for postpartum blues. However, approximately 80% of postpartum clients experience transient postpartum blues. (D, 3)

13. 3. Most authorities suggest that a woman in an early stage of labor should be allowed to walk if she wishes as long as no complications are present. Birthing cen-

ters and single-room maternity units allow women considerable latitude without much supervision at this stage of labor. Gravity and walking can assist the process of labor in some clients. If the client becomes tired, she can rest in bed in the left lateral recumbent position or sit in a comfortable chair. Resting in the left lateral recumbent position improves circulation to the fetus. (I, 3)

14. 1. Childbirth educators use various techniques and methods to prepare parents for labor and delivery. Active relaxation involves relaxing uninvolved muscle groups while contracting a specific group and using chest breathing techniques to lift the diaphragm off the contracting uterus. A deep, meditative, sleeplike state is a form of passive relaxation. Focusing on an object in the room is part of Lamaze technique for distraction. Breathing rapidly and deeply can lead to hyperventilation and is not recommended. (P, 3)

15. 3. Light stroking of the skin, or effleurage, is often used with the Lamaze method of childbirth preparation. Light abdominal massage with just enough pressure to avoid tickling is thought to displace the pain sensation during a contraction. Deep kneading and secure grasping are typically associated with relaxation massages to relieve stress. Prolonged pressure on specific sites is associated with acupressure. (I, 3)

16. 1. Some physicians do not allow clients with ruptured membranes to use a hot tub or jet hydrotherapy tub during labor for fear of infections. The temperature of the water should be between 98° and 100°F (36.7° to 37.8°C) to prevent hyperthermia. Jet hydrotherapy is not contraindicated for clients with multifetal gestation, diabetes mellitus, or hypotonic labor patterns. (I, 9)

17. 3. Cystic fibrosis and other inborn errors of metabolism are inherited as autosomal recessive traits. Such diseases do not occur unless there are two genes for the disease present. If one of the parents does not have the gene, the child will not have the disease. X-linked recessive genes can result in hemophilia A or color blindness. X-linked recessive genes are present only on the X chromosome and are typically manifested in the male child. X-linked dominant genes, which are located on and transmitted only by the female sex chromosome, can result in hypophosphatemia, an inborn error of metabolism marked by abnormally low serum alkaline phosphatase activity and excretion of phosphoethanolamine in the urine. This disorder is manifested as rickets in infants and children. Autosomal dominant gene disorders can result in muscular dystrophy, Marfan's syndrome, and osteogenesis imperfecta (brittle bone disease). Typically, a dominant gene for the disease trait is present along with a corresponding healthy recessive gene for the trait. (I, 3)

18. 4. To determine fetal lung maturity, the sample of amniotic fluid will be tested for the L/S ratio. When fetal lungs are mature, the ratio should be 2:1. Bilirubin indicates hemolysis and, if present in the fluid, suggests Rh disease. Red blood cells should not appear in the amniotic fluid because their presence suggests fetal bleeding. Barr body determination is a chromosome analysis of the sex chromosomes that is sometimes used when a child is born with ambiguous genitalia. (D, 3)

19. 2. Adolescent pregnancy carries an increased risk of pregnancy-induced hypertension, iron-deficiency anemia, and CPD. CPD is a concern because maturation of the skeletal bones (including the pelvis) is often not complete in adolescents. Adolescent labor does not differ from labor in the older woman if no CPD is present. A prolonged first stage of labor and poor fetal descent may indicate that CPD exists. Uterine inversion, a rapid third stage of labor, or decreased ability to push may occur regardless of the client's age. (A, 9)

20. 4. Delegation of duties and clients to ancillary personnel is often the responsibility of the registered nurse. The client who is a gravida II, para I with a history of hyperemesis gravidarum is the client with the least potential for labor complications. Hyperemesis gravidarum typically occurs and is treated in the first or second trimester of pregnancy and should be resolved by this point in the pregnancy. A gravida IV, para III client with a history of gestational diabetes may have cephalopelvic disproportion due to a large-for-gestational-age fetus requiring a cesarean section delivery. The gravida III, para I, Ab I client is preterm at 35 weeks' gestation and may require an intensive care neonatal team. In a gravida 1, para 0 client, leaking green amniotic fluid indicates that there has been fetal distress. (I, 1)

21. 3. Pushing during the first stage of labor, when the urge is felt but the cervix is not completely dilated, may produce cervical swelling, making labor more difficult. The client should be encouraged to use a pant-blow (or blow-blow) pattern of breathing to help overcome the urge to push. The McDonald procedure is used for cervical cerclage for an incompetent cervix and is inappropriate here. Increasing the rate of oxygen and intravenous fluids will not alleviate the pressure that the client is feeling. The client should not push even if she feels the urge to do so, because this may result in cervical edema at 7 cm dilation. (I, 3)

22. 4. The client is in the transition phase of the first stage of labor. During this phase, the client needs encouragement and support because this is a difficult and painful time, when contractions are especially strong. Usually, the client finds it difficult to maintain self control. Everything else seems secondary to her as she progresses into the second stage of labor and delivery. Although ice chips may be given, typically the client does not desire sips of water. Labor is hard work. Generally, the client is perspiring and does not desire additional warmth. Frequent perineal cleansing is not necessary unless there is excessive amniotic fluid leaking. (I, 3)

23. 1. The sagittal suture is the most readily felt during a vaginal examination. When the fetus is in the LOA position, the occiput faces the mother's left. The lambdoid suture is on the side of the skull. The coronal suture is a horizontal suture across the front portion of the fetal skull that forms the anterior fontanel. It may be felt with a brow presentation. The frontal suture may be felt with a brow or face presentation. (A, 3)

24. 2. Molding occurs with vaginal deliveries and is commonly seen in newborns. This is especially true with primigravid clients experiencing a lengthy labor process. Parents need to be reassured that it is not permanent and that it typically lasts a day or two before resolving. Molding rarely is present if the fetus is in a breech or brow presentation. Surgical intervention is not necessary. (I, 3)

25. 2. Avoidance, hostility, or low-key (passive) behavior toward the baby may be a cue to potential bonding problems. The nurse should encourage the client to give the baby the first feeding to begin the bonding process. Expressions of disappointment with the baby's gender may also signal problems with maternal–infant bonding. Comparing the baby's features to her own indicates identification of the neonate as belonging to her, suggesting bonding with neonate. Comparing the actual neonate with the "fantasized neonate" is a normal maternal reaction. Wanting to buy the newborn a blue outfit indicates an interest in and connection with the neonate and is a sign of bonding. (D, 9)

26. 4. According to the gate-control theory of pain perception, when the endings of small peripheral nerve fibers detect a stimulus, they transmit it to cells in the dorsal horn of the spinal cord. These impulses pass through a network of cells in the spinal cord called the *substantia gelatinosa,* and a synapse occurs that returns the transmission to the peripheral site through a motor nerve. The impulse is then transmitted through the spinal cord to the brain, where the impulse is perceived as pain. Gate-control mechanisms in the spinal cord are capable of halting these impulses (closing the gate), so that pain is not perceived. Input from the large sensory fibers closes the gate. Telling the client that labor pain is a matter of individual perception is not helpful and does not explain the gate-control theory. Deep chest breathing or other breathing techniques can help to keep the "gate" closed, not open. (P, 3)

27. 1. According to the gate-control theory of pain, a closed gate means that the client should feel no pain.

The gate-control theory of pain refers to the gate-control mechanisms in the substantia gelatinosa that are capable of halting an impulse at the level of the spinal cord so the impulse is never perceived at the brain level as pain (ie, a process similar to keeping a gate closed). (I, 3)

28. 4. The bladder status should be monitored throughout the labor process, but especially before the client begins pushing. A full bladder can impede the progress of labor and may result in injury to the client. Because she has had an epidural anesthetic, it is most likely that the client is receiving intravenous fluids, contributing to a full bladder. The client also does not feel the urge to void because of the anesthetic. Although it is important to monitor vital signs and fetal heart rate variability throughout labor, this does not affect the client's ability to push. There is no need to recheck cervical dilation. Furthermore, increasing the frequency of examinations can increase the client's risk for infection. (A, 9)

29. 1. The normal length of the latent stage of labor in a primigravid client is 6 hours. If the client is having prolonged labor, the nurse should monitor the client for signs of exhaustion as well as dehydration. Hypotonic contractions, which are painful but ineffective, may be occurring. Oxytocin augmentation may be necessary. Chills and fever are manifestations of an infection and are not associated with a prolonged latent phase of labor. Fluid overload can occur from rapid infusion of intravenous fluids administered if the client is experiencing hemorrhage or shock. It is not associated with prolonged latent phase. The client's membranes are intact, so it would be difficult to assess meconium staining of the fluid. Meconium-stained fluid is associated with fetal distress, and this fetus appears to be in a healthy state, as evidenced by a fetal heart rate within normal range and good variability. (A, 9)

30. 1. The client who has back pain during labor experiences marked discomfort because the fetus is in an LOP position. This pain is much greater than when the fetus is in the anterior position because the fetal head impinges on the sacrum in the course of rotating to the anterior position. Application of firm pressure to the sacral area can help to alleviate the pain. Complaints of severe back pain during labor do not typically require a cesarean delivery. The physician may elect to do an episiotomy, but it is not necessarily required. It is unlikely that a primigravid client with a fetus in an LOP position will have a precipitous delivery; rather, labor is usually more prolonged. A hands and knees position or a right side-lying position may help to rotate the fetal head and thus alleviate some of the back pain. (P, 3)

31. 1. The psychoprophylaxis method of childbirth suggests using slow chest breathing until it becomes inef-

fective during labor contractions, then switching to shallow chest breathing (mostly at the sternum) during the peak of a contraction. The rate is 50 to 70 breaths per minute. Deep chest breathing is appropriate for the early phase of labor, in which the client exhibits less frequent contractions. When transition nears, a rapid pant-blow pattern of breathing is used. Slow abdominal breathing is very difficult for clients in labor. (I, 3)

32. 3. The carbon dioxide insufficiency that occurs during hyperventilation will lead to respiratory alkalosis. Symptoms include confusion, unconsciousness, elevated plasma pH (greater than 7.45), and elevated urine pH (above 7). The nurse should try to calm the client and, if the hyperventilation persists, should ask the client to breathe into a paper bag. Metabolic alkalosis is associated with vomiting when a large amount of hydrochloric acid is lost. Metabolic acidosis is associated with loss of sodium ions through diarrhea. Respiratory acidosis is associated with shallow breathing and an inability to expire completely. (A, 9)

33. 3. Fetal scalp stimulation is often ordered when there is decreased fetal heart rate variability. Pressure is applied with the fingers to the fetal scalp through the dilated cervix. This should cause a tactile response in the fetus and increase the fetal heart rate and variability. However, if the fetus is in distress and becoming acidotic, fetal heart rate acceleration will not occur. The fetal hematocrit level can be measured by fetal blood sampling. Scalp stimulation does not increase the strength of the contractions. However, it can increase fetal heart rate and variability. Fetal position is assessed by identifying skull landmarks (sutures) during a vaginal examination. (I, 9)

34. 4. If the fetus is hypoxic, the pH will fall below 7.2 and be indicative of fetal distress. This finding typically requires immediate vaginal or cesarean delivery. A scalp pH reading of 7.21 to 7.25 should be repeated again in 30 minutes for assessment of hypoxia and acidosis. (D, 10)

35. 3. When a client complains of severe back pain during labor, the fetus is most likely in an occipitoposterior position. This means that the fetal head presses against the client's sacrum, causing marked discomfort during contractions. These sensations may be so intense, that the client requests medication for relief of the back pain rather than the contractions. (I, 3)

36. 3. The third maneuver involves facing the woman's head and using the tips of the fingers to palpate the uterine fundus. This maneuver is used to identify the part of the fetus that lies over the inlet to the pelvis. (A, 10)

37. 1. Leopold's maneuvers are performed to determine the presentation and position of the fetus. The third

maneuver determines whether the fetal presenting part is engaged in the maternal pelvis. The first maneuver distinguishes between a breech and a cephalic presentation through palpation of the top of the fundus. The second maneuver locates the fetal back, arms, and legs. The fetal heart rate monitoring device should be placed near the fetal skull and back for optimal fetal heart rate monitoring. The fourth maneuver is done to locate the fetal cephalic prominence if the fetus is in a cephalic position. (I, 3)

38. 4. The priority nursing diagnosis at this time is Pain related to LOP position and prolonged fetal descent. When the fetus is in this position, the fetal head presses against the client's sacrum, causing marked discomfort during contractions. Labor is usually longer and more uncomfortable when the fetus remains in an occipitoposterior position. Anxiety would be an appropriate nursing diagnosis if the client had stated that she was nervous, apprehensive, afraid, fearful, or restless. Ineffective Coping would be appropriate if the client exhibited a loss of control, screaming, crying, or thrashing around in the bed. Urinary Retention might be a related nursing diagnosis; however, if the nurse is vigilant in assessment of the client's bladder status, the client should void at least every 2 hours or have a catheterization performed. A full bladder can impair fetal descent and prolong labor. (D, 3)

39. 3. Small clots that are expressed during fundal examination in the immediate postpartum period are normal; however, large clots are indicative of retained placental tissue. A small trickle of bright red vaginal bleeding may indicate a laceration. The nurse should notify the physician immediately of these findings, because uterine atony may occur and the laceration, if present, needs to be repaired to prevent further blood loss. Methylergonovine is a powerful drug that contracts the uterus, but it usually is not administered to a client with a blood pressure of 136/92 mm Hg because of its hypertensive effects. Changing the perineal pads every 15 minutes is not helpful if the client is experiencing a hemorrhage. (I, 3)

The Multigravid Client in Labor

40. 1. When a client receives an epidural anesthetic, sympathetic nerves are blocked along with the pain nerves, possibly resulting in vasodilation and hypotension. Other adverse effects include bladder distention, prolonged second stage of labor, nausea and vomiting, pruritus, and delayed respiratory depression for up to 24 hours after administration. Diaphoresis and tremors are not usually associated with the administration of epidural anesthesia. Headache, a common adverse effect of many drugs, also is not associated with administration of epidural anesthesia. (I, 8)

41. 4. After an emergency delivery, the nurse suggests that the mother begin breast-feeding to contract the uterus. Breast-feeding stimulates the natural production of oxytocin. In a multiparous client, uterine atony is a potential complication because of the stretching of the uterine fibers following each subsequent pregnancy. Although breast-feeding does help to begin the parental-infant bonding process, this is not the primary reason for the nurse to suggest breast-feeding. Prevention of neonatal hypothermia is accomplished by placing blankets on both the neonate and the mother. Although colostrum in breast milk provides the neonate with nutrients and immunoglobulins, the primary reason for breast-feeding is to stimulate the natural production of oxytocin to contract the uterus. (I, 9)

42. 3. A chill shortly after delivery is a common and normal occurrence. Warm blankets can help provide comfort for the client. It has been suggested that the shivering response is caused by a difference between internal and external body temperatures. A different theory proposes that the woman is reacting to fetal cells that have entered the maternal bloodstream through the placental site. (I, 3)

43. 2. After an amniotomy, the nurse should plan to first assess the fetal heart rate for 1 full minute. One of the complications of amniotomy is cord compression and/or prolapsed cord, and a fetal heart rate of 100 bpm or less should be promptly reported to the physician. A cord prolapse requires prompt delivery by cesarean section. The client's contraction pattern should be monitored once labor has been established. The client's temperature, pulse, and respirations should be assessed every 2 to 4 hours after rupture of the membranes to detect an infection. The nurse should document the color, quantity, and odor of the amniotic fluid, but this can be done after the fetal heart rate is assessed and a reassuring pattern is present. (P, 3)

44. 3. The most appropriate diagnosis at this time is Risk for Injury related to the effects of the epidural anesthesia because the client may have no sensation in her lower abdomen and legs for several hours postpartum. Care should be taken to avoid injury, and ambulation should be delayed until sensation has returned. No information is presented in the scenario to suggest Pain due to episiotomy and exhaustive pushing. Multiparous clients often have shortened labors and may not require an episiotomy. If the client did have an episiotomy and the epidural anesthetic has worn off, then this nursing diagnosis would be appropriate. Anxiety would apply if the client expressed feelings of anxiety or nervousness because of a problem with moving her legs or toes. Excess Fluid Volume would apply if the client received excessive amounts of intravenous fluid or complained of oliguria, an early sign of pulmonary edema. (D, 8)

45. 1. Neonatal scalp edema is common after the use of a vacuum extractor to assist the client's expulsion efforts. This edema may persist up to 7 days. Vacuum extraction is not associated with uterine separation. Maternal lacerations may occur, but they are more common when forceps are used. Neonatal intracranial hemorrhage is a risk with both vacuum extraction and forceps deliveries, but it is not a common finding. (A, 3)

46. 1. Although breech presentations are rare, the most common is frank breech. In frank breech, there is flexion of the fetal thighs and extension of the knees. The feet rest at the side of the fetal head. Footling breech occurs when there is an extension of the fetal knees and one or both feet protrude through the pelvis. In complete breech, there is flexion of the fetal thighs and knees; the fetus appears to be squatting. Vertex presentation occurs in 95% of deliveries; here, the head is engaged in the pelvis. (D, 10)

47. 4. The nurse should assess the client's cervical dilation and station, because the client's symptoms are indicative of the transition phase of labor. Multiparous clients can proceed 5 to 9 cm per hour during the active phase of labor. Warming the temperature of the room is not helpful because the client will soon be ready to begin expulsive pushing. Increasing the intravenous fluid rate is not warranted unless the client is experiencing dehydration. Administration of an antiemetic at this point in labor is not warranted and may result in neonatal depression should a rapid delivery occur. (I, 3)

48. 4. To assess the frequency of the client's contractions, the nurse should assess the interval from the beginning of one contraction to the beginning of the next contraction. The duration of a contraction is the interval between the beginning and the end of a contraction. (A, 3)

49. 3. After spontaneous rupture of the amniotic fluid, the gushing fluid may carry the umbilical cord out of the birth canal. Sudden deceleration of the fetal heart rate often signifies cord compression and/or prolapse of the cord, which would require immediate delivery. This client is particularly at risk because the fetus is preterm and the fetal head may not be engaged. Turning the client to the right side is not a priority action. However, changing the client's position would be appropriate if variable decelerations are present. The nurse should assess the color, amount, and odor of the fluid, but this can be done once the fetal heart rate is assessed and no problems are detected. Cervical dilation should be checked but only after the fetal heart rate pattern is assessed. (I, 9)

50. 2. Spinal anesthesia is used less frequently today because of preference for epidural block anesthesia. One of the side effects of spinal anesthesia is a "spinal headache" caused by leakage of spinal fluid from the needle insertion. This can be treated by applying a cool cloth to the forehead, keeping the client in a flat position, or using a blood patch that can clot and seal off any further leakage of fluid. Another side effect of spinal anesthesia is hypotension caused by vasodilation. Spinal anesthesia is administered with the client in a sitting position. General anesthesia provides immediate anesthesia, whereas the full effects of spinal anesthesia may not be felt for 20 to 30 minutes. General anesthesia can be discontinued quickly when the anesthesiologist administers oxygen instead of nitrous oxide. Epidural anesthesia may take 1 to 2 hours to wear off. (E, 8)

51. 1. The drug of choice when hypotension occurs as a result of epidural anesthesia is ephedrine sulfate because it provides a quick reversal of the vasodilator effects of the anesthesia. Epinephrine is typically used to treat anaphylactic shock. Methylergonovine is a vasoconstrictor that is used for severe postpartum hemorrhage. Atropine sulfate is used to dry the oral and respiratory secretions and may be used during operative procedures. (P, 8)

52. 3. Cimetidine (Tagamet) is ordered by some anesthesiologists who will be giving a general anesthetic to reduce the level of acid in the stomach contents, altering the pH to reduce the risk of complications should aspiration of vomitus occur. Aspiration of vomitus is the fifth most common cause of maternal mortality. Most anesthesiologists insert an endotracheal tube to reduce the incidence of aspiration. Isoproterenol (Isuprel) is used to decrease the incidence of bronchospasm. Atropine sulfate is administered to dry oral and nasal secretions. Although cimetidine is useful for gastric ulcer therapy, gastric ulcers are not a common effect associated with operative deliveries. (I, 8)

53. 2. Lumbar epidural anesthesia is usually administered with the client in a sitting or a left side-lying position with shoulders parallel and legs slightly flexed. These positions expose the vertebrae to the anesthesiologist. Paracervical and local anesthetics are usually administered with the client in the lithotomy position. The knee-to-chest and prone positions are not used for anesthesia administration. (I, 8)

54. 1. Anterior–posterior slit occurs as the perineum flattens and is followed by an oval opening. As labor progresses, the perineum takes on a circular shape. Crowning occurs when the fetal head is visible. (A, 10)

55. 1. A neonate in good condition needs to be kept warm. This reduces cold stress and potential respiratory problems. Cold stress causes the neonate to burn much-needed brown fat. The infant can be evaluated under a radiant warmer or wrapped in dry, warm blankets on the mother's abdomen. Instilling erythromycin ointment, weighing the neonate, and applying identification bracelets can be done once the neonate has been placed under a radiant warmer and the temperature has stabilized. (I, 3)

The Intrapartal Client With Risk Factors

56. 1. Clients who are pregnant with two (or more) gestations are at greater risk for pregnancy-induced hypertension, hydramnios, placenta previa, preterm labor, and anemia. During delivery, occasionally the placenta of the second twin separates before that twin is delivered, causing profound bleeding. Urinary tract infections and chorioamnionitis are not more frequent in clients with multifetal gestation compared with women with single-fetus pregnancies. Although multiparous women frequently deliver more quickly than a nullipara does, precipitous delivery is not more common with twin gestations. (A, 9)

57. 3. The multigravid client with class II heart disease has a slight limitation of physical activity and may become fatigued with ordinary physical activity. A side-lying or semi-Fowler s position with the head elevated helps to ensure cardiac emptying and adequate oxygenation. In addition, oxygen by mask, analgesics and sedatives, diuretics, prophylactic antibiotics, and digitalis may be warranted. Although breathing slowly during a contraction may assist with oxygenation, it would have no effect on cardiac emptying. It is essential that the laboring woman with cardiac disease be relieved of discomfort and anxiety. Effective intrapartum pain relief with analgesia and epidural anesthesia may reduce cardiac workload as much as 20%. Local anesthetics are effective only during the second stage of labor. (P, 9)

58. 4. Assessing for signs and symptoms associated with cardiac decompensation is the priority. Class III heart disease during pregnancy has a 25% to 50% mortality. These clients are markedly compromised, with marked limitation of physical activity. They frequently experience fatigue, palpitations, dyspnea, or anginal pain. A pulse rate greater than 100 bpm or a respiratory rate greater than 25 breaths/minute may indicate cardiac decompensation that could result in cardiac arrest. Additional symptoms include dyspnea, peripheral edema, orthopnea, tachypnea, rales, and hemoptysis. (P, 9)

59. 2. Clients who have been diagnosed with class II heart disease and prosthetic valve replacement are most likely to have an order for antibiotic medications to prevent the development of bacterial endocarditis and bacteremia. Clients with valvular heart disease have a high susceptibility to subacute bacterial endocarditis. Anticoagulant therapy is usually discontinued during labor and delivery because of the potential for hemor-

rhage. Diuretic medications are generally not prescribed for clients with class I or class II heart disease. Diuretics usually are not necessary and may result in potassium depletion. Folic acid supplements are usually prescribed for clients with megaloblastic anemia. Folic acid is also included in many prenatal vitamins and can help to prevent neural tube defects in the fetus. (P, 8)

60. 1. Before administering prostaglandin E_2 gel, the nurse would assess the frequency and duration of any uterine contractions first, because prostaglandin E_2 gel is contraindicated if the client is having contractions. If there are no contractions, the client should be placed in a semi-Fowler s position to allow for vaginal insertion of the gel. Although determining whether the client s membranes have ruptured is part of the assessment of any client in labor, it is not specifically related to the administration of prostaglandin E_2 gel. If the membranes remain intact, an amniotomy may be performed once the client begins to dilate and the fetal head is engaged. However, it is not necessary for the nurse to prepare the client for this procedure at this time. (I, 8)

61. 4. One of the potential disadvantages of oxytocin induction is neonatal jaundice or hyperbilirubinemia. Oxytocin decreases the elimination of bilirubin from the neonate. Other side effects include maternal hypertension and frontal headache which disappears when the drug is discontinued. The drug has antidiuretic properties that can lead to maternal water intoxication. Dangerous effects of this powerful drug include uterine hyperstimulation or tetanic contractions, which can result in abruptio placenta and uterine rupture. Urinary frequency, maternal hypoglycemia, and preterm birth are not associated with oxytocin administration. Ultrasound procedures are used to estimate gestational age to prevent preterm delivery. Clients who are diabetic often are delivered before term because the placenta begins to deteriorate, possibly resulting in stillbirth. (I, 8)

62. 4. The highest priority nursing diagnosis for the client at this time is Risk for Injury, maternal or fetal, related to uterine hyperstimulation. Diabetic mothers have a higher incidence of pregnancy-induced hypertension, polyhydramnios, preterm birth, and larger-than-average fetuses and often have decreased placental perfusion. Infants of diabetic mothers may have polycythemia, congenital anomalies, and respiratory distress. Because of its antidiuretic properties, oxytocin infusion poses a risk of fluid overload, not fluid deficit. There is no information to support the diagnosis of Pain related to prolonged labor. For multigravidas, labor is often shorter than for primigravidas. A labor duration longer than 12 hours would indicate a prolonged labor. There is no indication that the client will require cesarean delivery at this time.

Signs of fetal distress or maternal complications (eg, abruptio placenta) would support the nursing diagnosis of Risk for Injury. (D, 8)

63. 4. A common sign of fetal distress related to an inadequate transfer of oxygen to the fetus is meconium-stained fluid. Because the fetus has suffered hypoxia, close fetal heart rate monitoring is necessary. If there are increasing signs of fetal distress (eg, late decelerations), the physician should be notified immediately. A cesarean delivery may be performed for fetal distress. Increasing the rate of the oxytocin infusion could lead to further fetal distress. Turning the client to a knee-to-chest position is not helpful if there is poor placental perfusion. The client should be turned to her left side to improve perfusion. The physician may wish to determine the extent of cervical dilation to make a decision about whether a cesarean delivery is warranted, but continuous fetal heart rate monitoring is essential to determine fetal status. (I, 9)

64. 3. Neonates born to mothers who smoke tend to have lower-than-average birth weights. Neonates born to mothers who smoke also are at higher risk for stillbirth, sudden infant death syndrome, bronchitis, allergies, delayed growth and development, and polycythemia. Maternal smoking is not related to higher neonatal hyperirritability, hyperbilirubinemia, or hypocalcemia. Rather, cocaine use during pregnancy is associated with neonatal hyperirritability and withdrawal symptoms. Hyperbilirubinemia is associated with Rh or ABO incompatibility or the administration of intravenous oxytocin during labor. Approximately 50% of neonates born to mothers with insulin-dependent diabetes experience hypocalcemia during the first 3 days of life. (A, 3)

65. 3. The client should be urged to push with an open glottis to prevent the Valsalva maneuver. Pushing with a closed glottis increases intrathoracic pressure, preventing venous return. Blood pressure also falls, and cardiac output decreases. Pushing for at least 1 to 3 minutes is too long; prolonged pushing can lead to reduced blood flow and fatigue. Pushing for 1 minute is sufficient. Pushing while holding the breath results in the Valsalva maneuver. Because the client has had an epidural anesthetic, she may not feel the urge to push and needs coaching. (P, 8)

66. 3. The American College of Obstetricians and Gynecologists has classified forceps applications into three categories: outlet, low, or middle. When the fetal skull is on the perineum with the scalp visible at the perineal floor or vaginal opening, this is considered outlet forceps application. When the head is higher in the pelvis but engaged and its greatest diameter has passed the inlet, the operation is termed midforceps. Midforceps deliveries are not recommended because they are extremely dangerous for the mother and fetus because of the possibility of uterine rupture. If the head is not engaged, at −1 station, this is termed high forceps. High forceps deliveries also are exceedingly dangerous for both the mother and fetus because of the possibility of uterine rupture and are not recommended. Cesarean delivery is preferred in these situations. The fetal head at station +2 or lower is termed low forceps. (D, 9)

67. 1. Oligohydramnios, or a decrease in the volume of amniotic fluid, is associated with variable fetal heart rate decelerations due to cord compression. Maintenance of an adequate amniotic fluid volume during labor provides protective cushioning of the umbilical cord and minimizes cord compression. Cord compression can result in fetal metabolic acidosis, not alkalosis. Amnioinfusion is used to minimize cord compression, not to increase the fetal heart rate accelerations during a contraction. The goal is to maintain the amniotic fluid index at 8 cm. This can be determined by ultrasound. (I, 9)

68. 4. A primigravid client diagnosed with pregnancy-induced hypertension has the potential for developing seizures (eclampsia). This client should be in a room with the least amount of stimulation possible to reduce the risk for seizures and as close to the nurse's station as possible in case the client requires immediate assistance. Bright lighting and sunshine can be a stimulant, possibly increasing the risk for seizures, as can being in a semiprivate room with roommate, visitors, conversation, and noise. (P, 1)

69. 4. The client is experiencing a precipitous delivery. The nurse should remain calm during a precipitous delivery. Explaining to the client what is happening as the birth progresses and how she can assist is likely to help her remain calm and cooperative. Maintaining eye contact is also beneficial. Telling the client that she is right and to just relax is inappropriate because the client may not be able to relax because of the strong urge to push the fetus out of the birth canal. Telling the client not to push because she may tear the cervix can instill fear, not cooperation. Saying that the physician will be there soon may not be an accurate statement and is not reassuring if the client is concerned about the delivery. (I, 5)

70. 2. During a precipitous delivery, after calling for assistance and checking for the umbilical cord around the neck, the nurse should hold the neonate's head lower than the trunk to promote drainage of secretions. It is not appropriate to tell the client to push between contractions because this may lead to lacerations. The shoulder should be delivered by applying downward traction until the anterior shoulder appears fully at the introitus, then upward pressure to lift out the other shoulder. Priority should be given to safe delivery of the infant over protecting the perineum by massage. (I, 9)

67

71. 2. Because delivery occurs so rapidly and the fetus is propelled quickly through the birth canal, the major complication of a precipitous delivery is a boggy fundus, or uterine atony. The neonate should be put to the breast, if the mother permits, to allow for the release of natural oxytocin. In a hospital setting, the physician will probably order administration of oxytocin. The nurse should gently massage the fundus to ensure that it is firm. There is no relationship between a precipitous delivery and postpartum blues or intrauterine infection. Postpartum blues usually does not occur until about 3 days postpartum, and symptoms of postpartum infection usually occur after the first 24 hours. There is no relationship between a precipitous delivery and urinary tract infection even though the delivery has been accomplished under clean rather than sterile technique. Symptoms of urinary tract infection typically begin on the first or second postpartum day. (A, 9)

72. 2. The fetal heart rate of a multipara diagnosed with Rh sensitization and probable fetal hydrops and anemia will most likely demonstrate a sinusoidal pattern that resembles a sine wave. It has been hypothesized that this pattern reflects an absence of autonomic nervous control over the fetal heart rate resulting from severe hypoxia. This client will most likely require a cesarean delivery to improve the fetal outcome. Early decelerations are associated with head compression; variable decelerations are associated with cord compression; and late decelerations are associated with poor placental perfusion. (D, 9)

73. 3. Oxytocin, given postpartum to contract the uterus, should be administered after delivery of the second placenta and after both twins have been delivered safely. If oxytocin is given any earlier—after the first twin, after the first placenta, or after the second twin—the uterus will contract and make delivery of the placenta or placentas difficult. (P, 8)

74. 1. A priority assessment for the nurse to make is to determine the estimated date of delivery or probable gestational age of the fetus. If the gestation is less than 37 weeks, the neonatal team should be called to begin resuscitative efforts if needed. Amniotic fluid status is not important at this point, because if the fetal skull is crowning delivery is imminent. Determination of gravida and parity is part of the normal nursing history, but the priority is the status of the fetus and safe delivery. Prenatal history is part of the nursing assessment, but this information is not especially relevant until the fetus is safely delivered and has been given immediate care. (A, 3)

75. 2. It is important that the parents be allowed to touch, hold, and participate in care of the twins whenever they desire. Ideally, this will be on a daily basis, to promote parent-infant bonding. It is not appropriate to discuss how the couple will cope with twin infants at home until they are ready to take the infants home. They are too overwhelmed at this point and are focused on the well-being of their infants while hospitalized. Having the couple visit the twins to provide care on a 24-hour basis is not warranted. Identifying complications that may occur is not appropriate. If complications arise, the parents should be well informed and given opportunities for discussion related to the care provided. (P, 5)

76. 4. The priority diagnosis is Risk for Infection related to birth trauma and prolonged ruptured membranes. Infection can be a serious postpartum complication. Although the client may be fatigued, she should not be experiencing activity intolerance. Clients with heart disease may experience activity intolerance due to excessive cardiac workload. Although the client may be experiencing sleep deprivation, most clients are alert and awake after delivery of a newborn. Situational Low Self-Esteem is not a priority. Clients who undergo a cesarean delivery often feel a sense of failure because of not delivering vaginally, but this is not the case for this client. (D, 9)

77. 2. Postmature neonates frequently have difficulty maintaining adequate glucose reserves and often develop hypoglycemia soon after birth. Other common problems include meconium aspiration syndrome, polycythemia, congenital anomalies, seizure activity, and cold stress. These complications result primarily from a combination of advanced gestational age, placental insufficiency, and continued exposure to amniotic fluid. Delayed meconium is not associated with post-term gestation. Hyperbilirubinemia occurs in term neonates as well as post-term neonates, but unless there is an Rh incompatibility it does not develop until after the first 24 hours of life. (A, 9)

78. 4. Polyhydramnios is an abnormally large amount of amniotic fluid in the uterus. The client has understood the instructions when the client states that polyhydramnios is associated with gastrointestinal disorders (eg, tracheoesophageal fistula). Polyhydramnios is also associated with maternal illnesses such as diabetes and anemia. Other fetal/neonatal disorders associated with this condition include congenital anomalies of the central nervous system (eg, anencephaly), upper gastrointestinal obstruction, and macrosomia. Polyhydramnios can lead to preterm labor, premature rupture of the membranes, and cord prolapse. Renal dysfunction and intrauterine growth retardation are associated with oligohydramnios, not polyhydramnios. Pulmonary hypoplasia (poorly developed lungs) is associated with prolonged oligohydramnios. (E, 9)

79. 1. If a client has been in active labor and there is no change in cervical dilation after 2 hours, the nurse should suspect cephalopelvic disproportion. This may be caused by an inadequate pelvis size of the mother or by a large-for-gestational-age fetus. The physician should be notified about the client's lack of progress. If the fetus cannot descend, a cesarean delivery is warranted. The client is not experiencing a prolonged latent phase (0 to 3 cm dilation), because her cervix is dilated to 6 cm. She has not reached the transitional phase, characterized by a cervical dilation of 8 to 10 cm. With a hypotonic labor pattern, contractions are painful but far apart and not very intense. This client's contractions are of moderate intensity. (D, 9)

80. 3. Preparation for cesarean delivery is similar to preparation for any abdominal surgery. The client must give informed consent. Another person may not sign for the client unless the client is unable to sign the form. If this is the case, only certain designated people can do so legally. The husband does not need to sign the form unless his wife is unable to do so. In an emergency situation, surgery may be performed without a written consent if it is done to save the life of the mother or the child, or both. (I, 1)

81. 4. Decreased variability may be seen in various conditions. However, it is most commonly caused by analgesic administration. Other factors that can cause decreased variability include anesthesia, deep fetal sleep, anencephaly, prematurity, hypoxia, tachycardia, brain damage, and arrhythmias. Maternal fatigue, fetal malposition, and small-for-gestational-age fetus are not commonly associated with decreased variability. (I, 3)

82. 4. It is not unusual for clients who undergo an emergency cesarean delivery to express thoughts of failure. Pain, hemorrhage, and anxiety may all occur, but the priority diagnosis at this time is Situational Low Self-Esteem. In this situation, the nurse should be supportive and should allow the client to verbalize any feelings of failure, guilt, or anger. Nursing care should include reviewing the events that occurred and clearing up any questions or misconceptions. (D, 5)

83. 4. Respiratory distress syndrome is more common in neonates delivered by cesarean section than in those delivered vaginally. During a vaginal delivery, pressure is exerted on the fetal chest, which aids in the fetal inhalation and exhalation of air and lung expansion. This pressure is not exerted on the fetus with a cesarean delivery. Congenital anomalies are not more common with cesarean delivery. Pulmonary hypertension occurs more commonly in infants with meconium aspiration syndrome, congenital diaphragmatic hernia, respiratory distress syndrome, or neonatal sepsis, not with cesarean delivery. Meconium aspiration syndrome occurs more commonly with vaginal delivery, post-term neonate, and prolonged labor, not with cesarean delivery. (I, 3)

84. 4. Congenital anomalies are not related to maternal urinary tract infections. A multigravida client with acute pyelonephritis is susceptible to preterm labor, premature rupture of the membranes, maternal sepsis, intrauterine growth retardation, and fetal loss. The most common organism responsible for the urinary tract infection is *Escherichia coli*. (E, 9)

85. 1. Conjunctivitis is a common complication of neonates who are born to mothers with untreated chlamydial infection. Neonatal pneumonia is another condition associated with chlamydial infection of the mother. Untreated chlamydial infection is not associated with heart disease or brain damage. Exposure to rubella may lead to neonatal heart defects, and brain damage may occur as a result of prolonged shoulder dystocia or difficulty delivering the fetal head during a vaginal breech delivery. Occasionally, because of the immature circulation, a neonate who has been lying on his or her side appears red on one side of the body. This "harlequin sign" is transient and is of no clinical significance. Presence of a harlequin sign is unrelated to untreated chlamydial infection. (I, 9)

86. 1. The purpose of the RHIG is to provide passive antibody immunity and prevent Rh-positive sensitization with the next pregnancy. It should be given within 72 hours after delivery of an Rh-positive neonate. Clients who are Rh negative and conceive an Rh-negative fetus do not need antibody protection. Rh-positive cells contribute to sensitization, not Rh-negative cells. The RHIG does not cross the placenta and destroy fetal Rh-positive cells. (I, 9)

87. 3. Because magnesium sulfate is a central nervous system depressant, the nurse should plan to assess the client's respiratory rate every hour. If the respiratory rate is less than 12 breaths/minute, the client may be experiencing magnesium sulfate overdose. Urinary output via an indwelling catheter should be assessed hourly and should be 25 to 30 mL/hour. Deep tendon reflexes and blood pressure also should be assessed every hour. At some institutions continuous electronic blood pressure monitoring will be performed. (A, 8)

88. 2. For a client diagnosed with probable placenta previa, hypovolemic shock is a complication. Continuous blood pressure monitoring with an electronic cuff is the priority assessment after the client's admission. Once the client is admitted, an ultrasound examination will be performed to determine the placement of the placenta. Whole blood replacement is not warranted at this time. However, it may be necessary if the client demonstrates signs and symptoms of hemorrhage or shock. Internal fetal heart rate monitoring is contraindicated because the monitoring device may puncture the placenta and place both the mother and fetus in jeopardy. An immediate cesarean delivery is not necessary until

there has been an assessment of the amount of bleeding and the location of the placenta previa. (P, 9)

89. 4. Dramatic vasoconstriction occurs as a result of sniffing crack cocaine. This can lead to increased respiratory and cardiac rates and hypertension. It can severely compromise placental circulation, resulting in abruptio placenta and preterm labor and delivery. Infants of these women can experience intracranial hemorrhage and withdrawal symptoms of tremulousness, irritability, and rigidity. Placenta previa, ruptured uterus, and maternal hypotension are not associated with cocaine use. Placenta previa may be associated with grand multiparity. Ruptured uterus may be associated with a large-for-gestational-age fetus. Hypertension may occur, because cocaine is a vasoconstrictor. (A, 9)

90. 2. Pregnant women who become infected with the rubella virus early in pregnancy risk having a neonate born with rubella syndrome. The symptoms include thrombocytopenia, cataracts, cardiac disorders, deafness, microcephaly, and motor and cognitive impairment. The most extensive neonatal effects occur when the mother is exposed during the first 2 to 6 weeks and up to 12 weeks' gestation, when critical organs are forming. Bulging fontanels are associated with increased intracranial pressure and meningitis, which can occur as the result of a β-hemolytic streptococcal infection. (A, 9)

91. 3. To stop the process of DIC, the underlying insult that began the phenomenon must be halted. Treatment includes fresh-frozen platelets or blood administration. The physician also may order heparin before the administration of blood products to restore the normal clotting mechanism. Immediate delivery of the fetus is essential. Magnesium sulfate is given for pregnancy-induced hypertension or preterm labor. Heparin, not warfarin sodium (Coumadin), is used to treat DIC. Meperidine hydrochloride (Demerol) is used for pain relief. (P, 8)

92. 2. The nurse determines that the medication has had a therapeutic effect when a decrease in the frequency and number of contractions is noted. Terbutaline (Brethine) is a tocolytic that is used to halt the preterm labor process. This medication is administered as a "piggyback" to the regular intravenous fluids. Side effects include tachycardia. It should not be given if the client's pulse rate is greater than 120 bpm. (E, 8)

93. 1. Although thioamides such as propylthiouracil and methimazole are considered teratogenic to the fetus and can lead to congenital hyperthyroidism (goiter) in the neonate, they still represent the treatment of choice. The client should be regulated on the lowest possible dose. Hyperthyroidism is associated with preterm labor and a low-birth-weight infant, so the client should contact the physician or health care provider if the contractions begin again. The client should not be urged to breast-feed, because medications such as propylthiouracil and methimazole are secreted in breast milk. Tachycardia (not bradycardia) is associated with thyroid storm, a medical emergency, and should be reported to physician. (I, 8)

94. 4. The first action by the nurse should be to call for immediate assistance in the client's room, because this is an emergency. Throughout the seizure, the nurse should note the time and length of the seizure and continue to monitor the status of both client and fetus. The side rails should have been padded at the time of the client's admission to the hospital as part of seizure precautions. The client should be turned to her left side to improve placental perfusion. Inserting a tongue blade is not recommended because it can further obstruct the airway or cause injury to the client's teeth. (I, 2)

95. 3. In an abusive situation, the client's safety is the priority. The nurse should refer the client to a social worker who can provide the client with options such as a safe shelter. Often clients who are battered feel powerless and fear that the batterer will kill them. As a result, they remain in the abusive situation. Telling the client to leave the boyfriend immediately is not helpful and reflects the values of the nurse. Although asking about fetal movement is important and is part of a routine assessment, a sonogram can be performed to detect and confirm fetal well-being. The referral is more important at this time. Although it may be part of the unit's policies and procedures to report any incidents such as this one to the unit supervisor, the client's immediate need for safety must be addressed first. (I, 1)

96. 1. The client's symptoms are indicative of amniotic fluid embolism, which is a medical emergency. After calling for assistance, the first action should be to administer oxygen by face mask or cannula to ensure adequate oxygenation of mother and fetus. If the client needs cardiopulmonary resuscitation, this can be started once oxygen has been administered. If the client survives, she will probably develop DIC and will need intravenous fibrinogen and heparin. Oxytocin, a vasoconstrictor, is not warranted for amniotic fluid embolism. (I, 10)

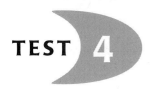

Postpartum Care

Select the best answer and indicate your choice by filling in the circle in front of the option.

The Postpartal Client With a Vaginal Birth

1. At which of the following locations would the nurse expect to palpate the fundus of a primiparous client immediately after delivery of a neonate?
   ○ 1. Halfway between the umbilicus and the symphysis pubis.
   ○ 2. At the level of the umbilicus.
   ○ 3. Just below the level of the umbilicus.
   ○ 4. Above the level of the umbilicus.

2. When instilling erythromycin ointment into the eyes of a neonate 1 hour old, the nurse would explain to the parents that the medication is used to prevent which of the following?
   ○ 1. Chorioretinitis from cytomegalovirus.
   ○ 2. Blindness secondary to gonorrhea.
   ○ 3. Cataracts from β-hemolytic streptococcus.
   ○ 4. Strabismus resulting from neonatal maturation.

3. The physician orders an intramuscular injection of phytonadione (AquaMEPHYTON) for a term neonate. The nurse explains to the mother that that this medication is used to prevent which of the following?
   ○ 1. Hypoglycemia.
   ○ 2. Hyperbilirubinemia.
   ○ 3. Hemorrhage.
   ○ 4. Polycythemia.

4. When developing the plan of care for a primiparous client during the first 12 hours after vaginal delivery, which of the following concerns of the client would be the nurse's primary focus of care?
   ○ 1. The neonate.
   ○ 2. The family.
   ○ 3. The client's own comfort.
   ○ 4. The client's significant other.

5. The nurse assesses a swollen ecchymosed area to the right of an episiotomy on a primiparous client 6 hours after a vaginal delivery. Which of the following would the nurse do next?
   ○ 1. Apply an ice pack to the perineal area.
   ○ 2. Assess the client's temperature.
   ○ 3. Have the client take a warm sitz bath.
   ○ 4. Contact the physician for orders for an antibiotic.

6. Two hours after vaginally delivering a viable male neonate under epidural anesthesia, the client with a midline episiotomy ambulates to the bathroom to void. After voiding, the nurse assesses the client's bladder, finding it distended. The nurse interprets this finding based on the understanding that the client's bladder distention is most likely caused by which of the following?
   ○ 1. Prolonged first stage of labor.
   ○ 2. Urinary tract infection.
   ○ 3. Pressure of the uterus on the bladder.
   ○ 4. Edema in the lower urinary tract area.

7. A primiparous client who is bottle-feeding her neonate at 12 hours after birth asks the nurse, "When will my menstrual cycle return?" Which of the following responses by the nurse would be *most* appropriate?
   ○ 1. Your menstrual cycle will return in 3 to 4 weeks.
   ○ 2. It will probably be 6 to 10 weeks before it starts again.
   ○ 3. You can expect your menses to start in 12 to 14 weeks.
   ○ 4. Your menses will return in 16 to 18 weeks.

8. While the nurse is preparing to assist the primiparous client to the bathroom to void 10 hours after a vaginal delivery under epidural anesthesia, the client says that she feels dizzy when sitting up on the side of the bed. The nurse explains that this is

most likely caused by which of the following?
- ○ 1. Effects of the anesthetic during labor.
- ○ 2. Hemorrhage during the delivery process.
- ○ 3. Effects of analgesics used during labor.
- ○ 4. Decreased blood volume in the vascular system.

9. The nurse delegates the care of a multipara client who delivered a viable term neonate vaginally 30 hours ago and is preparing to be discharged to a licensed practical nurse (LPN). The nurse expects to be notified by the LPN if the client exhibits which of the following?
- ○ 1. Pulse rate of 100 bpm.
- ○ 2. Oral temperature of 99°F (36.8°C).
- ○ 3. Excessive perspiration during the assessment.
- ○ 4. Frequent voiding in large amounts.

10. Which of the following would be a priority nursing diagnosis for a primipara client 4 hours after a low forceps vaginal delivery with a midline episiotomy and prolonged labor under epidural anesthesia who required catheterization during labor and once during the delivery?
- ○ 1. Risk for Infection related to prolonged labor and catheterization.
- ○ 2. Disturbed Body Image related to midline episiotomy.
- ○ 3. Risk for Imbalanced Fluid Volume related to prolonged labor and anesthesia.
- ○ 4. Urinary Retention related to trauma of delivery.

11. The nurse enlists the aid of an interpreter when caring for a primiparous client from Mexico who speaks very little English and delivered a viable term neonate 8 hours ago. When developing the postpartum dietary plan of care for the client, the nurse would encourage the client's intake of which of the following?
- ○ 1. Tomatoes.
- ○ 2. Potatoes.
- ○ 3. Corn products.
- ○ 4. Meat products.

12. Three hours postpartum, a primiparous client's fundus is firm and midline. On perineal inspection, the nurse observes a small, constant trickle of blood. For which of the following would the nurse suspect?
- ○ 1. Retained placental tissue.
- ○ 2. Uterine inversion.
- ○ 3. Bladder distention.
- ○ 4. Perineal lacerations.

13. While making a home visit to a postpartum client on day 10, the nurse would anticipate that the client's lochia would be which of the following colors?
- ○ 1. Dark red.
- ○ 2. Pink.
- ○ 3. Brown.
- ○ 4. White.

14. After instructing a primiparous client about episiotomy care, which of the following client statements indicates successful teaching?
- ○ 1. "I'll use hot, sudsy water to clean the episiotomy area."
- ○ 2. "I wipe the area from front to back using a blotting motion."
- ○ 3. "Before bedtime, I'll use a cold water sitz bath."
- ○ 4. "I can use ice packs for 3 to 4 days after delivery."

15. After explaining the procedure for using a portable sitz bath to a primiparous client who delivered 30 hours ago, which of the following would the nurse do *next*?
- ○ 1. Fill the collecting bag with water at a temperature of 107°F (41.25°C).
- ○ 2. Spray the perineal area with the ordered analgesic spray.
- ○ 3. Wash hands and don clean gloves for the procedure.
- ○ 4. Assess the client's perineum for swelling and redness.

16. A primiparous client, 20 hours after delivery, asks the nurse about starting postpartum exercises. Which of the following would be *most* appropriate to include in the nurse's instructions?
- ○ 1. Start with a sitting position, then lie back, and return to a sitting position, repeating this five times.
- ○ 2. Assume a prone position, then do push-ups by using the arms to lift the upper body.
- ○ 3. Flex the knees while supine, then inhale deeply and exhale while contracting the abdominal muscles.
- ○ 4. Flex the knees while supine, then bring chin to chest while exhaling and reach for the knees by lifting the head and shoulders while inhaling.

17. A multiparous client whose fundus is firm and midline at the umbilicus 8 hours after a vaginal delivery tells the nurse that when she ambulated to the bathroom after sleeping for 4 hours, her dark red lochia seemed heavier. Which of the following would the nurse include when explaining to the client about the increased lochia on ambulation?
- ○ 1. Her bleeding needs to be reported to the physician immediately.
- ○ 2. The increased lochia occurs from lochia pooling in the vaginal vault.
- ○ 3. The increase in lochia may be an early sign of postpartum hemorrhage.
- ○ 4. This increase in lochia usually indicates retained placental fragments.

18. Four hours after delivering a viable neonate by spontaneous vaginal delivery under epidural anes-

thesia, the client states she needs to urinate. Which of the following would the nurse anticipate doing *next*?
- ○ 1. Catheterize the client to obtain an accurate measurement.
- ○ 2. Palpate the bladder to determine distention.
- ○ 3. Assess the fundus to see if it is at the midline.
- ○ 4. Measure the first two voidings and record the amount.

19. A primiparous client who delivered vaginally 8 hours ago desires to take a shower. The nurse anticipates remaining nearby the client to assess for which of the following?
- ○ 1. Fatigue.
- ○ 2. Fainting.
- ○ 3. Diuresis.
- ○ 4. Hygiene needs.

20. A primiparous client who delivered 12 hours ago under epidural anesthesia with a midline episiotomy tells the nurse that she is experiencing a great deal of discomfort when she sits in the chair with the baby. Which of the following instructions would be *most* appropriate?
- ○ 1. "Ask for some pain medication before you sit in the chair."
- ○ 2. "Squeeze your buttocks muscles together before sitting down."
- ○ 3. "Keep a relaxed posture before sitting down with the full weight."
- ○ 4. "Ask the physician for some analgesic cream or spray."

21. Which of the following would the nurse include in the primiparous client's discharge teaching plan about measures to provide visual stimulation for the neonate?
- ○ 1. Maintain eye contact while talking to the baby.
- ○ 2. Paint the baby's room in bright colors accented with teddy bears.
- ○ 3. Use brightly colored animals and cartoon figures on the wall.
- ○ 4. Move a brightly colored rattle in front of the baby's eyes.

22. A primiparous client has just delivered a healthy male infant. The client and her husband are Muslim and the husband begins chanting a song in Arabic while holding the neonate. The nurse interprets the father's actions as indicative of which of the following?
- ○ 1. Thanking Allah for giving him a male heir.
- ○ 2. Singing to his son from the Koran in praise of Allah.
- ○ 3. Expressing appreciation that his wife and son are healthy.
- ○ 4. Performing a ritual similar to Baptism in other religions.

23. An adolescent primiparous client 24 hours postpartum asks the nurse how often she can hold her baby without "spoiling" him. Which of the following responses would be *most* appropriate?
- ○ 1. "Hold him when he is fussy or crying."
- ○ 2. "Hold him as much as you want to hold him."
- ○ 3. "Try to hold him infrequently to avoid over-stimulation."
- ○ 4. "You can hold him periodically throughout the day."

24. The nurse on the night shift finds a multiparous client, 8 hours postpartum, drenched in perspiration. The client's temperature is 99°F (36.8°C), the pulse is 68 bpm, and the blood pressure is 120/80 mm Hg. Which of the following nursing diagnoses would be *most* appropriate?
- ○ 1. Risk for Infection (postpartum) related to birth trauma.
- ○ 2. Ineffective Thermoregulation related to hormonal changes.
- ○ 3. Ineffective Tissue Perfusion: Renal, related to the status of multiparity.
- ○ 4. Excess Fluid Volume related to normal postpartal diuresis.

25. On the first postpartum day, the primiparous client complains of perineal pain that was unrelieved by ibuprofen 400 mg given 2 hours ago. The nurse would assess for which of the following?
- ○ 1. Puerperal infection.
- ○ 2. Vaginal lacerations.
- ○ 3. History of drug abuse.
- ○ 4. Perineal hematoma.

26. While the nurse is caring for a primiparous client on the first postpartum day, the client asks, "How is that woman doing who lost her baby from prematurity? We were in labor together." Which of the following responses by the nurse would be *most* appropriate?
- ○ 1. Ignore the client's question and continue with morning care.
- ○ 2. Tell the client that "I'm not sure how the other woman is doing today."
- ○ 3. Tell the client "I need to ask the woman's permission before discussing her well-being."
- ○ 4. Explain to the client that "Nurses are not allowed to discuss other clients on the unit."

27. A newly delivered primiparous client asks the nurse, "Can my baby see?" Which of the following statements about neonatal vision would the nurse include in the explanation?
- ○ 1. Neonates primarily focus on moving objects.
- ○ 2. They can see objects within a limited range.
- ○ 3. Usually by about 2 days after birth, they see clearly.
- ○ 4. Neonates primarily distinguish light from dark.

28. While assessing the fundus of a multipara 36 hours after delivery of a term neonate, the nurse notes a separation of the abdominal muscles. Which of the following would the nurse anticipate?
    ○ 1. A surgical repair at 6 weeks postpartum.
    ○ 2. Limited activity and bed rest until resolution occurs.
    ○ 3. Resolution on its own with the right posture and diet.
    ○ 4. Exercises involving head and shoulder raising in a lying position.

29. While the nurse is assessing the fundus of a multiparous client who delivered 24 hours ago, the client asks, "What can I do to get rid of these stretch marks?" Which of the following responses would be *most* appropriate?
    ○ 1. "As long as you don't get pregnant again, the marks will disappear completely."
    ○ 2. "They usually fade to a silvery-white color over a period of time."
    ○ 3. "You'll need to use a specially prescribed cream to help them disappear."
    ○ 4. "If you lose the weight you gained during pregnancy, the marks will fade to a pale pink."

30. A primipara who delivered a viable neonate 8 hours ago tells the nurse that she gained 26 pounds during pregnancy and asks how long it will take to return to her normal prepregnant weight. Which of the following would the nurse include as the usual time frame for returning to prepregnant weight?
    ○ 1. 4 weeks.
    ○ 2. 6 weeks.
    ○ 3. 8 weeks.
    ○ 4. 12 weeks.

31. An adolescent primiparous client at 24 hours postpartum tells the nurse that she and her baby will be living with her boyfriend's parents so that she can finish high school and go on to college. The client's boyfriend and parents have been supportive of the client and neonate. Which of the following would be an appropriate nursing diagnosis at this time?
    ○ 1. Anxiety related to return to high school and peer pressure.
    ○ 2. Ineffective Coping related to inability to view motherhood realistically.
    ○ 3. Readiness for Enhanced Family Coping, related to the addition of a new family member.
    ○ 4. Deficient Knowledge related to the financial and emotional costs of childrearing.

32. A primiparous client who delivered a viable term neonate vaginally 48 hours ago has a midline episiotomy and repair of a third-degree laceration. When preparing the client for discharge, which of the following assessments would be *most* important?
    ○ 1. Constipation.
    ○ 2. Diarrhea.
    ○ 3. Excessive bleeding.
    ○ 4. Rectal fistulas.

33. In preparation for discharge, the nurse discusses sexual issues with a primiparous client who had a routine vaginal delivery with a midline episiotomy. Which of the following would the nurse include as the *most* appropriate time for resuming sexual intercourse?
    ○ 1. In 6 weeks when the episiotomy is completely healed.
    ○ 2. After the physician has given the client a postpartum evaluation.
    ○ 3. Whenever the client is feeling amorous and desirable.
    ○ 4. When lochia flow and episiotomy pain have stopped.

34. The physician orders docusate sodium (Colace) 100 mg at bedtime for a primiparous client after vaginal delivery of a term neonate after a midline episiotomy. The nurse explains that this medication is used for which of the following reasons?
    ○ 1. Analgesia for episiotomy pain.
    ○ 2. Contraction of the uterus
    ○ 3. Softening of the stool.
    ○ 4. Aid in sleeping.

35. While caring for a multipara 4 hours after vaginal delivery of a term neonate, the nurse notes that the mother's temperature is 99.8°F (37.2°C), the pulse is 66 bpm, and the respirations are 18 breaths/minute. Her fundus is firm, midline, and at the level of the umbilicus. Which of the following actions would be *most* appropriate?
    ○ 1. Continue to monitor the client's vital signs.
    ○ 2. Assess the client's lochia for large clots.
    ○ 3. Notify the client's physician about the findings.
    ○ 4. Offer the mother an ice pack for her forehead.

36. While assessing the episiotomy site of a primiparous client on the first postpartum day, the nurse observes a fairly large hemorrhoid at the client's rectum. After instructing the client about measures to relieve hemorrhoid discomfort, which of the following client statements indicates the need for *additional* teaching?
    ○ 1. "I should try to gently manually replace the hemorrhoid."
    ○ 2. "Analgesic sprays and witch hazel pads can relieve the pain."
    ○ 3. "I should lie on my back as much as possible to relieve the pain."
    ○ 4. "I should drink lots of water and eat foods that have a lot of roughage."

37. A primiparous client, 24 hours postpartum, who is on a regular diet, is from Guatemala and speaks little English. The client's mother asks the nurse if she can bring her daughter some "special foods from

home." The nurse responds based on the understanding about which of the following?
- ○ 1. Foods from home are generally discouraged on the postpartum unit.
- ○ 2. The mother can bring the daughter any foods that she desires.
- ○ 3. This is permissible as long as the foods are nutritious and high in iron.
- ○ 4. The client's physician needs to give permission for the foods.

38. A primipara, 48 hours after a vaginal delivery, is to be discharged with a prescription for vitamins with iron because she is anemic. To maximize absorption of the iron, the nurse instructs the client to take the medication with which of the following?
- ○ 1. Orange juice.
- ○ 2. Herbal tea.
- ○ 3. Milk.
- ○ 4. Grape juice.

39. The nurse is caring for a multiparous client after vaginal delivery of a set of male twins 2 hours ago. Which of the following would the nurse encourage the mother and husband to do?
- ○ 1. Bottle-feed the twins to prevent exhaustion and fatigue.
- ○ 2. Plan for each parent to spend equal amounts of time with each twin.
- ○ 3. Avoid assistance from other family members until attachment occurs.
- ○ 4. Relate to each twin individually to enhance the attachment process.

40. Twelve hours after a vaginal delivery with epidural anesthesia, the nurse palpates the fundus of a primiparous client and finds it to be firm, above the umbilicus, and deviated to the right. Which of the following would the nurse do *next*?
- ○ 1. Document this as a normal finding in the client's record.
- ○ 2. Contact the physician for an order for methylergonovine.
- ○ 3. Encourage the client to ambulate to the bathroom and void.
- ○ 4. Gently massage the fundus to expel the clots.

The Postpartal Client Who Breast-Feeds

41. A primiparous client who delivered a viable neonate 48 hours ago experienced a third-degree laceration. In preparation for discharge, the nurse instructs the client, who is breast-feeding her neonate, about perineal care. Which of the following client statements indicates the need for *further* instructions?
- ○ 1. "I can take ibuprofen or acetaminophen every 3 to 4 hours for the discomfort."
- ○ 2. "Warm sitz baths three or four times a day for 20 minutes can offer relief."
- ○ 3. "I should try to prevent constipation by drinking plenty of fluids."
- ○ 4. "I can take an aspirin with codeine every 4 hours for the discomfort."

42. During the home visit, a breast-feeding client asks the nurse what contraception method she and her husband should use until she has her 6-week postpartum examination. Which of the following would be *most* appropriate for the nurse to suggest?
- ○ 1. Condom with spermicide.
- ○ 2. Oral contraceptives.
- ○ 3. Rhythm method.
- ○ 4. Cervical cap method.

43. A primiparous client who is beginning to breast-feed her neonate asks the nurse, "Is it important for my baby to get colostrum?" When instructing the client, the nurse would explain that colostrum provides the neonate with which of the following?
- ○ 1. More fat than breast milk.
- ○ 2. Vitamin K, which the neonate lacks.
- ○ 3. Delayed meconium passage.
- ○ 4. Passive immunity from maternal antibodies.

44. Which of the following forms the basis for the teaching plan about avoiding medication use unless prescribed for a primiparous client who is breast-feeding?
- ○ 1. Breast milk quality and richness are decreased.
- ○ 2. The mother's motivation to breast-feed is diminished.
- ○ 3. Medications may be excreted in breast milk to the nursing neonate.
- ○ 4. Medications interfere with the mother's let-down reflex.

45. A breast-feeding primiparous client with a midline episiotomy is prescribed ibuprofen 200 mg orally. The nurse instructs the client to take the medication at which of the following times?
- ○ 1. Before going to bed.
- ○ 2. Midway between feedings.
- ○ 3. Immediately after a feeding.
- ○ 4. When providing supplemental formula.

46. Which of the following would the nurse include in the teaching plan for a primiparous client about the frequency of breast-feeding the neonate during the first few days?
- ○ 1. Feeding the neonate whenever he or she cries.
- ○ 2. Restricting feedings to 1 to 2 minutes per side.
- ○ 3. Feeding the neonate for at least 10 minutes per side.
- ○ 4. Maintaining feeding for 20 to 30 minutes per side.

47. A multiparous client, 28 hours after cesarean delivery, who is breast-feeding complains of severe

cramps or afterpains. The nurse explains that these are caused by which of the following?

○ 1. Flatulence accumulation after a cesarean delivery.

○ 2. Healing of the abdominal incision after cesarean delivery.

○ 3. Side effects of the medications administered after delivery.

○ 4. Release of oxytocin during the breast-feeding session.

48. After the nurse counsels a primipara who is breast-feeding her neonate about diet and nutritional needs during the lactation period, which of the following client statements indicates a need for *additional* teaching?

○ 1. "I need to increase my intake of vitamin D."

○ 2. "I should drink at least five glasses of fluid daily."

○ 3. "I need to get an extra 650 calories per day."

○ 4. "I need to make sure I have enough calcium in my diet."

49. A breast-feeding primiparous client asks the nurse how breast milk differs from cow's milk. The nurse responds by saying that breast milk is higher in which of the following?

○ 1. Fat.

○ 2. Iron.

○ 3. Sodium.

○ 4. Calcium.

50. While assisting a primiparous client with her first breast-feeding session, which of the following actions would the nurse instruct the mother to do to stimulate the neonate to open the mouth and grasp the nipple?

○ 1. Pull down gently on the neonate's chin and insert the nipple.

○ 2. Squeeze both of the neonate's cheeks simultaneously.

○ 3. Place the nipple into the neonate's mouth on top of the tongue.

○ 4. Brush the neonate's lips lightly with the nipple.

51. A 25-year-old primipara who delivered a viable neonate 2 hours ago has decided to breast-feed her neonate. Which of the following would the nurse expect to address in the teaching plan about preventing nipple soreness?

○ 1. Keeping plastic liners in the brassiere to keep the nipple drier.

○ 2. Placing as much of the areola as possible into the baby's mouth.

○ 3. Smoothly pulling the nipple out of the mouth after 10 minutes.

○ 4. Removing any remaining milk left on the nipple with a soft washcloth.

52. Which of the following client statements indicates effective teaching about burping a breast-fed neonate?

○ 1. "Breast-fed babies who are burped frequently will take more on each breast."

○ 2. "If I supplement the baby with formula, I will rarely have to burp him."

○ 3. "I'll breast-feed my baby every 3 hours so I won't have to burp him."

○ 4. "When I switch to the other breast, I'll burp the baby."

53. After the nurse teaches a primiparous client planning to return to work in 6 weeks about storing breast milk, which of the following client statements indicates the need for *further* teaching?

○ 1. "I'll keep the milk stored in sterile plastic formula bottles."

○ 2. "I'll be sure to label the milk with the date, time, and amount."

○ 3. "I can safely store the milk for 48 hours in the refrigerator."

○ 4. "I should keep the milk frozen in clean glass bottles for up to 1 week."

54. During a home visit on the fourth postpartum day, a primiparous client tells the nurse that she is aware of a "let-down sensation" in her breasts and asks what causes it. The nurse explains that the let-down sensation is stimulated by which of the following?

○ 1. Adrenalin.

○ 2. Estrogen.

○ 3. Prolactin.

○ 4. Oxytocin.

55. A 19-year-old primiparous client delivered a viable male neonate 2 hours ago. She has decided to breast-feed, and her 22-year-old husband supports her decision. The neonate has a strong sucking reflex. Which of the following would be a *priority* nursing diagnosis?

○ 1. Ineffective Role Performance related to time involved in breast-feeding.

○ 2. Risk for Impaired Skin Integrity related to neonate's sucking needs.

○ 3. Deficient Knowledge related to inexperience with breast-feeding.

○ 4. Fear related to lack of motivation about breast-feeding.

56. During a home visit on the fourth postpartum day, a primiparous client tells the nurse that she has been experiencing breast engorgement. To relieve engorgement, the nurse teaches the client that before nursing her baby, the client should do which of the following?

○ 1. Apply an ice cube to the nipples.

○ 2. Rub her nipples gently with lanolin cream.

○ 3. Express a small amount of breast milk.

○ 4. Offer the neonate a small amount of formula.

57. A breast-feeding primiparous client who delivered 8 hours ago asks the nurse, "How will I know that my baby is getting enough to eat?" Which of the following would the nurse include in the teaching plan as evidence of adequate intake?
    ○ 1. Six to eight wet diapers by the fifth day.
    ○ 2. Three to four transitional stools on the fourth day.
    ○ 3. Ability to fall asleep easily after feeding on the first day.
    ○ 4. Regain of lost birth weight by the third day.

58. Which of the following would the nurse include in the teaching plan for a primiparous client who asks about weaning her neonate?
    ○ 1. "Wait until you have breast-fed for at least 4 months."
    ○ 2. "Eliminate the baby's favorite feeding times first."
    ○ 3. "Plan to omit the daytime feedings last."
    ○ 4. "Gradually eliminate one feeding at a time."

59. Two weeks after a breast-feeding primiparous client is discharged, she calls the birthing center and says that she is afraid she is "losing her breast milk. The baby had been nursing every 4 hours, but now she's crying to be fed every 2 hours." The nurse interprets the neonate's behavior as *most* likely caused by which of the following?
    ○ 1. Lack of adequate intake to meet maternal nutritional needs.
    ○ 2. The mother's fears about the baby's weight gain.
    ○ 3. Preventing the neonate from sucking long enough with each feeding.
    ○ 4. The neonate's temporary growth spurt, which requires more feedings.

60. During a home visit to a breast-feeding primiparous client at 1 week postpartum, the client tells the nurse that her nipples have become sore and cracked from the feedings. Which of the following would the nurse instruct the client to do?
    ○ 1. Wipe off any lanolin creams from the nipple before each feeding.
    ○ 2. Position the baby with the entire areola in the baby's mouth.
    ○ 3. Feed the baby less often for the next several days.
    ○ 4. Use a mild soap while in the shower to prevent an infection.

The Postpartal Client Who Bottle-Feeds

61. A 24-year-old primipara who has delivered a healthy neonate in the hospital's birthing center plans to bottle-feed her neonate. When developing the nutritional teaching plan for the mother about the neonate's daily calorie allotment, the nurse would determine that the number of calories required by the neonate each day per pound of body weight is which of the following?
    ○ 1. 30 to 35.
    ○ 2. 40 to 45.
    ○ 3. 50 to 55.
    ○ 4. 60 to 65.

62. A primiparous client with a neonate who is 36 hours old asks the nurse, "Why does my baby spit up a small amount of formula after feeding?" The nurse explains that the regurgitation is thought to result from which of the following?
    ○ 1. An immature cardiac sphincter.
    ○ 2. A defect in the gastrointestinal system.
    ○ 3. Too frequent burping of the infant.
    ○ 4. Moving the infant during the feeding.

63. A primiparous client who will be bottle-feeding her neonate asks, "What is the best position for the baby after feeding?" Which of the following positions would the nurse recommend as *best* to aid digestion?
    ○ 1. Supine position.
    ○ 2. On the left side.
    ○ 3. Prone without a pillow.
    ○ 4. Sitting on mom's lap for 20 minutes.

64. A primiparous client who is bottle-feeding her neonate asks, "When should I start giving the baby solid foods?" The nurse instructs the client to introduce solid foods no sooner than which of the following?
    ○ 1. 2 months of age.
    ○ 2. 6 months of age.
    ○ 3. 8 months of age.
    ○ 4. 10 months of age.

65. After instructing a primiparous client who is bottle-feeding about burping, which of the following client statements indicates that the client needs *further* teaching?
    ○ 1. "I'll burp him after 15 minutes of feeding him formula."
    ○ 2. "After he takes one-half ounce of formula, I'll burp him."
    ○ 3. "I'll burp him while he is in an upright position."
    ○ 4. " I'll gently pat his back to get him to burp."

66. When teaching a primiparous client about the growth and development of the neonate, which of the following would the nurse include as the usual age at which most babies are able to drink from a cup independently?
    ○ 1. 5 to 7 months.
    ○ 2. 8 to 10 months.
    ○ 3. 12 to 14 months.
    ○ 4. 15 to 16 months.

67. When preparing a 15-year-old primipara who is bottle-feeding her neonate for discharge, the nurse instructs the client not to "prop" the bottle while feeding the neonate because this can lead to which of the following?
    ○ 1. Overfeeding and obesity.
    ○ 2. Aspiration of the formula.
    ○ 3. Tooth decay in the formative months.
    ○ 4. Sudden infant death syndrome (SIDS).

The Postpartal Client With a Cesarean Birth

68. A 30-year-old woman, gravida IV, para IV, has delivered a healthy term female neonate by cesarean delivery due to a nonreassuring fetal heart rate tracing. At 2 hours postpartum, the nurse assesses the client's retention catheter and observes that the client's urine is slightly red tinged. Which of the following would the nurse do *next*?
    ○ 1. Continue to monitor the client's input and output.
    ○ 2. Palpate the client's fundus gently every 15 minutes.
    ○ 3. Assess the placement of the retention catheter.
    ○ 4. Contact the client's physician for further orders.

69. While changing the neonate's diaper, the client asks the nurse about some red-tinged drainage from the neonate's vagina. Which of the following responses would be *most* appropriate?
    ○ 1. "It's of no concern because it is such a small amount."
    ○ 2. "The cause is usually related to swallowing blood during the delivery."
    ○ 3. "Sometimes baby girls have this from hormones received from the mother."
    ○ 4. "This vaginal spotting is caused by hemorrhagic disease of the newborn."

70. Four hours after cesarean delivery of a neonate weighing 4000 g (8 pounds, 13 ounces), the primiparous client asks, "If I get pregnant again, will I need to have a cesarean?" When responding to the client, which of the following would the nurse need to keep in mind about vaginal birth after cesarean delivery (VBAC)?
    ○ 1. VBAC is possible if the client has not had a classic uterine incision.
    ○ 2. A history of rapid labor is a necessary criterion for VBAC.
    ○ 3. A low transverse incision contraindicates the possibility for VBAC.
    ○ 4. VBAC is not possible because the neonate was large for gestational age.

71. A client who had a cesarean delivery 24 hours ago complains of pain from abdominal distention. The client has been NPO for the past 36 hours. Which of the following actions would be *most* appropriate?
    ○ 1. Offer the client a carbonated beverage twice daily.
    ○ 2. Tell the client to use a straw when drinking fluids.
    ○ 3. Limit the client to a soft diet until more bowel sounds exist.
    ○ 4. Encourage ambulation in the hallway.

72. A primiparous client who underwent a cesarean delivery 30 minutes ago is a candidate for anti-Rh (D) immune globulin (RhoGAM). The nurse anticipates administering this ordered medication within which of the following time frames after delivery?
    ○ 1. 8 hours.
    ○ 2. 24 hours.
    ○ 3. 72 hours.
    ○ 4. 96 hours.

73. While the nurse is caring for a primipara after a cesarean delivery for cephalopelvic disproportion 4 hours ago, the client requests assistance in breast-feeding. To promote maximum maternal comfort, which of the following would be *most* appropriate for the nurse to suggest?
    ○ 1. Football hold.
    ○ 2. Scissors hold.
    ○ 3. Cross-cradle hold.
    ○ 4. Cradle hold.

The Postpartal Client With Complications

74. Which of the following would be *most* appropriate for the nurse to do after assessing a multiparous client at 24 hours postpartum who demonstrates a positive Homan's sign with discomfort?
    ○ 1. Place a cold pack on the client's perineal area.
    ○ 2. Place the client in a semi-Fowler's position.
    ○ 3. Notify the client's physician immediately.
    ○ 4. Ask the client to ambulate around the room.

75. Prophylactic heparin therapy is ordered to treat thrombophlebitis in a multiparous client who delivered 24 hours ago. After instructing the client about the medication, the nurse determines that the client understands the instructions when she states which of the following as the purpose of the drug?
    ○ 1. To thin the blood clots.
    ○ 2. To increase the lochial flow.
    ○ 3. To increase the perspiration for diuresis.
    ○ 4. To prevent further blood clot formation.

76. While caring for a primipara diagnosed with deep vein thrombosis at 48 hours postpartum who is

receiving treatment with bed rest and intravenous heparin therapy, the nurse would contact the client's physician immediately if the client exhibited which of the following?

○ 1. Pain in her calf.
○ 2. Dyspnea.
○ 3. Hypertension.
○ 4. Bradycardia.

77. A primiparous client 3 days postpartum is to be discharged on heparin therapy. After teaching her about possible side effects of heparin therapy, the nurse determines that the client needs *further* instruction when she states that the side effects include which of the following?

○ 1. Epistaxis.
○ 2. Bleeding gums.
○ 3. Slow pulse.
○ 4. Petechiae.

78. After being treated with heparin therapy for thrombophlebitis, a multiparous client who delivered 4 days ago is to be discharged on oral warfarin (Coumadin). After teaching the client about the medication and possible effects, which of the following client statements indicates successful teaching?

○ 1. "I can take two aspirin if I get uterine cramps."
○ 2. "Protamine sulfate should be available if I need it."
○ 3. "I should use a soft toothbrush to brush my teeth."
○ 4. "I can drink an occasional glass of wine if I desire."

79. Which of the following would the nurse include as the *most* common contributing factor when teaching a multipara who is 8 hours postpartum and diagnosed with a puerperal infection?

○ 1. Maternal age older than 30 years.
○ 2. Frequent vaginal examinations during labor.
○ 3. Spontaneous delivery of the placenta.
○ 4. Maternal blood loss of 300 mL during delivery.

80. A postpartum multiparous client diagnosed with endometritis is to receive intravenous antibiotic therapy with ampicillin sodium (Polycillin). Before administering this drug, the nurse *must* do which of the following?

○ 1. Ask the client if she has any drug allergies.
○ 2. Assess the client's pulse rate.
○ 3. Place the client in a side-lying position.
○ 4. Check the client's perineal pad.

81. Which of the following would be *most* important for the nurse to encourage in a primiparous client diagnosed with endometritis who is receiving intravenous antibiotic therapy?

○ 1. Ambulate to the bathroom frequently.
○ 2. Discontinue breast-feeding temporarily.

○ 3. Maintain bed rest in Fowler's position.
○ 4. Restrict visitors to prevent contamination.

82. Which of the following measures would the nurse expect to include in the teaching plan for a multiparous client who delivered 24 hours ago and is receiving intravenous antibiotic therapy for cystitis?

○ 1. Limiting fluid intake to 1 L daily to prevent overload.
○ 2. Emptying the bladder every 2 to 4 hours while awake.
○ 3. Washing the perineum with povidone iodine (Betadine) after voiding.
○ 4. Avoiding the intake of acidic fruit juices until the treatment is discontinued.

83. The nurse is caring for a primiparous client who is diagnosed with cystitis on the second postpartum day. The client has been requesting medication for back pain every 3 to 4 hours. Which of the following would be an appropriate nursing diagnosis for the client at this time?

○ 1. Fear related to intravenous therapy and outcome.
○ 2. Ineffective Coping related to prolonged hospitalization.
○ 3. Ineffective Role Performance related to prolonged bed rest.
○ 4. Pain related to dysuria and urinary frequency.

84. A primipara diagnosed with cystitis at 48 hours postpartum who is receiving intravenous ampicillin asks the nurse, "Can I still continue to breast-feed my baby?" Which of the following responses by the nurse would be *most* appropriate?

○ 1. "You can continue to breast-feed as long as you want to do so."
○ 2. "Alternate your breast-feeding with formula feeding to help you rest."
○ 3. "You'll need to discontinue breast-feeding until the antibiotic therapy is stopped."
○ 4. "You'll need to modify your technique by manually pumping your breasts."

85. Four days after a vaginal delivery, the client visits the clinic complaining of excessive lochia rubra with clots. The physician orders methylergonovine maleate (Methergine), 0.2 mg intramuscularly. Before administering this drug, which of the following would the nurse need to assess?

○ 1. Blood pressure.
○ 2. Pulse rate.
○ 3. Breath sounds.
○ 4. Bowel sounds.

86. During the first hour after delivery, assessment of a multiparous client who delivered a neonate weighing 4593 g (10 pounds, 2 ounces) by cesarean delivery reveals a soft fundus with excessive lochia rubra.

Which of the following would the nurse expect to include in the client's plan of care?
- ○ 1. Administration of intravenous oxytocin.
- ○ 2. Placement of the client in a side-lying position.
- ○ 3. Vigorous fundal massage every 5 minutes.
- ○ 4. Preparation for an emergency hysteromyomectomy.

87. A primipara client who was diagnosed with hydramnios and breech presentation while in early labor is diagnosed with early postpartum hemorrhage at 1 hour after a cesarean delivery. The client asks, "Why am I bleeding so much?" The nurse responds based on the understanding that the *most* likely cause of uterine atony in this client is which of the following?
- ○ 1. Trauma during labor and delivery.
- ○ 2. Moderate fundal massage after delivery.
- ○ 3. Lengthy and prolonged second stage of labor.
- ○ 4. Overdistention of the uterus from hydramnios.

88. Thirty-six hours after a vaginal delivery, a multiparous client is diagnosed with endometritis due to β-hemolytic streptococcus. When assessing the client, which of the following would the nurse expect to find?
- ○ 1. Profuse amounts of lochia.
- ○ 2. Abdominal distention.
- ○ 3. Nausea and vomiting.
- ○ 4. Odorless vaginal discharge.

89. A multiparous client visits the urgent care center 5 days after a vaginal delivery experiencing persistent lochia rubra in a moderate to heavy amount. The client asks the nurse, "Why am I continuing to bleed like this?" The nurse should instruct the client that this type of postpartum bleeding is usually caused by which of the following?
- ○ 1. Uterine atony.
- ○ 2. Cervical lacerations.
- ○ 3. Vaginal lacerations.
- ○ 4. Retained placental fragments.

90. A 26-year-old primipara client is seen in the urgent care clinic 2 weeks after delivering a viable female neonate. The client, who is breast-feeding, is diagnosed with infectious mastitis of the right breast. The client asks the nurse, "Can I continue breast-feeding?" Which of the following responses would be *most* appropriate?
- ○ 1. "You can continue to breast-feed, feeding your baby more frequently."
- ○ 2. "You can continue once your symptoms begin to decrease."
- ○ 3. "You must discontinue breast-feeding until antibiotic therapy is completed."
- ○ 4. "You must stop breast-feeding because the breast is contaminated."

91. A primiparous client who had a vaginal delivery 1 hour ago voices anxiety because she has a nephew with Down syndrome. After teaching the client about Down syndrome, which of the following client statements indicates the need for *additional* teaching?
- ○ 1. "Down syndrome is an abnormality that can result from a missing chromosome."
- ○ 2. "Down syndrome usually results in some degree of mental retardation."
- ○ 3. "There are several methods available to determine whether my baby has Down syndrome."
- ○ 4. "Older mothers are more likely to have a baby with chromosomal abnormalities."

92. A 15-year-old unmarried primipara is being cared for in the hospital's birthing center after vaginal delivery of a viable neonate. The neonate is being placed for adoption through a social service agency. Four hours postpartum, the client asks if she can feed her baby. Which of the following responses would be *most* appropriate?
- ○ 1. "I'll bring the baby to you for feeding."
- ○ 2. "I think we should ask your physician if this is a good idea."
- ○ 3. "It's not a good idea for you to have any contact with the baby."
- ○ 4. "I'll check with the social worker to see if the adopting parents will permit this."

93. After teaching a primiparous client about treatment and self-care of infectious mastitis of the right breast, the nurse determines that the client needs *further* instruction when she states which of the following?
- ○ 1. "I can apply localized heat to the infected area."
- ○ 2. "I should increase my fluid intake to 3000 mL per day."
- ○ 3. "I'll need to take antibiotics for 7 to 10 days before I am cured."
- ○ 4. "I should begin breast-feeding on the right side to decrease the pain."

94. During a home visit to a primiparous client who delivered vaginally 14 days ago, the client says, "I've been crying a lot the last few days. I just feel so awful. I am a rotten mother. I just don't have any energy. Plus, my husband just got laid off from his job." The nurse observes that the client's appearance is disheveled. Which of the following would be the nurse's *best* response?
- ○ 1. "These feelings often indicate symptoms of postpartum blues and are normal. They'll go away in a few days."
- ○ 2. "I think you're probably overreacting to the labor and delivery process. You're doing the best you can as a mother."
- ○ 3. "It's not unusual for some mothers to feel depressed after the birth of a baby. I think I should contact your doctor."
- ○ 4. "This may be a symptom of a serious mental illness. I think you should probably go to the hospital."

Correct Answers and Rationale

The letters in parentheses following the rationale identify the step of the nursing process (A, D, P, I, E) and client needs (1, 2, 3, 4, 5, 6, 7, 8, 9, 10). See the inside front cover for the key.

The Postpartal Client With a Vaginal Birth

1. 1. Immediately after delivery of the placenta, the nurse would expect to palpate the fundus halfway between the umbilicus and the symphysis pubis. Within 2 hours postpartum, the fundus should be palpated at the level of the umbilicus. The fundus remains at this level or may rise slightly above the umbilicus for approximately 12 hours. After the first 12 hours, the fundus should decrease one finger-breadth (1 cm) per day in size. By the 9th or 10th day, the fundus usually is no longer palpable. (I, 3)

2. 2. The instillation of erythromycin into the neonate's eyes provides prophylaxis for ophthalmia neonatorum, or neonatal blindness caused by gonorrhea in the mother. Erythromycin is also effective in the prevention of infection and conjunctivitis from *Chlamydia trachomatis*. The medication may result in redness of the neonate's eyes, but this redness will eventually disappear. Erythromycin ointment is not effective in treating neonatal chorioretinitis from cytomegalovirus. No effective treatment is available for a mother with cytomegalovirus. Erythromycin ointment is not effective in preventing cataracts. Additionally, neonatal infection with β-hemolytic streptococcus results in pneumonia, bacterial meningitis, or death. Cataracts in the neonate may be congenital or may result from maternal exposure to rubella. Erythromycin ointment is also not effective for preventing and treating strabismus (crossed eyes). Infants may exhibit strabismus until 6 months of age, when the condition spontaneously corrects itself without intervention. (I, 8)

3. 3. Phytonadione, vitamin K or AquaMEPHYTON, acts as a preventive measure against neonatal hemorrhagic disease. At birth, the neonate does not have the intestinal flora to produce vitamin K, which is necessary for coagulation. Hypoglycemia is prevented and treated by feeding the infant. Hyperbilirubinemia severity can be decreased by early feeding and passage of meconium to excrete the bilirubin. Hyperbilirubinemia is treated with phototherapy. Polycythemia may occur in neonates who are large for gestational age or post-term. Clamping of the umbilical cord before pulsations cease reduces the incidence of polycythemia. Generally, polycythemia is not treated unless it is extremely severe. (I, 8)

4. 3. The first 12 hours after delivery are part of the taking-in phase of maternal postpartum adjustment, which typically lasts from 1 to 3 days. During the taking-in phase, the client is primarily concerned with her own needs. After the first 1 to 3 days postpartum, the client is in the taking-hold phase and can focus more on the needs of the neonate. Although the family is an important unit of care and the significant other is important for the mother's emotional support, during the taking-in phase the mother is focused on herself. (P, 3)

5. 1. The client has a hematoma. During the first 24 hours postpartum, ice packs can be applied to the perineal area to reduce swelling and discomfort. Ice packs usually are not effective after the first 24 hours. After 24 hours, the client may obtain more relief by taking a warm sitz bath. This moist heat is an effective way to increase circulation to the perineum and provide comfort. Usually, hematomas resolve without further treatment within 6 weeks. Additionally, the nurse should measure the hematoma to provide a baseline for subsequent measurements and should notify the physician of its presence. Although vital signs, including temperature, are important assessments, taking the client's temperature is unrelated to the hematoma and would provide no additional information about swelling. An antibiotic is not warranted at this point because the client is not exhibiting any signs or symptoms of infection. (I, 3)

6. 4. Urinary retention soon after delivery is usually caused by edema and trauma of the lower urinary tract; this commonly results in difficulty with initiating voiding. Hyperemia of the bladder mucosa also commonly occurs. The combination of hyperemia and edema predisposes to decreased sensation to void, overdistention of the bladder, and incomplete bladder emptying. A prolonged first stage of labor can contribute to exhaustion and uterine atony, not urinary retention. If the client had a urinary tract infection, she would exhibit symptoms such as dysuria and a burning sensation. After delivery, the uterus is contracting, which leads to less pressure on the bladder. Pressure of the uterus on the bladder occurs during labor. (D, 3)

7. 2. For clients who are bottle-feeding, the menstrual flow should return in 6 to 10 weeks, after a rise in the production of follicle-stimulating hormone by the pituitary gland. Nonlactating mothers rarely ovulate before 4 to 6 weeks postpartum. Therefore, 3 to 4 weeks is too early for the menstrual cycle to resume. For women who are breast-feeding, the menstrual flow may not

return for 3 to 4 months (12 to 16 weeks) or, in some women, for the entire period of lactation, because ovulation is suppressed. (I, 3)

8. 4. The client's dizziness is most likely caused by orthostatic hypotension secondary to the decreased volume of blood in the vascular system resulting from the physiologic changes occurring in the mother after delivery. The client is experiencing dizziness because not enough blood volume is available to perfuse the brain. The nurse should first allow the client to "dangle" on the side of the bed for a few minutes before attempting to ambulate. By 10 hours postpartum, the effects of the anesthesia should be worn off completely. Typically, the effects of epidural anesthesia wear off by 1 to 2 hours postpartum, and the effects of local anesthesia usually disappear by 1 hour. The client scenario provides no information to indicate that the client experienced any postpartum hemorrhage. Normal blood loss during delivery should not exceed 500 mL. (I, 3)

9. 1. During the first week postpartum, the client's pulse rate should be slow, with an average of 60 to 70 bpm. A pulse of 100 bpm warrants further investigation to rule out a possible infectious process or postpartum hemorrhage. An oral temperature of 99°F (36.8°C) is within normal limits. Excessive perspiration and frequent voiding in large amounts are caused by the normal diuresis that occurs as the body returns to its prepregnant state. (E, 1)

10. 4. The priority nursing diagnosis at this time is Urinary Retention related to the trauma of delivery, particularly since forceps, which may result in trauma, were used during the delivery. The client is at some risk for infection, specifically urinary tract infection, from the repeated need for catheterization. However, this is not a priority at this time. With proper technique and adequate cleanliness and hygiene, infection can be prevented. Disturbed Body Image related to the episiotomy is not a priority at this time. The client may be feeling some discomfort from the episiotomy. There is no indication that the client is experiencing a risk for fluid volume imbalance related to the prolonged labor and anesthesia. Most likely, the client would be receiving intravenous fluid replacement. (D, 3)

11. 4. Because the diet of Hispanic Americans from Mexico and Central America commonly includes beans, corn products, tomatoes, chili peppers, potatoes, milk, cheeses, and eggs, the nurse needs to encourage an intake of meats, dark green leafy vegetables, and other high-protein products that are rich in iron. Doing so helps to compensate for the significant blood loss and subsequent iron loss that occurs during the postpartum period. Additionally, fresh fruits, meats, and green leafy vegetables may be scarce, possibly resulting in deficiencies of vitamin A, vitamin D, and iron. Toma-

toes are high in vitamin C, potatoes are good sources of carbohydrates and vitamin C, and corn products are high in thiamine, but these are not rich sources of iron. (P, 3)

12. 4. A small, constant trickle of blood and a firm fundus are usually indicative of a vaginal tear or cervical laceration. If the client had retained placental tissue, the fundus would fail to contract fully (uterine atony), exhibiting as a soft or boggy fundus. Also, vaginal bleeding would be evident. Uterine inversion occurs when the uterus is displaced outside of the vagina and is obvious on inspection. Bladder distention may result in uterine atony because the pressure of the bladder displaces the fundus, preventing it from fully contracting. In this case the fundus would be soft, possibly boggy, and displaced from midline. (A, 9)

13. 4. On about the 10th postpartum day, the lochia should be lochia alba, clear or white in color. Lochia rubra, which is dark red to red, may persist for the first 2 to 3 days postpartum. From day 3 to about day 10, lochia serosa, which is pink or brown, is normal. (D, 3)

14. 2. The nurse should instruct the client to cleanse the perineal area with warm water and to wipe from front to back with a blotting motion. Warm water is soothing to the tender tissue, and wiping from front to back reduces the risk of contamination. Hot, sudsy water may increase the client's discomfort and may even burn the client in a very tender area. After the first 24 hours, warm water sitz baths taken three or four times a day for 20 minutes can help increase circulation to the area. Ice packs are helpful for the first 24 hours. (E, 3)

15. 3. After explaining the procedure to the client, the nurse should wash hands and don clean gloves for the procedure. Washing the hands prevents the spread of infection. Standard precautions are necessary to protect both the client and the nurse. The temperature of the water should be between 100° and 105°F (37.4° and 40°C) to prevent burns. Spraying the perineal area with the ordered analgesic spray is done after the sitz bath to provide the greatest pain relief. Assessing the client's perineum for swelling and redness is part of the nursing assessment and needs to be done after hand washing and donning clean gloves. Also, the assessment would be done before the nurse explains the procedure. (I, 2)

16. 3. After an uncomplicated delivery, postpartum exercises may begin on the first postpartum day with exercises to strengthen the abdominal muscles. These are done in the supine position with the knees flexed, inhaling deeply while allowing the abdomen to expand and then exhaling while contracting the abdominal muscles. Exercises such as sit-ups (sitting, then lying back, and returning to a sitting position) and push-ups

or exercises involving reaching for the knees are ordinarily too strenuous for the first postpartum day. Sit-ups may be done later in the postpartum period, after approximately 3 to 6 weeks. (I, 3)

17. 2. Lochia can be expected to increase when the client first ambulates. Lochia tends to pool in the uterus and vagina when the client is recumbent and flows out when the client arises. If the client had reported that her lochia was bright red, the nurse would suspect bleeding. In this situation, the client would be put back in bed and the physician would be notified. Early postpartum hemorrhage occurs during the first 24 hours, but typically the fundus is soft or "boggy." The client's fundus here is firm and midline. Late postpartal hemorrhage, occurring after the first 24 hours, is usually caused by retained placental fragments or abnormal involution of the placental site. (I, 3)

18. 4. After delivery, the nurse should plan to measure the client's first two voidings and record the amount to make sure that the client is emptying the bladder. Frequent voidings of less than 150 mL suggest that the client is experiencing urinary retention. In addition, if urinary retention is occurring, the bladder may be palpable and the fundus may be displaced from midline. The client does not need to be catheterized unless there is evidence of urinary retention. Palpation of the bladder before voiding is unnecessary. However, if the client has difficulty voiding or exhibits signs of urinary retention, then bladder palpation is indicated. The fundus can be displaced by a full bladder and should be assessed after the client voids. (P, 3)

19. 2. Clients sometimes feel faint or dizzy when taking a shower for the first time after delivery because of the sudden change in blood volume in the body. Primarily for this reason, the nurse remains nearby while the client takes her first shower after delivery. If the client becomes dizzy or expresses symptoms of feeling faint, the nurse should get the client back to bed as soon as possible. If the client faints while in the shower, the nurse should cover the client to protect her privacy, stay with the client, and call for assistance. (I, 2)

20. 2. The nurse should instruct the client to squeeze or contract the muscles of the buttocks together before sitting down in the chair; this contracts the pelvic floor muscles, which reduces the tension on the tender perineal area. Then the client should put her full weight slowly down on the chair. Pain medication may only be ordered for every 3 to 4 hours, so the client may not be able to receive pain medication every time she desires to sit in the chair. The episiotomy pain usually fades by the fifth or sixth postpartum day. Maintaining a relaxed posture before sitting does not contract the pelvic floor muscles. Most physicians order an analgesic cream or

spray when a client has an episiotomy, but they provide only temporary relief. (I, 3)

21. 1. Neonates like to look at eyes, and eye-to-eye contact is a highly effective way to provide visual stimulation. The parent's eyes are circular, move from side to side, and become larger and smaller. Neonates have been observed to fix on them. In general, neonates prefer circular objects of darkness against a white background. Sharp black and white images of geometric figures are appropriate. Use of bright colors on the walls and moving a colorful rattle do not provide as much visual stimulation as eye-to-eye contact with talking. Brightly colored animals and cartoon figures are more appropriate at approximately 1 year of age. (I, 3)

22. 2. The father is praying to Allah because of the Muslim belief that the first sounds a child hears should be from the Koran in praise of and supplication to Allah. Although male children are revered in this culture, this practice is performed by Muslims whether the child is male or female. The father's actions are unrelated to his wife and son's being healthy. The nurse should allow the practice because doing so demonstrates cultural sensitivity and builds a trusting relationship with the family. The Muslim faith does not have a baptism rite whereby the child becomes a member of the faith. (D, 3)

23. 2. According to Erikson, infants are in the trust versus mistrust stage. Holding, talking to, singing to, and patting neonates helps them develop trust in caregivers. Tactile stimulation is important and should be encouraged. Holding neonates often is unlikely to spoil them because they are totally dependent on other human beings to meet their needs. Being held makes infants feel loved and cared for and should be encouraged. The mother can hold the neonate as often as she wants, not just when the baby is crying or fussy. Overstimulation typically does not result from holding an infant. (I, 3)

24. 4. Excessive perspiration and diuresis is common during the puerperium as the body attempts to return to its prepregnant state. The most appropriate nursing diagnosis is Excess Fluid Volume related to normal postpartal diuresis. A temperature of 99°F (37.2°C) is normal during the first 24 hours postpartum. Foul-smelling lochia and a temperature higher than 100.4°F (38°C) would suggest an infection. Although hormonal shifts occur during the postpartum period, the client's diaphoresis is related to diuresis, not to a problem with thermoregulation caused by hormonal changes. No evidence is presented to suggest altered renal tissue perfusion related to the client's multiparity status. Clients with renal disease or renal failure may exhibit painful urination, flank pain, or lack of urinary output. (D, 3)

25. 4. If the client continues to complain of perineal pain after an analgesic medication has been given, the nurse

should inspect the client's perineum for a hematoma, because this is the usual cause of such discomfort. Ibuprofen is a nonsteroidal anti-inflammatory medication used to relieve mild pain. Pain from a perineal hematoma can be moderate to severe, possibly requiring a stronger analgesic, such as acetaminophen with codeine (Tylenol with Codeine). Application of warm heat, such as a sitz bath three times daily for 20 minutes, also can help to relieve the discomfort. Typically hematomas resolve themselves within 6 weeks. A puerperal infection would be indicated if the client's temperature were 100.4°F (41°C) or higher. Also, lochia most likely would be foul smelling. A continuous trickle of lochia rubra would suggest a possible vaginal laceration. No evidence is presented to suggest a history of drug abuse. (A, 9)

26. 4. Ethical behavior requires that the nurse maintain confidentiality at all times. The nurse's best response is to explain to the client that nurses are not allowed to discuss other clients on the unit. Ignoring the client's question is inappropriate because doing so would interfere with the development of a trusting nurse-client relationship. Confidentiality must be maintained at all times. Telling the client that the nurse isn't sure may imply that the nurse will find out and then tell the client about the other woman. Asking the other woman's permission to discuss her with another client is inappropriate because confidentiality must be maintained at all times. (I, 1)

27. 2. The neonate has immature oculomotor coordination, an inability to accommodate for distance, and poorly developed eyes, visual nerves, and brain. However, the normal neonate can see objects clearly within a range of 9 to 12 inches, whether or not they are moving. Visual acuity at birth is 20/100 to 20/150, but it improves rapidly during infancy and toddlerhood. Newborns can distinguish colors and light from dark. (I, 3)

28. 4. The client is experiencing diastasis recti, a separation of the longitudinal muscles (recti) of the abdomen that usually is palpable on the third postpartum day. An exercise involving raising the head and shoulders about 8 inches with the client lying on her back with knees bent and hands crossed over the abdomen is preferred. This exercise helps to pull the abdominal muscles together. Typically, the client gradually works up to performing this exercise 50 times per day. However, until the diastasis has closed, the client should avoid exercises that rotate the trunk, twist the hips, or bend the trunk to one side, because further separation may occur. The condition does not need a surgical repair, and limited activity and bed rest are not necessary. (P, 9)

29. 2. Stretch marks or striae gravidarum are caused by stretching of the tissues, particularly over the abdomen. After delivery, the tissues atrophy, leaving silver scars. These skin pigmentations will not disappear completely. The striae gravidarum may reappear as pink streaks if the client becomes pregnant again. Special creams are not warranted because they are not helpful and may be expensive. Weight loss does not make the marks disappear. Straie gravidarum tend to run in families. (I, 3)

30. 2. In most cases, unless complications develop or the client has gained excessive weight during the antepartal period, she can expect to return to her prepregnant weight by 6 weeks. Many clients lose 14 to 20 pounds by 2 weeks postpartum, primarily because of the birth of the fetus, the placenta, and fluid losses. Diet and exercise can help the client return to her prepregnant weight. (I, 3)

31. 3. The most appropriate nursing diagnosis based on the information provided is Readiness for Enhanced Family Coping, related to the addition of a new family member. Based on the scenario, the client has the support of the boyfriend and his parents. A nursing diagnosis of Anxiety would be appropriate if the client verbalized anxious thoughts or feelings or worries about the situation. A nursing diagnosis of Ineffective Coping would be appropriate if the client showed little interest in the neonate or in mothering behaviors. A nursing diagnosis of Deficient Knowledge would be appropriate if the client expressed concerns about the financial and emotional costs of childrearing or questions about caring for the child. (D, 5)

32. 1. The client with a third-degree laceration should be assessed for constipation, because a third-degree laceration extends into a portion of the anal sphincter. Constipation, not diarrhea, is more likely because this condition is extremely painful, possibly causing the client to be reluctant to have a bowel movement. The laceration has been sutured and should not be bleeding at 48 hours postpartum. Rectal fistulas may develop at a later time, but not at 48 hours postpartum. (A, 9)

33. 4. For most clients, sexual intercourse can be resumed when the lochia has stopped flowing and episiotomy pain has ceased, usually about 3 weeks postpartum. Sexual intercourse may be painful until the episiotomy has healed. The client also needs instructions about the possibility that pregnancy may occur before the return of the client's menstrual flow. Typically, new mothers are exhausted and may not feel amorous or desirable for quite a while. In addition, the mother's physiologic responses may be diminished because of low hormonal levels, adjustments to the maternal role, and fatigue due to lack of rest and sleep. (I, 3)

34. 3. Docusate sodium (Colace) is a stool softener, used to assist in bowel elimination. The client is at risk for con-

stipation because of decreased food and fluid intake and pain from the episiotomy. Numerous analgesics, such as ibuprofen (Motrin) or acetaminophen (Tylenol), could be used to treat episiotomy pain, helping the client achieve comfort and thus fall asleep. Oxytocin is used to contract the uterus. (I, 8)

35. 1. The nurse needs to continue to monitor the client's vital signs. During the first 24 hours postpartum it is normal for the mother to have a slight temperature elevation because of dehydration. A temperature of 100.4°F (38°C) that persists after the first 24 hours may be indicative of an infection. Bradycardia during the first week postpartum is normal because of decreased blood volume, diuresis, and diaphoresis. The client's respiratory rate is within normal limits. Large clots are indicative of hemorrhage. However, the client's vital signs are within normal limits and her fundus is firm and midline. Therefore, large clots and possible hemorrhage can be ruled out. The physician does not need to be notified at this time. An ice pack is not necessary because the client's temperature is within normal limits. (I, 3)

36. 3. The client needs more teaching when she states, "I should lie on my back as much as possible to relieve the pain." Instead, the client should lie in the Sims position as much as possible to aid venous return to the rectal area and to reduce discomfort. Gentle manual replacement of the hemorrhoid is an appropriate measure to help relieve the discomfort and prevent enlargement. Analgesic sprays and witch hazel pads are helpful in reducing the discomfort of hemorrhoids. Drinking lots of water and eating roughage aid in bowel elimination, minimizing the risk for straining and subsequent hemorrhoidal development or enlargement. (E, 7)

37. 2. On most postpartum units, clients on regular diets are allowed to eat whatever kinds of food they desire. Generally, foods from home are not discouraged. The nurse does not need to obtain the physician's permission. Although it is preferred, the foods do not necessarily have to be high in iron. In many Latino cultures, there is a belief in the "hot-cold" theory of disease; certain foods (hot) are preferred during the postpartum period, and other foods (cold) are avoided. Therefore, the nurse should allow the mother to bring her daughter "special foods" from home. Doing so demonstrates cultural sensitivity and aids in developing a trusting relationship. (I, 7)

38. 1. Iron is best absorbed in an acid environment or with vitamin C. For maximum iron absorption, the client should take the medication with orange juice or a vitamin C supplement. Herbal tea has no effect on iron absorption. Milk decreases iron absorption. Grape juice is not acidic and therefore would have no effect on iron absorption. (I, 8)

39. 4. It is believed that the process of attachment is structured so that the parents become attached to only one infant at a time. Therefore, the nurse should encourage the parents to relate to each twin individually, rather than as a unit, to enhance the attachment process. Mothers of twins are usually able to breast-feed successfully because the milk supply increases on demand. However, possible fatigue and exhaustion require that the mother rest whenever possible. It would be highly unlikely and unrealistic that each parent would be able to spend equal amounts of time with both twins. Other responsibilities, such as employment, may prevent this. The parents should try to engage assistance from family and friends, because caring for twins or other multiple births (eg, triplets) can be exhausting for the family. (I, 5)

40. 3. At 12 hours postpartum, the fundus normally should be in the midline and at the level of the umbilicus. When the fundus is firm yet above the umbilicus, and deviated to the right rather than in the midline, the client's bladder is most likely distended. The client should be encouraged to ambulate to the bathroom and attempt to void, because a full bladder can prevent normal involution. A firm but deviated fundus above the level of the umbilicus is not a normal finding and should be reported to the physician. Methylergonovine (Methergine) is used to treat uterine atony. This client's fundus is firm, not boggy or soft, which would suggest atony. Gentle massage is not necessary because there is no evidence of atony or clots. (I, 9)

The Postpartal Client Who Breast-Feeds

41. 4. Postpartum clients who are breast-feeding need to be cautioned about taking various medications, many of which can be passed to the infant via breast milk. Aspirin and codeine products should be avoided because the drug can increase bleeding or cause sleepiness in the infant. Medications such as ibuprofen or acetaminophen can be used to help to relieve the discomfort without causing any apparent harm to the neonate. Warm sitz baths three to four times a day for 20 minutes can be helpful in relieving the client's discomfort. Application of moist heat is soothing and increases perineal circulation. Increased fluid (and fiber) intake promotes bowel elimination, thus preventing constipation, which can increase the client's discomfort. (E, 3)

42. 1. If not contraindicated for moral, cultural, or religious reasons, a condom with spermicide is often recommended for contraception after delivery until the client's 6-week postpartal examination. This method has no effect on the neonate who is breast-feeding. Oral contraceptives are not advised for women who are

breast-feeding because the hormones have been found in breast milk. Women who are not breast-feeding may use oral contraceptive agents. The rhythm method is not effective because the client is unlikely to be able to determine when ovulation has occurred until her menstrual cycle returns. Although breast-feeding is not considered an effective form of contraception, breast-feeding usually delays the return of both ovulation and menstruation. The length of the delay varies with the duration of lactation and the frequency of breast-feeding. After delivery, the mother's cervix is stretched and tender. A cervical cap may be difficult to insert and also may cause discomfort. (I, 3)

43. 4. Colostrum is a thin, watery, yellow fluid composed of protein, sugar, fat, water, minerals, vitamins, and maternal antibodies (eg, immunoglobulin A). It is important for the neonate to receive colostrum for passive immunity. Colostrum is lower in fat and lactose than mature breast milk. Colostrum does not contain vitamin K. The neonate will produce vitamin K once a feeding pattern is established. Colostrum may speed, rather than delay, the passage of meconium. (I, 3)

44. 3. Various medications can be excreted in the breast milk and affect the nursing neonate. The client should avoid all nonprescribed medications unless approved by the physician (eg, acetaminophen). Medications typically do not affect the quality of the mother's breast milk. Medications usually do not interfere with or diminish the mother's motivation to breast-feed, nor do they interfere with the mother's let-down reflex. (I, 3)

45. 3. Taking ibuprofen 200 mg orally immediately after breast-feeding helps minimize the neonate's exposure to the drug because drugs are most highly concentrated in the body soon after they are taken. Most mothers breast-feed on demand or every 2 to 3 hours, so the effects of the ibuprofen should be decreased by the next breast-feeding session. Taking the medication before going to bed is inappropriate because, although the mother may go to bed at a certain time, the neonate may wish to breast-feed soon after the mother goes to bed. If the mother takes the medication midway between feedings, then its peak action may occur midway between feedings. Breast milk is sufficient for the neonate's nutritional needs. Most breast-feeding mothers should not be encouraged to provide supplemental feedings to the infant because this may result in nipple confusion. (I, 8)

46. 3. During the first few days postpartum, the mother should be encouraged to nurse frequently. Breast-feeding for at least 10 minutes per side is recommended for the let-down reflex to begin. Feeding the infant whenever the infant cries is not appropriate and can lead to maternal exhaustion. Feeding for 1 to 2 minutes per side is insufficient for the let-down reflex.

Also, this short period of time prevents the neonate from latching on and obtaining the needed nutrition. Initially, feeding for 10 minutes per side is sufficient until the infant becomes more comfortable with breast-feeding. Then the mother can increase the breast-feeding time gradually to 20 to 30 minutes. (I, 3)

47. 4. Breast-feeding stimulates oxytocin secretion, which causes the uterine muscles to contract. These contractions account for the discomfort associated with afterpains. Flatulence may occur after a cesarean delivery. However, the mother typically would complain of abdominal distention and a bloating feeling, not a "cramplike" feeling. Stretching of the tissues or healing may cause slight tenderness or itching, not cramping feelings of discomfort. Medications such as mild analgesics or stool softeners, commonly administered postpartum, typically do not cause cramping. (I, 3)

48. 2. For the breast-feeding client, drinking at least 8 to 10 glasses of fluid a day is recommended. Breast-feeding women need an increased intake of vitamin D for calcium absorption. A breast-feeding woman requires an extra 650 calories per day to produce quality breast milk. Breast-feeding women need adequate calcium for blood clotting and strong bones and teeth. (E, 7)

49. 1. Breast milk has a higher fat content than cow's milk. Thirty percent to 55% of the calories in breast milk are from fat. Breast milk contains less iron than cow's milk does. However, the iron absorption from breast milk is greater in the neonate than with cow's milk. Breast milk contains less sodium and less calcium than cow's milk does. (I, 7)

50. 4. Lightly brushing the neonate's lips with the nipple causes the neonate to open the mouth and begin sucking. The neonate should be taught to open the mouth and grasp the nipple on his or her own. The neonate should not be forced to nurse. (I, 3)

51. 2. Several methods can be used to prevent nipple soreness. Placing as much of the areola as possible into the neonate's mouth is one method. This action prevents compression of the nipple between the neonate's gums, which can cause nipple soreness. Other methods include changing position with each feeding, avoiding breast engorgement, nursing more frequently, and feeding on demand. Plastic liners are not helpful because they prevent air circulation, thus promoting nipple soreness. Instead, air drying is recommended. Pulling the baby's mouth out smoothly after only 10 minutes may prevent the baby from getting the entire feeding. Any breast milk remaining on the nipples should not be wiped off, because the milk has healing properties. (P, 3)

52. 4. Breast-fed neonates do not swallow as much air as bottle-fed neonates, but they still need to be burped.

Good times to burp the neonate are when the mother switches from one breast to the other and at the end of the breast-feeding session. Neonates do not eat more if they are burped frequently. Breast-feeding mothers are advised not to supplement the feedings with formula because this may cause nipple confusion. If supplements are given, the baby still needs to be burped. Neonates who are fed every 3 hours still need to be burped. (E, 3)

53. 4. Breast milk should not be stored in glass containers because immunoglobulin tends to stick to glass bottles. Sterile plastic containers are recommended. The containers should be labeled with date, time, and amount to prevent inadvertent administration of spoiled milk. Stored breast milk can be safely kept in the refrigerator for 48 hours or in a freezer for 6 months at 0°F (−18°C). Frozen breast milk should be thawed in the refrigerator for a few hours, placed under warm tap water, then shaken. (E, 3)

54. 4. Oxytocin stimulates the let-down reflex when milk is carried to the nipples. A lactating mother can experience the let-down reflex suddenly when she hears her baby cry or when she anticipates a feeding. Some mothers have reported feeling the let-down reflex just by thinking about the baby. Adrenalin may increase if the mother is excited, but this hormone has no direct influence on breast feeding. Estrogen influences development of female secondary sex characteristics and controls menstruation. Prolactin stimulates milk production. (I, 3)

55. 3. The most appropriate initial nursing diagnosis for this client is Deficient Knowledge related to inexperience with breast-feeding. This is the client's first baby and first experience with breast-feeding. Also, as a young adult, the client needs guidance and education. Ineffective Role Performance would be indicated if the client had expressed concern about her role changes. Risk for Impaired Skin Integrity is not a priority at this time. With education and knowledge about proper positioning, the client's skin and nipple area should remain intact. Although this is the client's first experience with breast-feeding, there is no evidence that the client is fearful. The client also has the support of her husband. (D, 3)

56. 3. Although various measures such as ice, heat, and massage may be tried to relieve breast engorgement, prevention of breast engorgement by frequent feedings is the method of choice. Expressing a little milk before nursing, massaging the breasts gently, or taking a warm shower before feeding also may help to improve milk flow. Applying ice to the nipples does not relieve breast engorgement. However, it may temporarily relieve the discomfort associated with breast engorgement. Using lanolin on the nipples does not relieve

breast engorgement and is unnecessary. Use of lanolin may cause sensitivity and irritation. Having frequent breast-feeding sessions, rather than offering the neonate a small amount of formula, is the method of choice for preventing and relieving breast engorgement. In addition, offering the neonate small amounts of formula may result in nipple confusion. (I, 3)

57. 1. The nurse should instruct the client that the baby is getting enough to eat when there are six to eight wet diapers by the fifth day of age. Other signs include good suckling sounds during feeding, dripping breast milk at the mouth, and quiet rest or sleep after the feeding. By the fourth day of age, the infant should have soft yellow stools, not transitional (greenish) stools. Falling asleep easily after feeding on the first day is not a good indicator because most infants are sleepy during the first 24 hours. Most infants regain their lost birth weight in 7 to 10 days after birth. An infant who has gained weight during the first well-baby checkup (usually at 2 weeks) is getting sufficient breast milk at feedings. (I, 3)

58. 4. The client should wean the infant gradually, eliminating one feeding at a time. The baby can be weaned to a bottle (formula) anytime the mother desires; she does not have to breast-feed for 4 months. Most infants (and mothers) develop a "favorite feeding time," so this feeding session should be eliminated last. The client may wish to begin weaning with daytime feedings when the infant is busy. (I, 3)

59. 4. Neonates normally increase breast-feeding during periods of rapid growth (growth spurts). These can be expected at age 10 to 14 days, 5 to 6 weeks, 2.5 to 3 months, and 4.5 to 6 months. Each growth spurt is usually followed by a regular feeding pattern. Lack of adequate intake to meet maternal nutritional needs is not associated with the neonate's desire for more frequent breast-feeding sessions. However, an intake of adequate calories is necessary to produce quality breast milk. The mother's fears about weight gain, and preventing the neonate from sucking long enough, are not associated with the desire for more frequent breast-feeding sessions. (D, 3)

60. 2. The best method is to prevent cracked nipples before they occur. This can be done by feeding frequently and using proper positioning. Even if the nipples are sore and cracked, the mother should position the baby with the entire areola in the baby's mouth so that the nipple is not compressed between the baby's gums during feeding. Warm, moist tea bags can soothe cracked nipples because of tannic acid in the tea. Creams on the nipples should be avoided; wiping off any lanolin creams from the nipple before each feeding can cause further soreness. Feeding the baby less often for the next few days will cause engorgement (and possible neonatal weight loss), leading to additional problems. Soap use while in the shower should be avoided to prevent drying and removal of protective oils. (I, 9)

The Postpartal Client Who Bottle-Feeds

61. 3. As a general rule, most neonates require 50 to 55 calories per pound of body weight, or about 117 calories per kilogram of weight, each day. If the neonate receives less than this amount, malnutrition may occur. More than this amount can lead to obesity. (P, 7)

62. 1. Initial regurgitation in the neonate during the first 12 to 24 hours may be caused by excessive mucus and gastric irritation from foreign substances in the stomach. After the first 24 hours, regurgitation is thought to be caused by the neonate's immature cardiac sphincter. It represents an overflow of stomach contents and is probably a result of feeding the neonate too fast or too much. A small amount of regurgitation is normal, but vomiting or forceful fluid expulsion is not. Burping the infant often during a feeding can decrease the amount of air in the stomach from swallowing. However, burping too often can lead the neonate to become tired or fussy. Moving the infant usually does not result in regurgitation. (I, 3)

63. 1. To aid digestion, the neonate should be placed in a supine position or on the right side propped with a small blanket roll after a feeding. Placing the neonate on the right side promotes gastric emptying and digestion. Placing the neonate in a prone position has been associated with sudden infant death syndrome. Although the mother may desire to hold the infant in her lap after feeding, this is not necessary for the neonate's digestion. (I, 3)

64. 2. Pediatricians recommend that neonates be given either breast milk or formula until at least 6 months of age because of the neonate's difficulty digesting solid foods. Giving solid foods too early can lead to food allergies. Because chewing movements do not begin until 7 to 9 months of age, foods requiring chewing should be delayed until this time. (I, 3)

65. 1. The client needs further instruction when she says burping should be done after 15 minutes of formula feeding. The entire feeding should take only 15 to 20 minutes, and the neonate should be burped before that time. During initial feedings, the burping should be done after each half-ounce of formula with the neonate in an upright position, patting the neonate gently on the back. (E, 3)

66. 2. Most babies are developmentally ready to drink independently from a cup by the age of 8 to 10 months. If the child has not mastered drinking from a cup by this time, there may be a problem with motor development that requires further investigation. (I, 3)

67. 2. Bottle "propping" is not recommended because it can lead to aspiration, delayed bonding, feelings of mistrust (Erikson), and possible otitis media. The neonate will not be overfed during bottle propping but may suck too quickly, possibly resulting in aspiration of the formula. Putting the neonate to bed with a bottle can lead to tooth decay later in the formative years, but an infant cannot hold the bottle. The cause of SIDS has not been determined. However, it is associated with placing the infant in a prone position after eating. (I, 9)

The Postpartal Client With a Cesarean Birth

68. 4. Slightly red-tinged urine may indicate that the bladder was accidentally cut during the cesarean delivery. The nurse should notify the physician as soon as possible about the urine color. Continuing to monitor the client's input and output should be done after the physician is contacted. Palpating the fundus every 15 minutes is not necessary unless the client's fundus becomes soft or "boggy." Assessment of the retention catheter is a normal part of the elimination assessment by the nurse, but displacement is not the cause of the red-tinged urine. (I, 9)

69. 3. The most appropriate response would be to explain that the vaginal spotting in female neonates is associated with hormones received from the mother. Estrogen is believed to cause slight vaginal bleeding or spotting in the female neonate. The condition disappears spontaneously, so there is no need for concern. Telling the mother that it is of no concern does not allay the mother's worry. The vaginal spotting is related to hormones received from the mother, not to swallowing blood during the delivery or hemorrhagic disease of the neonate. However, anemia is associated with hemorrhagic disease. (I, 3)

70. 1. VBAC can be attempted if the client has not had a classic uterine incision. This type of incision carries a danger of uterine rupture. A physician must be available, and a cesarean delivery must be possible within 30 minutes. A history of rapid labor is not a criterion for VBAC. A low transverse incision is not a contraindication for VBAC. A classic (vertical) incision is a contraindication because the client has a greater possibility for uterine rupture. Estimated fetal weight greater than 4000 g by itself is not a contraindication if the mother is not diabetic. (I, 3)

71. 4. Abdominal distention, a major source of discomfort for the postoperative client, is best relieved by having the client ambulate more frequently. Ambulation stimulates circulation and peristalsis, thereby promoting the passage of flatus. Carbonated beverages contribute to additional gas formation, as can drinking through a straw, and should be avoided. The client can progress from full liquids to soft foods and then to a regular diet, once bowel sounds are present. The client does not need to limit her diet to soft foods, but she may wish to avoid foods that increase intestinal gas, such as beans or brussels sprouts. (I, 7)

72. 3. For maximum effectiveness, RhoGAM should be administered within 72 hours postpartum. Most Rh-negative clients also receive RhoGAM during the prenatal period at 28 weeks' gestation and then again after delivery. If there is doubt about the fetus's blood type after pregnancy is terminated, the mother should receive the medication. The drug is given to Rh-negative mothers who have a negative Coombs test and deliver Rh-positive neonates. (P, 8)

73. 1. After a cesarean delivery, most mothers have the greatest comfort when the neonate is positioned in the football hold with the mother in a side-lying position, supporting the neonate's head in her hand and resting the neonate's body on pillows alongside her hip. This position prevents pressure on the uterine incision yet allows the neonate easy access to the mother's breast. The scissors hold, where the mother places her hand well back on the breast to prevent touching the areola and interfering with the neonate's mouth placement, is used by the mother to hold the breast and support it during breast-feeding. The cross-cradle hold is done when the mother holds the neonate's head in the hand opposite from the breast on which the neonate will feed and the mother's arm supports the neonate's body across her lap. This position can be uncomfortable because of the pressure placed on the client's incision line. For the cradle hold, the mother cradles the infant alongside the arm at the breast on which the neonate will feed. This position also can be uncomfortable because of the pressure placed on the incision line. (I, 7)

The Postpartal Client With Complications

74. 3. A positive Homan's sign, discomfort behind the knee or in the upper calf area on dorsiflexion of the foot, may be indicative of thrombophlebitis. Other signs include edema and redness at the site and may be more reliable as an indicator of thrombophlebitis. The nurse should notify the physician immediately and ask the client to remain in bed to minimize the risk for pulmonary embolus, a serious consequence of thrombophlebitis should the clot dislodge. The Homan sign is observed on the client's legs, so placing an ice pack on the perineal area is inappropriate. However, ice to the perineum would be useful for episiotomy pain and swelling. The client does not need to be positioned in a semi-Fowler's position but should remain on bed rest to prevent dislodgement of a potential clot. (I, 9)

75. 4. Heparin therapy is ordered to prevent further clot formation by inhibiting further thrombus and clot formation. Heparin, an anticoagulant, does not make blood clots thinner. A side effect of heparin therapy during the puerperium is increased lochia flow, so the nurse must be observant for symptoms of hemorrhage, such as heavy lochial flow. Heparin does not increase diaphoresis, which is normal for the postpartum client. (E, 8)

76. 2. A major complication of deep vein thrombosis is pulmonary embolism. Signs and symptoms, which may occur suddenly and require immediate treatment, include dyspnea, severe chest pain, apprehension, cough (possibly accompanied by hemoptysis), tachycardia, fever, hypotension, diaphoresis, pallor, shortness of breath, and friction rub. Pain in the calf is common with a diagnosis of deep vein thrombosis. Hypotension, not hypertension, would suggest a possible pulmonary embolism. It also could suggest possible hemorrhage secondary to intravenous heparin therapy. Bradycardia for the first 7 days in the postpartum period is normal. (A, 9)

77. 3. A slowed pulse, bradycardia, is normal for the first 7 days postpartum as the body begins to adjust to the decrease in blood volume and return to the prepregnant state. Side effects of heparin therapy suggesting hemorrhage include hematuria, epistaxis, ecchymosis, increased lochial flow, and bleeding gums. Typically, tachycardia, not bradycardia, would be associated with hemorrhage. (E, 9)

78. 3. Successful teaching is demonstrated when the client says, "I should use a soft toothbrush to brush my teeth." Heparin therapy can cause the gums to bleed, so a soft toothbrush should be used to minimize this side effect. Use of aspirin and other nonsteriodal anti-inflammatory medications should be avoided because of the increased risk for possible hemorrhage. Protamine sulfate is the antidote for heparin therapy. Vitamin K is the antidote for Coumadin excess. Alcohol can inhibit the metabolism of oral anticoagulants and should be avoided. (E, 8)

79. 2. Frequent vaginal examination during labor results in deposits of pathogens in the cervix and later invasion of the decidua by the pathogens. Vaginal trauma (eg, laceration) also increases the risk of infection. Additionally, manual delivery of the placenta, delivery of a large infant, use of forceps or a vacuum extractor, and catheterization during labor can contribute to a puerperal infection. Furthermore, poor nutritional status during the prenatal period can interfere with resistance to infection during the postpartum period. Maternal age older than 30 years is not associated with puerperal infection. Maternal age older than 35 years is associated with a higher incidence of Down syndrome.

Hemorrhage or blood loss greater than 500 mL can contribute to infection because of the loss of leukocytes in the blood. (I, 9)

80. 1. Before administering ampicillin sodium (Polycillin) intravenously, the nurse must ask the client if she has any drug allergies, especially to penicillin. Antibiotic therapy can cause adverse side effects such as rash or even anaphylaxis. If the client is allergic to penicillin, the physician should be notified and ampicillin should not be given. Placing the client in a side-lying position and checking her pulse rate are not necessary. Assessing the amount of lochia by checking the perineal pad is important for all postpartum clients but is not necessary before antibiotic therapy. (I, 8)

81. 3. The nurse should encourage the client to maintain Fowler's position, which promotes comfort and facilitates drainage. Endometritis can make the client feel extremely uncomfortable and fatigued, so ambulation during intravenous therapy is not as important at this time. The client does not need to discontinue breast-feeding, although she may become quite fatigued and need assistance in caring for the neonate. Typically, breast-feeding would be discontinued only if the mother lacks the necessary energy. The institution's policy regarding visitors is to be followed. However, visitors do not need to be restricted to prevent contamination because the client is not considered to be contagious. The nurse should maintain the client's need for privacy and rest and should respect the client's wishes related to visitors. (I, 9)

82. 2. The client diagnosed with cystitis needs to void every 2 to 4 hours while awake to keep her bladder empty. In addition, she should maintain adequate fluid intake; 3000 mL per day is recommended. Intake of acidic fruit juices (eg, cranberry, apricot) is recommended because of their association with reducing the risk for infection. The client should wear cotton underwear and avoid tight-fitting slacks. She does not need to wash with povidone iodine (Betadine) after voiding. Plain warm water is sufficient to keep the perineal area clean. (P, 7)

83. 4. Because the client has been requesting medication for back pain every 3 to 4 hours, the priority nursing diagnosis at this time is Pain related to dysuria and urinary frequency. There are no data to suggest Fear as a diagnosis, which would be evidenced by expression of feelings such as, "I'm afraid of needles." There are no data to suggest Ineffective Coping as a diagnosis. This diagnosis would be appropriate if the client expressed concerns about her children or husband and their abilities related to functioning at home while the client is hospitalized. Ineffective Role Performance would be appropriate if the client expresses an inability to perform her normal roles at home. (D, 10)

84. 1. The client can continue to breast-feed as often as she desires. Continuation of breast-feeding is limited only by the client's discomfort or malaise. Antibiotics for treatment are chosen carefully so that they avoid affecting the neonate through breast milk. Drugs such as sulfonamides, nitrofurantoin, and cephalosporins usually are not prescribed for breast-feeding mothers. Manual pumping of the breasts is not necessary. (I, 3)

85. 1. Methylergonovine maleate (Methergine) can cause hypertension, so the nurse should assess the client's blood pressure before and after administration. This drug should not be administered to clients who are hypertensive. Assessing pulse, respiration, and temperature is important for all postpartum clients to provide evidence of possible complications, such as infection. Tachycardia and diminished breath sounds are associated with pulmonary embolism, but these signs are not specific to methylergonovine (Methergine) administration. Assessing breath sounds would be important for a client who has had pregnancy-induced hypertension and received magnesium sulfate before delivery. However, by the fourth postpartum day, the effects of magnesium sulfate should have disappeared. Bowel sounds should be assessed after an operative delivery to determine whether peristalsis has begun so that the client can begin to drink clear liquids or eat soft foods. (A, 8)

86. 1. The client is exhibiting signs of early postpartal hemorrhage, defined as blood loss greater than 500 mL in the first 24 hours postpartum. Rapid intravenous oxytocin infusion of 40 to 80 units in 1000 mL of normal saline, oxygen therapy, and gentle fundal massage to contract the uterus are usually effective. If bleeding persists, the nurse should inspect the cervix and vagina for lacerations. Intramuscular or intravenous methylergonovine may be administered, but this drug elevates the blood pressure. Severe uncontrolled hemorrhage may require bimanual uterine compression, a dilation and curettage to remove any retained placental tissue, or a hysterectomy to prevent maternal death from hemorrhage. The client should be placed in the supine position to allow evaluation of the fundus. The side-lying position is not helpful in controlling postpartum hemorrhage. Vigorous fundal massage every 5 minutes is unnecessary. In addition, it can be very painful for the mother. Rather, gentle massage along with oxytocin administration is used to stimulate the uterus to contract. A hysteromyomectomy is used to remove fibroid tumors. With massive hemorrhage, a hysterectomy (removal of the uterus) may be necessary to control the bleeding. (P, 3)

87. 4. The most likely cause of this client's uterine atony is overdistention of the uterus caused by the hydramnios. As a result, the stretched uterine musculature contracts

less vigorously. Besides hydramnios, a large infant, bleeding from abruptio placenta or placenta previa, and rapid labor and delivery can also contribute to uterine atony during the postpartum period. Trauma during labor and delivery is not a likely cause. In addition, no evidence of excessive trauma was described in the scenario. Moderate fundal massage helps to contract the uterus, not contribute to uterine atony. Although a lengthy or prolonged labor can contribute to uterine atony, this client had a cesarean delivery for breech presentation. Therefore, it is unlikely that she had a long labor. (I, 10)

88. 4. Scant and odorless vaginal discharge is associated with endometritis due to β-hemolytic streptococcus. The client also will exhibit "sawtooth" temperature spikes between 101° and 104°F (38.3° to 40°C), tachycardia, and chills. The classic symptom of foul-smelling lochia is not associated with this type of endometritis. Profuse and foul-smelling lochia is associated with classic endometritis from pathogens such as chlamydia or staphylococcus, not group B hemolytic streptococcus. Abdominal distention is associated with parametritis as the pelvic cellulitis advances and spreads, causing severe pain and distention. Nausea and vomiting are associated with parametritis resulting from an abscess and advancing pelvic cellulitis. (A, 9)

89. 4. The most likely cause of delayed postpartum hemorrhage is retained placental fragments. Methylergonovine 0.2 mg is typically ordered for these clients to maintain uterine tone and expel the placental fragments. In severe cases, the client may be scheduled for a dilation and curettage to remove any remaining placental fragments. Uterine atony, cervical lacerations, and vaginal lacerations are commonly associated with early, not late, postpartum hemorrhage. (I, 3)

90. 1. The client being treated for infectious mastitis should continue to breast-feed often, or at least every 2 to 3 hours. Treatment also includes bed rest, increased fluid intake, local heat application, analgesics, and antibiotic therapy. Continually emptying the breasts decreases the risk of engorgement or breast abscess. The client should not discontinue breast-feeding unless she chooses to do so. The client may continue breast-feeding while receiving antibiotic therapy. Generally, the breast milk is not contaminated by the offending organism and is safe for the neonate. (I, 10)

91. 1. Down syndrome is a genetic abnormality that is caused by an extra chromosome that results in mental retardation. The degree of mental retardation is difficult to predict in a neonate, although most children born with Down syndrome have some degree of mental retardation. Various methods can be used to determine whether a neonate has Down syndrome, which is commonly manifested by hypotonia, poor Moro reflex, flat facial profile, upslanting palpebral fissures, epicanthal folds, and hyperflexible joints. Genetic studies can be indicative of this disorder. Mothers older than 35 years of age are at a higher risk for having a child with Down syndrome. However, chromosomal abnormalities can occur regardless of the mother's age. (E, 9)

92. 1. After birth, the client should make the decision about how much she would like to participate in the neonate's care. Seeing and caring for the neonate often facilitates the grief process. The nurse should be nonjudgmental and should allow the client any opportunity to see, hold, and care for the neonate. The physician does not need to be contacted about the client's desire to see the baby, which is a normal reaction. The social worker and the adoptive parents do not need to give the client permission to feed the baby. (I, 3)

93. 4. The client needs further instruction when she says that she should begin feeding on the right (painful) breast to decrease the pain. Starting the feeding on the unaffected (left) breast can stimulate the milk ejection reflex in the right breast and thereby decrease the pain. For some mothers, mastitis is so painful that they choose to discontinue breast-feeding, so these mothers need a great deal of support. Applying heat to the infected area before starting to feed is appropriate because heat stimulates circulation and promotes comfort. Increasing fluid intake is advised to ensure adequate hydration. Antibiotics need to be taken until all medication has been used, usually 7 to 10 days to ensure eradication of the infection. (E, 9)

94. 3. The client is probably experiencing postpartum depression, and the doctor should be contacted. Postpartum depression is usually treated with psychotherapy, social support groups, and antidepressant medications. Contributing factors include hormonal fluctuations, a history of depression, and environmental factors (eg, job loss). An estimated 50% to 70% of women experience some degree of postpartum blues, but these feelings of sadness disappear within 1 to 2 weeks after birth. However, the client is voicing more than just sadness. Telling her that she is overreacting is not helpful and may make her feel even less worthy. She is not exhibiting symptoms of a serious mental illness (loss of contact with reality) and does not need hospitalization. (E, 3)

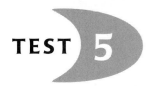

TEST 5

The Neonatal Client

- ▶ The Neonatal Client
- ▶ Physical Assessment of the Neonatal Client
- ▶ The Preterm Neonate
- ▶ The Post-term Neonate
- ▶ The Neonate With Risk Factors
- ▶ Correct Answers and Rationale

Select the one best answer, and indicate your choice by filling in the circle in front of the option.

The Neonatal Client

1. The nurse makes a home visit to a 3-day-old full-term neonate who weighed 3912 g (8 pounds, 10 ounces) at birth. Today the neonate, who is being bottle-fed, weighs 3572 g (7 pounds, 14 ounces). Which of the following instructions would the nurse *most* likely give to the mother?
   - ○ 1. Continue feeding every 3 to 4 hours since the weight loss is normal.
   - ○ 2. Contact the physician if the weight loss continues over the next few days.
   - ○ 3. Switch to a soy-based formula because the current one seems inadequate.
   - ○ 4. Change to a higher-calorie formula to prevent further weight loss.

2. A viable female neonate delivered vaginally at term has Apgar scores of 9 at 1 minute and 10 at 5 minutes after birth. Immediately postpartum, the nurse keeps the infant under a radiant warmer away from the cooling ducts in the room to prevent heat loss by which of the following mechanisms?
   - ○ 1. Evaporation.
   - ○ 2. Convection.
   - ○ 3. Conduction.
   - ○ 4. Radiation.

3. After explaining to the mother of a male neonate scheduled to receive an injection of vitamin K soon after birth about the rationale for the medication, which of the following statements by the mother indicates successful teaching?
   - ○ 1. "My baby doesn't have the normal bacteria in his intestines to produce this vitamin."
   - ○ 2. "My baby is at a high risk for a problem involving his blood's ability to clot."
   - ○ 3. "The red blood cells my baby formed during pregnancy are destroying the vitamin K."

   - ○ 4. "My baby's liver is not able to produce enough of this vitamin so soon after birth."

4. When developing the teaching plan for a new mother about the neonate's need for sensory and visual stimulation, information about which of the following as the most highly developed sense in the neonate would the nurse expect to include?
   - ○ 1. Taste.
   - ○ 2. Hearing.
   - ○ 3. Touch.
   - ○ 4. Vision.

5. While making a home visit to a primiparous client and her 3-day-old son, the nurse observes the mother changing the baby's disposable diaper. Before putting the clean diaper on the neonate, the mother begins to apply baby powder to the neonate's buttocks. Which of the following statements about baby powder would the nurse relate to the mother?
   - ○ 1. It may cause pneumonia to develop.
   - ○ 2. It helps prevent diaper rash.
   - ○ 3. It keeps the diaper from adhering to the skin.
   - ○ 4. It can result in allergies later in life.

6. After teaching a new mother about the care of her neonate after circumcision with a Gomco clamp, which of the following statements by the mother would indicate to the nurse that the mother needs *additional* instructions?
   - ○ 1. "The petroleum gauze may fall off into the diaper."
   - ○ 2. "A few drops of blood oozing from the site is normal."
   - ○ 3. "I'll leave the gauze in place for 24 hours."
   - ○ 4. "I'll remove any yellowish crusting gently with water."

7. After completing discharge instructions for a primipara who is bottle-feeding her term neonate, the

nurse determines that the mother understands the instructions when the mother says that she should contact the pediatrician if the neonate exhibits which of the following?
- ○ 1. Ability to fall asleep easily after each feeding.
- ○ 2. Spitting up of a tablespoon of formula after feeding.
- ○ 3. Passage of a liquid stool with a watery ring.
- ○ 4. Production of one to two light brown stools daily.

8. The nurse instructs a primiparous client about bottle-feeding her neonate. Which of the following demonstrates that the mother has understood the nurse's instructions?
- ○ 1. Placing the neonate on the back after the feeding.
- ○ 2. Bubbling the baby after 1 ounce of formula.
- ○ 3. Putting three fourths of the bottle nipple into the baby's mouth.
- ○ 4. Pointing the nipple toward the neonate's palate.

9. When caring for a term neonate during the first hour after birth, the nurse expects to assess the neonate's blood glucose level, obtaining the blood sample from the neonate's foot near which of the following areas?
- ○ 1. Lateral aspect of the heel.
- ○ 2. Middle of the heel.
- ○ 3. Middle of the foot.
- ○ 4. Base of the toes.

10. After circumcision with a Plastibell, the nurse instructs the neonate's mother to cleanse the circumcision site with which of the following?
- ○ 1. Antibacterial soap.
- ○ 2. Warm water.
- ○ 3. Povidone-iodine (Betadine) solution.
- ○ 4. Diluted hydrogen peroxide.

11. Approximately 90 minutes after birth, the nurse encourages the mother of a term neonate to do which of the following?
- ○ 1. Feed the neonate.
- ○ 2. Allow the neonate to sleep.
- ○ 3. Get to know the neonate.
- ○ 4. Change the neonate's diaper.

Physical Assessment of the Neonatal Client

12. After a vaginal delivery of a term neonate, the nurse observes that the neonate has one artery and one vein in the umbilical cord. The nurse notifies the pediatrician based on the analysis that this may be indicative of which of the following?
- ○ 1. Respiratory anomalies.
- ○ 2. Musculoskeletal anomalies.
- ○ 3. Cardiovascular anomalies.
- ○ 4. Facial anomalies.

13. While assessing a male neonate about 12 hours old after a vaginal delivery, the nurse notes a swelling on the neonate's scalp that crosses the suture line. The nurse interprets this finding as indicating which of the following?
- ○ 1. Cephalohematoma.
- ○ 2. Caput succedaneum.
- ○ 3. Cranial edema.
- ○ 4. Craniotabes.

14. Shortly after birth, the nurse measures the circumference of a term neonate's head and chest. When the two measurements are compared, which of the following would the nurse expect to find about the head circumference?
- ○ 1. Equal to the chest circumference.
- ○ 2. Approximately 2 cm larger than the chest.
- ○ 3. About 3 cm smaller than the chest.
- ○ 4. Approximately 4 cm larger than the chest.

15. After explaining to a primiparous client about the causes of her neonate's cranial molding, which of the following statements by the mother indicates the need for *further* instruction?
- ○ 1. "The molding was caused by an overlapping of the baby's cranial bones during my labor."
- ○ 2. "The amount of molding is related to the amount and length of pressure on the head."
- ○ 3. "The molding will usually disappear in a couple of days."
- ○ 4. "Brain damage may occur if the molding doesn't resolve quickly."

16. Initial assessment of a term female neonate about 4 hours old reveals a normal anterior fontanel. The nurse documents its shape as which of the following?
- ○ 1. Oval.
- ○ 2. Square.
- ○ 3. Diamond shaped.
- ○ 4. Triangular.

17. Which of the following observations would the nurse expect when assessing the gestational age of a neonate delivered at term?
- ○ 1. Ear lying flat against the head.
- ○ 2. Absence of rugae in the scrotum.
- ○ 3. Sole creases covering the entire foot.
- ○ 4. Square window sign angle of 90 degrees.

18. While performing a complete assessment of a term neonate, which of the following findings would alert the nurse to notify the pediatrician?
- ○ 1. Red reflex in the eyes.
- ○ 2. Expiratory grunt.
- ○ 3. Respiratory rate of 45 breaths/minute.
- ○ 4. Prominent xiphoid process.

19. After instructing a mother about normal reflexes of

term neonates, the nurse determines that the mother understands the instructions when she describes the tonic neck reflex as occurring when the neonate does which of the following?
- ○ 1. Steps briskly when held upright near a firm, hard surface.
- ○ 2. Pulls both arms and does not move the chin beyond the point of the elbows.
- ○ 3. Turns head to the left, extends left extremities, and flexes right extremities.
- ○ 4. Extends and abducts the arms and legs with the toes fanning open.

20. A primiparous client expresses concern, asking the nurse why her neonate's eyes are crossed. Which of the following would the nurse include when teaching the mother about neonatal strabismus?
- ○ 1. The neonate's eyes are unable to focus on light at this time.
- ○ 2. Neonates commonly lack eye muscle coordination.
- ○ 3. Congenital cataracts may be present.
- ○ 4. The neonate is able to fixate on distant objects immediately.

21. While performing a physical assessment on a term neonate shortly after birth, which of the following would cause the nurse to notify the pediatrician?
- ○ 1. Deep creases across the soles of the feet.
- ○ 2. Frequent sneezing during the assessment.
- ○ 3. Single crease on each of the palms.
- ○ 4. Absence of lanugo on the skin.

22. Assessment of a term neonate at 2 hours after birth reveals a heart rate of 110 bpm, periods of apnea approximately 25 to 30 seconds in length, and mild cyanosis around the mouth. The nurse notifies the pediatrician based on the interpretation that these findings may lead to which of the following?
- ○ 1. Respiratory arrest.
- ○ 2. Bronchial pneumonia.
- ○ 3. Intraventricular hemorrhage.
- ○ 4. Epiglottitis.

23. A new mother asks, "When will the soft spot near the front of my baby's head close?" Which of the following ages would the nurse include when responding to the mother about closure of the anterior fontanel?
- ○ 1. 2 to 3 months.
- ○ 2. 6 to 8 months.
- ○ 3. 9 to 10 months.
- ○ 4. 12 to 18 months.

24. Which of the following assessment findings in a term neonate would cause the nurse to notify the pediatrician?
- ○ 1. Absence of tears.
- ○ 2. Unequally sized corneas.
- ○ 3. Pupillary constriction to bright light.

- ○ 4. Red circle on pupils with ophthalmoscopic examination.

25. At 24 hours of age, assessment of the neonate reveals the following: eyes closed, skin pink, no sign of eye movements, heart rate of 120 bpm, and respiratory rate of 35 breaths/minute. The nurse interprets these findings as indicating that this neonate is *most* likely experiencing which of the following?
- ○ 1. Drug withdrawal.
- ○ 2. First period of reactivity.
- ○ 3. A state of deep sleep.
- ○ 4. Respiratory distress.

26. While assessing a male neonate whose mother desires him to be circumcised, the nurse observes that the neonate's urinary meatus appears to be located on the ventral surface of the penis. The physician is notified because the nurse suspects which of the following?
- ○ 1. Phimosis.
- ○ 2. Hydrocele.
- ○ 3. Epispadias.
- ○ 4. Hypospadias.

The Preterm Neonate

27. A neonate at 37 weeks' gestation is delivered by cesarean delivery because of placenta previa. Which of the following would the circulating nurse do *first* as soon as the neonate is delivered?
- ○ 1. Stimulate the neonate to cry vigorously.
- ○ 2. Aspirate mucus from the mouth with a bulb syringe.
- ○ 3. Begin resuscitation procedures with a bag and mask.
- ○ 4. Hold the neonate upright for the mother to view.

28. After a vaginal delivery, a preterm neonate is to receive oxygen via mask. While administering the oxygen, the nurse would place the neonate in which of the following positions?
- ○ 1. Left side, with the neck slightly flexed.
- ○ 2. Back, with the head turned to the left side.
- ○ 3. Abdomen, with the head down.
- ○ 4. Back, with the neck slightly extended.

29. Which of the following would the nurse do when performing external cardiac massage on a neonate born at 28 weeks' gestation?
- ○ 1. Alternate cardiac massage with ventilation.
- ○ 2. Compress the sternum with the palm of the hand.
- ○ 3. Compress the chest 70 to 80 times per minute.
- ○ 4. Displace the chest wall 1.5 inches.

30. A preterm neonate who has been stabilized is placed in a radiant warmer and is receiving oxygen via an

oxygen hood. While administering oxygen in this manner, the nurse would do which of the following?
- ○ 1. Humidify the air being delivered.
- ○ 2. Cover the neonate's scalp with a warm cap.
- ○ 3. Record the neonate's temperature every 3 to 4 minutes.
- ○ 4. Assess the neonate's blood glucose level.

31. Two hours ago, a neonate at 38 weeks' gestation and weighing 3175 g (7 pounds) was born to a primipara who tested positive for β-hemolytic streptococcus. Which of the following would alert the nurse to notify the pediatrician?
- ○ 1. Alkalosis.
- ○ 2. Increased muscle tone.
- ○ 3. Temperature instability.
- ○ 4. Bradycardia.

32. Which of the following would the nurse suspect when assessment of a 2-day-old neonate delivered at 34 weeks' gestation reveals absent apical pulse left of the midclavicular line, cyanosis, grunting, and diminished breath sounds?
- ○ 1. Diaphragmatic hernia.
- ○ 2. Pneumothorax.
- ○ 3. Coarctation of the aorta.
- ○ 4. Bacterial pneumonia.

33. Twenty-four hours after cesarean delivery, a neonate at 30 weeks' gestation is diagnosed with respiratory distress syndrome (RDS). When explaining to the parents about the cause of this syndrome, the nurse would include a discussion about an alteration in the body's secretion of which of the following?
- ○ 1. Somatotropin.
- ○ 2. Surfactant.
- ○ 3. Testosterone.
- ○ 4. Progesterone.

34. When caring for a neonate born at 30 weeks' gestation who is in an isolette and receiving continuous oxygen, which of the following would the nurse use as the *best* method to determine the effectiveness of this treatment?
- ○ 1. Evidence of cyanosis on mouth, hands, and feet.
- ○ 2. Continuous pulse rate monitoring.
- ○ 3. Arterial blood gas levels.
- ○ 4. Percentage of oxygen delivered.

35. A viable male neonate delivered to a 28-year-old multipara via cesarean delivery because of placenta previa is diagnosed with RDS. Which of the following would the nurse explain as the factor placing the neonate at the greatest risk for this syndrome?
- ○ 1. Mother's development of placenta previa.
- ○ 2. Neonate delivered preterm.
- ○ 3. Mother receiving analgesia 4 hours before delivery.
- ○ 4. Neonate with sluggish respiratory efforts after delivery.

36. While the nurse is caring for a neonate at 32 weeks' gestation in an isolette with continuous oxygen administration, the neonate's mother asks why the neonate's oxygen is humidified. Which of the following would be the nurse's *best* response?
- ○ 1. "The humidity promotes expansion of the neonate's immature lungs."
- ○ 2. "The humidity helps to prevent viral or bacterial pneumonia."
- ○ 3. "Oxygen is drying to the mucous membranes unless it is humidified."
- ○ 4. "Circulation to the baby's heart is improved with humidified oxygen."

37. A preterm neonate admitted to the neonatal intensive care nursery at about 30 weeks' gestation is placed in an oxygenated isolette. The neonate's mother tells the nurse that she was planning to breast-feed the neonate. Which of the following instructions about breast-feeding would be *most* appropriate?
- ○ 1. Breast-feeding is not recommended because the neonate needs increased fat in the diet.
- ○ 2. Once the neonate no longer needs oxygen and continuous monitoring, breast-feeding can be done.
- ○ 3. Breast-feeding is contraindicated because the neonate needs a high-calorie formula every 2 hours.
- ○ 4. Gavage feedings using breast milk can be given until the neonate can coordinate sucking and swallowing.

38. Which of the following *best* identifies the reason for assessing a neonate weighing 1500 g who was delivered vaginally at 32 weeks' gestation for retinopathy of prematurity (ROP)?
- ○ 1. The neonate is at risk because of multiple factors.
- ○ 2. Oxygen is being administered at a level of 28%.
- ○ 3. The neonate was alkalotic immediately after birth.
- ○ 4. Phototherapy is likely to be ordered by the pediatrician.

39. Which of the following would lead the nurse to suspect ROP when assessing a neonate at 32 weeks' gestation who weighs 2000 g?
- ○ 1. Sunken orbital sockets.
- ○ 2. Strabismus.
- ○ 3. Reaction to bright light.
- ○ 4. Constricted retinal vessels.

40. Which of the following would the nurse include when teaching the mother of a neonate diagnosed with ROP about possible treatment for complications?
- ○ 1. Cryotherapy.
- ○ 2. Cromolyn sodium (Intal) eye drops.

○ 3. Frequent testing for glaucoma.

○ 4. Corneal transplants.

41. Which of the following nursing diagnoses would be the *priority* for a neonate admitted to the neonatal intensive care nursery at 28 weeks' gestation weighing 1474 g (3 pounds, 4 ounces)?
    ○ 1. Risk for Impaired Skin Integrity related to gestational age.
    ○ 2. Imbalanced Nutrition: Less than Body Requirements, related to preterm gestational age.
    ○ 3. Impaired Gas Exchange related to immature pulmonary vasculature.
    ○ 4. Risk for Delayed Development related to prematurity.

42. Three days after admission of a neonate delivered at 30 weeks' gestation, the neonatologist plans to assess the neonate for periventricular-intraventricular hemorrhage (PIVH). The nurse would plan to assist the neonatologist by preparing the neonate for which of the following?
    ○ 1. Computed tomography scan.
    ○ 2. Arterial blood specimen collection.
    ○ 3. Radiographs of the skull.
    ○ 4. Complete blood count specimen collection.

43. Which of the following would the nurse expect to assess in a neonate delivered at 28 weeks' gestation who is diagnosed with PIVH?
    ○ 1. Increased muscle tone.
    ○ 2. Hyperbilirubinemia.
    ○ 3. Bulging fontanels.
    ○ 4. Hyperactivity.

44. While caring for a neonate delivered at 32 weeks' gestation, the nurse assesses the neonate daily for symptoms of necrotizing enterocolitis (NEC). Which of the following would alert the nurse to notify the neonatologist?
    ○ 1. The presence of 1 mL of gastric residual before a gavage feeding.
    ○ 2. Jaundice appearing on the face and chest.
    ○ 3. An increase in bowel peristalsis.
    ○ 4. Abdominal distention.

45. Which of the following statements by the mother of a neonate diagnosed with bronchopulmonary dysplasia (BPD) indicates effective teaching?
    ○ 1. "BPD is an acute disease that can be treated with antibiotics."
    ○ 2. "My baby may require permanent assisted ventilation."
    ○ 3. "Bronchodilators can cure my baby's condition."
    ○ 4. "My baby may have seizures later on in life because of this condition."

46. A neonate delivered at 34 weeks' gestation is diagnosed with a pneumothorax. Which of the following would the nurse expect the neonatologist to order?
    ○ 1. Placement of the neonate on a ventilator.
    ○ 2. Administration of bronchodilators through the nares.
    ○ 3. Suctioning of the neonate's nares with wall suction.
    ○ 4. Insertion of a chest tube into the neonate.

47. Which of the following would alert the nurse to suspect that a neonate delivered at 34 weeks' gestation who is currently in an isolette with humidified oxygen and receiving intravenous fluids has developed overhydration?
    ○ 1. Hypernatremia.
    ○ 2. Polycythemia.
    ○ 3. Hypoproteinemia.
    ○ 4. Increased urine specific gravity.

The Post-term Neonate

48. A neonate born by cesarean delivery at 42 weeks' gestation, weighing 4.1 kg (9 pounds, 1 ounce), with Apgar scores of 8 at 1 minute and 9 at 5 minutes after birth, develops an increased respiratory rate and tremors of the hands and feet 2 hours postpartum. Which of the following nursing diagnoses would be the *priority*?
    ○ 1. Ineffective Airway Clearance related to post-term gestational age.
    ○ 2. Hyperthermia related to large size and use of a radiant warmer.
    ○ 3. Decreased Cardiac Output related to difficult delivery.
    ○ 4. Imbalanced Nutrition: Less Than Body Requirements, related to depleted glycogen stores.

49. At a home visit, the nurse assesses a neonate delivered vaginally at 41 weeks' gestation 5 days ago, noting the following findings: frequent hiccups; loose, watery stool in diaper; red rash on face; and dry, peeling skin. Which of these findings warrants further assessment?
    ○ 1. Frequent hiccups.
    ○ 2. Loose, watery stool in diaper.
    ○ 3. Pink papular vesicles on the face.
    ○ 4. Dry, peeling skin.

50. When performing an initial assessment of a post-term male neonate weighing 4000 g (9 pounds) who was admitted to the observation nursery after a vaginal delivery with low forceps, the nurse detects Ortolani's sign. Which of the following would the nurse do next?
    ○ 1. Determine the length of the mother's labor.
    ○ 2. Notify the pediatrician immediately.
    ○ 3. Keep the neonate under the radiant warmer for 2 hours.
    ○ 4. Obtain a blood sample to check for hypoglycemia.

51. A neonate is admitted to the neonatal intensive care nursery for observation with a diagnosis of probable meconium aspiration syndrome (MAS). The neonate weighs 4650 g (10 pounds, 4 ounces) and is at 41 weeks' gestation. Which of the following nursing diagnoses would be the *priority* for this neonate?
    ○ 1. Impaired Skin Integrity related to post-term status.
    ○ 2. Imbalanced Nutrition: More than Body Requirements related to large size.
    ○ 3. Risk for Impaired Parent/Infant/Child Attachment related to transfer to the intensive care unit.
    ○ 4. Impaired Gas Exchange related to the effects of respiratory distress.

52. When developing the initial plan of care for a neonate born at 41 weeks' gestation and diagnosed with MAS, which of the following would the nurse include?
    ○ 1. Care of an umbilical arterial line.
    ○ 2. Frequent ultrasound scans.
    ○ 3. Orogastric feedings as soon as possible.
    ○ 4. Assessment for symptoms of hyperglycemia.

53. A post-term neonate diagnosed with persistent pulmonary hypertension is prescribed intravenous tolazoline (Priscoline). Which of the following would the nurse need to monitor while administering this drug?
    ○ 1. Feeding behaviors.
    ○ 2. Temperature.
    ○ 3. Skin color.
    ○ 4. Blood pressure.

The Neonate With Risk Factors

54. A multiparous client who has a neonate diagnosed with hemolytic disease of the newborn asks the nurse why the neonate has developed this problem. Which of the following responses by the nurse would be *most* appropriate?
    ○ 1. "You are Rh positive and the neonate's father is Rh negative."
    ○ 2. "You and the neonate's father are both Rh negative."
    ○ 3. "You are Rh negative and the neonate's father is Rh positive."
    ○ 4. "The fetus is Rh negative and you are Rh positive."

55. After teaching the multiparous mother about hemolytic disease of the newborn and Rh sensitization, the nurse determines that the client understands why she was not sensitized during her other pregnancy when she says which of the following?
    ○ 1. "My other baby had a different father."

○ 2. "Like most women, I have immunity against the Rh factor."
    ○ 3. "Antibodies are not usually formed until after exposure to an antigen."
    ○ 4. "My blood couldn't neutralize antibodies formed from my first pregnancy."

56. After teaching a multipara about the effects of hemolysis due to Rh sensitization on the neonate at delivery, the nurse determines that the client needs *further* instruction when the mother reports that the neonate may have which of the following?
    ○ 1. Cardiac decompensation.
    ○ 2. Polycythemia.
    ○ 3. Anemia.
    ○ 4. Splenic enlargement.

57. After delivery, a direct Coombs test is performed on the umbilical cord blood of a neonate with Rh-positive blood born to a mother with Rh-negative blood. The nurse explains to the client that this test is done to detect which of the following?
    ○ 1. Degree of anemia in the neonate.
    ○ 2. Electrolyte imbalances in the neonate.
    ○ 3. Antibodies coating the neonate's red blood cells.
    ○ 4. Antigens coating the neonate's red blood cells.

58. After teaching the mother of a neonate with erythroblastosis fetalis who is to receive an exchange transfusion, which of the following, if stated by the mother as the purpose of the transfusion, indicates effective teaching?
    ○ 1. To replenish the neonate's leukocytes.
    ○ 2. To restore the fluid and electrolyte balance.
    ○ 3. To correct the neonate's anemia.
    ○ 4. To replace Rh-negative blood with Rh-positive blood.

59. The nurse explains to the mother of a neonate diagnosed with erythroblastosis fetalis that the exchange transfusion is necessary to prevent damage *primarily* to which of the following organs in the neonate?
    ○ 1. Kidneys
    ○ 2. Brain.
    ○ 3. Lungs.
    ○ 4. Liver.

60. A neonate whose mother has insulin-dependent diabetes weighs 4564 g (10 pounds, 1 ounce), is large for gestational age, and is admitted to the neonatal intensive care unit. Which of the following would be a priority nursing diagnosis for this neonate?
    ○ 1. Hyperthermia related to size large for gestational age.
    ○ 2. Impaired Skin Integrity related to maternal diabetes.

○ 3. Risk for Disproportionate Growth related to excessive birth weight.

○ 4. Imbalanced Nutrition: Less Than Body Requirements related to increased glucose metabolism.

61. The nurse is caring for an infant of an insulin-dependent diabetic primiparous client. When the mother visits the neonate at 1 hour after birth, the nurse explains to the mother that the neonate is being closely monitored for symptoms of hypoglycemia because of which of the following?

○ 1. Increased use of glucose stores during a difficult labor and delivery process.

○ 2. Interrupted supply of maternal glucose and continued high neonatal insulin production.

○ 3. A normal response that occurs during transition from intrauterine to extrauterine life.

○ 4. Increased pancreatic enzyme production caused by decreased glucose stores.

62. When caring for the neonate of a diabetic mother weighing 4564 g (10 pounds, 1 ounce) who was delivered vaginally, the nurse would assess the neonate for fracture of which of the following?

○ 1. Clavicle.

○ 2. Skull.

○ 3. Wrist.

○ 4. Rib cage.

63. While caring for a neonate of a diabetic mother soon after delivery, after the neonate has received treatment for hypoglycemia, the nurse observes that the neonate's blood glucose level is 60 mg/dL but the neonate is still exhibiting jitteriness and tremors. The nurse notifies the physician because these symptoms may indicate which of the following?

○ 1. Phenylketonuria.

○ 2. Biliary duct obstruction.

○ 3. Viral infection.

○ 4. Hypocalcemia.

64. The nurse is caring for a neonate of a class B insulin-dependent diabetic primiparous client who weighs 4536 g (10 pounds). The infant was born via cesarean delivery 1 hour ago. The mother asks the nurse, "Why is my baby in the neonatal intensive care unit?" The nurse bases the response on the understanding that neonates of class B diabetic mothers frequently develop which of the following?

○ 1. Anemia.

○ 2. Persistent pulmonary hypertension.

○ 3. Hemolytic disease.

○ 4. Hypoglycemia.

65. While assessing a neonate weighing 3175 g (7 pounds) who was born at 39 weeks' gestation to a primipara who admits to cocaine use during pregnancy, which of the following would alert the nurse to possible cocaine withdrawal?

○ 1. Bradycardia.

○ 2. High-pitched cry.

○ 3. Sluggishness.

○ 4. Hypocalcemia.

66. After teaching a primiparous client who used cocaine during pregnancy about possible gastrointestinal signs and symptoms in her neonate, which of the following, if stated by the mother as common, indicates effective teaching?

○ 1. Colic.

○ 2. Constipation.

○ 3. Vomiting.

○ 4. Abdominal distention.

67. When teaching a primiparous client who used cocaine during pregnancy how to comfort her neonate when the neonate fussy, which of the following would the nurse suggest?

○ 1. Tightly swaddling the neonate.

○ 2. Feeding the neonate extra, high-calorie formula.

○ 3. Keeping the neonate in a brightly lit environment.

○ 4. Minimizing touching of the neonate (touching only when the neonate is crying).

68. A neonate born at 38 weeks' gestation is admitted to the neonatal nursery for observation. The neonate's mother, who is positive for human immunodeficiency virus (HIV) infection, has received no prenatal care. The mother asks the nurse if her neonate is positive for HIV. The nurse instructs the mother that

○ 1. more than 50% of neonates born to mothers who are positive for HIV will be positive at 18 months of age.

○ 2. an enlarged liver at birth generally means the neonate is HIV positive.

○ 3. a complete blood count analysis is the primary method for determining whether the neonate is HIV positive.

○ 4. most neonates are asymptomatic at birth and usually test positive for the HIV antibody at this time.

69. When caring for a multiparous client who is HIV positive and asking to breast-feed her neonate as soon as possible, which of the following instructions about breast milk would the nurse include in the teaching plan?

○ 1. It may help prevent the spread of the HIV virus.

○ 2. It contains antibodies that can protect the neonate from HIV.

○ 3. It can be beneficial for the bonding process.

○ 4. It has been found to contain the retrovirus HIV.

70. While caring for the neonate of an HIV-positive mother, the nurse prepares to administer an ordered hepatitis B intramuscular injection at 4 hours after

birth. Which of the following would the nurse do *first*?
- ○ 1. Bathe the neonate with an antibacterial soap.
- ○ 2. Place the neonate under a radiant warmer.
- ○ 3. Wash the injection site with povidone-iodine (Betadine) solution.
- ○ 4. Apply clean gloves before administering the medication.

71. A male neonate born at 38 weeks' gestation by cesarean delivery after prolonged rupture of the membranes and a maternal oral temperature of 102°F (38.8°C) is being observed for signs and symptoms of infection. Which of the following would alert the nurse to notify the physician?
- ○ 1. Leukocytosis.
- ○ 2. Apical heart rate of 132 bpm.
- ○ 3. Behavioral changes.
- ○ 4. Warm, moist skin.

72. The nurse is caring for a neonate shortly after birth when the neonate is diagnosed with sepsis and is to be treated with intravenous antibiotics. Which of the following will the nurse need to instruct the parents to do because of the neonate's infection?
- ○ 1. Use caution near the isolation incubator and equipment.
- ○ 2. Visit but do not touch the neonate.
- ○ 3. Wash their hands thoroughly before touching the neonate.
- ○ 4. Wear a mask when holding the neonate.

73. A female neonate delivered vaginally at term with a cleft lip and cleft palate is admitted to the regular nursery. Which of the following would the nurse do the first time that the parents visit the neonate in the nursery?
- ○ 1. Explain the surgical interventions that will be performed.
- ○ 2. Stress that this defect is not life-threatening.
- ○ 3. Emphasize the neonate's normal characteristics.
- ○ 4. Reassure the parents about the success rate of the surgery.

74. After teaching the parents of a neonate born with a cleft lip and cleft palate about appropriate feeding techniques, the nurse determines that the mother needs *further* instruction when the mother says which of the following?
- ○ 1. "I should clean her mouth with soapy water after feeding."
- ○ 2. "I should feed her in an upright position."
- ○ 3. "I need to remember to burp her often."
- ○ 4. "I may need to use a special nipple for feeding."

75. Which of the following would the nurse identify as a *priority* nursing diagnosis for a neonate diagnosed with a cleft palate at 1 hour postpartum?

- ○ 1. Activity Intolerance related to respiratory distress syndrome.
- ○ 2. Risk for Infection related to potential aspiration during feedings.
- ○ 3. Compromised Family Coping related to congenital malformation of the neonate.
- ○ 4. Impaired Skin Integrity related to frequent treatments and feedings.

76. A male neonate born at 36 weeks' gestation is admitted to the neonatal intensive care nursery with a diagnosis of probable fetal alcohol syndrome (FAS). The mother visits the nursery soon after the neonate is admitted. Which of the following would the nurse expect to include when developing the teaching plan for the mother about FAS?
- ○ 1. Withdrawal symptoms usually do not occur until 7 days postpartum.
- ○ 2. Large-for-gestational-age size is common with this condition.
- ○ 3. Facial deformities associated with FAS can be corrected by plastic surgery.
- ○ 4. Symptoms of withdrawal include tremors, sleeplessness, and seizures.

77. Which of the following would the nurse teach the mother about her neonate diagnosed with FAS?
- ○ 1. Neonates are often listless and lethargic.
- ○ 2. The IQ scores are usually average.
- ○ 3. Hyperactivity and speech disorders are common.
- ○ 4. The mortality rate is 70% unless treated.

78. Which of the following nursing diagnoses would be the *priority* for a neonate with FAS admitted to the special care nursery soon after birth?
- ○ 1. Delayed Growth and Development related to poor parenting abilities of the mother.
- ○ 2. Imbalanced Nutrition: Less Than Body Requirements related to hyperirritability.
- ○ 3. Impaired Swallowing related to FAS.
- ○ 4. Risk for Trauma related to immature parenting methods.

79. When developing the plan of care for a neonate diagnosed with gastroschisis, which of the following would the nurse expect to do *first*?
- ○ 1. Weigh the neonate.
- ○ 2. Insert an orogastric tube.
- ○ 3. Prepare for immediate blood transfusion.
- ○ 4. Cover the abdomen with a moistened sterile gauze.

80. The father of a neonate diagnosed with gastroschisis tells the nurse that his wife had planned on breastfeeding the neonate. Which of the following will the nurse include in the preoperative teaching plan about feeding the neonate?
- ○ 1. The neonate will remain NPO until after surgery.

○ 2. An iron-fortified formula will be given before surgery.

○ 3. The neonate will need total parenteral nutrition for nourishment.

○ 4. The mother may breast-feed the neonate before surgery.

81. After teaching the parents of a neonate diagnosed with gastroschisis, which of the following, if identified by the father as a major goal for the neonate, indicates the need for *additional* teaching?

○ 1. Prevention of hypothermia.

○ 2. Maintenance of fluid and electrolyte balance.

○ 3. Provision of time for parental bonding.

○ 4. Prevention of infection.

82. While caring for a male neonate diagnosed with gastroschisis, the nurse observes that the parents seem hesitant to touch the neonate because of the his appearance. The nurse determines that the parents are most likely experiencing which of the following stages of grief?

○ 1. Denial.

○ 2. Shock.

○ 3. Bargaining.

○ 4. Anger.

83. Which of the following instructions would the nurse give to the parents of a neonate diagnosed with hyperbilirubinemia who is receiving phototherapy?

○ 1. Keep the neonate's eyes completely covered.

○ 2. Do not put a diaper on the neonate.

○ 3. Offer feedings every 4 hours.

○ 4. Check the oral temperature every 8 hours.

84. While caring for a term neonate who has been receiving phototherapy for 8 hours, the nurse notifies the pediatrician if which of the following is noted?

○ 1. Bronze-colored skin.

○ 2. Maculopapular chest rash.

○ 3. Urine specific gravity of 1.018.

○ 4. Absent Moro reflex.

85. The nurse is caring for a neonate at 38 weeks' gestation when the nurse observes marked peristaltic waves on the neonate's abdomen. After this observation, the neonate exhibits projectile vomiting. The nurse notifies the pediatrician because these signs are indicative of which of the following?

○ 1. Esophageal atresia.

○ 2. Pyloric stenosis.

○ 3. Diaphragmatic hernia.

○ 4. Hiatal hernia.

86. The nurse is caring for a term neonate who is diagnosed with patent ductus arteriosus. While performing a physical assessment of the neonate, the nurse anticipates that the neonate will exhibit which of the following?

○ 1. Decreased cardiac output with faint peripheral pulses.

○ 2. Profound cyanosis over most of the body.

○ 3. Loud cardiac murmurs through systole and diastole.

○ 4. Harsh systolic murmurs with a palpable thrill.

87. Assessment of a term neonate at 8 hours after birth reveals tachypnea, dyspnea, sternal retractions, diminished femoral pulses, poor lower body perfusion, and cyanosis of the lower body and extremities, with a pink upper body. The nurse notifies the pediatrician based on the interpretation that these symptoms are associated with which of the following?

○ 1. Coarctation of the aorta.

○ 2. Atrioventricular septal defect.

○ 3. Pulmonary atresia.

○ 4. Transposition of the great arteries.

88. The nurse is caring for a 2-day-old neonate in the recovery room 30 minutes after surgical correction for the cardiac defect, transposition of the great vessels. Which of the following would alert the nurse to notify the physician?

○ 1. Oxygen saturation of 90%.

○ 2. Pale pink extremities.

○ 3. Warm, dry skin.

○ 4. Femoral pulse of 90 bpm.

89. A term neonate at 2 hours of life is diagnosed with tricuspid atresia. The nurse anticipates that the pediatrician will order which of the following medications intravenously?

○ 1. Indomethacin (Indocin).

○ 2. Digoxin (Lanoxin).

○ 3. Prostaglandin E (PGE$_1$ [Prostin VR Pediatric]).

○ 4. Hydrochlorothiazide (HydroDIURIL).

90. After the physician explains the prognosis and medical management for atrial septal defect to a primiparous client whose 2-day-old female neonate was diagnosed with this condition, the nurse determines that the mother needs *further* instructions when she says which of the following?

○ 1. "As my child grows, she may have increased fatigue and difficulty breathing."

○ 2. "My child may need to have antibiotics if she develops an infection."

○ 3. "This condition occurs more often in females than in males."

○ 4. "About half of the children born with this defect heal spontaneously."

Correct Answers and Rationale

The letters in parentheses following the rationale identify the step of the nursing process (A, D, P, I, E) and client needs (1, 2, 3, 4, 5, 6, 7, 8, 9, 10). See the inside front cover for the key.

The Neonatal Client

1. 1. This 3-day old neonate's weight loss falls within a normal range, and therefore no action is needed at this time. Full-term neonates tend to lose 5% to 10% of their birth weight during the first few days after birth, most likely because of minimal nutritional intake. With bottle-feeding, the neonate's intake varies from one feeding to another. Additionally, the neonate experiences a loss of extracellular fluid. Typically, neonates regain any weight loss by 7 to 10 days of life. If the weight loss continues after that time, the physician should be called. (I, 3)

2. 2. Keeping the neonate away from drafts and cooling ducts prevents heat loss by *convection* (flow of heat from the body surface to the cooler surrounding air). The neonate also loses heat through *evaporation* (conversion of a liquid to a vapor, as when a wet surface, such as the neonate's skin, is exposed to air); *conduction* (transfer of body heat to a cooler solid object in contact with the baby, as when the neonate comes in direct contact with a cold surface such as a scale or a cold stethoscope); and *radiation* (transfer of heat to cooler solid objects that are not in direct contact with the baby, as when the neonate is placed near a cold window surface or air conditioner). (I, 3)

3. 1. For vitamin K synthesis, which occurs in the intestines, to begin, food and normal intestinal flora are needed. However, at birth, the neonate's intestines are sterile. Therefore, vitamin K is administered via injection to prevent a vitamin K deficiency that may result in a bleeding tendency. When administered, vitamin K promotes formation in the liver of clotting factors II, VII, IX, and X. Neonates are not normally susceptible to clotting disorders, unless they are diagnosed with hemophilia or demonstrate a deficiency of or a problem with clotting factors. Hemolysis of fetal red blood cells does not destroy vitamin K. Hemolysis may be caused by Rh or ABO incompatibility, which leads to anemia and necessitates an exchange transfusion. (E, 8)

4. 3. Currently, the sense of touch is believed to be the most highly developed sense at birth. It is probably for this reason that neonates respond well to touch. Auditory sense typically is relatively immature in the neonate, as evidenced by the neonate's selective response to the human voice. By 4 months, the neonate should turn the eyes and head toward a sound coming from behind. Visual sense tends to be relatively immature. At birth, visual acuity is estimated at approximately 20/100 to 20/150, but it improves rapidly during infancy and toddlerhood. (P, 3)

5. 1. The nurse should inform the mother that baby powder can enter the neonate's lungs and result in pneumonia secondary to aspiration of the particles. The best prevention for diaper rash is frequent diaper changing and keeping the neonate's skin dry. The new disposable diapers have moisture-collecting materials and generally do not adhere to the skin unless the diaper becomes very saturated. Typically, allergies are not associated with the use of baby powder in neonates. (I, 9)

6. 4. The mother needs further instruction when she says that a yellowish crust should be removed with water. The yellowish crust is normal and indicates scar formation at the site. It should not be removed, because to do so might cause increased bleeding. The petroleum gauze prevents the diaper from sticking to the circumcision site, and it may fall off in the diaper. If this occurs, the mother should not attempt to replace it but should simply apply plain petroleum jelly to the site. The gauze should be left in place for 24 hours, and the mother should continue to apply petroleum jelly with each diaper change for 48 hours after the procedure. A few drops of oozing blood is normal, but if the amount is greater than a few drops the mother should apply pressure and contact the physician. Any bleeding after the first day should be reported. (E, 9)

7. 3. The mother demonstrates understanding of the discharge instructions when she says that she should contact the pediatrician if the baby has a liquid stool with a watery ring, because this indicates diarrhea. Infants can become dehydrated very quickly, and frequent diarrhea can result in dehydration. Normally, babies fall asleep easily after a feeding because they are satisfied and content. Spitting up a tablespoon of formula is normal. However, projectile or forceful vomiting in larger amounts should be reported. Bottle-feeding infants typically pass one to two light brown stools each day. (E, 9)

8. 1. Placing the infant on the back after the feeding is recommended to minimize the risk for sudden infant death syndrome (SIDS). Placing the infant on the

abdomen after feeding has been associated with SIDS. The mother should bubble or burp the baby after one-half ounce of formula has been taken and then again when the baby is finished. Waiting until the baby has eaten 1 ounce of formula can lead to regurgitation. The entire nipple should be placed on top of the baby's tongue and into the mouth to prevent excessive air from being swallowed. The nipple is pointed directly into the mouth, not toward the neonate's palate, to provide adequate sucking. (E, 9)

9. 1. In a neonate, the lateral aspect of the heel is the most appropriate site for obtaining a blood specimen. Using this area prevents damage to the calcaneus bone, which is located in the middle of the heel. The middle of the heel is to be avoided because of the increased risk for damaging the calcaneus bone located there. The middle of the foot contains the medial plantar nerve and the medial plantar artery, which could be injured if this site is selected. Because using the base of the toes as the site for specimen collection would cause a great deal of discomfort for the neonate, it is not the preferred site. (P, 9)

10. 2. After circumcision with a Plastibell, the most commonly recommended procedure is to cleanse the circumcision site with warm water with each diaper change. Other treatments are necessary only if complications, such as an infection, develop. Antibacterial soap or diluted hydrogen peroxide may cause pain and is not recommended. Povidone-iodine solution may cause stinging and burning, and therefore its use also is not recommended. (I, 3)

11. 2. As part of the neonate's physiologic adaptation to birth, at 90 minutes after birth the neonate typically is in the rest or sleep phase. During this time, the heart and respiratory rates slow and the neonate sleeps, unresponsive to stimuli. At this time, the mother should rest and allow the neonate to sleep. Feedings should be given during the first period of reactivity, considered the first 30 minutes after birth. During this period, the neonate's respirations and heart rate are elevated. Getting to know the neonate typically occurs within the first hour after birth and then when the neonate is awake and during feedings. Changing the neonate's diaper can occur at any time, but at 90 minutes after birth the neonate is usually in a deep sleep, unresponsive, and probably hasn't passed any meconium. (I, 3)

Physical Assessment of the Neonatal Client

12. 3. Normally, the umbilical cord has two umbilical arteries and one vein. When a neonate is born with only one artery and one vein, the nurse should notify the pediatrician for further evaluation of cardiac anomalies. Other common congenital problems associated with a missing artery include renal anomalies, central nervous system lesions, tracheoesophageal fistulas, trisomy 13, and trisomy 18. Respiratory anomalies are associated with dyspnea and respiratory distress; musculoskeletal anomalies include fractures or dislocated hip; and facial anomalies are associated with fetal alcohol syndrome or Down syndrome, not a missing umbilical artery. These conditions are not associated with a missing umbilical artery. (D, 9)

13. 2. Caused by pressure on the head during labor, caput succedaneum is an edematous area over the place where the scalp was encircled by the cervix, possibly crossing the suture line. It usually results from a difficult and long labor or from vacuum extraction. Caput succedaneum is usually reabsorbed within 12 hours to a few days after birth. Cephalohematoma is caused by blood between the bone and the periosteum. Because bleeding is under the periosteum, it cannot cross the suture line, whereas a caput succedaneum can. A cephalohematoma may take as long as a few weeks or months to disappear. Craniotabes refers to a reduction in mineralization of the skull with abnormal softness of the bones. (D, 3)

14. 2. Normally at birth, the neonate's head circumference is approximately 2 cm larger than the chest circumference. The average normal head circumference is 13 to 14 inches (33 to 35 cm); average normal chest circumference is 12.5 to 14 inches (31 to 35 cm). A head circumference that is equal to or smaller than the chest circumference may indicate microcephaly; a head that is larger than normal may indicate hydrocephalus. The presence of any of these conditions warrants further evaluation. (A, 3)

15. 4. The mother needs further instruction if she says the molding can result in brain damage. Brain damage is highly unlikely. Molding occurs during vaginal delivery when the cranial bones tend to override or overlap as the head accommodates to the size of the mother's birth canal. The amount and duration of pressure on the head influence the degree of molding. Molding usually disappears in a few days without any special attention. (E, 3)

16. 3. The anterior fontanel is normally diamond-shaped, approximately 2 to 3 cm wide and 3 to 4 cm long. This allows for brain growth during the early months of life. The posterior fontanel is small and triangular. (A, 3)

17. 3. Sole creases covering the entire foot are indicative of a term neonate. If the neonate's ear is lying flat against the head, the neonate is most likely preterm. An absence of rugae in the scrotum typically suggests a preterm neonate. A square window sign angle of 0 degrees occurs in neonates of 40 to 42 weeks' gestation. A 90-degree square window angle suggests an immature neonate of approximately 28 to 30 weeks' gestation. (A, 3)

18. 2. An expiratory grunt is significant and should be reported promptly, because it may indicate respiratory distress and the need for further intervention such as oxygen or resuscitation efforts. The presence of a red reflex in the eyes is normal. An absent red reflex may indicate congenital cataracts. A respiratory rate of 45 breaths/minute and a prominent xiphoid process are normal findings in a term neonate. (A, 9)

19. 3. The tonic neck reflex, also called the *fencing position,* is present when the neonate turns the head to the left side, extends the left extremities, and flexes the right extremities. This reflex disappears in a matter of months as the neonatal nervous system matures. The stepping reflex is demonstrated when the infant is held upright near a hard, firm surface. The prone crawl reflex is demonstrated when the infant pulls both arms but does not move the chin beyond the elbows. When the infant extends and abducts the arms and legs with the toes fanning open, this is a normal Babinski reflex. (E, 3)

20. 2. Convergent strabismus is common during infancy until about age 6 months because of poor oculomotor coordination. The neonate has peripheral vision and can fixate on close objects for short periods. The neonate can also perceive colors, shapes, and faces. Neonates can focus on light and should blink or close their eyes in response to light. However, this is not associated with strabismus. An absent red reflex or white areas over the pupils, not strabismus, may indicate congenital cataracts. Most neonates cannot focus well or accommodate for distance immediately after birth. (I, 3)

21. 3. A single crease across the palm (simian crease) is most often associated with chromosomal abnormalities, notably Down syndrome. Deep creases across the soles of the feet is a normal finding in a term neonate. Frequent sneezing in a term neonate is normal. This occurs because the neonate is a nose breather and sneezing helps to clear the nares. An absence of lanugo on the skin of a term neonate is a normal finding. (A, 9)

22. 1. Periods of apnea lasting longer than 20 seconds, mild cyanosis, and a heart rate of 110 bpm (bradycardia) are associated with a potentially life-threatening event and subsequent respiratory arrest. The neonate needs further evaluation by the pediatrician. Pneumonia is associated with tachycardia, anorexia, malaise, cyanosis, diminished breath sounds, and crackles. Intraventricular hemorrhage is associated with prematurity. Assessment findings include bulging fontanels and seizures. Epiglottitis is a bacterial form of croup. Assessment findings include inspiratory stridor,

cough, and irritability. It occurs most often in children age 3 to 7 years. (D, 9)

23. 4. Normally, the anterior fontanel closes between ages 12 and 18 months. Premature closure (craniostenosis or premature synostosis) prevents proper growth and expansion of the brain, resulting in mental retardation. The posterior fontanel typically closes by 2 to 3 months of age. (I, 3)

24. 2. Corneas of unequal size should be reported because this may indicate congenital glaucoma. An absence of tears is common because the neonate's lacrimal glands are not yet functioning. The neonate's pupils normally constrict when a bright light is focused on them. The finding implies that light perception and visual acuity are present, as they should be after birth. A red circle on the pupils seen when an ophthalmoscope's light is shining onto the retina is a normal finding. Called the red reflex, this indicates that the light is shining onto the retina. (A, 9)

25. 3. At 24 hours of age, the neonate is probably in a state of deep sleep, as evidenced by the closed eyes, lack of eye movements, normal skin color, and normal heart rate and respiratory rate. Jitteriness, a high-pitched cry, and tremors are associated with drug withdrawal. There is no evidence to suggest respiratory distress because the neonate's respiratory rate of 35 breaths/minute is normal. The first period of reactivity occurs in the first 30 minutes after birth, evidenced by alertness, sucking sounds, and rapid heart rate and respiratory rate. (D, 3)

26. 4. The condition in which the urinary meatus is located on the ventral surface of the penis, termed *hypospadias,* occurs in 1 of every 500 male infants. Circumcision is delayed until the condition is corrected surgically, usually between 6 and 12 months of age. Phimosis is an inability to retract the prepuce at an age when it should be retractable or by age 3 years. Phimosis may necessitate circumcision or surgical intervention. Hydrocele is a painless swelling of the scrotum that is common in neonates. It is not a contraindication for circumcision. Epispadias occurs when the urinary meatus is located on the dorsal surface of the penis. It is extremely rare and is often associated with bladder extrophy. (A, 9)

The Preterm Neonate

27. 2. The first step after cesarean delivery is to aspirate mucus from the neonate's mouth. If this is not done, the neonate will aspirate mucus when beginning to breathe. A patent airway is most important. Once mucus has been aspirated, the neonate may be stimulated to cry if necessary. If, once the airway has been established, the neonate does not begin breathing

efforts on his or her own, then resuscitation may be necessary. Although the mother will want to see the neonate, holding the neonate upright is inappropriate because the neonate's head should be kept lower than the rest of the body to aid in the expulsion of mucus or other fluids. (I, 3)

28. 4. When receiving oxygen by mask, the neonate is placed on the back with the neck slightly extended, in the sniffing or neutral position. This position optimizes lung expansion and places the upper respiratory tract in the best position for receiving oxygen. Placing a small rolled towel under the neonate's shoulders helps to extend the neck properly without overextending it. Once stabilized and transferred to an isolette in the intensive care unit, the neonate can be positioned in the prone position, which allows for lung expansion in the oxygenated environment. Placing the neonate on the left side does not allow for maximum lung expansion. Also, slightly flexing the neck interferes with opening the airway. Placing the neonate on the back with the head turned to the left side does not allow for lung expansion. Placing the neonate on the abdomen interferes with proper positioning of the oxygen mask. (I, 8)

29. 1. Cardiac massage should be alternated with ventilation to ensure breathing and circulation. Two fingers, not the palm of the hand, are used to compress a neonate's sternum. The chest is compressed 100 to 120 times per minute, and the chest wall is displaced 0.5 to 0.75 inch (1 to 1.5 cm). (I, 10)

30. 1. Whenever oxygen is administered, it should be humidified to prevent drying of the nasal passages and mucous membranes. Because the neonate is under a radiant warmer, a stocking cap is not necessary. Temperature, continuously monitored by a skin probe attached to the radiant warmer, is recorded every 30 to 60 minutes initially. Although the oxygen concentration in the hood requires close monitoring and measurement of blood gases, checking the blood glucose level is not necessary. (I, 8)

31. 3. The neonate is at high risk for sepsis due to exposure to the mother's infection. Temperature instability in a neonate at 38 weeks' gestation is an early sign of sepsis. Other signs include tachycardia, decreased muscle tone, acidosis, apnea, respiratory distress, hypotension, poor feeding behaviors, vomiting, and diarrhea. Late signs of infection include jaundice, seizures, enlarged liver and spleen, respiratory failure, and shock. Alkalosis is not typically seen in neonates who develop sepsis. Acidosis and respiratory distress may develop unless treatment such as antibiotics is started. Also, bradycardia is common in low-birth-weight preterm neonates, not in neonates at 38 weeks weighing 3175 g (7 pounds). (A, 9)

32. 2. With an absent apical pulse left of the midclavicular line accompanied by cyanosis, grunting, and diminished breath sounds, the neonate is most likely experiencing pneumothorax. Pneumothorax occurs when alveoli are overdistended and subsequently the lung collapses, compressing the heart and lung and compromising the venous return to the right side of the heart. This condition can be confirmed by x-ray or ultrasound studies. Diaphragmatic hernia is associated with respiratory distress soon after birth, not typically 2 days later. Bowel sounds also may be auscultated in the chest. Coarctation of the aorta is associated with poor lower body perfusion exhibited as cyanosis, metabolic acidosis, and congestive heart failure. Assessment findings include absent or diminished femoral pulses, increased brachial pulses, and a late systolic murmur. Commonly, bacterial pneumonia is associated with fever, diminished breath sounds, and crackles. (A, 9)

33. 2. RDS, previously called *hyaline membrane disease*, is a developmental condition involving a decrease in lung surfactant leading to improper expansion of the lung alveoli. Surfactant contains a group of surface-active phospholipids, of which one component—lecithin—is the most critical for alveolar stability. Surfactant production peaks at about 35 weeks' gestation. This syndrome primarily attacks preterm neonates, although it can also affect term and post-term neonates. Altered somatotropin secretion is associated with growth disorders such as gigantism or dwarfism. Altered testosterone secretion is associated with masculinization. Altered progesterone secretion is associated with spontaneous abortion during pregnancy. (I, 10)

34. 3. The best way to determine the adequacy of oxygen therapy is to monitor the neonate's arterial blood gas values. These results quantitatively measure oxygen and carbon dioxide tensions. Cyanosis, a late sign, can validate laboratory findings, but without laboratory results it is not a reliable indicator of the effectiveness of oxygen therapy. Pulse rate likewise does not serve as a good index because there is poor correlation between it and extreme hyperoxia. The percentage of oxygen received is not a good indicator of the arterial blood gas level of oxygen. Even with high levels of oxygen, the preterm neonate may continue to have poor perfusion because of immature development of the heart and lungs. The percentage delivered is based on the analysis of the neonate's arterial blood gases. (E, 9)

35. 2. RDS is a developmental condition that primarily affects preterm infants before 35 weeks' gestation because of inadequate lung development from deficient surfactant production. The development of placenta previa has little correlation with the development of RDS. Although excessive analgesia can depress the neonate's respiratory condition if it is given shortly

before birth, the scenario presents no information that this has occurred. The neonate's sluggish respiratory activity postpartum is not the likely cause of RDS but may be a sign that the neonate has the condition. (I, 9)

36. 3. Oxygen should be humidified before administration to help prevent drying of the mucous membranes in the respiratory tract. Drying impedes the normal functioning of cilia in the respiratory tract and predisposes to mucous membrane irritation. Humidification of oxygen does not promote expansion of the immature lungs. Expansion is promoted by placing the infant in a prone position or providing the preterm infant with surfactant medication. Humidified oxygen does not prevent viral or bacterial pneumonia. In fact, in some nurseries, *Staphylococcus aureus* has been detected in moist environments and on the hands and nails of staff members, predisposing the neonate to pneumonia. Humidified oxygen does not improve blood circulation in the cardiac system. (I, 8)

37. 4. Many intensive care units that care for high-risk neonates recommend that the mother pump her breasts, store the milk, and bring it to the unit so the neonate can be fed with it, even if the neonate is being fed by gavage. As soon as the neonate has developed a coordinated suck-and-swallow reflex, breast-feeding can begin. Secretory immunoglobulin A, found in breast milk, is an important immunoglobulin that can provide immunity to the mucosal surfaces of the gastrointestinal tract. It can protect the neonate from enteric infections, such as those caused by *Escherichia coli* and *Shigella* species. Some studies have also shown that breast-fed preterm neonates maintain transcutaneous oxygen pressure and body temperature better than bottle-fed neonates. There is some evidence that breast milk can decrease the incidence of necrotizing enterocolitis. The preterm neonate does not need additional fat in the diet. However, some neonates may need an increased caloric intake. In such cases, breast milk can be fortified with an additive to provide additional calories. Neonates who are receiving oxygen can breast-feed. During feedings, supplemental oxygen can be delivered by nasal cannula. (I, 3)

38. 1. ROP, previously called *retrolental fibroplasia*, is associated with multiple risk factors, including high arterial blood oxygen levels, prematurity, and very low birth weight (less than 1500 g). In the early acute stages of ROP, the neonate's immature retinal vessels constrict. If vasoconstriction is sustained, vascular closure follows, and irreversible capillary endothelial damage occurs. Oxygen levels of 28% are not excessively high; normal room air is at 21%. Acidosis, not alkalosis, is frequently seen in preterm neonates, but this is not related to the development of ROP. Phototherapy is not related to the development of ROP. However, during phototherapy,

the neonate's eyes should be constantly covered to prevent damage from the lights. (A, 9)

39. 4. Constricted retinal vessels may indicate the degree of ROP. In ROP, immature blood vessels in the retina constrict and become permanently occluded. New vessels proliferate to reestablish circulation. If the new vessels extend into the vitreous humor of the eye, hemorrhage can occur, resulting in scarring and retinal detachment. Sunken orbital sockets would be suggestive of dehydration, not ROP. Strabismus ("crossed eyes") is common in all neonates because of poor oculomotor coordination. A reaction to bright light is a normal finding. (A, 9)

40. 1. Because the retina may become detached with ROP, laser therapy and cryotherapy have been used successfully in some medical centers to treat ROP. Cromolyn sodium (Intal) is used to treat seasonal allergies. ROP is not associated with glaucoma, so frequent testing is not necessary. Because the vessels of the eye are affected, not the corneas, corneal transplantation is not used. (I, 10)

41. 3. The priority nursing diagnosis for a preterm neonate is Impaired Gas Exchange related to immature pulmonary vasculature. RDS is a primary problem for preterm neonates and a particular problem for neonates of 28 weeks' gestation because of the lack of surfactant in the lungs. Risk for Impaired Skin Integrity related to gestational age is not a priority at this time. The immediate problem is related to breathing and oxygenation. The priority is to establish an airway and adequate respirations. (D, 3)

42. 1. Neonates who weigh less than 1500 g or are born at less than 34 weeks' gestation are susceptible to PIVH. Computed tomography scanning or ultrasound scanning can confirm the diagnosis. The spinal fluid will show an increased number of red blood cells. Arterial blood gas specimen collection is done to evaluate the neonate's oxygen saturation level. Skull radiographs are not commonly used because of the danger of radiation. Additionally, computed tomography scans have replaced the use of skull x-ray films because they can provide more definitive results. Complete blood count specimen collection is usually performed to determine the hemoglobin, hematocrit, and white blood cell count. The results are not specific for PIVH. (P, 9)

43. 3. A common finding of PIVH is a bulging fontanel. The most common site of hemorrhage is the periventricular subependymal germinal matrix, where there is a rich blood supply and where the capillary walls are thin and fragile. Rapid volume expansion, hypercarbia, and hypoglycemia contribute to the development of PIVH. Other common manifestations include neurologic signs such as hypotonia, lethargy, temperature instability, nystagmus, apnea, bradycardia, decreased

hematocrit, and increasing hypoxia. Seizures also may occur. Hyperbilirubinemia refers to an increase in bilirubin in the blood and is not associated with PIVH. (A, 10)

44. 4. Indications of NEC include abdominal distention with gastric retention and vomiting. Other signs may include lethargy, irritability, positive blood culture in stool, absent or diminished bowel sounds, apnea, diarrhea, metabolic acidosis, and unstable temperature. A gastric residual of 1 mL is not significant. Jaundice of the face and chest is associated with the neonate's immature liver function and increased bilirubin, not NEC. Typically with NEC, the neonate would exhibit absent or diminished bowel sounds, not increased peristalsis. (A, 10)

45. 2. BPD is a chronic illness that may require prolonged hospitalization and permanent assisted ventilation. The disease typically occurs in compromised very-low-birth-weight neonates who require oxygen therapy and assisted ventilation for treatment of RDS. The cause is multifactorial, and the disease has four stages. The neonate's activities may be limited by the disease. Antibiotics may be ordered, and bronchodilators may be used, but these medications will not cure the chronic disease state. Seizure activity is associated with PIVH, not BPD. (E, 10)

46. 4. Pneumothorax is an accumulation of air in the thoracic cavity between the parietal and visceral pleurae. A life-threatening situation, it requires immediate removal of the accumulated air. Initially, the air is aspirated with a syringe attached to an 18-gauge catheter or a 23-gauge butterfly drain inserted into the second or third intercostal space at the midclavicular line with the neonate in a supine position. Complete resolution of pneumothorax requires a size 10F chest tube connected to continuous negative pressure. The neonate does not need to be placed on a ventilator unless there is evidence of severe respiratory distress. The goal of treatment is to reinflate the collapsed lung. Administering bronchodilators through the nares or suctioning the neonate's nares would do nothing to aid in lung reinflation. (I, 10)

47. 3. Decreased protein or hypoproteinemia is a sign of overhydration, which can lead to patent ductus arteriosus or congestive heart failure. Bulging fontanels, decreased serum sodium, decreased urine specific gravity, and decreased hematocrit are other signs of overhydration. Hypernatremia (increased serum sodium concentration) or increased urine specific gravity would suggest dehydration, not overhydration. Polycythemia evidenced by an elevated hematocrit would suggest hypoxia or congenital heart disorder. (A, 9)

The Post-term Neonate

48. 4. Increased respiratory rate and tremors are indicative of hypoglycemia, which frequently affects the post-term neonate because of depleted glycogen stores. There is no indication that the neonate has ineffective airway clearance, which would be evidenced by excessive amounts of mucus or visualization of meconium on the vocal cords. Lethargy, not tremors, would suggest infection or hyperthermia. Furthermore, the post-term neonate typically has difficulty maintaining temperature, hypothermia, not hyperthermia, is usually more of a problem. Decreased cardiac output is not indicated, particularly because the neonate was delivered by cesarean delivery, which is not considered a difficult delivery. (D, 3)

49. 2. A loose, watery stool in the diaper is indicative of diarrhea and needs immediate attention. The infant may become severely dehydrated quickly because of the higher percentage of water content per body weight in the neonate, compared with the adult. Frequent hiccups are considered normal in a neonate and do not warrant additional investigation. Pink papular vesicles (erythema toxicum) on the face are considered normal in a neonate and disappear without treatment. Dry, peeling skin is normal in a post-term neonate. (D, 3)

50. 2. Ortolani's maneuver involves flexing the neonate's knees and hips at right angles and bringing the sides of the knees down to the surface of the examining table. A characteristic click or "clunk," felt or heard, represents a positive Ortolani's sign, suggesting a possible hip dislocation. The nurse should notify the physician promptly because treatment is needed, while maintaining the dislocated hip in a position of flexion and abduction. Determining the length of the mother's labor provides no useful information related to the nurse's finding. Keeping the infant under the radiant warmer is necessary only if the neonate's temperature is low or unstable. Checking for hypoglycemia is not indicated at this time, unless the neonate is exhibiting jitteriness. (I, 9)

51. 4. The priority nursing diagnosis for the neonate with probable MAS is Impaired Gas Exchange related to the effects of respiratory distress. Obstruction of the airways may be complete or partial. Meconium aspiration may lead to pneumonia or pneumothorax. Establishing adequate respirations is the primary goal. Although nutrition may be altered, oxygenation takes priority over nutrition. If the parents do not express interest or concern for the neonate, then Risk for Impaired Parent/Infant/Child Attachment may be appropriate once the airway is established. (D, 10)

52. 1. Care of an umbilical arterial line would be included in the neonate's plan of care because an umbilical arte-

rial line often is inserted to monitor arterial blood pressures, blood pH, blood gases, and infusion of intravenous fluids, blood, or medications. Frequent ultrasound scans are not indicated at this time. However, chest radiographs may be used to detect lung densities, because pneumonia is a major complication of this disorder. Orogastric feeding may not be feasible while the health care team focuses on interventions to establish adequate oxygenation. The neonate with MAS frequently experiences hypoglycemia, not hyperglycemia. Hypoglycemia occurs because of depletion of glucose stores related to hypothermia. (P, 10)

53. 4. Tolazoline (Priscoline) can cause profound hypotension. Therefore, the nurse should monitor the neonate's blood pressure when giving this drug. Adverse side effects of the medication include petechiae, dark stools, bleeding, and diarrhea. Plasma expanders are often used with tolazoline to prevent dramatic changes in blood pressure. Feeding behaviors, temperature, and skin color are routine assessments for all neonates, unrelated to the use of tolazoline. (I, 8)

The Neonate With Risk Factors

54. 3. Hemolytic disease of the newborn is associated with Rh problems. Hemolytic disease of the newborn occurs most often when the mother is Rh negative and the father is Rh positive. About 13% of white Americans, 7% to 8% of African Americans, and 1% of Asian Americans are Rh negative. Rh-positive cells enter the mother's Rh-negative bloodstream, and antibodies to the Rh-positive cells are produced. In a subsequent pregnancy, the antibodies cross the placenta to the Rh-positive fetus and begin the destruction of Rh-positive cells through hemolysis. This results in severe fetal anemia. (I, 10)

55. 3. The problem of Rh sensitivity arises when the mother's blood develops antibodies after fetal red blood cells enter the maternal circulation. In cases of Rh sensitivity, this usually does not occur until after the first pregnancy. Hence, hemolytic disease of the newborn is rare in a primipara. A mismatched blood transfusion in the past or an unrecognized spontaneous abortion could also result in hemolytic disease because the transfusion or abortion would have the same effects on the client. The statement about the other baby having a different father may be true. However, if both fathers were Rh positive, then sensitization could occur. Most women do not have immunity against the antibodies formed when Rh-positive cells enter the mother's bloodstream. Antibodies are not neutralized by the mother's system. (E, 9)

56. 2. The Rh-sensitized neonate generally does not have problems related to polycythemia. Therefore, the client

needs additional teaching. In general, moderate to severe Rh sensitization can cause anemia, enlarged spleen, and cardiac decompensation. Cardiac decompensation (eg, heart failure) occurs because of severe anemia. Anemia is caused by the destruction of red blood cells by antibodies as the severity of hemolytic disease of the neonate increases. Splenic enlargement is caused by the excessive destruction of fetal red blood cells. (E, 10)

57. 3. A direct Coombs test is done on umbilical cord blood to detect antibodies coating the neonate's red blood cells. (I, 9)

58. 3. An exchange transfusion is done to reduce the blood concentration of bilirubin and correct the anemia. The exchange transfusion does not replenish the white blood cells or restore the fluid and electrolyte balance. The neonate's Rh-positive blood is replaced by Rh-negative blood. (E, 9)

59. 2. The organ most susceptible to damage from uncontrolled hemolytic disease is the brain. Bilirubin levels increase as the red blood cells are destroyed. Bilirubin crosses the blood-brain barrier and damages the cells of the central nervous system. This condition, called *kernicterus*, and is potentially fatal. (I, 9)

60. 4. A priority nursing diagnosis is Impaired Nutrition: Less Than Body Requirements related to increased glucose metabolism. The increased glucose metabolism is a result of the hyperinsulinemia. Maternal hyperglycemia is accompanied by fetal hyperglycemia. On delivery, the neonate is no longer dependent on maternal glucose, and a hypoglycemic state soon develops. Hyperthermia is not a priority at this time; large-for-gestational-age neonates tend to become hypothermic as they deplete their glucose stores. (D, 3)

61. 2. Glucose crosses the placenta, but insulin does not. Hence, a high maternal blood glucose level causes a high fetal blood glucose level. This causes the fetal pancreas to secrete more insulin. At birth, the neonate loses the maternal glucose source but continues to produce much insulin, which often causes a drop in blood glucose levels (hypoglycemia), usually at 30 to 60 minutes postpartum. Most neonates do not develop hypoglycemia if their mothers are not insulin dependent unless they are preterm. Therefore, hypoglycemia is not a normal response as the neonate transitions to extrauterine life. (I, 9)

62. 1. Infants born to diabetic mothers tend to be larger than average, and this neonate weighs 4564 g (10 pounds, 1 ounce). The most common fractures are those of the clavicle and long bones, such as the femur. (A, 9)

63. 4. Tremors occurring after therapy for hypoglycemia are clinical signs of hypocalcemia. At term, diabetic women tend to have higher calcium levels, which can cause secondary hypoparathyroidism in their neonates. Other factors that can contribute to hypocalcemia in neonates include hypophosphatemia from tissue metabolism, vitamin D antagonism from increased cortisol levels, and decreased serum magnesium levels. (D, 9)

64. 4. Hypoglycemia is caused by the rapid depletion of glucose stores. In addition, neonates born to class B diabetic women suffer from respiratory distress syndrome about seven times more often than neonates born to nondiabetic women. This neonate should be closely monitored for symptoms of hypoglycemia and respiratory distress. Neonates of diabetic mothers frequently have polycythemia, not anemia. Anemia and hemolytic disease are associated with erythroblastosis fetalis. Persistent pulmonary hypertension is associated with meconium aspiration syndrome. (D, 9)

65. 2. Manifestations of cocaine withdrawal in the neonate include a shrill, high-pitched cry, tachycardia, muscular rigidity, irritability, restlessness, fist-sucking, and an exaggerated startle reflex. These signs usually appear within 72 hours and persist for several days. These neonates are difficult to console, have poor feeding behaviors, and have diarrhea. Bradycardia is associated with preterm neonates. Sluggishness and lethargy are associated with neonates whose mothers received analgesia shortly before delivery. Hypocalcemia occurs most often in infants of diabetic mothers, premature infants, and low-birth-weight infants. (A, 9)

66. 3. Neonates experiencing cocaine withdrawal have gastrointestinal problems similar to those of adults withdrawing from cocaine. The neonates exhibit poor sucking, vomiting, drooling, diarrhea, regurgitation, and anorexia. In addition, they are difficult to console and difficult to feed. Because of these problems, the neonate withdrawing from cocaine needs to be monitored carefully to prevent dehydration. Abdominal distention is associated with necrotizing enterocolitis, not cocaine withdrawal. (E, 9)

67. 1. A neonate undergoing cocaine withdrawal is irritable, often restless, difficult to console, and often in need of increased activity. It is often helpful to swaddle the neonate tightly with a blanket, offer a pacifier, and cuddle and rock the neonate. Offering extra nourishment is not advised because overfeeding tends to increase gastrointestinal problems such as vomiting, regurgitation, and diarrhea. Environmental stimuli such as bright lights and loud noises should be kept to a minimum to decrease agitation. Minimizing touching of the neonate to only when he or she is crying will not aid the bonding process between mother and neonate. Frequent holding and touching are permissible. (I, 9)

68. 4. Although most neonates are asymptomatic, they do test positive for HIV at birth because of the mother's antibodies. It may take several months before an accurate diagnosis can be made. It is estimated that 20% to 40% of all HIV-positive mothers deliver HIV-positive infants. With appropriate drug intervention to the mother during pregnancy, 95% of these neonates can be born unaffected. An enlarged liver at birth is associated with erythroblastosis fetalis, not HIV infection. Virologic testing, such as DNA polymerase chain reaction, viral culture, or RNA plasma assay, can diagnose HIV infection by 6 months of age and often in the first month. (I, 9)

69. 4. Breast milk has been found to contain the retrovirus HIV. In general, mothers are discouraged from breast-feeding if they are HIV positive because of the risk of possible transmission of the virus if the neonate is HIV negative. Breast milk does contain some immunoglobulins, but it does not protect the neonate from HIV infection. (I, 3)

70. 4. As part of standard precautions, the nurse should don a pair of clean gloves. Additionally, the site is cleansed thoroughly with an alcohol swab before the skin is injected. Sterile gloves are not necessary. Bathing the neonate is not necessary before giving the injection. Some research suggests that bathing removes the neonate's protective skin oils. Placing the neonate under the radiant warmer is not necessary unless the neonate's temperature is subnormal. The neonate's temperature has usually stabilized by 4 hours of age. Washing the injection site with povidone-iodine before giving the injection is not necessary because of the risk for possible allergy to iodine preparations. (I, 2)

71. 3. Symptoms of infection in a neonate include subtle behavioral changes, such as lethargy and irritability, and color changes such as pallor or cyanosis. Other symptoms include temperature instability, poor feeding, gastrointestinal disorders, hyperbilirubinemia, and apnea. Leukocytosis, an elevated white blood cell count possibly as high as 30,000 cells/mm^3 or more, may be normal during the first 24 hours. An apical heart rate of 132 bpm is normal. Warm, moist skin is not a typical sign of infection in neonates. Typically, temperature instability is common. The neonate's temperature is low and the skin is cool and dry. (A, 3)

72. 3. The parents of a neonate with an infection should be allowed to participate in daily care as long as they use good handwashing technique. This includes touching and holding the neonate. The parents need to be careful around the intravenous site so that it is not dislodged. However, the parents can be instructed in this. Restricting parental visits has not been shown to have any effect on the infection rate and may have detrimental effects on the neonate's psychological development. Normally, the neonate does not need to be isolated. It is not necessary for the parents to wear a mask

while holding the neonate. The neonate is not contagious and is receiving treatment for the infection. (I, 2)

73. 3. On the initial visit, the parents may be shocked, fearful, and anxious. Nursing care should include spending time with the parents to allow them to express their emotions. The nurse should initially emphasize the neonate's normal characteristics. After the parents have had sufficient time to adjust to the neonate's special needs, surgical interventions can be discussed. Telling the parents that this is not a life-threatening defect or that everything will be all right after the surgery is not helpful. Doing so discounts their feelings. Reassuring the parents about the success rate of the surgery can be done once the parents have had time to adjust to the neonate and express their emotions. (I, 5)

74. 1. After feeding, the mouth should be cleaned with sterile water, not soapy water, to reduce the risk for aspiration. The cleft lip should be cleaned with sterile water to prevent crusting before surgical repair. The neonate needs to be fed in an upright position to prevent aspiration. The neonate with a cleft lip and palate frequently swallows large amounts of air during feeding. Therefore, the neonate needs to be burped frequently to help eliminate the air and decrease the risk for regurgitation. The neonate with a cleft lip and palate should be fed with a special soft nipple that fills the cleft and facilitates sucking. (E, 9)

75. 2. One hour after birth, the priority nursing diagnosis for the neonate with a cleft palate is Risk for Infection related to potential aspiration. Feeding difficulties are the primary problem before surgical repair. Activity Intolerance may occur, but this is not a primary problem and there is no evidence of the neonate's having been diagnosed with respiratory distress syndrome. There is no evidence presented to suggest Compromised Family Coping. However, this nursing diagnosis may be appropriate later on since the infant may require frequent health care follow-up visits and surgeries. Impaired Skin Integrity is not a problem for this neonate, who is allowed to engage in normal activity without restraint before surgery. After surgery the infant may have restraints to prevent damage to the suture line, thus requiring frequent position changes. (D, 9)

76. 4. The long-term prognosis for neonates with FAS is poor. Symptoms of withdrawal include tremors, sleeplessness, seizures, abdominal distention, hyperactivity, and inconsolable crying. Symptoms of withdrawal often occur within 6 to 12 hours or, at the latest, within the first 3 days of life. The neonate with FAS is usually growth deficient at birth. Most neonates with FAS are mildly to severely mentally retarded. The facial deformities, such as short palpebral fissures, epicanthal folds, broad nasal bridge, flattened midfacies, and

short, upturned nose are not easily corrected with plastic surgery. (P, 9)

77. 3. Central nervous system disorders are common in neonates with FAS. Speech and language disorders and hyperactivity are common manifestations of central nervous system dysfunction. Mild to severe mental retardation and feeding problems also are common. Delayed growth and development is expected. These neonates feed poorly and often have persistent vomiting until age 6 to 7 months. These neonates do not have a 70% mortality rate, and there is no treatment. (I, 9)

78. 2. The priority nursing diagnosis for the neonate with FAS is Imbalanced Nutrition: Less Than Body Requirements related to hyperirritability. The neonate's hyperirritability interferes with the ability to ingest adequate nutrients. There are no data to suggest that growth and development will be altered because of poor parenting abilities, although the mother's alcohol use may continue once the neonate arrives home. If it does, then this does become a potential problem. The neonate has poor feeding behaviors, but this is caused by exaggerated mouthing behaviors and hyperirritability, not impaired swallowing. Although the neonate may be at an increased risk for abuse and neglect if the mother's alcohol use continues once at home, the priority at this time is the neonate's nutritional status. (D, 9)

79. 4. Gastroschisis is a rare anomaly characterized by the evisceration of abdominal contents through a full-thickness defect in the abdominal wall. The nurse should first protect the abdominal contents with a sterile gauze moistened with sterile saline. Immediate surgery is required. Weighing the neonate is not a priority at this time, but it may need to be done before surgery to determine the appropriate amount of anesthesia. An orogastric tube is not necessary because the infant will not be fed before surgery. An immediate blood transfusion is not needed at this time. (P, 9)

80. 1. The parents need to know that the neonate will be kept NPO and will receive intravenous therapy before surgery. After surgery, feeding will depend on the neonate's condition. Total parenteral nutrition may be ordered after surgery, but not before. Breast-feeding may be started after surgery if the neonate's condition is stable. The mother can pump the breasts until that time. (I, 9)

81. 3. The major goals for the neonate include maintaining fluid and electrolyte balance, preventing infection, and preventing hypothermia. The neonate needs immediate surgery, so bonding is not a priority at this time. (E, 9)

82. 2. The physical appearance of the anomaly and the life-threatening nature of the disorder may result in shock to the parents. The parents may hesitate to form

a bond with the neonate because of the guarded prognosis. Denial would be evidenced if the parents acted as if nothing were wrong. Bargaining would be evidenced by parental statements involving "if–then" phrasing, such as, "If the surgery is successful, I will go to church every Sunday." Anger would be evidenced if the parents attempted to blame someone, such as health care personnel, for the neonate's condition. (A, 5)

83. 1. To prevent eye damage from phototherapy, the eyes must remain covered at all times while under the lights. The eye patches can be removed when the neonate is held out of the lights by the parents for feeding. The diaper is kept on to prevent damage to the genitalia from the phototherapy. Feeding formula or breast milk every 2 to 3 hours is recommended to prevent hypoglycemia and to encourage gastrointestinal motility. Because the phototherapy lights can overheat the neonate, the temperature should be checked by the axillary route every 2 to 4 hours. (I, 9)

84. 4. An absent Moro reflex, lethargy, opisthotonos, and seizures are symptoms of bilirubin encephalopathy, which, although rare, can be life-threatening. Bronze discoloration of the skin and maculopapular chest rash are normal and are caused by the phototherapy. They will disappear once the phototherapy is discontinued. A urine specific gravity of 1.001 to 1.020 is normal in term neonates. (A, 9)

85. 2. Marked visible peristaltic waves in the abdomen and projectile vomiting are signs of pyloric stenosis. If the condition progresses without surgical intervention, the neonate will become dehydrated and develop metabolic alkalosis. Signs of esophageal atresia include coughing and regurgitation with feedings. Diaphragmatic hernia, a life-threatening event in which the abdominal contents herniate into the thoracic cavity, may be evidenced by breath sounds being heard over the abdomen and significant respiratory distress with cyanosis. Signs of hiatal hernia include vomiting, failure to thrive, and short periods of apnea. (A, 9)

86. 3. With a patent ductus arteriosus, a cardiac defect marked by a failure of the patent ductus arteriosus to close completely at birth, blood from the aorta flows into the pulmonary arteries to be reoxygenated in the lungs and returned to the left atrium and ventricle. The effect of this altered circulation includes increased workload on the left side of the heart and increased pulmonary vascular congestion. Term infants are often asymptomatic, but a loud, machinery-like murmur may be heard throughout systole and diastole. This murmur may be accompanied by a suprasternal thrill, and the heart may be enlarged. Decreased cardiac output with faint peripheral pulses, poor peripheral perfusion, feeding difficulties, and severe congestive heart failure are symptoms associated with severe aortic

stenosis. With this defect, the aortic valve is thickened and rigid, leading to decreased cardiac output and reduced myocardial blood flow. Profound cyanosis over most of the body, fatigue on exertion, feeding difficulties, and chronic hypoxemia are associated with tetralogy of Fallot. With this defect, malalignment of the ventricular system results in nonrestricted ventral septal defects, pulmonic stenosis, overriding of the aorta, and hypertrophy of the left ventricle. The heart appears boot shaped. A harsh systolic murmur with a palpable thrill is associated with truncus arteriosus. It is marked by incomplete division of the great vessel. This is caused by a ventral septal defect. Bounding pulses and a widening pulse pressure may also be present. (A, 9)

87. 1. Coarctation of the aorta accounts for 5% to 7% of congenital heart disease. There is localized constriction of the aorta, at or near the insertion site of the ductus arteriosus, that increases afterload and decreases cardiac output. The infant with coarctation of the aorta presents with symptoms of poor lower body perfusion, metabolic acidosis, and congestive heart failure. Cyanosis is present in the lower part of the body because of decreased cardiac output. The child with a partial atrioventricular septal defect may be asymptomatic at birth. The symptoms in a child with a complete defect depend on the pulmonary artery pressure. If the pressure is high, the child will experience cyanosis on exertion; if it is low, congestive heart failure, manifested by tachypnea, dyspnea, and sternal retractions, may be present. The child with pulmonary atresia has profound (complete) cyanosis. On auscultation, the second heart sound (S_2) is heard as a single sound. This is caused by failure of the pulmonary valve to develop and is accompanied by hypoplastic development of the pulmonary artery and right ventricle. Transposition of the great arteries is associated with complete cyanosis during the first few hours of life. These infants demonstrate hypoxemia with a minimal response to oxygen. In this defect, the pulmonary and systemic systems exist in parallel. Systemic blood (unoxygenated) travels to the right atrium and right ventricle, then into the aorta. Pulmonary venous blood (oxygenated) recirculates through the left side of the heart and through the lungs. (D, 9)

88. 4. The normal pulse rate in a neonate is 120 to 160 bpm. Therefore, a femoral pulse rate of 90 bpm is too low. Diminished peripheral pulses, coolness and mottling of the extremities, delayed capillary refill, hypotension, and decreased urine output are indicative of low cardiac output and poor perfusion. The neonate may be experiencing a complication of the surgery, such as blood loss or leaking of fluid into the interstitial space. The surgeon should be notified immediately to

correct the diminished pulse, through either medications or transfusions. An oxygen saturation between 85% and 100% is considered normal. The surgeon does not need to be notified unless the oxygen saturation falls below 85%. Pale pink extremities are considered a normal finding. If mottling or cyanosis develops, the surgeon should be notified immediately. Warm, dry skin is also a normal finding. If the skin becomes cool or appears cyanotic, the surgeon should be notified. (A, 9)

89. 3. Continuous PGE_1 infusion is necessary for the infant diagnosed with tricuspid atresia to reestablish pulmonary blood flow. This medication maintains a patent ductus arteriosus, which is necessary for the oxygenation of the neonate before surgical intervention. Absence of the tricuspid valve forces all of the blood entering the right atrium to be shunted through the foramen ovale into the left atrium, bypassing the lungs. Oxygenation takes place by retrograde blood flow through a persistent patent ductus arteriosus. Indomethacin (Indocin) is used to allow ductal closure when a patent ductus arteriosus is present in the neonate. It is a prostaglandin inhibitor that promotes ductal closure. Digoxin (Lanoxin) is used for children diagnosed with patent ductus arteriosus or atrioventricular septal defects. This medication helps to control the symptoms of congestive heart failure associated with these defects. Hydrochlorothiazide (HydroDIURIL) is used for children diagnosed with patent ductus arteriosus, ventricular septal defects, or atrioventricular septal defects. This medication helps to control the symptoms of congestive heart failure associated with these defects. (P, 8)

90. 4. A child with atrial septal defect will be monitored by a cardiologist. Nonsurgical closure may be attempted via cardiac catheterization. Surgical closure, using either a prosthetic patch or sutures, is performed on an elective basis early in childhood. Children diagnosed with this disorder do not have spontaneous healing or closure. About 20% to 60% of children born with a ventricular septal defect, an abnormal opening between the right and left ventricles, have spontaneous closure. Atrial septal defect accounts for approximately 10% of all congenital heart disease and is seen in more female than male neonates. This lesion consists of an abnormal opening between the atria. Ostium secundum, a defect located in the middle of the atrial septum, is the most common type seen. As the child grows, she may experience fatigue and dyspnea on exertion. A large defect may result in congestive heart failure if the lesion is unrepaired. Bacterial endocarditis prophylaxis with antibiotics may be ordered if the child develops an infection. (E, 9)

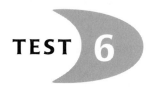

TEST 6

General Client Needs

▶ **Pharmacologic and Parenteral Therapies**

▶ **Growth and Development**

▶ **Management of Care**

▶ **Correct Answers and Rationale**

Select the one best answer, and indicate your choice by filling in the circle in front of the option.

Pharmacologic and Parenteral Therapies

1. A 20-year-old client visiting the clinic requests the use of oral contraceptives. When reviewing the client's history, which of the following would alert the nurse to a possible contraindication to using these agents?
   ○ 1. Thrombophlebitis.
   ○ 2. Urinary tract infections.
   ○ 3. Ulcerative colitis.
   ○ 4. Menorrhagia.

2. A 30-year-old multipara has been prescribed oral contraceptives as a method of birth control. The nurse instructs the client that decreased effectiveness may occur if the client is prescribed which of the following?
   ○ 1. Indomethacin (Indocin).
   ○ 2. Amitriptyline (Elavil).
   ○ 3. Ampicillin.
   ○ 4. Omeprazole (Prilosec).

3. A primigravid client in active labor has just received an epidural block for pain. After administration of the epidural block, for which of the following would the nurse frequently assess the client?
   ○ 1. Spinal headache.
   ○ 2. Hypotension.
   ○ 3. Hyperreflexia.
   ○ 4. Uterine relaxation.

4. One hour after receiving intravenous meperidine (Demerol) for pain during labor, a primigravid client delivers a full-term neonate with symptoms of respiratory depression. The nurse anticipates that the neonate will require the administration of which of the following?
   ○ 1. Betamethasone (Celestone).
   ○ 2. Naltrexone (Trexan).
   ○ 3. Promethazine (Phenergan).
   ○ 4. Naloxone (Narcan).

5. A physician has ordered nalbuphine hydrochloride (Nubain) 10 mg intravenously for a client in active labor. The pharmacy supplies a vial labeled as 50 mg in a 5-mL vial. Which of the following amounts would the nurse administer?
   ○ 1. 0.5 mL.
   ○ 2. 1.0 mL.
   ○ 3. 1.5 mL.
   ○ 4. 2.0 mL.

6. After several hours of induction with intravenous oxytocin administered along with a primary intravenous solution of lactated Ringer's solution, assessment of a primigravid client at 42 weeks' gestation reveals a fetal heart rate near the baseline at 120 bpm and strong contractions occurring every 2 to 2.5 minutes and lasting 90 to 100 seconds. Which of the following would the nurse do *first*?
   ○ 1. Position the client in a supine position.
   ○ 2. Contact the physician for further orders.
   ○ 3. Stop the intravenous flow of oxytocin.
   ○ 4. Administer oxygen at a rate of 5 L/minute.

7. During the immediate postpartum period, the nurse is caring for a primipara who delivered a post-term neonate after oxytocin induction. When developing the client's plan of care, which of the following would the nurse expect to assess for frequently?
   ○ 1. Respiratory depression.
   ○ 2. Increased pulse rate.
   ○ 3. Hypertension.
   ○ 4. Uterine atony.

8. The nurse is preparing to administer a rubella vaccine to a postpartum client before discharge. Which of the following would the nurse caution the client to avoid?
   ○ 1. Breast-feeding the newborn for at least 2 weeks.
   ○ 2. Becoming pregnant for at least 3 months.
   ○ 3. Taking prescription oral contraceptives for at least 1 month.
   ○ 4. Using anti-inflammatory medications for at least 6 weeks.

9. Twenty-four hours after delivery of a term neonate,

113

a primiparous client receives acetaminophen with codeine (Tylenol with Codeine) for complaints of perineal pain. One hour after administering the medication, observation of which of the following would alert the nurse to the development of a possible side effect?

- ○ 1. Dizziness.
- ○ 2. Hypertension.
- ○ 3. Diarrhea.
- ○ 4. Urinary frequency.

10. A primigravid client in active labor has been diagnosed with severe pregnancy-induced hypertension. The client has been receiving intravenous magnesium sulfate for several hours. Which of the following assessments would lead the nurse to notify the physician?
- ○ 1. Urinary output of 45 mL/hour.
- ○ 2. Respiratory rate of 14 breaths/minute.
- ○ 3. Fetal heart rate of 126 bpm.
- ○ 4. Serum magnesium level of 9 mg/dL.

11. A primigravida at 32 weeks' gestation with ruptured membranes is ordered to receive betamethasone (Celestone) 12 mg intramuscularly for two doses 24 hours apart. When teaching the client about the medication, which of the following would the nurse include as the purpose of this drug?
- ○ 1. To prevent potential infection.
- ○ 2. To accelerate fetal lung maturity.
- ○ 3. To reduce contraction frequency.
- ○ 4. To improve the fetal heart rate pattern.

12. The nurse is preparing to administer vitamin K (AquaMEPHYTON) intramuscularly to a term neonate of a primipara who has just delivered. After explaining the purpose of the drug to the mother, which of the following statements by the mother indicates effective teaching?
- ○ 1. "Vitamin K will help my baby to breathe easier."
- ○ 2. "Vitamin K will prevent my baby from becoming jaundiced."
- ○ 3. "Vitamin K will help my baby's blood to clot properly."
- ○ 4. "Vitamin K will prevent my baby from developing an infection."

13. The nurse is preparing to administer erythromycin ophthalmic ointment to a neonate soon after delivery. The nurse would explain to the parents that this medication, in addition to preventing blindness caused by gonococcal organisms, also prevents neonatal blindness caused by which of the following?
- ○ 1. β-Hemolytic streptococcus.
- ○ 2. *Escherichia coli.*
- ○ 3. *Chlamydia trachomatis.*
- ○ 4. *Staphylococcus aureus.*

14. The physician orders oral terbutaline (Brethine) for a primigravid client with symptoms of preterm labor at 35 weeks' gestation after her contractions have stopped. After administering the first dose, for which of the following would the nurse assess the client?
- ○ 1. Tachycardia.
- ○ 2. Hypertension.
- ○ 3. Hyperkalemia.
- ○ 4. Facial edema.

15. While caring for a post-term multigravid client who is being induced with intravenous oxytocin (Pitocin) solution, which of the following maternal assessments would the nurse interpret as indicative of a possible complication?
- ○ 1. Convulsions.
- ○ 2. Jaundice.
- ○ 3. Depressed deep tendon reflexes.
- ○ 4. Hypotension.

Growth and Development

16. While caring for a newly delivered female term neonate, the nurse observes that the neonate's clitoris is enlarged and there is some fusion of the posterior labia majora. The nurse should notify the pediatrician, because these findings are associated with which of the following?
- ○ 1. Renal disorders.
- ○ 2. Potter's syndrome.
- ○ 3. Ambiguous genitalia.
- ○ 4. Turner's syndrome.

17. On the first postpartum day, a primiparous client asks the nurse, "Why are my baby's breasts so swollen?" The nurse explains that breast enlargement in neonates is caused by which of the following transferred from the mother?
- ○ 1. Prolactin.
- ○ 2. Estrogen.
- ○ 3. Progesterone.
- ○ 4. Growth hormone.

18. When developing the teaching plan for a primiparous client and her term neonate on the first postpartum day, the nurse expects to discuss neonatal reflexes. After describing the rooting reflex, which of the following, if stated by the mother as the age at which the reflex disappears, indicates effective teaching?
- ○ 1. 2 weeks to 1 month.
- ○ 2. 6 weeks to 2 months.
- ○ 3. 3 to 4 months.
- ○ 4. 5 to 6 months.

19. The nurse is assigned to care for a newly delivered primiparous client and her term neonate 1 hour

after a vaginal delivery. The nurse observes that the neonate's Apgar score at 5 minutes was 9. The nurse interprets this as indicating which of the following about the neonate?
- ○ 1. Vigorous resuscitation was needed.
- ○ 2. The neonate was cyanotic at birth.
- ○ 3. Oxygen administration was necessary at birth.
- ○ 4. The neonate is in stable condition.

20. When performing Ortolani's maneuver to assess a 1-day-old term neonate for congenital hip dysplasia, which of the following would the nurse do?
- ○ 1. Compare the symmetry of the gluteal folds on the right and left legs with the neonate prone.
- ○ 2. Measure the legs to determine whether one leg is longer than the other with the neonate supine.
- ○ 3. Flex both of the knees and adduct the legs until the examiner's thumbs touch one another.
- ○ 4. Flex the knees while holding the thumbs at midthigh and the fingers over the greater trochanters.

21. A newly immigrated multiparous client from Africa who delivered a term neonate a short time ago requests that a "special bracelet" be placed on the baby's wrist. Which of the following would be the nurse's *most* appropriate action?
- ○ 1. Tell the mother that the bracelet is not recommended for cleanliness reasons.
- ○ 2. Apply the bracelet on the neonate's wrist as the mother requests.
- ○ 3. Place the bracelet on the neonate, limiting its use to when the neonate is with the mother.
- ○ 4. Recommend that the mother wait until she is discharged to apply the bracelet.

22. On the first postpartum day, the nurse instructs a primipara who has delivered a term neonate about the neonate's senses. Which of the following statements by the mother indicates successful teaching?
- ○ 1. "My baby will not be able to hear very well for a few weeks."
- ○ 2. "My baby has very good peripheral vision and can see shapes."
- ○ 3. "My baby's eye color will be established by 1 month of age."
- ○ 4. "My baby can distinguish the color red from the color blue."

23. When teaching a primiparous client who delivered a term male neonate 1 hour ago about the characteristics of her neonate, which of the following would the nurse include?
- ○ 1. Obligatory nose breather.
- ○ 2. Testes probably undescended.
- ○ 3. Kidneys typically nonpalpable.
- ○ 4. Oozing at the cord insertion site.

24. A primipara calls the birthing unit 3 days after a vaginal delivery. She tells the nurse that she is bottle-feeding and her breasts are swollen and painful. Which of the following instructions would be *most* appropriate?
- ○ 1. Wear a tight breast binder for the next 24 hours.
- ○ 2. Avoid wearing a bra to allow the engorgement to subside.
- ○ 3. Refrain from taking a shower with the water on the breasts.
- ○ 4. Use ice packs for 20 minutes every 3 to 4 hours.

25. On the first postpartum day, a neonate diagnosed with an ABO incompatibility has a bilirubin level of 10 mg/dL. After teaching the parents about this condition, which of the following statements by the parents about the neonate indicates the need for *additional* teaching?
- ○ 1. "Phototherapy causes the baby's stools to be bright green."
- ○ 2. "Breast feeding may need to be stopped temporarily."
- ○ 3. "The baby will need an exchange transfusion with type A blood."
- ○ 4. "The baby may become anemic over the next 2 weeks."

26. When assessing a neonate 1 hour after birth, the nurse observes that the neonate exhibits slight cyanosis when quiet but becomes pink when crying. The nurse is unable to pass a catheter through the left nostril. The nurse notifies the pediatrician because the neonate most likely is exhibiting symptoms of which of the following?
- ○ 1. Esophageal reflux disorder.
- ○ 2. Unilateral choanal atresia.
- ○ 3. Respiratory distress syndrome.
- ○ 4. Tracheoesophageal fistula.

27. After delivery of a male neonate at 38 weeks' gestation, the nurse dries the neonate and places him under the radiant warmer. The nurse performs this action based on the understanding that one neonatal response to cold stress involves which of the following?
- ○ 1. Metabolism of brown adipose tissue.
- ○ 2. Decreased utilization of glycogen stores.
- ○ 3. Decreased utilization of calorie stores.
- ○ 4. Increased shivering to keep warm.

28. When developing the teaching plan for a primipara who is bottle-feeding her term neonate for the first feeding, which of the following instructions would the nurse expect to include?
- ○ 1. Fill the entire nipple of the bottle with formula.
- ○ 2. All term babies have well developed sucking skills.
- ○ 3. Bubble the baby after 2 ounces of formula have been taken.
- ○ 4. Propping of the bottle results in too much air being taken in by the baby.

29. A primiparous client at 4 hours after a vaginal delivery and manual removal of the placenta voids for the first time. The nurse palpates the fundus, noting it to be 1 cm above the umbilicus, slightly firm, and deviated to the left side and notes a moderate amount of lochia rubra. The nurse notifies the physician based on the interpretation that the assessment indicates which of the following?
○ 1. Perineal lacerations.
○ 2. Retained placental fragments.
○ 3. Cervical lacerations.
○ 4. Urinary retention.
30. While performing a gestational age assessment for a newly delivered male neonate who was delivered vaginally at 37 weeks' gestation, which of the following would the nurse expect to find?
○ 1. An anterior transverse crease on the soles.
○ 2. Extensive rugae on the scrotum.
○ 3. Some cartilage in the ear lobes.
○ 4. Coarse and silky scalp hair.

Management of Care

31. A neonate of a primipara client delivered at 36 weeks' gestation in a small, rural hospital is to be transferred by ambulance to a level III nursery. To prepare the parents for the transfer, which of the following would the nurse include in the plan of care?
○ 1. Instruct the parents that the neonate is in critical condition.
○ 2. Obtain the mother's consent for the neonate's transfer.
○ 3. Allow the parents to touch the neonate before transfer.
○ 4. Ask the father if he desires to ride in the ambulance during the transfer.
32. A multiparous client delivers a neonate at 24 weeks' gestation. After 12 hours, the neonate's condition deteriorates, and death appears likely within the next few minutes. The parents are Roman Catholic, and they request that the neonate be baptized. Which of the following actions would be *most* appropriate?
○ 1. Contact the hospital chaplain to perform the baptism.
○ 2. Alert the hospital's director that a neonatal death is imminent.
○ 3. Find a health care provider who is Roman Catholic to perform the baptism.
○ 4. Baptize the neonate, regardless of the nurse's own religious beliefs.
33. The nurse on the postpartum unit has delegated the care of a multiparous client and her term neonate at 4 hours postpartum to the licensed practical nurse. Which of the following assessments should the licensed practical nurse report to the nurse immediately?
○ 1. Neonatal regurgitation of 1 tablespoon after feeding.
○ 2. Maternal pulse rate of 100 bpm at rest.
○ 3. Neonatal heart rate of 140 bpm while at rest.
○ 4. Increased maternal lochia rubra with initial ambulation.
34. A multiparous client and her neonate, who has been cared for in the intensive care nursery for the past 3 days because of being small for gestational age, are to be discharged. Before their release, the mother tells the nurse "I've been living in my car for the past 2 weeks." Which of the following would the nurse do *next*?
○ 1. Notify the director of the birthing unit.
○ 2. Contact the hospital's social worker.
○ 3. Contact the client's physician.
○ 4. Notify any of the client's family members.
35. A multiparous client at 16 weeks' gestation is diagnosed as having a fetus with probable anencephaly. The client is a devout Baptist and has decided to continue the pregnancy and donate the neonatal organs after the death of the neonate. Which of the following actions would be *most* appropriate?
○ 1. Explore nurse's own feelings about the issues of anencephaly and organ donation.
○ 2. Contact the client's minister to discuss the client's options related to the pregnancy.
○ 3. Advise the client that the prolonged neonatal death will be very painful for her.
○ 4. Ask the client if she has discussed this with her family members.
36. Assessment of a primigravid client in active labor reveals cervical dilation at 9 cm with complete effacement and the fetus at +1 station. Which of the following would the nurse do when the physician orders meperidine (Demerol) 50 mg intramuscularly (IM) for the client?
○ 1. Administer the medication in the left ventrogluteal muscle.
○ 2. Be certain that naloxone (Narcan) is at the client's bedside.
○ 3. Ask the physician to validate the dosage of the drug.
○ 4. Refuse to administer the medication to the client.
37. A 17-year-old unmarried primigravida client at 10 weeks' gestation tells the nurse that her family doesn't have much money and her dad just got laid off from his job. Which of the following would be the nurse's most appropriate action?
○ 1. Instruct the client in methods for low-cost, highly nutritious meal preparation.
○ 2. Determine whether the client qualifies for state assistance programs.

○ 3. Refer the client to a social worker for enrollment in the Women, Infants, and Children (WIC) program.

○ 4. Ask the client if she has a job and the amount of income earned.

38. The nurse has been assigned to care for several postpartum clients and their neonates on a birthing unit. Which of the following clients would the nurse assess *first*?

○ 1. A multipara at 48 hours postpartum who is being discharged.

○ 2. A primipara at 2 hours postpartum who delivered a term neonate vaginally.

○ 3. A multipara at 24 hours postpartum whose infant is in the special care nursery.

○ 4. A primipara at 48 hours after cesarean delivery of a term neonate.

39. A 16-year-old primipara has decided to place her baby for adoption. The adoptive parents are on their way to the hospital when the mother says, "I want to see the baby one last time." Which of the following would the nurse do?

○ 1. Tell the client that it would be best if she didn't see the baby.

○ 2. Allow the client to see the baby through the nursery window.

○ 3. Contact the physician for advice related to the client's visitation.

○ 4. Allow the client to see and hold the baby for as long as she desires.

40. Assessment of a primigravid client in active labor reveals a cervix dilated to 5 cm and completely effaced, with the fetus at −1 station. The client has indicated that she wants a "natural childbirth" with no analgesia or anesthesia. The client's husband has been present since their arrival at the birthing unit. The physician enters the room and tells the client that it is time for an epidural anesthetic. Which of the following would be the nurse's *best* action at this time?

○ 1. Ask the client if she desires an epidural anesthetic.

○ 2. Tell the physician that the client desires a "natural childbirth."

○ 3. Tell the client that her labor will be more comfortable with an anesthetic.

○ 4. Ask the client to discuss this with her husband and then make a decision.

41. The nurse is working on a hospital's birthing unit when a primigravid client in active labor is ordered to receive meperidine (Demerol) 75 mg IM. As the nurse enters the medication room, the nurse observes a female coworker slipping a vial of morphine into the side pocket of her uniform. Which of the following actions would be *most* appropriate?

○ 1. Contact the hospital's security chief.

○ 2. Notify the supervisor of the unit.

○ 3. Tell the coworker of the incident.

○ 4. Notify the federal drug agents about the incident.

42. The nurse is working on a birthing unit that has several unlicensed assistive personnel (UAP). The nurse expects the UAP assigned to several clients in labor to notify the nurse if the UAP notes which of the following about one of the clients?

○ 1. An episode of nausea after administration of an epidural anesthetic.

○ 2. Contractions 3 minutes apart and lasting 40 seconds.

○ 3. Evidence of spontaneous rupture of the membranes.

○ 4. Sleeping after administration of intravenous nalbuphine (Nubain).

43. Two hours after a vaginal delivery, the nurse has transferred a primiparous client and her term neonate to the mother-baby unit. Which of the following observations by the nurse is a *priority* assessment to be related to the nurse receiving the client on the mother–baby unit?

○ 1. Firm fundus when gentle massage is used.

○ 2. Evidence of bonding well with the neonate.

○ 3. Labor that lasted 12 hours with a 1-hour second stage.

○ 4. Temperature of 99°F (37.4°C) and pulse rate of 80 bpm.

44. The nurse is working in a newborn nursery and caring for several neonates. Precautions that should be taken to prevent an infant abduction include which of the following?

○ 1. Notifying the hospital's security staff about anyone who appears unusual.

○ 2. Taking several neonates to their mothers at the same time.

○ 3. Placing the infant near the doorway of the mother's room.

○ 4. Contacting the hospital's security staff if an exit alarm is triggered.

45. The nurse has provided an in-service presentation to ancillary staff about standard precautions on the birthing unit. The nurse determines that one of the staff members needs *further* instructions when the nurse observes which of the following?

○ 1. Use of protective goggles during a cesarean delivery.

○ 2. Placement of bloody sheets in a container designated for contaminated linens.

○ 3. Wearing of sterile gloves to bathe a newly delivered neonate at 1 hour of age.

○ 4. Disposal of used scalpel blades in a puncture-resistant container.

Correct Answers and Rationale

The letters in parentheses following the rationale identify the step of the nursing process (A, D, P, I, E) and client needs (1, 2, 3, 4, 5, 6, 7, 8, 9, 10). See the inside front cover for the key.

Pharmacologic and Parenteral Therapies

1. 1. Oral contraceptives are contraindicated for clients with a history of thrombophlebitis because a serious side effect of oral contraceptives is thrombus formation. Other contraindications include stroke and liver disease. Oral contraceptives are used cautiously in clients with migraines, hypertension, or diabetes. Close follow-up of these clients is essential. (A, 8)

2. 3. Oral contraceptives may interact with other medications and the effectiveness may be decreased if the client is prescribed ampicillin, tetracycline, or anticonvulsants, such as phenytoin (Dilantin). Indomethacin (Indocin), an anti-inflammatory agent; amitriptyline (Elavil), an antidepressant agent; and omeprazole (Prilosec), a drug used to suppress gastric acid secretion do not decrease the effectiveness of oral contraceptives. (I, 8)

3. 2. One of the most common maternal side effects after epidural anesthesia is hypotension. Therefore, the blood pressure must be assessed frequently after administration of this type of anesthesia. Other side effects include bladder distention, a prolonged second stage of labor, pruritus, nausea and vomiting, and delayed respiratory depression. Uterine relaxation is associated with general anesthesia, not epidural anesthesia. (A, 8)

4. 4. The drug of choice to reverse opioid-induced respiratory depression in a neonate is naloxone (Narcan). Naloxone reverses the effects of opioids. Betamethasone (Celestone) is administered to enhance surfactant production in preterm neonates. Naltrexone (ReVia) is used to relieve pruritus from epidural narcotics. Promethazine (Phenergan) is used to control nausea and vomiting in the mother. (P, 8)

5. 2. The nurse should administer 1 mL of the solution, calculated as follows:

$$\frac{10 \text{ mg}}{50 \text{ mg}} = \frac{x}{5 \text{ mL}} \qquad \frac{1}{5} = \frac{x}{5 \text{ mL}}$$
$$5\,x = 5 \text{ mL} \qquad x = 1 \text{ mL}$$

(I, 8)

6. 3. The nurse should stop the intravenous flow of oxytocin, because the client is exhibiting a hypertonic uter-ine contraction pattern caused by the oxytocin. Once the oxytocin infusion is stopped, the client should be placed in side-lying or lateral position to improve placental blood flow to the fetus, and the nurse should contact the physician to report this finding and obtain further orders. Oxygen may be administered, but at a rate of 8 to 10 L/minute, not 5 L/minute. (I, 8)

7. 4. Uterine atony is more common in clients who have received oxytocin during labor because the uterine muscle becomes fatigued and does not contract effectively to compress the vessels at the placental site. Respiratory depression, not typically associated with oxytocin induction, may occur with narcotic overdose or excessive magnesium sulfate administration. Increased pulse rate and hypertension are not typically associated with oxytocin induction during labor. (P, 9)

8. 2. The rubella vaccine is a live virus and can result in serious fetal anomalies if the client becomes pregnant soon after it is administered. Therefore, the client should not become pregnant for at least 3 months. The rubella vaccine is not passed in breast milk and has no effect on the neonate. Therefore, breast-feeding is not contraindicated. (I, 8)

9. 1. Analgesics with narcotics have numerous side effects, including respiratory depression, dizziness, lightheadedness, hypotension, and fainting. Other side effects include constipation, nausea and vomiting, and urinary retention. (A, 8)

10. 4. The physician should be notified immediately if the client's serum magnesium level is 9 mg/dL because this suggests hypermagnesemia. The normal therapeutic range is 4 mg/dL to 8 mg/dL. Typically, urinary output should be greater than 30 mL/hour. Therefore, a urinary output of 45 mL/hour is acceptable. A respiratory rate should not fall below 12 breaths/minute; a respiratory rate of 14 breaths/minute is acceptable. A fetal heart rate of 126 bpm is within the normal range of 120 to 160 bpm. (D, 8)

11. 2. Corticosteriods, such as betamethasone, are prescribed for clients who are preterm to accelerate fetal lung maturity and reduce the incidence and severity of respiratory distress syndrome. Betamethasone is contraindicated if an infection is present. (I, 8)

12. 3. At birth, the vitamin K–dependent blood clotting factors are significantly decreased and there is a transitory deficiency in blood coagulation during the second and fifth days of life. As a preventive measure, 0.5 to 1 mg of vitamin K is administered to the newborn during the first day of life to aid in blood clotting. (E, 8)

13. 3. The use of erythromycin ophthalmic ointment prevents blindness from the gonococcal organisms and *C. trachomatis.* This ointment usually is less expensive than tetracycline. β-Hemolytic streptococcus, *E. coli,* and *S. aureus* can cause a generalized infection in the neonate. However, these organisms typically are not responsible for causing neonatal blindness. (I, 8)

14. 1. Terbutaline (Brethine) is used as a tocolytic agent to prevent preterm labor contractions. Side effects include maternal and fetal tachycardia, hypotension, hypokalemia, nervousness, emesis, headache, and pulmonary edema. Facial edema is associated with the use of steroids, not terbutaline. (A, 8)

15. 1. Severe water intoxication with convulsions and coma can occur when clients are induced with oxytocin. Other serious adverse effects include hypertension, uterine rupture, tetanic contractions, neonatal jaundice, and postpartum hemorrhage. Depression of deep tendon reflexes is a possible complication of magnesium sulfate therapy. (D, 8)

Growth and Development

16. 3. An enlarged clitoris with fusion of the posterior labia majora is associated with ambiguous genitalia. Ultrasound examination will reveal whether ovaries are present. Renal disorders are associated with absence of a kidney and oliguria. Potter's syndrome is a fatal condition involving renal agenesis and facial deformities. Turner's syndrome is an autosomal anomaly in which there are 45 chromosomes. This syndrome also involves mental retardation, a long spine, and delayed or absent sexual maturity. (D, 9)

17. 2. Temporary breast enlargement in neonates is caused by maternal estrogen. The breast enlargement should subside within a few days. Prolactin is the hormone involved in the production of maternal breast milk. Progesterone is the hormone responsible for the development of the vascular endometrium during the menstrual cycle. Growth hormone is responsible for neonatal growth and may be increased in infants of insulin-dependent diabetic mothers. (I, 3)

18. 3. The rooting reflex, stimulated by touching the upper lip or cheek before a feeding, disappears by the age of 3 to 4 months. A rooting reflex that disappears before 2 months of age or persists beyond 4 months of age requires further evaluation of neurologic capabilities. (E, 3)

19. 4. Apgar scores are generally determined at 1 minute and at 5 minutes after birth by someone who has not delivered the neonate. The maximum score is 2 on each of five signs, including heart rate (greater than 100 bpm); color (completely pink); respiratory effort (good,

crying); reflex irritability (cough, sneeze, cry); and muscle tone (well-flexed). A total score lower than 4 requires vigorous resuscitation; a score of 4 to 6 means that the infant required some stimulation and oxygenation; and a score of 7 to 10 is considered good, indicating that the neonate is in stable condition. There is a high correlation between a low Apgar score and neonatal morbidity and mortality, primarily because of neurologic morbidity. (D, 3)

20. 4. To perform Ortolani's maneuver, the nurse should flex the knees while holding the thumbs at midthigh and the fingers over the greater trochanters. When the infant's leg is held with the fingers on the greater and lesser trochanters and the hip is abducted, subluxation, if present, will cause a "clunk" when the femur head strikes the shallow acetabulum. (A, 3)

21. 2. The nurse should abide by the mother's request and place the bracelet on the neonate. In some cultures, amulets and other special objects are viewed as good luck symbols. By allowing the bracelet, the nurse demonstrates culturally sensitive care, promoting trust. The neonate can wear the bracelet while with the mother or in the nursery. The bracelet can be removed while the neonate is being bathed and replaced afterward. (I, 3)

22. 2. The nurse determines that the mother has understood the instructions when she says "My baby has very good peripheral vision and can see shapes." At birth, the neonate has good peripheral vision but poorly developed central vision. Most neonates, unless born with congenital deafness, have excellent hearing abilities. The eye (iris) color is usually established by 3 to 4 months of age. Most babies cannot distinguish color until about 8 months of age. Neonates respond well to black-and-white geometric shapes. (E, 3)

23. 1. The nurse should instruct the mother that the neonate is an obligatory nose breather. Care must be taken to keep the infant's nares free from obstruction. The testes of a term male neonate should be in the scrotal sac. If they are undescended, further evaluation is required. Both kidneys should be palpable, each approximately the size of a walnut. Oozing at the cord insertion site is not normal and may indicate an infection. (I, 3)

24. 4. Ice packs cause vasoconstriction and can provide temporary relief of breast engorgement for the bottle-feeding mother. Breast engorgement is transitory and usually disappears within a few days. A tight breast binder is not recommended because it can worsen the engorgement and restrict blood flow. A supportive bra should be worn at all times by both bottle-feeding and breast-feeding mothers. Taking a warm shower may help relieve some of the discomfort of the breast engorgement. (I, 3)

25. 3. ABO incompatibility occurs when the mother has type O blood, and the neonate is A, B, or AB. This condition is not as serious as Rh incompatibility. The mother needs further instructions when she says the neonate will require an exchange transfusion with type A blood. Unless the bilirubin concentration reaches the dangerous level (approximately 20 mg/dL), an exchange transfusion is not usually performed. If an exchange transfusion does become necessary, type O blood is used. Phototherapy is the common treatment for ABO incompatibility. The neonate may have bright green stools as bilirubin is broken down and excreted in the stool. The mother may need to temporarily halt breast-feeding, but she may pump the breasts and continue feeding after the first 48 hours. The destruction of the neonate's red blood cells occurs after birth, so the neonate may become anemic until the hemolysis ceases, usually within 2 weeks. (E, 9)

26. 2. Infants are obligatory nose breathers except when crying. The observation that the infant has slight cyanosis when quiet but becomes pink when crying and the inability to pass a catheter through the left nostril suggest that the neonate is exhibiting symptoms of unilateral choanal atresia. With this condition, one of the nasal passages is blocked by an abnormality of the septum. Surgical intervention is necessary to open the nostril. Typically, a neonate with esophageal reflux disorder exhibits episodes of apnea and vomiting after eating. Respiratory distress syndrome commonly occurs in preterm neonates who lack surfactant to maintain lung expansion. Common findings include sternal retractions, tachypnea, grunting respirations, nasal flaring, cyanosis, pallor, hypotonia, and bradycardia. A neonate with tracheoesophageal fistula commonly exhibits cyanosis during feedings and vomiting. (D, 9)

27. 1. Neonates burn brown adipose tissue (fat) as a response to cold stress. In addition, there is increased utilization of glycogen and calorie stores. Hypoglycemia may result from becoming stressed by a cold environment. Neonates do not have the ability to shiver. (D, 3)

28. 1. Formula should fill the entire nipple of the bottle while the baby is sucking. This decreases the amount of air taken by the baby, which can lead to regurgitation. Not all babies at term are born with well-developed sucking skills. Some neonates are sleepy and do not suck well. For the first feeding, the baby should be bubbled after taking one-fourth to one-half ounce of formula and then again when the infant has finished the feeding. Bottle propping can lead to aspiration, decreased infant bonding, and aspiration of formula. However, it is not associated with the intake of too much air. (P, 3)

29. 2. At 4 hours postpartum, the fundus should be midline and at the level of the umbilicus. Whenever there is manual removal of the placenta, there is a possibility that all of the placenta has not been removed after the delivery. Sometimes small pieces of the placenta are retained, a common cause of late postpartum hemorrhage. The client is exhibiting signs associated with retained placental fragments. The client will continue to bleed until the fragments are expelled. Perineal and cervical lacerations are characterized by bright red bleeding and a firmly contracted fundus at the level that is expected. Urinary retention is characterized by a full bladder, which can be observed by a bulge or fullness just above the symphysis pubis. Also, the client's fundus would be deviated to one side and boggy to the touch. (D, 9)

30. 3. A neonate born at 37 weeks' gestation will have some cartilage in the ear lobes, fine and fuzzy hair, scant to moderate rugae in the scrotum, and a breast nodule diameter of 4 mm. Neonates born before 36 weeks' gestation will have only an anterior transverse crease on the soles of the feet. Extensive rugae on the scrotum are a typical finding in neonates born at 39 weeks' gestation or later. Coarse and silky scalp hair typically is found in neonates that are born at 39 weeks' gestation or later. (A, 3)

Management of Care

31. 3. When a neonate is being transferred to a neonatal care center (level III nursery), the parents should be allowed to see and touch the neonate, if possible, before transfer. The parents should be given the location and telephone number of the unit to which the neonate is being transferred. This helps to keep the parents informed. The parents are already aware of the neonate's condition and should recognize that it is critical if the neonate is being transferred to a neonatal care center. The parents have signed consent for treatment on admission, and in most states another consent is not necessary. Asking whether the father would like to ride in the ambulance with the neonate during the transfer is inappropriate. Most ambulances or transferring vehicles (eg, helicopters, airplanes) do not allow family members to accompany the ill client. Space in the motor vehicle, helicopter, or plane is limited. In addition, most transferring vehicles do not have insurance to cover family members should an accident occur during transfer. (P, 1)

32. 4. Tenets of the Roman Catholic Church hold that it is acceptable for anyone, regardless of his or her religious beliefs, to baptize a neonate. For Roman Catholic families, baptism ensures entry into heaven. Local practice may vary, and in some situations the parents may pre-

fer to have a Roman Catholic person perform the rites; however, the priest may not be available until after the death. The parents may wish to have a priest contacted for grief support. Notification of the hospital's director is not necessary. (I, 1)

33. 2. The practical nurse should report a maternal pulse rate of 100 bpm at rest because it could potentially indicate shock or hemorrhage. Typically, the pulse rate of a postpartum client slows after delivery and continues to be slow for about 1 week because of an increase in central circulation that results in increased stroke volume to provide adequate maternal circulation. The normal pulse rate is 60 to 70 bpm. Neonatal regurgitation of 1 tablespoon after feeding, a neonatal heart rate of 140 bpm at rest, and increased maternal lochia rubra when the mother initially ambulates are normal findings. (I, 1)

34. 2. When a client is being released from the hospital with her neonate and the nurse learns that the client is homeless, the nurse should contact the hospital's or unit's social worker. Social workers have access to resources to assist the client to find temporary shelter in emergency situations. The director of the birthing unit does not need to be notified. The director's responsibilities are primarily administrative. The client's physician can be notified once the social worker has offered assistance to the client. The physician may cancel the release of the neonate until temporary housing is located. Notifying any of the client's family members is inappropriate. The client may not have any immediate family members, or there may be some stress between the client and family members. (I, 1)

35. 1. Anencephaly is a neural tube defect that is not compatible with life, although some of these infants live for several days before death occurs. When the client has decided to continue the pregnancy and donate the neonatal organs after the death of the neonate, the nurse should remain nonjudgmental. The nurse should explore his or her feelings about the issue of anencephaly and organ donation. The nurse should not make judgments about the client's position, nor should the nurse try to persuade the client to terminate the pregnancy. Contacting the client's minister to explore the client's options is not appropriate. As a devout Baptist, the client probably has already discussed the matter with her minister. Telling the client that the neonatal death will be prolonged and painful to her is not helpful. Death may occur very soon after birth. Contacting the client's family members is not appropriate. The client may wish to maintain confidentiality and privacy related to the birth. (I, 1)

36. 4. The nurse should refuse to administer the medication to the client because of the risk of respiratory depression in the neonate. Meperidine, given IM, peaks in 30 to 60 minutes and lasts 2 to 4 hours. Based on the assessment findings, the client most likely will be delivering within that time frame, increasing the risk for respiratory depression in the neonate, a serious consequence. Therefore, the nurse should not administer the drug. Naloxone (Narcan) should be readily available whenever narcotics that can result in respiratory depression are used. Asking the physician to validate the dosage is not necessary. For clients in early labor, meperidine can be given IM in dosages ranging from 50 mg to 100 mg. (I, 1)

37. 3. The nurse should refer the client to a social worker for assistance in enrolling in the WIC program. This program provides assistance for foods such as milk, cereal, and infant formula. Instructing the client in low-cost, highly nutritious meal preparation will not meet the client's needs for additional funds for food. Determining whether the client qualifies for state assistance is part of the role of the social worker, not the nurse. Asking the client if she has a job and the amount of income earned is not within the role of the nurse. The social worker can determine whether the family income guidelines are met for state and federal assistance. (I, 1)

38. 2. The primipara at 2 hours postpartum who delivered a term neonate vaginally should be assessed first, because this client is at risk for postpartum hemorrhage. Early postpartum hemorrhage typically occurs during the first 24 hours postpartum. Once the nurse has assessed the client's fundus, lochia, and vital signs, a determination about the stability of the client can be made. After this assessment, the nurse can provide care to the other clients, who are of lesser priority than the newly delivered primipara. (I, 1)

39. 4. The nurse should allow the client to see and hold the baby for as long as she desires. Such activities provide memories for the mother and assist in the grieving process. There is a possibility that the client may change her mind about the adoption. In most states, there is a defined period (6 months to 1 year or longer) before an adoption becomes final. If the client changes her mind about the adoption, the nurse should accept the client's decision and notify the physician and social worker. Telling the client that it would be best if she didn't see the baby is imposing the nurse's value system on the client. Allowing the client to see the baby through the nursery window is inappropriate, because the client should be allowed to touch and hold the baby. Contacting the physician for advice related to the client's visitation is not necessary. (I, 1)

40. 1. To be a true client advocate, the nurse should ask the client if she desires an epidural anesthetic even though the client has indicated a desire for "natural childbirth." The client has a right to change her mind and also a right to refuse treatment. The client, not the nurse, should be the one to tell the physician that she does not want an epidural anesthetic; the nurse should support the client's decision. Although telling the client that her labor will be more comfortable with an anesthetic provides the client with information, a statement such as this can be viewed as an attempt to change the client's mind. The client may wish to discuss this situation with her husband, but she does not have to do so. (I, 1)

41. 2. When a nurse observes the theft of a narcotic, it is the responsibility of the nurse to report the incident to the supervisor of the unit. The supervisor of the unit can confront the coworker and notify the hospital's chief of security about the incident. In some situations, the drug-abusing coworker may be offered drug counseling. In situations where the drugs are being sold, the police should be notified. The nurse should not confront the coworker, because this may put the nurse in danger. It is not the responsibility of the nurse to notify federal drug agents about the incident. (I, 1)

42. 3. The nurse expects the UAP assigned to several clients in labor to notify the nurse if the UAP observes that one of the clients has evidence of spontaneous rupture of the membranes. When the membranes rupture spontaneously there is danger of a prolapsed cord, a medical emergency requiring a cesarean delivery. Nausea may occur after administration of an epidural anesthetic, but this is not a priority or emergency situation. Having contractions that are 3 minutes apart and last for 40 seconds is normal during active labor. Because nalbuphine (Nubain) is an analgesic, it is normal for a client to fall asleep after intravenous administration of this drug. (I, 1)

43. 1. The priority assessment is that the client has a firm fundus when gentle massage is used. This indicates that the client's fundus may be soft or "boggy" when it is not massaged. The receiving nurse should assess the client's fundus soon after admission and continue to monitor the client's fundus, lochia, and pulse rate. Postpartum hemorrhage is associated with uterine atony. (A, 1)

44. 1. The nurse should notify the hospital's security staff about anyone who appears unusual. Typically the abductor is an older woman who wishes to have a baby. The nurse should take only one baby at a time to a mother to prevent the neonate's being taken to the wrong mother. Infants should never be left in the hallway. When in the mother's room, the infant should be placed away from the doorway to prevent or minimize the risk of abduction of the neonate. If an exit alarm is triggered, it is possible that an abductor is running away with an infant. Staff members should investigate the alarm immediately and stop the potential abductor. Hospital security can be alerted if someone is seen exiting the unit carrying a large bag or an infant. (I, 1)

45. 3. One of the staff members needs further instructions when the nurse observes the staff member wearing sterile gloves to bathe a newly delivered neonate at 1 hour of age. Clean gloves should be worn, not sterile gloves. Sterile gloves are more expensive than clean gloves and are not necessary when bathing a newly delivered neonate. (E, 2)

Bibliography

Gorrie, T.M., McKinney, E.S., & Murray, S.S. (1998). *Foundations of maternal newborn nursing.* (2nd ed.). Philadelphia: WB Saunders.

May, K.A., & Mahlmeister, L.R. (1994). *Maternal and neonatal nursing.* (3rd ed.). Philadelphia: J.B. Lippincott.

Pillitteri, A. (1999). *Maternal and child health nursing: Care of the childbearing and childrearing family.* (3rd ed.). Philadelphia: Lippincott Williams & Wilkins.

Reeder, S.J., Martin, L.L., and Koniak-Griffin, D. (1997). *Maternity nursing: Family, newborn, and women's health care.* (18th ed.). Philadelphia: Lippincott–Raven.

The Nursing Care of Children

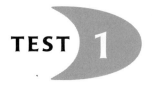
Health Promotion

Select the one best answer, and indicate your choice by filling in the circle in front of the option.

Health Promotion of the Infant and Family

1. A mother who brings her 4-month-old infant to the clinic for a regular check-up is concerned that her infant is not developing appropriately. When assessing the infant, which of the following would the nurse expect to find?
   ○ 1. Ability to sit up with support.
   ○ 2. Fine motor finger-to-thumb grasp.
   ○ 3. Ability to reach for a toy.
   ○ 4. Ability to say mama or dada.

2. In addition to immunizing for diphtheria, tetanus, and pertussis (DTaP) during the first 6 months of life, the nurse should administer which of the following immunizations?
   ○ 1. Mumps.
   ○ 2. Measles.
   ○ 3. Tuberculosis.
   ○ 4. Hepatitis B.

3. The parents of a 9-month-old bring the infant to the clinic for a regular checkup. The infant has received no immunizations. Which of the following would be appropriate for the nurse to administer at this visit?
   ○ 1. DTaP, Hib, IPV, and PPD.
   ○ 2. DTaP, Hib, OPV, and MMR.
   ○ 3. PPD, MMR, Hep B, and OPV.
   ○ 4. HEP B, IPV, Hib and varicella.

4. A mother of a 1-month-old infant states that she is curious as to whether her infant is developing normally. Which of the following developmental milestones would the nurse expect the infant to perform?
   ○ 1. Smiling and laughing out loud.
   ○ 2. Rolling from back to side.
   ○ 3. Holding a rattle briefly.
   ○ 4. Turning the head from side to side.

5. The mother of a 6-month-old states that she has started her infant on 2% milk. Which of the following would be the nurse's *best* response?
   ○ 1. "Your baby will probably be fine with this milk."
   ○ 2. "The baby should be switched to whole milk."
   ○ 3. "You need to keep the infant on formula."
   ○ 4. "You need to switch to formula right now."

6. The nurse notes that an infant stares at an object placed in her hand and takes it to her mouth, coos and gurgles when talked to, and sustains part of her own weight when held in a standing position. The nurse correctly interprets these findings as characteristic of an infant at which of the following ages?
   ○ 1. 2 months.
   ○ 2. 4 months.
   ○ 3. 7 months.
   ○ 4. 9 months.

7. A parent seems concerned about the fact that the infant's soft spot is still open. Which of the following would the nurse include when explaining about the usual age for closure of the soft spot near the front of the infant's head?
   ○ 1. 2 to 4 months.
   ○ 2. 5 to 8 months.
   ○ 3. 9 to 11 months.
   ○ 4. 12 to 18 months.

8. A mother states that she thinks her 9-month-old "is developing slowly." When assessing the infant's development, the nurse is also concerned because the infant should be demonstrating which of the following characteristics?
   ○ 1. Vocalizing single syllables.
   ○ 2. Standing alone.
   ○ 3. Building a tower of two cubes.
   ○ 4. Drinking from a cup with little spilling.

Health Promotion of the Toddler and Family

9. A mother brings her 18-month-old to the clinic because the child "eats ashes, crayons, and paper." Which of the following about the toddler would the nurse assess *first*?
   - ○ 1. Evidence of eruption of large teeth.
   - ○ 2. Amount of attention from the mother.
   - ○ 3. Any changes in the home environment.
   - ○ 4. Intake of a soft, low-roughage diet.

10. When assessing a 2-year-old child brought by his mother to the clinic for a routine checkup, which of the following would the nurse expect the child to be able to do?
   - ○ 1. Ride a tricycle.
   - ○ 2. Tie his shoelaces.
   - ○ 3. Kick a ball forward.
   - ○ 4. Use blunt scissors.

11. A 2$\frac{1}{2}$-year-old brought to the clinic by her parents is uncooperative when the nurse tries to look in her ears. Which of the following would the nurse try *first*?
   - ○ 1. Ask another nurse to assist.
   - ○ 2. Allow a parent to assist.
   - ○ 3. Wait until the child calms down.
   - ○ 4. Restrain the child's arms.

12. When observing the parent instilling prescribed ear drops ordered twice a day for a toddler, the nurse decides that the teaching about positioning of the pinna for instillation of the drops is effective when the parent pulls the toddler's pinna in which of the following directions?
   - ○ 1. Up and forward.
   - ○ 2. Up and backward.
   - ○ 3. Down and forward.
   - ○ 4. Down and backward.

13. The mother asks the nurse for advice about discipline for her 18-month-old. Which of the following would the nurse suggest that the mother use *first*?
   - ○ 1. Structured interactions.
   - ○ 2. Spanking.
   - ○ 3. Reasoning.
   - ○ 4. Time out.

14. When assessing for pain in a toddler, which of the following methods would be the *most* appropriate?
   - ○ 1. Ask the child about the pain.
   - ○ 2. Observe the child for restlessness.
   - ○ 3. Use a numeric pain scale.
   - ○ 4. Assess for changes in vital signs.

15. When planning a 15-month-old toddler's daily diet with the parents, which of the following amounts of milk would the nurse include?
   - ○ 1. $\frac{1}{2}$ to 1 cup.
   - ○ 2. 2 to 3 cups.
   - ○ 3. 3 to 4 cups.
   - ○ 4. 4 to 5 cups.

Health Promotion of the Preschooler and Family

16. The mother of a 4-year-old expresses concern that her child may be hyperactive. She describes the child as always in motion, constantly dropping and spilling things. Which of the following actions would be *most* appropriate at this time?
   - ○ 1. Determine whether there have been any changes at home.
   - ○ 2. Explain that this is not unusual behavior.
   - ○ 3. Explore the possibility that the child is being abused.
   - ○ 4. Suggest that the child be seen by a pediatric neurologist.

17. The mother of a preschooler reports that her child creates a scene every night at bedtime. The nurse and the mother decide that the *best* course of action would be to do which of the following?
   - ○ 1. Allow the child to stay up later one or two nights a week.
   - ○ 2. Establish a set bedtime and follow a routine.
   - ○ 3. Encourage active play before bedtime.
   - ○ 4. Give the child a cookie if bedtime is pleasant.

18. After teaching a group of parents of preschoolers attending a well-child clinic about oral hygiene and teeth brushing, the nurse determines that the teaching has been successful when the parents state that children can begin to brush their teeth without help at which of the following ages?
   - ○ 1. 3 years.
   - ○ 2. 5 years.
   - ○ 3. 7 years.
   - ○ 4. 9 years.

19. After having a blood sample drawn, a 5-year-old child insists that the site be covered with an adhesive bandage strip. When the mother tries to remove the bandage before leaving the office, the child screams that all the blood will come out. The nurse interprets this behavior as indicating a fear of which of the following?
   - ○ 1. Injury.
   - ○ 2. Compromised body integrity.
   - ○ 3. Pain.
   - ○ 4. Loss of control.

20. A mother is concerned because her 5-year-old son seems prone to minor accidents such as skinning his elbows and knees and falling off his scooter. The nurse explains to the mother that childhood accidents are more likely to occur in which of the following situations?
   - ○ 1. The child is the sole child in the family.
   - ○ 2. The family has limited formal education.
   - ○ 3. The family is experiencing changes.
   - ○ 4. The child and family live in the suburbs.

21. When developing the teaching plan for the mother of a preschooler about illness, which of the following would the nurse expect to include about how a preschooler perceives illness?
    ○ 1. A necessary part of life.
    ○ 2. Test of self-worth.
    ○ 3. Punishment for wrongdoing.
    ○ 4. The will of God.

Health Promotion of the School-Aged Child and Family

22. The nurse asks a 9-year-old child and mother about the child's best friend to assess which of the following about the child?
    ○ 1. Language development.
    ○ 2. Motor development.
    ○ 3. Neurologic development.
    ○ 4. Social development.

23. A 10-year-old child proudly tells the nurse that brushing and flossing her teeth is her responsibility. The nurse interprets this statement as indicating which of the following about the child?
    ○ 1. She is too young to be given this responsibility.
    ○ 2. She is most likely capable of this responsibility.
    ○ 3. She should have assumed this responsibility much sooner.
    ○ 4. She is probably just exaggerating the responsibility.

24. The mother tells the nurse that her 8-year-old child is continually telling jokes and riddles to the point of driving the other family members crazy. The nurse explains that this behavior is a sign of which of the following?
    ○ 1. Inadequate parental attention.
    ○ 2. Mastery of language ambiguities.
    ○ 3. Inappropriate peer influence.
    ○ 4. Excessive television watching.

25. The mother asks the nurse about her 9-year-old child's apparent need for between-meal snacks, especially after school. When developing a sound nutritional plan for the child with the mother, which of the following would the nurse need to keep in mind?
    ○ 1. The child does not need to eat between-meal snacks.
    ○ 2. The child should eat the snacks the mother thinks are appropriate.
    ○ 3. The child should help with preparing his or her own snacks.
    ○ 4. The child will instinctively select nutritional snacks.

26. When a child's height and weight are compared with standard growth charts, the child is found to be in the 85th percentile for height and in the 45th percentile for weight. The nurse interprets these findings as indicating which of the following?
    ○ 1. Average height and weight.
    ○ 2. Overweight for height.
    ○ 3. Underweight for height.
    ○ 4. Abnormal in height.

27. When preparing a teaching plan for the parents of a group of 4- to 6-year-old children about recommended immunizations for school entrance, the nurse would expect to include which of the following?
    ○ 1. Diphtheria, tetanus, pertussis, and polio.
    ○ 2. Measles, mumps, rubella, and polio.
    ○ 3. Polio, measles, and pertussis.
    ○ 4. Tetanus, diphtheria, and rubella.

Health Promotion of the Adolescent and Family

28. The school nurse develops a plan with an adolescent to provide relief of dysmenorrhea to aid in her development of which of the following?
    ○ 1. Positive peer relations.
    ○ 2. Positive self-identity.
    ○ 3. A sense of autonomy.
    ○ 4. A sense of independence.

29. An adolescent tells the school nurse that she would like to use tampons during her period. Which of the following would be *most* appropriate for the nurse to do?
    ○ 1. Assess her usual menstrual flow pattern.
    ○ 2. Determine whether she is sexually active.
    ○ 3. Provide information about preventing toxic shock syndrome.
    ○ 4. Refer her to a specialist in adolescent gynecology.

30. The school nurse is invited to attend a meeting with several parents who express frustration with the amount of time their adolescents spend in front of the mirror and the length of time it takes them to get dressed. The nurse explains that this behavior is indicative of which of the following?
    ○ 1. An abnormal narcissism.
    ○ 2. A method of procrastination.
    ○ 3. A way of testing the parents' limit-setting.
    ○ 4. A result of developing self-concept.

31. Several high-school seniors are referred to the school nurse because of suspected alcohol misuse. When the nurse assesses the situation, which of the following would be *most* important to determine?
    ○ 1. What they know about the legal implications of drinking.
    ○ 2. The type of alcohol they usually drink.
    ○ 3. The reasons they choose to use alcohol.
    ○ 4. When and with whom they use alcohol.

Common Childhood and Adolescent Health Problems

32. A parent asks the nurse about head lice (pediculosis capitis) infestation during a visit to the clinic. Which of the following symptoms would the nurse tell the parent is *most* common in a child infected with head lice?
    - ○ 1. Itching of the scalp.
    - ○ 2. Scaling of the scalp.
    - ○ 3. Serous weeping on the scalp surface.
    - ○ 4. Pinpoint hemorrhagic spots on the scalp surface.

33. A parent asks, "Can I get head lice too?" The nurse indicates that adults can also be infested with head lice but that pediculosis is more common among school children, primarily for which of the following reasons?
    - ○ 1. An immunity to pediculosis usually is established by adulthood.
    - ○ 2. School-aged children tend to be more neglectful of frequent handwashing.
    - ○ 3. Pediculosis usually is spread by close contact with infested children.
    - ○ 4. The skin of adults is more capable of resisting the invasion of lice.

34. After teaching the parents about the cause of ringworm of the scalp (tinea capitis), which of the following, if stated by the father, indicates successful teaching?
    - ○ 1. Overexposure to the sun.
    - ○ 2. Infestation with a mite.
    - ○ 3. Fungal infection of the scalp.
    - ○ 4. An allergic reaction.

35. Griseofulvin (Grisactin) was ordered to treat a child's ringworm of the scalp. The nurse instructs the parents to use the medication for several weeks for which of the following reasons?
    - ○ 1. A sensitivity to the drug is less likely if it is used over a period of time.
    - ○ 2. Fewer side effects occur as the body slowly adjusts to a new substance over time.
    - ○ 3. Fewer allergic reactions occur if the drug is maintained at the same level long-term.
    - ○ 4. The growth of the causative organism into new cells is prevented with long-term use.

36. A mother asks the nurse, "How did my children get pinworms?" The nurse explains that pinworms are most commonly spread by which of the following when contaminated?
    - ○ 1. Food.
    - ○ 2. Hands.
    - ○ 3. Animals.
    - ○ 4. Toilet seats.

37. A mother tells the nurse that one of her children has chicken pox and asks what she should do to care for that child. When teaching the mother, which of the following would be *most* important to prevent?
    - ○ 1. Acid-base imbalance.
    - ○ 2. Malnutrition.
    - ○ 3. Skin infection.
    - ○ 4. Respiratory infection.

38. A mother calls the clinic to talk to the nurse. The mother states that a physician described her daughter as having 20/60 vision and asks the nurse what this means. The nurse responds based on the interpretation that the child is experiencing which of the following?
    - ○ 1. A loss of approximately one third of her visual acuity.
    - ○ 2. Ability to see at 60 feet what she should see at 20 feet.
    - ○ 3. Ability to see at 20 feet what she should see at 60 feet.
    - ○ 4. Visual acuity three times better than average.

39. After teaching a group of mothers about temper tantrums, the nurse knows the teaching has been effective when one of the mothers states which of the following?
    - ○ 1. "I will ignore the temper tantrum."
    - ○ 2. "I should pick up the child during the tantrum."
    - ○ 3. "I'll talk to my daughter during the tantrum."
    - ○ 4. "I should put my child in time out."

40. The nurse discusses the eating habits of school-aged children with their parents, explaining that these habits are most influenced by which of the following?
    - ○ 1. Food preferences of their peers.
    - ○ 2. Smell and appearance of foods offered.
    - ○ 3. Examples provided by parents at mealtimes.
    - ○ 4. Parental encouragement to eat nutritious foods.

41. When discussing the onset of adolescence with parents, the nurse explains that it occurs at which of the following times?
    - ○ 1. Same age for both boys and girls.
    - ○ 2. 1 to 2 years earlier in boys than in girls.
    - ○ 3. 1 to 2 years earlier in girls than in boys.
    - ○ 4. 3 to 4 years later in boys than in girls.

42. Parents report that they think their 15-year-old son is moody and rude. The nurse develops a plan with the parents that includes which of the following *initially*?
    - ○ 1. Limiting involvement in nonschool activities.
    - ○ 2. Discussing their feelings with him.
    - ○ 3. Obtaining family counseling.
    - ○ 4. Talking with other parents of adolescents.

43. A mother has heard that several children have been diagnosed with mononucleosis. She asks the nurse

what precautions should be taken to prevent this from occurring in her child. Which of the following would the nurse advise the mother to do?

○ 1. Take no particular precautionary measures.

○ 2. Sterilize the child's eating utensils before they are reused.

○ 3. Wash the child's linens separately in hot, soapy water.

○ 4. Wear masks when providing direct personal care.

44. A father asks the nurse how he would know if his child had developed mononucleosis. The nurse explains that in addition to fatigue, which of the following would be *most* common?

○ 1. Liver tenderness.

○ 2. Enlarged lymph glands.

○ 3. Persistent nonproductive cough.

○ 4. A blush-like generalized skin rash.

45. A parent asks why it is recommended that the second dose of the measles, mumps, rubella (MMR) vaccine be given by 12 years of age? The nurse responds based on which of the following as the *most* important reason?

○ 1. The risks to a fetus are high if a girl receiving the vaccine becomes pregnant.

○ 2. The chance of contracting the disease is much lower after puberty than before it.

○ 3. The dangers associated with a strong reaction to the vaccine are increased after puberty.

○ 4. The changes that occur in the immunologic system may affect the rhythm of the menstrual cycle.

Correct Answers and Rationale

The letters in parentheses following the rationale identify the step of the nursing process (A, D, P, I, E) and client needs (1, 2, 3, 4, 5, 6, 7, 8, 9, 10). See the inside front cover for the key.

Health Promotion of the Infant and Family

1. 1. Typically, a 4-month-old infant should be able to sit with support from a person holding the infant lightly in the area of the hips or lower chest. Fine pincer grasp, finger-to-thumb grasp, usually develops at about 9 months of age. Typically, an infant can reach for a toy at about 8 months of age. Saying recognizable syllables like mama or dada occurs at about 7 months of age. (A, 3)

2. 4. According to the guidelines developed by the American Academy of Pediatrics for immunization of children (*Report of the Committee on Infectious Diseases*, 1999), a series of three injections of diphtheria, tetanus, and acellular pertussis (DTaP) and a series of three injections of *Haemophilus influenzae* type B (Hib) vaccine are recommended during the first year of life. In addition, the infant should receive three immunizations for hepatitis B. Poliomyelitis protection is administered twice during the first year, unless the disease is prevalent in the area where the child lives, in which case another dose may be given. Measles, mumps, and rubella (MMR) vaccine and Hib vaccine are recommended when the child is between 12 and 15 months of age. An immunization for tuberculosis is not used. However, infants are tested for tuberculosis. The tuberculin skin test (PPD) is not administered until the infant is at least 9 months of age. (I, 4)

3. 1. The American Academy of Pediatrics recommends that infants who are delayed in receiving their immunizations or have not started their series by 9 months of age begin with DTaP, inactivated poliomyelitis vaccine (IPV), Hib, and PPD. Oral polio vaccine (OPV) is not used because cases of polio have been reported with use of the vaccine. MMR and varicella vaccines are not administered until 12 months of age. (I, 4)

4. 4. A 1-month-old infant usually is able to lift the head and turn it from side to side when lying prone. The full-term infant with no abnormalities or complications probably has been able to do this since birth. Smiling and laughing aloud are expected behaviors for a 2- to 3-month-old infant. Rolling from the back to the side is a characteristic behavior of a 4-month-old infant. Holding a rattle for a brief time is characteristic behavior of a 4-month old infant. (A, 3)

5. 2. The mother has already changed the infant from formula to cow's milk, so she probably will not change the infant back to formula. Therefore, the best the nurse can hope for is that the mother will switch to whole milk. Because cow's milk causes microscopic blood loss in the intestine, it is best for the infant to remain on formula until 1 year of age and then be switched to whole milk, which has a higher fat content than 2% milk. The fat is needed for brain growth. (I, 4)

6. 2. Holding the head erect when sitting, staring at an object placed in the hand, taking the object to the mouth, cooing and gurgling, and sustaining part of her body weight when in a standing position are behaviors characteristic of a 4-month old infant. A 2-month-old typically vocalizes, follows objects to the midline, and smiles. A 7-month-old typically is able to sit without support, turns toward the voice, and transfers object from hand to hand. Usually, a 9-month-old can crawl, stand while holding on, and initiate speech sounds. (D, 3)

7. 4. The anterior fontanel, the soft spot near the front of the infant's head, usually closes between age 12 and 18 months. The small posterior fontanel usually closes by 6 to 8 weeks of age. (I, 3)

8. 1. Normally, a 9-month-old infant should have been voicing single syllables since 6 months of age. Absence of this finding would be a cause for concern. An infant usually is able to stand alone at about 10 months of age. An infant usually is able to build a tower of 2 cubes at about 15 months of age. An infant usually is able to drink from a cup with little spilling at about 15 months of age. (A, 9)

Health Promotion of the Toddler and Family

9. 3. A craving to eat nonfood substances is known as *pica*. Toddlers use oral gratification as a means to cope with anxiety. Therefore, the nurse should first assess whether the child is experiencing any change in the home environment that could cause anxiety. Teething or the eruption of large teeth and the amount of attention from the mother are unlikely causes of pica. Nutritional deficiencies, especially iron deficiency, were once thought to cause pica, but research has not substantiated this theory. The intake of a soft, low-roughage diet is an unlikely cause. (A, 3)

10. 3. A 2-year-old usually can kick a ball forward. Riding a tricycle is characteristic of a 3-year-old. Tying shoelaces is a behavior to be expected of a 5-year-old. Using blunt scissors is characteristic of a 3-year-old. (A, 3)

11. 2. Parents can be asked to assist when their child becomes uncooperative during a procedure. Most commonly, the child's difficulty in cooperating is caused by fear. In most situations, the child will feel more secure with a parent present. Other methods may be necessary, but obtaining a parent's assistance is the recommended first action. Restraints should be use only as a last resort, after all other attempts have been made to encourage cooperation. (A, 35)

12. 4. In a child younger than 3 years of age, the pinna is pulled back and down, because the auditory canals are almost straight in children. In an adult, the pinna is pulled up and backward because the auditory canals are directed inward, forward, and down. (E, 8)

13. 4. Time out is the most appropriate discipline for toddlers. It helps to remove them from the situation and allows them to regain control. Structuring interactions with 3-year-olds helps minimize unacceptable behavior. This approach involves setting clear and reasonable rules and calling attention to unacceptable behavior as soon as it occurs. Physical punishment, such as spanking, does cause a dramatic decrease in a behavior but has serious negative effects. However, slapping a child's hand is effective when the child refuses to listen to verbal commands. Reasoning is more appropriate for older children, such as preschoolers and those older, especially when moral issues are involved. Unfortunately, reasoning combined with scolding often takes the form of shame or criticism and children take such remarks seriously, believing that they are "bad." (I, 3)

14. 2. Toddlers usually express pain through such behaviors as restlessness, facial grimaces, irritability, and crying. It is not particularly helpful to ask toddlers about pain. In most instances, they would be unable to understand or describe the nature and location of their pain because of their lack of verbal and cognitive skills. However, preschool and older children have the verbal and cognitive skills to be able to respond appropriately. Numeric pain scales are more appropriate for children who are of school age or older. Changes in vital signs do occur as a result of pain, but behavioral changes usually are noticed first. (A, 3)

15. 2. Toddlers around the age of 15 months need 2 to 3 cups of milk per day to supply necessary nutrients such as calcium. A daily intake of more than 3 cups of milk may interfere with the ingestion of other necessary nutrients. (P, 4)

Health Promotion of the Preschooler and Family

16. 2. Preschool-aged children have been described as powerhouses of gross motor activity who seem to have endless energy. A limitation of their motor ability is that in moving as quickly as they do, they are not always able to judge distances, nor are they able to estimate the amount of strength and balance needed for activities. As a result, they have frequent mishaps. This level of activity typically is not associated with changes at home. However, if the behavior intensifies, a referral to a pediatric neurologist would be appropriate. Children who have been abused usually demonstrate withdrawn behaviors, not endless energy. (I, 3)

17. 2. Bedtime is often a problem with preschoolers. Recommendations for reducing conflicts at bedtime include establishing a set bedtime; having a dependable routine, such as story reading; and conveying the expectation that the child will comply. Allowing the child to stay up late one or two nights interferes with establishing the needed bedtime rituals. Excitement, such as active play, just before bedtime should be avoided because it stimulates the child, making it difficult for the child to calm down and prepare for sleep. Using food such as a cookie as a reward if bedtime is pleasant should be avoided because it places too much importance on food. Other rewards, such as stickers, could be used as an alternative. (I, 3)

18. 3. Children younger than 7 years of age do not have the manual dexterity needed for tooth brushing. Therefore, parents need to help with this task until that time. (E, 4)

19. 2. The preschool-aged child does not have an accurate concept of skin integrity and can view medical and surgical treatments as hostile invasions that can destroy or damage the body. The child does not understand that exsanguination will not occur from an injection site. Fear of pain would be manifested if the child thought that bodily harm would occur. If the child thought that he would urinate in his pants, then he would be demonstrating a fear of loss of control. (D, 3)

20. 3. Family changes and stresses (eg, moving, having company, taking vacations, adding new members) can distract parental attention and contribute to accidents. Because only children tend to receive more attention than children with siblings, the risk for accidents would be less. The parents' limited formal education is unrelated to a child's risk for accidents. Because it costs money to maintain a home so as to minimize the risk of accidents and families living in the suburbs usually are more affluent, they therefore are better able financially to maintain a home that is less conducive to accidents. (I, 3)

21. 3. Preschool-aged children may view illness as punishment for their fantasies. At this age children do not have the cognitive ability to separate fantasies from reality and may expect to be punished for their "evil thoughts." Viewing illness as a necessary part of life requires a higher level of cognition than preschoolers possess. This view is seen in children of middle school age and older. Perceiving illness as a test of self-worth or as the will of God is more characteristic of adults. (P, 5)

Health Promotion of the School-Aged Child and Family

22. 4. During the school-aged years, a child learns to socialize with children of the same age. Therefore, the nurse is assessing the child's social development. The "best friend" stage, which occurs at about 9 or 10 years of age, is very important in providing a foundation for self-esteem and later relationships. Language development is best assessed by having the child read and participate in conversations. Motor development usually is assessed with a neurologic examination. Neurologic development is assessed by testing deep tendon reflexes and having the child tandem walk and perform visual-perceptual activities. (A, 3)

23. 2. Children are capable of mastering the skills required for flossing when they reach 9 years of age. By age 9 or 10 years, many children are able to assume responsibility for personal hygiene. (D, 3)

24. 2. School-aged children delight in riddles and jokes. Mastery of the ambiguities of language and of sentence structure allows the school-aged child to manipulate words, and telling riddles and jokes is a way of practicing this skill. (I, 3)

25. 3. Snacks are necessary for school-aged children because of their high energy level. School-aged children are in a stage of cognitive development in which they can learn to categorize or classify and can also learn cause and effect. By preparing their own snacks, children can learn the basics of nutrition (e.g., what carbohydrates are and what happens when they are eaten). The mother and child should make the decision about appropriate foods together. School-aged children learn to make decisions based on information, not instinct. Some knowledge of nutrition is needed to make appropriate choices. (P, 7)

26. 1. The values of height and weight percentiles are usually similar for an individual child. Measurements between the 5th and 95th percentiles are considered normal. Marked discrepancies identify overweight or underweight children. (D, 4)

27. 1. According to the American Academy of Pediatrics Committee on Infectious Disease, boosters of diphtheria, tetanus, and pertussis (DTaP) and polio vaccine (IPV) are the immunizations recommended for children between ages 4 and 6 years before entering school. The recommended ages for measles, mumps, and rubella (MMR) immunization are 15 months and 4 to 6 years or 11 to 12 years. (P, 4)

Health Promotion of the Adolescent and Family

28. 2. Relieving dysmenorrhea in adolescence is crucial for the female's development of positive self-identity, of which positive body image and sexual identity are important components. Menstruation should not be viewed as painful and debilitating. Positive peer relations and a sense of independence would develop with a positive self-identity. Sense of autonomy, according to Erikson, is the developmental task of toddlers that, if successfully mastered, leads to a sense of self-control. (I, 3)

29. 3. The nurse needs to provide the adolescent with information about toxic shock syndrome because of the identified relationship between tampon use and the syndrome's development. Additionally, about 95% of cases of toxic shock syndrome occur during menses. Most adolescent females can use tampons safely if they change them frequently. (I, 3)

30. 4. An adolescent's body is undergoing rapid changes. Adolescence is a time of integrating these rapidly occurring physical changes into the self-concept to achieve the developmental task of a positive self identity. Thus, most adolescents spend much time worrying about their personal appearance. This behavior is not a method of procrastination or a way of testing the parents' limits. (I, 3)

31. 3. Information about why adolescents choose to use alcohol or other drugs can be used to determine whether they are becoming responsible users or problem users. A person may use alcohol out of simple curiosity or as a means of escape. (A, 6)

Common Childhood and Adolescent Health Problems

32. 1. The most common characteristic of head lice infestation (pediculosis capitis) is severe itching. Itching also occurs when lice infest other parts of the body. Scratch marks are almost always found when lice are present. The head is the most common site of lice infestation. If the child scratches, scaling may occur. (A, 10)

33. 3. Lice are spread by close personal contact and by contact with infested clothing, bed and bathroom linens, and combs and brushes. Lice are more common in school-aged children than in adults because of the close contact in school and the common practice of sharing possessions. Lice are not commonly spread by hand contact. (I, 10)

34. 3. Ringworm of the scalp is caused by a fungus of the dermatophyte group of the species. Overexposure to the sun would result in sunburn. An allergic reaction commonly is manifested by hives, rash, or anaphylaxis. (E, 10)

35. 4. Griseofulvin is an antifungal agent that acts by binding to the keratin that is deposited in the skin, hair, and nails as they grow. This keratin is then resistant to the fungus. But as the keratin is normally shed, the fungus enters new, uninfected cells unless drug therapy continues. Long-term administration of griseofulvin does not prevent sensitivity or allergic reactions. As the body adjusts to a new substance over time, side effects are variable and do not necessarily decrease. (I, 8)

36. 2. The adult pinworm emerges from the rectum and colon at night onto the perianal area to lay its eggs. Itching and scratching introduces the eggs to the hands, from where they can easily reinfect the child or infect others. Nightclothes and bed linens can be sources of infection. The eggs can also be transmitted by dust in the home. Although transmission through contaminated food and water supplies is possible, it is rare. Contaminated animals can spread histoplasmosis and salmonella. The spread of infections by toilet seats has not been supported by research. (I, 10)

37. 3. The care of a child with chicken pox focuses primarily on preventing infection in the lesions. The lesions cause severe itching, and organisms are ordinarily introduced into the lesion through scratching. Acid-base imbalance rarely occurs with chicken pox. Malnutrition is a chronic problem associated with the ingestion of an inadequate diet over a long period. It is not associated with chicken pox. Secondary infection in the lesions, not the respiratory tract, is most common. (I, 2)

38. 3. A child with 20/60 vision sees at 20 feet what those with 20/20 vision see at 60 feet. A visual acuity of 20/200 is considered to be the boundary of legal blindness. (D, 4)

39. 1. Children who have temper tantrums should be ignored as long as they are safe. They should not receive either positive or negative reinforcement to avoid perpetuating the behavior. Temper tantrums are a toddler's way of achieving independence. (E, 3)

40. 3. Although children may be influenced by their peers and smell and appearance may be important, children are most likely to be influenced by the example and atmosphere provided by their parents. Coaxing and badgering a child to eat most likely will aggravate poor eating habits. (I, 3)

41. 3. Girls experience the onset of adolescence about 1 to 2 years earlier than boys. The reason for this is not understood. (I, 3)

42. 2. Mood swings and rudeness are not abnormal for adolescents. Parents should first discuss their feelings with their adolescent. Restricting activities may make the situation worse because the adolescent is more likely to rebel or act out. Family counseling is not indicated as a first intervention. However, it may be necessary later on. Talking with other parents of adolescents may or may not be helpful. (P, 3)

43. 1. The cause of infectious mononucleosis is thought to be the Epstein-Barr virus. No precautionary measures are recommended for patients with mononucleosis. The virus is believed to be spread only by direct intimate contact. (I, 2)

44. 2. Mononucleosis usually has an insidious onset, with fatigue and the inability to maintain usual activity levels as the most common symptoms. The lymph nodes are typically enlarged, and the spleen also may be enlarged. Fever and a sore throat often accompany mononucleosis. A persistent nonproductive cough can follow an upper respiratory tract infection. A blush-like generalized skin rash is more characteristic of rubella. (I, 10)

45. 1. After receiving the rubella vaccine, the person develops a mild form of the disease, stimulating the body to develop an immunity. Administration to a woman early in pregnancy puts the fetus at risk for deformity or spontaneous abortion. Some authorities recommend withholding the immunization for rubella after puberty because a woman does not always know when she is pregnant and a fetus could be placed in jeopardy. However, the risk of contracting the disease is not lower after puberty. There is no difference in the reaction to the vaccine before or after puberty. Changes in the immunologic system do not affect the rhythm of the menstrual cycle. (I, 4)

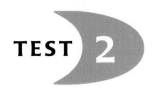

TEST 2

The Child With Respiratory Health Problems

Select the one best answer, and indicate your choice by filling in the circle in front of the option.

The Client With Tonsillitis

1. Which of the following would the nurse identify as a priority nursing diagnosis when preparing the preoperative plan of care for a 4-year-old undergoing a tonsillectomy and adenoidectomy (T&A)?
   ○ 1. Anxiety related to surgery.
   ○ 2. Impaired Parenting related to surgery.
   ○ 3. Pain related to surgery.
   ○ 4. Imbalanced Nutrition: Less Than Body Requirements related to surgery.

2. The nurse identifies a nursing diagnosis of Risk for Perioperative-Positioning Injury related to the surgical procedure for a school-aged child scheduled for a tonsillectomy. Which of the following would be the most appropriate expected outcome for this nursing diagnosis?
   ○ 1. The child is able to tell about the surgery and recovery.
   ○ 2. The child remains NPO for the designated preoperative period.
   ○ 3. The child and family demonstrate an understanding of the procedure.
   ○ 4. The child knows the parents will not leave.

3. After a T&A, which of the following findings would alert the nurse to suspect early hemorrhage in a 5-year-old child?
   ○ 1. Drooling of bright red secretions.
   ○ 2. Pulse rate of 95 bpm.
   ○ 3. Vomiting of 25 mL of dark brown emesis.
   ○ 4. Blood pressure of 95/56 mm Hg.

4. After teaching the parents of a preschooler who has undergone a T&A about appropriate foods to give the child after discharge, which of the following, if stated by the parents as appropriate foods, indicates successful teaching?
   ○ 1. Meat loaf and uncooked carrots.
   ○ 2. Pork and noodle casserole.
   ○ 3. Cream of chicken soup and orange sherbet.
   ○ 4. Hot dog and potato chips.

5. The nurse teaches the parents about the possibility of postoperative hemorrhage after a T&A, explaining that the risk is greatest at which of the following times?
   ○ 1. 2 to 4 days after surgery.
   ○ 2. 5 to 7 days after surgery.
   ○ 3. 8 to 10 days after surgery.
   ○ 4. 11 to 13 days after surgery.

The Client With Chronic Otitis Media

6. When determining the parents' compliance with treatment for their toddler who has recurrent otitis media, which of the following measures would the nurse expect the parents to describe?
   ○ 1. Cleansing the child's ear canals with hydrogen peroxide.
   ○ 2. Administering continuous, small-dose antibiotic therapy.

3. Instilling ear drops regularly to prevent cerumen accumulation.
4. Holding the child upright when feeding with a bottle.

7. A toddler is scheduled to have tympanostomy tubes inserted. When approaching the toddler for the first time, which of the following would the nurse do?
   1. Talk to the mother first so that the toddler can get used to the new person.
   2. Hold the toddler so that the toddler becomes more comfortable.
   3. Walk over and pick the toddler up right away so that the mother can relax.
   4. Pick up the toddler and take the child to the play area so that the mother can rest.

8. After insertion of bilateral tympanostomy tubes, which of the following instructions would the nurse include in a child's discharge plan for the parents?
   1. Insert ear plugs into the canals when the child bathes.
   2. Blow the nose forcibly during a cold.
   3. Administer the prescribed antibiotic while the tubes are in place.
   4. Disregard any drainage from the ear after 1 week.

The Client With Foreign Body Aspiration

9. A child brought to the emergency department by his parents is diagnosed with a foreign body aspiration. Which of the following nursing diagnoses would the nurse identify as the priority for this child?
   1. Ineffective Airway Clearance related to foreign body aspiration.
   2. Risk for Injury related to foreign body aspiration.
   3. Impaired Parenting related to foreign body aspiration.
   4. Ineffective Health Maintenance related to foreign body aspiration.

10. The mother asks the nurse why peanuts are one of the worst things a child can aspirate. Which of the following would the nurse include in the explanation as the *main* reason for the problem associated with aspirating peanuts?
    1. They swell when wet.
    2. They contain a fixed oil.
    3. They decompose when wet.
    4. They contain sodium.

11. After teaching the parents of a toddler 2 years of age about commonly aspirated foods, which of the following foods, if identified by the parents as easily aspirated, would indicate the need for *additional* teaching?
    1. Popcorn.
    2. Raw vegetables.
    3. Round candy.
    4. Crackers.

12. A toddler who has been treated for a foreign body aspiration begins to fuss and cry when the parents attempt to leave the hospital for an hour. The parents will be returning to take the toddler home. As the nurse tries to take the child out of the crib, the child pushes the nurse away. The nurse interprets this behavior as indicating separation anxiety involving which of the following?
    1. Protest.
    2. Despair.
    3. Regression.
    4. Detachment.

13. After teaching the parents of an 18-month-old who was treated for a foreign body obstruction about the three cardinal signs indicative of choking, the nurse determines that the teaching has been successful when the parents state that a child is choking when he or she cannot speak, turns blue, and does which of the following?
    1. Vomits.
    2. Gasps.
    3. Gags.
    4. Collapses.

The Client With Asthma

14. When preparing the teaching plan for the mother of a child with asthma, which of the following would the nurse include as signs to alert the mother that her child is having an asthma attack?
    1. Secretion of thin, copious mucus.
    2. Tight, productive cough.
    3. Wheezing on expiration.
    4. Temperature of 99.4°F (37.4°C).

15. A 10-year-old child with a history of asthma who is 5 feet 4 inches (138 cm) tall uses an inhaled bronchodilator only when needed. He takes no other medications routinely. His best peak expiratory flow rate is 270 L/minute. The child's current peak flow reading is 180 L/minute. The nurse interprets this reading as indicating which of the following?
    1. The child's asthma is under good control, so the routine treatment plan should continue.
    2. The child needs to start a short-acting inhaled β_2-agonist medication.
    3. This is medical emergency requiring a trip to the emergency department for treatment.

○ 4. The child needs to begin treatment with inhaled cromolyn sodium (Intal) for asthma control.

16. An adolescent complains of chest pain and goes to the school nurse. The nurse determines that the teenager also has a history of asthma but has had no problems for years. Which of the following would the nurse do *next*?
    ○ 1. Call the adolescent's parent.
    ○ 2. Have the adolescent lie down for 30 minutes.
    ○ 3. Obtain a peak flow reading.
    ○ 4. Give two puffs of a short-acting bronchodilator.

17. A 7-year-old with a history of asthma controlled without medications is referred to the school nurse by the teacher because of persistent coughing. Which of the following would the nurse do *first*?
    ○ 1. Obtain the child's heart rate.
    ○ 2. Give the child a nebulizer treatment.
    ○ 3. Call a parent to obtain more information.
    ○ 4. Have a parent come and pick up the child.

18. When developing a teaching plan for the mother of an asthmatic child concerning measures to reduce allergic triggers, which of the following suggestions would the nurse expect to include?
    ○ 1. Keep the humidity in the home between 50% and 60%.
    ○ 2. Have the child sleep in the bottom bunk bed.
    ○ 3. Use a scented room deodorizer to keep the room fresh.
    ○ 4. Vacuum the carpet once or twice a week.

19. After discussing asthma as a chronic condition, which of the following statements by the father of a child with asthma best reflects the family's positive adjustment to this aspect of the child's disease?
    ○ 1. "We try to keep him happy at all costs; otherwise he has an asthma attack."
    ○ 2. "We keep our child away from other children to help cut down on infections."
    ○ 3. "Although our child's disease is serious, we try not to let it be the focus of our family."
    ○ 4. "I'm afraid that when my child gets older, he won't be able to care for himself like I do."

20. An 8-year old child with asthma states, "I want to play some sports like my friends. What can I do?" The nurse responds to the child based on the understanding of which of the following?
    ○ 1. Physical activities are inappropriate for children with asthma.
    ○ 2. Children with asthma must be excluded from team sports.
    ○ 3. Vigorous physical exercise frequently precipitates an asthmatic episode.
    ○ 4. Most children with asthma can participate in sports if the asthma is controlled.

The Client With Cystic Fibrosis and Bronchopneumonia

21. When developing the plan of care for a child with cystic fibrosis (CF) who is scheduled to receive postural drainage, the nurse would anticipate performing postural drainage at which of the following times?
    ○ 1. After meals.
    ○ 2. Before meals.
    ○ 3. After rest periods.
    ○ 4. Before inhalation treatments.

22. When teaching the parents of an older infant with CF about the type of diet the child should consume, which of the following would be *most* appropriate?
    ○ 1. Low-protein diet.
    ○ 2. High-fat diet.
    ○ 3. Low-carbohydrate diet.
    ○ 4. High-calorie diet.

23. At a follow-up appointment after being hospitalized, an adolescent with a history of CF describes his stools to the nurse. Which of the following descriptions would the nurse interpret as indicative of continued problems with malabsorption?
    ○ 1. Soft with little odor.
    ○ 2. Large and foul-smelling.
    ○ 3. Loose with bits of food.
    ○ 4. Hard with streaks of blood.

24. When developing a recreational therapy plan of care for a 3-year-old child hospitalized with pneumonia and CF, which of the following toys would be *most* supportive?
    ○ 1. 100-piece jigsaw puzzle.
    ○ 2. Child's favorite doll.
    ○ 3. Fuzzy stuffed animal.
    ○ 4. Scissors, paper, and paste.

25. Which of the following, if described by the parents of a child with CF, indicates that the parents understand the underlying problem of the disease?
    ○ 1. An abnormality in the body's mucus-secreting glands.
    ○ 2. Formation of fibrous cysts in various body organs.
    ○ 3. Failure of the pancreatic ducts to develop properly.
    ○ 4. Reaction to the formation of antibodies against streptococcus.

26. Which of the following outcome criteria would the nurse develop for a child with CF who has a nursing diagnosis of Ineffective Airway Clearance related to increased pulmonary secretions and inability to expectorate?
    ○ 1. Respiratory rate and rhythm within expected range.

○ 2. Absence of chills and fever.

○ 3. Ability to engage in age-related activities.

○ 4. Ability to tolerate usual diet without vomiting.

27. A school-aged child with CF asks the nurse what sports she can become involved in as she becomes older. Which of the following activities would be *most* appropriate for the nurse to suggest?

○ 1. Swimming.

○ 2. Track.

○ 3. Baseball.

○ 4. Javelin throwing.

The Client With Sudden Infant Death Syndrome

28. After the parents bring their male infant to the emergency department, the nurse obtains a brief history of events occurring before and after the parents found the infant not breathing. Which of the following questions would be *most* appropriate for the nurse to ask the parents?

○ 1. "Was the infant sleeping while wrapped in a blanket?"

○ 2. "Was the infant lying on his stomach?"

○ 3. "What did the infant look like when you found him?"

○ 4. "When had you last checked on the infant?"

29. When planning a visit to the parents of an infant who died of sudden infant death syndrome (SIDS) at home, the community health nurse would expect to visit the parents at which of the following times?

○ 1. A few days after the funeral.

○ 2. Two weeks after the funeral.

○ 3. As soon as the parents are ready to talk.

○ 4. As soon after the infant's death as possible.

30. When developing the ongoing plan of care for the parents whose infant died of SIDS, the community health nurse would expect to accomplish which of the following on the second home visit?

○ 1. Allow the parents to express their feelings.

○ 2. Have the parents gain an understanding of the disease.

○ 3. Assess the impact of the infant's death on their other children.

○ 4. Deal with issues such as having other children.

The Client Who Requires Cardiopulmonary Resuscitation

31. On finding a child who is not breathing, which of the following would the nurse do *first*?

○ 1. Clear the airway.

○ 2. Begin mouth-to-mouth resuscitation.

○ 3. Initiate oxygen therapy.

○ 4. Start chest compressions.

32. Which of the following rates would the nurse use when performing rescue breathing during cardiopulmonary resuscitation (CPR) for a 5-year-old?

○ 1. 10 breaths/minute.

○ 2. 12 breaths/minute.

○ 3. 15 breaths/minute.

○ 4. 20 breaths/minute.

33. At which of the following rates would the nurse deliver external chest compressions to a 5-year-old child who is pulseless?

○ 1. 40 to 60 compressions/minute.

○ 2. 60 to 80 compressions/minute.

○ 3. 80 to 100 compressions/minute.

○ 4. 100 to 120 compressions/minute.

34. As part of a health education program, the nurse teaches a group of parents of preschoolers how to perform chest compressions during CPR. The nurse determines that the teaching has been effective when the parents state that the child's chest should be compressed to which of the following depths?

○ 1. 1 to 1.5 inches.

○ 2. 1.5 to 2 inches.

○ 3. 2 to 2.5 inches.

○ 4. 2.5 to 3 inches.

35. When performing CPR, which of the following assessments would indicate to the nurse that external chest compressions are effective?

○ 1. Mottling of the skin.

○ 2. Pupillary dilation.

○ 3. Palpable pulse.

○ 4. Cool, dry skin.

36. A nurse walks into the room just as a 10-month-old infant places an object in his mouth and starts to choke. After opening the infant's mouth, which of the following would the nurse do *next* to clear the airway?

○ 1. Use blind finger sweeps.

○ 2. Deliver four back blows.

○ 3. Apply four subdiaphragmatic abdominal thrusts.

○ 4. Attempt to visualize the object.

37. When preparing to deliver back blows to an infant who is choking on a foreign body, in which of the following positions would the nurse position the infant?

○ 1. Head down and lower than the trunk.

○ 2. Head up and raised above the trunk.

○ 3. Head to one side and even with the trunk lower than the head.

○ 4. Head parallel to the nurse and supported at the buttocks.

38. When teaching the parents of an infant how to perform back blows to dislodge a foreign body, which of the following would the nurse tell the parents to use to deliver the blows?
    ○ 1. Palm of the hand.
    ○ 2. Heel of the hand.
    ○ 3. Fingertips.
    ○ 4. Entire hand.

39. While the nurse is delivering abdominal thrusts to a 6-year old who is choking on a foreign body, the child begins to cry. Which of the following would the nurse do *next*?
    ○ 1. Tap or gently shake the shoulders.
    ○ 2. Deliver four back blows.
    ○ 3. Perform a blind finger sweep of the mouth.
    ○ 4. Observe the child closely.

The Client With Croup

40. The father of a 16-month-old calls the clinic because the child has a low-grade fever, cold symptoms, and a hoarse cough. Which of the following would the nurse suggest that the father do?
    ○ 1. Offer extra fluids frequently.
    ○ 2. Bring the child to the clinic immediately.
    ○ 3. Count the child's respiratory rate.
    ○ 4. Use a hot air vaporizer.

41. A 21-month-old admitted with the diagnosis of croup now has a respiratory rate of 48 breaths/minute, a heart rate of 120 bpm, and a temperature of 100.8°F (38.2°C) rectally. The nurse is having difficulty calming the child. Which of the following would the nurse do *next*?
    ○ 1. Administer acetaminophen (Tylenol).
    ○ 2. Notify the physician immediately.
    ○ 3. Allow the toddler to continue to cry.
    ○ 4. Offer clear fluids every few minutes.

The Client With Bronchiolitis

42. A father brings his 3-month-old infant to the clinic, reporting that the infant has a cold, is having trouble breathing, and "just doesn't seem to be acting right." Which of the following actions would the nurse do *first*?
    ○ 1. Check the infant's heart rate.
    ○ 2. Weigh the infant.
    ○ 3. Assess the infant's oxygen saturation.
    ○ 4. Obtain more information from the father.

43. While the nurse is working in a homeless shelter, assessment of a 6-month-old infant reveals a respiratory rate of 52 breaths/minute, retractions, and wheezing. The mother states that her infant was doing fine until yesterday. Which of the following actions would be *most* appropriate?
    ○ 1. Administer a nebulizer treatment.
    ○ 2. Send the infant for a chest radiograph.
    ○ 3. Refer the infant to the emergency department.
    ○ 4. Provide teaching about cold care to the mother.

44. In preparation for discharge, the nurse teaches the mother of an infant diagnosed with bronchiolitis about the condition and its treatment. Which of the following statements by the mother indicates successful teaching?
    ○ 1. "I need to be sure to take my child's temperature every day."
    ○ 2. "I hope I don't get a cold from my child."
    ○ 3. "Next time my child gets a cold I need to listen to the chest."
    ○ 4. "I need to wash my hands more often."

Correct Answers and Rationale

The letters in parentheses following the rationale identify the step of the nursing process (A, D, P, I, E) and client needs (1, 2, 3, 4, 5, 6, 7, 8, 9, 10). See the inside front cover for the key.

The Client With Tonsillitis

1. 1. A 4-year-old child is aware of what is happening and would be anxious in a new environment when not sure of what may happen or what is expected. The parents also would be anxious about how the child will tolerate the surgery and any complications that may occur. The child will pick up on the parents' anxiety. There are no data provided to support the nursing diagnosis of Impaired Parenting. During the preoperative period, the child is not in any pain. However, pain may be a priority in the postoperative period. Even though the child will be NPO preoperatively, intravenous fluids will be initiated once surgery begins, minimizing the risk of harm or problems. (D, 3)

2. 2. The most appropriate outcome for a nursing diagnosis of Risk for Perioperative-Positioning Injury related to the surgical procedure would be that the child remains NPO for the designated period of time before surgery, thereby minimizing the risk of aspiration during the surgery. Ability to tell about the surgery and demonstrating an understanding of the procedure are appropriate outcomes for a nursing diagnosis of Deficient Knowledge. Knowing that the parents will not leave is associated with a nursing diagnosis of Anxiety or Fear related to separation from support systems or an unfamiliar environment. (P, 9)

3. 1. After a T&A, drooling bright red blood is considered an early sign of hemorrhage. Often, because of discomfort in the throat, children tend to avoid swallowing; instead, they drool. Frequent swallowing would also be an indication of hemorrhage because the child attempts to clear the airway of blood by swallowing. Secretions may be slightly blood-tinged because of a small amount of oozing after surgery. However, bright red secretions indicate bleeding. A pulse rate of 95 bpm is within the normal range for a 5-year-old child, as is a blood pressure of 95/56 mm Hg. A small amount of blood that is partially digested, and therefore dark brown, is often present in postoperative emesis. (A, 9)

4. 3. For the first few days after a T&A, liquids and soft foods are best tolerated by the child while the throat is sore. Children typically do not chew their food thoroughly, and solid foods are to be avoided because they are difficult to swallow. Although meat loaf would be considered a soft food, uncooked carrots would not be. Pork is frequently difficult to chew. Foods that have sharp edges, such as pieces of potato chips, are contraindicated because they are hard to chew and may cause more throat discomfort. (E, 7)

5. 3. The risk for hemorrhage is greatest about 1 week after surgery as tissue sloughing occurs during the healing process. (I, 9)

The Client With Chronic Otitis Media

6. 4. Sitting or holding a child upright for formula feedings helps prevent pooling of formula in the pharyngeal area. When the vacuum in the middle ear opens into the pharyngeal cavity, formula (along with bacteria) is drawn into the middle ear. Cleansing the ears does not reduce the incidence of otitis media because the pathogenic bacteria are in the nasopharynx, not the external area of the ears. Continuous low-dose antibiotic therapy is used only in cases of recurrent otitis media, when the child finishes a course of antibiotics but then develops another ear infection a few days later. Although accumulation of cerumen makes it difficult to visualize the tympanic membrane, it does not promote inner ear infections. (E, 3)

7. 1. Toddlers should be approached slowly, because they are wary of strangers and need time to get used to someone they do not know. The best approach is to ignore them initially and to focus on talking to the parents. (I, 3)

8. 1. Placing ear plugs in the ears will prevent contaminated bathwater from entering the middle ear through the tympanostomy tube and causing an infection. Blowing the nose forcibly during a cold causes organisms to ascend through the eustachian tube, possibly leading to otitis media. It is not necessary to administer antibiotics continuously to a child with a tympanostomy tube. Antibiotics are appropriate only when an ear infection is present. Drainage from the ear may be a sign of middle ear infection and should be reported to the health care provider. (I, 9)

The Client With Foreign Body Aspiration

9. 1. The child with a foreign body aspiration is experiencing an airway obstruction and requires imme-

diate intervention to ensure adequate ventilation. Therefore, the priority is Ineffective Airway Clearance. Risk for Injury related to foreign body aspiration may be important once the child's airway patency has been established. Impaired Parenting related to foreign body aspiration requires obtaining additional data about how the aspiration occurred. (D, 10)

10. 1. Peanuts swell and become soft when moistened with bronchial secretions, making them difficult to remove. Although peanuts contain a fixed oil that can cause lipoid pneumonia, begin to decompose when wet, and contain calcium, these factors do not make them particularly dangerous when aspirated. (I, 4)

11. 4. Crackers, because they crumble and easily dissolve, are not commonly aspirated. Because children commonly eat popcorn hulls or pieces that have not popped, popcorn can be easily aspirated. Toddlers frequently do not chew their food well, making raw vegetables a commonly aspirated food. Round candy is often difficult to chew and comes in large pieces, making it easily aspirated. (E, 4)

12. 1. Young children have specific reactions to separation and hospitalization. In the protest stage, the toddler physically and verbally attacks anyone who attempts to provide care. Here, the child is fussing and crying and visibly pushes the nurse away. In the despair stage, the toddler becomes withdrawn and obviously depressed (eg, not engaging in play activities, sleeping more than usual). Denial or detachment occurs if the toddler's stay in the hospital without the parent is prolonged because the toddler settles in to the hospital life and denies the parents' existence (eg, not reacting when the parents come to visit). Regression is a return to a developmentally earlier phase because of stress or crisis (eg, a toddler who could feed himself before this event now is not doing so). (D, 5)

13. 4. The three cardinal signs indicating that a child is truly choking and requires immediate life-saving interventions include inability to speak, blue color (cyanosis), and collapse. Vomiting does not occur while a child is unable to breathe. Once the object is dislodged, however, vomiting may occur. Gasping, a sudden intake of air, indicates that the child is still able to inhale. When a child is choking, air is not being exchanged, so gagging will not occur. (E, 9)

The Client With Asthma

14. 3. The child who is experiencing an asthma attack typically demonstrates wheezing on expiration initially. This results from air moving through narrowed airways secondary to bronchoconstriction. The child's expiratory phase is normally longer than the inspiratory phase. Expiration is passive as the diaphragm relaxes. During an asthma attack, secretions are thick and are not usually expelled until the bronchioles are more relaxed. At the beginning of an asthma attack the cough will be tight but not productive. Fever is not always present unless there is an infection that may have triggered the attack. (P, 10)

15. 2. The peak flow of 180 L/minute is in the yellow zone, or 50% to 80% of the child's personal best. This means that the child's asthma is not well controlled, thereby necessitating the use of a short-acting β_2-agonist medication to relieve the bronchospasm. A peak flow reading greater than 80% of the child's personal best (in this case, 220 L/minute or better) would indicate that the child's asthma is in the green zone or under good control. A peak flow reading in the red zone, or less than 50% of the child's personal best (135 L/minute or less), would require notification of the health care provider or a trip to the emergency department. Cromolyn sodium (Intal) is not used for short-term treatment of acute bronchospasm. It is used as part of a long-term therapy regimen to help desensitize mast cells and thereby help to prevent symptoms. (D, 9)

16. 3. Complaints of chest pain in children and adolescents are rarely cardiac. With a history of asthma, the most likely cause of the chest pain is related to the asthma. Therefore, the nurse should check the adolescent's peak flow reading to evaluate the status of the air flow. Calling the adolescent's parent would be appropriate, but this would be done after the nurse obtains the peak flow reading and additional assessment data. Having the adolescent lie down may be an option, but more data need to be collected to help establish a possible cause. Because the adolescent has not experienced any asthma problems for a long time, it would be inappropriate for the nurse to administer a short-acting bronchodilator at this time. (I, 9)

17. 3. Because persistent coughing may indicate an asthma attack and a 7-year-old would be able to provide only minimal history information, it would be important to obtain information from the parent. Although determining the child's heart rate is an important part of the assessment, it would be done after the history is obtained. More information needs to be obtained before giving the child a nebulizer treatment. Although it may be necessary for the parent to come and pick up the child, a thorough assessment including history information should be obtained first. (I, 9)

18. 1. To help reduce allergic triggers in the home, the nurse should recommend that the humidity level be kept between 50% and 60%. Doing so keeps the air

moist and comfortable for breathing. When air is dry, the risk for respiratory infections increase. Too high a level of humidity increases the risk for mold growth. Typically, the child with asthma should sleep in the top bunk bed to minimize the risk of exposure to dust mites. The risk of exposure to dust mites increases when the child sleeps in the bottom bunk bed because dust mites fall from the top bed, settling in the bottom bed. Scented sprays should be avoided because they may trigger an asthmatic episode. Ideally, carpeting should be avoided in the home if the child has asthma. However, if it is present, carpeting in the child's room should be vacuumed often, possibly daily, to remove dust mites and dust particles. (P, 9)

19. 3. Positive adjustment to a chronic condition requires placing the child's illness in its proper perspective. Children with asthma need to be treated as normally as possible within the scope of the limitations imposed by the illness. They also need to learn how to manage exacerbations and then resume as normal as life as possible. Trying to keep the child happy at all costs is inappropriate and can lead to the child's never learning how to accept responsibility for behavior and get along with others. Although minimizing the child's risk for exposure to infections is important, the child needs to be with his or her peers to ensure appropriate growth and development. Children with a chronic illness need to be involved in their care so that they can learn to manage it. Some parents tend to overprotect their child with a chronic illness. This overprotectiveness may cause a child to have an exaggerated feeling of importance or later, as an adolescent, to rebel against the overprotectiveness and the parents. (E, 5)

20. 4. Physical activities are beneficial to asthmatic children, physically and psychosocially. Most children with asthma can engage in school and sports activities that are geared to the child's condition and within the limits imposed by the disease. The coach and other team members need to be aware of the child's condition and know what to do in case an attack occurs. Those children who have exercise-induced asthma usually use a short-acting bronchodilator before exercising. (I, 3)

The Client With Cystic Fibrosis and Bronchopneumonia

21. 2. Postural drainage, which aids in mobilizing the thick, tenacious secretions commonly associated with CF, usually is performed before meals to avoid the possibility of vomiting or regurgitating food. Although the child with CF needs frequent rest periods, this is not an important factor in scheduling

postural drainage. However, the nurse would not want to interrupt the child's rest period to perform the treatment. Inhalation treatments are usually given before postural drainage to help loosen secretions. (P, 9)

22. 4. Cystic fibrosis affects the exocrine glands. Mucus is thick and tenacious, sticking to the walls of the pancreatic and bile ducts and eventually causing obstruction. Because of the difficulty with digestion and absorption, a moderate-fat, high-protein, high-calorie diet is indicated. (I, 10)

23. 2. In children with CF, poor digestion and absorption of foods, especially fats, results in frequent bowel movements that are bulky, large, and foul-smelling. The stools also contain abnormally large quantities of fat, which is called *steatorrhea*. An adolescent experiencing good control of the disease would describe soft stools with little odor. Stool described as loose with bits of food indicates diarrhea. Stool described as hard with streaks of blood may indicate constipation. (D, 10)

24. 2. The child's favorite doll would be a good choice of toys. The doll provides support and is familiar to the child. Although a 3-year-old may enjoy puzzles, a 100-piece jigsaw puzzle is too complicated for an ill 3-year-old child. In view of the child's lung pathology, a fuzzy stuffed animal would not be advised because of its potential as a reservoir for dust and bacteria, possibly predisposing the child to additional respiratory problems. Scissors, paper, and paste are not appropriate for a 3-year-old unless the child is supervised closely. (P, 3)

25. 1. Cystic fibrosis is characterized by a dysfunction in the body's mucus-producing exocrine glands. The mucus secretions are thick and sticky rather than thin and slippery. The mucus obstructs the bronchi, bronchioles, and pancreatic ducts. Mucus plugs in the pancreatic ducts can prevent pancreatic digestive enzymes from reaching the small intestine, resulting in poor digestion and poor absorption of various food nutrients. Fibrous cysts do not form in various organs. Cystic fibrosis is an autosomal recessive inherited disorder and does not involve any reaction to the formation of antibodies against streptococcus. (E, 10)

26. 1. After treatment, the client outcome would be that respiratory status would be within normal limits, as evidenced by a respiratory rate and rhythm within expected range. Absence of chills and fever, although related to an underlying problem causing the respiratory problem (ie, the infection), do not specifically relate to the respiratory problem of ineffective airway clearance. The child's ability to engage in age-related activities may provide some evidence of improved respiratory status. However, this outcome criterion is

more directly related to a nursing diagnosis of Activity Intolerance. Although the child's ability to tolerate his or her usual diet may indirectly relate to respiratory function, this outcome is more specifically related to a nursing diagnosis of Imbalanced Nutrition: Less Than Body Requirements, which may or may not be related to the child's respiratory status. (P, 10)

27. 1. Swimming would be the most appropriate suggestion because it coordinates breathing and movement of all muscle groups and can be done on an individual basis or as a team sport. Because track events, baseball, and javelin throwing usually are performed outdoors, the child would be breathing in large amounts of dust and dirt, which would be irritating to her mucous membranes and pulmonary system. The strenuous activity and increased energy expenditure associated with track events, in conjunction with the dust and possible heat, would play a role in placing the child at risk for an upper respiratory tract infection and compromising her respiratory function. (I, 4)

The Client With Sudden Infant Death Syndrome

28. 3. Because this is an especially disturbing and upsetting time for the parents, they must be approached in a sensitive manner. Asking what the infant looked like when found allows the parents to verbalize what they saw and felt, thereby helping to minimize their feelings of guilt without implying any blame, neglect, wrongdoing, or abuse. Asking if the child was wrapped in a blanket or lying on his stomach, or when the parents last checked on the infant, implies that the parents did something wrong or failed in their care of the infant, thus blaming them for the event. (A, 10)

29. 4. The community health nurse should visit as soon after the death as possible, because the parents may need help to deal with the sudden, unexpected death of their infant. Parents often have a great deal of guilt in these situations and need to express their feelings to someone who can provide counseling. (P, 5)

30. 1. The goal of the second home visit is to help the parents express their feelings more openly. Many parents are reluctant to express their grief and need help. The goal of the first visit is to help the parents understand the disease and what happened. The first visit also provides time to help the parents understand that they are not to blame. Although it is important to assess the impact of SIDS on siblings, this is not the primary goal for the second visit. However, the nurse must be flexible in case problems involving this area arise. Typically, parents are unable to deal with decisions such as having other children during the second visit because they are grieving for the child that they lost. This topic may be discussed later on in the course of care. (P, 5)

The Client Who Requires Cardiopulmonary Resuscitation

31. 1. When breathlessness is determined, the priority nursing action is to clear the airway. This action alone may reestablish spontaneous respiration. If the client does not begin breathing, mouth-to-mouth resuscitation is initiated. Oxygen therapy would not be initiated at this time, because the child is not breathing. Also, administering oxygen therapy would interfere with providing mouth-to-mouth resuscitation. Chest compressions are begun only after the client is determined to be pulseless. (I, 10)

32. 3. Rescue breaths should be delivered slowly at a volume that makes the chest rise and fall. For a 5-year-old child, the rate is one breath every 4 seconds, or 15 times per minute. Typically, the rate of rescue breathing for an adult is 10 to 12 breaths per minute. (I, 10)

33. 3. For a 5-year-old child, external chest compressions should be delivered at a rate of 80 to 100 times per minute. This rate approximates the resting minimum pulse, which allows for adequate brain perfusion. A rate less than 80 per minute does not provide adequate brain perfusion for a 5-year-old child. A rate of 100 to 120 times per minute is too fast. (I, 10)

34. 1. For preschoolers, aged 3 to 5 years, the chest is compressed to a depth of 1 to 1.5 inches. This depth forces blood out of the heart and into the vital organs (lungs and brain). Deeper compressions could damage the liver, lungs, or other underlying structures. Shallower compressions would not provide adequate circulation to the vital organs. The chest is compressed to a depth of 1.5 to 2 inches for adults. (E, 10)

35. 3. With CPR, effectiveness of external chest compressions is indicated by palpable peripheral pulses, the disappearance of mottling and cyanosis, the return of pupils to normal size, and warm, dry skin. To determine whether the victim of cardiopulmonary arrest has resumed spontaneous breathing and circulation, chest compressions must be stopped for 5 seconds at the end of the first minute and every few minutes thereafter. (E, 10)

36. 4. After opening the infant's mouth, the nurse attempts to find and remove the object. The nurse should attempt to remove only a visible object. If the nurse sees the object, then it can be removed. If the nurse cannot see the foreign body, mechanical force—back blows and chest thrusts—should be used in an attempt to dislodge the object. Blind finger sweeps are not appropriate in infants and children because the foreign body may be pushed back into the airway. Sub-diaphragmatic abdominal thrusts are not used for infants age 1 year or younger because of the risk of injury to abdominal organs. (I, 9)

37. 1. To deliver back blows, the nurse would place the infant face down, straddled over the nurse's arm, with the head lower than the trunk and the head supported. This position, together with the back blows, facilitates dislodgement and removal of a foreign object and minimizes aspiration if vomiting occurs. Placing the infant with the head up and raised above the trunk would not aid in dislodging and removing the foreign object. In addition, this position places the infant at risk for aspiration should vomiting occur. Placing the head to one side may minimize the risk for aspiration. However, it would not help with removal of an object that is dislodged by the back blows. Placing the infant with the head parallel to the nurse and supported at the buttocks is more appropriate for burping the infant. (I, 10)

38. 2. Back blows are delivered rapidly and forcefully with the heel of the hand between the infant's shoulder blades. Slowly delivered back blows are less likely to dislodge the object. Using the heel of the hand allows more force to be applied than when using the palm or the whole hand, increasing the likelihood of loosening the object. The fingertips would be used to deliver chest compressions to an infant younger than 1 year of age. (I, 10)

39. 4. Crying indicates that the airway obstruction has been relieved. No additional thrusts are needed. However, the child needs to be observed closely for complications, including respiratory distress. Tapping or shaking the shoulders is used initially to determine unresponsiveness in someone who appears unconscious. Delivering chest or back blows could jeopardize the child's now-patent airway. Because the obstruction has been relieved, there is no need to sweep the child's mouth. Additionally, blind finger sweeps are contraindicated because the object may be pushed further back, possibly causing a complete airway obstruction. (I, 10)

The Client With Croup

40. 1. The toddler is exhibiting cold symptoms. A hoarse cough may be part of the upper respiratory tract infection. The best suggestion is to have the father offer the child additional fluids at frequent intervals to help keep secretions loose and membranes moist. There is no evidence presented to suggest that the child needs to be brought to the clinic immediately. Although having the father count the child's respiratory rate may provide some additional information,

it may lead the father to suspect that something is seriously wrong, possibly leading to undue anxiety. A hot air vaporizer is not recommended. However, a cool mist vaporizer would cause vasoconstriction of the respiratory passages, making it easier for the child to breathe and loosening secretions. (I, 4)

41. 2. The nurse may be having difficulty calming the child because the child is experiencing increasing respiratory distress. The normal respiratory rate for a 21-month-old is 25 to 30 breaths/minute. The child's respiratory rate is 48 breaths/minute. Therefore the physician needs to be notified immediately. Typically, acetaminophen is not given to a child unless the temperature is 101°F (38.6°C) or higher. Letting the toddler cry is inappropriate with croup. Crying increases respiratory distress. Offering fluids every few minutes to a toddler experiencing increasing respiratory distress would do little, if anything, to calm the child. Also, the child would have difficulty coordinating breathing and swallowing, possibly increasing the risk for aspiration. (I, 10)

The Client With Bronchiolitis

42. 3. In an infant with these symptoms, the first action by the nurse would be to obtain an oxygen saturation reading to determine how well the infant is oxygenating, which is valuable information for an infant with trouble breathing. Because the father probably can provide no other information, checking the heart rate would be the second action done by the nurse. Then the nurse would obtain the infant's weight. (I, 4)

43. 3. Based on the assessment findings of increased respiratory rate, retractions, and wheezing, this infant needs further evaluation, which could be obtained in an emergency department. Without a definitive diagnosis, administering a nebulizer treatment would be outside the nurse's scope of practice unless there was an order for such a treatment. Sending the infant for a radiograph may not be in the nurse's scope of practice. The findings need to be reported to a physician who can then determine whether or not a chest radiograph is warranted. The infant is exhibiting signs and symptoms of respiratory distress and is too ill to send out with just instructions on cold care for the mother. (I, 10)

44. 4. Handwashing is the best way to prevent respiratory illnesses and the spread of disease. Bronchiolitis, a viral infection primarily affecting the bronchioles, causes swelling and mucus accumulation of the lumina and subsequent hyperinflation of the lung with air trapping. It is transmitted primarily by direct contact with respiratory secretions as a result of eye-to-hand or

nose-to-hand contact or from contaminated fomites. Therefore, handwashing minimizes the risk for transmission. Taking the child's temperature is not appropriate in most cases. As long as the child is getting better, taking the temperature will not be helpful. The mother's statement that she hopes she doesn't get a cold from her child does not indicate understanding of what to do after discharge. For most parents, listening to the child's chest would not be helpful because the parents would not know what they were listening for. Rather, watching for an increased respiratory rate, fever, or evidence of not eating or drinking well would be more helpful in alerting the parent to the child's being ill. (E, 10)

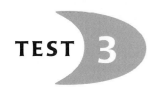

TEST 3

The Child With Cardiovascular and Hematologic Health Problems

Select the one best answer, and indicate your choice by filling in the circle in front of the option.

The Client Undergoing a Cardiac Catheterization

1. Which of the following nursing diagnoses would the nurse identify as the *priority* for a 4-year-old child diagnosed with a ventricular septal defect who will be undergoing a cardiac catheterization?
   ○ 1. Pain related to the structural defect.
   ○ 2. Deficient Knowledge (parental) related to cardiac catheterization.
   ○ 3. Risk for Infection related to decreased oxygenation.
   ○ 4. Decreased Cardiac Output related to the structural defect.

2. When developing the plan of care for a 3-year-old diagnosed with ventricular septal defect, the nurse would include actions that foster the development of which of the following psychosocial tasks according to Erikson?
   ○ 1. Autonomy versus shame and doubt.
   ○ 2. Identity versus role diffusion.
   ○ 3. Initiative versus guilt.
   ○ 4. Industry versus guilt.

3. When teaching the parents of a child with a ventricular septal defect who is scheduled for a cardiac catheterization, the nurse explains that this procedure involves the use of which of the following?
   ○ 1. Ultra-high-frequency sound waves.
   ○ 2. Catheter placed in the right femoral vein.

   ○ 3. Cutdown procedure to place a catheter.
   ○ 4. General anesthesia.

4. When developing the discharge teaching plan for the parents of a child who has undergone a cardiac catheterization for ventricular septal defect, which of the following would the nurse expect to include?
   ○ 1. Restriction of the child's activities for the next 3 weeks.
   ○ 2. Use of sponge baths until the stitches are removed.
   ○ 3. Use of prophylactic antibiotics before receiving any dental work.
   ○ 4. Maintenance of a pressure dressing until a return visit with the physician.

The Client With Tetralogy of Fallot

5. A child diagnosed with tetralogy of Fallot becomes upset, crying and thrashing around when a blood specimen is obtained. The child's color becomes blue and the respiratory rate increases to 44 breaths/minute. Which of the following actions would the nurse do *first*?
   ○ 1. Obtain an order for sedation for the child.
   ○ 2. Assess for an irregular heart rate and rhythm.
   ○ 3. Explain to the child that it will only hurt for a short time.
   ○ 4. Place the child in a knee-to-chest position.

6. When teaching a child how to perform coughing and deep-breathing exercises before corrective surgery for tetralogy of Fallot, which of the following teaching and learning principles would the nurse address *first*?
   ○ 1. Organizing information to be taught in a logical sequence.
   ○ 2. Arranging to use actual equipment for demonstrations.
   ○ 3. Building the teaching on the child's current level of knowledge.
   ○ 4. Presenting the information in order from simplest to most complex.

7. When planning care for a child before corrective surgery for tetralogy of Fallot, which of the following would the nurse identify as the *priority* nursing diagnosis?
   ○ 1. Ineffective Coping related to upcoming surgery and complications.
   ○ 2. Pain related to surgical incision required to correct the defect.
   ○ 3. Deficient Knowledge related to upcoming surgery and postoperative events.
   ○ 4. Impaired Gas Exchange related to structural cardiac defect.

8. When assessing a child after heart surgery to correct tetralogy of Fallot, which of the following would alert the nurse to suspect a low cardiac output?
   ○ 1. Bounding pulses and mottled skin.
   ○ 2. Altered level of consciousness and thready pulse.
   ○ 3. Capillary refill of 2 seconds and blood pressure of 96/67 mm Hg.
   ○ 4. Extremities warm to the touch and pale skin.

9. When developing the teaching plan for the parents of a child who has had open heart surgery to repair tetralogy of Fallot with a patch, which of the following would the nurse expect to include?
   ○ 1. Antibiotic therapy administration before any invasive procedures.
   ○ 2. Intake of at least 10 glasses of water per day before the next appointment.
   ○ 3. Need for frequent nap and rest periods for the first 4 weeks at home.
   ○ 4. Restriction of ingestion of bananas and citrus fruits.

10. Which of the following would the nurse expect to include in the plan of care for a child diagnosed with tetralogy of Fallot who has undergone corrective surgery?
    ○ 1. Two to 3 g of sodium in the diet each day.
    ○ 2. Physical activity restrictions.
    ○ 3. Visits limited to a selected few.
    ○ 4. Assignment to an isolation room.

11. After surgery to correct tetralogy of Fallot, the child's

parents express concern to the nurse that their 4-year-old child wants to be held more frequently than usual. The nurse interprets the child's behavioral response to stress as which of the following?
    ○ 1. Repression.
    ○ 2. Depression.
    ○ 3. Regression.
    ○ 4. Discomfort.

12. The mother of a child diagnosed with tetralogy of Fallot who is hospitalized tells the nurse that the child's 3-year-old sibling has become quiet and shy and demonstrates more than the usual amount of sexual curiosity since her other child has been hospitalized. The nurse responds to the mother based on the interpretation that these behaviors reflect which of the following?
    ○ 1. Usual behavior for a 3-year-old.
    ○ 2. Need for more attention.
    ○ 3. Exposure to a sexual experience.
    ○ 4. Indication of depression.

The Client With Rheumatic Fever

13. Which of the following would the nurse expect to include in the plan of care for a child who is diagnosed with rheumatic fever and carditis and admitted to the hospital?
    ○ 1. Ensuring continuous parental presence at the child's bedside.
    ○ 2. Providing the child with periods of rest.
    ○ 3. Encouraging participation in age-appropriate activities.
    ○ 4. Advising the child to eat as much as possible.

14. Which of the following outcomes indicates that the activity restriction necessary for a 7-year-old child with rheumatic fever during the acute phase has been effective?
    ○ 1. Joints demonstrate absence of permanent injury.
    ○ 2. The resting heart rate is between 60 and 100 bpm.
    ○ 3. The child exhibits a decrease in chorea movements.
    ○ 4. The subcutaneous nodules over the joints are no longer palpable.

15. Which of the following initial physical findings would indicate the development of carditis in a child with rheumatic fever?
    ○ 1. Heart murmur.
    ○ 2. Low blood pressure.
    ○ 3. Irregular pulse.
    ○ 4. Anterior chest wall pain.

16. The physician orders pulse assessment several times

through the night for a child with rheumatic fever who has a daytime heart rate of 120 bpm. The nurse explains to the mother that the primary reason for obtaining a sleeping pulse rate is to ensure that the elevation in the child's pulse rate is unrelated to which of the following?
- ○ 1. Morning dose of digitalis.
- ○ 2. Normal activity during waking hours.
- ○ 3. Warmer environment during the day than at night.
- ○ 4. Variations in pulse rates obtained during day and evening hours.

17. Which of following would the nurse perform to help alleviate a child's joint pain associated with rheumatic fever?
- ○ 1. Maintaining the joints in an extended position.
- ○ 2. Applying gentle traction to the child's affected joints.
- ○ 3. Supporting proper alignment with rolled pillows.
- ○ 4. Using a bed cradle to avoid the weight of bed linens on joints.

The Client With Kawasaki Disease

18. When developing the plan of care for a newly admitted 2-year-old with the diagnosis of Kawasaki disease (KD), which of the following would be the *priority*?
- ○ 1. Taking vital signs every 6 hours.
- ○ 2. Monitoring intake and output every hour.
- ○ 3. Minimizing skin discomfort.
- ○ 4. Providing passive range of motion exercises.

19. A 16-month-old diagnosed with KD is very irritable, refuses to eat, and exhibits peeling skin on the hands and feet. Which of the following would the nurse interpret as the *priority*?
- ○ 1. Applying lotion to the hands and feet.
- ○ 2. Offering foods the toddler likes.
- ○ 3. Placing the toddler in a quiet environment.
- ○ 4. Encouraging the parents to get some rest.

20. Which of the following would the nurse include when completing discharge instructions for the parents of a 12-month-old diagnosed with KD being discharged to home?
- ○ 1. Offer the child extra fluids every 2 hours for 2 weeks.
- ○ 2. Take the child's temperature daily for several days.
- ○ 3. Check the child's blood pressure daily until the follow-up appointment.
- ○ 4. Call the physician if the irritability lasts for 2 more weeks.

The Client With Sickle Cell Anemia

21. The nurse explains to the parents of a 1-year-old admitted to the hospital in sickle cell crisis that the local tissue damage the child has on admission is caused by which of the following?
- ○ 1. Autoimmune reaction complicated by hypoxia.
- ○ 2. Lack of oxygen in the red blood cells.
- ○ 3. Obstruction to circulation.
- ○ 4. Elevated serum bilirubin concentration.

22. The mother asks the nurse why her child's hemoglobin was normal at birth but now the child has S hemoglobin. Which of the following responses by the nurse would be *most* appropriate?
- ○ 1. "The placenta bars passage of the hemoglobin S from the mother to the fetus."
- ○ 2. "The red bone marrow does not begin to produce hemoglobin S until several months after birth."
- ○ 3. "Antibodies transmitted from you to the fetus provide the newborn with temporary immunity."
- ○ 4. "The newborn has a high concentration of fetal hemoglobin in the blood for some time after birth."

23. Which of the following would the nurse identify as the *priority* nursing diagnosis during a toddler's vasoocclusive sickle cell crisis?
- ○ 1. Ineffective Coping related to presence of a life-threatening disease.
- ○ 2. Decreased Cardiac Output related to abnormal hemoglobin formation.
- ○ 3. Pain related to tissue anoxia.
- ○ 4. Excess Fluid Volume related to infection.

The Client With Iron-Deficiency Anemia

24. A mother asks the nurse if her child's iron-deficiency anemia is related to the child's frequent infections. The nurse responds based on the understanding of which of the following?
- ○ 1. Little is known about iron-deficiency anemia and its relationship to infection in children.
- ○ 2. Children with iron-deficiency anemia are more susceptible to infection than are other children.
- ○ 3. Children with iron-deficiency anemia are less susceptible to infection than are other children.
- ○ 4. Children with iron-deficiency anemia are equally as susceptible to infection as are other children.

25. Which of the following foods would the nurse encourage the mother to offer to her child with iron-deficiency anemia?

○ 1. Rice cereal, whole milk, and yellow vegetables.
○ 2. Potato, peas, and chicken.
○ 3. Macaroni, cheese, and ham.
○ 4. Pudding, green vegetables, and rice.

The Client With Hemophilia

26. The physician has ordered several laboratory tests to help diagnose an infant's bleeding disorder. Which of the following tests, if abnormal, would the nurse interpret as most likely to indicate hemophilia?
○ 1. Bleeding time.
○ 2. Tourniquet test.
○ 3. Clot retraction test.
○ 4. Partial thromboplastin time (PTT).

27. A diagnosis of hemophilia A is confirmed in an infant. With which of the following instructions would the nurse provide the parents as the infant becomes more mobile and starts to crawl?
○ 1. Administer one half of a children's aspirin for a temperature higher than 101°F (38.3°C).
○ 2. Sew thick padding into the elbows and knees of the child's clothing.
○ 3. Check the color of the child's urine every day.
○ 4. Expect the eruption of the primary teeth to produce moderate to severe bleeding.

28. Which of the following assessments in a child with hemophilia would lead the nurse to suspect early hemarthrosis?
○ 1. Child's reluctance to move a body part.
○ 2. Cool, pale, clammy extremity.
○ 3. Ecchymosis formation around a joint.
○ 4. Instability of a long bone on passive movement.

29. Because of the risks associated with administration of factor VIII concentrate, the nurse would teach the child's family to recognize and report which of the following?
○ 1. Yellowing of the skin.
○ 2. Constipation.
○ 3. Abdominal distention.
○ 4. Puffiness around the eyes.

30. The mother tells the nurse she will be afraid to allow her child with hemophilia to participate in sports because of the danger of injury and bleeding. After explaining that physical fitness is important for children with hemophilia, which of the following activities would the nurse suggest as *ideal*?
○ 1. Snow skiing.
○ 2. Swimming.
○ 3. Basketball.
○ 4. Gymnastics.

The Client With Leukemia

31. After teaching the parents of a child newly diagnosed with leukemia about the disease, which of the following descriptions given by the mother best indicates that she understands the nature of leukemia?
○ 1. "The disease is an infection resulting in increased white blood cell production."
○ 2. "The disease is a type of cancer characterized by an increase in immature white blood cells."
○ 3. "The disease is an inflammation associated with enlargement of the lymph nodes."
○ 4. "The disease is an allergic disorder involving increased circulating antibodies in the blood."

32. Laboratory findings indicate that a child with leukemia is also anemic. The nurse interprets this finding as *most* likely resulting from which of the following?
○ 1. Inadequate dietary folic acid intake.
○ 2. Decreased red blood cell production.
○ 3. Increased destruction of red blood cells by lymphocytes.
○ 4. Progressive replacement of bone marrow with scar tissue.

33. Which of the following statements would the nurse use to describe to the parents why their child with leukemia is at risk for infections?
○ 1. Play activities are too strenuous.
○ 2. Vitamin C intake is reduced over a period of time.
○ 3. The number of red blood cells is inadequate for carrying oxygen.
○ 4. Immature white blood cells are incapable of handling an infectious process.

34. Which of the following beverages would the nurse plan to give a child with leukemia if nausea should occur?
○ 1. Orange juice.
○ 2. Weak tea.
○ 3. Plain water.
○ 4. A carbonated beverage.

35. Which of the following medication orders to help relieve discomfort in a child with leukemia would the nurse question?
○ 1. Acetaminophen (Tylenol).
○ 2. Acetaminophen with codeine (Tylenol with Codeine).
○ 3. Ibuprofen (Motrin).
○ 4. Propoxyphene hydrochloride (Darvon).

36. After teaching a child with leukemia scheduled for a bone marrow aspiration about the procedure, the nurse determines that the teaching has been suc-

cessful when the child identifies which of the following as the puncture site?
- ○ 1. Right lateral side of the right wrist.
- ○ 2. Middle of the chest.
- ○ 3. Distal end of the thigh.
- ○ 4. Back of the hipbone.

37. Which of the following nursing diagnoses would the nurse identify as the *priority* when dealing with a child newly diagnosed with leukemia and the child's family?
- ○ 1. Risk for Injury related to malignant process.
- ○ 2. Pain related to treatment modalities.
- ○ 3. Imbalanced Nutrition: Less Than Body Requirements, related to loss of appetite.
- ○ 4. Anticipatory Grieving related to diagnosis and potential loss of child.

38. The nurse and parents are planning for the discharge of a child with leukemia who is receiving dactinomycin (actinomycin D) and vincristine (Oncovin). Which of the following would the nurse expect to teach the parents to do?

- ○ 1. Encourage increased fluid intake.
- ○ 2. Keep the child out of the sun.
- ○ 3. Monitor the child's heart rate.
- ○ 4. Observe the child for drowsiness.

39. After doing well for a period of time, a child with leukemia develops an overwhelming infection. The child's death is imminent. Which of the following statements offers the nurse the best guide in making plans to assist the parents in dealing with their child's imminent death?
- ○ 1. Knowing that the prognosis is poor helps prepare relatives for the death of children.
- ○ 2. Relatives are especially grieved when a child does well at first but then declines rapidly.
- ○ 3. Trust in health care personnel is most often destroyed by a death that is considered untimely.
- ○ 4. It is more difficult for relatives to accept the death of an older child than that of a toddler.

Correct Answers and Rationale

The letters in parentheses following the rationale identify the step of the nursing process (A, D, P, I, E) and client needs (1, 2, 3, 4, 5, 6, 7, 8, 9, 10). See the inside front cover for the key.

The Client Undergoing a Cardiac Catheterization

1. 2. Before the procedure, the child and family would need to know what cardiac catheterization is, what to expect, why it is being performed, and what care will be provided both before and after the procedure. Deficient Knowledge, not Decreased Cardiac Output, is the priority. Pain might be a priority nursing diagnosis after the catheterization because the procedure is invasive. A 4-year-old with a ventricular septal defect would not be at risk for infection related to decreased oxygenation. With this condition, blood flow increases through the pulmonary system, allowing the blood to become oxygenated before going on to the systemic circulation. (D, 9)

2. 3. Erikson maintained that the chief psychosocial task of the preschool period is acquiring a sense of initiative. The child's activities center around energetic learning and seeking accomplishment and satisfaction in these activities. The conflict of guilt arises when the child oversteps the limits of abilities and behaves or acts inappropriately. Autonomy versus shame and doubt is the psychosocial task of toddlers. Identity versus identity diffusion is the psychosocial task of early adolescents. Industry versus inferiority is the psychosocial task of school-aged children. (P, 3)

3. 2. In children, cardiac catheterization usually involves a right-sided approach because septal defects permit entry into the left side of the heart. The catheter is usually inserted into the femoral vein through a percutaneous puncture. A cutdown procedure is rarely used. Echocardiography involves the use of ultra-high-frequency sound waves. The catheterization is usually performed under local, not general, anesthesia with sedation. (I, 9)

4. 3. Prophylactic antibiotics are suggested for children with heart defects before dental work is done to reduce the risk of bacterial infection. Typically, activities are not restricted after a cardiac catheterization. A percutaneous approach is used to insert the catheter, so stitches are not necessary. Showering or bathing is allowed as usual. The pressure dressing will be removed before the child is discharged. (P, 9)

The Client With Tetralogy of Fallot

5. 4. The child is experiencing a tet or hypoxic episode. Therefore the nurse should place the child in a knee-to-chest position. Flexing the legs reduces venous flow of blood from the lower extremities and reduces the volume of blood being shunted through the interventricular septal defect and the overriding aorta in the child with tetralogy of Fallot. As a result, the blood then entering the systemic circulation has a higher oxygen content, and dyspnea is reduced. Flexing the legs also increases vascular resistance and pressure in the left ventricle. An infant often assumes a knee-to-chest position in the crib, or the mother learns to put the infant over her shoulder while holding the child in a knee-to-chest position to relieve dyspnea. If this position is ineffective, then the child may need a sedative. Once the child is in the position, the nurse may assess for an irregular heart rate and rhythm. Explaining to the child that it will only hurt for a short time does nothing to alleviate the hypoxia. (I, 10)

6. 3. Before developing any teaching program for a child, the nurse's first step is to assess the child to determine what is already known. Most older preschool children have some understanding of a condition present since birth. However, the child's interest will soon be lost if familiar material is repeated too often. (I, 10)

7. 3. When planning care for a child with tetralogy of Fallot who is to undergo corrective surgery, Deficient Knowledge would be the priority nursing diagnosis. The child and parents would need to be prepared for what occurs before and after surgery. Pain would be a priority nursing diagnosis after surgery. However, pain management would be addressed in the preoperative period, with teaching to correct the knowledge deficit. The child with tetralogy of Fallot has experienced cyanosis from birth. Therefore, Impaired Gas Exchange would not be a priority diagnosis. (D, 10)

8. 2. With a low cardiac output and subsequently poor tissue perfusion, signs and symptoms would include pale, cool extremities; cyanosis; weak, thready pulses; delayed capillary refill; and decrease in level of consciousness. (A, 10)

9. 1. Children who have undergone open heart surgery to repair tetralogy of Fallot with a patch as part of the correction are at risk for infections, specifically subacute bacterial endocarditis (SBE). Therefore the parents need instruction about SBE precautions, including the

need for antibiotic therapy administration before any invasive procedure. Having the child drink a large amount of fluid before a follow-up appointment is not necessary. Also, too great a fluid intake could possibly lead to overload, increasing the workload of the heart. Children gear their rest schedule to their activities. Therefore, frequent rest and nap periods are not necessary. No evidence is provided to indicate that the child has a high serum potassium concentration that would necessitate the restriction of foods high in potassium, such as bananas and citrus fruits. (P, 10)

10. 1. Because of the hemodynamic changes that occur with open heart surgical repair, particularly with septal defects, transient congestive heart failure may develop. Therefore, the child's sodium intake typically is restricted to 2 to 3 g/day. Activity restrictions are inappropriate. Typically, the child is encouraged to walk in the halls of the unit. Visitors are not restricted unless the pediatric unit has restrictive visiting policies. The child can be placed in a room with other children who are not contagious. Placement in an isolation room is not warranted. After correction of the defect, the risk for infection in the child is the same as for any postoperative client. (P, 10)

11. 3. The child's behavior suggests *regression*, defined as the act of moving backward. In psychology, the term is used to describe a person who reverts to an earlier stage of behavior or emotion. *Repression* is a defense mechanism by which an unacceptable or painful experience is put out of the conscious mind. For example, months later, the child does not recall having the surgery or being hospitalized. *Depression* is characterized by feelings of sadness, gloom, and dispiritedness, manifested by behaviors such as crying or whining. *Discomfort* is a negative feeling state often evidenced by squirming. (D, 5)

12. 2. The central psychosocial task for the preschool-aged child is to develop a sense of initiative versus guilt, according to Erikson's theory. Any environmental change may affect a child. In this situation, the sibling is probably feeling less attention from the mother and is attempting to resolve the conflict with inappropriate behavior. (D, 3)

The Client With Rheumatic Fever

13. 2. The nurse would encourage and plan to provide periods of rest for the child with rheumatic fever and carditis to allow the heart to rest. The parents should be made to feel that they can come and go as they need to. The child is not in critical condition, so the parents do not need to be present at the child's bedside continuously. The child should be allowed to participate in nonstrenuous activities that avoid overtaxing the heart, thus allowing the heart time to rest. There is no reason to encourage the child to eat as much as possible; in fact, overeating should be discouraged because it taxes the heart muscle. (P, 10)

14. 2. During the acute phase of rheumatic fever, the heart is inflamed and every effort is made to reduce the work of the heart. Bedrest with limited activity is necessary to prevent heart failure. Therefore, the most reliable indicator that activity restriction has been effective is a resting heart rate between 60 and 100 bpm, normal for a 7-year-old. No permanent damage to the joints occurs with rheumatic fever. The chorea movements associated with rheumatic fever are self-limited and usually disappear in 1 to 3 months. They are unrelated to activity restrictions. Subcutaneous nodules that occur over joint surfaces also resolve over time with no treatment. Therefore, they are not appropriate for evaluating the effectiveness of activity restrictions. (E, 10)

15. 1. In rheumatic fever, the connective tissue of the heart becomes inflamed, leading to carditis. The most common signs of carditis are heart murmurs, tachycardia during rest, cardiac enlargement, and changes in the electrical conductivity of the heart. Heart murmurs are present in about 75% of all clients during the first week of carditis and in 85% of clients by the third week. (A, 10)

16. 2. An above-average pulse rate that is out of proportion to the degree of activity is an early sign of cardiac failure in a client with rheumatic fever. The sleeping pulse is used to determine whether mild tachycardia continues during sleep (inactivity) or whether it is the result of daytime activity. Digitalis lowers the heart rate, so the heart rate would be decreased during the daytime. The environmental temperature would need to be quite warm before it could influence the heart rate. (I, 9)

17. 4. For a child with arthritis associated with rheumatic fever, the joints are usually so tender that even the weight of bed linens can cause pain. Use of a bed cradle is recommended to help remove the weight of the linens on painful joints. Joints need to be maintained in good alignment, not positioned in extension, to ensure that they remain functional. Applying gentle traction to the joints is not recommended because traction is usually used to relieve muscle spasms, not typically associated with rheumatic fever. Supporting the body in good alignment and changing the client's position are recommended, but these measures are not likely to relieve pain. (I, 9)

The Client With Kawasaki Disease

18. 2. Cardiac status must be monitored carefully in the initial phase of KD because the child is at high risk

for congestive heart failure. Therefore, the nurse needs to assess the child frequently for signs of congestive heart failure (CHF), which would include respiratory distress and decreased urine output. Vital signs would be obtained more often than every 6 hours because of the risk of CHF. Although minimizing skin discomfort would be important, it is does not take priority over monitoring the child's hourly intake and output. Passive range-of-motion exercises would be done if the child develops arthritis. (P, 10)

19. 3. One of the characteristics of children with KD is irritability. They are often inconsolable. Placing the child in a quiet environment may help quiet the child and reduce the workload of the heart. Although peeling of the skin occurs with KD, the child's irritability takes priority. Children with KD usually are not hungry and do not eat well regardless of what is served. There is no indication that the parents need rest. Additionally, in this situation, the child takes priority over the parents. (P, 10)

20. 2. The child's temperature should be taken for several days after discharge, because recurrent fever may develop. Offering the child fluids every 2 hours is not necessary. Doing so increases the child's risk for CHF. Checking the child's blood pressure at home usually is not included as part of the discharge instructions because, by the time of discharge, the child is considered stable and the risk for cardiac problems is minimal. Most children with KD recover fully. Irritability may last for 2 months after discharge. (I, 10)

The Client With Sickle Cell Anemia

21. 3. Characteristic sickle cells tend to cause "log jams" in capillaries. This results in poor circulation to local tissues, leading to ischemia and necrosis. The basic defect in sickle cell disease is an abnormality in the structure of the red blood cells. The erythrocytes are sickle-shaped, rough in texture, and rigid. Sickle cell disease is an inherited disease, not an autoimmune reaction. Elevated serum bilirubin concentrations are associated with jaundice, not sickle cell disease. (I, 10)

22. 4. Sickle cell disease is an inherited disease that is present at birth. However, 60% to 80% of a newborn's hemoglobin is fetal hemoglobin, which has a structure different from that of hemoglobin S or hemoglobin A. Sickle cell symptoms usually occur about 4 months after birth, when hemoglobin S begins to replace the fetal hemoglobin. The gene for sickle cell disease is transmitted at the time of conception, not passed through the placenta. Some hemoglobin S is produced by the fetus near term. The fetus produces all its own

hemoglobin from the earliest production in the first trimester. Passive immunity conferred by maternal antibodies is not related to sickle cell disease, but this transmission of antibodies is important to protect the infant from various infections during early infancy. (I, 10)

23. 3. For the child in sickle cell crisis, Pain is the priority nursing diagnosis because the sickled cells clump and obstruct the blood vessels, leading to occlusion and subsequent tissue ischemia. Although Ineffective Coping may be important, it is not the priority. Decreased Cardiac Output is not a problem with this type of vasoocclusive crisis. Typically, a sickle cell crisis can be precipitated by a fluid volume deficit or dehydration. (D, 10)

The Client With Iron-Deficiency Anemia

24. 2. Children with iron-deficiency anemia are more susceptible to infection because of marked decreases in bone marrow functioning with microcytosis. (D, 10)

25. 2. Potato, peas, chicken, green vegetables, and rice cereal contain significant amounts of iron and therefore would be recommended. Milk and yellow vegetables are not good iron sources. Rice by itself also is not a good source of iron. (I, 10)

The Client With Hemophilia

26. 4. PTT measures the activity of thromboplastin, which is dependent on intrinsic clotting factors. In hemophilia, the intrinsic clotting factor VIII (antihemophilic factor) is deficient, resulting in a prolonged PTT. Bleeding time reflects platelet function; the tourniquet test measures vasoconstriction and platelet function; and the clot retraction test measures capillary fragility. All of these are unaffected in people with hemophilia. (D, 9)

27. 2. As the hemophilic infant begins to acquire motor skills, the risk of bleeding increases because of falls and bumps. Such injuries can be minimized by padding vulnerable joints. Aspirin is contraindicated because of its antiplatelet properties, which increase the infant's risk for bleeding. Because genitourinary bleeding is not a typical problem in children with hemophilia, urine testing is not indicated. Although some bleeding may occur with tooth eruption, it does not normally cause moderate to severe bleeding episodes in children with hemophilia. (I, 2)

28. 1. Bleeding into the joints in the child with hemophilia leads to pain and tenderness, resulting in restricted movement. Therefore, an early sign of hemarthrosis

would be the child's reluctance to move a body part. If the bleeding into the joint continues, the area becomes hot, swollen, and immobile—not cool, pale, and clammy. Ecchymosis formation around a joint would be difficult to assess. Instability of a long bone on passive movement is not associated with joint hemarthrosis. (A, 10)

29. 1. Because factor VIII concentrate is derived from large pools of human plasma, the risk of hepatitis is always present. Clinical manifestations of hepatitis include yellowing of the skin, mucous membranes, and sclera. Use of factor VIII concentrate is not associated with constipation, abdominal distention, or puffiness around the eyes. (I, 8)

30. 2. Swimming is an ideal activity for a child with hemophilia because it is a noncontact sport. Many noncontact sports and physical activities that do not place excessive strain on joints are also appropriate. Such activities strengthen the muscles surrounding joints and help control bleeding in these areas. Noncontact sports also enhance general mental and physical well-being. Falls and subsequent injury to the child may occur with snow skiing. Basketball is a contact sport and therefore increases the child's risk for injury. Gymnastics is a very strenuous sport. Gymnasts frequently have muscle and joint injuries that result in bleeding episodes. (I, 4)

The Client With Leukemia

31. 2. Leukemia is a neoplastic, or cancerous, disorder of blood-forming tissues that is characterized by a proliferation of immature white blood cells. (E, 10)

32. 2. The anemia seen in children with leukemia is caused by the bone marrow's overproduction of immature white blood cells at the expense of producing red blood cells and platelets. In this client, anemia is not caused by an inadequate intake of iron but rather by insufficient red blood cells. (D, 9)

33. 4. In leukemia, the number of normal white blood cells that are capable of fighting an infection is decreased. Although there is an increased number of immature white blood cells, they are unable to combat infection. Therefore, a child with leukemia is subject to infection. The major morbidity and mortality factor associated with leukemia is infection resulting from the presence of granulocytopenia. (I, 9)

34. 4. Carbonated beverages ordinarily are the best tolerated when a child feels nauseated. Many children find cola drinks especially easy to tolerate, but noncola beverages are also recommended. Orange juice usually is not tolerated well because of its high acid content. (I, 9)

35. 3. Ibuprofen prolongs bleeding time and is contraindicated in clients with leukemia. Non-narcotic drugs other than ibuprofen or aspirin, such as acetaminophen (Tylenol), may be prescribed to control pain. Narcotic analgesics, such as acetaminophen with codeine or propoxyphene hydrochloride, may be required when pain is severe. (I, 8)

36. 4. Although bone marrow specimens may be obtained from various sites, the most commonly used site in children is the posterior iliac crest, the back of the hipbone. This area is close to the body's surface but removed from vital organs. The area is large, so specimens can easily be obtained. For infants, the proximal tibia and the posterior iliac crest are used. The middle of the chest or sternum is the usual site for bone marrow aspiration in an adult. (E, 9)

37. 4. Most often, the newly diagnosed child and parents are overwhelmed when first informed of the diagnosis. The family and child go through the beginning stages of grieving in anticipation of what may occur. The priority nursing diagnosis initially would be Anticipatory Grieving. (D, 5)

38. 1. Dactinomycin and vincristine both cause nausea and vomiting. Oral fluids are encouraged, and antiemetics are given to prevent dehydration. Avoiding sun exposure is not necessary because photosensitivity is not associated with these drugs. Heart rate changes and drowsiness also are not associated with either of these two drugs. (P, 8)

39. 2. It has been found that parents are more grieved when optimism is followed by defeat. The nurse should recognize this when planning various ways to help the parents of a dying child. It is not necessarily true that knowing about a poor prognosis for years helps prepare parents for a child's death. Death is still a shock when it occurs. Trust in health care personnel is not necessarily destroyed when a death is untimely if the family views the personnel as having done all that was possible. It is not more difficult for parents to accept the death of an older child than that of a younger child. (P, 5)

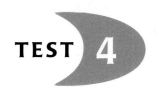

TEST 4

The Child With Health Problems of the Upper Gastrointestinal Tract

Select the one best answer, and indicate your choice by filling in the circle in front of the option.

The Client With Cleft Lip and Palate

1. When developing the plan of care for an infant with a cleft lip before corrective surgery is performed, which of the following would be a *priority*?
   - ○ 1. Maintaining skin integrity in the oral cavity.
   - ○ 2. Using techniques to minimize crying.
   - ○ 3. Altering the usual method of feeding.
   - ○ 4. Preventing the infant from putting fingers in the mouth.

2. Which of the following measures would be *most* effective in helping the infant with a cleft lip and palate to retain oral feedings?
   - ○ 1. Bubble the infant at frequent intervals.
   - ○ 2. Feed the infant small amounts at one time.
   - ○ 3. Place the end of the nipple far to the back of the infant's tongue.
   - ○ 4. Maintain the infant in a lying position while feeding.

3. When teaching the mother of an infant who has undergone surgical repair of a cleft lip how to care for the suture line, the nurse demonstrates how to remove formula and drainage. Which of the following solutions would the nurse use?
   - ○ 1. Mouthwash.
   - ○ 2. Povidone-iodine (Betadine) solution.

   - ○ 3. A mild antiseptic solution.
   - ○ 4. Half-strength hydrogen peroxide.

4. After teaching the mother of an infant who has had a surgical repair for a cleft lip about the use of elbow restraints at home, the nurse determines that the teaching has been successful when the mother states which of the following?
   - ○ 1. "We will keep the restraints on continuously except when checking the skin under them for redness."
   - ○ 2. "We will keep the restraints on during the day while he is awake, but take them off when we put him to bed at night."
   - ○ 3. "After we get home, we won't have to use the restraints because our child does not suck on his hands or fingers."
   - ○ 4. "We will be sure to keep the restraints on all the time until we come to see the physician for a follow-up visit."

5. The mother of an infant with a cleft lip and palate asks the nurse when her infant's cleft palate will be repaired. The nurse responds by stating that the first repair of a cleft palate is usually done at which of the following times?
   - ○ 1. Before the eruption of teeth.
   - ○ 2. When the child weighs approximately 10 kg (22 pounds).

159

○ 3. Before the development of speech.

○ 4. After the child learns to drink from a cup.

6. On the second postoperative day after repair of a cleft palate, which of the following would the nurse expect as *most* appropriate to use with a toddler?

   ○ 1. Cup.

   ○ 2. Straw.

   ○ 3. Rubber-tipped syringe.

   ○ 4. Large-holed nipple.

7. Immediately on return to the nursing unit after surgical repair of a cleft palate, in which of the following positions would the nurse place the child?

   ○ 1. On the back with the head in a position of comfort.

   ○ 2. In low Fowler's position with the head turned to the side.

   ○ 3. Lying on the abdomen with the head turned to the side.

   ○ 4. In reverse Trendelenburg with the head tilted forward.

The Client With Tracheoesophageal Fistula

8. The parents of a child with a tracheoesophageal fistula (TEF) express feelings of guilt about their baby's anomaly. Which of the following approaches by the nurse would *best* support the parents?

   ○ 1. Helping the parents accept their feelings as a normal reaction.

   ○ 2. Explaining that the parents did nothing to cause the newborn's defect.

   ○ 3. Encouraging the parents to concentrate on planning their baby's care.

   ○ 4. Urging the parents to visit their newborn as often as possible.

9. After teaching the parents of a neonate diagnosed with TEF about this anomaly, the nurse determines that the teaching was successful when the father describes the condition as which of the following?

   ○ 1. "The muscle below the stomach is too tight, causing the baby to vomit forcefully."

   ○ 2. "There is a blind upper pouch and an opening from the esophagus into the airway."

   ○ 3. "The lower bowel is lacking certain nerves to allow normal function."

   ○ 4. "A part of the bowel is on the outside without anything covering it."

10. Which of the following nursing diagnoses would the nurse identify as a priority for the infant with TEF?

    ○ 1. Impaired Parenting related to newborn's illness.

    ○ 2. Risk for Injury related to increased potential for aspiration.

○ 3. Ineffective Breathing Pattern related to a weak diaphragm.

○ 4. Imbalanced Nutrition: Less Than Body Requirements, related to poor sucking ability.

11. Which of the following would indicate that the infant with TEF needs suctioning?

    ○ 1. Brassy cough.

    ○ 2. Substernal retractions.

    ○ 3. Decreased activity level.

    ○ 4. Increased respiratory rate.

12. When administering gastrostomy feedings to an infant after surgery to correct a TEF, which of the following would be *most* appropriate to prevent air from entering the stomach once the syringe barrel is attached to the gastrostomy tube?

    ○ 1. Unclamp the tube after pouring the complete amount of formula to be administered into the syringe barrel.

    ○ 2. Pour all of the formula to be administered into the syringe barrel after opening the clamp.

    ○ 3. Maintain a continuous flow of formula down the side of the syringe barrel once the clamp is opened.

    ○ 4. Allow a small amount of formula to enter the stomach before pouring more formula into the syringe barrel.

13. After surgery to repair a TEF, an infant receives gastrostomy tube feedings. After feeding the infant by this method, the nurse cradles and rocks the infant for about 15 minutes, primarily to help accomplish which of the following?

    ○ 1. Promote intestinal peristalsis.

    ○ 2. Prevent regurgitation of formula.

    ○ 3. Relieve pressure on the surgical site.

    ○ 4. Associate eating with a pleasurable experience.

14. A newborn who had a surgical repair of a TEF is started on oral feedings. Which of the following would the nurse include in the teaching plan for the mother about oral feedings?

    ○ 1. They are better tolerated when small, frequent feedings are offered.

    ○ 2. They should be offered on a feeding schedule to help the infant accept the feedings more readily.

    ○ 3. They are best accepted by the infant when offered by the same nurse or by the infant's mother.

    ○ 4. They are best planned in conjunction with observations of the infant's behavior.

The Client With an Anorectal Anomaly

15. A newborn with the diagnosis of imperforate anus is to be scheduled for a radiographic examination.

The nurse explains to the parents that this examination is done to determine the distance between the anal dimple and which of the following?
○ 1. Perineum.
○ 2. Closed end of the rectum.
○ 3. Colon.
○ 4. Rectovesical pouch.

16. While caring for a neonate with an imperforate anus, the nurse assesses the neonate's urine output for which of the following?
○ 1. Meconium.
○ 2. Blood.
○ 3. Bile.
○ 4. Acetone.

17. After teaching the mother of a neonate who has successfully undergone surgery to repair a low anorectal anomaly, the mother indicates that she understands her child's prognosis when she states which of the following?
○ 1. "My child will need to wear protective pads until puberty."
○ 2. "My child will need extra fluids to prevent constipation."
○ 3. "My child will probably always need a high-fiber diet."
○ 4. "My child has a good chance of being potty trained."

18. When the infant returns to the unit after imperforate anus repair, the nurse places the infant in which of the following positions?
○ 1. On the abdomen, with legs pulled up under the body.
○ 2. On the back, with legs extended straight out.
○ 3. Lying on the side with the hips elevated.
○ 4. Lying on the back in a position of comfort.

19. The father of a neonate scheduled for gastrointestinal surgery asks the nurse how newborns respond to painful stimuli. Which of the following would be the nurse's *best* response?
○ 1. "Newborns cry and cannot be distracted to stop crying."
○ 2. "When faced with a pain, newborns try to roll away from it."
○ 3. "Newborns typically move their whole body in response to pain."
○ 4. "Pain causes the newborn to withdraw the affected part."

20. When developing the plan of care for a neonate who was diagnosed with an anorectal malformation and who subsequently underwent surgery, which of the following would be *most* helpful in facilitating parent–infant bonding?
○ 1. Explaining to the parents that they can visit at any time.
○ 2. Encouraging the parents to hold their infant.
○ 3. Asking the parents to help monitor the infant's intake and output.
○ 4. Helping the parents plan for their infant's discharge.

The Client With Pyloric Stenosis

21. A 4-week-old infant admitted with the medical diagnosis of hypertrophic pyloric stenosis presents with a history of vomiting. The nurse would anticipate that the infant's vomitus would contain gastric contents and which of the following?
○ 1. Bile and streaks of blood.
○ 2. Mucus and bile.
○ 3. Mucus and streaks of blood.
○ 4. Stool and bile.

22. A 6-year-old is admitted to the pediatric unit with a diagnosis of hypertrophic pyloric stenosis after vomiting for several days. Which of the following nursing diagnoses would be the *priority*?
○ 1. Deficient Fluid Volume related to prolonged vomiting.
○ 2. Ineffective Airway Clearance to impaired swallowing.
○ 3. Imbalanced Nutrition: Less Than Body Requirements related to prolonged vomiting.
○ 4. Bowel Incontinence related to abdominal pain.

23. When an infant with pyloric stenosis is admitted to the hospital, which of the following would the nurse do *first*?
○ 1. Weigh the infant.
○ 2. Begin an intravenous infusion.
○ 3. Switch the infant to an oral electrolyte solution.
○ 4. Orient the mother to the hospital unit.

24. After teaching the mother of an infant with pyloric stenosis about the disease, which of the following, if stated by the mother as a cause, indicates effective teaching?
○ 1. "An enlarged muscle below the stomach sphincter."
○ 2. "A telescoping of the large bowel into the smaller bowel."
○ 3. "A result of giving the baby more formula than is necessary."
○ 4. "My baby taking the formula too quickly."

25. Fluid replacement therapy is ordered for an infant diagnosed with pyloric stenosis. In addition to dextrose, water, and sodium chloride, which of the following would the nurse anticipate the physician to order as an additive to the intravenous solution?
○ 1. Calcium chloride.
○ 2. Bicarbonate chloride.
○ 3. Potassium chloride.
○ 4. Magnesium chloride.

26. When developing the plan of care for an infant with pyloric stenosis, the nurse identifies a nursing diagnosis of Deficient Fluid Volume related to prolonged vomiting. Which of the following parameters would the nurse expect to use when evaluating the client outcome?
    ○ 1. Abdominal distention.
    ○ 2. Weight loss.
    ○ 3. Vomiting.
    ○ 4. Respiratory effort.

27. After undergoing surgical correction of pyloric stenosis, an infant is returned to the room in stable condition. While standing by the crib, the mother says, "Perhaps if I had brought my baby to the hospital sooner, the surgery could have been avoided." Which of the following would be the nurse's *best* response?
    ○ 1. "Surgery is the most effective treatment for pyloric stenosis."
    ○ 2. "Try not to worry; your baby will be fine."
    ○ 3. "Do you feel that this problem indicates that you are not a good mother?"
    ○ 4. "Do you think that earlier hospitalization could have avoided surgery?"

28. After surgery to correct pyloric stenosis, the nurse instructs the parents about the postoperative feeding schedule for their infant. The parents exhibit understanding of these instructions when they state that they can start feeding the child within which of the following time frames?
    ○ 1. 6 hours.
    ○ 2. 8 hours.
    ○ 3. 10 hours.
    ○ 4. 12 hours.

29. Immediately after the first oral feeding after corrective surgery for pyloric stenosis, a 4-week-old infant is fussy and restless. Which of the following actions would be *most* appropriate at this time?
    ○ 1. Encourage the parents to hold the infant.
    ○ 2. Hang a mobile over the infant's crib.
    ○ 3. Give the infant more to eat.
    ○ 4. Give the infant a pacifier to suck on.

30. Which of the following behaviors exhibited by the parents of an infant with pyloric stenosis would the nurse correctly interpret as a positive indication of parental coping?
    ○ 1. Telling the nurse that they have to get away for a while.
    ○ 2. Discussing the infant's care realistically.
    ○ 3. Repeatedly asking if their child is normal.
    ○ 4. Exhibiting fear that they will disturb the infant.

The Client With Intussusception

31. When assessing a 4-month-old diagnosed with possible intussusception, the nurse would expect the mother to relate which of the following about the infant's crying and episodes of pain?
    ○ 1. Constant accompanied by leg extension.
    ○ 2. Intermittent with knees drawn to the chest.
    ○ 3. Shrill during ingestion of solids.
    ○ 4. Intermittent while being held in the mother's arms.

32. When obtaining the nursing history from the mother of an infant with suspected intussusception, which of the following questions would be *most* helpful?
    ○ 1. "What do the stools look like?"
    ○ 2. "When was the last time your child urinated?"
    ○ 3. "Is your child eating normally?"
    ○ 4. "Has your child had any episodes of vomiting?"

33. A nasogastric tube inserted during surgery to correct an infant's intussusception is no longer freely removing gastric secretions. Which of the following would the nurse do *next*?
    ○ 1. Aspirate the tube with a syringe.
    ○ 2. Irrigate the tube with distilled water.
    ○ 3. Increase the level of suction.
    ○ 4. Rotate the tube.

34. Which of the following assessments would be the priority for an infant who has had surgery to correct an intussusception and is now at risk for development of a paralytic ileus postoperatively?
    ○ 1. Measurement of urine specific gravity.
    ○ 2. Auscultation of bowel sounds.
    ○ 3. Inspection of the first stool passed.
    ○ 4. Measurement of gastric output.

35. An infant is to be discharged after surgery for intussusception. Which of the following would the nurse expect to include in the discharge teaching plan for the mother?
    ○ 1. The infant will experience a change in the normal home routine.
    ○ 2. The infant can return to the prehospital routine immediately.
    ○ 3. The infant needs to ingest more calories at home than what was consumed in the hospital.
    ○ 4. The infant will continue to experience abdominal cramping for a few days.

The Client With Inguinal Hernia

36. When assessing an infant with suspected inguinal hernia, which of the following findings would be *most* significant?
    ○ 1. The inguinal swelling is reddened, and the abdomen is distended.
    ○ 2. The infant is irritable, and a thickened spermatic cord is palpable.

○ 3. The inguinal swelling can be reduced, and the infant has a stool in the diaper.

○ 4. The infant's diaper is wet with urine, and the abdomen is nontender.

37. The physician is able to reduce an infant's hernia and schedules the infant for a herniorrhaphy in 2 days. The mother asks the nurse why the surgery is not performed now. Which of the following responses indicates that the nurse understands the rationale for delaying the surgery?

○ 1. "Delaying the surgery ensures that your infant will receive the proper preoperative preparation."

○ 2. "We need to make sure that your infant receives nothing by mouth for at least 24 hours before the surgery."

○ 3. "Waiting these 2 days helps to allow any edema and inflammation in the area to subside."

○ 4. "Your infant needs to wear a truss for at least 24 hours before any surgery can be attempted."

38. Preoperatively, the nurse develops a plan to prepare a 7-month-old infant psychologically for a scheduled herniorrhaphy the next day. Which of the following would the nurse expect to implement to accomplish this goal?

○ 1. Explaining the preoperative and postoperative procedures to the mother.

○ 2. Having the mother stay with the infant.

○ 3. Making sure the infant's favorite toy is available.

○ 4. Allowing the infant to play with surgical equipment.

39. Which of the following instructions would the nurse expect to include in the discharge teaching plan for the mother of an infant who has had an inguinal herniorrhaphy?

○ 1. Change diapers as soon as they become soiled.

○ 2. Apply an abdominal binder.

○ 3. Keep the incision covered with a sterile dressing.

○ 4. Restrain the infant's hands.

40. A mother asks, "How should I bathe my baby now that he's had surgery for his inguinal hernia?" Which of the following instructions would the nurse give the mother?

○ 1. "Cleanse his face and diaper area for 2 weeks."

○ 2. "Use sterile sponges to cleanse the inguinal incision."

○ 3. "Give him a sponge bath daily for 1 week."

○ 4. "Give the infant full tub baths every day."

41. A male adolescent who underwent repair of an inguinal hernia earlier today and is getting ready to go home receives instructions about resuming physical activities. Which of the following statements would indicate that he has understood the instructions?

○ 1. "I can start riding my bike next week."

○ 2. "I have to skip physical education classes for 2 weeks."

○ 3. "I can start wrestling again in 3 weeks."

○ 4. "I can return to my weight-lifting class in 2 weeks."

The Client With Hirschsprung's Disease

42. During physical assessment of a 4-month-old with Hirschsprung's disease, the nurse would most likely note which of the following?

○ 1. Scaphoid-shaped abdomen.

○ 2. Weight less than expected for height and age.

○ 3. Clubbing and cyanosis of the fingers and toes.

○ 4. Hyperactive deep tendon reflexes.

43. An infant diagnosed with Hirschsprung's disease is scheduled to receive a temporary colostomy. When initially discussing the diagnosis and treatment with the parents, which of the following would be *most* appropriate?

○ 1. Assessing the adequacy of their coping skills.

○ 2. Reassuring them that their child will be fine.

○ 3. Encouraging them to ask questions.

○ 4. Giving them printed material on the procedure.

44. After teaching the parents of an infant diagnosed with Hirschsprung's disease, the nurse determines that the parents understand the diagnosis when the father states which of the following?

○ 1. "There is no rectal opening for stool to pass."

○ 2. "There is a tube between the trachea and esophagus."

○ 3. "The nerves to the end of the large colon are missing."

○ 4. "The muscle below the stomach is too tight."

45. When developing the preoperative plan of care for an infant with Hirschsprung's disease, which of the following would the nurse expect to include?

○ 1. Administering a tapwater enema.

○ 2. Inserting a gastrostomy tube.

○ 3. Restricting oral intake to clear liquids.

○ 4. Using povidone-iodine solution to prepare the perineum.

46. An infant diagnosed with Hirschsprung's disease undergoes surgery with the creation of a temporary colostomy. Which of the following statements by the mother about her child's colostomy indicates the need for *further* teaching?

○ 1. "My child should be able to care for the colostomy by the time he's 8 years old."

○ 2. "The colostomy will give the intestine time to shrink to its normal size."

○ 3. "The colostomy may include two separate abdominal openings."

○ 4. "Right after the procedure, the stoma will appear big and red."

47. When teaching the mother of an infant who has received a temporary colostomy for treatment of Hirschsprung's disease about how the stoma should normally appear, which of the following descriptions about the stoma's appearance would the nurse include in the teaching?

○ 1. Becoming dark brown in 2 months.

○ 2. Staying deep red in color.

○ 3. Changing to several shades of pink.

○ 4. Turning almost purple in color.

48. When teaching the mother of an infant with Hirschsprung's disease who received a temporary colostomy about the types of foods her infant will be able to eat, which of the following would the nurse recommend?

○ 1. High-fiber diet.

○ 2. Low-fat diet.

○ 3. High-residue diet.

○ 4. Regular diet.

49. Eight hours ago, an infant with Hirschsprung's disease had surgery to create a colostomy. Which of the following findings would alert the nurse to notify the physician immediately?

○ 1. A 3-cm increase in abdominal circumference.

○ 2. Periods of occasional fussiness.

○ 3. Absence of bowel sounds since surgery.

○ 4. Evidence of the infant's returning appetite.

50. An infant with Hirschsprung's disease is to be discharged 1 or 2 days after surgery to create a colostomy. After teaching the infant's parents about the overall effects of their infant's surgery, the nurse determines that the teaching has been effective when the parents state which of the following?

○ 1. "His abdomen will be large for awhile."

○ 2. "When he's ready, toilet training may be difficult."

○ 3. "We need to limit his intake of dairy products."

○ 4. "We will give him vitamin supplements until he is an adolescent."

The Client With Diarrhea or Gastroenteritis

51. Which of the following would be an important assessment finding for an 8-month-old infant admitted with severe diarrhea?

○ 1. Absent bowel sounds.

○ 2. Pale yellow urine.

○ 3. Normal skin elasticity.

○ 4. Depressed anterior fontanel.

52. Which of the following would be the *best* activity for the nurse to include in the plan of care for an infant experiencing severe diarrhea?

○ 1. Monitoring the total 8-hour formula intake.

○ 2. Weighing the infant each day.

○ 3. Checking the anterior fontanel every shift.

○ 4. Monitoring abdominal skin turgor every shift.

53. Which of the following would be most appropriate for the nurse to teach the mother of a 6-month-old infant hospitalized with severe diarrhea to help her comfort her infant who is fussy?

○ 1. Offering a pacifier.

○ 2. Placing a mobile above the crib.

○ 3. Sitting at crib side talking to the infant.

○ 4. Turning the television on to cartoons.

54. Which of the following nursing diagnoses would be appropriate for the nurse to identify as a *priority* diagnosis for an infant just admitted to the hospital with a diagnosis of gastroenteritis?

○ 1. Pain related to repeated episodes of vomiting.

○ 2. Deficient Fluid Volume related to excessive losses from severe diarrhea.

○ 3. Impaired Parenting related to infant's loss of fluid.

○ 4. Impaired Urinary Elimination related to increased fluid intake feeding pattern.

55. Which of the following would the nurse use to determine achievement of the expected outcome for an infant with severe diarrhea and a nursing diagnosis of Deficient Fluid Volume related to passage of profuse amounts of watery diarrhea?

○ 1. Moist mucous membranes.

○ 2. Passage of a soft, formed stool.

○ 3. Absence of diarrhea for a 4-hour period.

○ 4. Ability to tolerate intravenous fluids well.

56. Which of the following would the nurse include when teaching the father of an infant just admitted with gastroenteritis about initial treatment for his infant?

○ 1. The infant will receive no liquids by mouth.

○ 2. Intravenous antibiotics will be started.

○ 3. The infant will be placed in a mist tent.

○ 4. An iron-fortified formula will be used.

57. The nurse teaches the father of an infant hospitalized with gastroenteritis about the next step of the treatment plan once the infant's condition has been controlled. The nurse would determine that the father understands when he explains that which of the following will occur with his infant?

○ 1. The infant will receive clear liquids for a period of time.

○ 2. Formula and juice will be offered.

○ 3. Blood will be drawn daily to test for anemia.

○ 4. The infant will be allowed to go to the playroom.

58. The mother of a toddler who has just been admitted with severe dehydration secondary to gastroenteritis says that she cannot stay with her child because she has to take care of her other children at home. Which of the responses by the nurse would be *most* appropriate?
    - ○ 1. "You really shouldn't leave right now. Your child is very sick."
    - ○ 2. "I understand, but feel free to visit or call anytime to see how your child is doing."
    - ○ 3. "It really isn't necessary to stay with your child. We'll take very good care of him."
    - ○ 4. "Can you find someone to stay with your children? Your child needs you here."

59. A child is admitted to the pediatric unit with the diagnosis of severe gastroenteritis. Which of the following would be *most* appropriate for the nurse to do?
    - ○ 1. Institute standard precautions.
    - ○ 2. Place the child in a semiprivate room.
    - ○ 3. Use regular eating utensils.
    - ○ 4. Single-bag all linens.

60. Which of the following would *most* likely alert the nurse to the possibility that a preschooler is experiencing moderate dehydration?
    - ○ 1. Vomiting.
    - ○ 2. Diaphoresis.
    - ○ 3. Absence of tear formation.
    - ○ 4. Decreased urine specific gravity.

61. The physician orders intravenous fluid replacement therapy with potassium chloride to be added for a child with severe gastroenteritis. Before adding the potassium chloride to the intravenous fluid, which of the following assessments would be *most* important?
    - ○ 1. Ability to void.
    - ○ 2. Passage of stool today.
    - ○ 3. Baseline electrocardiogram.
    - ○ 4. Serum calcium level.

62. Which of the following would *first* alert the nurse to suspect that a child with severe gastroenteritis who has been receiving intravenous therapy for the past several hours may be developing circulatory overload?
    - ○ 1. A drop in blood pressure.
    - ○ 2. Change to slow, deep respirations.
    - ○ 3. Auscultation of moist crackles.
    - ○ 4. Marked increase in urine output.

63. The stool culture of a child with profuse diarrhea reveals *Salmonella* bacilli. After teaching the mother about the course of *Salmonella* enteritis, which of the following statements by the mother indicates effective teaching?
    - ○ 1. "Some people become carriers and stay infectious for a long time."

    - ○ 2. "After the acute stage passes, the organism is usually not present in the stool."
    - ○ 3. "Although the organism may be alive indefinitely, in time it will be of no danger to anyone."
    - ○ 4. "If my child continues to have the organism in the stool, an antitoxin can help destroy the organism."

64. The child is started on a soft diet after having been on clear liquids following an episode of severe gastroenteritis. When helping the mother choose foods for her child, which of the following foods would be *most* appropriate?
    - ○ 1. Muffins and eggs.
    - ○ 2. Bananas and rice cereal.
    - ○ 3. Bran cereal and a bagel.
    - ○ 4. Pancakes and sausage.

65. When assessing a child diagnosed with diarrhea due to *Salmonella,* for which of the following possible sources would the nurse be alert during history taking?
    - ○ 1. Nonrefrigerated custard.
    - ○ 2. A pet canary.
    - ○ 3. Undercooked eggs.
    - ○ 4. Unwashed fruit.

66. On a home visit following discharge from the hospital after treatment for severe gastroenteritis, the mother tells the nurse that her toddler answers "No!" and is difficult to manage. After discussing this further with the mother, the nurse explains that the child's behavior is most probably the result of which of the following?
    - ○ 1. Beginning leadership skills.
    - ○ 2. Inherited personality trait.
    - ○ 3. Expression of individuality.
    - ○ 4. Usual lack of interest in everything.

67. The mother of a toddler hospitalized for episodes of diarrhea reports that when her toddler cannot have things the way she wants, she throws her legs and arms around, screams, and cries. The mother says, "I don't know what to do!" After teaching the mother about ways to manage this behavior, which of the following statements indicates that the nurse's teaching was successful?
    - ○ 1. "Next time she screams and throws her legs, I'll ignore the behavior."
    - ○ 2. "I'll allow her to have what she wants once in a while."
    - ○ 3. "I'll explain why she cannot have what she wants."
    - ○ 4. "When she behaves like this, I'll tell her that she is being a bad girl."

68. The mother of a potty-trained toddler who was admitted to the hospital for severe gastroenteritis and subsequent dehydration and is now at home

asks the nurse why the child still wets the bed. Which of the following would be the nurse's *best* response?

- ○ 1. "Hospitalization is a traumatic experience for children. Regression is common and it takes time for them to return to their former behavior."
- ○ 2. "The stress of hospitalization is hard for many children, but usually they have no problems when they return home."
- ○ 3. "After returning home from being hospitalized, children still feel they should be the center of attention."
- ○ 4. "Children do not feel comfortable in their home surroundings once they return home from being hospitalized."

The Client With Appendicitis

69. When obtaining the initial health history from a 10-year-old child with abdominal pain and suspected appendicitis, which of the following questions would be *most* helpful in eliciting data to help support the diagnosis?
    - ○ 1. "Where did the pain start?"
    - ○ 2. "What did you do for the pain?"
    - ○ 3. "How often do you have a bowel movement?"
    - ○ 4. "Is the pain continuous, or does it let up?"

70. When developing the plan of care for a school-aged child with a suspected diagnosis of appendicitis who is complaining of severe abdominal pain, which of the following measures would the nurse expect to include in the child's plan of care?
    - ○ 1. Application of a heating pad.
    - ○ 2. Insertion of a rectal tube.
    - ○ 3. Application of an ice bag.
    - ○ 4. Administration of an intravenous narcotic.

71. Which of the following assessment findings would alert the nurse to suspect appendicitis in an male adolescent complaining of severe abdominal pain?
    - ○ 1. Abdomen appears slightly rounded.
    - ○ 2. Bowel sounds are heard twice in 2 minutes.
    - ○ 3. All four abdominal quadrants reveal tympany.
    - ○ 4. The patient demonstrates a cremasteric reflex.

72. An adolescent male client scheduled for an emergency appendectomy is to be transferred directly from the emergency room to the operating room. Which of the following statements by the client would the nurse interpret as *most* significant?
    - ○ 1. "All of a sudden it doesn't hurt at all."

- ○ 2. "The pain is centered around my navel."
- ○ 3. "I feel like I'm going to throw up."
- ○ 4. "It hurts when you press on my stomach."

73. Which of the following would be the *priority* assessment for an adolescent on return to the nursing unit after an appendectomy?
    - ○ 1. The dressing on the surgical site.
    - ○ 2. Intravenous fluid infusion site.
    - ○ 3. Nasogastric (NG) tube function.
    - ○ 4. Amount of pain.

74. An adolescent who has had an appendectomy and developed peritonitis complains of nausea. Which of the following would the nurse do *first*?
    - ○ 1. Administer an antiemetic.
    - ○ 2. Irrigate the NG tube.
    - ○ 3. Notify the surgeon.
    - ○ 4. Take the blood pressure.

75. When developing the postoperative plan of care for an adolescent who has undergone an appendectomy for a ruptured appendix, in which of the following positions would the nurse expect to place the client during the early postoperative period?
    - ○ 1. The semi-Fowler's position.
    - ○ 2. Supine.
    - ○ 3. Lithotomy position.
    - ○ 4. Prone.

76. Which of the following would a nurse expect to hear from an adolescent who has just returned to her room after an appendectomy?
    - ○ 1. "I'll need plastic surgery for this scar."
    - ○ 2. "I'm worried about the size of my scar."
    - ○ 3. "I don't want to have any pain."
    - ○ 4. "What will my boyfriend say about the scar?"

77. Which of the following client actions would the nurse judge to be a healthy coping behavior for a male adolescent after an appendectomy?
    - ○ 1. Insisting on wearing a T-shirt and gym shorts rather than pajamas.
    - ○ 2. Avoiding interactions with other adolescents on the nursing unit.
    - ○ 3. Refusing to fill out the menu, and allowing the nurse to do so.
    - ○ 4. Not taking telephone calls from friends so he can rest.

78. When teaching an adolescent scheduled for an appendectomy about what to expect, which of the following approaches would be *most* effective?
    - ○ 1. Providing the primary essential information.
    - ○ 2. Offering advice and opinions as needed.
    - ○ 3. Using diagrams when explaining procedures.
    - ○ 4. Using age-appropriate jargon with explanations.

Correct Answers and Rationale

The letters in parentheses following the rationale identify the step of the nursing process (A, D, P, I, E) and client needs (1, 2, 3, 4, 5, 6, 7, 8, 9, 10). See the inside front cover for the key.

The Client With Cleft Lip and Palate

1. 3. Before corrective surgery for a cleft lip, the infant needs to consume formula. Methods for feeding may need to be adjusted to fit the infant's needs, because the infant with a cleft lip experiences a decreased ability to suck, which interferes with the infant's ability to compress the nipple. Commonly, a rubber-tipped syringe or medicine dropper is used to feed the infant to ensure adequate caloric intake. Problems with infection and skin integrity in the mouth are uncommon because the areas of the defect are not open areas. Although crying may cause the infant to swallow more air because of the defect, crying poses no harm to the infant. There is no need to keep the infant's fingers out of the mouth preoperatively. The fingers will not harm the defect or cause an infection. (P, 9)

2. 1. An infant with a cleft lip and palate typically swallows large amounts of air while being fed and therefore should be bubbled frequently. The soft palate defect allows air to be drawn into the pharynx with each swallow of formula. The stomach becomes distended with air, and regurgitation, possibly with aspiration, is likely if the infant is not bubbled frequently. Feeding frequently, even in small amounts, would not prevent swallowing of large amounts of air. A nipple placed in the back of the mouth is likely to cause the infant to gag and aspirate. Holding the infant in a lying position during feedings can also lead to regurgitation and aspiration of formula. The infant should be fed in an upright position. (I, 10)

3. 4. Half-strength hydrogen peroxide is recommended for cleansing the suture line after cleft lip repair. The bubbling action of the hydrogen peroxide is effective for removing debris. Normal saline also may be used. Mouthwashes frequently contain alcohol, which can be irritating. Also, mouthwashes are not as effective in removing debris as half-strength peroxide solutions are. Povidone-iodine solution is not used because the iodine contained in the solution can be absorbed through the skin, leading to toxicity. A mild antiseptic solution has some antibacterial properties but is ineffective in removing suture-line debris. (I, 10)

4. 1. To keep the infant from disturbing the suture line by placing fingers or other objects in the mouth, either intentionally or accidentally, the restraints should be in place at all times. They should be removed for a short period, however, so that the underlying skin can be checked for any redness or breakdown. While the restraints are removed, the parents should be instructed to manually restrain the hands and arms. (E, 2)

5. 3. The optimal time for cleft palate repair depends on many factors. However, it is best done before speech develops and the child learns faulty speech habits as a result of the defect, usually at about 12 to 15 months of age. Tooth eruption usually begins at about 6 months of age. An infant may learn to start drinking from a cup as early as 6 to 7 months of age, possibly up to the first birthday. (I, 10)

6. 1. A cup is the preferred drinking or eating utensil after repair of a cleft palate. At the age when repair is done, the child is ordinarily able to drink from a cup. Use of a cup avoids having to place a utensil in the mouth, which would increase the potential for injury to the suture lines. (P, 10)

7. 3. Immediately after a surgical repair of a cleft palate, the child is placed on the abdomen with the head turned to the side to lessen the chance of aspiration by allowing secretions to drain out. Positioning the child on the back places the child at risk for aspiration should any regurgitation or vomiting occur, even in low Fowler's position with the head to the side or in reverse Trendelenburg position with the head tilted forward. (I, 10)

The Client With Tracheoesophageal Fistula

8. 1. The parents of children born with defects often have feelings of guilt and ask what they might have done to cause the condition or how they might have avoided it. It is important to allow parents to express their feelings and to accept these feelings as normal reactions. Explaining that the parents are not at fault would not be appropriate until they have dealt with their feelings of guilt. Encouraging long-term planning generally is of little benefit to parents who are emotionally distraught. Additionally, the parents may interpret this as ignoring their feelings and confirming that they played a role in causing their child's anomaly. Urging the parents to visit their infant as often as possible would generally be of little help and could appear to the parents

as though they are being "talked out" of their feelings. (I, 5)

9. 2. Although TEF includes several different structural anomalies, the most common type involves a blind upper pouch and a fistula from the esophagus into the trachea. Other types include a blind pouch at the end of the esophagus with no connection to the trachea and a normal trachea and esophagus with an opening that connects them. A tightened muscle below the stomach and projectile vomiting of normal amounts of formula are characteristic of pyloric stenosis. Aganglionic megacolon is a lack of autonomic parasympathetic ganglion cells in a portion of the lower intestine. Gastroschisis occurs when the bowel herniates through a defect in the abdominal wall and no membrane covers the exposed bowel. (E, 10)

10. 2. Because the blind pouch associated with TEF fills quickly with fluids, the child is at high risk for aspiration. Therefore, the priority nursing diagnosis would be Risk for Injury. Children with TEF frequently develop aspiration pneumonia. Prevention of aspiration by suctioning or positioning is essential. Impaired Parenting may occur any time there is an infant with an obvious defect. Parents often have difficulty accepting that their child is not perfect. If the infant did aspirate, then Ineffective Breathing Pattern would be appropriate. However, care focuses on preventing aspiration. Infants with TEF do not experience poor sucking as a result of the defect. Poor sucking ability may be related to something else, such as prematurity. (D, 10)

11. 2. With TEF, overflow of secretions into the larynx leads to laryngospasm. This obstruction to inspiration stimulates the strong contraction of accessory muscles of the thorax to assist the diaphragm in breathing. This produces substernal retractions. The laryngospasm that occurs with TEF resolves quickly when secretions are removed from the oropharynx area. A brassy cough is related to a relatively constant laryngeal narrowing, usually caused by edema. It is not an indication of the need to suction. A decreased activity level and an increased respiratory rate in an infant with TEF are usually the result of hypoxia, a relatively long-term and constant phenomenon in infants with TEF. (A, 10)

12. 1. The best way to prevent air from entering the stomach when feeding an infant through a gastrostomy tube is to open the clamp after all the formula has been placed in the syringe barrel. Doing so prevents air from mixing with the formula and thus being introduced into the stomach. Pouring all the formula into the barrel after opening the clamp, maintaining a continuous flow of formula down the side of the barrel after unclamping the tube, and allowing a small amount of formula to enter the stomach before adding more formula to the barrel permit air to enter the stomach. (I, 9)

13. 4. The nurse can help meet the psychological needs of an infant being fed through a gastrostomy tube by rocking the infant after a feeding. The infant soon learns to associate eating with a pleasurable experience and learns to trust the caregiver. (I, 5)

14. 4. When initiating oral feedings after surgical repair of a TEF, it is best to follow a plan of care in conjunction with observation of the infant's needs and behavior. When the infant's needs and behavior are overlooked, plans are likely to be unsatisfactory and are more likely to meet the nurse's needs rather than the infant's needs. After a surgical procedure, infants initially tolerate small amounts of fluids offered more frequently better than larger amounts offered less often. Smaller amounts cause less bloating as the infant becomes used to feeding again. Although infants accept feedings more readily from their mother or from someone who feeds the infant repeatedly, the priority is to meet the infant's nutritional needs based on the infant's behavior. (P, 10)

The Client With an Anorectal Anomaly

15. 2. For the child with an imperforate anus, the purpose of the radiographic examination is to ascertain the distance between the anal dimple and the closed end of the rectum. (I, 9)

16. 1. Passage of meconium in the urine is a sign of rectourinary fistula, in which the rectum and bladder communicate. Blood in the urine would suggest an infection. Acetone in the urine would indicate excessive fat catabolism. Bile is not found in the urine. (A, 10)

17. 4. Children who undergo surgical correction for low anorectal anomalies as infants usually are continent. Fecal continence can be expected after successful correction of anal membrane atresia. Therefore, this child probably has a good chance of being potty trained and will not need to wear protective pads. Extra fluids and a high-fiber diet are not required to prevent constipation. Children with high anomalies may or may not achieve continence. (E, 10)

18. 3. After surgical repair for an imperforate anus, the infant should be positioned either supine with the legs suspended at a 90-degree angle or on either side with the hips elevated to prevent pressure on the perineum. A neonate who is placed on the abdomen pulls the legs up under the body, which puts tension on the perineum, as does positioning the neonate with the legs extended straight out. (I, 10)

19. 3. The neonate responds to pain with total body movement and brief, loud crying that ceases with distraction. After age 6 months, an infant reacts to pain with intense physical resistance and tries to escape by rolling away. A toddler reacts to pain by withdrawing the affected part. (I, 3)

20. 2. Encouraging the parents to hold their neonate promotes parent–infant attachment. Parent–infant bonding is based on a relationship that begins when the parent first touches the infant. Both the parents and the infant have predictable steps that they go through in this process. Explaining that the parents can visit at any time promotes bonding only if they do visit with, talk to, and hold the newborn. Asking the parents to help monitor intake and output at this time may be too anxiety-producing, thus interfering with bonding. Helping the parents plan for the infant's discharge involves them in the newborn's care and is important. However, it is not the first step in the development of bonding. (I, 5)

The Client With Pyloric Stenosis

21. 3. The vomitus of an infant with hypertrophic pyloric stenosis contains gastric contents, mucus, and streaks of blood. The vomitus does not contain bile because the pyloric constriction is proximal to the ampulla of Vater. (A, 10)

22. 1. Infants with pyloric stenosis usually have some degree of dehydration because of vomiting of the stomach contents. Therefore, a priority nursing diagnosis would be Deficient Fluid Volume related to prolonged vomiting. A nursing priority would be to restore fluid and electrolyte imbalances. Pyloric stenosis involves the pyloric valve distal to the stomach, not the respiratory tract. In addition, even though vomiting occurs, a normal 6-year-old should be able to protect the airway. Therefore, Ineffective Airway Clearance would be inappropriate. Impaired Nutrition: Less Than Body Requirements could be applicable but would not be the priority diagnosis. Bowel Incontinence and abdominal pain are not typically associated with pyloric stenosis. (D, 10)

23. 1. Unless the infant is in hypovolemic shock, obtaining a baseline weight is an important first action because the weight is used to calculate the child's fluid and electrolyte needs. The intravenous fluid rate and the amounts of electrolytes to be added to the fluid are based on the infant's weight. The weight also helps determine the infant's degree of dehydration. The intravenous infusion is initiated once the weight has been obtained. The child with pyloric stenosis typically experiences vomiting and is at risk for fluid volume deficit and metabolic acidosis. As a result, oral food and fluids are withheld and the infant is allowed nothing by mouth. Fluid replacement is given intravenously. Orientation can wait until treatment is under way. (I, 10)

24. 1. Pyloric stenosis involves hypertrophy of the pylorus muscle distal to the stomach and obstruction of the gastric outlet resulting in vomiting, metabolic acidosis, and dehydration. Telescoping of the bowel is called intussusception. Overfeeding, feeding too quickly, or underfeeding is not associated with pyloric stenosis. (E, 10)

25. 3. The child with pyloric stenosis experiences vomiting. The major electrolyte lost during vomiting is potassium. Infants with pyloric stenosis typically have low or low-normal serum potassium levels. Therefore, potassium chloride would be added to the intravenous solution. Vomiting also causes loss of hydrochloric acid, leading to metabolic alkalosis. Therefore, bicarbonate replacement would not be indicated. Typically, magnesium and calcium levels in the child with pyloric stenosis are within normal limits. (P, 8)

26. 2. For the client with a nursing diagnosis of Deficient Fluid Volume related to vomiting, the outcome would focus on restoration of fluid balance. Typically, the nurse would evaluate the client for evidence of dehydration. Parameters would include assessment of the client's weight for loss or decreased skin turgor. (P, 10)

27. 4. Restating or rephrasing a mother's response provides the opportunity for clarification and validation. It also helps to focus on what the mother is saying and address her concerns and feelings. Although surgery is the most effective treatment for pyloric stenosis, stating this ignores the mother's feelings and does not give her an opportunity to express them. Telling the mother not to worry also ignores the mother's feelings. Additionally, this type of statement gives the mother premature reassurance, which may turn out to be false. Asking the mother if she thinks the problem indicates that she is not a good mother implies such an idea. It does not allow her to express her concerns and feelings and therefore is not a therapeutic response. (I, 10)

28. 1. Clear liquids containing glucose and electrolytes are usually prescribed 4 to 6 hours after surgery. If vomiting does not occur, formula or breast milk then can be gradually substituted for clear liquids until the infant is taking normal feedings. (E, 10)

29. 4. Giving the infant a pacifier would help meet non-nutritive sucking needs and ensure oral gratification. Additionally, sucking aids in calming the infant. Holding the infant to decrease fussiness and restlessness is more effective in an older infant. Also, the reason for the infant's fussiness needs to be explored. Hanging a mobile over the crib frequently does not decrease fussiness. After surgery to correct pyloric stenosis, feeding the infant more formula would lead to vomiting, putting additional stress on the operative site. (I, 9)

30. 2. The parents' ability to verbalize the infant's care realistically indicates that they are working through their fears and concerns. This behavior demonstrates an understanding of the infant's condition and needs. Without further data, the fact that the parents "have to get away" could be interpreted as ineffective coping, possibly suggesting that they are unable to handle the situation. Continuing to ask about the child's general condition even after answers have been given does not suggest effective coping. The parents are demonstrating that they are unsure of themselves as parents or are hoping for positive information. Exhibiting fear that they will disturb the infant does not suggest effective coping. This behavior indicates that they are uncertain or lack knowledge about infants. (D, 5)

The Client With Intussusception

31. 2. The infant with intussusception experiences acute episodes of colic-like abdominal pain. Typically, the infant screams and draws the knees to the chest. Between these episodes of acute abdominal pain, the infant appears comfortable and normal. Feeding does not precipitate episodes of pain. Additionally, a 4-month-old typically would not be ingesting solid foods. Pain exhibited by crying that occurs when the infant is placed in a reclining position, as in the mother's arms, is not associated with intussusception. This type of cry may indicate that the infant wants attention, wants to be held, or needs to have a diaper change. (A, 10)

32. 1. For the infant with intussusception, stools characteristically have the appearance of currant jelly because of the intestinal inflammation and hemorrhage resulting from intestinal obstruction. These stools occur later in the course of the disease process. (A, 10)

33. 1. The first action is to check the placement of the tube to ensure that it is in the correct position. To check tube position, the nurse should aspirate the tube with a syringe. A return of gastric contents indicates that the end of the tube is in the stomach. Another method is to inject a small amount of air while auscultating with a stethoscope over the epigastric area. The tube is irrigated with normal saline, not distilled water, and only after the position of the tube is confirmed. The suction level should not be increased, because doing so could damage the mucosa. Rotating the tube could irritate or traumatize the nasal mucosa. (I, 9)

34. 2. Development of a paralytic ileus postoperatively is a functional obstruction of the bowel. Bowel sounds initially may be hyperactive, but then they diminish and cease. The first stool and the amount of gastric output provide information about the return of gastric function. Measurement of urine specific gravity provides information about fluid and electrolyte status. (A, 10)

35. 1. Infants who have had an interruption in their normal routine and experiences, such as hospitalization and surgery, typically manifest behavior changes when discharged. The infant's normal routine has been significantly altered, so it will take time to reestablish another routine. Calorie requirements at home will continue to be the same as those in the hospital. The infant does not need more calories at home. The surgical procedure corrected the problems, so the infant should not continue to have abdominal cramping. (P, 10)

The Client With Inguinal Hernia

36. 1. Abdominal distention and a redness of the inguinal swelling are significant findings. Their presence in conjunction with area tenderness and inability to reduce the hernia indicate an incarcerated hernia. An incarcerated hernia can lead to strangulation, necrosis, and gangrene of the bowel. Other findings associated with strangulation include irritability, anorexia, and difficulty in defecation. Irritability is nonspecific and could be caused by various factors. A palpable, thickened spermatic cord on the affected side is diagnostic of inguinal hernia and would be an expected finding. A wet diaper indicates that urine is being excreted, a finding unrelated to inguinal hernia. (A, 10)

37. 3. If nonoperative reduction is successful, delaying surgery for 2 to 3 days allows the edema and inflammation in the inguinal area to subside. Thus, the area to be operated will appear more normal, helping to decrease the risk of complications. The preoperative preparation for a herniorrhaphy is minimal and is not the reason for delaying the surgery. Typically, the infant is fed until a few hours before surgery to prevent dehydration. Trusses do not prevent incarceration, and there is no reason to use a truss preoperatively. (D, 10)

38. 2. The best way to prepare a 7-month-old infant psychologically for surgery is to have the primary caretaker stay with the child. Infants in the second 6 months of life commonly develop separation anxiety. Therefore, the priority in this case is to support the child by having the parent present. Teaching the mother what to expect may decrease her anxiety; this is important because infants sense anxiety and distress in parents, but the priority in this case is to have the parent present. Actual play and acting out life experiences are appropriate for preschool-aged children. Allowing

an infant to play with surgical equipment would be inappropriate and dangerous. (P, 5)

39. 1. Changing a diaper as soon as it becomes soiled helps prevent wound infection, the most common complication after inguinal hernia repair in an infant secondary to possible wound contamination with urine and stool. Because the surgical wound is unlikely to separate, an abdominal binder is unnecessary. The incision may or may not be covered with a dressing. If a dressing is not used, the physician may apply a topical spray to protect the wound. Restraining the infant's hands is unnecessary if the diaper is applied tightly. The infant would be unable to get the hands into the diaper close to the surgical site. (P, 10)

40. 3. The incision must be kept as clean and dry as possible. Therefore, daily sponge baths are given for about 1 week postoperatively. Cleansing the infant's face and diaper area should occur at least daily and continuously, not limited to a 2-week period. Because this type of surgery results in a wound that heals through primary intention, the skin will heal and cover the wound in 2 to 3 days. Therefore, it is not necessary to use sterile gauze to cleanse the incision. Clean technique is acceptable. Because the incision must be kept as clean and dry, full tub baths are inappropriate. (I, 9)

41. 3. Because of possible stress on the suture line, physical activities such as bicycle riding, physical education classes, weight-lifting, and wrestling are contraindicated for about 3 weeks. (E, 7)

The Client With Hirschsprung's Disease

42. 2. Infants with Hirschsprung's disease typically display failure to thrive, with poor weight gain due to malabsorption of nutrients. Therefore, the nurse would expect to see a child who weighs less than that which is expected for height and age. A distended, rather than a scaphoid-shaped, abdomen would be noted. Clubbing and cyanosis of fingers and toes are associated with congenital heart disease. Hyperactive deep tendon reflexes are associated with upper motor neuron problems, such as cerebral palsy. (A, 10)

43. 3. By encouraging parents to ask questions during information-sharing sessions, the nurse can clarify misconceptions and determine the parents' understanding of information. A better understanding of what is happening allows the parents to feel some control over the situation. Assessing the adequacy of the parents' coping skills is important but secondary to encouraging them to express their concerns. The questions they ask and their interactions with the nurse may provide clues to the adequacy of their coping skills. The nurse should

never give false reassurance to parents. At this point, there is no way for the nurse to know whether the child will be fine. Written materials are appropriate for augmenting the nurse's verbal communication. However, these are secondary to encouraging questions. (I, 5)

44. 3. The primary defect in Hirschsprung's disease is an absence of autonomic parasympathetic ganglion cells in the distal portion of the colon. Thus, the nerves to the end of the large colon are missing. Absence of a rectal opening refers to an imperforate anus. A tube between the trachea and esophagus refers to a tracheoesophageal fistula. Presence of a tight muscle below the stomach refers to pyloric stenosis. (E, 10)

45. 3. Before intestinal surgery, dietary intake is limited to clear liquids for 24 to 48 hours. A clear liquid diet meets the child's fluid needs and avoids the formation of fecal material in the intestine. Typically, repeated saline enemas, not tapwater enemas, are given to empty the bowel. Soapsuds enemas are contraindicated for infants, as are tapwater enemas. A nasogastric tube may be inserted for gastric decompression. Insertion of a gastrostomy tube is outside the scope of nursing practice. Because the perineal area is not involved in the surgery, it does not need to be prepared. (P, 10)

46. 1. The goal of surgery is to remove the aganglionic bowel and to improve functioning of the internal sphincter. A temporary loop or double-barreled colostomy is usually created to rest the bowel. This enables the normal distal bowel to regain its original tone and size. Final corrective surgery is done when the child is age 6 to 12 months or weighs about 10 kg. The colostomy probably will be reversed before the child is old enough to be responsible for its care. In the immediate postoperative period, a new stoma is swollen and erythematous. (E, 10)

47. 2. Typically, the stoma should remain deep red in color as long as the infant has the colostomy. A dark-red to purplish color may indicate impaired circulation to the stoma. (I, 10)

48. 4. A regular diet would be recommended for the child with a colostomy; no special diet is needed. High-fiber foods, such as fruits and vegetables, should be minimized because they increase the bulk in the stool. Fat is necessary for brain growth in the first year of life. A high-residue diet would result in bulkier stools and increased gas production, which will collect in the colostomy bag. Therefore, a high-residue diet is not indicated. (I, 7)

49. 1. Abdominal circumference is measured to monitor for abdominal distention. An increase of 3 cm in 8 hours would require notification of the physician; it would indicate a substantial degree of abdominal distention, possibly from fluid or gas accumulation. Nor-

mally, after surgery, an infant experiences occasional periods of fussiness. However, as long as the infant is able to be quiet by himself or with the aid of a pacifier, the physician does not need to be contacted. Absence of bowel sounds would be expected after surgery because of the effects of anesthesia. It takes approximately 48 hours for gastric motility to resume. Even if the infant displays evidence that he is hungry, fluids will not be offered until bowel sounds are heard, indicating a functioning gastrointestinal tract. (A, 9)

50. 2. Toilet-training is commonly more difficult for children who have undergone surgery for Hirschsprung's disease than it is for other children. This is because of the trauma to the area and the associated psychological implications. Abdominal distention is an early sign of infection and therefore the parents need to report it to the physician. Typically, dietary restrictions are not required. Usually the infant is placed on an age-appropriate diet. Vitamin supplementation is not necessary if the infant's dietary intake is adequate. (E, 10)

The Client With Diarrhea or Gastroenteritis

51. 4. An infant with severe diarrhea will experience some degree of dehydration. In an 8-month-old child, the anterior fontanel has not closed. Therefore, a depressed anterior fontanel would be an important finding. Additionally, the infant would exhibit dry mucous membranes, lethargy, hyperactive bowel sounds, dark urine, and sunken eyeballs. Skin turgor would be decreased or delayed (ie, slow to return when pinched). (A, 9)

52. 2. Because an infant experiencing severe diarrhea is at high risk for Deficient Fluid Volume, the nurse needs to evaluate the infant's fluid balance status by weighing the infant at least every day. Body weight is the best indicator of hydration status because a higher proportion of an infant's body weight is water, compared with an adult. Initially, the infant with severe diarrhea is not allowed liquids but is given fluids intravenously. Therefore, monitoring the oral intake of formula is inappropriate. Although checking the anterior fontanel for depression or bulging provides information about hydration status, this method is not considered the best indicator of the infant's fluid balance. Monitoring skin turgor can provide information about fluid volume status. The abdomen is commonly used to assess skin turgor in an infant because it is a large surface area and can be accessed quickly. However, weight is the best indicator of fluid balance. (P, 10)

53. 1. Typically, an infant hospitalized with severe diarrhea would be receiving fluid replacement intravenously rather than orally. Oral fluids and food are usually withheld. Although activities such as placing a mobile over the crib, speaking to the infant, or turning on the television may provide distraction for or help in calming the infant, a fussy infant receiving nothing by mouth is usually best comforted by providing a pacifier to satisfy sucking needs. (I, 3)

54. 2. Given this infant's history of gastroenteritis, the priority nursing diagnosis would be Deficient Fluid Volume. With gastroenteritis, vomiting and diarrhea occur, leading to the loss of fluids. This loss of fluids is problematic in infants because a higher proportion of their body weight is water. Impaired Urinary Elimination is related to the infant's fluid volume deficit resulting from vomiting and diarrhea associated with gastroenteritis. If the infant's fluid volume deficit is not corrected, then this nursing diagnosis may become the priority. (D, 10)

55. 1. The outcome of moist mucous membranes indicates adequate hydration and fluid balance, showing that the problem of fluid volume deficit has been corrected. Although a normal bowel movement, ability to tolerate intravenous fluids, and an increasing time interval between bowel movements are all positive signs, they do not specifically address the problem of deficient fluid volume. (E, 10)

56. 1. Children hospitalized with gastroenteritis are usually not allowed fluids by mouth to allow the gastrointestinal tract time to rest. Antibiotics are not indicated unless there is a bacterial infection. A mist tent would be used to treat respiratory disorders, not gastroenteritis. Once the infant is allowed oral intake, clear fluids are used initially. (I, 3)

57. 1. The usual way to treat an infant hospitalized with gastroenteritis is to keep the infant NPO to rest the gastrointestinal tract. The resultant fluid volume deficit is treated with intravenous fluids. When the infant's condition is controlled (ie, when vomiting subsides), clear liquids are then started slowly. Formula and juice will be started once the infant's vomiting has subsided and the infant has demonstrated the ability to tolerate clear liquids for a period of time. In this situation, there is no need to test the infant's blood every day for anemia. Most likely, the infant's serum electrolyte levels would be monitored closely. Typically, an infant is placed in a private room because gastroenteritis is most commonly caused by a virus that is easily transmitted to others. (E, 10)

58. 2. The nurse's best course of action would be to support the mother. This is best done by conveying understanding and encouraging the mother to visit or call. Telling the mother that she shouldn't leave and that the child is very sick is critical and insensitive. Additionally, it implies guilt should the mother leave. Commenting that the child does not need anyone is not

appropriate or true. Toddlers in particular need family members present because of the stresses associated with hospitalization. They experience separation anxiety, a normal aspect of development, and need constancy in their environment. Asking the mother to find someone else to stay with her children is inappropriate. The children at home also need the support of the mother and/or other family members to minimize the disruptions in family life resulting from the toddler's hospitalization and to maintain consistency. (I, 5)

59. 1. For the child with severe gastroenteritis, diarrhea is a problem; it exposes all persons caring for the child to possibly infectious body fluids. Subsequently, any other clients being cared for by these individuals are also at risk. Therefore, the nurse would institute standard precautions, including good handwashing and use of appropriate personal protective equipment (gowns, gloves, eye protection) to minimize the risk for exposure. Typically, the child with severe gastroenteritis is placed in a private room until the causative organism is determined, to prevent transmission and protect others, including clients, families, and staff, from to acquiring the infection. Because gastroenteritis is usually viral in origin and highly contagious, disposable eating utensils would be used to prevent transmission. For the child with gastroenteritis, double-bagging all linens is appropriate to prevent possible transmission from contaminated linens. (I, 2)

60. 3. The absence of tears is typically found when moderate dehydration is observed as the body attempts to conserve fluids. Other typical findings associated with moderate dehydration include a dry mouth, sunken eyes, poor skin turgor, and an increased pulse rate. Decreased perspiration, not diaphoresis, would be seen with moderate dehydration. The specific gravity of urine increases with decreased output in the presence of dehydration. (A, 9)

61. 1. Potassium chloride is readily excreted in the urine. Before adding potassium chloride to the intravenous fluid, the nurse should ascertain whether the child can void; if not, potassium chloride may build up in the serum and cause hyperkalemia. An electrocardiogram could be done during intravenous potassium replacement therapy to evaluate for these changes. (A, 8)

62. 3. An early sign of circulatory overload is moist rales or crackles heard when auscultating over the chest wall. Elevated blood pressure, engorged neck veins, a wide variation between fluid intake and output (with a higher intake than output), shortness of breath, increased respiratory rate, dyspnea, and cyanosis occur later. (A, 9)

63. 1. After having *Salmonella* enteritis, some patients become chronic carriers of the causative organism and remain infectious for a long time as the organism continues to be shed from the body. No antitoxin is available to treat or prevent salmonella infections. (E, 10)

64. 2. After clear liquids, the foods of choice are soft foods. These foods should be easily digested and low in fat. Additionally, the foods should be non–bulk forming. Bananas and rice cereal are low in fat and easy to digest. Muffins and eggs, as well as sausage and pancakes, are typically high in fat and would be avoided. Although a bagel is low in fat, bran cereal is high in fiber and would be avoided because it may cause more diarrhea. (I, 7)

65. 3. Diarrhea related to *Salmonella* bacilli is commonly spread by raw or undercooked fowl and eggs, pet turtles, and kittens. Food poisoning caused by *Staphylococcus* species is commonly spread by inadequately cooked or refrigerated custards, cream fillings, or mayonnaise. Psittacosis, a respiratory illness, may be spread by canaries. Contaminated, unwashed fruit is associated with typhoid fever (caused by *Salmonella typhi*), a disorder rarely seen in the United States. (A, 10)

66. 3. The "no" behavior demonstrated by a toddler is typical of this age group as the child attempts to be self-assertive as an individual. The negativism does not demonstrate an inherited personality trait or disinterest. Rather, it reflects the developmental task of establishing autonomy. The toddler is attempting to exert control over the environment. It is too early to assess leadership qualities in a toddler. (I, 3)

67. 1. The child is demonstrating behavior associated with temper tantrums, which are relatively frequent normal occurrences during toddlerhood as the child attempts to develop a sense of autonomy. The development of autonomy requires opportunities for the child to make decisions and express individuality. Ignoring the outbursts is probably the best strategy. Doing so avoids rewarding the behavior and helps the child to learn limits, promoting the development of self-control. However, the mother should intervene in a temper tantrum if the child is likely to injure herself. Allowing the child to have what she wants occasionally would typically add to the problems associated with temper tantrums, because doing so rewards the behavior and prevents the child from developing self-control. Toddlers do not possess the capacity to understand explanations about behavior. Expressing disappointment in the child's behavior or telling her that she is being a bad girl reinforces feelings of guilt and shame, thus interfering the child's ability to develop a sense of autonomy. (E, 3)

68. 1. Hospitalization is a traumatic time for a child, and it takes some time to readjust to the home environment.

The child may regress at home for a period until she feels comfortable. Children normally do not dislike their home environment; in fact, they usually are anxious to get home to familiar surroundings where they feel safe. (I, 3)

The Client With Appendicitis

69. 1. The most helpful question would be to determine the location of the pain when it started. The pain associated with appendicitis usually begins in the periumbilical area, then progresses to the right lower quadrant. After the nurse has determined the location of the pain, asking about what was done for the pain would be appropriate. Asking about the child's usual bowel movement pattern is a general question unrelated to child's condition. Children with appendicitis may have diarrhea or constipation. Additionally, knowledge about the child's usual pattern would not be a priority because the child with appendicitis typically is not hospitalized long enough to reestablish the normal pattern. Although the characteristics of the pain are important, asking if the pain is continuous or intermittent is vague and general because the pain could be associated with numerous conditions. With appendicitis, the client's pain may begin as intermittent, but it eventually becomes continuous. (A, 10)

70. 3. Application of an ice bag may help to relieve pain by decreasing circulation to the area. A heating pad is contraindicated because heat may increase circulation to the appendix, possibly leading to rupture. Rectal tubes are contraindicated because they stimulate bowel motility and can exacerbate abdominal pain. Also, they would be ineffective, because accumulation of gas in the lower bowel is not likely to be the cause of the child's discomfort. Because narcotics can mask the child's symptoms, such as pain and discomfort, and they also decrease bowel motility, they are not given until after a definitive diagnosis has been made. (P, 10)

71. 2. Manifestations of appendicitis include decreased or absent bowel sounds. Normally, bowel sounds are heard every 10 to 30 seconds. Therefore, bowel sounds heard twice in 2 minutes suggests appendicitis. Normally, the contour of the male adolescent abdomen is flat to slightly rounded, and tympany is typically heard when auscultating over most of the abdomen. A cremasteric reflex is normal for male adolescents. (A, 10)

72. 1. Sudden relief of pain in a client with appendicitis may indicate that the appendix has ruptured. Rupture relieves the pressure within the appendix but spreads the infection to the peritoneal cavity. Periumbilical pain (pain centered around the navel), vomiting, and abdom-

inal tenderness on palpation are common findings associated with appendicitis. (D, 10)

73. 1. The priority assessment after an appendectomy would be the dressing over the surgical site to determine whether there is any drainage or bleeding. The surgical dressing should be clean, dry, and intact. Once the dressing has been assessed, the nurse would assess the intravenous infusion site, assess the NG tube to be sure it is functioning, and finally, determine the degree of pain the client is experiencing. (A, 10)

74. 2. After an appendectomy, the client who develops peritonitis typically has an NG tube in place. When a client complains of nausea, the nurse would first check to ensure that the NG tube is functioning correctly, because the client's nausea may be related to a blockage of the NG tube. If the tube is clogged, it can be irrigated with normal saline. An antiemetic may be given, but only after the nurse has determined that the NG tube is functioning properly. Postoperative orders usually include an order for an antiemetic. Typically, the nurse would notify the surgeon if the client did not obtain relief from irrigation of the NG tube or administration of an ordered antiemetic. Although taking the client's blood pressure is an important postoperative nursing activity, it is unrelated to relieving the client's nausea. (I, 10)

75. 1. After an appendectomy for a ruptured appendix, assuming the semi-Fowler's or a right side-lying position helps localize the infection. These positions promote drainage from the peritoneal cavity and decrease the incidence of subdiaphragmatic abscess. (P, 10)

76. 2. Typically, adolescents are concerned about the immediate state and functioning of their bodies. The adolescent needs to know whether any changes (eg, illness, trauma, surgery) will alter her lifestyle or interfere with her quest for physical perfection. Having a scar may be devastating to the adolescent. The need for plastic surgery cannot be determined at this point. The adolescent has just returned from surgery and has yet to see the scar. Healing has yet to occur. Typically scars become smaller and fade over time. The desire for no pain is unrealistic. Although adolescents are worried about pain and how they will respond, they typically are discharged within 24 hours after an appendectomy with pain well controlled by oral analgesics. The immediate concern of adolescents is the state and functioning of their bodies. After concerns about themselves, then adolescents are concerned about their peer group and their responses. Although the boyfriend's response will matter, this concern would be more common later in the course of the adolescent's recovery. (A, 3)

77. 1. Adolescents struggle for independence and identity, needing to feel in control of situations and to con-

form with peers. Control and conformity are often manifested in appearance, including clothing, and this carries over into the hospital experience. The adolescent feels best when he is able to look and act as he normally does—for example, wearing a T-shirt and gym shorts. Adolescents normally want to interact with peers and commonly seek every opportunity to do so. Avoiding other adolescents on the nursing unit or not taking phone calls from friends might suggest ineffective coping behavior. Refusing to fill out the menu and allowing the nurse to do so demonstrates dependent behavior, not a healthy coping mechanism. (E, 5)

78. 3. Adolescents can comprehend scientific rationale and complexity. They appreciate detailed descriptions and explanations using charts, diagrams, and models. Adolescents want to know more than the essential information. They have questions and want to know what to expect. They dislike lectures and unsolicited advice and opinions. They need to feel that they have some control, fostered by allowing the adolescent to participate in the conversation rather than be lectured to or given advice. Participation helps to foster decision-making skills. Jargon is a means to establish the identity of the peer group. An adult's use of adolescent jargon may be viewed as false or dishonest. (I, 3)

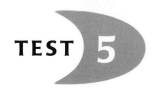

TEST 5

The Child With Health Problems Involving Ingestion, Nutrition, or Diet

Select the one best answer, and indicate your choice by filling in the circle in front of the option.

The Client With Ingestion of Toxic Substances

1. While conducting a medication inventory, the emergency department nurse of a pediatric hospital checks to ensure that syrup of ipecac is readily available. This action is based on the nurse's knowledge that this drug is used primarily to accomplish which of the following?
   ○ 1. Induce vomiting.
   ○ 2. Promote diuresis.
   ○ 3. Control seizure activity.
   ○ 4. Stimulate the heart.

2. A toddler is brought to the emergency room after ingesting an undetermined amount of drain cleaner. The nurse would expect to prepare to assist with which of the following *first*?
   ○ 1. Administering an emetic.
   ○ 2. Performing a tracheostomy.
   ○ 3. Performing gastric lavage.
   ○ 4. Inserting an indwelling urinary (Foley) catheter.

3. After the acute stage following an ingestion of drain cleaner by a child, the nurse would be alert for the development of which of the following as a likely complication?
   ○ 1. Tracheal stenosis.
   ○ 2. Tracheal varices.
   ○ 3. Esophageal strictures.
   ○ 4. Esophageal diverticula.

4. A child presents to the emergency room with the history of ingesting a large amount of acetaminophen. For which of the following would the nurse assess?
   ○ 1. Hypertension.
   ○ 2. Frequent urination.
   ○ 3. Right upper quadrant pain.
   ○ 4. Headache.

5. When developing the plan of care for a toddler who has taken an acetaminophen overdose, which of the following would the nurse expect to include as part of the *initial* treatment?
   ○ 1. Frequent blood level determinations.
   ○ 2. Gastric lavage.
   ○ 3. Tracheostomy.
   ○ 4. Electrocardiogram.

6. While assessing a preschooler brought by her parents to the emergency department after ingestion of kerosene, the nurse would be alert for which of the following?
   ○ 1. Uremia.
   ○ 2. Hepatitis.
   ○ 3. Carditis.
   ○ 4. Pneumonitis.

The Client With Lead Poisoning

7. Which of the following statements by the mother of an 18-month-old would indicate to the nurse that the child needs laboratory testing for lead levels?
   ○ 1. "My child does not always wash after playing outside."

○ 2. "My child drinks 2 cups of milk every day."

○ 3. "My child has more temper tantrums than other kids."

○ 4. "My child is smaller than other kids of the same age."

8. A child's blood lead concentration is 17 μg/dL, and it has been higher than 10 μg/dL for several months. Which of the following would the nurse anticipate?
   ○ 1. Need for no further follow-up.
   ○ 2. Immediate initiation of chelation therapy.
   ○ 3. Investigation of the child's environment.
   ○ 4. Prompt admission to the hospital.

9. When teaching the mother of a toddler diagnosed with lead poisoning, which of the following would the nurse include as the *most* serious complication if the condition goes untreated?
   ○ 1. Cirrhosis of the liver.
   ○ 2. Stunted growth rate.
   ○ 3. Neurologic deficits.
   ○ 4. Heart failure.

10. When teaching a mother about measures to prevent lead poisoning in her children, which of the following would the nurse include as the *most* effective preventive measure?
    ○ 1. Condemning of old housing developments.
    ○ 2. Educating the public on common sources of lead.
    ○ 3. Educating the public on the importance of good nutrition.
    ○ 4. Keeping pregnant women out of old homes that are being remodeled.

11. Which of the following would be the nurse's best response to a mother who asks about the outcome for her child with lead poisoning?
    ○ 1. "Many children suffer brain damage from lead poisoning."
    ○ 2. "Many of its effects require the child to receive special schooling."
    ○ 3. "Most children with lead poisoning experience problems with the law."
    ○ 4. "Most effects of lead poisoning are reversible if diagnosed early."

The Client With Celiac Disease

12. Which of the following statements by a mother would suggest to the nurse that her child has celiac disease?
    ○ 1. "His urine is so dark in color."
    ○ 2. "His stools are large and smelly."
    ○ 3. "His belly is so small."
    ○ 4. "He is so short."

13. During assessment of a child with celiac disease, the nurse would most likely note which of the following physical findings?
    ○ 1. Enlarged liver.
    ○ 2. Protuberant abdomen.
    ○ 3. Tender inguinal lymph nodes.
    ○ 4. Periorbital edema.

14. After teaching the mother of a child with celiac disease about dietary management, which of the following statements by the mother indicates successful teaching?
    ○ 1. "I will feed my child foods that contain wheat products."
    ○ 2. "I will be sure to give my child lots of milk."
    ○ 3. "I will plan to feed my child foods that contain rice."
    ○ 4. "I will be sure my child gets oatmeal every day."

15. Which of the following foods would be appropriate for a 12-month-old child with celiac disease?
    ○ 1. Cheerios.
    ○ 2. Pancakes.
    ○ 3. Rice Chex.
    ○ 4. Waffles.

16. The mother of a child with celiac disease asks, "How long must he stay on this diet?" Which of the following would be the nurse's *best* response?
    ○ 1. "Until the jejunal biopsy is normal."
    ○ 2. "When his stools appear normal."
    ○ 3. "For the next 6 months."
    ○ 4. "For the rest of his life."

The Client With Phenylketonuria

17. When preparing to obtain a neonatal screening test for phenylketonuria (PKU), the neonate must have received which of the following to ensure reliable results?
    ○ 1. A feeding of an iron-rich formula.
    ○ 2. Nothing by mouth for 4 hours before the test.
    ○ 3. Cow's or breast milk for 24 hours before the test.
    ○ 4. A loading dose of glucose water.

18. When developing the plan of care for a child diagnosed with PKU, which of the following would the nurse expect to include as an appropriate goal of care?
    ○ 1. Meeting the child's nutritional needs for optimal growth.
    ○ 2. Ensuring that the special diet is started at age 3 weeks.
    ○ 3. Maintaining serum phenylalanine level higher than 12 mg/100 mL.
    ○ 4. Maintaining serum phenylalanine level lower than 2 mg/100 mL.

19. When taking a diet history from the mother of a 7-year-old child with PKU, a report of an intake of which of the following would cause the nurse to become concerned?
    ○ 1. Cola.
    ○ 2. Carrots.
    ○ 3. Orange juice.
    ○ 4. Bananas.

20. When teaching the mother of a child diagnosed with PKU about its transmission, the nurse would use knowledge of which of the following as the basis for the discussion?
    ○ 1. Chromosome translocation.
    ○ 2. Chromosome deletion.
    ○ 3. Autosomal recessive gene.
    ○ 4. X-linked recessive gene.

21. A newborn diagnosed with PKU is placed on a milk substitute, Lofenalac. The mother asks the nurse how long her infant will be taking this. Which of the following responses would be *most* appropriate?
    ○ 1. "Until the infant is taking solid foods well."
    ○ 2. "Until the child has stopped growing."
    ○ 3. "When the phenylalanine level remains below normal for 6 months."
    ○ 4. "Probably for a long time, but its not definitely known."

22. Even though several teaching sessions have been documented in the client's health record, the mother asks the nurse again what caused her child's PKU. Which of the following statements would *best* reflect the nurse's interpretation of why the mother keeps asking for information that she has already received?
    ○ 1. Because the child's condition is chronic, parents often want very detailed explanations about the causes of and treatments for their child's disease.
    ○ 2. Parents of a chronically ill child often require a long time to work through the grieving process for their child's disease.
    ○ 3. The parents often test a health worker's knowledge about the causes of and treatments for their child's disease.
    ○ 4. Parents often deal with their guilt about possibly causing their child's disease by asking challenging questions.

The Client With Colic

23. When performing the nursing history, which of the following would be *most* important for the nurse to obtain from the mother of an infant with suspected colic?
    ○ 1. The type of formula the infant is taking.

○ 2. The infant's crying pattern.
○ 3. The infant's sleep position.
○ 4. The position of the infant during burping.

24. The parents of a child with colic are asked to describe the infant's bowel movements. Which of the following descriptions would the nurse expect?
    ○ 1. Soft, yellow stools.
    ○ 2. Frequent watery stools.
    ○ 3. Ribbon-like stools.
    ○ 4. Foul-smelling stools.

25. The mother tells the nurse that the diagnosis of colic upsets her because she knows her infant will continue to have colicky pain. Which of the following responses by the nurse would be *most* appropriate?
    ○ 1. "I know that your baby's crying upsets you, but she needs your undivided attention for the next few months."
    ○ 2. "It can be difficult to listen to your baby cry so loud and so long, so try to make sure that you get some free time."
    ○ 3. "It's must be distressing to see your baby in pain, but at least she doesn't have an intestinal obstruction."
    ○ 4. "The next 3 months will be a difficult time for you, but your daughter will outgrow the colic by this time."

26. The nurse judges that the mother has understood the teaching about care of an infant with colic when the nurse observes the mother doing which of the following?
    ○ 1. Holding the infant prone while feeding.
    ○ 2. Holding the infant in her lap to burp.
    ○ 3. Placing the infant prone after the feeding.
    ○ 4. Burping the infant during and after the feeding.

The Client With Obesity

27. Which of the following methods would the nurse use to provide the *most* accurate assessment of an adolescent's status in regard to obesity?
    ○ 1. A food intake diary for 1 week.
    ○ 2. Body mass index.
    ○ 3. A 4-hour dietary history.
    ○ 4. Skinfold thickness measurements.

28. When counseling an obese adolescent, the nurse would advise the client that which of the following is the *most* common complication?
    ○ 1. Lifelong obesity.
    ○ 2. Gastrointestinal problems.
    ○ 3. Orthopedic problems.
    ○ 4. Psychosocial problems.

29. When developing the teaching plan for the mother of an infant about introducing solid foods into the

diet, which of the following would the nurse expect to include in the plan as a measure to help prevent obesity?

- ○ 1. Decreasing the amount of formula or breast milk intake as solid food intake increases.
- ○ 2. Introducing the infant to the taste of vegetables by mixing then with formula or breast milk.
- ○ 3. Mixing cereal and fruit in a bottle when offering solid food for the first few times.
- ○ 4. Using a large-bowled spoon for feeding solid foods during the first several months.

30. A pregnant mother who has brought her toddler to the clinic for a check-up asks the nurse how she can keep her next baby from becoming fat. The mother plans to bottle-feed her next child. Which of the following would the nurse include in the teaching plan as a means to avoid overnourishing her infant?

- ○ 1. Recognizing clues indicating that a baby is full.
- ○ 2. Establishing a regular feeding schedule.
- ○ 3. Supplementing feedings with sterile water.
- ○ 4. Adding more water than directed when preparing formula.

The Client With Cow's Milk Sensitivity

31. A father tells the nurse that he has heard of cow's milk allergy but knows nothing about cow's milk sensitivity. The nurse would explain this condition as which of the following?

- ○ 1. Hereditary disorder of carbohydrate metabolism.
- ○ 2. Adverse reaction to cow's milk protein.
- ○ 3. Acquired lactose intolerance.
- ○ 4. Existence of a lifelong allergy.

32. After teaching the parents of a child with lactose intolerance about the disorder, the nurse determines that the teaching was effective when hearing the mother describe the condition to a visitor as which of the following?

- ○ 1. "The lack of an enzyme to break down lactose."
- ○ 2. "An allergy to lactose found in milk."
- ○ 3. "Inability to digest proteins completely."
- ○ 4. "Inability to digest fats completely."

33. After teaching the mother of a 2-year-old child with lactose intolerance about which dairy products to include in the child's diet, which of the following if stated by the mother indicates effective teaching?

- ○ 1. Ice cream.
- ○ 2. Creamed soups.
- ○ 3. Pudding.
- ○ 4. Cheese.

34. The mother of a 1-month-old diagnosed with cow's milk sensitivity who is breast-feeding her infant asks the nurse what she should do about feeding her infant. Which of the following recommendations would be *most* appropriate?

- ○ 1. Continue to breast-feed but eliminate all milk products from your own diet.
- ○ 2. Discontinue breast-feeding and start using a predigested formula.
- ○ 3. Limit breast-feeding to once per day and begin feeding an iron-fortified formula.
- ○ 4. Change to a soy-based formula exclusively and begin solid foods.

Correct Answers and Rationale

The letters in parentheses following the rationale identify the step of the nursing process (A, D, P, I, E) and client needs (1, 2, 3, 4, 5, 6, 7, 8, 9, 10). See the inside front cover for the key.

The Client With Ingestion of Toxic Substances

1. 1. Syrup of ipecac is an emetic that exerts its action by stimulating the vomiting center directly and producing irritating effects on the stomach mucosa. It is given with one to two glasses of water or fruit juice. If the child does not vomit within 20 minutes after taking syrup of ipecac, a second dose may be administered. Diuretics such as furosemide (Lasix) would promote diuresis. Drugs such as phenobarbital, diazepam (Valium), or phenytoin (Dilantin) are used to control seizures. Drugs such as epinephrine may be used to stimulate the heart. (I, 8)

2. 2. Drain cleaner almost always contains lye, which can burn the mouth, pharynx, and esophagus on ingestion. The nurse would be prepared to assist with a tracheostomy, which may be necessary because of swelling around the area of the larynx. An emetic is contraindicated because, as the substance burns on ingestion, so too would it burn when vomiting. Additionally, the mucosa becomes necrotic and vomiting could lead to perforations. Gastric lavage is contraindicated because the mucosa is burned from the ingestion of the caustic lye, causing necrosis. Gastric lavage also could lead to perforation of the necrotic mucosa. Insertion of an indwelling urinary (Foley) catheter would be indicated after the measures to remove the caustic substance have been started. (P, 9)

3. 3. As the burn from the lye ingestion heals, scar tissue develops and can lead to esophageal strictures, a common complication of lye ingestion. Tracheal stenosis would occur if the child had vomited and aspirated. Tracheal varices do not commonly occur after the ingestion of lye or other substances. Although very rare, esophageal diverticula may occur. Diverticula are commonly found in the colon of adults. (A, 10)

4. 3. After ingesting a large amount of acetaminophen, the child would complain of right upper quadrant pain due to hepatic damage from glutathione combining with the metabolite of acetaminophen being broken down. Hypertension is not associated with acetaminophen ingestion. Frequent urination occurs as a result of intravenous fluid administration, not acetaminophen ingestion. Headache is not an expected finding with acetaminophen overdose. (A, 10)

5. 2. Initial management of a child who has ingested a large amount of acetaminophen would include inducing vomiting or performing gastric lavage with or without activated charcoal to aid in the removal of the substance. Frequent blood level determinations may be obtained during the follow-up phase, but they are not done as part of the initial treatment. Tracheostomy is not typically part of the initial treatment for acetaminophen overdose. However, it may be necessary later if respiratory distress develops. Acetaminophen primarily affects the liver, not the heart. Therefore, an electrocardiogram would not be considered part of the initial treatment plan. (P, 9)

6. 4. Chemical pneumonitis is the most common complication of ingestion of hydrocarbons, such as in kerosene. The pneumonitis is caused by irritation from the hydrocarbons aspirated into the lungs. Uremia is the result of renal insufficiency, which causes nitrogenous wastes products to build up in the blood rather than being excreted. Hepatitis is caused by a viral infection. Carditis in a preschooler may be the result of rheumatic fever. (A, 10)

The Client With Lead Poisoning

7. 1. Eating with dirty hands, especially after playing outside, can lead to lead poisoning because lead is often present in soil surrounding homes. Also, children who eat lead-containing paint chips commonly develop lead poisoning. Drinking 2 cups of milk per day is less than that which is recommended for this age group, so more nutritional information would need to be obtained. Temper tantrums are characteristic of 18-month-old children as they try to assert themselves. Determining whether the child is smaller than other children the same age requires measuring height and weight and plotting them on growth charts. In addition, inadequate growth could be a result of numerous causes, such as genetics, chronic illness, or chronic drug use (eg, prednisone). (A, 10)

8. 3. The child is considered to be at moderate risk, because the increased blood level concentration has persisted. When blood levels reach 15 to 19 μg/dL, an investigation of the child's environment will be initiated. Oral chelation therapy is started when blood lead levels reach 45 μg/dL. When they reach 70 μg/dL, the child usually is hospitalized for intravenous chelation therapy. (P, 9)

9. 3. The most serious and irreversible consequence of lead poisoning is mental retardation due to neurologic changes. It can be expected if lead poisoning is long-standing and goes untreated. Lead poisoning also affects the hematologic and renal systems. Cirrhosis is the end stage of several chronic liver diseases, such as biliary atresia and hepatitis. Lead poisoning is not associated with stunted growth. Chronic illnesses, such as cystic fibrosis, cause slowing of the growth velocity. Heart failure is associated with congenital heart disease and rheumatic fever. (I, 10)

10. 2. Public education about the sources of lead that could cause poisoning has been found to be the most effective measure to prevent lead poisoning. This includes recent efforts to alert the public to lead in certain types of window blinds. Condemning old housing developments has been ineffective because lead paint still exists in many other dwellings. Providing education about good nutrition, although important, is not an effective preventive measure. Pregnant women and children should not remain in an older home that is being remodeled because they may breathe in lead in the dust, but this is not the most effective preventive measure. (I, 2)

11. 4. Most of the pathologic effects of lead poisoning are reversible as long as the problem is diagnosed early. The most serious effects are those on the central nervous system (eg, brain damage, mental retardation, behavior changes), not problems with the law. However, because of screening programs, many children with lead poisoning are diagnosed and treated early. As a result, little if any brain damage occurs that would require children to receive special schooling. (I, 10)

The Client With Celiac Disease

12. 2. Celiac disease is a disorder involving intolerance to the protein gluten, which is found in wheat, rye, oats, and barley. The stools of a child with celiac disease are characteristically malodorous, pale, large (bulky), and soft (loose). Excessive flatus is common, and bouts of diarrhea may occur. Dark urine is commonly associated with concentrated urine, such as when a child has dehydration. The belly of a child with celiac disease, a malabsorption disorder, typically is protuberant. A small belly may be associated with a child who is thin. Short stature is not associated with this malabsorption disorder. (D, 10)

13. 2. The intestines of a child with celiac disease fill with accumulated undigested food and flatus, causing the characteristic protuberant abdomen. Celiac disease is not usually associated with any liver dysfunction, including poor liver functioning leading to liver enlarge-

ment. Tender inguinal lymph nodes are often associated with an infection. Periorbital edema, swelling around the eyes, is associated with nephritis. (A, 10)

14. 3. Damage to intestinal mucosa in celiac disease is caused by gliadin, a part of the protein found in wheat, rye, barley, and oats. Foods containing these grains must be eliminated entirely from the diet of children with celiac disease. Foods containing rice and corn are a good substitute. Although an adequate intake of milk is important for any child, children with celiac disease do not need an increased milk intake. (E, 10)

15. 3. The child with celiac disease should not eat foods containing wheat, oats, rye, or barley. Foods containing rice, such as Rice Chex cereal, or corn are appropriate. Because Cheerios are made from oats, this cereal should be avoided. Pancakes and waffles are made from flour that typically is derived from wheat and therefore should be avoided. (I, 10)

16. 4. Most children with celiac disease have a lifelong sensitivity to gluten, which requires that they maintain some type of diet restriction for the rest of their lives. (I, 10)

The Client With Phenylketonuria

17. 3. PKU is an autosomal recessive genetic disorder involving the absence of an enzyme needed to metabolize the essential amino acid, phenylalanine, to tyrosine. To ensure reliable results, the neonate must have ingested a diet high in phenylalanine, such as cow's or breast milk, for at least 24 hours. Testing of the neonate before that time, excessive vomiting, or poor intake can yield false-negative results. The infant does not need to be in a fasting state for 4 hours before the test. A loading dose of glucose water is not necessary. (P, 9)

18. 1. The goal of care is to prevent mental retardation by adjusting the diet to meet the infant's nutritional needs for optimal growth. The diet needs to be started as soon as the infant is diagnosed, ideally within a few days of birth. Serum phenylalanine level should be maintained between 3 and 7 mg/100 mL. Significant brain damage usually occurs if the serum phenylalanine level exceeds 10 to 15 mg/100 mL. If the level drops below 2 mg/100 mL, the body begins to catabolize its protein stores, causing growth retardation. (P, 10)

19. 1. Foods with low phenylalanine levels include vegetables, fruits, and juices. Foods high in phenylalanine include meats and dairy products, which must be restricted or eliminated. Colas are higher in phenylalanine than the fruits listed. (A, 10)

20. 3. PKU is caused by an inborn error of metabolism. It is an autosomal recessive disorder that inhibits the conversion of phenylalanine to tyrosine. A form of Down syndrome, trisomy 21, is an example of a disorder caused by chromosomal translocation. Cri-du-chat is an example of a disorder caused by chromosomal deletion. Hemophilia A is an example of a disorder caused by an X-linked recessive gene. (I, 20)

21. 4. Although it is not known how long diet therapy must continue for children with PKU, many experts suggest continuing it indefinitely because of academic difficulties and lower intelligence quotients in older children who have stopped the restrictive diet. For women it is necessary to resume the diet before conception to lower the phenylalanine levels in the fetus and prevent complications. (I, 10)

22. 2. PKU is considered a chronic illness. Parents typically grieve about the loss of health in their child afflicted with a chronic disease. Many times, they repeat questions, as though trying to deny what is really happening. This type of behavior represents an attempt to integrate the experience and their feelings with their self-image as they pass through the grieving process. Asking for detailed explanations, testing the competence of health workers, and expressing impatience with health workers may explain the parents' behavior, but viewing the behavior as a part of the grieving process is the most plausible explanation. (D, 10)

The Client With Colic

23. 2. Information on the crying pattern of the infant is most helpful in confirming the diagnosis of colic. Typically the colic attack begins abruptly, with the infant crying loudly and continuously, possibly for hours. The attack may end when the child becomes exhausted. The child also may attain some relief after passing stool or flatus. Often, in an attempt to alleviate the infant's crying, parents try to feed the infant, resulting in over-feeding leading to discomfort and distention. (A, 10)

24. 1. Infants with colic usually pass normal stools, typically soft and yellowish. Frequent watery stools might indicate diarrhea. Ribbon-like stools are suggestive of a narrowing of the colon or rectum. Foul-smelling stools by themselves are related to diet. With other symptoms such as large size and protuberant abdomen are present, malabsorption may be possible. (A, 10)

25. 2. The nurse needs to provide the parents with support because of the infant's crying. The parents are stressed and need to be encouraged to get out of the house and arrange for some free time. Although infants need lots of attention and care for the first few months, they do not need the mother's undivided attention. Comparing colic with other problems is inappropriate. Parents have the right to be upset. Although colic usually disappears spontaneously by age 3 months, the nurse should not make any guarantees. (I, 5)

26. 4. Infants with colic should be burped frequently during and after the feeding. Much of the discomfort of colic appears to be associated with the presence of air in the stomach and intestines. Frequent burping helps to relieve the air. Infants with colic should be held fairly upright while being fed, to help air rise. The preferred position for burping the infant with colic is to hold the infant at the mother's shoulder so that the infant's abdomen lies on the shoulder. This position causes more pressure to be exerted on the infant's abdomen, leading to a more forceful burp. The child should be placed in an infant seat after feedings. (E, 10)

The Client With Obesity

27. 2. The most accurate way to determine whether an adolescent has a problem with obesity is to calculate the body mass index (BMI). The BMI indicates a relationship between height and weight. Numbers obtained through calculation are then applied to a BMI table for interpretation. Measuring skinfold thickness with skinfold calipers is a common method used to assess obesity. The skinfold thickness test, which determines the amount of subcutaneous fat, determines obesity more accurately than does a height and weight chart. However, it is not the most accurate method and is not routinely performed by nurses. (A, 4)

28. 1. The most common complication of adolescent obesity is its persistence into adulthood. However, the incidence of Legg-Calvé-Perthes disease and of genu valgum (knock knees) is greater for obese adolescents. Although psychosocial problems do occur, they are not the most common complication. (I, 9)

29. 1. Decreasing the amount of formula given as the infant begins to take solids helps prevent excess caloric intake. Because the infant is receiving calories from the solid foods, the formula no longer needs to provide the infant's total caloric requirements. Mixing vegetables with formula or breast milk does not allow the child to become accustomed to new textures or tastes. Solid foods should be given with a spoon, not in a bottle. Using a bottle with food allows the infant to ingest more food than is needed. Also, the infant needs to learn to eat from a spoon. A small-bowled spoon is recommended for infants because infants have a tendency to push food out with the tongue. The small bowled spoon helps in placing the food at the back of the infant's tongue when feeding. (P, 7)

30. 1. Infants generally do not overeat unless they are urged to do so. Parents should watch for clues indicating that the infant is full; for example, stopping sucking and pushing the nipple out of the mouth. Bottle-feeding instead of breast-feeding is more likely to lead to excessive caloric intake. A demand schedule, rather

than a regulated schedule, allows the infant to regulate intake according to individual needs. Normally, giving an infant a regular supplementation of water is unnecessary; the infant's sucking needs can be met by providing a pacifier. Adding more water to the formula than as directed decreases the caloric intake and also places the infant at risk for hyponatremia due to decreased sodium and increased water intake. (P, 7)

The Client With Cow's Milk Sensitivity

31. 2. Cow's milk sensitivity is an adverse local and systemic gastrointestinal reaction to cow's milk protein. This is the most common nutritional allergy in infants. Almost all sensitive children can tolerate cow's milk by 2 years of age. Lactose intolerance involves a deficiency of the enzyme lactase, which is needed for digestion of lactose. (I, 7)

32. 1. Lactose intolerance is not an allergy. Rather, it is caused by the lack of the digestive enzyme lactase. This enzyme, found in the intestines, is necessary for the digestion of lactose, the primary carbohydrate in cow's milk. Protein and fat digestion are not affected. (E, 10)

33. 4. People who are lactose-intolerant usually are able to tolerate dairy products in which lactose has been fermented, such as yogurt, cheese, and buttermilk. Pudding, ice cream, and creamed soups contain lactose that has not been fermented. (E, 10)

34. 1. Mothers of infants with a cow's milk allergy can continue to breast-feed if they eliminate cow's milk from their diet. It is important to encourage mothers to continue to breast-feed because breast milk is usually the least allergenic and most easily digested food for an infant. In addition, the infant is able to obtain protein through the mother's milk. If the mother stops breast-feeding, then a predigested protein hydrolysate formula would be the first choice. An iron-fortified formula is a cow's milk-based formula. A soy-based formula is not used because approximately 20% of infants with cow's milk sensitivity are also sensitive to soy. Solid foods are not introduced until the infant is 4 to 6 months of age. (I, 7)

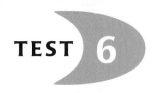

TEST 6

The Child With Health Problems of the Urinary System

Select the one best answer, and indicate your choice by filling in the circle in front of the option.

The Client With Cryptorchidism

1. A father brings his 4-week-old son to the clinic for a checkup, stating that he is afraid that his son's testicle is missing. Which of the following explanations would be *most* appropriate?
   - ○ 1. "Although the testes should have descended by now, it is not a cause for worry."
   - ○ 2. "The testes often do not descend until age 6 months, but let's check to see whether the testes are present."
   - ○ 3. "The testes are present in the scrotal sac at birth, but surgery can remedy the situation."
   - ○ 4. "Although the testes normally descend by 6 weeks of age, I can understand your concern."

2. While preparing to examine a 6-week old infant's scrotal sac and testes for possible undescended testes, which of the following would be *most* important for the nurse to do?
   - ○ 1. Check the diaper for recent urination.
   - ○ 2. Give the infant a pacifier.
   - ○ 3. Ensure that the room is kept warm.
   - ○ 4. Tap lightly on the left inguinal ring.

3. While the nurse is examining the infant for presence of testes, the father paces around the room shaking his head. Which of the following would be the most appropriate response by the nurse?
   - ○ 1. "I'm sure everything will work out for the best, and he'll be fine."
   - ○ 2. "You seem upset; please tell me how you're feeling."

   - ○ 3. "Don't worry; his testes will probably descend on their own."
   - ○ 4. "Would you like to talk with a parent of a child who has the same problem?"

4. When assessing an infant with an undescended testis, the nurse also would be alert for which of the following?
   - ○ 1. Abnormal lower extremity reflexes.
   - ○ 2. A history of frequent emesis.
   - ○ 3. A bulging in the inguinal area.
   - ○ 4. Poor weight gain.

5. When developing the plan of care for an infant with undescended testis, the nurse would expect to include which of the following as a nonsurgical treatment method?
   - ○ 1. A trial of human chorionic gonadotrophic hormone.
   - ○ 2. A trial of adrenocorticotropic hormone.
   - ○ 3. Frequent stimulation of the cremasteric reflex.
   - ○ 4. Use of several warm baths each day.

6. When developing the preoperative teaching plan for a 14-month-old with undescended testis who is scheduled to have surgery, which of the following methods would the nurse anticipate using?
   - ○ 1. Telling the child that his penis and scrotum will be "fixed."
   - ○ 2. Explaining to the parents how the defect will be corrected.
   - ○ 3. Telling the child that he will not see any incisions after surgery.
   - ○ 4. Using an anatomically correct doll to show the child what will be "fixed."

7. An adolescent with a history of surgical repair for undescended testis comes to the clinic for a sports physical. Anticipatory guidance for the parents and adolescent would focus on which of the following as *most* important?
   ○ 1. The adolescent's sterility.
   ○ 2. The adolescent's future plans.
   ○ 3. Technique for monthly testicular self-examinations.
   ○ 4. Need for a lot of psychological support.

The Client With Hydrocele

8. When explaining to the parents of a child with a hydrocele about the possible cause of the condition, the nurse bases this explanation on the interpretation that a hydrocele is most likely the result of which of the following?
   ○ 1. Blockage in the inguinal canal that allows fluid to accumulate in epididymis and ductus deferens.
   ○ 2. Failure of the upper part of the processus vaginalis to atrophy, allowing accumulation of fluid in the testicle and the peritoneal cavity.
   ○ 3. A patent processus vaginalis that results in the collection of fluid along the spermatic cord or tunica vaginalis of the testicle.
   ○ 4. An obliterated processus vaginalis that allows fluid to accumulate in the scrotal sac.

9. During a clinic visit, the mother of an infant with hydrocele states that the infant's scrotum is smaller now than when he was born. After teaching the mother about the infant's condition, which of the following statements by the mother indicates that the teaching had been effective?
   ○ 1. "I guess keeping his bottom up has helped."
   ○ 2. "Massaging his groin area is working."
   ○ 3. "It seems like the fluid is being reabsorbed over time."
   ○ 4. "Keeping him quiet and in an infant seat has really helped."

10. Shortly after an infant is returned to his room following hydrocele repair, the infant's mother tells the nurse that the child's scrotum looks swollen and bruised. Which of the following responses by the nurse would be *most* appropriate?
    ○ 1. "Let me see if the doctor has ordered aspirin for him. If he did, I'll get it right away."
    ○ 2. "Why don't you wait in his room. Then you can ask me any questions when I get there?"
    ○ 3. "What you are describing is unusual after this type of surgery. I'll let the doctor know."
    ○ 4. "This is normal after this type of surgery. Let's look at it together just to be sure."

The Client With Hypospadias

11. The parents of a neonate with hypospadias and chordee wish to have him circumcised. Which of the following rationales would the nurse incorporate into the discussion with the parents concerning the recommendation to delay circumcision?
    ○ 1. The associated chordee is difficult to remove during circumcision.
    ○ 2. The foreskin is used to repair the deformity surgically.
    ○ 3. The meatus can become stenosed, leading to urinary obstruction.
    ○ 4. The infant is too small to have a circumcision.

12. A 1-year-old child is scheduled for surgery to correct hypospadias and chordee. The nurse explains to the parents that this is the preferred time for surgical repair based on which of the following?
    ○ 1. At this age, the child will experience less pain.
    ○ 2. The child is too young to have developed castration anxiety.
    ○ 3. The child will not remember the surgical experience.
    ○ 4. The repair is easier to perform before the child is toilet trained.

13. After a surgical repair of a hypospadias, a 12-month-old child returns to the nursing unit with an intravenous line, a urethral catheter, and a suprapubic catheter in place. Which of the following would the nurse explain to the parents is the primary purpose for the suprapubic catheter?
    ○ 1. To ensure an accurate measurement of urine output.
    ○ 2. To provide an alternative urinary elimination route.
    ○ 3. To provide an entry port for bladder irrigation.
    ○ 4. To allow assessment for blood clots in the urine.

14. After teaching the parents about the urethral catheter placed after surgical repair of their son's hypospadias, the nurse determines that the teaching was successful when the mother states that the catheter in her child's penis accomplishes which of the following?
    ○ 1. Decreases pain at the surgical site.
    ○ 2. Keeps the new urethra from closing.
    ○ 3. Measures his urine correctly.
    ○ 4. Prevents bladder spasms.

15. While preparing the parents of a child undergoing the first of two surgeries for repair of a hypospadias, the nurse describes the appearance of the surgical site, including swelling of the penis. The nurse also would describe the penis as having which of the following appearances?
    ○ 1. Bright red in color.
    ○ 2. Dusky blue at the tip.

○ 3. Somewhat misshapen.

○ 4. Pale pink.

16. When developing the teaching plan for the parents of a 12-month-old infant with hypospadias and chordee repair, which of the following would the nurse expect to include as *most* important?
    ○ 1. Assisting the child to become familiar with his dressings so he will leave them alone.
    ○ 2. Encouraging the child to ambulate as soon as possible by using a favorite push toy.
    ○ 3. Forcing fluids to at least 2500 mL/day by offering his favorite juices.
    ○ 4. Preventing the child from disrupting the catheters by using soft restraints.

17. The physician orders a urinalysis for a child who has undergone surgical repair of a hypospadias. Which of the following results would the nurse report to the physician?
    ○ 1. Urine specific gravity of 1.017.
    ○ 2. Ten red blood cells per high-powered field.
    ○ 3. Twenty-five white blood cells per high-powered field.
    ○ 4. Urine pH of 6.0.

The Client With Urinary Tract Infection

18. A recent history of which of the following would alert the nurse to suspect a urinary tract infection in a 2-year-old child who is exhibiting fever and fussiness?
    ○ 1. Abdominal pain.
    ○ 2. Swollen lymph glands.
    ○ 3. Skin rash.
    ○ 4. Back pain.

19. A father of a child with a urinary tract infection calls the clinic and explains, "My wife and I are concerned because our child refuses to obey us concerning the preventions you told us about. Our child refuses to take the medication unless we buy a present. We don't want to use discipline because of the illness, but we're worried about the behavior." Which of the following would be the nurse's *best* response?
    ○ 1. "I sympathize with your difficulties, but just ignore the behavior for now."
    ○ 2. "I understand it's hard to discipline a child who is ill, but things need to be kept as normal as possible."
    ○ 3. "I understand that things are difficult for you right now, but your child is ill and deserves special treatment."
    ○ 4. "I understand your concern, but this type of behavior happens all the time; your child will get over it when feeling better."

20. When teaching the parents of a child diagnosed with a urinary tract infection secondary to vesicoureteral reflux, which of the following would the nurse incorporate into the explanation about how the reflux contributes to the infection?
    ○ 1. It prevents complete emptying of the bladder.
    ○ 2. It causes urine backflow into the kidney.
    ○ 3. It results in painful bladder spasms.
    ○ 4. It causes painful urination.

The Client With Glomerulonephritis

21. Which of the following questions would the nurse ask *first* when obtaining a history from the mother of a 10-year-old with a fever, complaints of not feeling well, and swelling around the eyes?
    ○ 1. "Has the child had a sore throat recently?"
    ○ 2. "Is the child playing with friends as usual?"
    ○ 3. "Does the child urinate as much as usual?"
    ○ 4. "Is the urine pale in color?"

22. A school-aged client admitted to the hospital because of decreased urine output and periorbital edema is diagnosed with glomerulonephritis. Which of the following interventions would receive the *highest* priority?
    ○ 1. Assessing vital signs every 4 hours.
    ○ 2. Monitoring intake and output every 12 hours.
    ○ 3. Obtaining daily weight measurements.
    ○ 4. Obtaining serum electrolyte levels daily.

23. When developing the plan of care for a school-aged child with glomerulonephritis who has a fluid restriction of 1000 mL/day, which of the following fluids would the nurse consider as *most* appropriate for the client's condition and effective for preventing excessive thirst?
    ○ 1. Diet cola.
    ○ 2. Ice chips.
    ○ 3. Lemonade.
    ○ 4. Tap water.

24. During hospitalization, a 10-year-old with glomerulonephritis and oliguria asks for food from home. After teaching the mother and child about diet, the nurse determines that the teaching had been effective when the mother brings in which of the following?
    ○ 1. Pizza and cola.
    ○ 2. Hamburger and fries.
    ○ 3. Ice cream sundae.
    ○ 4. Strawberries and kiwi.

25. The nurse is planning interventions for the nursing diagnosis Deficient Diversional Activity for a school-aged child. Which of the following activities would the nurse expect to include?
    ○ 1. Playing a card game with someone the same age.

○ 2. Putting together a puzzle with mother.

○ 3. Playing video games with a 4-year-old.

○ 4. Watching a movie with a younger brother.

26. A 10-year old child hospitalized with glomerulone-phritis during the acute stage has elevated blood pressure and low urine output for 14 hours. Which of the following would the nurse do *next*?

○ 1. Assess the child's neurologic status.

○ 2. Encourage the child to drink more water.

○ 3. Advise the child to eat a low-sodium breakfast.

○ 4. Help the client to ambulate in the hallway.

27. When developing the discharge plan for a school-aged child diagnosed with glomerulonephritis, which of the following would the nurse expect to discuss?

○ 1. Restricting dietary protein.

○ 2. Monitoring pulse rate and rhythm.

○ 3. Preventing respiratory infections.

○ 4. Restricting foods high in potassium.

28. An older adolescent with a history of losing weight and feeling tired and irritable has been admitted to the hospital with a diagnosis of chronic glomeru-lonephritis. Which of the following laboratory results would the nurse most likely see?

○ 1. Serum sodium of 133 mEq/L.

○ 2. Blood urea nitrogen (BUN) of 7 mg/dL.

○ 3. Serum potassium of 3.8 mEq/L.

○ 4. Blood pH of 7.43.

The Client With Nephrotic Syndrome

29. The urinalysis of a toddler diagnosed with neph-rotic syndrome reveals +4 for protein. The nurse interprets this result as indicating which of the fol-lowing?

○ 1. Decreased secretion of aldosterone.

○ 2. Increased glomerular permeability to albumin.

○ 3. Inhibited tubular reabsorption of sodium and water.

○ 4. Loss of red blood cells in the urine.

30. Which of the following statements by the mother of a toddler diagnosed with nephrotic syndrome indi-cates that the mother has understood the nurse's teaching about this disease?

○ 1. "My child really likes chips and bologna. I guess we'll have to find something else."

○ 2. "We'll have to encourage lots of liquids. Did you say about 4 liters every day?"

○ 3. "We worry about the surgery. Do you think we should do direct donation of blood?"

○ 4. "We understand the need for antibiotics. I just wish the antibiotics could be given by mouth."

31. A toddler diagnosed with nephrotic syndrome has a nursing diagnosis of Excess Fluid Volume related to

fluid accumulation in the tissues. Which of the fol-lowing would the nurse anticipate including in the child's plan of care?

○ 1. Limiting visitors to 2 to 3 hours a day.

○ 2. Maintaining strict bed rest.

○ 3. Testing urine specific gravity every shift.

○ 4. Weighing the child before breakfast.

32. The mother of a toddler with nephrotic syndrome asks the nurse what can be done about the child's swollen eyes. Which of the following would the nurse suggest?

○ 1. Applying cool compresses to the child's eyes.

○ 2. Elevating the head of the child's bed.

○ 3. Applying eye drops every 8 hours.

○ 4. Limiting the child's television watching.

33. The nurse determines that interventions for decreas-ing fluid retention have been effective when the child with nephrotic syndrome demonstrates evi-dence of which of the following?

○ 1. Decreased abdominal girth.

○ 2. Increased caloric intake.

○ 3. Increased respiratory rate.

○ 4. Decreased heart rate.

34. The toddler with nephrotic syndrome exhibits gen-eralized edema. Which of the following measures would the nurse institute for this child with a nurs-ing diagnosis of Impaired Skin Integrity related to edema?

○ 1. Ambulate every shift while awake.

○ 2. Apply lotion on opposing skin surfaces.

○ 3. Apply powder to skinfolds.

○ 4. Separate opposing skin surfaces with soft cloth.

35. The toddler with nephrotic syndrome responds to treatment and is ready to go home. When helping the family plan for home care, which of the following instructions would the nurse include in the teaching?

○ 1. Administer pain medication as needed.

○ 2. Keep the child away from others with an infec-tion.

○ 3. Notify the physician if there is an increase in the child's urine output.

○ 4. Administer acetaminophen (Tylenol) daily.

The Client With Acute or Chronic Renal Failure

36. When explaining the advantages of peritoneal dial-ysis versus hemodialysis to an adolescent with chronic renal failure, the nurse states that continu-ous peritoneal dialysis involves which of the fol-lowing?

○ 1. Fewer dietary restrictions.

○ 2. Less chance of infection.

○ 3. More protein loss.

○ 4. More rapid fluid removal.

37. While performing daily peritoneal dialysis and catheter exit site care with the mother of a child with chronic renal failure, which of the following would be an important step to stress to the mother?
    ○ 1. Applying an occlusive dressing after cleansing the site.
    ○ 2. Changing the dressing when the peritoneal space is dry.
    ○ 3. Examining the site for signs of infection while cleansing the area.
    ○ 4. Pulling on the catheter to hold taut while cleansing the skin.

38. When developing the discharge teaching plan for a child with chronic renal failure and the family, the nurse would emphasize restriction of which of the following nutrients?
    ○ 1. Ascorbic acid.
    ○ 2. Calcium.
    ○ 3. Magnesium.
    ○ 4. Phosphorus.

39. After emphasizing to an adolescent with renal failure the importance of maintaining a positive self-concept, which of the following behaviors by the adolescent would the nurse identify as an indicator that the plan is working?
    ○ 1. Complaints about headaches, abdominal pain, and nausea.
    ○ 2. Insistence on making diet choices even if the foods chosen are restricted.
    ○ 3. Verbalization of plans to quit all after-school activities when returning home.
    ○ 3. Demonstration of desire to do the dressing changes and take care of the medications.

40. Which of the following diet plans would be appropriate for the nurse to discuss with the family of a child with acute renal failure?
    ○ 1. High carbohydrate and protein.
    ○ 2. High fat and carbohydrate.
    ○ 3. Low fat and protein.
    ○ 4. Low in carbohydrate and fat.

41. An adolescent with chronic renal failure is scheduled to go home with a peritoneal dialysis catheter in place. When developing the discharge teaching plan for the client and family focusing on psychosocial needs, which of the following areas would be a top priority to include?
    ○ 1. Advantages of limiting social activities and contacts for the first few months.
    ○ 2. Not disclosing information about the peritoneal dialysis to people outside the family.
    ○ 3. Possible effect on body image of the presence of an abdominal catheter.
    ○ 4. Importance of relying on parents to do the dialysis and dressing changes.

42. During a home visit, the public health nurse assesses the peritoneal catheter exit site of a child with chronic renal failure. Which of the following findings would lead the nurse to formulate the nursing diagnosis Risk for Infection?
    ○ 1. Dialysate leakage.
    ○ 2. Granulation tissue.
    ○ 3. Increased time for drainage.
    ○ 4. Tissue swelling.

43. After teaching the mother of a young child with a peritoneal catheter about the signs and symptoms of peritonitis, the nurse determines that the mother has understood the teaching when she identifies which of the following as an important sign?
    ○ 1. Cloudy dialysate drainage return.
    ○ 2. Distended abdomen.
    ○ 3. Shortness of breath.
    ○ 4. Weight gain of 3 pounds in 2 days.

44. The nurse assesses the child with chronic renal failure who is receiving peritoneal dialysis for edema. Which of the following would the nurse expect to find?
    ○ 1. Absence of pulmonary crackles.
    ○ 2. Increased dialysate outflow.
    ○ 3. Normal blood pressure.
    ○ 4. Pallor.

45. The mother of a child with chronic renal failure who is receiving peritoneal dialysis at home asks the public health nurse what she can do if both inflow and drain times are increased. Which of the following instructions would be *most* appropriate for the nurse to include when responding to the mother?
    ○ 1. Assess the child for constipation.
    ○ 2. Decrease the amount of dialysate infused for each dwell.
    ○ 3. Incorporate the increased inflow and drain times into the dialysis schedule.
    ○ 4. Monitor the child for shoulder pain during inflow and drain times.

46. The nurse judges that the mother understands the diet restrictions for her child with chronic renal failure who is receiving peritoneal dialysis when she reports providing a diet involving which of the following?
    ○ 1. Sodium and water restrictions.
    ○ 2. High protein and carbohydrates.
    ○ 3. High potassium and iron.
    ○ 4. Protein and phosphorus restrictions.

The Client With Wilms' Tumor

47. When assessing a child admitted to the pediatric unit with the diagnosis of Wilms' tumor, which of the following findings would the nurse expect?
    ○ 1. Hypotension.
    ○ 2. Proteinemia.

○ 3. Pallor.

○ 4. Petechiae.

48. When assessing a 2-year-old child with Wilms' tumor, the nurse should keep in mind that it is *most* important to avoid which of the following?

○ 1. Measuring the child's chest circumference.

○ 2. Palpating the child's abdomen.

○ 3. Placing the child in an upright position.

○ 4. Measuring the child's occipitofrontal circumference.

49. The nurse determines that the mother of a child with Wilms' tumor understands what *stage II tumor* means when she states which of the following?

○ 1. "The tumor has extended beyond the kidney but was completely removed."

○ 2. "Although the tumor was in the kidney, it has spread to the lung, liver, and bone."

○ 3. "The tumor has extended outside the kidney to the lungs and the liver."

○ 4. "The tumor was solely located in the kidney but it was totally removed."

50. A child diagnosed with Wilms' tumor undergoes successful surgery for removal of the diseased kidney. On return to the room, the nurse would place the child in which of the following positions?

○ 1. Modified Trendelenburg.

○ 2. Sims'.

○ 3. Semi-Fowler's.

○ 4. Supine.

51. After a nephrectomy for a Wilms' tumor, the nurse continues to assess the child postoperatively for which of the following as an early sign of a complication?

○ 1. Increased abdominal distention.

○ 2. Elevated blood pressure.

○ 3. Increased respiratory rate.

○ 4. Increased urine output.

52. When developing the discharge plan for a child who had a nephrectomy for a Wilms' tumor, the nurse identifies outcomes to prevent damage to the child's remaining kidney and accomplish which of the following?

○ 1. Minimize pain.

○ 2. Prevent dependent edema.

○ 3. Prevent urinary tract infection.

○ 4. Minimize sodium intake.

Correct Answers and Rationale

The letters in parentheses following the rationale identify the step of the nursing process (A, D, P, I, E) and client needs (1, 2, 3, 4, 5, 6, 7, 8, 9, 10). See the inside front cover for the key.

The Client With Cryptorchidism

1. 4. Normally the testes descend by age 6 weeks; failure to do so may indicate a problem with patency or a hormonal imbalance. By age 4 weeks, descent may not have occurred. However, telling the father that lack of descent is not a cause for worry is inappropriate and uncaring. Additionally, a statement such as this may be false reassurance. By acknowledging the father's concern, the nurse indicates acceptance of his feelings. If the testes have not descended, then they will not be palpable in the scrotal sac. Surgery is not discussed until after a full assessment is completed. (I, 3)

2. 3. A cold environment can cause the testes to retract. Cold and touch stimulate the cremasteric reflex, which causes a normal retraction of the testes toward the body. Therefore, the nurse should warm the hands and make sure that the environment also is warm. Checking the diaper for urination provides information about the infant's voiding and urinary function, not information about the testes. Giving the infant a pacifier may help to calm the infant and possibly make the examination easier, but the concern here is with the temperature of the environment. Tapping on the inguinal ring would not be helpful in assessing the infant. (A, 4)

3. 2. The nurse needs more information about the father's perceptions and feelings before providing any information or taking action. Determining the exact nature of the father's concern rather than making an assumption about it is essential. Therefore, the nurse should identify what is observed and ask the father how he is feeling. Telling the father that everything will be fine or not to worry is inappropriate and provides false reassurance. It also devalues the father's concern. Later on it may be appropriate for the father to talk to a parent of a child with the same problem for support. (I, 5)

4. 3. When an anomaly is found in one system, such as the genitourinary system, that system requires a more focused assessment to reveal other conditions that also may be occurring. A bulging in the inguinal area may suggest an inguinal hernia. Also, hydrocele or an upper urinary tract anomaly may occur on the same side as the undescended testis. A neuromuscular problem, not a genitourinary problem such as undescended testes, would most likely be the cause of abnormal lower extremity reflexes. A history of frequent emesis may be caused by pyloric stenosis or viral gastroenteritis. Poor weight gain might suggest a metabolic or feeding problem. (A, 4)

5. 1. A trial of human chorionic gonadotrophin may be given to stimulate descent of the affected testis. A trial of adrenocorticotropic hormone will not cause the testis to descend. The cremasteric reflex results in the testis' being drawn up, the opposite of the intended effect. Application of warmth, such as warm baths, although soothing and relaxing for the infant, would have little or no effect on stimulating the testis to descend. (P, 8)

6. 2. Preoperative teaching would be directed at the parents, because the child is too young to understand the teaching. Telling the child that his penis and scrotum will be fixed, telling the child about not seeing incisions after surgery, and using a doll to illustrate the surgery are appropriate methods for a preschool-aged child. (P, 10)

7. 3. Because the incidence of testicular cancer is increased in adulthood among children who have had undescended testes, it is extremely important to teach the adolescent how to perform the testicular self-examination monthly. The undescended testicle is removed to reduce the risk of cancer in that testicle. Removal of a testis would not necessarily make the adolescent sterile because the other testicle remains. Although discussing the adolescent's future plans is important, it is not the priority at this time. Because the adolescent has been dealing with the situation for a long time, the need for a sports physical at this time should not be a cause of emotional distress requiring a lot of psychological support. (I, 4)

The Client With Hydrocele

8. 3. A hydrocele is a collection of fluid in the tunica vaginalis of the testicle or along the spermatic cord that results from a patent processus vaginalis. Failure of the upper part of the processus vaginalis to atrophy allows the accumulation of fluid in the testicle and peritoneal cavity, causing an inguinal hernia. (D, 10)

9. 3. A hydrocele is a collection of fluid in the tunica vaginalis of the testicle or along the spermatic cord that results from a patent processus vaginalis. Because scro-

tal size is decreasing, the fluid is being absorbed. Elevation of the infant's bottom, massage, or keeping the infant quiet or in an infant seat would have no effect in promoting fluid reabsorption in hydrocele. (E, 10)

10. 4. Some swelling and bruising are normal postoperatively. By assessing the area with the mother, the nurse is conveying acceptance of the mother's concern. In addition, the nurse needs to inspect the area to determine if indeed what the mother is describing is accurate. Doing so also provides an opportunity for teaching. Aspirin is not usually prescribed for children because of the link between aspirin and Reye's syndrome. Acetaminophen is commonly administered for fever or pain relief. Asking the mother to wait in the child's room ignores the mother's concerns. There is no need to notify the doctor at this time. (I, 10)

The Client With Hypospadias

11. 2. The condition in which the urethral opening is on the ventral side of the penis or below the glans penis is referred to as *hypospadias. Chordee* refers to a ventral curvature of the penis that results from a fibrous band of tissue that has replaced normal tissue. Circumcision is delayed because the foreskin, which is removed with a circumcision, often is used to reconstruct the urethra. The chordee is corrected when the hypospadias is repaired. Circumcision is performed at the same time. Urethral meatal stenosis, which can occur in circumcised infants, results from meatal ulceration, possibly leading to urinary obstruction. It is not associated with hypospadias or circumcision. The infant is not too small to have a circumcision, which is commonly performed on the first or second day of life. (D, 9)

12. 2. The preferred time for surgery is between the ages of 6 to 18 months, before the child develops castration and body image anxiety. Children learn early on about society's emphasis on the importance of genitals. Pain is different for each child and is not related to the preferred time for repair of the hypospadias or chordee. Although the child will probably not remember the experience, this is not the basis for having the surgery at this age. If the condition is not repaired, the child will have difficulty with toilet training because urine is not eliminated through the tip of the penis. (I, 10)

13. 2. Surgical repair of a hypospadias involves use of the skin from the prepuce to extend the urethra to the tip of the penis. An alternative urinary elimination route is needed because the surgical site needs to be kept dry, clean, and free from the pressure of a full bladder. Pressure from a full bladder might cause fluid to leak around the urethral catheter or possibly disrupt the delicate plastic surgery. Although the suprapubic catheter does aid in providing an accurate measure-

ment of urine output, its primary purpose is to provide an alternative route for urinary elimination. After surgical repair of a hypospadias, the bladder does not need to be irrigated. (I, 9)

14. 2. The main purpose of the urethral catheter is to maintain patency of the reconstructed urethra. The catheter prevents the new tissue inside the urethra from healing on itself. However, the urethral catheter can cause bladder spasms. Recently, stents have been used instead of catheters. The urethral catheter will have no effect on the child's pain level. In fact, because bladder spasms are associated with its use, the child's complaints of pain may actually increase. Urine output can be measured through the suprapubic catheter because it provides an alternative route for urinary elimination, thus keeping the bladder empty and pressure-free. (E, 9)

15. 3. Because this is the first of two surgeries, the penis may appear somewhat misshapen or bumpy because of the intermediate phase of reconstruction. The penis is unlikely to look entirely normal even after reconstruction. Swelling and local bruising would be normal. The penis may appear red, but it should not be bright red in color. After the first surgery for hypospadias, blood supply to the area is still adequate. The penis should appear pale pink. A dusky blue color at the tip of the penis may indicate a problem with circulation. (I, 10)

16. 4. The most important consideration for a successful outcome of this surgery is maintenance of the catheters or stents. A 12-month-old likes to explore his environment but must be prevented from manipulating his dressings or catheters through the use of soft restraints. Allowing the infant to become familiar with the dressings will not prevent him from pulling at them. After surgery the child is allowed limited activity, possibly with sitting in the parent's lap. A 12-month-old may or may not be walking. If he is, most likely he will be clumsy and possibly injure himself. Although increasing fluids is important, 2500 mL/day is an excessive amount for a 12-month-old child. Fluid requirements would be 115 mL/kg. (P, 10)

17. 3. A normal white blood cell count in a urinalysis is 1 to 2 cells/mL. A white blood cell count of 25 per high-powered field indicates a urinary tract infection. A urine specific gravity of 1.017 is within the normal range of 1.002 to 1.030. After urologic surgery, it is not unusual for a small number of red blood cells to appear in the urine. The child's urine pH is within the normal range of 4.6 to 8. (D, 9)

The Client With Urinary Tract Infection

18. 1. Abdominal pain frequently accompanies urinary tract infection in children 2 years of age and older. Other asso-

ciated signs and symptoms include decreased appetite, vomiting, fever, and irritability. The presence of swollen lymph glands (lymphadenopathy) is unrelated to urinary tract infections. Lymphadenopathy is associated with a systemic infection or possibly cancer. Skin rash is associated with exposure to allergens or irritants (eg, poison ivy, harsh soaps); prolonged contact with urine (eg, diaper dermatitis); or illnesses such as measles, rheumatic fever, or juvenile rheumatoid arthritis. Flank or back pain is associated with urinary tract infection in children older than 2 years of age and in adults. (D, 10)

19. 2. To ensure appropriate psychosocial development, a child needs to have normal patterns maintained as much as possible during illness. It is tempting to give ill children extra treatment and hard to discipline them. However, family routines and discipline should be kept as normal as possible. The child needs to know the limits to ensure feelings of security. When they are ill, children commonly attempt to stretch the rules and limits. If this occurs, returning to the previous well-behavior patterns will take time. (I, 3)

20. 1. The reason that urinary tract infections are a problem in children with vesicoureteral reflux is that urine flows back up the ureter, past the incompetent valve, and back into the bladder after the child has finished voiding. This incomplete emptying of the bladder results in stasis of urine, providing a good medium for bacterial growth and subsequent infection. Vesicoureteral reflux does not cause bladder spasms or painful urination. However, the child may experience painful urination with a urinary tract infection. (I, 10)

The Client With Glomerulonephritis

21. 3. Most likely, the nurse suspects that the child is exhibiting signs and symptoms of glomerulonephritis, such as periorbital edema and fever. Other signs and symptoms include loss of appetite, dark-colored urine, pallor, headaches, and abdominal pain. To confirm this suspicion, the nurse would ask about the child's urinary elimination patterns. Typically the child with glomerulonephritis experiences a decrease in urine output. Asking about any recent sore throat would provide additional information to confirm the suspicion of glomerulonephritis, because the most common type is acute poststreptococcal glomerulonephritis, which follows a strep throat by 10 to 14 days. Frequently, the children have only mild cold symptoms and do not realize they have a streptococcal infection. Asking whether the child plays with friends as usual is important and gives the nurse information about how the child feels in general. However, this is a general question that would be appropriate to ask later on in the history. Although asking the mother about the color of

the child's urine is important, the nurse needs to determine whether there is any change in the child's urinary output first. (A, 10)

22. 3. The child with glomerulonephritis experiences a problem with renal function that ultimately affects fluid balance. Because weight is the best indicator of fluid balance, obtaining daily weights would be the highest priority. (I, 10)

23. 2. The most appropriate and effective choice would be ice chips, because they help moisten the mouth and lips while keeping fluid intake low. However, ice chips must still be counted as intake with the fluid restriction. Sweet beverages, such as diet cola or lemonade, commonly increase thirst. Tap water effectively relieves thirst but does not help keep fluid intake low. (P, 10)

24. 4. The best choice would be fruits such as strawberries and kiwi because they are low in sodium and potassium. Typically, diet is related to the stage and severity of the disease. In children with uncomplicated disease, a regular diet is offered but sodium is usually restricted. In children with hypertension and edema, moderate restriction of sodium is instituted. Pizza and cola, hamburgers and fries, and ice cream are high in sodium and should be avoided. Children with oliguria usually also have potassium restricted. Therefore, foods such as bananas and oranges would be avoided. (E, 10)

25. 1. Generally, school-aged children enjoy activities with their peers first, then family members, and lastly younger children. School-aged children like to be busy but also to accomplish something. This helps to meet their task of industry versus inferiority, feeling good about what they are able to accomplish. (P, 3)

26. 1. The nurse should assess the child's neurologic status, because hypertensive encephalopathy is a major potential complication of the acute phase of glomerulonephritis. Seizure precautions also should be instituted. Hypertensive encephalopathy can result in transient loss of vision, hemiparesis, disorientation, and grand mal seizures. Encouraging the child to drink more water is inappropriate because the child has had a low urine output for 14 hours. Typically, in this situation, fluids would be restricted. Although a low-sodium diet is encouraged, it is not the priority action at this time. Initially, bed rest, not ambulation, is advocated during the acute phase of glomerulonephritis. (I, 9)

27. 3. Children recovering from glomerulonephritis need to avoid exposure to all types of infections. Glomerulonephritis is caused by group A β-hemolytic streptococcus, a common cause of sore throat. As the child recovers, he or she may be susceptible to a recurrence if exposed to the organism again. During convalescence from glomerulonephritis, fluid and dietary restrictions are no longer indicated because the kidneys are now

functioning normally. There is no need for the parents to assess the child's vital signs. (P, 10)

28. 1. Because the client with chronic glomerulonephritis is in a permanent salt-losing state, the sodium level would be on the low end of normal range of 138 to 145 mEq/L. The blood urea nitrogen level is usually increased above the normal range of 5 to 18 mg/dL. The serum potassium level is usually increased above the normal range of 3.5 to 5.0 mEq/L. Acidosis is usually present. A blood pH of 7.43 is within the normal range of 7.35 to 7.45. (A, 10)

The Client With Nephrotic Syndrome

29. 2. Nephrotic syndrome involves altered glomerular permeability, which results in increased permeability to albumin, leading to the excretion of large amounts of protein in the urine. Aldosterone secretion is increased, resulting in sodium and water reabsorption. Red blood cells are not lost in the urine in nephrotic syndrome. (D, 9)

30. 1. Children with nephrotic syndrome usually require sodium restriction. Because potato chips and bologna are high in sodium, the mother's statement about finding something else reflects understanding of this need. Although fluid intake is not restricted in children with nephrotic syndrome, 4 liters is an excessive amount for a toddler. The typical fluid requirement for a toddler is 115 mL/kg. Surgical intervention and antibiotic therapy are not parts of the treatment plan for nephrotic syndrome. (E, 10)

31. 4. The best indicator of fluid balance is weight. Therefore, daily weight measurements help determine fluid losses and gains. Although limiting visitors to 2 to 3 hours per day or maintaining strict bed rest would help to ensure that the child gets adequate rest, this is unrelated to the child's fluid balance. In nephrotic syndrome, urine is tested for protein, not specific gravity. (P, 10)

32. 2. The child's swollen eyes are caused by fluid accumulation. Elevating the head of the bed allows gravity to increase the downward flow of fluids in the body, away from the face. Applying cool compresses or eye drops, or limiting television, may be comforting but will not relieve the swelling. (I, 10)

33. 1. Fluid accumulates in the abdomen and interstitial spaces owing to hydrostatic pressure changes. Increased abdominal fluid is evidenced by an increase in abdominal girth. Therefore, decreased abdominal girth is a sign of reduced fluid in the third spaces and tissues. When fluid accumulates in the abdomen and interstitial spaces, the child does not feel hungry and does not eat well. Although increased caloric intake may indicate decreased intestinal edema, it is not the best and most accurate indicator of fluid retention. Increased respiratory rate may be an indication of increasing fluid in the abdomen (ascites) causing pressure on the diaphragm. Heart rate usually stays in the normal range even with excessive fluid volume. (E, 10)

34. 4. Placing soft cloth between opposing skin surfaces absorbs moisture and keeps the area dry, thus preventing any further breakdown. The child with nephrotic syndrome and severe edema is usually maintained on bed rest. Therefore, ambulation is not appropriate. Applying lotion or powder to edematous surfaces that touch increases moisture and can lead to maceration, causing further breakdown. (I, 7)

35. 2. A child recovering from nephrotic syndrome should be protected from infection. Therefore, the nurse would teach the parents to keep the child away from others with an infection. Because pain is not associated with this disorder, pain medication typically is not needed. The physician should be notified if urine output decreases, not increases. In children recovering from nephrotic syndrome, there is no reason to administer acetaminophen daily. (I, 9)

The Client With Acute or Chronic Renal Failure

36. 1. A client receiving continuous peritoneal dialysis usually requires few dietary restrictions, whereas a client receiving hemodialysis usually has fluid and food restrictions. With continuous peritoneal dialysis, fluid excesses and increased body wastes are removed continuously. With hemodialysis, which is performed two or three times per week, fluid and wastes accumulate between treatments. Although infection is associated with both hemodialysis and peritoneal dialysis, the risk of peritonitis is the major disadvantage of peritoneal dialysis. During peritoneal dialysis, plasma proteins, amino acids, and polypeptides diffuse into the dialysate because of the permeability of the peritoneal membrane. Peritoneal dialysis removes fluid less rapidly than does hemodialysis because peritoneal dialysis uses the peritoneal membrane for diffusion and there is no direct vascular access. (I, 9)

37. 3. Until it heals, the catheter exit site is particularly vulnerable to invasion by pathogenic organisms. Therefore, the site must be monitored for signs of infection. An occlusive dressing is not needed because there is no danger of air being sucked in or out of the peritoneal space. Furthermore, the catheter used is designed with a cuff, so that the skin grows around the catheter, sealing off the area. Site care may be done at any time, but the child may experience abdominal discomfort if the peritoneal space is dry during site care. Holding the catheter taut or pulling on it may cause irritation of the skin at the exit site, which could lead to infection. (I, 2)

38. 4. With minimal or absent kidney function, the serum phosphate level rises, and the ionized calcium level falls in response. This causes increased secretion of parathyroid hormone, which releases calcium from the bones. Therefore, the intake of foods high in phosphorus is restricted. Because renal failure results in decreased erythropoietin production, an increase in ascorbic acid intake is needed. Because magnesium is minimally affected by renal failure, its intake need not be restricted. (P, 10)

39. 4. Demonstration of desire to do the dressing changes and manage medications implies compliance with the medical regimen and acceptance of the condition, thereby indicating a positive self-image. Diffuse somatic complaints could indicate anxiety or problems with coping, with a negative affect on self-concept. Insistence on choosing restricted foods implies that the adolescent has not accepted the diagnosis and is noncompliant, possibly indicating a negative self-concept. Social withdrawal from activities may indicate depression, possibly negatively affecting the self-concept. (E, 10)

40. 2. The child with acute renal failure needs extra calories to reduce tissue catabolism, metabolic acidosis, and uremia. Using a high-fat and carbohydrate diet helps to supply the necessary extra calories. If the child is able to tolerate oral foods, concentrated food sources that are high in carbohydrate and fat but low in protein, potassium, and sodium may be provided. (I, 10)

41. 3. For an adolescent, body image is a major concern. The presence of an abdominal catheter can greatly affect the client's body image. The adolescent needs opportunities to discuss feelings about altered body image due to the catheter. Adolescents need to be with their peers and to maintain social activities and contacts in order to meet the development tasks for this age group. The adolescent client may choose to confide in friends for both psychological health and physical safety. Because peers are most important to adolescents, they will confide in their peers before confiding in family members. Another major developmental need of the adolescent is achieving independence. Relying on the parents would interfere with the adolescent's ability to do so. (P, 5)

42. 4. Tissue swelling, pain, redness, and exudate indicate infection. Dialysate leakage is associated with improper catheter function, incomplete healing at the insertion site, or excessive instillation of dialysate. Granulation tissue indicates healing around the exit site, not infection. Increased time for drainage may indicate that the tube is kinked, suggesting an obstruction. (D, 9)

43. 1. Normally, dialysate drainage return should be clear. With peritonitis, large numbers of bacteria, white blood cells, and fibrin cause the dialysate to appear cloudy. Abdominal distention is unrelated to peritonitis. However, it might suggest an obstruction. Weight gain and shortness of breath are associated with fluid excess, not infection. (E, 10)

44. 4. With edema, pallor can occur owing to hemodilution as intestinal fluid moves to the vascular space. The child would exhibit pulmonary crackles secondary to pulmonary congestion and edema. Dialysate outflow would decrease, not increase, as the body attempts to conserve fluid. The child's blood pressure would be increased because of excessive fluid volume. (A, 10)

45. 1. Accumulation of hard stool in the bowel can cause the distended intestine to block the holes of the catheter. Consequently, the dialysate cannot flow freely through the catheter. Decreasing the dialysate infusion may make the dialysis less effective. Altering fluid, electrolyte, and waste product removal can cause fluid and electrolyte imbalance and increased levels of blood urea nitrogen and creatinine. Incorporating the increased times into the dialysis may make the dialysis less effective because fewer cycles can be scheduled. Shoulder pain, which may occur occasionally, can be caused by air in the peritoneal space and diaphragmatic irritation. However, it is unrelated to inflow and drain times. (I, 10)

46. 4. Regulation of the diet is the most effective means, besides dialysis, for reducing renal excretion. Dietary phosphorus is restricted, which reduces the protein load on the kidneys. Clients are also given substances to bind phosphorus in the intestines to prevent absorption. Limited protein in the diet should include foods high in essential amino acids. Foods high in fat and carbohydrate are used to increase caloric intake. Sodium and water may not be restricted because of the continual loss of sodium and water through the dialysate. Iron-rich foods are commonly high in protein. (E, 10)

The Client with Wilms' Tumor

47. 3. Wilms' tumor, or nephroblastoma, is the most common intra-abdominal tumor of childhood and the most common type of renal cancer. It is highly malignant. Anemia, which is secondary to hemorrhage within the tumor, causes pallor, anorexia, and lethargy. The most common presenting sign is an abdominal mass. Other signs and symptoms are the result of compression from the tumor mass, metabolic alterations secondary to the tumor, or metastasis. Hypertension occurs occasionally, probably owing to excessive excretion of renin by the tumor. Proteinemia and petechiae are not associated with Wilms' tumor. Generally, proteinemia is associated with renal disorders such as nephrotic syndrome and glomerulonephritis. Petechiae are seen with hematologic problems such as idiopathic thrombocytopenia and leukemias. (A, 10)

48. 2. The abdomen of the child with Wilms' tumor should not be palpated because of the danger of disseminating tumor cells. Techniques such as measuring the occipitofrontal circumference (which is done in children younger than 18 months of age because the anterior fontanel closes between 12 to 18 months of age), upright positioning, and measuring chest circumference are not necessarily contraindicated; however, the child with Wilms' tumor should always be handled gently and carefully. (A, 10)

49. 1. A stage II tumor is one that extends beyond the kidney but is completely resected. The tumor staging is verified during surgery to maximize treatment protocols. The following criteria for staging are commonly used: *stage I*, tumor is limited to the kidney and completely resected; *stage II*, tumor extends beyond the kidney but is completely resected; *stage III*, residual nonhematogenous tumor is confined to the abdomen; *stage IV*, hematogenous metastasis occurs, with deposits beyond stage III (lung, bone and brain, liver); *stage V*, bilateral renal involvement is present at diagnosis. (E, 10)

50. 3. The child who has undergone abdominal surgery is usually placed in a semi-Fowler's position to facilitate draining of abdominal contents and promote pulmonary expansion. The modified Trendelenburg position is used for clients in shock. The Sims position is likely to be uncomfortable for this child because of the large transabdominal incision. The supine position, without the head elevated, puts the child at increased risk for aspiration. (I, 9)

51. 1. Children who have undergone abdominal surgery are at risk for intestinal obstruction from adynamic ileus. Indications of intestinal obstruction include abdominal distention, decreased or absent bowel sounds, and vomiting. Later signs of intestinal obstruction include tachycardia, fever, hypotension, shock, and decreased urinary output. (A, 9)

52. 3. Because the child has only one kidney, measures should be recommended to prevent urinary tract infection and injury to the remaining kidney. Severe pain and dependent edema are not associated with surgery for Wilms' tumor. Dietary sodium is not restricted because function in the remaining kidney is not impaired. (P, 4)

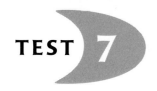

TEST 7

The Child With Neurologic Health Problems

- ▶ The Client With Myelomeningocele
- ▶ The Client With Hydrocephalus
- ▶ The Client With Down Syndrome
- ▶ The Client With a Seizure Disorder
- ▶ The Client With Meningitis
- ▶ The Client With Near-Drowning
- ▶ The Client With Guillain-Barré Syndrome (Infectious Polyneuritis)
- ▶ The Client With a Head Injury
- ▶ The Client With a Brain Tumor
- ▶ The Client With a Spinal Cord Injury
- ▶ Correct Answers and Rationale

Select the one best answer, and indicate your choice by filling in the circle in front of the option.

The Client With Myelomeningocele

1. When assessing a newborn admitted to the pediatric unit with upper lumbar myelomeningocele, which of the following would the nurse anticipate finding?
   - ○ 1. Minimal movement of the lower extremities.
   - ○ 2. Upper extremity paralysis.
   - ○ 3. Urinary bladder prolapse.
   - ○ 4. Respiratory problems.

2. When developing the plan of care for an infant diagnosed with myelomeningocele and the parents who have just been informed of the infant's diagnosis, which of the following would the nurse include as the *priority* when the parents visit the infant for the first time?
   - ○ 1. Emphasizing the infant's normal and positive features.
   - ○ 2. Encouraging the parents to discuss their fears and concerns.
   - ○ 3. Reinforcing the doctor's explanation of the defect.
   - ○ 4. Having the parents feed their infant.

3. The mother of a newborn with myelomeningocele asks if her baby is likely to have any other defects. The nurse responds based on the understanding that myelomeningocele is frequently associated with which of the following?
   - ○ 1. Excessive cerebrospinal fluid within the cranial cavity.

   - ○ 2. Abnormally small head.
   - ○ 3. Congenital absence of the cranial vault.
   - ○ 4. Overriding of the cranial sutures.

4. The parents of an infant with myelomeningocele ask the nurse about their child's future mental ability. Which of the following would be the nurse's *best* response?
   - ○ 1. "About one third are mentally retarded, but it's too early to tell about your child."
   - ○ 2. "About two thirds are significantly retarded, and you'll know soon if this will occur."
   - ○ 3. "Your child will probably be of normal intelligence since he demonstrates signs of it now."
   - ○ 4. "You'll need to talk with the doctor about that, but you can ask later."

5. After placing an infant with myelomeningocele in an isolette shortly after birth, which of the following would the nurse use as the *best* indicator to determine the effectiveness of this intervention?
   - ○ 1. The arterial PO$_2$ remains between 94 and 100 mm Hg.
   - ○ 2. The axillary temperature remains between 97° and 98°F (36.1° and 36.7°C).
   - ○ 3. The bilirubin level remains stable.
   - ○ 4. Weight increases by about 1 ounce per day.

6. When positioning the neonate with an unrepaired myelomeningocele, which of the following positions would be *most* appropriate?
   - ○ 1. Supine with the hips at 90-degree flexion.

○ 2. Right side-lying position with the knees flexed.
○ 3. Prone with hips in abduction.
○ 4. Semi-Fowler's position with chest and abdomen elevated.

7. After surgical repair of a myelomeningocele, which of the following would the nurse use to prevent musculoskeletal deformity in the infant?
    ○ 1. Placing the feet in flexion.
    ○ 2. Allowing the hips to be abducted.
    ○ 3. Maintaining knees in the neutral position.
    ○ 4. Placing the legs in adduction.

8. Which of the following would alert the nurse initially to suspect hydrocephalus in an infant who has undergone surgical repair of a myelomeningocele?
    ○ 1. Seizures and vomiting.
    ○ 2. Frontal bossing and sunset eyes.
    ○ 3. Increased head circumference and bulging fontanel.
    ○ 4. Irritability and shrill cry.

9. When developing the discharge plan for the parents of an infant who has undergone a myelomeningocele repair, which of the following would the nurse include as *most* important?
    ○ 1. A list of available hospital services.
    ○ 2. Schedule for daily home health care.
    ○ 3. Chaplain referral for psychological support.
    ○ 4. Daily care required by the infant.

10. Which of the following statements by the mother of an infant with a repaired upper lumbar myelomeningcele indicates that she understands the nurse's teaching at the time of discharge?
    ○ 1. "I can apply a heating pad to his lower back."
    ○ 2. "I'll be sure to keep him away from other infants."
    ○ 3. "I will call the doctor if his urine has a funny smell."
    ○ 4. "I will prop him with pillows to prevent him from rolling over."

11. A preschooler with a history of repaired lumbar myelomeningocele is in the emergency department with wheezing and skin rash. Which of the following questions would the nurse ask the mother *first*?
    ○ 1. "Is your child taking any medications?"
    ○ 2. "Who brought your child to the emergency department?"
    ○ 3. "Is your child allergic to bananas or milk products?"
    ○ 4. "What are you doing to treat your child's skin rash?"

The Client With Hydrocephalus

12. Before placement of a ventriculoperitoneal shunt for hydrocephalus, an infant is irritable, lethargic, and difficult to feed. To maintain the infant's nutritional status, which of the following actions would be *most* appropriate?
    ○ 1. Feeding the infant just before doing any procedures.
    ○ 2. Giving the infant small, frequent feedings.
    ○ 3. Feeding the infant in a horizontal position.
    ○ 4. Scheduling the feedings for every 6 hours.

13. A 4-year-old with hydrocephalus is scheduled to have a ventroperitoneal shunt in the right side of the head. When developing the child's postoperative plan of care, the nurse would expect to place the preschooler in which of the following positions immediately after surgery?
    ○ 1. On the right side, with the foot of the bed elevated.
    ○ 2. On the left side, with the head of the bed elevated.
    ○ 3. Prone, with the head of the bed elevated.
    ○ 4. Supine, with the head of the bed flat.

14. Which of the following would the nurse do when providing postoperative nursing care to a child after insertion of a ventriculoperitoneal shunt?
    ○ 1. Administer narcotics for pain control.
    ○ 2. Check the urine for glucose and protein.
    ○ 3. Monitoring for increased temperature.
    ○ 4. Test cerebrospinal fluid leakage for protein.

15. The nurse evaluates the discharge teaching as successful when the parents of a school-aged child with a ventriculoperitoneal shunt insertion identify which of the following as signaling a blocked shunt?
    ○ 1. Decreased urine output with stable intake.
    ○ 2. Tense fontanel and increased head circumference.
    ○ 3. Elevated temperature and reddened incisional site.
    ○ 4. Irritability and increasing difficulty with eating.

The Client With Down Syndrome

16. After talking with the parents of a child with Down syndrome, which of the following would the nurse identify as an appropriate goal for care of the child?
    ○ 1. Encouraging self-care skills in the child.
    ○ 2. Teaching the child something new each day.
    ○ 3. Encouraging more lenient behavior limits for the child.
    ○ 4. Achieving age-appropriate social skills.

17. The nurse discusses with the parents how best to raise the IQ of their child with Down syndrome. Which of the following would be *most* appropriate?
    ○ 1. Serving hearty, nutritious meals.
    ○ 2. Giving vasodilator medications as prescribed.

○ 3. Letting the child play with more able children.

○ 4. Providing stimulating, nonthreatening life experiences.

18. Which of the following would alert the nurse to suspect a physical problem commonly associated with Down syndrome?

○ 1. Weight loss.

○ 2. Irregular heart rate.

○ 3. Rapid respirations.

○ 4. Increased blood pressure.

19. When developing a teaching plan for the parents of a child with Down syndrome, the nurse focuses on activities to increase which of the following for the parents?

○ 1. Affection for their child.

○ 2. Responsibility for their child's welfare.

○ 3. Understanding of their child's disability.

○ 4. Confidence in their ability to care for their child.

20. The nurse mentions that a group meeting for mothers of mentally retarded children is to be held soon. "Not retarded!" the child's mother angrily blazes, "Exceptional." When responding to this outburst, which of the following replies by the nurse would be *most* appropriate?

○ 1. "'Retarded' is the commonly used and accepted term."

○ 2. "I'm sorry if I offended you by my thoughtless remark."

○ 3. "No matter what it's called, the condition is still the same, isn't it?"

○ 4. "I'd like to hear more of your thoughts and feelings on that."

The Client With a Seizure Disorder

21. After teaching a group of school teachers about seizures, the teachers role-play a scenario involving a child experiencing a generalized tonic-clonic seizure. Which of the following actions, when performed *first*, indicates that the nurse's teaching has been successful?

○ 1. Asking the other children what happened before the seizure.

○ 2. Moving the child to the nurse's office for privacy.

○ 3. Removing any nearby objects that could harm the child.

○ 4. Placing a padded tongue blade between the child's teeth.

22. When developing a plan of care focusing on promoting growth and development for the parents of a 6-year-old girl diagnosed with a seizure disorder, which of the following would the nurse expect to include?

○ 1. Need for activity limitation and inability to perform as others do in the child's class.

○ 2. Existence of a learning disability and need for tutoring to help the child reach her grade level.

○ 3. Most often, demonstration of normal intelligence and ability to attend regular school.

○ 4. Problems associated with social stigma and inability to attend public school.

23. The parents of a child with occasional generalized seizures want to send the child to summer camp. The parents contact the nurse for advice on planning for the camping experience. Which of the following activities would the nurse and family decide is *most* important for the child to avoid?

○ 1. Rock climbing.

○ 2. Hiking.

○ 3. Swimming.

○ 4. Tennis.

24. Which of the following statements obtained from the nursing history of a toddler would alert the nurse to suspect that the child has had a febrile seizure?

○ 1. The child has had a low-grade fever for several weeks.

○ 2. The family history is negative for convulsions.

○ 3. The seizure resulted in respiratory arrest.

○ 4. The seizure occurred when the child had a respiratory infection.

25. After teaching the parents of a child with febrile seizures about methods to lower temperature other than medication, which of the following statements indicates successful teaching?

○ 1. "We'll add extra blankets when he complains of being cold."

○ 2. "We'll wrap him in a blanket if he starts shivering."

○ 3. "We'll make the bath water cold enough to make him shiver."

○ 4. "We'll use a solution of half alcohol and half water when sponging him."

26. An adolescent girl with a seizure disorder controlled with phenytoin (Dilantin) and carbamazepine (Tegretol) asks the nurse about getting married and having children. Which of the following responses by the nurse would be *most* appropriate?

○ 1. "You probably shouldn't consider having children until your seizures are cured."

○ 2. "Your children won't necessarily have an increased risk of seizure disorder."

○ 3. "When you decide to have children, talk to the doctor about changing your medication."

○ 4. "Women who have seizure disorders commonly have a difficult time conceiving."

27. When teaching an adolescent with a seizure disorder who is receiving valproic acid (Depakene), which of the following would the nurse instruct the client to report to the health care provider?
    ○ 1. Three episodes of diarrhea.
    ○ 2. Loss of appetite.
    ○ 3. Jaundice.
    ○ 4. Sore throat.

The Client With Meningitis

28. During the acute stage of meningitis, a 3-year-old child is restless and irritable. Which of the following would be *most* appropriate to institute?
    ○ 1. Limiting conversation with the child.
    ○ 2. Keeping extraneous noise to a minimum.
    ○ 3. Allowing the child to play in the bathtub.
    ○ 4. Performing treatments quickly.

29. Which of the following would lead the nurse to suspect that a child with meningitis has developed disseminated intravascular coagulation?
    ○ 1. Hemorrhagic skin rash.
    ○ 2. Edema.
    ○ 3. Cyanosis.
    ○ 4. Dyspnea on exertion.

30. When interviewing the parents of a 2-year-old child, a history of which of the following illnesses would lead the nurse to suspect pneumococcal meningitis?
    ○ 1. Bladder infection.
    ○ 2. Middle ear infection.
    ○ 3. Fractured clavicle.
    ○ 4. Septic arthritis.

31. A preschooler with pneumonococci meningitis is receiving intravenous antibiotic therapy. When discontinuing the intravenous therapy, the nurse allows the child to apply a dressing to the area where the needle is removed. The nurse's rationale for doing so is based on the interpretation that a child in this age group has a need to accomplish which of the following?
    ○ 1. Trust those caring for her.
    ○ 2. Find diversional activities.
    ○ 3. Protect the image of an intact body.
    ○ 4. Relieve the anxiety of separation from home.

32. A hospitalized preschooler with meningitis who is to be discharged becomes angry when the discharge is delayed. Which of the following play activities would be *most* appropriate at this time?
    ○ 1. Reading the child a story.
    ○ 2. Painting with watercolors.
    ○ 3. Pounding on a pegboard.
    ○ 4. Stacking a tower of blocks.

The Client With Near-Drowning

33. The nurse caring for a toddler just admitted with the diagnosis of near-drowning in a neighbor's swimming pool is *most* concerned about which of the following?
    ○ 1. Hypothermia.
    ○ 2. Hypoxia.
    ○ 3. Fluid aspiration.
    ○ 4. Cutaneous capillary paralysis.

34. When assessing a toddler with near-drowning, which of the following acid-base imbalances would the nurse expect to find?
    ○ 1. Respiratory acidosis and metabolic acidosis.
    ○ 2. Respiratory acidosis and metabolic alkalosis.
    ○ 3. Respiratory alkalosis and metabolic acidosis.
    ○ 4. Respiratory alkalosis and metabolic alkalosis.

35. The parents of a child tell the nurse that they feel guilty because their child almost drowned. Which of the following remarks by the nurse would be *most* appropriate?
    ○ 1. "I can understand why you feel guilty, but these things happen."
    ○ 2. "Tell me a little bit more about your feelings of guilt."
    ○ 3. "You should not have taken your eyes off of your child."
    ○ 4. "You really shouldn't feel guilty; you're lucky because your child will be all right."

The Client With Guillain-Barré Syndrome (Infectious Polyneuritis)

36. Which of the following assessments would be *most* important for the nurse to make initially in a school-aged child being seen in the clinic for complaints of a sore throat, muscle tenderness, arms feeling weak, and generally not feeling well?
    ○ 1. Difficulty swallowing.
    ○ 2. Diet intake for the last 24 hours.
    ○ 3. Exposure to illnesses.
    ○ 4. Difficulty urinating.

37. Which of the following actions would be the priority when caring for a school-aged child admitted to the pediatric unit with the diagnosis of Guillain-Barré syndrome?
    ○ 1. Assessing the child's ability to follow simple commands.
    ○ 2. Evaluating the child's bilateral muscle strength.
    ○ 3. Making a game of the range-of-motion exercises.
    ○ 4. Providing the child with a diversional activity.

38. The nurse asks a school-aged child with Guillain-Barré syndrome to cough and also assesses the child's speech for decreased volume and clarity. The underlying rationale for these assessments is to determine which of the following?
    - ○ 1. Inflammation of the larynx and epiglottis.
    - ○ 2. Increased intracranial pressure.
    - ○ 3. Involvement of facial and cranial nerves.
    - ○ 4. Regression to an earlier developmental phase.

39. Assessment of a school-aged child with Guillain-Barré syndrome reveals absent gag and cough reflexes. Which of the following nursing diagnoses would receive the highest priority during the acute phase?
    - ○ 1. Risk for Infection due to altered immune system.
    - ○ 2. Ineffective Breathing Pattern related to neuromuscular impairment.
    - ○ 3. Impaired Swallowing related to neuromuscular impairment.
    - ○ 4. Total Urinary Incontinence related to fluid losses.

40. A 9-year-old child with Guillain-Barré syndrome requires mechanical ventilation. Which of the following would the nurse do?
    - ○ 1. Maintain the child in a supine position to prevent unnecessary nerve stimulation.
    - ○ 2. Transfer the child to a bedside chair three times a day to prevent orthostatic hypotension.
    - ○ 3. Engage the child in vigorous passive range-of-motion exercises to prevent loss of muscle function.
    - ○ 4. Turn the child slowly and gently from side to side to prevent respiratory complications.

41. The mother brings her child to the clinic after discharge from the hospital for Guillain-Barré syndrome. Which of the following statements by the mother indicates that she is following the discharge plan?
    - ○ 1. "She and her sister argue all day."
    - ○ 2. "I have to bribe her to get her to do her exercises."
    - ○ 3. "I take her to the pool where she can exercise with other children."
    - ○ 4. "She's missed a few of her therapy sessions because she often sleeps."

The Client With a Head Injury

42. For a child with serious head trauma, the nurse anticipates inserting a nasogastric tube *initially* to accomplish which of the following?
    - ○ 1. Administer medications.
    - ○ 2. Decompress the stomach.

○ 3. Obtain gastric specimens for analysis.
○ 4. Provide adequate nutrition.

43. A nasogastric tube is ordered to be inserted for a child with severe head trauma. Diagnostic testing reveals that the child has a basilar skull fracture. Which of the following would the nurse do *next*?
    - ○ 1. Ask for the order to be changed to oral gastric tube.
    - ○ 2. Attempt to place the tube into the duodenum.
    - ○ 3. Test the gastric aspirate for blood.
    - ○ 4. Use extra lubrication when inserting the nasogastric tube.

44. The parents of a child with a serious head injury ask the nurse if the child is going to be all right. Which of the following responses by the nurse would be *most* appropriate?
    - ○ 1. "Children usually don't do very well after head injuries like this."
    - ○ 2. "Children usually recover rapidly from head injuries."
    - ○ 3. "It's hard to tell this early, but we'll keep you informed of the progress."
    - ○ 4. "That's something you'll have to talk to the doctor about."

45. When developing the plan of care for a child who is unconscious after a serious head injury, in which of the following positions would the nurse expect to place the child?
    - ○ 1. Prone with hips and knees slightly elevated.
    - ○ 2. Lying on the side, with the head of the bed elevated.
    - ○ 3. Lying on the back, in the Trendelenburg position.
    - ○ 4. In the semi-Fowler's position, with arms at the side.

46. The parents ask the nurse why the physician ordered mannitol to be given to their child with a serious head injury. The nurse's response is based on the understanding that mannitol acts in which of the following ways?
    - ○ 1. It helps hold fluid in the vascular bed, to prevent shock.
    - ○ 2. It aids in decreasing fluid, to decrease swelling in the brain.
    - ○ 3. It increases caloric intake, to aid wound healing.
    - ○ 4. It fights off bacteria, to prevent infections.

The Client With a Brain Tumor

47. A 13-year-old has seen the school nurse several times with complaints of headache, vomiting, and difficulty walking. When calling the adolescent's

mother about the complaints, which of the following would the nurse suggest the mother do *first*?
○ 1. Schedule an appointment with the eye doctor.
○ 2. Begin psychological counseling for her adolescent.
○ 3. Make an appointment with the adolescent's physician.
○ 4. Meet with the adolescent's teachers to determine academic progress.

48. A school-aged child is admitted to the hospital with the diagnosis of probable infratentorial brain tumor. During the child's admission to the pediatric unit, which of the following would the nurse anticipate doing?
○ 1. Eliminating the child's anxiety.
○ 2. Implementing seizure precautions.
○ 3. Introducing the child to other clients of the same age.
○ 4. Preparing the child and parents for diagnostic procedures.

49. After a child undergoes a craniotomy for an infratentorial brain tumor, the nurse positions the child in which of the following positions to prevent undue strain on the sutures?
○ 1. Prone.
○ 2. Semi-Fowler's.
○ 3. Side-lying.
○ 4. Trendelenburg.

50. A child who was intubated after a craniotomy now shows signs of decreased level of consciousness. The physician orders manual hyperventilation to keep the $PaCO_2$ between 25 and 29 mm Hg and the PaO_2 between 80 and 100 mm Hg. The nurse interprets this order based on the understanding that this action will accomplish which of the following?
○ 1. Decrease intracranial pressure.
○ 2. Ensure a patent airway.
○ 3. Lower the arousal level.
○ 4. Produce hypoxia.

51. Which of the following would the nurse do *first* when noting clear drainage on the child's dressing and bed linen after a craniotomy for a brain tumor?
○ 1. Change the dressing.
○ 2. Elevate the head of the bed.
○ 3. Test the fluid for glucose.
○ 4. Notify the physician.

52. An 8-year-old does well after infratentorial tumor removal and is transferred back to the pediatric unit. Although she had been told about having her head shaved for surgery, she is very upset. After exploring the child's feelings, which of the following would the nurse do?
○ 1. Ask the child if she'd like to wear a hat.
○ 2. Reassure the child that her hair will grow back.

○ 3. Explain to the child's parents that her reaction is normal.
○ 4. Suggest that the parents buy the child a wig as a surprise.

53. Which of the following statements made by the mother of a school-aged child who has had a craniotomy for a brain tumor would warrant further exploration by the nurse?
○ 1. "After this, I'll never let her out of my sight again."
○ 2. "I hope that she'll be able to go back to school soon."
○ 3. "I wonder how long it will be before she can ride her bike."
○ 4. "Her best friend is anxious to see her; I hope she won't be upset."

The Client With a Spinal Cord Injury

54. A nurse who witnesses an accident involving an adolescent riding a motorcycle, hitting a tree, and being thrown 30 feet into a field stops to help. The adolescent reports that he is now unable to move his legs. While waiting for the emergency medical service to arrive, which of the following would the nurse do?
○ 1. Flex the adolescent's knees to relieve stress on his back.
○ 2. Leave the adolescent as he is, staying close by.
○ 3. Remove the adolescent's helmet as soon as possible.
○ 4. Assess the adolescent for abdominal trauma.

55. An adolescent sustains a T3 spinal cord injury. After insertion of an intravenous line, a nasogastric tube, and an indwelling urinary (Foley) catheter, the adolescent is admitted to the intensive care unit. Which of the following would the nurse do *next* when assessment reveals that the adolescent's feet and legs are cool to the touch?
○ 1. Cover the adolescent's legs with blankets.
○ 2. Report this finding to the physician immediately.
○ 3. Reposition the adolescent's legs.
○ 4. Lay the adolescent flat to aid circulation.

56. During assessment of an adolescent who has sustained a recent thoracic spinal injury, the nurse auscultates the adolescent's abdomen. The nurse explains to the parents that this is necessary because clients with spinal cord injury often develop which of the following?
○ 1. Abdominal cramping.
○ 2. Hyperactive bowel sounds.
○ 3. Paralytic ileus.
○ 4. Profuse diarrhea.

57. Which of the following findings would lead the nurse to decide that spinal shock was resolving in the adolescent with a spinal cord injury?
    ○ 1. Atonic urinary bladder.
    ○ 2. Flaccid paralysis.
    ○ 3. Hyperactive reflexes.
    ○ 4. Widened pulse pressure.

58. A school-aged boy with a spinal cord injury is moved to the rehabilitation unit. The nurse notes that the child tends to refuse to cooperate in care and to be hostile. The nurse interprets this behavior as indicative of which of the following?
    ○ 1. A stage of grief reaction.
    ○ 2. A phase of rebellion.
    ○ 3. A reaction to sensory overload.
    ○ 4. A response to too much attention.

59. Two months after an adolescent's thoracic spinal cord injury, he complains of a pounding headache. The nurse notes that the client's arms and face are flushed and he is diaphoretic. Which of the following would the nurse do *next*?
    ○ 1. Check the patency of the urinary catheter.
    ○ 2. Lower the adolescent's head below his knees.
    ○ 3. Place the adolescent flat on his back.
    ○ 4. Prepare to administer epinephrine subcutaneously.

Correct Answers and Rationale

The letters in parentheses following the rationale identify the step of the nursing process (A, D, P, I, E) and client needs (1, 2, 3, 4, 5, 6, 7, 8, 9, 10). See the inside front cover for the key.

The Client With Myelomeningocele

1. 1. Clinical manifestations of myelomeningocele are related to the anatomic level of the defect and the nerves involved. An upper lumbar (L1 to L2) myelomeningocele is associated with minimal movement of the lower extremities and dribbling of urine and feces. The upper lumbar area of the spinal cord controls leg flexion at the hip and adduction of the thigh. The sacral area of the spinal cord controls foot and toe movement as well as sphincter and perineal muscle contraction. Upper extremity paralysis would be seen with a cervical spine injury. Rectal prolapse, not urinary bladder prolapse, may occur with myelomeningocele due to lack of innervation to the rectum. Respiratory problems are not associated with an upper level myelomeningocele. (A, 10)

2. 1. The parents should see the neonate as soon as possible, because the longer they must wait to see the neonate, the more anxiety they will feel. Because the parents are acutely aware of the deficit, the nurse should emphasize the neonate's normal and positive features during the visit. All parents, but especially those with a child who has a disability or defect, need to hear positive comments and comments that reflect how the infant is normal. Although the parents need to discuss their fears and concerns, the priority on the first visit is to emphasize the neonate's normal and positive features. Reinforcing the doctor's explanation of the defect may be necessary later. Reinforcing the explanation at this initial visit emphasizes the defect, not the child. The parents should spend time with or care for the neonate after birth because parent-infant contact is necessary for attachment. The parents cannot feed the neonate before the defect is repaired because the repair typically occurs within 24 hours. The infant will be prone in an isolette or warmed and watched closely. However, the parents can fondle and stroke the neonate. (P, 5)

3. 1. Excessive cerebrospinal fluid in the cranial cavity, hydrocephalus, is the most common anomaly associated with myelomeningocele. Microencephaly, an abnormally small head, is associated with maternal exposure to rubella or cytomegalovirus. Anencephaly, a congenital absence of the cranial vault, is a different type of neural tube defect. Overriding of the sutures, possibly a normal finding after a vaginal delivery, is not associated with myelomeningocele. (I, 9)

4. 1. Approximately one third of infants diagnosed with myelomeningocele are mentally retarded, but the degree of retardation is variable and it is difficult to predict intellectual functioning in neonates. The parents are asking for an answer now and should not be told to talk with the physician later. (I, 10)

5. 2. The nurse places the neonate with myelomeningocele in an isolette shortly after birth to help to maintain the infant's temperature. Because of the defect, the neonate cannot be bundled in blankets. Therefore, it may be difficult to prevent cold stress. The isolette can be maintained at higher than room temperature, helping to maintain the temperature of a neonate who cannot be dressed or bundled. Body temperature readings, not arterial oxygen levels, are the best indicator. Typically, an infant loses 5% to 10% of body weight before beginning to regain the weight. (E, 9)

6. 3. Before surgery, the infant is kept flat in the prone position to decrease tension on the sac. This allows for optimal positioning of the hips, knees, and feet because orthopedic problems are common. The supine position is unacceptable because it causes pressure on the defect. (I, 10)

7. 2. Because of the potential for hip dislocation, the neonate's legs should be slightly abducted, hips maintained in slight to moderate abduction, and feet maintained in a neutral position. The infant's knees are flexed to help maintain the hips in abduction. (P, 10)

8. 3. In a neonate with open cranial sutures, increasing head circumference is the predominant and earliest sign of increased intracranial pressure. Bulging fontanels also are seen. However, some neonates may exhibit bulging fontanels without head enlargement. Seizures and vomiting are associated with hydrocephalus, but most often these are seen in an older child with closed cranial sutures. Shortly after increasing head circumference and bulging fontanels occur, other signs and symptoms, such as frontal bossing or enlargement with depressed eyes and the sunset sign (sclera visible above the iris), may develop. Although irritability is an early sign, a brief, shrill cry is a later sign of increasing intracranial pressure associated with the development of hydrocephalus. (A, 9)

9. 4. The most important aspect of the discharge plan is to ensure that the parents understand what the daily care of their infant involves and to provide teaching related to carrying out this daily care. In addition to the routine care required by the infant, care also may include physical therapy to the lower extremities. Providing a list of available hospital services may be helpful to the parents, but it is not the most important aspect to include in the discharge plan. Usually, home health care is not needed because the parents are able to care for their child. A referral for counseling is initiated whenever the need arises, not just at discharge. (P, 10)

10. 3. All children with myelomeningocele are prone to urinary tract infections. Because of the level of the defect, sensory impairment is present and the child is unaware of bladder discomfort. Similarly, the child is insensitive to pressure and other sources of tissue damage, such as heat. Using a heating pad could lead to thermal injury. The immune system is not affected with a myelomeningocele. Keeping the infant away from other infants would be unnecessary. Additionally, the infant needs the stimulation of others for adequate growth and development. Activities that encourage body consciousness, such as rolling over, are encouraged. Because the defect has been repaired, there is no need to keep the infant off his back. (E, 9)

11. 3. Children with myelomeningocele are at high risk for development of latex allergy because of repeated exposure to latex products during surgery and bladder catheterizations. Cross-reactions to food items such as bananas, kiwi, milk products, chestnuts, and avocados also occur. These allergic reactions vary in severity ranging from mild such as sneezing to severe anaphylaxis. (A, 9)

The Client With Hydrocephalus

12. 2. An infant with hydrocephalus is difficult to feed because of poor sucking, lethargy, and vomiting, which are associated with increased intracranial pressure. Small, frequent feedings given at times when the infant is relaxed and calm are tolerated best. Feeding an infant before any procedure is inappropriate because the stress of the procedure may lead to vomiting. Ideally, the infant should be held in a slightly vertical position when feeding to prevent backflow of formula into the eustachian tubes and subsequent development of ear infections. Most infants are fed on demand every 3 to 4 hours. (I, 7)

13. 4. For at least the first 24 hours after insertion of a ventriculoperitoneal shunt, the child is positioned supine with the head of the bed flat to prevent too rapid a decrease in cerebrospinal fluid pressure. Although elevating the head increases cerebrospinal fluid drainage and reduces intracranial pressure, a rapid reduction in the size of the ventricles can cause subdural hematoma. Positioning on the operative or right side is avoided because it places pressure on the shunt valve, possibly blocking desired drainage of the cerebrospinal fluid. Elevating the foot of the bed could increase intracranial pressure. With continued increased intracranial pressure, the child would be positioned with the head of the bed elevated to allow gravity to aid drainage. The child should be kept off the nonoperative side (side opposite the shunt), or the left side, to help prevent rapid decompression leading to a cerebral hematoma. (P, 10)

14. 3. Monitoring the temperature allows the nurse to assess for infection, the most common and most hazardous postoperative complication after ventroperitoneal shunt placement. Typically, pain after insertion of a ventriculoperitoneal shunt is mild, requiring the use of mild analgesics. Usually narcotics are not administered because they alter the level of consciousness, making assessment of cerebral function difficult. Neither proteinuria nor glycosuria is associated with shunt placement. Cerebrospinal fluid leakage commonly occurs with head injury. It is not usually associated with shunt placement. (I, 10)

15. 4. In a school-aged child, irritability, lethargy, vomiting, difficulty with eating, and decreased level of consciousness are signs of increased intracranial pressure caused by a blocked shunt. Decreased urine output with stable fluid intake indicates fluid loss from a source other than the kidneys. A tense fontanel and increased head circumference would be signs of a blocked shunt in an infant. Elevated temperature and redness around incisions might suggest an infection. (E, 9)

The Client With Down Syndrome

16. 1. The goal in working with mentally retarded children is to train them to be as independent as possible, focusing on developmental skills. The child may not be capable of learning something new every day but needs to repeat what has been taught previously. Rather than encouraging more lenient behavior limits, the parents need to be strict and consistent when setting limits for the child. Most children with Down syndrome are unable to achieve age-appropriate social skills due to their mental retardation. Rather, they are taught socially appropriate behaviors. (P, 4)

17. 4. Nonthreatening experiences that are stimulating and interesting to the child have been observed to help raise IQ. Practices such as serving nutritious meals or letting the child play with more able children have not been supported by research as beneficial in increasing intelligence. Vasodilator medications act to increase oxygenation to the tissues, including the brain. However, these medications do not increase the child's IQ. (I, 3)

18. 3. It is especially important to observe the nature of the child's respirations because children with Down syndrome are prone to develop respiratory infections. Weight loss usually is not a problem for children with Down syndrome. An irregular heart rate and increased blood pressure may be associated with children with Down syndrome and cardiac problems. (A, 10)

19. 4. When teaching the parents of a child with Down syndrome, activities should focus on increasing the parents' confidence in their ability to care for the child. The parents must continue to work daily with their child. Most parents feel affection and a sense of responsibility for their child regardless of the child's limitations. Parents usually understand the child's disability on the cognitive level but have difficulty accepting it on the emotional level. As the parents' confidence in their caring abilities increases, their understanding of the child's disability also increases on all levels. (P, 5)

20. 4. When responding to a mother who becomes angry when someone calls her child mentally retarded instead of exceptional, the nurse should give the mother a chance to explore her feelings on the subject. Because the mother obviously has difficulty with the term "retarded," stressing the use of this term would cause further angry feelings. Apologizing, trying to use logic, and defending the comment are not effective ways to handle the situation because the mother's feelings need to be addressed. (I, 5)

The Client With a Seizure Disorder

21. 3. During a generalized tonic-clonic seizure, the first priority is to keep the child safe and protect the child by removing any nearby objects that could cause injury. Although obtaining information about events surrounding the seizure is important, this information can be obtained later, once the child's safety is ensured. During a seizure, the child should not be moved. Although providing privacy is important, the child's safety is the priority. Once a seizure begins and during a seizure, nothing should be forced into the client's mouth because this can cause severe damage to the teeth and mouth. (E, 10)

22. 3. Most children who develop seizures after infancy are intellectually normal. A child with seizure disorders needs the same experiences and opportunities to develop intellectual, emotional, and social abilities as

any other child. Activity limitation is not needed. Learning disabilities are not associated with seizures. The child is able to attend public school, and social stigma is a rarity. (I, 3)

23. 1. A child who has generalized seizures should not participate in activities that are potentially hazardous. Even if accompanied by a responsible adult, the child could be seriously injured if a seizure were to occur during rock climbing. Someone also should accompany the child during activities in or on the water. At summer camp, hiking and swimming would occur most commonly as group activities, so someone would be with the child. Tennis would be considered an appropriate, nonhazardous activity for a child with generalized seizures. (P, 2)

24. 4. Most febrile seizures occur in the presence of an upper respiratory infection, otitis media, or tonsillitis. Febrile seizures typically occur during a temperature rise rather than after prolonged fever. There appears to be increased susceptibility to febrile seizures within families. Infrequently, febrile seizures may lead to respiratory arrest. (D, 10)

25. 2. Shivering, the body's defense against rapid temperature decrease, results in an increase in body temperature. Therefore the parents need to take measures to stop the shivering (and increase body temperature) by increasing the room temperature or the temperature of the child's immediate environment (such as with blankets) until the shivering stops. Then, attempts are made to lower the temperature more slowly. Shivering does not necessarily correlate with being cold. Alcohol, a toxic substance, can be absorbed through the skin. Its use is to be avoided. (E, 10)

26. 3. Phenytoin sodium (Dilantin) is a known teratogenic agent, causing numerous fetal problems. Therefore the adolescent should be advised to talk to the doctor about changing the medication. Additionally, anticonvulsant requirements usually increase during pregnancy. Seizures can be controlled but cannot be cured. There is a familial tendency for seizure disorders. Seizure disorders and infertility are not related. (I, 8)

27. 3. A toxic effect of valproic acid (Depakene) is liver toxicity, which may manifest with jaundice and abdominal pain. If jaundice occurs, the client needs to notify the health care provider as soon as possible. Diarrhea and sore throat are not common side effects of this drug. Increased appetite is common with this drug. (I, 8)

The Client With Meningitis

28. 2. A child in the acute stage of meningitis is irritable and hypersensitive to loud noise and light. Therefore,

extraneous noise should be minimized and bright lights avoided as much as possible. There is no need to limit conversations with the child. However, the nurse should speak in a calm, gentle, reassuring voice. The child needs gentle and calm bathing. Because of the acuteness of the infection, sponge baths would be more appropriate than tub baths. Although treatments need to be completed as quickly as possible to prevent overstressing the child, any treatments should be performed carefully and at a pace that avoids sudden movements to prevent startling the child and subsequently increasing intracranial pressure. (I, 7)

29. 1. Disseminated intravascular coagulation is characterized by skin petechiae and a purpuric skin rash caused by spontaneous bleeding into the tissues. An abnormal coagulation phenomenon causes the condition. Heparin therapy is often used to interrupt the clotting process. Edema would suggest a fluid volume excess. Cyanosis would indicate decreased tissue oxygenation. Dyspnea on exertion would suggest respiratory problems, such as pulmonary edema. (A, 10)

30. 2. Organisms that cause bacterial meningitis, such as pneumococci or meningococci, are commonly spread in the body by vascular dissemination from a middle ear infection. The meningitis may also be a direct extension from the paranasal and mastoid sinuses. The causative organism is a pneumococcus. A chronically draining ear is frequently also found. Bladder infections commonly are caused by *Escherichia coli*, unrelated to the development of pneumococcal meningitis. Pneumococcal meningitis is unrelated to a fractured clavicle or to septic arthritis, which is commonly caused by *Staphylococcus aureus*, group A streptococci, or *Haemophilus influenzae*. (A, 10)

31. 3. Preschool-aged children worry about having an intact body and become fearful of any threat to body integrity. Allowing the child to participate in required care helps protect her image of an intact body. Development of trust is the task typically associated with infancy. Additionally, allowing the child to apply a dressing over the intravenous insertion site is unrelated to the development of trust. Finding diversional activities is not a priority need for a child in this age group. Separation anxiety is more common in toddlers than in preschoolers. (D, 3)

32. 3. The child is angry and needs a positive outlet for expression of feelings. An emotionally tense child with pent-up hostilities needs a physical activity that will release energy and frustration. Pounding on a pegboard offers this opportunity. Listening to a story does not allow the child to express emotions. It also places the child in a passive role and does not allow the child to deal with feelings in a healthy and positive way. Activities such as painting and stacking a tower of

blocks require concentration and fine movements, which could add to frustration. However, if the child then knocks the tower over, doing so may help to dispel some of the anger. (I, 3)

The Client With Near-Drowning

33. 2. Hypoxia is the primary problem because it results in brain cell damage. Irreversible brain damage occurs after 4 to 6 minutes of submersion. Hypothermia occurs rapidly in infants and children because of their large body surface area. Hypothermia is more of a problem when the child is in cold water. Although fluid aspiration occurs in most drownings and results in atelectasis and pulmonary edema further aggravating hypoxia, hypoxia is the primary problem. Cutaneous capillary paralysis is not a problem. (A, 10)

34. 1. When a child experiences near-drowning, respiratory acidosis occurs secondary to the retention of carbon dioxide from inadequate pulmonary ventilation, and metabolic acidosis occurs secondary to the buildup of acid metabolites from anaerobic metabolism resulting from tissue hypoxia. (A, 9)

35. 2. Guilt is a common parental response. The parents need to be allowed to express their feelings openly in a nonthreatening, nonjudgmental atmosphere. Telling the parents that these things happen does not allow them to verbalize their feelings. Telling the parents that they should not have taken their eyes off the child blames them, possibly further contributing to their guilt. Telling the parents that they shouldn't feel guilty denies the parents' feelings of guilt and is inappropriate. Telling the parents that they are lucky that the child will be okay does not remove the feelings of guilt. (I, 5)

The Client With Guillain-Barré Syndrome (Infectious Polyneuritis)

36. 1. Most children with sore throat have some difficulty swallowing, so it is important for the nurse to determine the extent of difficulty to aid in determining what action is necessary. Typically a sore throat precedes the paralysis of this disorder. Muscle tenderness is an initial symptom. Distal muscle weakness follows proximal muscle weakness, ultimately progressing to paralysis. (A, 4)

37. 2. With Guillain-Barré syndrome, progressive ascending paralysis occurs. Therefore, the nurse should assess the child's muscle strength bilaterally to determine the extent of involvement and progression of the illness. Assessing the child's ability to follow simple commands evaluates brain function. Range-of-motion exercises are an important part of treatment, but they are not a priority initially. Although the child may need

diversional activities later, they also are not a priority initially. (A, 10)

38. 3. In a child with Guillain-Barré syndrome, decreased volume and clarity of speech and decreased ability to cough voluntarily indicate ascending progression of neural inflammation, specifically affecting the cranial nerves. Inflammation of the larynx and epiglottis is manifested by hoarseness, stridor, and dyspnea. A child with laryngeal inflammation still retains the ability to cough. Irritability, behavior changes, headache, and vomiting are common signs of increased intracranial pressure in a school-aged child. Regression would be manifested by being more dependent and less able to care for self. (D, 10)

39. 2. Ineffective Breathing Pattern caused by the ascending paralysis of the disorder interferes with the child's ability to maintain an adequate oxygen supply. Therefore, this nursing diagnosis takes precedence. Additionally, as the neurologic impairment progresses, it will probably have an effect on the child's ability to maintain respirations. Risk for Infection related to an altered immune system is not involved with Guillian-Barré syndrome. Although impaired swallowing and incontinence may occur with the ascending paralysis of this disorder, oxygenation is the priority. (D, 10)

40. 4. Even in the absence of respiratory problems or distress, the child must be turned frequently to help prevent the cardiopulmonary complications associated with immobility, such as atelectasis and pneumonia. Maintaining the child in a supine position is unnecessary. Doing so does not prevent unnecessary nerve stimulation. In addition, maintaining a supine position may lead to stasis of secretions, placing the child at risk for pneumonia. Transferring the child to a chair will not prevent orthostatic hypotension. However, doing so will increase vascular tone and help prevent respiratory and skin complications. During the acute disease phase, vigorous physiotherapy is contraindicated because the child may experience muscle pain and be hypersensitive to touch. Careful and gentle handling is essential. (I, 10)

41. 3. Developmentally appropriate activities and therapeutic play should be used as rehabilitation modalities. Taking the child to the pool to exercise with other children indicates that the child is participating in exercise as well as engaging with other children, thus fostering development. Arguing with the sister does not address the discharge plan. Inappropriate rewards or threats should not be used to coerce a child into compliance. Although the mother is attempting to comply with the discharge plan, bribery is an inappropriate technique to foster compliance. Missing therapy sessions delays recovery. The parents need to help set the child's sched-

ule to ensure that she gets adequate rest to be able to follow her treatment plan. (E, 10)

The Client With a Head Injury

42. 2. For the child with serious head trauma, a nasogastric tube is inserted initially to decompress the stomach and to prevent vomiting and aspiration. Medications would be administered intravenously in the initial period. Nutrition is not a priority initially. Later on, the tube may be used to administer feedings. (P, 9)

43. 1. Because a basilar skull fracture can involve the frontal and ethmoid bones, inserting a nasogastric tube carries the risk of introducing the tube into the cranial cavity through the fracture. An oral gastric tube is preferred for a client with a basilar skull fracture. The tube would not be placed into the duodenum. Gastric aspirate is not routinely tested for blood unless there is an indication to suggest bleeding, such as a falling hemoglobin or visible blood in the drainage. (I, 9)

44. 3. As a rule, children demonstrate more rapid and more complete recovery from coma than do adults. However, it is extremely difficult to predict a specific outcome. Reassuring the parents that they will be kept informed helps open lines of communication and establish trust. Telling the parents that children do not do well would be extremely negative, destroying any hope that the parents might have. Telling the parents that children recover rapidly may give the parents false hopes. Telling the parents to talk to the doctor ignores the parents' concerns and interferes with trust-building. (I, 10)

45. 2. The unconscious child is positioned to prevent aspiration of saliva and minimize intracranial pressure. The head of the bed should be elevated, and the child should be in either the semiprone or the side-lying position. Lying prone with hips and knees slightly elevated increases intracranial pressure, as does lying on the back in the Trendelenburg position. The semi-Fowler's position with arms at the side is not the best choice. (P, 10)

46. 2. Mannitol is an osmotic diuretic used to help decrease intracranial pressure by decreasing cerebral edema. Fluid would be eliminated, not held in the vascular bed. Although mannitol does contribute to the calorie intake of the child, it is used for its diuretic effect. Mannitol has no effect on bacteria. (I, 8)

The Client With a Brain Tumor

47. 3. A child who has symptoms of vomiting, headaches, and problems walking needs to be evaluated by a health care provider to determine the cause. Unex-

plained headaches and vomiting along with complaints of difficulty walking (eg, ataxia) may suggest a brain tumor. Evaluation by an eye doctor would be appropriate once a complete medical evaluation has been accomplished. Psychological counseling may be indicated for this adolescent, but only after medical evaluation to determine that she is physically healthy. Meeting with the child's teachers would be appropriate after medical evaluation. (I, 10)

48. 4. When a brain tumor is suspected, the child and parents are likely to be very apprehensive and anxious. It is unrealistic to expect to eliminate their fears; rather, the nurse's goal is to decrease them. Preparing both the child and family during hospitalization can help them cope with some of their fears. Although the nurse may be able to decrease some of the child's anxiety, it would be impossible to eliminate it. Children with infratentorial tumors seldom have seizures, so seizure precautions are not indicated. Although introducing the child to other children is a positive action, this action would be more appropriate once the nurse has decreased some of the child's and parents' anxiety by preparing them. (I, 5)

49. 3. After surgery for an infratentorial tumor, the child is usually positioned flat on either side, with the head and neck in midline and the body slightly extended. Pillows against the back, not the head, help maintain position. Such a position helps avoid pressure on the operative site. The Trendelenburg position is usually contraindicated because keeping the head below the level of the heart increases intracranial pressure as well as the risk of hemorrhage. (I, 10)

50. 1. Hypercapnia, hypoxia, and acidosis are potent cerebral vasodilating mechanisms that can cause increased intracranial pressure. Lowering the carbon dioxide level and increasing the oxygen level through hyperventilation is the most effective short-term method of reducing intracranial pressure. Although ensuring a patent airway is important, this is not accomplished by manual hyperventilation. Manual hyperventilation does not lower the arousal level; in fact, the arousal level may increase. Manual hyperventilation is used to reduce hypoxia, not produce it. (D, 9)

51. 3. Glucose in this clear, colorless fluid indicates the presence of cerebrospinal fluid. Excessive fluid leakage should be reported to the physician. The nurse should not change the dressing of a postoperative craniotomy client unless instructed to do so by the surgeon. Ordinarily, the head of the bed would not be elevated because this would put pressure on the sutures. The nurse should notify the physician after testing the fluid for glucose. (I, 9)

52. 1. It is not uncommon for a child to be concerned about a change in appearance when the entire head or only

part of the head has been shaved. The child should be encouraged to participate in decisions about her care when possible. Asking her if she would like to wear a hat is one way to encourage this participation. Reassuring the child that her hair will grow back does not address the immediate change in appearance, and it ignores the child's current feelings. Explaining that this type of reaction is normal does not address the child's feelings. The child needs to be able to express feelings and be involved in care as much as possible. Buying the child a wig as a surprise does not address the child's feelings and does not allow her to participate in decision making. Rather, the parents should ask the child if she would like a wig and then work with the child to determine what kind of wig she would like. (I, 5)

53. 1. Parents of a child who has undergone neurosurgery can easily become overprotective. Yet the parents must foster independence in the convalescing child. It is important for the child to resume age-appropriate activities, and parents play an important role in encouraging this. Statements about going back to school would be expected. Parents want the child to return to normal activities after a serious illness or injury as a sign that the child is doing well. (D, 5)

The Client With a Spinal Cord Injury

54. 2. The adolescent's signs and symptoms suggest a spinal cord injury. A client with suspected spinal cord injury should not be moved until the spine has been immobilized. Removing the helmet could further aggravate a spinal cord injury. The nurse could assess for abdominal trauma, but only if it can be done without moving the adolescent. (I, 9)

55. 1. In spinal cord injury, temperature regulation is lost below T3. Body temperature must be maintained by adjusting room temperature or bed linens, such as covering the client's legs with blankets. Coolness of the extremities is an expected finding. Therefore, it is not necessary to notify the physician immediately. Repositioning the client's legs does not alleviate the temperature regulation problem and could be harmful, considering the client's diagnosis. Moving the legs before the spine is stabilized could lead to further cord damage. Laying the client flat will not increase the warmth to the legs and feet. (I, 10)

56. 3. A thoracic spinal cord injury involves the muscles of the lower extremities, bladder, and rectum. Paralytic ileus often occurs as a result of decreased gastrointestinal muscle innervation. The nurse evaluates this by auscultating the abdomen. Because the client has a thoracic spinal cord injury, the client may not feel abdominal cramping. Additionally, auscultation would provide no evidence of cramping. Hyperactive bowel

sounds would be evidenced with increased peristalsis; peristalsis would probably be diminished with this injury. Profuse diarrhea, resulting from increased peristalsis, would not be an expected finding. Diarrhea would be more commonly associated with a gastrointestinal infection. (I, 10)

57. 3. Spinal shock causes a loss of reflex activity below the level of the injury, resulting in bladder atony and flaccid paralysis. When the reflex arc returns, it tends to be overactive, resulting in spasticity. The reflexes and bladder becomes hypertonic during this phase of spinal shock resolution; sensation does not return. A widened pulse pressure is not associated with resolution of spinal shock. (A, 10)

58. 1. After a catastrophic injury, individuals commonly experience grief. Initially, the person experiences denial, the most common response. With gradual awareness of the situation, anger commonly occurs. The child is demonstrating anger, not rebellion, as he gradually becomes aware of his situation. Rebellion is the child's way to maintain autonomy and individuality. It is a reaction to rigid rules. Examples include refusing to follow a treatment protocol when the child had no input and running away. Sensory overload would cause the child to be irritable and tired and to have difficulty sleeping. Too much attention usually would lead to irritability, difficulty sleeping, and mood swings. (D, 5)

59. 1. The adolescent is exhibiting signs of autonomic dysreflexia, a generalized sympathetic response usually caused by bladder or bowel distention. Immediate treatment involves eliminating the cause. Because bladder distention is a common cause of this problem, the nurse should immediately determine the patency of the indwelling (Foley) catheter. Lying flat will not decrease blood pressure. Epinephrine is contraindicated because it elevates blood pressure and therefore can exacerbate the problem. (I, 10)

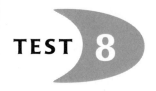
The Child With Musculoskeletal Health Problems

Select the one best answer, and indicate your choice by filling in the circle in front of the option.

The Client With Musculoskeletal Dysfunction

1. A child who limps and complains of pain has been found to have Legg-Calvé-Perthes disease. Which of the following would the nurse expect to include in the child's plan of care?
   - ○ 1. Initiation of pain control measures, especially at night when acute.
   - ○ 2. Promotion of ambulation despite child's discomfort in the affected hip.
   - ○ 3. Prevention of flexion in the affected hip and knee.
   - ○ 4. Avoidance of weight bearing on the head of the affected femur.

2. When planning home care for the child with Legg-Calvé-Perthes disease, which of the following would be the primary focus for family teaching?
   - ○ 1. Need for intake of protein-rich foods.
   - ○ 2. Gentle stretching exercises for both legs.
   - ○ 3. Management of the corrective appliance.
   - ○ 4. Relaxation techniques for pain control.

3. A characteristic abnormality in which of the following would lead the nurse to suspect that an infant has torticollis (wry neck)?
   - ○ 1. Quadriceps.
   - ○ 2. Cervical vertebrae.
   - ○ 3. Trapezius muscle.
   - ○ 4. Sternocleidomastoid muscle.

4. When assessing a female adolescent for scoliosis, the nurse would ask the client to do which of the following?
   - ○ 1. Bend forward at the waist with arms hanging freely.
   - ○ 2. Lie flat on the floor and extend her legs straight from the trunk.
   - ○ 3. Sit in a chair while lifting her feet and legs to a right angle with the trunk.
   - ○ 4. Stand against a wall while pressing the length of her back against the wall.

5. After teaching the family of a child with scoliosis who needs to wear a Boston brace, which of the following activities, if stated by the child and family as occasions appropriate for removal of the brace, indicates successful teaching?
   - ○ 1. When bathing, for about 1 hour per day.
   - ○ 2. While eating, for a total of 3 hours a day.
   - ○ 3. During school, for about 8 hours a day.
   - ○ 4. When sleeping, for a total of 10 hours a day.

6. When teaching the child with scoliosis being treated with a Boston brace about exercises, the nurse explains that the exercises are performed *primarily* for which of the following purposes?
   - ○ 1. To decrease back muscle spasms.
   - ○ 2. To improve the brace's traction effect.
   - ○ 3. To prevent spinal contractures.
   - ○ 4. To strengthen the back and abdominal muscles.

7. An adolescent tells the school nurse that the area below his knee has been hurting for several weeks. The nurse would obtain history information about participation in which of the following?
   - ○ 1. Soccer.
   - ○ 2. Golf.
   - ○ 3. Diving.
   - ○ 4. Swimming.

8. An adolescent is on the football team and practices

in the morning and afternoon before school starts for the year. The temperature on the field has been high. The school nurse has been called to the practice field because the adolescent is now complaining of muscle cramps, nausea, and dizziness. Which of the following actions would the school nurse do *next*?
- ○ 1. Administer cold water with ice cubes.
- ○ 2. Take the adolescent's temperature.
- ○ 3. Have the adolescent go to the swimming pool.
- ○ 4. Move the adolescent to a cool environment.

The Client With Cerebral Palsy

9. The mother of a toddler with cerebral palsy comes to the clinic for developmental screening. The nurse explains that the *major* reason that these tests are done is to recognize primary delays early so as to accomplish which of the following?
   - ○ 1. Encourage health maintenance.
   - ○ 2. Facilitate communication.
   - ○ 3. Prevent secondary developmental delays.
   - ○ 4. Maintain current development.
10. The nurse judges that the mother understands the term *cerebral palsy* when she describes it as a term applied to impaired movement resulting from which of the following?
    - ○ 1. Injury to the cerebrum caused by viral infection.
    - ○ 2. Malformed blood vessels in the ventricles caused by inheritance.
    - ○ 3. Nonprogressive brain damage caused by injury.
    - ○ 4. Inflammatory brain disease caused by metabolic imbalances.
11. When assessing the development of a 15-month-old with cerebral palsy, which of the following milestones would the nurse expect a toddler of this age to have achieved?
    - ○ 1. Walking up steps.
    - ○ 2. Using a spoon.
    - ○ 3. Copying a circle.
    - ○ 4. Putting a block in cup.
12. The mother asks the nurse whether her child with hemiparesis due to spastic cerebral palsy will be able to walk normally because he can pull himself to a standing position. Which of the following responses by the nurse would be *most* appropriate?
    - ○ 1. "Ask the doctor what he thinks at your next appointment."
    - ○ 2. "Maybe, maybe not. How old were you when you first walked?"
    - ○ 3. "It's difficult to predict, but his ability to bear weight is a positive factor."

- ○ 4. "If he really wants to walk, and works hard, he probably will eventually."
13. The nurse assesses the family's ability to cope with the child's cerebral palsy. Which of the following would alert the nurse to the possibility of their inability to cope with the disease?
    - ○ 1. Limiting interaction with extended family and friends.
    - ○ 2. Learning measures to meet the child's physical needs.
    - ○ 3. Requesting teaching about cerebral palsy in general.
    - ○ 4. Not seeking financial help to pay for medical bills.

The Client With Duchenne's Muscular Dystrophy

14. The mother of a child with Duchenne's muscular dystrophy asks about the chance that her next child will have the disease. The nurse responds based on the understanding of which of the following?
    - ○ 1. Sons have a 50% chance of being affected.
    - ○ 2. Daughters have a 1 in 4 chance of being carriers.
    - ○ 3. Each child has a 25% chance of developing the disease.
    - ○ 4. Each child has a 50% chance of being a carrier.
15. A home health nurse is making an initial visit to a family with a 3-year-old with early Duchenne's muscular dystrophy. Which of the following would the nurse *most* likely expect to assess with this child?
    - ○ 1. Contractures of the large joints.
    - ○ 2. Enlarged calf muscles.
    - ○ 3. Difficulty riding a tricycle.
    - ○ 4. Small, weak muscles.
16. The nurse observes as a child with Duchenne's muscular dystrophy attempts to rise from a sitting position on the floor. After attaining a kneeling position, the child "walks" his hands up his legs to stand. The nurse documents this as which of the following?
    - ○ 1. Galeazzi's sign.
    - ○ 2. Goodell's sign.
    - ○ 3. Goodenough's sign.
    - ○ 4. Gower's sign.
17. When developing the plan of care for a child with early Duchenne's muscular dystrophy, which of the following would the nurse identify as the *primary* nursing goal for the child?
    - ○ 1. Encouraging early wheelchair use.
    - ○ 2. Fostering social interactions.
    - ○ 3. Maintaining function of unaffected muscles.
    - ○ 4. Prevent circulatory impairment.

18. When interacting with the mother of a child who has Duchenne's muscular dystrophy, the nurse observes behavior indicating that the mother may feel guilty about her child's condition. The nurse interprets this behavior as guilt stemming from which of the following?
    ○ 1. The terminal nature of the disease.
    ○ 2. The dependent behavior of the child.
    ○ 3. The genetic mode of transmission.
    ○ 4. The sudden onset of the disease.

19. The nurse teaches the mother of a young child with Duchenne's muscular dystrophy about the disease and its management. Which of the following statements by the mother indicates successful teaching?
    ○ 1. "My son will probably be unable to walk independently by the time he is 9 to 11 years old."
    ○ 2. "Muscle relaxants are effective for some children; I hope they can help my son."
    ○ 3. "When my son is a little older, he can have surgery to improve his ability to walk."
    ○ 4. "I need to help my son be as active as possible to prevent progression of the disease."

The Client With Developmental Dysplasia of the Hip

20. A 16-month-old is seen in the clinic for a check-up for the first time. The nurse notices that the toddler limps when walking. Which of the following would be appropriate to use when assessing this toddler for developmental dysplasia of the hip?
    ○ 1. Ortolani's maneuver.
    ○ 2. Barlow's maneuver.
    ○ 3. Adam's position.
    ○ 4. Trendelenburg's sign.

21. The nurse is assessing the infant shown in Figure 1. On observing the client from this angle, the nurse should document that this infant has which of the following?

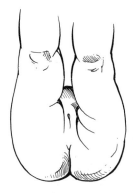

Figure 1.

○ 1. Ortolani's "click."
○ 2. Limited abduction.
○ 3. Galeazzi's sign.
○ 4. Asymmetric gluteal folds.

22. The nurse teaches the parents of an infant with developmental dysplasia of the hip how to handle their child in a Pavlik harness. Which of the following interventions would be *most* appropriate?
    ○ 1. Fitting the diaper under the straps.
    ○ 2. Leaving the harness off while the infant sleeps.
    ○ 3. Checking for skin redness under straps every other day.
    ○ 4. Putting powder on the skin under the straps every day.

23. When developing the teaching plan for parents using the Pavlik harness with their child, which of the following would be the nurse's *initial* step?
    ○ 1. Assessing the parents' current coping strategies.
    ○ 2. Determining the parents' knowledge about the device.
    ○ 3. Providing the parents with written instructions.
    ○ 4. Giving the parents a list of community resources.

24. When teaching the family of an older infant who has had a hip spica cast applied for developmental dysplasia of the hip, which of the following would the nurse include when describing the abduction stabilizer bar?
    ○ 1. It can be adjusted to a position of comfort.
    ○ 2. It is used to lift the child.
    ○ 3. It adds strength to the cast.
    ○ 4. It is necessary to turn the child.

25. The mother asks the nurse about using a car seat for her toddler who is in a hip spica cast. Which of the following would be the nurse's *best* reply?
    ○ 1. "You can use a seat belt because of the spica cast."
    ○ 2. "You will need a specially designed car seat for your toddler."
    ○ 3. "You can still use the car seat you already have."
    ○ 4. "You'll need to get a special release from the police so that a car seat won't be needed."

The Client With Congenital Clubfoot

26. The parents of a neonate born with congenital clubfoot express feelings of helplessness and guilt, exhibiting anxiety about how the neonate will be treated. Which of the following actions by the nurse would be *most* appropriate initially?
    ○ 1. Ask them to share these concerns with the physician.

213

○ 2. Arrange a meeting with other parents whose infants have had successful clubfoot treatment.

○ 3. Discuss with them the problem and the current feelings that the parents are experiencing.

○ 4. Suggest that they make an appointment to talk things over with a counselor.

27. After teaching the parents of an infant with clubfoot requiring application of a plaster cast how to care for the cast, which of the following statements would indicate that the parents have understood the teaching?

○ 1. "If the cast becomes soiled, we'll clean it with soap and water."

○ 2. "We'll elevate the leg with the cast on pillows, so the leg is above heart level."

○ 3. "We will check the color and temperature of the toes of the casted leg frequently."

○ 4. "The petals on the edge of the cast can be removed after the first 24 hours."

The Client With Juvenile Rheumatoid Arthritis

28. The father of a preschool-aged child with a tentative diagnosis of juvenile rheumatoid arthritis (JRA) asks about a test to definitively diagnose JRA. The nurse's response is based on knowledge of which of the following?

○ 1. The latex fixation test is diagnostic.

○ 2. An increased erythrocyte sedimentation rate is diagnostic.

○ 3. A positive synovial fluid culture is diagnostic.

○ 4. No specific laboratory test is diagnostic.

29. The parents of a child just diagnosed with JRA tell the nurse that the diagnosis frightens them because they know nothing about the prognosis. Which of the following would the nurse include when teaching the parents about the disease?

○ 1. Half of affected children recover without joint deformity.

○ 2. Many affected children go into long remissions but have severe deformities.

○ 3. The disease usually progresses to crippling rheumatoid arthritis.

○ 4. Most affected children recover completely within a few years.

30. The mother of a 4-year-old with JRA is worried that her child will have to stop attending preschool because of the illness. Which of the following responses by the nurse would be *most* appropriate?

○ 1. "It may be difficult for your child to attend school because of the side effects of the medications he will be prescribed."

○ 2. "You child should be encouraged to attend school, but he'll need extra time to work out early-morning stiffness."

○ 3. "You should keep your child at home from school whenever he experiences discomfort or pain in his joints."

○ 4. "Your child will probably need to wear splints and braces so that his joints will be supported properly."

31. A preschool-aged child with JRA has become withdrawn, and the mother asks the nurse what she should do. Which of the following suggestions by the nurse would be *most* appropriate?

○ 1. Introduce the child to other children her age who also have JRA.

○ 2. Tell the mother to spend extra time with the child and less time with her other children.

○ 3. Recommend that the mother send the child to see a counselor for therapy.

○ 4. Encourage the mother to be supportive and understanding of the child.

32. Which of the following would the nurse include when developing the teaching plan for the parents of a child with JRA who is being treated with aspirin?

○ 1. Anti-inflammatory effect will occur in approximately 8 weeks.

○ 2. Within 24 hours, the child will have anti-inflammatory relief.

○ 3. The nurse should be called before giving the child any over-the-counter medications.

○ 4. If a dose is forgotten or missed, that dose is not made up.

The Client With a Fracture

33. A child is admitted with a fracture of the femur and placed in skeletal traction. Which of the following would the nurse assess *first*?

○ 1. The pull of traction on the pin.

○ 2. The Ace bandage.

○ 3. The pin sites for signs of infection.

○ 4. The dressings for tightness.

34. An infant with a fractured femur of the left leg is placed in traction, as shown in Figure 2. The nurse should

○ 1. place a pillow under the infant's buttocks to provide support.

○ 2. remove the weight from the left leg.

○ 3. assess the feet for signs of neuromuscular impairment.

○ 4. reposition the pulleys so the traction occurs at a 45-degree angle.

35. The nurse in the emergency department is caring for a 3-year-old with a fractured humerus. The child is crying and screaming, "I hate you." Which of the following would be *most* appropriate?

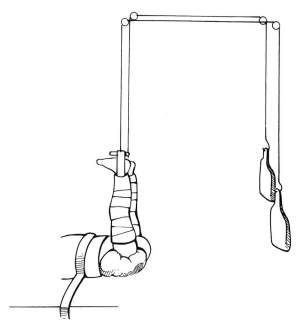

Figure 2.

○ 1. Tell the parents they will need to wait out in the lobby.

○ 2. Ask the charge nurse to assign this client to another nurse.

○ 3. Reassure the parents that this a normal behavior under the circumstances.

○ 4. Ask the parents to discipline the child so that the physician can treat her.

36. After a plaster cast has been applied to the arm of a child with a fractured right humerus, the nurse completes discharge teaching. The nurse would evaluate the teaching as successful when the mother agrees to seek medical advice if the child experiences which of the following?

○ 1. Inability to extend the fingers on the right hand.

○ 2. Vomiting after the cast is applied.

○ 3. Coolness and dampness of the cast after 5 hours.

○ 4. Fussiness with complaints that the cast is heavy.

37. The nurse would teach the mother of a child who has a new cast for a fractured radius to do which of the following for the first few days at home?

○ 1. Use a hair dryer to dry the cast more quickly.

○ 2. Have the child refrain from strenuous activities.

○ 3. Check movement and sensation of the child's fingers once a day.

○ 4. Administer acetaminophen every 8 to 12 hours for discomfort.

38. While assessing a 3-year-old who has had an injury to the leg, complains of pain, and refuses to walk, the nurse notes that the child's left thigh is swollen. Which of the following would the nurse do *next*?

○ 1. Assess the neurologic status of the toes.

○ 2. Determine the circulatory status of the upper thigh.

○ 3. Obtain the child's vital signs.

○ 4. Notify the physician immediately.

39. Anticipating that a 3-year-old in traction will have need for diversion, which of the following would the nurse expect to offer the child?

○ 1. A video game.

○ 2. Blocks.

○ 3. Hand puppets.

○ 4. Marbles.

40. The parents of a child who requires skeletal traction are unable to visit their child for more than 1 hour a day because there are five other children at home and both parents work outside of the home. The nurse recognizes expressions of guilt in both parents. To help alleviate this guilt, the nurse would make which of the following remarks?

○ 1. "I'm sure you feel guilty about not being able to visit often."

○ 2. "It's important that you visit even if for 1 hour."

○ 3. "Not all parents can stay all the time."

○ 4. "Perhaps you could take turns visiting for a bit longer."

41. The child in a new hip spica cast seems to be adjusting to the cast, except that after each meal the child complains that the cast is too tight. Which of the following would the nurse plan to do?

○ 1. Give the enema that was ordered PRN.

○ 2. Offer smaller, more frequent meals.

○ 3. Give the child a mechanical soft diet.

○ 4. Offer the child more fruits and grains.

42. The nurse is helping a family plan for the discharge of their child, who will be going home in a spica cast. Which of the following points of information would be *most* important for the nurse to consider?

○ 1. The bathrooms are all on the second floor.

○ 2. The child's bedroom is on the second floor.

○ 3. A 16-year-old sister will care for the child during the day.

○ 4. There are three steps up to the front door.

The Client With Osteomyelitis

43. During the initial assessment of a child admitted to the pediatric unit with osteomyelitis of the left tibia, the nurse would expect the area over the tibia to exhibit which of the following?

○ 1. Diffuse tenderness.

○ 2. Decreased pain.

○ 3. Increased warmth.

○ 4. Localized edema.

44. After receiving orders for laboratory tests and antibiotics for a child with osteomyelitis, the nurse would expect to start the antibiotic after blood is drawn for which of the following?
    ○ 1. Creatinine.
    ○ 2. Culture.
    ○ 3. Hemoglobin.
    ○ 4. White blood cell count.

45. On reviewing the preliminary laboratory results for a child with osteomyelitis, which of the following findings would lead the nurse to suspect osteomyelitis?
    ○ 1. Hematocrit, 30%.
    ○ 2. Erythrocyte sedimentation rate, 35 mm/hour.
    ○ 3. Serum potassium concentration, 5.7 mEq/L.
    ○ 4. White blood cell count, 12,000/mm^3.

46. The home health nurse is caring for a child with osteomyelitis who will be receiving high-dose intravenous antibiotic therapy for 3 to 4 weeks. The nurse would plan to monitor which of the following?
    ○ 1. Blood glucose level.
    ○ 2. Thrombin times.
    ○ 3. Urine glucose level.
    ○ 4. Urine specific gravity.

47. To meet the developmental needs of an 8-year-old who is confined to home with osteomyelitis, the home health nurse would expect to include which of the following?
    ○ 1. Encouraging the child to communicate with schoolmates.
    ○ 2. Encouraging the parents to stay with the child.
    ○ 3. Allowing siblings to visit freely throughout the day.
    ○ 4. Talking to the child about his interests twice daily.

48. Which of the following meals would be appropriate for the child with osteomyelitis to choose?
    ○ 1. Beef and bean burrito with cheese, carrot and celery sticks, and an orange.
    ○ 2. Buttered wheat bread, cream of broccoli soup, tossed salad with dressing, and an apple.
    ○ 3. Potato soup; bacon, lettuce, and tomato sandwich; and an orange.
    ○ 4. Tomato soup, grilled cheese sandwich, and banana.

Correct Answers and Rationale

The letters in parentheses following the rationale identify the step of the nursing process (A, D, P, I, E) and client needs (1, 2, 3, 4, 5, 6, 7, 8, 9, 10). See the inside front cover for the key.

The Client with Musculoskeletal Dysfunction

1. 4. Legg-Calvé-Perthes disease, also known as *coxa plana* or *osteochondrosis,* is characterized by aseptic necrosis at the head of the femur when the blood supply to the area is interrupted. Avoidance of weight bearing is especially important to prevent the head of the femur from leaving the acetabulum, thus preventing hip dislocation. Devices such as an abduction brace, a leg cast, or a harness sling are used to protect the affected joint while revascularization and bone healing occur. Surgical procedures are used in some cases. Although pain control measures may be appropriate, pain is not necessarily more acute at night. Initial therapy involves rest and non–weight bearing to help restore motion. Preventing flexion is not necessary. (P, 10)

2. 3. Because most of the child's care takes place at home, the primary focus of family teaching would be on the care and management of the corrective device. Devices such as an abduction brace, a leg cast, or a harness sling are used to protect the affected joint while revascularization and bone healing occur. As long as the child is eating a well-balanced diet, there is no need for an intake of protein-rich foods. Once therapy has been initiated, pain is usually not a problem. The key is management of the corrective device. (P, 9)

3. 4. In torticollis, the sternocleidomastoid muscle appears contracted or shortened, and range of motion in the neck is limited. This causes the neck to turn laterally to one side, with the chin directed to the opposite side. (A, 10)

4. 1. Scoliosis, a lateral deviation of the spine, is assessed by having the client bend forward at the waist with arms hanging freely, then looking for lateral curvature of the spine and a rib hump. (A, 4)

5. 1. One of the most effective spinal braces for correcting scoliosis, the Boston brace should be worn for at least 16 to 23 hours a day, except when carrying out personal hygiene measures. (E, 9)

6. 4. Exercises are prescribed for the child with scoliosis wearing a Boston brace to help strengthen spinal and abdominal muscles and provide support. Typically, children wearing a Boston brace do not complain of muscle spasms. Performing exercises provides no effect on the brace's traction ability. Spinal contractures do not occur when a Boston brace is worn. (I, 10)

7. 1. The adolescent's complaint should alert the nurse to the possibility of Osgood-Schlatter disease. This disease, found primarily in boys 10 to 15 years of age and in girls 8 to 13 years of age, occurs when the infrapatellar ligament of the quadriceps muscle is not well anchored to the tibial tubercle. Excessive activity of the quadriceps muscle results in microtrauma, which causes swelling and pain. Track, soccer, and football commonly produce this condition. Osgood-Schlatter disease is self-limited and usually responds to rest and application of ice. (A, 10)

8. 4. The adolescent is most likely experiencing heat exhaustion or heat collapse, which are common after vigorous exercise in a hot environment. Symptoms result from loss of fluids and include nausea, vomiting, dizziness, headache, and thirst. Treatment consists of moving the adolescent to a cool environment and giving cool liquids. Cool liquids are easier to drink than cold liquids. Taking the adolescent's temperature would be appropriate once these actions have been completed. However, the adolescent's temperature is likely to be normal or only mildly elevated. The water in a swimming pool would be too cool, possibly causing the adolescent to shiver and thus raising his temperature. (I, 7)

The Client With Cerebral Palsy

9. 3. The major goal of early recognition of primary developmental delays in children with cerebral palsy is to prevent secondary and tertiary delays. For example, a young infant who is unable to reach or focus on objects would be unable to attain various levels of sensory-perceptual development described by Piaget. (I, 4)

10. 3. The term *cerebral palsy* refers to a group of nonprogressive disorders of upper motor neuron impairment that result in motor dysfunction due to injury. In addition, a child may have speech or ocular difficulties, seizures, hyperactivity, or cognitive impairment. The condition of congenital malformed blood vessels in the ventricles is known as arteriovenous malformations. (E, 10)

11. 4. Delay in achieving developmental milestones is a characteristic of children with cerebral palsy. Ninety percent of 15-month-old children can put a block in a

cup. Walking up steps typically is accomplished at 18 to 24 months. A child usually is able to use a spoon at 18 months. The ability to copy a circle is achieved at approximately 3 to 4 years of age. (A, 3)

12. 3. The nurse needs to respond honestly to the mother. Most children with hemiparesis due to spastic cerebral palsy are able to walk because the motor deficit is usually greater in the upper extremity. There is no need to refer the mother to the physician. The age at which the mother walked may be important to elicit, but this does not influence when the child will walk. The will to walk is important, but without neurologic stability the child may be unable to do so. (I, 10)

13. 1. Limited interaction or lack of interaction with friends and family may lead the nurse to suspect a possible problem with the family's inability to cope with others' reactions and responses to a child with cerebral palsy. Learning measures to meet the child's physical needs demonstrates some understanding and acceptance of the disease. Requesting teaching about the disease suggests curiosity or a desire for understanding, thus demonstrating the family's dealing with the situation. Although not seeking financial help to pay for medical bills may be problem, it does not indicate the type of response the family is having to the child's problems. (A, 5)

The Client With Duchenne's Muscular Dystrophy

14. 1. Duchenne's muscular dystrophy is an X-linked recessive disorder. The gene is transmitted through female carriers to affected sons 50% of the time. Daughters have a 50% chance of being carriers. (D, 10)

15. 3. Usually the first clinical manifestations of Duchenne's muscular dystrophy include difficulty with typical age-appropriate physical activities such as running, riding a bicycle, and climbing stairs. Contractures of the large joints typically occur much later in the disease process. Occasionally enlarged calves may be noted, but they are not typical findings in a child with Duchenne's muscular dystrophy. Muscular atrophy and development of small, weak muscles are later signs. (A, 10)

16. 4. With Gower's sign, the child walks the hands up the legs in an attempt to stand, a common approach used by children with Duchenne's muscular dystrophy when rising from a sitting to a standing. position. Galeazzi's sign refers to the shortening of the affected limb in congenital hip dislocation. Goodell's sign refers to the softening of the cervix, considered a sign of probable pregnancy. Goodenough's sign refers to a test of mental age. (D, 10)

17. 3. The primary nursing goal is to maintain function in unaffected muscles for as long as possible. There is no effective treatment for childhood muscular dystrophy. Children who remain active are able to forestall being confined in wheelchair. Remaining active also minimizes the risk for social isolation. Preventing rather than encouraging wheelchair use by maintaining function for as long as possible is an appropriate nursing goal. Children with muscular dystrophy become socially isolated as their condition deteriorates and they can no longer keep up with friends. Maintaining function helps prevent social isolation. Circulatory impairment is not associated with muscular dystrophy. (P, 10)

18. 3. The guilt feelings that mothers of children with muscular dystrophy commonly experience frequently result from the fact that the disease is genetic and the mother transmitted the defective gene to her son. Although many children do die from the disease, the disease is considered chronic and progressive. As the disease progresses, the child becomes more dependent. However, guilt typically stems from the knowledge that the mother transmitted the disease to her son rather than the dependency of the child. The disease onset is usually gradual, not sudden. (D, 5)

19. 1. Muscular dystrophy is a progressive disease. Children who are affected by this disease usually are unable to walk independently by age 9 to 11 years. There is no effective treatment for childhood muscular dystrophy. Although children who remain active are able to avoid wheelchair confinement for a longer period, activity does not prevent disease progression. (E, 10)

The Client With Developmental Dysplasia of the Hip

20. 4. In a toddler, weight bearing causes the pelvis to tilt downward on the unaffected side instead of upward as it would normally. This is Trendelenburg's sign, and it indicates developmental dysplasia of the hip. Ortolani's maneuver is used during the neonatal period to assess developmental dysplasia of the hip in infants. With the infant quiet, relaxed, and lying on the back, the hips and knees are flexed at right angles. The knees are moved to abduction and pressure is exerted. If the femoral head moves forward, then it is dislocated. Barlow's maneuver is used to assess developmental dysplasia of the hip in infants. As the femur is moved into or out of the acetabulum, a clunk is heard, indicating dislocation. Adam's position is used to evaluate for structural scoliosis. The child bends forward with feet together and arms hanging freely or with palms together. (A, 9)

21. 4. This infant with congenital hip dysplasia has asymmetric gluteal folds. The Ortolani "click" occurs when the nurse feels the femur sliding into the acetabulum with a "click." Limited abduction may be observed during an attempt to abduct the infant's thighs. Galeazzi's sign reveals femoral foreshortening and is observed by flexing the thighs. (D, 4)

22. 1. The Pavlik harness is worn over a diaper. Knee socks are also worn to prevent the straps and foot and leg pieces from rubbing directly on the skin. For maximum results, the infant needs to wear the harness continuously. The skin should be inspected several times a day, not every other day, for signs of redness or irritation. Lotions and powders are to be avoided because they can cake and irritate the skin. (I, 9)

23. 2. Assessing the learner's knowledge level is the initial step in any teaching plan to promote the maximum amount of learning. This assessment also provides the nurse with a starting point for teaching. Assessing coping strategies can provide important information to the development of the teaching plan but is not the initial step. Giving parents written instructions or a list of community resources is appropriate once the parents' knowledge level has been determined and teaching has begun. (P, 9)

24. 3. The abduction bar is incorporated into the cast to increase the cast's strength and maintain the legs in alignment. The bar cannot be removed or adjusted, unless the cast is removed and a new cast is applied. The bar should never be used to lift or turn the client, because doing so may weaken the cast. (I, 9)

25. 2. The toddler in a hip spica cast needs a specially designed car seat. The one that the mother already has will not be appropriate because of the need for the car seat to accommodate the cast and abductor bar. Legally, all children younger than 4 years of age are required to be restrained in a car seat. (I, 2)

The Client With Congenital Clubfoot

26. 3. When an infant is born with an unexpected anomaly, parents are faced with questions, uncertainties, and possible disappointments. They may feel inadequate, helpless, and anxious. The nurse can help the parents initially by assessing their concerns and providing appropriate information to help them clarify or resolve the immediate problems. Having them talk with other parents would be helpful a little bit later, once the nurse assesses their concerns and discusses the problem and the parents' current feelings. If the parents continue to have difficulties expressing and working through their feelings, referral to a counselor would be appropriate. (I, 5)

27. 3. A cast that is too tight can cause a tourniquet effect, compromising the neurovascular integrity of the extremity. Manifestations of neurovascular impairment include pain, edema, pulselessness, coolness, altered sensation, and inability to move the distal exposed extremity. The toes of the casted extremity should be assessed frequently to evaluate for changes in neurovascular integrity. Wetting a plaster cast with water and soap softens the plaster, which may alter the cast's effectiveness. There is no reason to elevate the casted extremities when a child with clubfoot is being treated with nonsurgical measures. The legs would be elevated if swelling were present. Petals, which are applied to cover the rough edges of the cast, are to be left in place to minimize the risk for skin irritation from the cast edges. (E, 9)

The Client With Juvenile Rheumatoid Arthritis

28. 4. The nurse's response to the father is based on the knowledge that there is no definitive test for JRA. The latex fixation test, which is commonly used to diagnose arthritis in adults, is negative in 90% of children. The erythrocyte sedimentation rate may or may not be increased during active disease. This test identifies the presence of inflammation only. Synovial fluid cultures are done to rule out septic arthritis, not to diagnose JRA. (D, 9)

29. 1. In half of the children diagnosed with JRA, recovery occurs without joint deformity. Approximately one third of the children will continue to have the disease into adulthood, and approximately one sixth will experience severe, crippling deformities. (I, 10)

30. 2. Socialization is important for this preschool-aged child, and activity is important to maintain function. Because children with JRA commonly experience the most problems in the early morning after arising, they need more time to "warm up." Side effects may or may not occur. The child's normal routine needs to be maintained as much as possible. Although splints and braces may be needed, they are worn during periods of rest, not activity, to maintain function. (I, 10)

31. 4. Because the child is dealing with grief and loss associated with a chronic illness, parents need to be supportive and understanding. The child needs to feel valued and worthwhile. Introducing the child to others of the same age who also have JRA most probably would be ineffective because preschoolers are developmentally egocentric. Although the child needs to feel valued, the mother's spending more time with the child and less time with her other children is inappropriate because the child with JRA may experience secondary gain from the illness if the family interaction patterns are altered. Also, this action reinforces the child's with-

drawal behavior. Psychological counseling is not needed at this time because the child's reaction is normal. (I, 5)

32. 3. The first group of drugs typically prescribed is the nonsteroidal anti-inflammatory drugs, which include aspirin. Aspirin is also present in some over-the-counter medications, so the family should check with the nurse before giving any over-the-counter medication. Once aspirin therapy is started, it takes hours or days for relief from pain to occur. However, it takes 3 to 4 weeks for the anti-inflammatory effects to occur, including reduction in swelling and less pain with movement. The missed dose will need to be made up to maintain the serum level of aspirin and to maintain therapeutic effectiveness of the drug. (P, 8)

The Client With a Fracture

33. 1. Skeletal traction applies the pull directly to the skeletal structure by tongs, pin, or wire. The nurse should assess the pull of the traction on the pin first. This is critical to the success of the traction. Once this is assessed, then the pin sites are assessed for signs of infection. The dressings would be examined after the pull of the traction, neurovascular status, and pin sites were assessed. The Ace wrap is used to anchor skin traction nonadherent straps, not skeletal traction. (A, 9)

34. 3. The traction is set up correctly. The buttocks should remain slightly elevated from the bed; traction should be applied to both legs at a 90-degree angle. The nurse should assess the client frequently for signs of neurovascular impairment of the feet such as pallor, coldness, numbness, or tingling. (I, 7)

35. 3. Explaining to the parents that this is a normal reaction under the circumstances is most appropriate. The child's outburst is related to the child's fears of the unknown. The child is scared and anxious and needs the parents for support. Asking the parents to wait outside would only add to the child's fear and anxiety. The reaction is normal for a child her age and does not usually call for a change in staff assignments. Asking the parents to discipline their child for her behavior is inappropriate. The nurse needs to handle the situation. (I, 3)

36. 1. Inability to extend the fingers of the involved arm may indicate neurologic impairment caused by pressure on soft tissue. It is not unusual for a child to vomit after experiencing a traumatic injury. It may take up to 72 hours for a plaster cast to dry. Until the cast dries, the dampness causes the sensation of coolness. The cast will seem heavy until the child adjusts to the extra weight. The child may exhibit fussiness, such as whining, crying or clinging, as a result of numerous causes,

such placement of the cast, the hospital experience, or pain. (A, 9)

37. 2. For the first few days after application of a plaster or Fiberglas cast, the child should not engage in strenuous activities, to minimize swelling that would cause the cast to become too tight. Use of a hair dryer to complete the drying of the cast is not encouraged because the hair dryer only dries the outside of the cast. Movement and sensation of the fingers need to be checked several times a day for the first few days. Typically, the mother would be instructed to administer acetaminophen every 4 to 6 hours, not every 8 to 12 hours, for discomfort. (I, 9)

38. 1. Because the nurse suspects a possible fracture based on the child's presentation, assessing the neurologic and circulatory status of the toes, the tissues distal to the fracture, is important. Soft tissue contusions, which accompany femur fractures, can result in severe hemorrhage into the tissue and subsequent circulatory and neurologic impairment. Once this information has been obtained, vital signs can be assessed and the nurse can notify the physician and report the findings. (I, 10)

39. 3. Hand puppets would enable a 3-year-old child in traction to act out feelings within the constraints imposed by the traction. A 3-year-old needs creative play. The video game would make the child too active in bed and does not meet the child's developmental need for creative play. Blocks would be more appropriate for a younger child. Marbles are unsafe at this age because they can be swallowed. (P, 3)

40. 2. Stressing the importance of the parents' visiting when they can helps to alleviate the guilt they feel. It allows the parents to feel that they are doing what they can. Acknowledging the guilt gives the parents an opportunity to talk about it but does not help alleviate it. Comparing the parents with other parents does not alleviate guilt feelings. The parents need reinforcement that what they are doing is appropriate. Suggesting that the parents take turns visiting implies that they should feel guilty because they may not be doing all they could. (I, 5)

41. 2. A hip spica cast encircles the abdomen. When the child eats a large meal, abdominal pressure increases, causing the cast to feel tight. Therefore, the nurse would plan to offer smaller, more frequent meals to minimize abdominal distention. If the child's appetite were decreased in conjunction with a feeling of fullness, the nurse might suspect that the child was becoming constipated and plan to use laxatives or a higher-fiber diet. A mechanical soft diet is indicated when the child has difficulty chewing food adequately. Giving the child more fruits and grains would contribute to abdominal distention and complaints of the cast tightness after eating. (P, 9)

42. 2. The child with a hip spica cast who is going home and has a bedroom on the second floor of the home needs to have the bed moved to an area that is more central to family life. Negotiating a flight of steps at least twice a day (on awakening in the morning and before going to bed at night) with a child in hip spica cast would be difficult and most likely dangerous. Because the child in a hip spica cast will need to use a bedpan or urinal, the bathrooms can be on any floor. Because the family is involved in the discharge, the 16-year-old should be taught appropriate care along with the rest of the family. The child can be carried up and down the three steps to the house the few times necessary after discharge. (P, 2)

The Client With Osteomyelitis

43. 3. Findings associated with osteomyelitis commonly include pain over the area, increased warmth, localized tenderness, and diffuse swelling over the involved bone. The area over the affected bone is red. (A, 10)

44. 2. Antibiotic therapy starts after blood for culture is drawn. The blood cultures determine the causative organism. (P, 9)

45. 2. In osteomyelitis, the erythrocyte sedimentation rate is increased (for a child, the normal range is 0 to 13 mm/hour). The erythrocyte sedimentation rate rises in the presence of severe localized or systemic inflammation. The hematocrit level would be normal in a child with osteomyelitis. This child's hematocrit is lower than the normal level, which typically is greater than 33%. The serum potassium concentration would be normal in a child with osteomyelitis; in this child it is higher than the normal range of 3.5 to 5.5 mEq/L. The leukocyte count in osteomyelitis is increased, usually 15,000 to 25,000/mm^3. This child's leukocyte level is low in light of the diagnosis of osteomyelitis. Normally, the white blood cell count ranges from 5000 to 10,000/mm^3. (D, 10)

46. 4. Long-term, high-dose antibiotic therapy can adversely affect renal, hepatic, and hematopoietic function. Urine specific gravity would provide valuable information about the kidneys' ability to concentrate or dilute urine, thereby suggesting renal impairment. Blood glucose levels reveal how well the client's body is using glucose. Thrombin times reveal information about the clotting mechanism. Urine glucose levels reveal information about the body's use and excretion of glucose. (I, 8)

47. 1. Encouraging contact with schoolmates allows the school-aged child to maintain and develop socialization with peers, an important developmental task of this age group. Although having family visits and interacting with the child are important, they do not meet the child's developmental needs. Talking to the child about his interests is important, but encouraging contact with schoolmates is crucial to maintain and develop socialization with peers. (P, 3)

48. 1. Children with osteomyelitis need a diet that is high in protein and calories. Milk, eggs, cheese, meat, fish, and beans are the best sources of these nutrients. (I, 10)

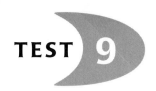
The Child With Dermatologic, Endocrine, and Other Health Problems

Select the one best answer, and indicate your choice by filling in the circle in front of the option.

The Client With Atopic Dermatitis

1. A 9-month-old infant with eczema has lesions that are secondarily infected. Which of the following interventions would be *most* appropriate to help the father best meet the needs of his child?
   ○ 1. Preventing siblings from being in close contact.
   ○ 2. Sending the child to day care as usual.
   ○ 3. Playing video cartoons for several hours each evening.
   ○ 4. Playing with the child every day.

2. After the nurse teaches the mother of a child with atopic dermatitis how to bathe her child, which of the following statements by the mother indicates effective teaching?
   ○ 1. "I let my child play in the tub for 30 minutes every night."
   ○ 2. "My child loves the bubble bath I put in the tub."
   ○ 3. "When my child gets out of the tub I just pat the skin dry."
   ○ 4. "I make sure my child has a bath every night."

The Client With Burns

3. The nurse is assessing a 9-year-old child who has third-degree burns as shown in Figure 1. Using the "rule of nines" adapted for children, the nurse estimates that the extent of burns in this child is

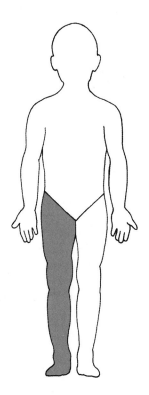

Figure 1

   ○ 1. 9%.
   ○ 2. 14%.
   ○ 3. 18%.
   ○ 4. 24%.

4. Which of the following would be *most* appropriate to institute when a school-aged child with burns becomes angry and combative when it is time to change the dressings and apply mafenide acetate (Sulfamylon)?
   ○ 1. Ensure parental support during the dressing changes.
   ○ 2. Allow the child to assist in removing the dressings and applying the cream.
   ○ 3. Give the child permission to cry during the procedure.
   ○ 4. Allow the child to schedule the time for dressing changes.

5. A 5-year-old child with burns on the trunk and arms has no appetite. The nurse and mother develop a plan of care to stimulate the child's appetite. Which of the following suggestions made by the mother would indicate that she needs additional teaching?
   ○ 1. Deciding that the mother will feed the child.
   ○ 2. Withholding dessert and treats unless meals are eaten.
   ○ 3. Offering the child finger foods that the child likes.
   ○ 4. Serving smaller and more frequent meals.

6. After teaching the mother of a child with severe burns about the importance of specific nutritional support in burn management, which of the following, if chosen by the mother from the child's diet menu, indicates the need for further instruction?
   ○ 1. Bacon, lettuce, and tomato sandwich; milk; and celery and carrot sticks.
   ○ 2. Cheeseburger, cottage cheese and pineapple salad, chocolate milk, and a brownie.
   ○ 3. Chicken nuggets, orange and grapefruit sections, and a vanilla milkshake.
   ○ 4. Beef, bean, and cheese burrito; a banana; fruit-flavored yogurt; and skim milk.

7. When caring for a child with moderate burns from the waist down, which of the following should the nurse do when positioning the child?
   ○ 1. Place the child in a position of comfort.
   ○ 2. Allow the child to lie on the abdomen.
   ○ 3. Ensure the application of leg splints.
   ○ 4. Have the child flex the hips and knees.

The Client With Hyperthyroidism

8. An 11-year-old has been diagnosed with Grave's disease and is to start drug therapy. Which of the following instructions would the school nurse include in the teaching plan for the child's mother and teacher?
   ○ 1. Continue with the same amount of schoolwork and homework.

   ○ 2. Understand that mood swings are rare with this disorder.
   ○ 3. Limit the amount of food that is offered to the child.
   ○ 4. Provide the child with a calm, nonstimulating environment.

The Client With Insulin-Dependent Diabetes Mellitus

9. After a school-aged child with insulin-dependent diabetes mellitus attends a nutritional teaching class, the nurse determines that the teaching has been effective when the child states which of the following?
   ○ 1. "If I don't eat all my meal, I can make up the carbohydrates at the next meal."
   ○ 2. "If I'm not hungry for a meal, I can eat the carbohydrates for a snack later."
   ○ 3. "When I don't finish a meal, I must make up the carbohydrates right then."
   ○ 4. "When I don't finish a meal, I just need to take more insulin."

10. The nurse talks to an adolescent about how she can tell her friends about her new diagnosis of diabetes. Which of the following behaviors by the adolescent indicates that the adolescent has responded positively to the discussion?
    ○ 1. She asks the nurse for material on diabetes for a school paper.
    ○ 2. She introduces the nurse to her friends as "the one who taught me all about my diabetes."
    ○ 3. She says, "I'll try to tell my friends, but they'll probably quit hanging out with me."
    ○ 4. She asks her friends what they think about someone who has a lifelong illness.

11. When developing the teaching plan for the mother and a child with insulin-dependent diabetes about sick-day management, which of the following instructions would the nurse expect to include?
    ○ 1. Adhere to the same schedule and type and amount of insulin.
    ○ 2. Immediately call the physician for information about what to do.
    ○ 3. Adjust insulin based on more frequent testing of blood glucose levels.
    ○ 4. Take the child to the emergency room for immediate care.

12. An adolescent with insulin-dependent diabetes is being taught the importance of rotating the sites of insulin injections. The nurse would judge that the teaching was successful when the adolescent identifies which of the following as a result of using the same site?
    ○ 1. Destruction of the fat tissue and poor absorption.

○ 2. Destruction of nerves and painful neuritis.

○ 3. Destruction of the tissue and too-rapid insulin uptake.

○ 4. Development of resistance to insulin and need for increased amounts.

13. Which of the following tests would the nurse expect to be performed as a follow-up measure to periodically assess the effectiveness of treatment for a child with insulin-dependent diabetes?
    ○ 1. Hemoglobin electrophoresis.
    ○ 2. Glycosylated hemoglobin.
    ○ 3. Glucose tolerance test.
    ○ 4. Post-postprandial blood test.

The Client Who Is Abused

14. When obtaining a nursing history from parents who are suspected of abusing their child, which of the following characteristics about the parents would the nurse typically find?
    ○ 1. Attentiveness to the child's needs.
    ○ 2. Self-blame for the injury to the child.
    ○ 3. Ability to relate child's developmental achievements.
    ○ 4. Evidence of little concern about the extent of the injury.

15. A 3-year-old child with a history of being abused has blood drawn. The child lies very still and makes no sound during the procedure. Which of the following comments by the nurse would be *most* appropriate?
    ○ 1. "It's okay to cry when something hurts."
    ○ 2. "That really didn't hurt, did it?"
    ○ 3. "We're mean to hurt you that way, aren't we?"
    ○ 4. "You were very good not to cry with the needle."

16. Which of the following nursing diagnoses would the nurse include as the priority in the plan of care for a preschooler who has been physically abused?
    ○ 1. Risk for Trauma related to the characteristics of the child and caregiver.
    ○ 2. Impaired Physical Mobility related to physical maltreatment.
    ○ 3. Self-Care Deficit related to child's developmental level.
    ○ 4. Anticipatory Grieving related to the cycle of abuse.

17. While interviewing a 3-year-old girl who has been sexually abused, which of the following would the nurse ask the child to do?
    ○ 1. Describe what happened during the abusive act.
    ○ 2. Draw a picture and explain what it means.
    ○ 3. "Play out" the event using anatomically correct dolls.
    ○ 4. Use puppets to recreate the sexual abuse, observing the child's reactions.

18. Which of the following observations by the nurse would strongly suggest that a 15-month-old toddler has been abused?
    ○ 1. The child appears happy when personnel work with him.
    ○ 2. The child plays alongside others contentedly.
    ○ 3. The child is underdeveloped for his age.
    ○ 4. The child sucks his thumb.

19. When planning interventions for parents who are abusive, the nurse would incorporate knowledge about which of the following as a common parental indicator into the plan of care?
    ○ 1. Lower socioeconomic group.
    ○ 2. Unemployment.
    ○ 3. Low self-esteem.
    ○ 4. Loss of emotional family attachments.

The Client Who Is Septic

20. The father of a 3-week-old infant who has developed sepsis says that he feels guilty because he did not realize his infant was sick. Which of the following responses by the nurse would be *most* appropriate?
    ○ 1. "You should have realized something was wrong; he is your son."
    ○ 2. "Did you read the booklet on newborns that was sent home with you from the hospital?"
    ○ 3. "What you are feeling is normal; next time, you will know what to look for."
    ○ 4. "Babies can get sick quickly, and parents do not always realize it."

21. When developing the plan of care for a 1-month-old infant with sepsis, which of the following instructions would the nurse expect to include?
    ○ 1. Monitor vital signs every 6 hours.
    ○ 2. Use the intravenous line solely for antibiotics.
    ○ 3. Withhold formula feedings.
    ○ 4. Weigh the infant every other day.

22. Assessment of a 3-week-old infant with sepsis reveals that the infant is using abdominal muscles to breathe and has a respiratory rate of 50 breaths/minute. Which of the following would the nurse do *next*?
    ○ 1. Document the findings.
    ○ 2. Check oxygen saturation with a pulse oximeter.
    ○ 3. Notify the physician of the findings.
    ○ 4. Apply oxygen immediately to the infant.

The Client With Failure to Thrive

23. The nurse formulates the nursing diagnosis Imbalanced Nutrition: Less than Body Requirements related to negative feeding patterns for a 5-month old infant

diagnosed with failure to thrive. To meet the short-term goals of the infant's plan of care, the nurse would expect to do which of the following?

○ 1. Instruct the parents in proper feeding techniques.

○ 2. Give infant formula that has 24 calories/ounce.

○ 3. Provide consistent staff to care for the infant.

○ 4. Allow the infant sit in a high chair during feedings.

24. The health care team determines that the family of an infant with failure to thrive who is to be discharged will need follow-up care. Which of the following would be the *most* effective method of follow-up?

○ 1. Daily phone calls from the hospital nurse.

○ 2. Enrollment in community parenting classes.

○ 3. Twice-weekly clinic appointments.

○ 4. Weekly visits by a community health nurse.

The Client With Various Health Problems

25. The nurse judges that more teaching is necessary for the father of a child with conjunctivitis on hearing the father say which of the following?

○ 1. "Use your brother's towel until I can get the others washed."

○ 2. "Remember to wash your hands after touching your eyes."

○ 3. "It will not take long for your eye infection to get better."

○ 4. "Use a tissue to clean your eyes and then throw it away."

26. A mother calls the clinic to report that her toddler has pinworms. Which of the following instructions would be appropriate for the nurse to give to the mother?

○ 1. Bring the child in after treatment to check for a recurrence.

○ 2. Check the child's stool every day for presence of pinworms.

○ 3. Wash the toddler's hands after the child has played outside.

○ 4. Administer doses of the medication until all of it is finished.

27. A 5-year-old brought to the clinic with several superficial sores on the front of the left leg is diagnosed with impetigo. Which of the following instructions would the nurse give the mother?

○ 1. Wash the child's legs gently every day with a mild soap.

○ 2. Wash the crusts off the sores every day.

○ 3. Allow the child to go back to school after 24 hours of treatment.

○ 4. Have the child return to the clinic the next week for a follow-up examination.

28. When developing the teaching plan for the mother of a 2-year-old diagnosed with scabies, which of the following points would the nurse expect to include?

○ 1. The house should be thoroughly cleaned.

○ 2. The child should frequently be held for long periods of time.

○ 3. Itching should cease in a few days.

○ 4. The entire family should be treated.

Correct Answers and Rationale

The letters in parentheses following the rationale identify the step of the nursing process (A, D, P, I, E) and client needs (1, 2, 3, 4, 5, 6, 7, 8, 9, 10). See the inside front cover for the key.

The Client With Atopic Dermatitis

1. 4. The father can best meet the needs of his 9-month-old infant by playing with the child every day. All infants need time with their parents to develop trust and thus attain optimal development. The parents of a child with a chronic problem may need more guidance to meet the child's needs because of the focus on medical problems. The child's lesions are secondarily infected and therefore should not be contagious. Siblings do not need to stay away. Even with lesions that are infected, the child can still attend day care. Watching cartoon videos for several hours is not appropriate for a 9-month-old. Infants need interactive contact for optimal development. (I, 3)

2. 3. Atopic dermatitis is a chronic pruritic dermatitis that usually begins in infancy. Many of the children diagnosed with it have a family history of eczema, allergies, or asthma. Atopic dermatitis is best treated with hydrating the skin, controlling the pruritus, and preventing secondary infection. Patting the skin dry removes less natural skin moisturizer and thus maintains skin hydration. Water has a drying effect on the skin. Playing in the tub for 30 minutes each night would deplete the skin of its natural moisturizers, thereby leading to increased pruritus and dry skin. Bubble baths are to be avoided in children with atopic dermatitis because they may act as a irritant, possibly exacerbating the condition. Also, bubble baths deplete the skin of its natural moisturizers. The issue is not whether the child bathes every night. Rather, the goal is to decrease dryness and itching. (E, 10)

The Client With Burns

3. 2. The child has burns of the entire leg. Because of the smaller size of children's legs, the estimate of 14% is used instead of 18%, which is used with adults. The arms of children are estimated at 9%, and the anterior and posterior trunk at 18% each. The head of the child is estimated at 18%, rather than the 9% used for adults. (D, 10)

4. 2. Expressions of anger and combativeness are often the result of loss of control and a feeling of powerless-

ness. Some control over the situation is regained by allowing the child to participate in care. Although having parental support during the dressing changes may be helpful, this action does nothing to allow the child control. Giving the child permission to cry may help with verbalizing feelings, but doing so does nothing to provide the child with control over the situation. Although allowing the child to determine the time for dressing changes may provide a sense of control over the situation, doing so is inappropriate because the dressing changes need to be performed as ordered to ensure effectiveness and healing. (I, 10)

5. 2. Allowing the mother to feed the child, serving smaller and more frequent meals, and offering finger foods are all acceptable interventions for a 5-year-old child. This is true whether the child is well or ill. Withholding certain foods until the child complies is punitive and rarely successful. (E, 7)

6. 1. Hypoproteinemia is common after severe burns. The child's diet should be high in protein to compensate for protein loss and to promote tissue healing. The child will also require a diet that is high in calories and rich in iron. The menu of bacon, lettuce, and tomato sandwich; milk; and celery sticks is lacking in sufficient protein and calories. (E, 10)

7. 3. A child with moderate burns is at high risk for contractures. A position of comfort would encourage contracture formation. Therefore, splints need to be applied to maintain proper positioning and joint function, thereby preventing contractures and loss of function. Allowing the child to lie on the abdomen or with hips and knees flexed often encourages contracture formation. (I, 9)

The Client With Hyperthyroidism

8. 4. Because it takes approximately 2 weeks before the response to drug treatment occurs, much of the child's care focuses on managing the child's physical symptoms. Signs and symptoms of the disorder include inability to sit still or concentrate, increased appetite with weight loss, emotional lability, and fatigue. Nursing care is directed toward ensuring that the mother and teacher know how to handle the child, suggesting a shortened school day, a nonstimulating environment, and decreased stress and workload. The child should be encouraged to eat a well-balanced diet. (P, 10)

The Client With Insulin-Dependent Diabetes Mellitus

9. 3. The diabetic diet usually is based on an exchange system that takes into account the fact that some foods have similar fat, carbohydrate, and protein components and therefore can be exchanged one for another. The meal or snack must be eaten in its entirety because it is calculated together with the dose of insulin. If a child does not eat all the meal or snack, then a make-up meal should be given. (E, 10)

10. 2. The ability to talk about her diabetes indicates that the adolescent feels good enough about herself to share her problem with her peers. Asking for reference material does not specifically indicate that the client's self-esteem has improved or that she has accepted her diagnosis. Saying that her friends will probably desert her if she tells them about the illness indicates that the adolescent still needs to work on her self-esteem and her feelings about the disease. Asking her friends what they think of someone with a lifelong illness would not indicate that the nurse's interventions targeted toward improving self-esteem have been successful. Rather, this statement demonstrates the adolescent's uncertainty about herself. (E, 5)

11. 3. Sick-day management requires more frequent monitoring of the child's blood glucose to evaluate for changes associated with a decreased intake and absorption of food, commonly associated with illness. Based on the child's glucose levels, insulin adjustments may be needed. In this case, regular insulin is used. Adhering to the same schedule, type, and amount of insulin is inappropriate because the child's ability to take in food and absorb nutrients can change rapidly. Typically, the child and parents are provided with specific instructions about sick-day management rules. Commonly the physician will prescribe adjustments to insulin (eg, on a sliding scale) based on the child's blood glucose levels. Therefore, calling the physician to report that the child is ill and ask what to do is inappropriate. However, the parents do need to notify the physician should any problems arise with management of the child's blood glucose levels. The child who can tolerate oral feedings of simple sugars can be kept at home as long as the parents monitor the child's blood glucose levels frequently for changes. (P, 10)

12. 1. Repeated use of the same injection site can result in atrophy of the fat in the subcutaneous tissue and lead to poor insulin absorption. The neuritis that develops from diabetes is related to microvascular changes that occur. Resistance to insulin is caused by an immune response to the insulin protein. (E, 8)

13. 2. Glycosylated hemoglobin, which reflects the average blood glucose level for the past 2 to 3 months, provides a good indication of how well the blood glucose level has been controlled. Hemoglobin electrophoresis is indicated for differentiation among types of thalassemias, evaluation of hemolytic anemia, and differentiation of sickle cell trait from sickle cell disease; it provides no information about the effectiveness of diabetic treatment. A glucose tolerance test is used to evaluate the client's response to the ingestion of a specific amount of glucose. This test may be used to diagnose diabetes. A post-postprandial blood test reflects the body's metabolic response to the ingestion of a specific amount of glucose. It may be used to help make the medical diagnosis of diabetes. (P, 9)

The Client Who Is Abused

14. 4. Parents of an abused child are typically unconcerned or show little concern about the child's injury. They may blame the child or others for the injury, may not ask questions about treatment, and may not know developmental information. (A, 6)

15. 1. It is not normal for a preschooler to be totally passive during a painful procedure. Typically a preschooler reacts to a painful procedure by crying or pulling away because of the fear of pain. However, an abused child may become "immune" to pain and may find that crying can bring on more pain. The child needs to learn that appropriate emotional expression is acceptable. Telling the child that it really didn't hurt is inappropriate because it is untrue. (I, 6)

16. 1. A child who is abused would have as a priority nursing diagnosis Risk for Trauma because the child is at risk for continued abuse or a recurrence of the abuse. Although Impaired Physical Mobility related to physical maltreatment or Self-Care Deficit related to developmental level may be appropriate after serious abuse has occurred, the priority nursing diagnosis is Risk for Trauma. A 3-year-old would not experience anticipatory grieving because of the child's cognitive level of development at this age. (D, 6)

17. 3. A 3-year-old child has limited verbal skills and should not be asked to describe an event, explain a picture, or respond verbally or nonverbally to questions. More appropriately, the child can act out an event using dolls. (A, 6)

18. 3. An almost universal finding in descriptions of abused children is underdevelopment for age. This may be reflected in small physical size or in poor psychosocial development. The child should be evaluated further until a plausible diagnosis can be established. A child who appears happy when personnel work with him is exhibiting normal behavior. Children who are abused often are suspicious of others, especially adults.

A child who plays alongside others is exhibiting normal behavior, that of parallel play. A child who sucks his thumb contentedly is exhibiting normal behavior. (A, 6)

19. 3. Parents who are abusive often suffer from low self-esteem, commonly because of the way they were parented, including not being able to develop trust in caretakers and not being encouraged or offered emotional support by parents. Therefore, the nurse works to bolster the parents' self-esteem. This can be achieved by praising the parents for appropriate parenting. Employment and socioeconomic status are not indicators of abusive parents. Abusive parents usually are attached to their children and do not want to give them up to foster care. Parents who are abusive love their children and feel close to them emotionally. (D, 6)

The Client Who Is Septic

20. 4. The signs and symptoms of sepsis in a neonate, such as changes in appearance and behavior, are almost imperceptible. Often, the parents' only complaint is that the neonate does not look "right." Fever and localized response, which are clues to infections in older children, are often absent in the neonate. Telling the father that he should have realized something was wrong is condescending and serves only to further the father's guilt feelings. Asking the father whether he read the booklet from the hospital implies that the father is at fault. One experience would not necessarily ensure that the father would be able to detect sepsis another time. (I, 5)

21. 3. The infant who is septic with lethargy and tachycardia is NPO. Feeding places too much stress on the infant. For an infant with sepsis, close monitoring is essential. Therefore, vital signs are typically monitored at least every 4 hours, and possibly more frequently, depending on the infant's condition. An intravenous line is inserted to administer antibiotics and also to administer fluid and electrolyte replacement. Weight is obtained every day to evaluate the infant's hydration status. (P, 10)

22. 1. It is normal for a young infant to breathe using the abdominal muscles. A respiratory rate of 50 breaths/minute is high for an infant of this age. Therefore, the nurse needs to check the infant's oxygen saturation level with a pulse oximeter. Once this is done, then the nurse would institute oxygen therapy if the infant's oxygen saturation level is low and notify the physician. After these actions, then the nurse would document the findings. (I, 9)

The Client With Failure to Thrive

23. 3. In the short-term care of this infant, it is important that the same person feed the infant at each meal and that this person be able to assess for negative feeding patterns and replace them with positive patterns. Once the infant is gaining weight and shows progress in the feeding patterns, the parents can be instructed in proper feeding techniques. This is a long-term goal of nursing care. Because there is no organic reason for the failure to thrive, it should not be necessary to increase the formula calorie content from 20 to 24 calories/ounce. A 5-month-old infant is too young to be expected to sit in a high chair for feedings and should still be bottle-fed. (P, 10)

24. 4. The most effective follow-up care would occur in the home environment. The community health nurse can be supportive of the parents and will be able to observe parent-infant interactions in a natural environment. The community health nurse can evaluate the infant's progress in gaining weight, offer suggestions to the parents, and help the family solve problems as they arise. (P, 10)

The Client With Various Health Problems

25. 1. Conjunctivitis is very contagious, so using a sibling's towel is not recommended because of the danger of spreading the infection. Careful and frequent handwashing is necessary to reduce the risk of transmission. Typically, the child can return to school 24 hours after starting treatment. Medication for conjunctivitis is used for approximately 5 days. Teaching for the parents and the child with conjunctivitis should also include instructions to wash the hands after touching the eyes, dispose of tissue used to clean the eyes after use, and launder washcloths and towels in hot water. (E, 10)

26. 3. Pinworm infection is the most common parasite infection in children. The eggs, which can live in house dust for 2 weeks, come from contaminated fingers, mouth, and anus and are easily transmitted to persons in close contact. Therefore, the nurse needs to emphasize the need for washing the toddler's hands after the child has played outside. Treatment involves one dose of medication, such as mebendazole (Vermox) or pyrantel pamoate (Antiminth), and there is no need for follow-up. Parents do not need to check their child's stool once treatment has been given. (I, 10)

27. 3. Impetigo involving several superficial lesions is usually treated topically, including washing the affected areas, removing crusts, and applying antibiotic ointment several times a day. The child can return to day care or school after being treated for 24 hours. There is no need for follow-up unless the lesions have not resolved or have become more severe. (I, 10)

28. 4. Scabies is caused by the scabies mite, *Sarcoptes scabiei*. The mite burrows into the stratum corneum of

the epidermis, where the female deposits eggs and fecal material. These burrows are linear. Scabies is highly contagious. The length of time from infestation to physical symptoms is 30 to 60 days, so everyone in close contact with the child will need to be treated. The bed linens and the child's clothing should be washed in hot water and dried on the hot setting. The child should be held minimally until treatment is completed. Family members should wash their hands after contact with the child. Itching lasts for 2 to 3 weeks until the stratum corneum is replaced. (P, 10)

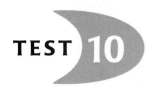

TEST 10

General Client Needs

▶ **Pharmacology and Parenteral Therapies**
▶ **Growth and Development**
▶ **Management of Care**
▶ **Correct Answers and Rationale**

Select the one best answer, and indicate your choice by filling in the circle in front of the option.

Pharmacology and Parenteral Therapies

1. A child is receiving methylprednisolone (Solu-Medrol) intravenously as treatment for a severe asthmatic attack. The nurse closely monitors the flow rate of the intravenous infusion to prevent the development of which of the following?
   ○ 1. Hypertension.
   ○ 2. Nausea.
   ○ 3. Flushing of the skin.
   ○ 4. Seizures.

2. A child with asthma continues to have a heart rate of 160 bpm and a respiratory rate of 36 breaths/minute. The child appears restless and anxious. The child is given albuterol (Ventolin) via nebulizer. Which of the following would indicate that the nebulizer treatment has been effective?
   ○ 1. Pulse oximeter reading of 91%.
   ○ 2. Nonproductive cough.
   ○ 3. Expiratory wheezing.
   ○ 4. Increase in peak expiratory flow rate.

3. The nurse teaches the parents of a 2-year-old how to instill antibiotic ear drops. Which of the following statements about the direction to pull on the earlobe indicates that the child's father has understood the teaching?
   ○ 1. Up and forward.
   ○ 2. Up and backward.
   ○ 3. Down and outward.
   ○ 4. Down and backward.

4. Which of the following techniques would be *most* appropriate to use when determining whether the parental teaching about how to administer ear drops correctly has been successful?
   ○ 1. Observing the parents instilling the drops in the child's ear.
   ○ 2. Listening to the parents as they describe the procedure.
   ○ 3. Asking the parents to list the steps in the procedure.

   ○ 4. Asking the parents whether they have read the handout on the procedure.

5. Which of the following statements by the mother of a child who is receiving pancreatic enzymes for treatment of cystic fibrosis indicates that the mother understands the teaching?
   ○ 1. "I should give the medicine about 1 hour before meals."
   ○ 2. "I can sprinkle the enzymes on food."
   ○ 3. "I'll give the enzymes when my child is sick."
   ○ 4. "I'll give the medication when my child has diarrhea."

6. When developing a teaching plan for the parents of a child who is receiving digoxin (Lanoxin), which of the following would be *most* important for the nurse to include?
   ○ 1. Telling the parents about the side effects.
   ○ 2. Discussing why the child is receiving this medicine.
   ○ 3. Explaining the difference between milligrams and micrograms.
   ○ 4. Showing the mother the correct prescribed dosage.

7. Which of the following would the nurse explain to the mother of a child receiving digoxin (Lanoxin) as the primary reason for giving this drug?
   ○ 1. To relax the walls of the heart's arteries.
   ○ 2. To improve the strength of the heartbeat.
   ○ 3. To prevent irregularities in ventricular contractions.
   ○ 4. To decrease inflammation of the heart wall.

8. Which of the following signs and symptoms would indicate to the nurse that the child is experiencing mercaptopurine (Purinethol) toxicity?
   ○ 1. Anorexia, nausea, and vomiting.
   ○ 2. Skin rash, constipation, and polyuria.
   ○ 3. Dry mouth, blurred vision, and headache.
   ○ 4. Drowsiness, malaise, and low blood pressure.

9. Which of the following nursing measures would be carried out for a child who is receiving chemotherapy and allopurinol (Zyloprim)?

○ 1. Encouraging a high fluid intake.
○ 2. Omitting carbonated fluids.
○ 3. Giving foods that are high in potassium.
○ 4. Limiting foods that are high in natural sugar.

10. Which of the following would the nurse expect to do for the child who is receiving high-dose methotrexate (amethopterin) therapy?
    ○ 1. Keep the child in a fasting state.
    ○ 2. Obtain a white blood cell count.
    ○ 3. Prepare for radiography of the spinal canal.
    ○ 4. Collect a specimen for urinalysis.

11. A child has an order to receive 250 mL of intravenous fluids every 4 hours. The nurse would set the infusion pump using microdrip tubing to run at which of the following flow rates?
    ○ 1. 10 mL/hour.
    ○ 2. 25 mL/hour.
    ○ 3. 42 mL/hour.
    ○ 4. 63 mL/hour.

12. A child is to receive intravenous fluids at a rate of 95 mL/hour. The tubing for the infusion delivers 10 drops/mL. At which of the following rates would the nurse infuse the solution?
    ○ 1. 10 drops/minute.
    ○ 2. 14 drops/minute.
    ○ 3. 16 drops/minute.
    ○ 4. 20 drops/minute.

13. Which of the following statements by an adolescent receiving gentamicin sulfate (Garamycin) would the nurse interpret as indicating toxicity of the drug?
    ○ 1. "I'm feeling dizzy."
    ○ 2. "I have no appetite."
    ○ 3. "I urinate a lot now."
    ○ 4. "I haven't moved my bowels in 3 days."

14. Which of the following laboratory test results would the nurse assess in a child with nephrotic syndrome who is receiving cyclophosphamide (Cytoxan)?
    ○ 1. Glucose.
    ○ 2. Protein.
    ○ 3. Platelets.
    ○ 4. White cell count.

15. The mother of an infant who has an order for 40 mg of acetaminophen every 4 hours for pain states that she will use the infant drops, which come in a concentration of 80 mg/0.8 mL. Which of the following amounts would the nurse tell the mother to give the infant?
    ○ 1. One dropperful.
    ○ 2. One-half dropperful.
    ○ 3. 0.78 mL, using a 1-mL syringe.
    ○ 4. 1.5 mL, using a 3-mL syringe.

Growth and Development

16. The grandmother of a 7-month-old brings the infant to the clinic because she thinks the child is slow.

Which of the following developmental milestones would the nurse normally expect to assess in an infant of this age?
    ○ 1. Playing pat-a-cake.
    ○ 2. Sitting alone.
    ○ 3. Saying two words.
    ○ 4. Waving bye-bye.

17. A parent asks the nurse about the nutritional needs of her toddler. Which of the following responses by the nurse would be *most* appropriate?
    ○ 1. "Toddlers usually do not have a good appetite."
    ○ 2. "Toddlers have definite food preferences."
    ○ 3. "Toddlers usually consume large quantities of milk."
    ○ 4. "Toddlers are inquisitive, willing to try new foods."

18. The nurse visits a day care center and assesses several 18-month-old toddlers. Which of the following would the nurse expect a child in this age group to be able to accomplish?
    ○ 1. Build a tower of four cubes.
    ○ 2. Say three words.
    ○ 3. Use spoon with little spilling.
    ○ 4. Throw a ball overhand.

19. When talking with the grandparents of a toddler, which of the following would the nurse recommend as the *most* appropriate toy?
    ○ 1. Tricycle.
    ○ 2. Wheelbarrow.
    ○ 3. Sled.
    ○ 4. Blocks.

20. The parent of a preschool-aged child has been told the child has sleep terrors. Which of the following would the nurse include when teaching the parents about sleep terrors?
    ○ 1. The dreams are real to the child.
    ○ 2. Sleep terrors require psychological counseling.
    ○ 3. It is appropriate to intervene only if it is necessary to protect the child..
    ○ 4. Getting the child back to sleep may be difficult.

21. When teaching a group of parents of school-aged children about growth and development, which of the following characteristics would the nurse include about children of this age?
    ○ 1. Desire to carry a task to completion.
    ○ 2. Ability to imagine possibilities.
    ○ 3. Feeling that others are focused on them.
    ○ 4. Ability to consider hypothetical risks and benefits.

22. When assessing a 13-year-old adolescent, which of the following would the nurse expect to find?
    ○ 1. Tanner stage I of development.
    ○ 2. Decision about a career.
    ○ 3. Primarily one friend.
    ○ 4. Subjective judgments of right and wrong.

23. A babysitter calls the clinic nurse because she is concerned about a school-aged child's constant swearing. Which of the following suggestions would be *most* appropriate?
    ○ 1. Put hot sauce on the child's tongue.
    ○ 2. Ground the child to the bedroom.
    ○ 3. Embarrass the child in front of friends.
    ○ 4. Tell the parents so that they can punish the child.

24. Which of the following responses by the nurse would be *most* appropriate for the mother of a 4-year-old son who voices concern about her child's stuttering?
    ○ 1. "This behavior is normal and the child probably will stop soon."
    ○ 2. "The child needs to see a speech therapist before school starts."
    ○ 3. "The majority of children do this until they are about 6 years of age."
    ○ 4. "You need to help the child complete the words giving him problems."

25. The mother of a 7-year-old child comes to the clinic very upset, having just learned that her child has stolen a computer game from a store. The nurse expects to respond to the mother based on understanding of which of the following?
    ○ 1. The child needs to receive serious punishment for the stealing behavior.
    ○ 2. The child needs to apologize and return the game to the store.
    ○ 3. The mother needs to have a long talk with the child to explain why the behavior was wrong.
    ○ 4. This is an indication of something is seriously wrong with the child.

26. The nurse in a homeless clinic has an opportunity to teach parents of toddlers. Which of the following would be *most* important to include when teaching the parents how to promote overall toddler development?
    ○ 1. Language is the most important achievement.
    ○ 2. Discipline is critical to appropriate development.
    ○ 3. Safety is a priority concern for this age group.
    ○ 4. Eating habits that follow into adulthood begin now.

27. During a home visit, the nurse notices that a 1-month-old infant has esotropia. The nurse would advise the parent to do which of the following?
    ○ 1. Call the baby's health care provider immediately.
    ○ 2. Mention this finding at the baby's 6-month checkup.
    ○ 3. Do nothing, because this condition is normal for the infant's age.
    ○ 4. Call the clinic for a referral to an optometrist.

28. The mother of a 4-year-old is concerned about her child's masturbating. When responding to the mother, which of the following would the nurse need to keep in mind?
    ○ 1. The child needs counseling for the abnormal behavior.
    ○ 2. Masturbation is normal in children of this age.
    ○ 3. The child is expressing some unmet needs.
    ○ 4. Masturbation at this age provides sexual release.

29. At the day care center, one of the toddlers bites another child. Which of the following actions by the teacher would be *most* appropriate?
    ○ 1. Bite the child who did the biting.
    ○ 2. Place the child who did the biting in "time out."
    ○ 3. Spank the child who did the biting.
    ○ 4. Call the parents to pick up the child who did the biting.

Management of Care

30. Which of the following would the nurse do when suspecting that a child has been abused by the mother?
    ○ 1. Continue to collect information until there is no doubt in the nurse's mind that abuse has occurred.
    ○ 2. Ensure that any and all findings are reported to the proper state and legal authorities.
    ○ 3. Keep the findings confidential, because they represent legal privileged communication between the nurse and the mother.
    ○ 4. Report the findings to the physician because that falls within the responsibilities of medical practice.

31. When preparing to admit an infant diagnosed with diarrhea to the pediatric unit, the nurse would expect to assign the infant to which of the following rooms?
    ○ 1. A four-bed room with postoperative clients.
    ○ 2. A two-bed room with an infant with respiratory disease.
    ○ 3. A two-bed room with no roommate.
    ○ 4. A room with other infants younger than 1 year of age.

32. After receiving report, the nurse is making out assignments. Which of the following clients would be appropriate to assign to unlicensed nursing personnel?
    ○ 1. A 6-year-old with a femur fracture and a fever.
    ○ 2. A 13-year-old with fluctuating vital signs and a new central line.
    ○ 3. A 7-year-old transferred from the cardiac intensive care unit.
    ○ 4. An 8-month-old with pneumonia who will be discharged today.

33. When making rounds on assigned clients, which of the following clients would the nurse assess *first*?
    ○ 1. A 16-month-old with periorbital cellulitis who is to be discharged today.
    ○ 2. A 7-year-old who had an appendectomy yesterday and developed peritonitis.
    ○ 3. A 10-year-old who has just been admitted in sickle cell crisis.
    ○ 4. A 16-year-old receiving a third day of chemotherapy.

34. Which of the following families would the nurse determine as *most* in need of follow-up?
    ○ 1. A single mother with a 7-month-old child whose immunizations are delayed.
    ○ 2. A two-parent family whose 3-year-old has a fractured leg from an automobile accident.
    ○ 3. A single parent with a toddler who has third-degree burns over 20% of the body.
    ○ 4. A two-parent family with a foster child who has a history of caustic liquid ingestion.

35. The grandmother has brought an infant to the clinic for a checkup and has signed the consent for immunization administration. Which of the following would the nurse do *first*?
    ○ 1. Ask who is the infant's legal guardian.
    ○ 2. Notify the physician immediately.
    ○ 3. Administer the immunizations as ordered.
    ○ 4. Call the infant's mother for verbal consent.

36. The charge nurse for the pediatric unit is making client care assignments for the staff which includes LPN/LVN and unlicensed assistive personnel. Which of the following children would be *most* appropriate to assign to the LPN/LVN?
    ○ 1. An 8-year-old with a concussion whose hourly vital signs are stable.
    ○ 2. A 9-year-old with a week-old fractured femur who is in traction.
    ○ 3. A 13-year-old who has just returned from surgery for repair of internal injuries.
    ○ 4. A 15-year-old who is just beginning to awaken from a drug overdose.

37. Which of the following actions would be *most* appropriate for a charge nurse to do *first* when finding that a nurse who is caring for a very sick infant is making inappropriate remarks and acting in a bizarre manner?
    ○ 1. Report this nurse to the supervisor.
    ○ 2. Remove this nurse from the client assignment.
    ○ 3. Call the nurse's family to have someone take the nurse home.
    ○ 4. Talk with the nurse to determine why this behavior is occurring.

38. The parents of an infant with congenital defects tell the nurse they will not come back to take their baby home. Which of the following would the nurse do *next*?
    ○ 1. Determine why the parents will not pick their baby up.
    ○ 2. Notify the physician so the physician can contact the parents.
    ○ 3. Call the police to report an abandoned infant.
    ○ 4. Refer the family to a social service agency.

39. A nurse is explaining the pediatric unit's quality improvement (QI) program to a newly employed nurse. Which of the following would the nurse include as one of the primary purposes of QI programs?
    ○ 1. Evaluation of staff members' performances.
    ○ 2. Evaluation of the system and client outcomes.
    ○ 3. Improvement in efficiency of care.
    ○ 4. Preparation for accreditation of the organization by the Joint Commission on Accreditation of Healthcare Organizations (JCAHO).

40. The nurse manager of the pediatric unit notices that vital signs are frequently not being documented on children returning from surgery. According to total quality management (TQI), to correct this problem, the manager would do which of the following?
    ○ 1. Talk to staff members individually to determine why this is occurring.
    ○ 2. Call a meeting of all staff members to discuss the issue.
    ○ 3. Have a group of staff nurses review the established standards of care for postoperative patients.
    ○ 4. Document which staff members are not recording vital signs and reprimand them.

41. A nurse overhears a fellow staff member talking about the mother of a child for whom the staff nurse is caring. The nurse is telling others private information that the mother had shared. Which of the following responses by the nurse overhearing the conversation would be *best*?
    ○ 1. Reporting this incident to their nurse manager.
    ○ 2. Telling the mother what was being said about her.
    ○ 3. Talking to the staff member privately about this.
    ○ 4. Talking to the staff in general about confidentiality.

42. A father who is very upset about something the staff nurse said to him is in his child's room yelling and saying he will take his child home. Which of the following actions by the nurse manager would be *most* appropriate?
    ○ 1. Notifying the physician that the father is taking the child home.
    ○ 2. Calling the social worker who knows the father well.

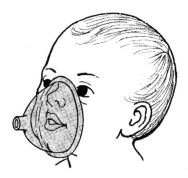

Figure 1.

○ 3. Asking the father to come to the conference room to discuss the problem.

○ 4. Calling the child's mother to let her know what the situation is.

43. Two parents who are arguing in their infant's room, with voices raised and getting louder, start to hit each other. The infant is crying. Which of the following would the staff nurse do *next*?

○ 1. Try to reason with both of the parents.

○ 2. Ask one of the parents to leave the room.

○ 3. Call security to come and break up the fight.

○ 4. Remove the infant from the room.

44. A neonate is experiencing respiratory distress and is using a neonatal oxygen mask. An unlicensed assistive personnel has positioned the oxygen mask as shown in Figure 1. The nurse is assessing the neonate and determines that the mask

○ 1. is appropriate for the neonate.

○ 2. is too large, because it covers the neonate's eyes.

○ 3. is too small, because it obstructs the nose.

○ 4. should be covered with a soft cloth before being placed against the skin.

Correct Answers and Rationale

The letters in parentheses following the rationale identify the step of the nursing process (A, D, P, I, E) and client needs (1, 2, 3, 4, 5, 6, 7, 8, 9, 10). See the inside front cover for the key.

Pharmacology and Parenteral Therapies

1. 1. A serious side effect of intravenous administration of methylprednisolone is hypertension, which occurs more frequently when the infusion is administered at too rapid a flow rate. Although nausea may occur with this drug, it is not as serious a problem as hypertension is. Flushing is not associated with methylprednisolone administration. Seizures may occur if an infusion of ampicillin is given too rapidly. (I, 8)

2. 4. The best indicator of the effectiveness of the albuterol is an increase in peak expiratory flow rate. Albuterol, a bronchodilator, opens and relaxes the airways, allowing a greater exchange of air, which is reflected as a higher peak expiratory flow rate. As the airways open, the child should begin to have a productive cough. Pulse oximetry reflects how well the client is oxygenating: the higher the reading, the better the client's oxygenation. Typically, a pulse oximeter reading of 95% or greater is the goal. Furthermore, a pulse oximeter reading of 91% is meaningless unless previous readings are available for comparison. Wheezing may or may not be a reliable indicator for determining the effectiveness of the albuterol treatment. The nebulizer treatment may increase wheezing by opening the airways enough so that air can travel through the excessively mucus-filled bronchioles. Because this child is still experiencing respiratory distress, some wheezing would be expected. However, wheezing in a child with asthma who is in acute distress may indicate an improvement, demonstrating the movement of air through the airways that were previously blocked. (E, 8)

3. 4. For children aged 3 years and younger, the external auditory canal is straightened by gently pulling the earlobe down and backward. For an older child or an adult, the earlobe is gently pulled up and backward. (E, 9)

4. 1. Return demonstrations are the best way to evaluate a person's ability to perform a skill. This technique enables the teacher to observe not only the learner's sequencing of steps of the procedure but also the learner's ability to perform the skill. (E, 9)

5. 2. One problem associated with cystic fibrosis is poor digestion and absorption of foods, especially fats. Pancreatic enzymes can help improve digestion and absorption of nutrients. Therefore, they are given with meals and can be sprinkled on food. They must be taken regularly, not just when the child is sick. (E, 8)

6. 4. Although all of the responses should be included in the teaching plan, the most important thing is to show the mother what the correct dose of digoxin should look like. Too much of the medication can cause significant slowing of the heart. The drug is toxic and can be harmful, perhaps even fatal, if an overdose is taken. (P, 8)

7. 2. Digitalis preparations, such as digoxin (Lanoxin), act to improve and strengthen the heartbeat. They increase cardiac output by increasing the strength of the heart's contraction and decreasing the heart rate. Digoxin does not relax the heart's arterial walls, prevent irregularities in ventricular contractions, or decrease inflammation of the heart wall. (I, 8)

8. 1. Toxic doses of mercaptopurine would most likely produce anorexia, nausea, vomiting, and diarrhea. This drug is associated with bone marrow suppression. Therefore, blood counts are especially important. Dry mouth, blurred vision, headache, drowsiness, malaise, and low blood pressure are side effects associated with antihistamine use. (I, 8)

9. 1. Destruction of malignant cells during chemotherapy produces large amounts of uric acid. The client's kidneys may not be able to eliminate the uric acid, and tubular obstruction from the crystals could result in renal failure and uremia. Allopurinol (Zyloprim) interrupts the process of purine degradation to reduce uric acid buildup. The client should be encouraged to increase fluid intake to further assist in eliminating uric acid. Carbonated fluids need not be omitted when allopurinol is administered. An intake of foods high in potassium is not necessary, nor is limiting foods high in natural sugar. (I, 8)

10. 2. Methotrexate is not highly toxic in low doses but may cause severe leukopenia at higher doses. It is customary and recommended for blood tests to be done before therapy to provide a baseline from which to study the effects of the drug on white blood cell levels. Maintaining a fasting state, radiography of the spinal canal, and urinalysis are not necessary when this drug is administered. (D, 8)

11. 4. The rate set on the pump equals the number of milliliters to be delivered in 1 hour: 250 mL in 4 hours is equal to about 63 mL to be infused each hour. (I, 8)

12. 3. To determine the number of drops per minute, multiply 95 mL/hour by 10 (drop factor). This equals 950 mL/hour. Dividing 950 mL/hour by 60 minutes yields 15.8 drops/minute. Therefore, 16 drops/minute should be infused. (I, 8)

13. 1. Gentamicin sulfate is a broad-spectrum aminoglycoside antibiotic that can cause nephrotoxicity and ototoxicity. Manifestations of ototoxicity include hearing problems and vestibular disturbances, such as dizziness. Anorexia may occur; however, it is not indicative of gentamicin toxicity. Frequent urination is more commonly associated with diuretic therapy. If nephrotoxicity were occurring, the client probably would report a decrease in urination. No bowel movement in 3 days suggests constipation. More commonly, constipation is related to the use of narcotic analgesics. (D, 8)

14. 4. Children with nephrotic syndrome who are sensitive to steroids or have frequent relapses are candidates for therapy with cyclophosphamide. Common side effects include decreased white blood cell count, increased susceptibility to infections, cystitis (from bladder irritation when the drug accumulates in the bladder before excretion), and possibly hair loss and sterility. Because a child with nephrotic syndrome is susceptible to infection, it is important to monitor the white blood cell count and institute precautions if it is low. (A, 8)

15. 2. The correct amount is one-half dropperful, or 0.4 mL: 80 mg = 0.8 mL; 40 mg = 0.4 mL. One dropperful is 0.8 mL; one-half of a dropperful is 0.4 mL. (I, 8)

Growth and Development

16. 2. The majority of infants (90%) can sit without support by 7 months of age. Approximately 75% of infants at 10 months of age are able to play pat-a-cake. The ability to say two words occurs in 90% of children by 16 months. A child typically can wave bye-bye at about 14 months of age. (A, 3)

17. 2. Toddlers have definite food preferences, typically wanting the same food item for several days in a row. Because toddlers experience a slow and steady growth rate, they usually have a good appetite. Toddlers should consume 2 to 3 cups of milk per day. The majority of their nutrients should come from table foods. Toddlers typically are not interested in trying new foods. (I, 3)

18. 2. By 18 months, 90% of children can say three words. Typically a child 23 months of age can build a tower of four cubes. The ability to use a spoon or fork with little spilling is accomplished by the age of 20 months. Throwing a ball overhand typically is achieved by 3 years of age. (A, 3)

19. 4. As toddlers begin imaginative play, blocks are an excellent toy choice. Children can use blocks any way they desire, thus fostering imaginative play. A tricycle, wheelbarrow, or sled is an appropriate toy for a preschooler because it requires the use of specific motor skills developed during the preschool period. These motor skills are lacking in a toddler. (I, 3)

20. 3. Sleep terrors typically start within a few hours after the child falls asleep. The child has no memory of the dream and returns to sleep rapidly. Also, it is difficult to keep the child awake. Sleep terrors are very common and rarely require intervention. The dreams are real to the child experiencing nightmares, not sleep terrors. Comforting to return to sleep is needed when the child experience nightmares. (I, 3)

21. 1. School-aged children typically desire to carry a task to completion to achieve a sense of personal accomplishment. Adolescents have more abstract thought, including the ability to imagine possibilities or consider hypothetical risks and benefits, and also feelings that others are focused on them. (I, 3)

22. 4. For the adolescent, moral development occurs as abstract reasoning develops. Moral issues are seen to differ based on opinions. Many adolescents at 13 years of age have reached at least Tanner stage II, an assessment of the development of secondary sex characteristics. Many adolescents at this age do not have a career choice in mind yet. Typically adolescents have more than one friend. (A, 3)

23. 2. The most appropriate action for the babysitter is to ground the child to the bedroom. By doing so, the babysitter is indicating to the child that the child's behavior is unacceptable and that unacceptable behavior results in consequences. The babysitter also should tell the parents about the incident once the parents get home. Putting hot sauce on the child's tongue does not teach the child appropriate behavior. Embarrassing the child also is not appropriate because it does not teach the child to control behavior. (I, 3)

24. 1. Stuttering is considered a normal behavior during preschool years. Children know what they want to say but hesitate or repeat sounds as they search for the correct words. The child would not need to see a speech therapist unless the stuttering continues beyond the preschool years. The parent is advised never to help a child by finishing a word for him. Rather, the child needs plenty of time to finish. (I, 3)

25. 2. In most situations, children 5 to 8 years of age have not yet developed respect for others' property. They may take something such as money or a game because they are attracted to it. This usually is not an indication of a serious problem in the child. Serious punishment is inappropriate. A long talk is not warranted in this situation because the child is unable to maintain attention for a long period. (P, 3)

26. 3. Because of toddlers' high energy and poor impulse control, safety is a priority concern for this age group.

Additionally, the family's homeless situation further underscores the need for safety because the family has less control over the environment. (P, 2)

27. 3. The nurse should advise the parents to do nothing, because esotropia, inward turning of the eyes, is a normal finding in infants of this age. If the condition continues past the age of 4 months, more aggressive treatment will be advised. Waiting until the infant's 6-month checkup to mention the finding is inappropriate. (I, 3)

28. 2. Most boys and girls masturbate, most commonly at about 4 years of age and then again during adolescence. It is not considered abnormal behavior. Masturbation at this age is part of sexual exploration and curiosity; it does not express unmet needs or release sexual tension. Parents need to ensure privacy for the child. (I, 3)

29. 2. Biting is an unacceptable aggressive behavior that should not be allowed. Placing the child who did the biting in "time out" is most appropriate because it removes the child from the situation and the other children and also teaches the child that the behavior is inappropriate. When a child bites another, the child who did the biting should never be bitten. Doing so teaches the child that biting is an acceptable behavior. Spanking the child is inappropriate because doing so reinforces the hitting behavior as appropriate. Calling the parents to pick up the child is inappropriate because the teacher should be able to handle this situation properly. However, the parents should be informed of the incident. (I, 3)

Management of Care

30. 2. Evidence of child abuse is legally reportable by anyone who works with children. The nurse should ensure that the findings are reported to the proper authorities. Laws ordinarily provide immunity from legal actions for people who are required to report suspicion of child abuse, if the report is done in good faith. Suspicion, not absolute proof, is necessary for reporting abuse. The nurse's primary responsibility is to the primary client, the child, and not the mother. (I, 1)

31. 3. To reduce the risk of infection transmission, a infant with diarrhea of undetermined origin should be placed in a room alone until a causative organism can be identified. Additionally, because infants do not have bowel control, the risk for transmission increases. (P, 1)

32. 4. The most appropriate client to assign to unlicensed nursing personnel would be the client who is stable. RNs have the responsibility for assessment, evaluation, and making nursing judgments. (P, 1)

33. 3. Of the clients listed, the newly admitted client should be assessed first. This is the client who is likely to be unstable and in pain. The child to be discharged today would be considered the most stable and therefore would be assessed last. (A, 1)

34. 3. A toddler has burns usually as the result of not being closely supervised. Toddlers are very inquisitive and need constant supervision. Therefore, close follow-up is necessary. In addition, the child probably will need some type of wound care requiring involvement of the parent and possibly others. The amount of support available to the single parent is not known. Although immunization schedules need to be adhered to, it is very possible for a 7-month-old to be delayed in receiving immunizations because of illness or other conflicts. An automobile accident can happen to anyone and does not indicate a lack of safety or supervision. A history of ingestion in a foster child may have been from a time before the child began living with the foster parents; it does not indicate a lack of safety or supervision. (A, 1)

35. 1. The first question to ask is who is the infant's legal guardian. The legal guardian gives consent for treatments, procedures, and immunizations. Once this is determined and consent is obtained, then the nurse may administer the immunizations as ordered. Notifying the physician would be done if the nurse determined that the grandmother was not the infant's legal guardian. If the nurse determined that the infant's legal guardian was the mother, then calling the mother for consent would be appropriate. (I, 1)

36. 1. The most appropriate client to assign to the LPN/LVN is the client with stable vital signs and a predictable outcome. The 9-year-old would be assigned to unlicensed assistive nursing personnel because this client is stable. The adolescent just returning from surgery requires frequent, close assessment and monitoring for possible complications, which is inappropriate for the LPN/LVN level. The adolescent just beginning to awaken from a drug overdose is not stable and requires close, frequent assessment for changes. (P, 1)

37. 2. Because client safety is the priority, the most appropriate first action by the charge nurse would be to remove the nurse who is acting bizarrely from the client assignment. The charge nurse would next report the behavior to the supervisor. Then the charge nurse might try talking to the nurse and calling someone to take the nurse home. (I, 1)

38. 1. The first action by the nurse would be to determine why the parents stated they would not pick up their baby. Parents who are upset, anxious, or having difficulty coping may say things they do not mean. Notifying the physician would be appropriate, but more information needs to be obtained before doing so. A

referral to a social service agency may be needed once the nurse determines why the parents stated that they would not be picking up their baby. Calling the police would be done last. (I, 1)

39. 2. The goal of QI is to ensure that the best care is delivered to clients and families. This can be achieved by attention to client outcomes. Staff performance evaluations, completed according to institutional policy, focus on staff, not client outcomes. Improved care efficiency may be an aspect of quality client care, but it is not the goal. JCAHO has strict parameters to which an institution must adhere to ensure accreditation. QI is but one aspect to demonstrate adherence to the parameters. The goal of QI is to ensure that the best care is delivered to clients and families, not to ensure JCAHO accreditation. (I, 1)

40. 3. According to TQI—a proactive, participative approach to improving all aspects of client care—the manager would have a group of staff members review the established patient care standards and make suggestions. (I, 1)

41. 3. The best approach is to talk to the staff member privately about the information that the mother shared. This information is confidential and should not be disclosed. Reporting the incident to the nurse manager is appropriate once the nurse has spoken to the staff member privately. Although it may be tempting to tell the mother, talking to the staff member privately is the best approach, because trust between the staff nurse and mother needs to be maintained. Talking to the staff in general about confidentiality may be beneficial. However, the nurse needs to speak with the staff member in private first. (I, 1)

42. 3. The situation needs to be defused immediately. Therefore, removal of the father from the child's room, such as to a conference room, is the best approach to resolve the situation. The physician needs to be notified, but not until after the manager has attempted resolution. Calling the social worker or the mother may be helpful after the situation is defused. (I, 1)

43. 4. The situation is escalating, and the nurse's priority is to protect the infant from harm. Therefore, removal of the infant from this situation would be the first action by the nurse. Reasoning at this point or asking one of the parents to leave the room would be ineffective and may serve to further escalate the situation. Calling security is necessary, but only after the nurse has removed the child from the room. (I, 1)

44. 2. The mask is too large and is covering the neonate's eyes. The correct size covers the nose but not the eyes. Masks that are too small may pinch the nose. Masks should fit snugly against the cheeks and chin. (E, 1)

Bibliography

American Academy of Pediatrics, Committee on Infectious Disease. (2000). *Red Book: Report of the Committee on Infectious Disease.* Elk Grove Village, IL: Author.

Bowden, V., Dickey, S., & Greenberg, C. (1998). *Children and their families.* Philadelphia: W. B. Saunders.

Broome, M., & Rollins, J., (Eds.). (1998). *Core curriculum for nursing care of children and their families.* Jannetti Publishers.

Curley, M., & Moloney-Harmon, P. (Eds.). (2001). *Critical care nursing of infants and children.* Philadelphia: W. B. Saunders.

Fischbach, F. (1998). *Nurses' quick reference to common laboratory and diagnostic tests.* (2nd ed.) Philadelphia: Lippincott Williams & Wilkins.

Pillitteri, A. (1998). *Maternal and child health nursing: Care of the childbearing and childbearing family* (3rd ed.). Philadelphia: Lippincott Williams & Wilkins.

Slota, M. C. (Ed.).(1998). *Core curriculum for pediatric critical care nursing.* Philadelphia: W. B. Saunders.

Whaley, L. F., & Wong, D. L. (1999). *Nursing care of infants and children* (6th ed.). St. Louis: Mosby–Year Book.

PART III

The Nursing Care of Adults With Medical and Surgical Health Problems

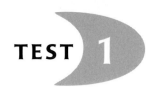
The Client With Cardiac Health Problems

▶ **The Client With Myocardial Infarction**

▶ **The Client With Heart Failure**

▶ **The Client With Valvular Heart Disease**

▶ **The Client With Hypertension**

▶ **The Client With Angina**

▶ **The Client With a Permanent Pacemaker**

▶ **The Client Requiring Cardiopulmonary Resuscitation**

▶ **Correct Answers and Rationale**

Select the one best answer, and indicate your choice by filling in the circle in front of the option.

The Client With Myocardial Infarction

1. A 60-year-old male client comes into the emergency department with complaints of crushing substernal chest pain that radiates to his shoulder and left arm. The admitting diagnosis is acute myocardial infarction (MI). Immediate admission orders include oxygen by nasal cannula at 4 L/minute, blood work, a chest radiograph, a 12-lead electrocardiogram (ECG), and 2 mg of morphine sulfate given intravenously. The nurse should first
   ○ 1. administer the morphine.
   ○ 2. obtain a 12-lead ECG.
   ○ 3. obtain the blood work.
   ○ 4. order the chest radiograph.
2. When administering a thrombolytic drug to the client experiencing an MI, the nurse explains to him that the purpose of the drug is to
   ○ 1. help keep him well hydrated.
   ○ 2. dissolve clots that he may have.
   ○ 3. prevent kidney failure.
   ○ 4. treat potential cardiac dysrhythmias.
3. The nurse is assessing a client who has had an MI. The nurse notes the cardiac rhythm shown on the ECG strip in Figure 1. The nurse identifies this rhythm as which of the following?
   ○ 1. Atrial fibrillation.
   ○ 2. Ventricular tachycardia.
   ○ 3. Premature ventricular contractions (PVCs).
   ○ 4. Third-degree heart block.
4. The nurse is assessing a client who has had an MI. The nurse notes the cardiac rhythm shown on the ECG strip in Figure 2. The nurse identifies this rhythm as which of the following?

   ○ 1. Atrial fibrillation.
   ○ 2. Ventricular tachycardia.
   ○ 3. PVCs.
   ○ 4. Sinus tachycardia.
5. The nurse is assessing a client who has had an MI. The nurse notes the cardiac rhythm shown on the ECG strip in Figure 3. The nurse identifies this rhythm as which of the following?
   ○ 1. Atrial fibrillation.
   ○ 2. Ventricular tachycardia.
   ○ 3. PVCs.
   ○ 4. Third-degree heart block.
6. If the client who was admitted for MI develops cardiogenic shock, which characteristic sign should the nurse expect to observe?
   ○ 1. Oliguria.
   ○ 2. Bradycardia.
   ○ 3. Elevated blood pressure.
   ○ 4. Fever.
7. The physician orders continuous intravenous nitroglycerin infusion for the client with MI. Essential nursing actions include which of the following?
   ○ 1. Obtaining an infusion pump for the medication.
   ○ 2. Monitoring blood pressure every 4 hours.
   ○ 3. Monitoring urine output hourly.
   ○ 4. Obtaining serum potassium levels daily.
8. When teaching the client with MI, the nurse explains that the pain associated with MI is caused by
   ○ 1. left ventricular overload.
   ○ 2. impending circulatory collapse.
   ○ 3. extracellular electrolyte imbalances.
   ○ 4. insufficient oxygen reaching the heart muscle.

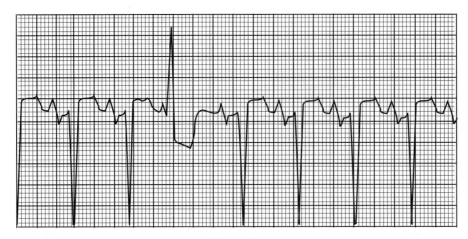

Figure 1.

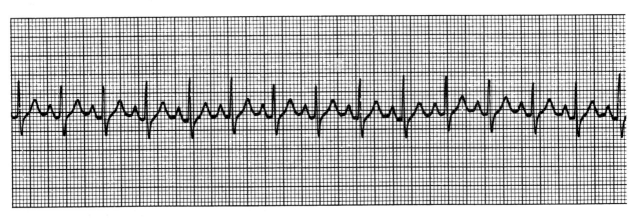

Figure 2.

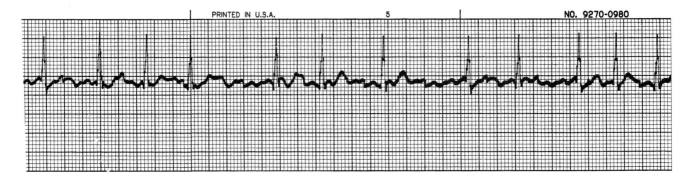

Figure 3.

9. Aspirin is administered to the client experiencing an MI because of its
   - ○ 1. antipyretic action.
   - ○ 2. antithrombotic action.
   - ○ 3. antiplatelet action.
   - ○ 4. analgesic action.

10. While caring for a client who has sustained an MI, the nurse notes eight PVCs in 1 minute on the cardiac monitor. The client is receiving an intravenous infusion of 5% dextrose in water and oxygen at 2 L/minute. The nurse's *first* course of action should be to
    - ○ 1. increase the intravenous infusion rate.
    - ○ 2. notify the physician promptly.
    - ○ 3. increase the oxygen concentration.
    - ○ 4. administer a prescribed analgesic.

11. Which of the following is an expected outcome for a client on the second day of hospitalization after an MI? The client
    - ○ 1. has minimal chest pain.
    - ○ 2. can identify risk factors for MI.
    - ○ 3. agrees to participate in a cardiac rehabilitation program.

○ 4. can perform personal self-care activities without pain.

12. When teaching a client about the expected outcomes after intravenous administration of furosemide, the nurse would include which outcome?
○ 1. Increased blood pressure.
○ 2. Increased urine output.
○ 3. Decreased pain.
○ 4. Decreased PVCs.

13. After an MI, the hospitalized client is taught to move the legs about while resting in bed. This type of exercise is recommended primarily to help
○ 1. prepare the client for ambulation.
○ 2. promote urinary and intestinal elimination.
○ 3. prevent thrombophlebitis and blood clot formation.
○ 4. decrease the likelihood of decubitus ulcer formation.

14. Which of the following reflects the principle on which a client's diet will most likely be based during the acute phase of MI?
○ 1. Liquids as desired.
○ 2. Small, easily digested meals.
○ 3. Three regular meals per day.
○ 4. Nothing by mouth.

15. Of the following controllable risk factors for coronary artery disease (CAD) appears most closely linked to the development of the disease?
○ 1. Age.
○ 2. Medication usage.
○ 3. High cholesterol levels.
○ 4. Gender.

16. Which of the following is an uncontrollable risk factor that has been linked to the development of CAD?
○ 1. Exercise.
○ 2. Obesity.
○ 3. Stress.
○ 4. Heredity.

17. If a client displays risk factors for CAD such as smoking cigarettes, eating a diet high in saturated fat, or leading a sedentary lifestyle, techniques of behavior modification may be used to help the client change behavior. The nurse can best reinforce new adaptive behaviors by
○ 1. explaining how the old behavior leads to poor health.
○ 2. withholding praise until the new behavior is well established.
○ 3. rewarding the client whenever the acceptable behavior is performed.
○ 4. instilling mild fear into the client to extinguish the behavior.

18. Alteplase recombinant, or tissue plasminogen activator (t-PA), a thrombolytic enzyme, is administered during the first 6 hours after onset of MI to

○ 1. control chest pain.
○ 2. reduce coronary artery vasospasm.
○ 3. control the dysrhythmias associated with MI.
○ 4. revascularize the blocked coronary artery.

19. After the administration of t-PA, the nurse understands that a nursing assessment priority is to
○ 1. observe the client for chest pain.
○ 2. monitor for fever.
○ 3. monitor the 12-lead ECG every 4 hours.
○ 4. monitor breath sounds.

20. When monitoring a client who is receiving t-PA, the nurse understands it is important to monitor vital signs and have resuscitation equipment available because reperfusion of the cardiac tissue can result in which of the following?
○ 1. Cardiac dysrhythmias.
○ 2. Hypertension.
○ 3. Seizure.
○ 4. Hypothermia.

21. Contraindications to the administration of t-PA include which of the following?
○ 1. Age greater than 60 years.
○ 2. History of cerebral hemorrhage.
○ 3. History of heart failure.
○ 4. Cigarette smoking.

22. A client has driven himself into the emergency room. He is 50 years old, has a history of hypertension, and informs the nurse that his father died from a heart attack at 60 years of age. The client is presently complaining of indigestion. The nurse connects him to an ECG monitor and begins administering oxygen at 2 L/minute per nasal cannula. The nurse's next action would be to
○ 1. call for the doctor.
○ 2. start an intravenous line.
○ 3. obtain a portable chest radiograph.
○ 4. draw blood for laboratory studies.

23. Crackles heard on lung auscultation indicate which of the following?
○ 1. Cyanosis.
○ 2. Bronchospasm.
○ 3. Airway narrowing.
○ 4. Fluid-filled alveoli.

24. A 68-year-old female client on day 2 after hip surgery has no cardiac history but starts to complain of chest heaviness. The first nursing action should be to
○ 1. inquire about the onset, duration, severity, and precipitating factors of the heaviness.
○ 2. administer oxygen via nasal cannula.
○ 3. offer pain medication for the chest heaviness.
○ 4. inform the physician of the chest heaviness.

25. The nurse receives emergency laboratory results for a client with chest pain and immediately informs the physician. An increased myoglobin level suggests which of the following?

○ 1. Cancer.
○ 2. Hypertension.
○ 3. Liver disease.
○ 4. Myocardial damage.

26. An older, sedentary adult may not respond to emotional or physical stress as well as a younger individual because of
   ○ 1. left ventricular atrophy.
   ○ 2. irregular heart beats.
   ○ 3. peripheral vascular occlusion.
   ○ 4. pacemaker placement.

The Client With Heart Failure

27. A 69-year-old woman has a history of heart failure. She is admitted to the emergency department with heart failure complicated by pulmonary edema. On admission of this client, which of the following should be assessed *first*?
   ○ 1. Blood pressure.
   ○ 2. Skin breakdown.
   ○ 3. Serum potassium.
   ○ 4. Urine output.

28. In which of the following positions should the nurse place a client with suspected heart failure?
   ○ 1. Semi-sitting (low Fowler's position).
   ○ 2. Lying on the right side (Sims' position).
   ○ 3. Sitting almost upright (high Fowler's position).
   ○ 4. Lying on the back with the head lowered (Trendelenburg position).

29. Which of the following would be a priority nursing diagnosis for the client with heart failure and pulmonary edema?
   ○ 1. Risk for Infection related to line placements.
   ○ 2. Impaired Skin Integrity related to pressure.
   ○ 3. Activity Intolerance related to imbalance between oxygen supply and demand.
   ○ 4. Constipation related to immobility.

30. The major goal of therapy for a client with heart failure and pulmonary edema would be to
   ○ 1. increase cardiac output.
   ○ 2. improve respiratory status.
   ○ 3. decrease peripheral edema.
   ○ 4. enhance comfort.

31. Digoxin is administered intravenously to a client with heart failure, primarily because the drug acts to
   ○ 1. dilate coronary arteries.
   ○ 2. increase myocardial contractility.
   ○ 3. decrease cardiac dysrhythmias.
   ○ 4. decrease electrical conductivity in the heart.

32. Captopril, an angiotensin-converting enzyme (ACE) inhibitor, may be administered to a client with heart failure because it acts as a
   ○ 1. vasopressor.
   ○ 2. volume expander.
   ○ 3. vasodilator.
   ○ 4. potassium-sparing diuretic.

33. Furosemide is administered intravenously to a client with heart failure. How soon after administration should the nurse begin to see evidence of the drug's desired effect?
   ○ 1. 5 to 10 minutes.
   ○ 2. 30 to 60 minutes.
   ○ 3. 2 to 4 hours.
   ○ 4. 6 to 8 hours.

34. The nurse teaches a client with heart failure to take oral furosemide in the morning. The primary reason for this is to help
   ○ 1. prevent electrolyte imbalances.
   ○ 2. retard rapid drug absorption.
   ○ 3. excrete excessive fluids accumulated during the night.
   ○ 4. prevent sleep disturbances during the night.

35. Clients with heart failure are prone to atrial fibrillation. During physical assessment, the nurse would suspect atrial fibrillation when palpation of the radial pulse reveals
   ○ 1. two regular beats followed by one irregular beat.
   ○ 2. an irregular pulse rhythm.
   ○ 3. pulse rate below 60 bpm.
   ○ 4. a weak, thready pulse.

36. When teaching the client about complications of atrial fibrillation, the nurse understands that the complications can be caused by
   ○ 1. stasis of blood in the atria.
   ○ 2. increased cardiac output.
   ○ 3. decreased pulse rate.
   ○ 4. elevated blood pressure.

37. The nurse should teach the client that signs of digitalis toxicity include which of the following?
   ○ 1. Skin rash over the chest and back.
   ○ 2. Increased appetite.
   ○ 3. Visual disturbances such as seeing yellow spots.
   ○ 4. Elevated blood pressure.

38. The nurse should be especially alert for signs and symptoms of digitalis toxicity if serum levels indicate that the client has a
   ○ 1. low sodium level.
   ○ 2. high glucose level.
   ○ 3. high calcium level.
   ○ 4. low potassium level.

39. Which of the following foods should the nurse teach a client with heart failure to avoid or limit when following a 2-g sodium diet?
   ○ 1. Apples.
   ○ 2. Tomato juice.
   ○ 3. Whole wheat bread.
   ○ 4. Beef tenderloin.

40. To help maintain a normal blood serum level of potassium, the client receiving a loop diuretic should be encouraged to eat such foods as bananas, orange juice, and
   ○ 1. spinach.
   ○ 2. skimmed milk.
   ○ 3. baked chicken.
   ○ 4. brown rice.

41. The nurse finds the apical impulse below the fifth intercostal space. The nurse suspects
   ○ 1. left atrial enlargement.
   ○ 2. left ventricular enlargement.
   ○ 3. right atrial enlargement.
   ○ 4. right ventricular enlargement.

42. The nurse is admitting a 69-year-old man to the clinical unit. The client has a history of left ventricular enlargement. During the assessment, the nurse notes +3 pitting edema of the ankles bilaterally. The client does not have chest pain. The nurse observes that the client does have dyspnea at rest. The nurse infers that the client may have
   ○ 1. arteriosclerosis.
   ○ 2. congestive heart failure.
   ○ 3. chronic bronchitis.
   ○ 4. acute myocardial infarction.

43. The nurse's discharge teaching plan for the client with congestive heart failure would stress the significance of which of the following?
   ○ 1. Maintaining a high-fiber diet.
   ○ 2. Walking 2 miles every day.
   ○ 3. Obtaining daily weights at the same time each day.
   ○ 4. Remaining sedentary for most of the day.

The Client With Valvular Heart Disease

44. A 70-year-old woman is scheduled to undergo mitral valve replacement for severe mitral stenosis and mitral regurgitation. Although the diagnosis was made during childhood, she did not have symptoms until 4 years ago. Recently, she noticed increased symptoms, despite daily doses of digoxin and furosemide. During the initial interview with the client, the nurse would most likely learn that the client's childhood health history included
   ○ 1. chicken pox.
   ○ 2. poliomyelitis.
   ○ 3. rheumatic fever.
   ○ 4. meningitis.

45. A client experiences some initial signs of excitation after having an intravenous infusion of lidocaine hydrochloride started. The nurse would assess that the client is demonstrating a typical adverse reaction to lidocaine hydrochloride when the client complains of

○ 1. palpitations.
○ 2. tinnitus.
○ 3. urinary frequency.
○ 4. lethargy.

46. A woman with severe mitral stenosis and mitral regurgitation has a pulmonary artery catheter inserted. The physician orders pulmonary artery pressure monitoring, including pulmonary capillary wedge pressures. The purpose of this is to help assess the
   ○ 1. degree of coronary artery stenosis.
   ○ 2. peripheral arterial pressure.
   ○ 3. pressure from fluid within the left ventricle.
   ○ 4. oxygen and carbon dioxide concentrations in the blood.

47. Which of the following signs and symptoms would most likely be found in a client with mitral regurgitation?
   ○ 1. Exertional dyspnea.
   ○ 2. Confusion.
   ○ 3. Elevated creatine phosphokinase concentration.
   ○ 4. Chest pain.

48. The nurse expects that a client with mitral stenosis would demonstrate symptoms associated with congestion in the
   ○ 1. aorta.
   ○ 2. right atrium.
   ○ 3. superior vena cava.
   ○ 4. pulmonary circulation.

49. Because a client has mitral stenosis and is a prospective valve recipient, the nurse preoperatively assesses the client's past compliance with medical regimens. Lack of compliance with which of the following regimens would pose the greatest health hazard to this client?
   ○ 1. Medication therapy.
   ○ 2. Diet modification.
   ○ 3. Activity restrictions.
   ○ 4. Dental care.

50. In preparing the client and the family for a postoperative stay in the intensive care unit after open heart surgery, the nurse should explain that
   ○ 1. the client will remain in the intensive care unit for 5 days.
   ○ 2. the client will sleep most of the time while in the intensive care unit.
   ○ 3. noise and activity within the intensive care unit are minimal.
   ○ 4. the client will receive medication to relieve pain.

51. A client who has undergone a mitral valve replacement experiences persistent bleeding from the surgical incision during the early postoperative period. Which of the following pharmaceutical agents

should the nurse be prepared to administer to this client?

○ 1. Vitamin C.
○ 2. Protamine sulfate.
○ 3. Quinidine sulfate.
○ 4. Warfarin sodium (Coumadin).

52. The most effective measure the nurse can use to prevent wound infection when changing a client's dressing after coronary artery bypass surgery is to
○ 1. observe careful handwashing procedures.
○ 2. cleanse the incisional area with an antiseptic.
○ 3. use prepackaged sterile dressings to cover the incision.
○ 4. place soiled dressings in a waterproof bag before disposing of them.

53. For a client who excretes excessive amounts of calcium during the postoperative period after open heart surgery, which of the following measures should the nurse institute to help prevent complications associated with excessive calcium excretion?
○ 1. Ensure a liberal fluid intake.
○ 2. Provide an alkaline-ash diet.
○ 3. Prevent constipation.
○ 4. Enrich the client's diet with dairy products.

54. The nurse teaches the client who is receiving warfarin sodium that
○ 1. partial thromboplastin time values determine the dosage of warfarin sodium.
○ 2. protamine sulfate is used to reverse the effects of warfarin sodium.
○ 3. the international normalized ratio (INR) is used to assess effectiveness.
○ 4. warfarin sodium will facilitate clotting of the blood.

55. Good dental care is an important measure in reducing the risk of endocarditis. A teaching plan to promote good dental care in a client with mitral stenosis should include demonstration of the proper use of
○ 1. a manual toothbrush.
○ 2. an electric toothbrush.
○ 3. an irrigation device.
○ 4. dental floss.

56. Before a client's discharge after mitral valve replacement surgery, the nurse should evaluate the client's understanding of postsurgery activity restrictions. Which of the following should the client not engage in until after the 1-month postdischarge appointment with the surgeon?
○ 1. Showering.
○ 2. Lifting anything heavier than 10 pounds.
○ 3. A program of gradually progressive walking.
○ 4. Light housework.

57. Three days after mitral valve surgery, a 45-year-old woman comments that she hears a "clicking" noise coming from her chest and her "rather large" chest

incision. The nurse's response should reflect the understanding that the client may be experiencing which of the following?
○ 1. Anxiety related to altered body image.
○ 2. Anxiety related to altered health status.
○ 3. Altered tissue perfusion.
○ 4. Lack of knowledge regarding the postoperative course.

The Client With Hypertension

58. An industrial health nurse at a large printing plant finds a male employee's blood pressure to be elevated on two occasions 1 month apart and refers him to his private physician. The employee is about 25 pounds overweight and has smoked a pack of cigarettes daily for more than 20 years. The client's physician prescribes atenolol for the hypertension. The nurse should instruct the client to
○ 1. avoid sudden discontinuation of the drug.
○ 2. monitor the blood pressure annually.
○ 3. follow a 2-g sodium diet.
○ 4. discontinue the medication if severe headaches develop.

59. The nurse teaches her client, who has recently been diagnosed with hypertension, about his dietary restrictions: a low-calorie, low-fat, low-sodium diet. Which of the following menu selections would best meet the client's needs?
○ 1. Mixed green salad with blue cheese dressing, crackers, and cold cuts.
○ 2. Ham sandwich on rye bread and an orange.
○ 3. Baked chicken, an apple, and a slice of white bread.
○ 4. Hot dogs, baked beans, and celery and carrot sticks.

60. A client's job involves working in a warm, dry room, frequently bending and crouching to check the underside of a high-speed press, and wearing eye guards. Given this information, the nurse should assess the client for which of the following?
○ 1. Muscle aches.
○ 2. Thirst.
○ 3. Lethargy.
○ 4. Postural hypotension.

61. An exercise program is prescribed for the client with hypertension. Which intervention would be most likely to assist the client in maintaining an exercise program?
○ 1. Giving the client a written exercise program.
○ 2. Explaining the exercise program to the client's spouse.
○ 3. Reassuring the client that he or she can do the exercise program.

○ 4. Tailoring a program to the client's needs and abilities.

62. The client realizes the importance of quitting smoking, and the nurse develops a plan to help the client achieve this goal. Which of the following nursing interventions should be the initial step in this plan?
○ 1. Review the negative effects of smoking on the body.
○ 2. Discuss the effects of passive smoking on environmental pollution.
○ 3. Establish the client's daily smoking pattern.
○ 4. Explain how smoking worsens high blood pressure.

63. Essential hypertension would be diagnosed in a 40-year-old man whose blood pressure readings were consistently at or above which of the following?
○ 1. 120/90 mm Hg.
○ 2. 130/85 mm Hg.
○ 3. 140/90 mm Hg.
○ 4. 160/80 mm Hg.

64. When teaching a client about propranolol hydrochloride, the nurse should base the information on the knowledge that propranolol hydrochloride
○ 1. blocks β-adrenergic stimulation and thus causes decreased heart rate, myocardial contractility, and conduction.
○ 2. increases norepinephrine secretion and thus decreases blood pressure and heart rate.
○ 3. is a potent arterial and venous vasodilator that reduces peripheral vascular resistance and lowers blood pressure.
○ 4. is an angiotensin-converting enzyme (ACE) inhibitor that reduces blood pressure by blocking the conversion of angiotensin I to angiotensin II.

65. The nurse understands that a priority nursing diagnosis for the client with hypertension would be
○ 1. Pain.
○ 2. Deficient Fluid Volume.
○ 3. Impaired Skin Integrity.
○ 4. Ineffective Health Maintenance.

66. The most important long-term goal for a client with hypertension would be to
○ 1. learn how to avoid stress.
○ 2. explore a job change or early retirement.
○ 3. make a commitment to long-term therapy.
○ 4. control high blood pressure.

67. The client with hypertension is prone to long-term complications of the disease. Which of the following is a long-term complication of hypertension?
○ 1. Renal insufficiency and failure.
○ 2. Valvular heart disease.
○ 3. Endocarditis.
○ 4. Peptic ulcer disease.

68. Hypertension is known as the silent killer. This phrase is associated with the fact that hypertension often goes undetected until symptoms of other system failures occur. This may occur in the form of
○ 1. cerebrovascular accidents (CVAs).
○ 2. liver disease.
○ 3. myocardial infarction.
○ 4. pulmonary disease.

The Client With Angina

69. During the past few months, a 56-year-old woman has felt brief twinges of chest pain while working in her garden and has had frequent episodes of indigestion. She comes to the hospital after experiencing severe anterior chest pain while raking leaves. Her evaluation confirms a diagnosis of stable angina pectoris. After stabilization and treatment, the client is discharged from the hospital. At her follow-up appointment, she is discouraged because she is experiencing pain with increasing frequency. She states that she visits an invalid friend twice a week and now cannot walk up the second flight of steps to the friend's apartment without pain. Which of the following measures that the nurse could suggest would most likely help the client deal with this problem?
○ 1. Visit her friend early in the day.
○ 2. Rest for at least an hour before climbing the stairs.
○ 3. Take a nitroglycerin tablet before climbing the stairs.
○ 4. Lie down once she reaches the friend's apartment.

70. The client who experiences angina has been told to follow a low-cholesterol diet. Which of the following meals should the nurse tell the client would be best on her low-cholesterol diet?
○ 1. Hamburger, salad, and milkshake.
○ 2. Baked liver, green beans, and coffee.
○ 3. Spaghetti with tomato sauce, salad, and coffee.
○ 4. Fried chicken, green beans, and skim milk.

71. Which of the following symptoms should the nurse teach the client with unstable angina to report immediately to her physician?
○ 1. A change in the pattern of her pain.
○ 2. Pain during sexual activity.
○ 3. Pain during an argument with her husband.
○ 4. Pain during or after an activity such as lawn-mowing.

72. The physician refers the client with unstable angina for a cardiac catheterization. The nurse explains to the client that this procedure is being used in this specific case to

○ 1. open and dilate blocked coronary arteries.
○ 2. assess the extent of arterial blockage.
○ 3. bypass obstructed vessels.
○ 4. assess the functional adequacy of the valves and heart muscle.

73. The client is scheduled for a percutaneous transluminal coronary angioplasty (PTCA) to treat angina. Priority goals for the client immediately after PTCA would include
○ 1. minimizing dyspnea.
○ 2. maintaining adequate blood pressure control.
○ 3. decreasing myocardial contractility.
○ 4. preventing fluid volume deficit.

74. Which of the following is not generally considered to be a risk factor for the development of atherosclerosis?
○ 1. Family history of early heart attack.
○ 2. Late onset of puberty.
○ 3. Total blood cholesterol level greater than 220 mg/dL.
○ 4. Elevated fasting blood sugar concentration.

75. Many more men than women younger than 50 years of age have coronary artery disease as a result of atherosclerosis. The leading cause of death in women is
○ 1. acquired immunodeficiency syndrome.
○ 2. breast cancer.
○ 3. coronary artery disease.
○ 4. chronic obstructive pulmonary disease.

76. A client with angina asks the nurse, "What information does an ECG provide?" The nurse would respond that an electrocardiogram (ECG) primarily gives information about the
○ 1. electrical conduction of the myocardium.
○ 2. oxygenation and perfusion of the heart.
○ 3. contractile status of the ventricles.
○ 4. physical integrity of the heart muscle.

77. As an initial step in treating a client with angina, the physician prescribes nitroglycerin tablets, 0.3 mg given sublingually. This drug's principal effects are produced by
○ 1. antispasmodic effects on the pericardium.
○ 2. causing an increased myocardial oxygen demand.
○ 3. vasodilation of peripheral vasculature.
○ 4. improved conductivity in the myocardium.

78. The nurse teaches the client with angina about the common expected side effects of nitroglycerin, including
○ 1. headache.
○ 2. high blood pressure.
○ 3. shortness of breath.
○ 4. stomach cramps.

79. Sublingual nitroglycerin tablets begin to work within 1 to 2 minutes. How should the nurse instruct the client to use the drug when chest pain occurs?
○ 1. Take one tablet every 2 to 5 minutes until the pain stops.
○ 2. Take one tablet and rest for 10 minutes. Call the physician if pain persists after 10 minutes.
○ 3. Take one tablet, then an additional tablet every 5 minutes for a total of three tablets. Call the physician if pain persists after three tablets.
○ 4. Take one tablet. If pain persists after 5 minutes, take two tablets. If pain still persists 5 minutes later, call the physician.

80. The nurse interprets the rhythm strip in Figure 4 from a client's bedside monitor as which of the following?
○ 1. Normal sinus rhythm.
○ 2. Sinus tachycardia.
○ 3. Atrial fibrillation.
○ 4. Ventricular fibrillation.

81. The nurse interprets the rhythm strip in Figure 5 from a client's bedside monitor as which of the following?
○ 1. Normal sinus rhythm.
○ 2. Sinus tachycardia.
○ 3. Atrial fibrillation.
○ 4. Pacemaker rhythm.

82. The nurse interprets the rhythm strip in Figure 6 from a client's bedside monitor as which of the following?
○ 1. Normal sinus rhythm.
○ 2. Sinus tachycardia.
○ 3. Atrial fibrillation.
○ 4. Ventricular tachycardia.

83. A client with angina has been taking nifedipine. The client should be taught to
○ 1. monitor blood pressure monthly.
○ 2. perform daily weights.
○ 3. inspect gums daily.
○ 4. limit intake of green leafy vegetables.

The Client With a Permanent Pacemaker

84. A 74-year-old woman is admitted to the telemetry unit for placement of a permanent pacemaker because of sinus bradycardia. A priority goal for the client within 24 hours after insertion of a permanent pacemaker would be to
○ 1. maintain skin integrity.
○ 2. maintain cardiac conduction stability.
○ 3. decrease cardiac output.
○ 4. increase activity level.

85. The client who had a permanent pacemaker implanted 2 days earlier is being discharged from the hospital. Outcome criteria include that the client

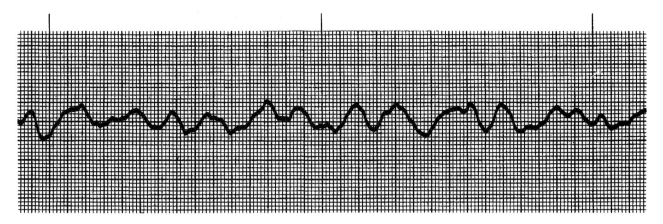

Figure 4.

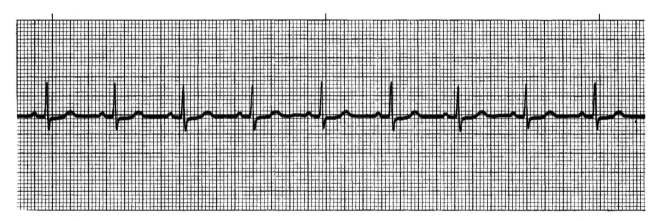

Figure 5.

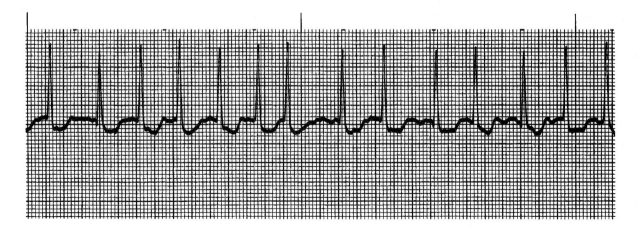

Figure 6.

○ 1. selects a low-cholesterol diet to control coronary artery disease.
○ 2. states a need for bed rest for 1 week after discharge.
○ 3. verbalizes safety precautions needed to prevent pacemaker malfunction.
○ 4. explains signs and symptoms of myocardial infarction.

The Client Requiring Cardiopulmonary Resuscitation

86. A rescuer is called to a neighbor's home after a 56-year-old man collapses. After quickly assessing the victim, the rescuer determines that the victim is unresponsive. To determine unresponsiveness, the rescuer can
   ○ 1. call the victim's name and gently shake the victim.
   ○ 2. perform the chin-tilt to open the victim's airway.
   ○ 3. feel for any air movement from the victim's nose or mouth.
   ○ 4. watch the victim's chest for respirations.

87. Proper hand placement for chest compressions during cardiopulmonary resuscitation (CPR) is essential to reduce the risk of which of the following complications?
   ○ 1. Gastrointestinal bleeding.
   ○ 2. Myocardial infarction.
   ○ 3. Emesis.
   ○ 4. Rib fracture.

88. The American Heart Association guidelines urge greater availability of automated external defibrillators (AEDs) and people trained to use them. AEDs are used in cardiac arrest situations for
   ○ 1. early defibrillation in cases of atrial fibrillation.
   ○ 2. cardioversion in cases of atrial fibrillation.
   ○ 3. pacemaker placement.
   ○ 4. early defibrillation in cases of ventricular fibrillation.

89. A client who has been given CPR is transported by ambulance to the hospital's emergency department, where the admitting nurse quickly assesses the client's condition. Of the following observations, the one most often recommended for determining the effectiveness of CPR is noting whether the
   ○ 1. pulse rate is normal.
   ○ 2. pupils are reacting to light.
   ○ 3. mucous membranes are pink.
   ○ 4. systolic blood pressure is at least 80 mm Hg.

90. The client receives epinephrine during resuscitation in the emergency department. This drug is administered primarily because of its ability to

   ○ 1. dilate bronchioles.
   ○ 2. constrict arterioles.
   ○ 3. free glycogen from the liver.
   ○ 4. enhance myocardial contractility.

91. The rescuer understands that the compression-to-ventilation ratio for one-rescuer adult CPR is
   ○ 1. 5:1.
   ○ 2. 15:1.
   ○ 3. 5:2.
   ○ 4. 15:2.

92. During CPR, the xiphoid process at the lower end of the sternum should not be compressed when performing cardiac compressions. Which of the following organs would be most likely at risk for laceration by forceful compressions over the xiphoid process?
   ○ 1. Lung.
   ○ 2. Liver.
   ○ 3. Stomach.
   ○ 4. Diaphragm.

93. When performing external chest compressions on an adult during CPR, the rescuer should depress the sternum
   ○ 1. 0.5 to 1 inch.
   ○ 2. 1 to 1.5 inches.
   ○ 3. 1.5 to 2 inches.
   ○ 4. 2 to 2.5 inches.

94. The American Heart Association guidelines for Basic Cardiac Life Support recommend that the rescuer, after first establishing unresponsiveness, should
   ○ 1. perform CPR for 2 minutes on the adult victim, then place a call for emergency assistance.
   ○ 2. place a call for emergency assistance immediately.
   ○ 3. begin rescue breathing for the victim.
   ○ 4. begin CPR on the adult victim and wait until help comes on the scene.

95. If the victim's chest wall fails to rise with each inflation when rescue breathing is administered during CPR, the most likely reason is that the
   ○ 1. airway is not opened properly.
   ○ 2. victim is beyond resuscitation.
   ○ 3. inflations are being given at too rapid a rate.
   ○ 4. rescuer is using inadequate force for cardiac compression.

96. During rescue breathing in CPR, the victim will exhale by
   ○ 1. normal relaxation of the chest.
   ○ 2. gentle pressure of the rescuer's hand on the upper chest.
   ○ 3. the pressure of cardiac compressions.
   ○ 4. turning the head to the side.

97. The nurse understands that the estimated maximum time a person can be without cardiopulmonary function and still not experience permanent brain damage is

○ 1. 1 to 2 minutes.
○ 2. 4 to 6 minutes.
○ 3. 8 to 10 minutes.
○ 4. 12 to 15 minutes.

98. The nurse knows to perform the Heimlich maneuver on a suspected choking victim when the victim
○ 1. starts to become cyanotic.
○ 2. cannot speak due to airway obstruction.
○ 3. can make only minimal vocal noises.
○ 4. is coughing vigorously.

99. When performing the Heimlich maneuver on a conscious adult victim, the rescuer delivers inward and upward thrusts specifically

○ 1. above the umbilicus.
○ 2. at the level of the xiphoid process.
○ 3. over the victim's midabdominal area.
○ 4. below the xiphoid process and above the umbilicus.

100. The monitor technician informs the nurse that the client has started having premature ventricular contractions every other beat. What is the *priority* nursing action?
○ 1. Call a "code blue" emergency situation.
○ 2. Assess the client's orientation and vital signs.
○ 3. Call the physician.
○ 4. Give the client a bolus of lidocaine.

Correct Answers and Rationale

The letters in parentheses following the rationale identify the step of the nursing process (A, D, P, I, E) and client needs (1, 2, 3, 4, 5, 6, 7, 8, 9, 10). See the inside front cover for the key.

The Client With Myocardial Infarction

1. 1. Although obtaining the ECG, chest radiograph, and blood work are all important, the nurse's priority action should be to relieve the crushing chest pain. Therefore, administering morphine sulfate is the priority action. (I, 10)

2. 2. Thrombolytic drugs are administered within the first 6 hours after onset of a myocardial infarction to lyse clots and reduce the extent of myocardial damage. (I, 8)

3. 3. PVCs are characterized by a QRS of longer than 0.10 seconds and by a wide, notched, or slurred QRS complex. There is no P wave related to the QRS complex, and the T wave is usually inverted. (D, 9)

4. 4. Sinus tachycardia is characterized by normal conduction and a regular rhythm, but with a rate exceeding 100 bpm. A P wave precedes each QRS, and the QRS is usually normal. (D, 9)

5. 1. Atrial fibrillation is characterized by an atrial rate of 350 bpm or greater and a ventricular rate of 120 bpm or greater. There are no P waves, but there are F waves (fibrillatory) waves that can be identified. The QRS is usually normal. (D, 9)

6. 1. Oliguria occurs during cardiogenic shock because there is reduced blood flow to the kidneys. Typical signs of cardiogenic shock include low blood pressure, rapid and weak pulse, decreased urine output, and signs of diminished blood flow to the brain, such as confusion and restlessness. Cardiogenic shock is a serious complication of MI, with a mortality rate approaching 90%. Fever is not a typical sign of cardiogenic shock. (A, 4)

7. 1. Intravenous nitroglycerin infusion requires an infusion pump for precise control of the medication. Blood pressure monitoring would be done with a continuous system, and more frequently than every 4 hours. Hourly urine outputs are not always required. Obtaining serum potassium levels is not associated with nitroglycerin infusion. (I, 8)

8. 4. An MI interferes with or blocks blood circulation to the heart muscle. Decreased blood supply to the heart muscle causes ischemia, or poor myocardial oxygena-

tion. Diminished oxygenation or lack of oxygen to the cardiac muscle results in ischemic pain or angina. (I, 10)

9. 2. Aspirin does have antipyretic, antiplatelet, and analgesic actions, but the primary reason aspirin is administered to the client experiencing an MI is its antithrombotic action. In clinical trials, the antithrombotic action of aspirin has been thought to account for improved outcomes in clients with MI. (P, 8)

10. 2. PVCs are often a precursor of life-threatening dysrhythmias, including ventricular tachycardia and ventricular fibrillation. An occasional PVC is not considered dangerous, but if PVCs occur at a rate greater than five or six per minute in the post-MI client, the physician should be notified immediately. More than six PVCs per minute is considered serious and usually calls for decreasing ventricular irritability by administering medications such as lidocaine hydrochloride. Increasing the intravenous infusion rate would not decrease the number of PVCs. Increasing the oxygen concentration should not be the nurse's first course of action; rather, the nurse should notify the physician promptly. Administering a prescribed analgesic would not decrease ventricular irritability. (I, 10)

11. 4. By day 2 of hospitalization after an MI, clients are expected to be able to perform personal care without chest pain. Day 2 of hospitalization may be too soon for clients to be able to identify risk factors for MI or to be able to agree to participate in a cardiac rehabilitation program. (E, 7)

12. 2. Furosemide is a loop diuretic that acts to increase urine output. Furosemide does not increase blood pressure, decrease pain, or decrease dysrhythmias. (E, 8)

13. 3. Although this type of exercise may decrease the likelihood of heel decubitus ulcer formation, it is taught to the MI client to prevent thrombophlebitis and blood clot formation. Movement of the lower extremities provides muscular action and aids venous return. As a result, the activity helps prevent stasis of blood, which predisposes the client to thrombophlebitis and blood clot formation. This type of exercise is not associated with promoting urinary and intestinal elimination. (I, 9)

14. 2. Recommended dietary principles in the acute phase of MI include avoiding large meals because small, easily digested foods are better tolerated. Fluids are given according to the client's needs, and sodium restrictions may be prescribed, especially for clients with manifestations of heart failure. Cholesterol restrictions may be ordered as well. Clients are not prescribed diets of

liquids only or restricted to nothing by mouth unless their condition is very unstable. (P, 7)

15. 3. High cholesterol levels are considered a controllable risk factor for CAD and appear most closely linked to the development of the disease. High cholesterol levels can be modified through diet, exercise, and medication. Age and gender are uncontrollable risk factors for CAD. Medication usage is not considered a risk factor for CAD. (A, 4)

16. 4. Heredity has been linked to CAD and is an uncontrollable risk factor. Exercise, obesity, and stress are controllable risk factors for CAD. (A, 4)

17. 3. A basic principle of behavior modification is that behavior that is learned and continued is behavior that has been rewarded. Other reinforcement techniques have not been found to be as effective as reward. (I, 4)

18. 4. The thrombolytic agent t-PA, administered intravenously, lyses the clot blocking the coronary artery. The drug is most effective when administered within the first 6 hours after onset of MI. (I, 8)

19. 1. Although monitoring the 12-lead ECG and monitoring breath sounds are important, observing the client for chest pain is the nursing assessment priority, because closure of the previously obstructed coronary artery may recur. Clients who receive t-PA frequently receive heparin to prevent closure of the artery after t-PA. Careful assessment for signs of bleeding and monitoring of partial thromboplastin time are essential to detect complications. Administration of t-PA should not cause fever. (A, 8)

20. 1. Cardiac dysrhythmias are commonly observed with administration of t-PA. Cardiac dysrhythmias are associated with reperfusion of the cardiac tissue. Hypotension is commonly observed with administration of t-PA. Seizures and hypothermia are not generally associated with reperfusion of the cardiac tissue. (D, 10)

21. 2. A past history of cerebral hemorrhage is a contraindication to administration of t-PA because the risk of hemorrhage may be further increased. Age greater than 60 years, history of heart failure, and cigarette smoking are not contraindications. (P, 8)

22. 2. Advanced cardiac life support recommends that at least one or two intravenous lines be inserted in one or both of the antecubital spaces. Calling the physician, obtaining a portable chest radiograph, and drawing blood for the laboratory are important but secondary to starting the intravenous line. (I, 10)

23. 4. Crackles are auscultated over fluid-filled alveoli. Crackles heard on lung auscultation do not have to be associated with cyanosis. Bronchospasm and airway narrowing generally are associated with wheezing sounds. (A, 10)

24. 1. Further assessment is needed in this situation. It is premature to initiate other actions until further data have been gathered. Inquiring about the onset, duration, location, severity, and precipitating factors of the chest heaviness will provide pertinent information to convey to the physician. (A, 10)

25. 4. Detection of myoglobin is one diagnostic tool to determine whether myocardial damage has occurred. Myoglobin is generally detected about 1 hour after a heart attack is experienced and peaks within 4 to 6 hours after infarction. (I, 10)

26. 1. In older adults who are less active and do not exercise the heart muscle, atrophy can result. Disuse or deconditioning can lead to abnormal changes in the myocardium of the older adult. As a result, under sudden emotional or physical stress, the left ventricle is less able to respond to the increased demands on the myocardial muscle. Decreased cardiac output, cardiac hypertrophy, and heart failure are examples of the chronic conditions that may develop in response to inactivity, rather than in response to the aging process. Irregular heartbeats are generally not associated with an older sedentary adult's lifestyle. Peripheral vascular occlusion or pacemaker placement should not affect response to stress. (I, 10)

The Client With Heart Failure

27. 1. It is a priority to assess the blood pressure first, because people with pulmonary edema typically experience severe hypertension that requires early intervention. (A, 10)

28. 3. Sitting almost upright in bed with the feet and legs resting on the mattress decreases venous return to the heart, thus reducing myocardial workload. Also, the sitting position allows maximum space for lung expansion. Low Fowler's position would be used if the client could not tolerate high Fowler's position for some reason. Lying on the right side would not be a good position for the client in heart failure. The client in heart failure would not tolerate the Trendelenburg position. (I, 10)

29. 3. Activity Intolerance is a primary problem for clients with heart failure and pulmonary edema. The decreased cardiac output associated with heart failure leads to reduced oxygen and fatigue. Clients frequently complain of dyspnea and fatigue. The client could be at risk for infection related to line placements or impaired skin integrity related to pressure. However, these are not the priority nursing diagnoses for the client with heart failure and pulmonary edema, nor is constipation related to immobility (D, 10)

30. 1. Increasing cardiac output is the main goal of therapy for the client with heart failure or pulmonary edema.

Pulmonary edema is an acute medical emergency requiring immediate intervention. Respiratory status and comfort will be improved when cardiac output increases to an acceptable level. Peripheral edema is not typically associated with pulmonary edema. (P, 10)

31. 2. Digoxin is a cardiac glycoside with positive inotropic activity. This inotropic activity causes increased strength of myocardial contractions and thereby increases output of blood from the left ventricle. Digoxin does not dilate coronary arteries. Although digoxin can be used to treat dysrhythmias and does decrease the electrical conductivity of the myocardium, this is not the primary reason for its use in clients with heart failure and pulmonary edema. (P, 8)

32. 3. ACE inhibitors have become the vasodilators of choice in the client with mild to severe congestive heart failure. Vasodilator drugs are the only class of drugs clearly shown to improve survival in overt heart failure. (P, 8)

33. 1. After intravenous injection of furosemide, diuresis normally begins in about 5 minutes and reaches its peak within about 30 minutes. Medication effects last 2 to 4 hours. When furosemide is given intramuscularly or orally, drug action begins more slowly and lasts longer than when it is given intravenously. (E, 8)

34. 4. When diuretics are given early in the day, the client will void frequently during the daytime hours and will not need to void frequently during the night. Therefore, the client's sleep will not be disturbed. Taking furosemide in the morning has no effect on preventing electrolyte imbalances or retarding rapid drug absorption. The client should not accumulate excessive fluids throughout the night. (I, 8)

35. 2. Characteristics of atrial fibrillation include pulse rate greater than 100 bpm, totally irregular rhythm, and no definite P waves on the ECG. During assessment, the nurse is likely to note the irregular rate and should report it to the physician. A weak, thready pulse is characteristic of a client in shock. (A, 10)

36. 1. Atrial fibrillation occurs when the sinoatrial node no longer functions as the heart's pacemaker and impulses are initiated at sites within the atria. Because conduction through the atria is disturbed, atrial contractions are reduced and stasis of blood in the atria occurs, predisposing to emboli. Some estimates predict that 30% of clients with atrial fibrillation develop emboli. Atrial fibrillation is not associated with increased cardiac output, elevated blood pressure, or decreased pulse rate; rather, it is associated with an increased pulse rate. (E, 10)

37. 3. Colored vision and seeing yellow spots are symptoms of digitalis toxicity. Abdominal pain, anorexia, nausea, and vomiting are other common symptoms of digitalis toxicity. Additional signs of toxicity include dysrhythmias, such as atrial fibrillation or bradycardia. Skin rash, increased appetite, and elevated blood pressure are not associated with digitalis toxicity. (E, 8)

38. 4. A low serum potassium level (hypokalemia) predisposes the client to digitalis toxicity. Because potassium inhibits cardiac excitability, a low serum potassium level would mean that the client would be prone to increased cardiac excitability. (I, 8)

39. 2. Canned foods and juices, such as tomato juice, are typically high in sodium and should be avoided in a sodium-restricted diet. Canned foods and juices in which sodium has been removed or limited are available. The client should be taught to read labels carefully. Apples and whole wheat breads are not high in sodium. Beef tenderloin would have less sodium than canned foods or tomato juice. (I, 7)

40. 1. Foods rich in potassium include bananas, orange juice, and green leafy vegetables such as spinach. Honeydew melon, cantaloupe, and watermelons are also rich in potassium. Other good sources of potassium are grapefruit juice, nectarines, potatoes, dried prunes, raisins, and figs. Skimmed milk, baked chicken, and brown rice are not considered high in potassium. (I, 7)

41. 2. A normal apical impulse is found over the apex of the heart and is typically located and auscultated in the left fifth intercostal space in the midclavicular line. An apical impulse located or auscultated below the fifth intercostal space or lateral to the midclavicular line may indicate left ventricular enlargement. (A, 10)

42. 2. Peripheral edema is a symptom of congestive heart failure. Congestive heart failure results when the heart chronically pumps against increased resistance or is unable to contract forcefully to pump the blood out into the systemic circulation. As a result, the ventricles become overfilled and there is an accumulation of volume within the closed system. The client's symptoms do not indicate arteriosclerosis, chronic bronchitis, or acute myocardial infarction. (D, 10)

43. 3. Congestive heart failure is a complex and chronic condition. Education should focus on health promotion and preventive care in the home environment. Signs and symptoms can be monitored by the client. Instructing the client to obtain daily weights at the same time each day is very important. The client should be told to call the physician if there has been a weight gain of 2 pounds or more. This may indicate fluid overload, and treatment can be prescribed early and on an outpatient basis, rather than waiting until the symptoms become life-threatening. Following a high-fiber diet is beneficial, but it is not relevant to the teaching needs of the client with congestive heart failure. Prescribing an exercise program for the client, such as walking 2 miles

every day, would not be appropriate at discharge. The client's exercise program would need to be planned in consultation with the physician and based on the history and the physical condition of the client. The client may require exercise tolerance testing before an exercise plan is laid out. Although the nurse does not prescribe an exercise program for the client, a sedentary lifestyle should not be recommended. (I, 3)

The Client With Valvular Heart Disease

44. 3. Most clients with mitral stenosis have a history of rheumatic fever or bacterial endocarditis. Chicken pox, poliomyelitis, and meningitis are not associated with mitral stenosis. (A, 10)

45. 2. Common adverse effects of lidocaine hydrochloride include dizziness, tinnitus, blurred vision, tremors, numbness and tingling of extremities, excessive perspiration, hypotension, convulsions, and finally coma. Cardiac effects include slowed conduction and cardiac arrest. Palpitations, urinary frequency, and lethargy are not considered typical adverse reactions to lidocaine hydrochloride. (E, 8)

46. 3. The pulmonary artery pressures are used to assess the heart's ability to receive and pump blood. The pulmonary capillary wedge pressure reflects the left ventricular end-diastolic pressure and guides the physician in determining fluid management for the client. The degree of coronary artery stenosis is assessed during a cardiac catheterization. The peripheral arterial pressure is assessed with an arterial line. The oxygen and carbon dioxide concentrations in the arterial blood can be measured by an arterial blood gas determination. (P, 9)

47. 1. Weight gain due to fluid retention and worsening heart failure cause exertional dyspnea in clients with mitral regurgitation. The rise in left atrial pressure that accompanies mitral valve disease is transmitted backward to the pulmonary veins, capillaries, and arterioles and eventually to the right ventricle. Signs and symptoms of pulmonary and systemic venous congestion follow. Confusion, elevated creatine phosphokinase concentration, and chest pain are not typically associated with mitral regurgitation. (A, 10)

48. 4. When mitral stenosis is present, the left atrium has difficulty emptying its contents into the left ventricle. Hence, because there is no valve to prevent backward flow into the pulmonary vein, the pulmonary circulation is under pressure. Functioning of the aorta, right atrium, and superior vena cava is not immediately influenced by mitral stenosis. (A, 10)

49. 1. Preoperatively, anticoagulants may be prescribed for the client with advanced valvular heart disease to prevent emboli. Postoperatively, all clients with mechanical valves and some clients with bioprostheses are maintained indefinitely on anticoagulant therapy. Adhering strictly to a dosage schedule and observing specific precautions are necessary to prevent hemorrhage or thromboembolism. Some clients are maintained on lifelong antibiotic prophylaxis to prevent recurrence of rheumatic fever. Episodic prophylaxis is required to prevent infective endocarditis after dental procedures or upper respiratory, gastrointestinal, or genitourinary tract surgery. Diet modification, activity restrictions, and dental care are important; however, they do not have as much significance postoperatively as medication therapy does. (A, 4)

50. 4. Management of postoperative pain is a priority for the client after surgery, including valve replacement surgery, according to the Agency for Health Care Policy and Research. The client and family should be informed that pain will be assessed by the nurse and medications will be given to relieve the pain. The client will stay in the intensive care unit as long as monitoring and intensive care are needed. Sensory deprivation and overload, high noise levels, and disrupted sleep and rest patterns are some environmental factors that affect recovery from valve replacement surgery. (I, 5)

51. 2. Protamine sulfate is used to help combat persistent bleeding in a client who has had open heart surgery. Vitamin C and quinidine sulfate do not influence blood clotting. Warfarin sodium is an anticoagulant, as is heparin, and these two agents would tend to cause the client to bleed even more. (I, 8)

52. 1. Many factors help prevent wound infections, including washing hands carefully, using sterile prepackaged supplies and equipment, cleansing the incisional area well, and disposing of soiled dressings properly. However, most authorities say that the single most effective measure in preventing wound infections is to wash the hands carefully before and after changing dressings. Careful handwashing is also important in helping reduce other infections often acquired in hospitals, such as urinary tract and respiratory system infections. (I, 2)

53. 1. In an immobilized client, calcium leaves the bone and concentrates in the extracellular fluid. When a large amount of calcium passes through the kidneys, calcium can precipitate and form calculi. Nursing interventions that help prevent calculi include ensuring a liberal fluid intake (unless contraindicated). A diet rich in acid should be provided to keep the urine acidic, which increases the solubility of calcium. Preventing constipation is not associated with excessive calcium excretion. Limiting foods rich in calcium, such as dairy products, will help in preventing renal calculi. (I, 7)

54. 3. The INR is the value used to assess effectiveness of the warfarin sodium therapy. INR is the prothrombin time ratio that would be obtained if the thromboplastin reagent from the World Health Organization was used for the plasma test. It is now the recommended method to monitor effectiveness of warfarin sodium. Generally, the INR for clients administered warfarin sodium should range from 2 to 3. In the past, prothrombin time was used to assess effectiveness of warfarin sodium and was maintained at 1.5 to 2.5 times the control value. Partial thromboplastin time is used to assess the effectiveness of heparin therapy. Fresh frozen plasma or vitamin K is used to reverse warfarin sodium's anti-coagulant effect, whereas protamine sulfate reverses the effects of heparin. Warfarin sodium will help to prevent blood clots. (I, 8)

55. 1. Daily dental care and frequent checkups by a dentist who is informed about the client's condition are required to maintain good oral health. Use of an electric toothbrush, an irrigation device, or dental floss may cause gums to bleed and allow bacteria to enter mucous membranes and the bloodstream, increasing the risk of endocarditis. (I, 9)

56. 2. Most cardiac surgical clients have median sternotomy incisions, which take about 3 months to heal. Measures that promote healing include avoiding heavy lifting, performing muscle reconditioning exercises, and using caution when driving. Showering or bathing is allowed as long as the incision is well approximated with no open areas or drainage. Activities should be gradually resumed on discharge. (I, 7)

57. 1. Verbalized concerns from this client may stem from her anxiety over the changes her body has gone through after open heart surgery. Although the client may experience anxiety related to her altered health status or may have a lack of knowledge regarding her postoperative course, she is pointing out the changes in her body image. The client is not concerned about altered tissue perfusion. (A, 5)

The Client With Hypertension

58. 1. Atenolol is a β-adrenergic antagonist indicated for management of hypertension. Sudden discontinuation of this drug is dangerous because it may exacerbate symptoms. The medication should not be discontinued without a doctor's order. Blood pressure needs to be monitored more frequently than annually in a client who is newly diagnosed and treated for hypertension. Clients are not usually placed on a 2-g sodium diet for hypertension. (I, 8)

59. 3. Processed and cured meat products, such as cold cuts, ham, and hot dogs, are all high in both fat and sodium and should be avoided on a low-calorie, low-fat, low-salt diet. Dietary restrictions of all types are complex and difficult to implement with clients who are basically asymptomatic. (I, 7)

60. 4. Possible dizziness from postural hypotension when rising from a crouched or bent position increases the client's risk of being injured by the equipment. The nurse should assess the client's blood pressure in all three positions (lying, sitting, and standing) at all routine visits. The client may experience muscle aches, or thirst from working in a warm, dry room, but these are not as potentially dangerous as postural hypotension. The client should not be experiencing lethargy. (A, 10)

61. 4. Tailoring or individualizing a program to the client's lifestyle has been shown to be an effective strategy for changing health behaviors. Providing a written program, explaining the program to the client's spouse, and reassuring the client that he or she can do the program may be helpful but are not as likely to promote adherence as individualizing the program. (P, 4)

62. 3. A plan to reduce or stop smoking begins with establishing the client's personal daily smoking pattern and activities associated with smoking. It is important that the client understands the associated health and environmental risks, but this knowledge has not been shown to help clients change their smoking behavior. (I, 4)

63. 3. American Heart Association standards define hypertension as a consistent systolic blood pressure level greater than 140 mm Hg and a consistent diastolic blood pressure level greater than 90 mm Hg. (A, 10)

64. 1. Propranolol is a β-adrenergic blocking agent. Actions of propranolol hydrochloride include reducing heart rate, decreasing myocardial contractility, and slowing conduction. (I, 8)

65. 4. Managing hypertension is a priority for the client with hypertension. Clients with hypertension frequently do not experience other signs and symptoms, such as pain, deficient fluid volume, or impaired skin integrity. It is the asymptomatic nature of hypertension that makes it so difficult to treat, because clients may not recognize they are hypertensive or may not perceive the need for aggressive management of the disease. (D, 10)

66. 3. Compliance is the most critical element of hypertension therapy. In most cases, hypertensive clients require lifelong treatment and their hypertension cannot be managed successfully without drug therapy. Stress management and weight management are important components of hypertension therapy, but the priority goal is related to compliance. (P, 9)

67. 1. Renal disease, including renal insufficiency and failure, is a complication of hypertension. Effective treatment of hypertension assists in preventing this complication.

Valvular heart disease, endocarditis, and peptic ulcer disease are not complications of hypertension. (D, 10)

68. 1. Hypertension is referred to as the silent killer for adults, because until the adult has significant damage to other systems, the hypertension may go undetected. CVAs can be related to long-term hypertension. Liver or pulmonary disease is not generally associated with hypertension. Myocardial infarction is generally related to coronary artery disease. (D, 9)

The Client With Angina

69. 3. Nitroglycerin may be used prophylactically before stressful physical activities such as stair-climbing to help the client remain pain free. Visiting her friend early in the day would have no impact on decreasing pain episodes. Resting before or after an activity is not as likely to help prevent an activity-related pain episode. (I, 8)

70. 3. Pasta, tomato sauce, salad, and coffee would be the best selection for the client following a low-cholesterol diet. Hamburgers, milkshakes, liver, and fried foods tend to be high in cholesterol. (I, 7)

71. 1. The client should report a change in the pattern of chest pain. It may indicate increasing severity of coronary artery disease. Pain occurring during stress or sexual activity would not be unexpected, and the client may be instructed to take nitroglycerin to prevent this pain. Pain during or after an activity such as lawn-mowing also would not be unexpected; the client may be instructed to take nitroglycerin to prevent this pain or may be restricted from doing such activities. (I, 10)

72. 2. Cardiac catheterization is done in clients with angina primarily to assess the extent and severity of the coronary artery blockage. A decision about medical management, angioplasty, or coronary artery bypass surgery will be based on the catheterization results. Coronary bypass surgery would be used to bypass obstructed vessels. Although cardiac catheterization can be used to assess the functional adequacy of the valves and heart muscle, in this case the client has unstable angina and therefore would need the procedure to assess the extent of arterial blockage. (I, 9)

73. 4. Because the contrast medium used in PTCA acts as an osmotic diuretic, the client may experience diuresis with resultant fluid volume deficit after the procedure. Additionally, potassium levels must be closely monitored because the client may develop hypokalemia due to the diuresis. Dyspnea would not be anticipated after this procedure. Maintaining adequate blood pressure control should not be a problem after the procedure. Increased myocardial contractility would be a goal, not decreased contractility. (P, 9)

74. 2. Late onset of puberty is not generally considered to be a risk factor for the development of atherosclerosis. Risk factors for atherosclerosis include cigarette smoking, hypertension, high blood cholesterol level, male gender, family history of atherosclerosis, diabetes mellitus, obesity, and physical inactivity. (A, 4)

75. 3. Coronary artery disease is the leading cause of death in women as well as men. Although it is generally agreed that estrogen helps protect women from atherosclerotic changes before menopause, women are still at risk for coronary artery disease. Much attention has been focused on the lack of research studies dealing with cardiac disease in women and minorities, and work is under way to gain a better understanding of cardiac disease in these populations. (A, 4)

76. 1. An ECG directly reflects the transmission of electrical cardiac impulses through the heart. This information makes it possible to evaluate indirectly the functional status of the heart muscle and the contractile response of the ventricles. However, these elements are not measured directly. The ECG does not give information about the oxygenation and perfusion of the heart. (I, 9)

77. 3. Nitroglycerin produces peripheral vasodilation, which reduces myocardial oxygen consumption and demand. Vasodilation in coronary arteries and collateral vessels may also increase blood flow to the ischemic areas of the heart. Nitroglycerin decreases myocardial oxygen demand. Nitroglycerin does not have an effect on pericardial spasticity or conductivity in the myocardium. (I, 8)

78. 1. Because of its widespread vasodilating effects, nitroglycerin often produces such side effects as headache, hypotension, and dizziness. The client should sit or lie down to avoid fainting. Nitroglycerin does not cause shortness of breath or stomach cramps. (I, 8)

79. 3. The correct protocol for nitroglycerin use involves immediate administration, with subsequent doses taken at 5-minute intervals as needed, for a total dose of three tablets. Sublingual nitroglycerin appears in the bloodstream within 2 to 3 minutes and is metabolized within about 10 minutes. (I, 8)

80. 4. This rhythm is ventricular fibrillation, which is characterized by the absence of any definite pattern. Ventricular fibrillation causes pulselessness and complete cardiac arrest in the victim, and treatment is defibrillation. Lidocaine hydrochloride may be administered after defibrillation to suppress additional ventricular ectopi. (D, 9)

81. 1. This rhythm is normal sinus rhythm. It is characterized by a regular ventricular rate of 60 to 100 bpm, and each QRS complex is preceded by a P wave. The PR and QRS intervals are within normal limits. (D, 9)

82. 3. This rhythm is atrial fibrillation. It is characterized by an irregular QRS interval, no definite P waves before the QRS waves, and a ventricular rate greater than 100 bpm. (D, 9)

83. 3. The client taking nifedipine should inspect the gums daily to monitor for gingival hyperplasia. This is an uncommon side effect but one that requires monitoring and intervention if it occurs. The client taking nifedipine might be taught to monitor blood pressure, but more often than monthly. These clients would not generally need to perform daily weights or limit intake of green leafy vegetables. (I, 8)

The Client With a Permanent Pacemaker

84. 2. Maintaining cardiac conduction stability to prevent dysrhythmias is a priority immediately after artificial pacemaker implantation. The client should have continuous electrocardiographic (ECG) monitoring until proper pacemaker functioning is verified. (P, 9)

85. 3. Education is a major component of the discharge plan for a client with an artificial pacemaker. The client with a permanent pacemaker needs to be able to state specific information about safety precautions necessary to maintain proper pacemaker function. (E, 9)

The Client Requiring Cardiopulmonary Resuscitation

86. 1. Calling the victim's name and gently shaking the victim is used to establish unresponsiveness. The head-tilt, chin-lift maneuver is used to open the victim's airway. Feeling for any air movement from the victim's nose or mouth indicates whether the victim is breathing on his own. The rescuer can watch the victim's chest for respirations to see if the victim is breathing. (I, 10)

87. 4. Proper hand placement during chest compressions is essential to reduce the risk of rib fractures, which may lead to pneumothorax and other internal injuries. Gastrointestinal bleeding and myocardial infarction are generally not considered complications of CPR. Although the victim may vomit during CPR, this is not associated with poor hand placement, but rather with distention of the stomach. (I, 10)

88. 4. AEDs are used for early defibrillation in cases of ventricular fibrillation. The American Heart Association places major emphasis on early defibrillation for ventricular fibrillation and use of the AED as a tool to increase sudden cardiac arrest survival rates. (I, 10)

89. 2. Pupillary reaction is the best indication of whether oxygenated blood has been reaching the client's brain. Pupils that remain widely dilated and do not react to light probably indicate that serious brain damage has occurred. The pulse rate may be normal, mucous membranes may still be pink, and systolic blood pressure may be 80 mm Hg or higher, and serious brain damage may still have occurred. (E, 10)

90. 4. Epinephrine is administered during resuscitation efforts primarily for its ability to improve cardiac activity. Epinephrine has great affinity for adrenergic receptors in cardiac tissue and acts to strengthen and speed the heart rate as well as to increase impulse conduction from atria to ventricles. Epinephrine dilates bronchioles and constricts arterioles, but these are not the primary reasons for administering it during resuscitation. Epinephrine is not associated with freeing glycogen from the liver. (I, 8)

91. 4. With one-rescuer CPR, the compression-to-ventilation ratio is 15:2. (I, 10)

92. 2. Because of its location near the xiphoid process, the liver is the organ most easily damaged from pressure exerted over the xiphoid process during CPR. The pressure on the victim's chest wall should be sufficient to compress the heart but not so great as to damage internal organs. Injury may result, however, even when CPR is performed properly. (I, 10)

93. 3. An adult's sternum must be depressed 1.5 to 2 inches with each compression to ensure adequate heart compression. (I, 10)

94. 2. The American Heart Association guidelines for Basic Cardiac Life Support now recommends that the rescuer call for emergency assistance immediately after establishing unresponsiveness in the adult victim. A call for emergency assistance takes precedence over initiating CPR in the adult victim, in an effort to get emergency personnel and an AED to the scene. Early defibrillation and prompt bystander CPR have increased sudden cardiac arrest survival rates. (I, 10)

95. 1. If the airway is not opened properly, it is impossible to inflate the lungs during CPR. A common sign of airway obstruction is failure of the victim's chest wall to rise with each inflation. The victim should not be considered beyond resuscitation; rather, the airway should be opened properly. Inflations may be being given too rapidly. However, this is not the usual cause of not being able to adequately ventilate the victim. If the rescuer is using inadequate force for cardiac compression, it should not interfere with how ventilations are delivered. (E, 10)

96. 1. The exhalation phase of ventilation is a passive activity that occurs during CPR as part of the normal relaxation of the victim's chest. No action by the rescuer is necessary. (E, 10)

97. 2. After a person is without cardiopulmonary function for 4 to 6 minutes, permanent brain damage is almost certain. To prevent permanent brain damage, it is important to begin CPR promptly after a cardiopulmonary arrest. (E, 10)

98. 2. The Heimlich maneuver should be administered only to a victim who cannot make *any* sounds due to airway obstruction. If the victim can whisper words or cough, some air exchange is occurring and the emergency medical system should be called instead of attempting the Heimlich maneuver. (A, 10)

99. 4. The thrusts should be delivered below the xiphoid process, but above the umbilicus, to minimize the risk of internal injuries. (I, 10)

100. 2. The priority action is to assess the client and determine whether the rhythm is life-threatening. More information, including vital signs, should be obtained and the physician should be quickly notified. A bolus of lidocaine may be ordered to treat this dysrhythmia. This is not a code-type situation unless the client has been determined to be in a life-threatening situation. (A, 10)

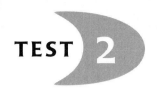

TEST 2

The Client With Vascular Disease

Select the one best answer, and indicate your choice by filling in the circle in front of the option.

The Client With Peripheral Vascular Disease

1. Peripheral blood flow is dependent on which of the following variables?
   ○ 1. Blood viscosity and diameter of vessels.
   ○ 2. Diameter and resistance of vessels.
   ○ 3. Force of contraction of the heart and resistance of vessels.
   ○ 4. Pressure differences in the arterial and venous systems and resistance.

2. Blood pressure in the systemic circulation is highest in the
   ○ 1. arterioles.
   ○ 2. capillaries.
   ○ 3. aorta.
   ○ 4. venules.

3. Which of the following factors is the *most* important in determining the resistance of a vessel?
   ○ 1. Length of the vessel.
   ○ 2. Diameter of the vessel.
   ○ 3. Blood being too thin.
   ○ 4. Blood being too thick.

4. A common abnormality associated with the development of peripheral vascular disease (PVD) is
   ○ 1. high serum calcium.
   ○ 2. high serum lipids.
   ○ 3. low serum potassium.
   ○ 4. low serum lipids.

5. Which of the following is an important regulator of blood flow in the peripheral circulation of the human body?

   ○ 1. Autonomic nervous system.
   ○ 2. Central nervous system.
   ○ 3. Parasympathetic nervous system.
   ○ 4. Sympathetic nervous system.

6. The nurse has been assigned to a client with a history of PVD who has symptoms of claudication. These symptoms result when
   ○ 1. oxygen demand by the muscle exceeds the supply.
   ○ 2. oxygen demand and supply of the working muscle are in balance.
   ○ 3. the oxygen supply exceeds the demand of the working muscle.
   ○ 4. oxygen is absent.

7. To assess the client's pedal pulses, the nurse would palpate the
   ○ 1. medial aspect of the foot and the ventral aspect of the ankle.
   ○ 2. top of the foot and inner side of each foot.
   ○ 3. popliteal space and the medial aspect of the ankle.
   ○ 4. posterior aspect of the foot and anterior aspect of the ankle.

8. Which of the following explains the influence of aging on the development of PVD?
   ○ 1. Decreased resistance.
   ○ 2. Increased resistance.
   ○ 3. Decreased viscosity.
   ○ 4. Increased viscosity.

9. The client admitted with PVD asks the nurse why her legs hurt when she walks. The nurse bases a

response on the knowledge that the main character-istic of PVD is
- ○ 1. decreased blood flow.
- ○ 2. increased blood flow.
- ○ 3. slow blood flow.
- ○ 4. thrombus formation.

10. The nurse notes on the client's chart that he has PVD and a history of heart failure. The nurse must plan care and anticipate that the client may have a low tolerance for exercise related to
- ○ 1. decreased blood flow.
- ○ 2. increased blood flow.
- ○ 3. decreased pain.
- ○ 4. increased blood viscosity.

11. When assessing the lower extremities of a client with PVD, the nurse notes bilateral ankle edema. The edema is related to
- ○ 1. competent venous valves.
- ○ 2. decreased blood volume.
- ○ 3. increase in muscular activity.
- ○ 4. increased venous pressure.

12. When assessing lower-extremity pulses in older adults with PVD, the nurse first notes whether or not the pulses are palpable. The nurse then assesses for which of the following characteristics?
- ○ 1. Rhythm.
- ○ 2. Quality.
- ○ 3. Rate.
- ○ 4. Pattern.

13. Atherosclerosis results in stenosis of the arteries. Which of the following vascular problems is also a result of atherosclerosis?
- ○ 1. Thickened endothelial lining of the vessels walls.
- ○ 2. Formation of aneurysm.
- ○ 3. Hardening of the arteries.
- ○ 4. Formation of varicose veins.

14. The nurse realizes that the underlying etiology for the nursing diagnosis of Pain related to PVD is atherosclerotic lesions resulting from
- ○ 1. atheromas.
- ○ 2. calcium plaques and hardening.
- ○ 3. thickened intima and calcium plaques.
- ○ 4. fibrous plaque and fatty streaks.

15. The nurse reviews with the client the risk factors associated with atherosclerosis. Nonmodifiable risk factors that the nurse instructs the client about include
- ○ 1. diabetes.
- ○ 2. age.
- ○ 3. exercise level.
- ○ 4. dietary preferences.

16. The nurse is assessing the lower extremities of the client with PVD. The nurse would expect to find which of the following signs of PVD?
- ○ 1. Hairy legs.
- ○ 2. Mottled skin.
- ○ 3. Pink, cool skin.
- ○ 4. Warm, moist skin.

17. The client complains of experiencing midcalf pain when walking a block or more. The patient states that the discomfort is relieved with rest. The nurse suspects that this client may be experiencing intermittent claudication. Intermittent claudication occurs when arterial occlusion reaches which of the following percentages?
- ○ 1. 20%.
- ○ 2. 40%.
- ○ 3. 50%.
- ○ 4. 100%.

18. The nurse is unable to palpate the client's left pedal pulses. Which of the following actions would the nurse take next?
- ○ 1. Auscultate the pulses with a stethoscope.
- ○ 2. Call the physician.
- ○ 3. Use a Doppler ultrasound device.
- ○ 4. Inspect the left lower extremity.

19. When using a Doppler instrument to assess peripheral pulses, the nurse understands that correct placement of the transducer is important because it is difficult to differentiate between
- ○ 1. arterial and capillary blood flow.
- ○ 2. arterial and venous blood flow.
- ○ 3. arterial and arteriole blood flow.
- ○ 4. capillary and venous blood flow.

20. Which of the following lipid abnormalities is a risk factor for the development of atherosclerosis and PVD?
- ○ 1. Low concentration of triglycerides.
- ○ 2. High levels of high-density lipid (HDL) cholesterol.
- ○ 3. High levels of low-density lipid (LDL) cholesterol.
- ○ 4. Low levels of LDL cholesterol.

21. When assessing an individual with PVD, which clinical manifestation would indicate complete arterial obstruction in the lower left leg?
- ○ 1. Aching pain in the left calf.
- ○ 2. Burning pain in the left calf.
- ○ 3. Numbness and tingling in the left leg.
- ○ 4. Coldness of the left foot and ankle.

22. One goal of care for a client with PVD is to decrease anxiety, so as to decrease or prevent vasoconstriction of the
- ○ 1. arteries.
- ○ 2. capillaries.
- ○ 3. lymphatics.
- ○ 4. veins.

23. A 70-year-old man with the diagnosis of claudication has been hospitalized for an evaluation of his

increasingly impaired mobility and complaints of pain. The client tells the nurse that he can no longer walk a block without having severe pain in his left calf and foot. Based on these data, which nursing diagnosis would be most appropriate for this client?
- ○ 1. Activity Intolerance related to decrease blood supply and pain.
- ○ 2. Self-Care Deficit Level II related to increased leg pain.
- ○ 3. Ineffective Coping related to chronic pain.
- ○ 4. Impaired Skin Integrity related to poor circulation.

24. A client with PVD returns to the surgical care unit after having femoral-popliteal bypass grafting. Of the following interventions, which is the nurse's *first* priority?
- ○ 1. Assess the client for postoperative pain.
- ○ 2. Assess the client's peripheral pulses.
- ○ 3. Assess the client's urinary output.
- ○ 4. Initiate measures to prevent wound infection.

25. A client with a history of heart failure has bilateral +4 edema of her right ankle that extends up to mid-calf. She is sitting out of bed and has her legs in a dependent position. The nurse will choose interventions to obtain which of the following outcomes?
- ○ 1. Decrease venous congestion.
- ○ 2. Maintain normal respirations.
- ○ 3. Maintain body temperature.
- ○ 4. Prevent injury to lower extremities.

26. The nurse is assessing an older Caucasian man who has a history of PVD. The nurse observes that the man's left great toe is black. The discoloration is probably a result of
- ○ 1. atrophy.
- ○ 2. contraction.
- ○ 3. gangrene.
- ○ 4. rubor.

27. The nurse uses a Doppler ultrasound device to assess the client's lower extremities. In addition, the nurse calculates the ankle-brachial index to estimate stenosis of the
- ○ 1. arteries.
- ○ 2. aorta.
- ○ 3. carotid.
- ○ 4. veins.

28. A client is scheduled for an arteriogram. The nurse should explain to the client that the arteriogram will confirm the diagnosis of occlusive arterial disease by
- ○ 1. showing the location of the obstruction and the collateral circulation.
- ○ 2. scanning the affected extremity and identifying the areas of volume changes.
- ○ 3. using ultrasound to estimate the velocity changes in the blood vessels.
- ○ 4. determining how long the client can walk.

29. A client is scheduled to have an arteriogram. During the arteriogram, the client complains of nausea, tingling, and dyspnea. The nurse's *immediate* action should be to
- ○ 1. administer epinephrine.
- ○ 2. inform the physician.
- ○ 3. administer oxygen.
- ○ 4. inform the client that the procedure is almost over.

30. A client with PVD has chronic, severe pretibial and ankle edema bilaterally. Because the client is on complete bed rest and circulation is compromised, one goal is to maintain tissue integrity. Which of the following interventions will help achieve this outcome?
- ○ 1. Administering pain medication.
- ○ 2. Encouraging fluids.
- ○ 3. Turning the client every 1 to 2 hours.
- ○ 4. Maintaining hygiene.

31. A client who has been diagnosed with PVD is being discharged. The client needs *further* instruction if she says she will
- ○ 1. avoid heating pads.
- ○ 2. not cross her legs.
- ○ 3. wear leather shoes.
- ○ 4. use iodine on a injured site.

32. A client with PVD has bypass surgery. The *primary* goal of the plan of care after surgery is to
- ○ 1. maintain circulation.
- ○ 2. prevent infection.
- ○ 3. relieve pain.
- ○ 4. provide education.

33. A client has been admitted with the diagnosis of occlusion of the left subclavian artery. The nurse anticipates that which of the following procedures will be done?
- ○ 1. Amputation.
- ○ 2. Bypass grafting.
- ○ 3. Coronary artery bypass grafting.
- ○ 4. Percutaneous transluminal angioplasty (PTA).

34. A client is scheduled to undergo a right axillary–to–axillary artery bypass surgery. Which of the following interventions is *most* important for the nurse to implement in the preoperative period?
- ○ 1. Assess the temperature in the affected arm.
- ○ 2. Monitor the radial pulse in the affected arm.
- ○ 3. Protect the extremity from cold.
- ○ 4. Avoid using the arm for a venipuncture.

The Client With Peripheral Vascular Disease Having an Amputation

35. A client is admitted to the hospital with peripheral vascular disease of the lower extremities. He is

scheduled for an amputation of the left leg. The client says, "I've really tried to manage my condition well." Which of the following routines would the nurse evaluate as having been appropriate for him?

○ 1. Resting with his legs elevated above the level of his heart.

○ 2. Walking slowly but steadily for 30 minutes twice a day.

○ 3. Minimizing activity.

○ 4. Wearing antiembolism stockings at all times when out of bed.

36. While the nurse is providing preoperative teaching, the client says, "I hate the idea of being an invalid after they cut off my leg." The nurse's most therapeutic response would be

○ 1. "You'll still have one good leg to use."

○ 2. "Tell me more about how you're feeling."

○ 3. "Let's finish the preoperative teaching."

○ 4. "You're fortunate to have a wife who can take care of you."

37. The client asks the nurse, "Why can't the doctor tell me exactly how much of my leg they're going to take off? Don't you think I should know that?" The nurse responds knowing that the final decision on the level of the amputation will depend *primarily* on

○ 1. the need to remove as much of the leg as possible.

○ 2. the adequacy of the blood supply to the tissues.

○ 3. the ease with which a prosthesis can be fitted.

○ 4. the client's ability to walk with a prosthesis.

38. A client has undergone an amputation of several toes and a femoral-popliteal bypass. The nurse should teach the client that after surgery which of the following leg positions is contraindicated for her while sitting in a chair?

○ 1. Crossing her legs.

○ 2. Elevating her legs.

○ 3. Flexing her ankles.

○ 4. Extending her knees.

39. The room for the client who has had an amputation should contain which emergency equipment when the client returns from surgery?

○ 1. Suction equipment.

○ 2. Emergency cart.

○ 3. Airway.

○ 4. Tourniquet.

40. The client has had a below-the-knee amputation secondary to arterial occlusive disease. The nurse is instructing the client in stump care. Which of the following statements by the client indicates that she understands how to implement her plan of care?

○ 1. "I should inspect the incision carefully when I change the dressing every other day."

○ 2. "I should wash the incision, dry it, and apply moisturizing lotion daily."

○ 3. "I should rewrap the stump as often as needed."

○ 4. "I should elevate the stump on pillows to decrease swelling."

41. One goal in caring for a client with arterial occlusive disease is to promote vasodilation in the affected extremity. To achieve this goal, the nurse encourages the client to

○ 1. avoid eating low-fat foods.

○ 2. elevate the legs above the heart.

○ 3. stop smoking.

○ 4. begin a jogging program.

42. The client complains of aching, weakness, and a cramping sensation in both of his lower extremities while walking. The nurse knows that exercise enhances blood circulation and utilization of oxygen by the tissues. To promote health and maintain the client's level of activity, the nurse suggests that the client try

○ 1. cross-country skiing.

○ 2. jogging.

○ 3. golfing.

○ 4. riding a stationary bike.

43. The client with peripheral vascular disease (PVD) has been prescribed diltiazem (Cardizem). The purpose of using diltiazem for this client would be to promote

○ 1. relief of anxiety.

○ 2. sedation.

○ 3. vasoconstriction.

○ 4. vasodilation.

44. Pentoxifylline (Trental) is a drug used to decrease platelet aggregation and blood viscosity. The nurse would anticipate that pentoxifylline would be useful in the treatment of clients with which of the following conditions?

○ 1. Angina.

○ 2. Gastric reflux.

○ 3. Intermittent claudication.

○ 4. Transient ischemic attacks.

45. A client with PVD and chronic obstructive pulmonary disease takes Theo-dur (200 mg twice daily) every day. The doctor now prescribes pentoxifylline (Trental). To prevent problematic side effects the nurse should monitor the client's

○ 1. digoxin level.

○ 2. partial thromboplastin time (PTT).

○ 3. serum cholesterol level.

○ 4. theophylline level.

46. A client with a history of coronary artery disease has been diagnosed with PVD. The physician started the client on pentoxifylline once daily. Approximately 1 hour after receiving the initial dose of pentoxifylline, the client complained of chest pain, which he stated he had not experienced before. Which of the

following interventions represents the most appropriate nursing action?

- ○ 1. Advise the client to rest.
- ○ 2. Inform the physician.
- ○ 3. Encourage the client to relax.
- ○ 4. Document the episode in the chart.

47. A client with PVD is recovering from an aortofemoral-popliteal bypass graft. When developing a postoperative education plan, the nurse would consider which of the following questions most essential?
- ○ 1. "How did you manage your health before admission?"
- ○ 2. "How far could you walk without pain before surgery?"
- ○ 3. "What is your home environment like?"
- ○ 4. "Do you have problems with urinary retention?"

48. The client with PVD and a history of hypertension is to be discharged on a low-fat, low-cholesterol, low-sodium diet. What would be the nurse's *first* step in planning the dietary instructions?
- ○ 1. Determine the client's knowledge level about cholesterol.
- ○ 2. Ask the client to name foods high in fat, cholesterol, and salt.
- ○ 3. Explain the importance of complying with the diet.
- ○ 4. Assess the family's food preferences.

The Client With Buerger's Disease (Thromboangiitis Obliterans)

49. The nurse has been assigned to a client with Buerger's disease (thromboangiitis obliterans). Which of the following anatomic areas are most often affected by this vascular condition?
- ○ 1. Hands and fingers.
- ○ 2. Lower legs and feet.
- ○ 3. Head and neck.
- ○ 4. Lower back.

50. A 30-year-old male client is admitted with Buerger's disease. Which of the following factors has increased the client's risk for development of Buerger's disease?
- ○ 1. History of cigarette smoking.
- ○ 2. Occupational exposure to radiation.
- ○ 3. Age and gender.
- ○ 4. History of hypertension.

51. The primary goal for the client with Buerger's disease is to prevent
- ○ 1. embolus formation.
- ○ 2. fat embolus formation.
- ○ 3. thrombus formation.
- ○ 4. thrombophlebitis.

52. A client with Buerger's disease smokes two packs of cigarettes a day. Smoking cessation is critical or the client may lose the affected extremity. When helping a client change behavior it is important to know the client's
- ○ 1. ability to attend support groups.
- ○ 2. goals of the treatment.
- ○ 3. perception of the behavior.
- ○ 4. motivation.

53. Because smoking cessation is a critical strategy for the client diagnosed with Buerger's disease, the nurse anticipates that the client will go home with a prescription for which of the following medications?
- ○ 1. Nicotine (Nicotrol).
- ○ 2. Nitroglycerin.
- ○ 3. Furosemide (Lasix).
- ○ 4. Ibuprofen.

54. The client with Buerger's disease experiences which of the following signs or symptoms?
- ○ 1. Thickening of the intima and media of the artery.
- ○ 2. Inflammation and fibrosis of arteries, veins, and nerves.
- ○ 3. Vasospasm lasting several minutes.
- ○ 4. Pain, pallor, and pulselessness.

The Client With Raynaud's Disease

55. Raynaud's disease is known as arteriospastic disease and is seen most often in
- ○ 1. young women.
- ○ 2. old women.
- ○ 3. old men.
- ○ 4. young men.

56. The nurse has been assigned to a client with Raynaud's disease. The nurse realizes that the underlying etiology of Raynaud's disease is unknown but that it is characterized by
- ○ 1. episodic vasospastic disorder of the small arteries.
- ○ 2. episodic vasospastic disorder of the small veins.
- ○ 3. episodic vasospastic disorder of the capillaries.
- ○ 4. episodic vasospastic disorder of the aorta.

57. The client with Raynaud's disease complains of cold and numbness in her fingers. The nurse assesses the client for effects of vasoconstriction. Which of the following is an early sign of vasoconstriction?
- ○ 1. Cyanosis.
- ○ 2. Gangrene.
- ○ 3. Pallor.
- ○ 4. Rubor.

58. A female client has Raynaud's disease. During the initial assessment, the nurse notes that the client is

experiencing a vasospastic episode. The nurse will immediately assess the
○ 1. brachial artery.
○ 2. carotid artery.
○ 3. femoral artery.
○ 4. radial artery.

59. The nurse should instruct a client who has been diagnosed with Raynaud's disease to
○ 1. immerse her hands in cold water during an episode.
○ 2. wear light garments when the temperature gets below 50°F (10°C).
○ 3. wear gloves when handling ice or frozen foods.
○ 4. live in a cold climate.

60. Stress can produce vasospasm in clients with Raynaud's disease. The client states she is worried about making the necessary behavioral changes to control the vasospastic episodes. Which of the following nursing diagnoses is appropriate?
○ 1. Activity Intolerance related to Raynaud's disease.
○ 2. Anxiety related to change in health status.
○ 3. Disturbed Body Image related to illness treatment.
○ 4. Impaired Social Interaction related to self-concept disturbance.

61. The physician has prescribed a β-adrenergic blocking medication for the client with Raynaud's disease. An example of a β-adrenergic blocker is
○ 1. tamsulosin hydrochloride (Flomax).
○ 2. terazosin hydrochloride (Hytrin).
○ 3. propranolol (Inderal).
○ 4. labetalol hydrochloride (Trandate).

62. When giving discharge instructions to the client with Raynaud's disease, the nurse will explain that the expected outcome of taking a β-adrenergic blocking medication is to control the symptoms by
○ 1. decreasing the influence of the sympathetic nervous system on the tissues in the hands and feet.
○ 2. decreasing the pain by producing analgesia.
○ 3. increasing the blood supply to the affected area.
○ 4. increasing monoamine oxidase.

63. A client with Raynaud's disease is scheduled for sympathectomy. This surgery is performed
○ 1. in the early stages of the disease to prevent further circulatory disturbances.
○ 2. when the disease is controlled by medication.
○ 3. when the client is unable to control stress-related vasospasm.
○ 4. when all other treatment alternatives have failed.

The Client With Thrombophlebitis and Embolus Formation

64. A client is discharged after being hospitalized for thrombophlebitis. She will be driving home with her daughter, who lives 2 hours away. During the 2-hour ride the client should
○ 1. perform arm circles while riding in the car.
○ 2. perform active ankle and foot range-of-motion exercises.
○ 3. elevate her legs while riding in the car.
○ 4. take an ambulance home.

65. A client is admitted from a nursing home with an acute onset of shortness of breath. A diagnosis of pulmonary embolism is made. One common cause of pulmonary embolism is
○ 1. arteriosclerosis.
○ 2. aneurysm formation.
○ 3. deep vein thrombosis.
○ 4. varicose veins.

66. A client receives a thrombolytic agent. The expected outcome of this drug therapy includes
○ 1. improved cerebral perfusion.
○ 2. decreased vascular permeability.
○ 3. dissolved emboli.
○ 4. prevention of further cerebral hemorrhage.

67. The nurse understands that a client on complete bed rest is at risk of developing which of the following complications involving the venous system?
○ 1. Air embolus.
○ 2. Fat embolus.
○ 3. Stress fractures.
○ 4. Thrombophlebitis.

68. The client has an intravenous (IV) catheter in the left antecubital space. The nurse notes that the area is swollen and red, and the client complains of discomfort at the site. The nurse realizes that 65% of the clients receiving IV therapy will develop
○ 1. deep vein thrombus (DVT).
○ 2. deep vein thrombophlebitis.
○ 3. superficial vein thrombus.
○ 4. superficial vein thrombophlebitis.

69. A client is receiving an IV infusion of 5% dextrose in water (D5W). The skin around the IV insertion site is red, warm to touch, and painful. The nurse should *first*
○ 1. administer acetaminophen (Tylenol).
○ 2. change the D5W to normal saline.
○ 3. discontinue the IV.
○ 4. place a warm compress on the area.

70. Bed rest is related to an increased incidence of thrombophlebitis. The plan of care for a client on bed rest would *not* include
○ 1. Turning every 2 hours.
○ 2. Passive and active range-of-motion exercises.

○ 3. Use of thromboembolytic disease support (TED) hose.

○ 4. Maintaining the client in the supine position.

71. The client is admitted with left lower leg pain, a positive Homans sign, and temperature greater than 100.4°F (38°C). The nurse suspects
○ 1. an aortic aneurysm.
○ 2. DVT in the left leg.
○ 3. IV drug abuse.
○ 4. intermittent claudication.

72. The nurse understands that certain risk factors are related to DVT. Which of the following is one such risk factor?
○ 1. The client exercises on a regular basis.
○ 2. The client lives alone at home.
○ 3. The client recently had abdominal surgery.
○ 4. The client wears antithrombotic hose on a regular basis.

73. A client is admitted to the unit with a diagnosis of thrombophlebitis and DVT of the right leg. A loading dose of heparin has been given in the emergency room, and IV heparin will be continued for the next several days. Care of this client will involve
○ 1. administering aspirin as ordered.
○ 2. encouraging green leafy vegetables in the diet.
○ 3. monitoring the client's prothrombin time (PT).
○ 4. monitoring the client's activated partial thromboplastin time (aPTT) and international normalized ratio (INR).

74. With a client who has undergone abdominal or pelvic surgery, the nurse implements strategies to prevent a DVT. Interventions for promoting the circulation in the lower extremities include
○ 1. avoiding fluids.
○ 2. encouraging deep breathing.
○ 3. remaining sedentary.
○ 4. using pneumatic compression stockings.

75. A client with DVT has an edematous right lower extremity. The client lies on her right side frequently. Rubor is noted on the lateral aspect of the right ankle. From the data collected, the appropriate nursing diagnosis for this client would be
○ 1. Activity Intolerance related to complaints of pain in lower right extremity.
○ 2. Altered Health Maintenance related to lack of knowledge about DVT.
○ 3. Pain related to edema.
○ 4. Risk for Impaired Skin Integrity related to impaired tissue perfusion and increased capillary compression.

76. The nurse interviews a 22-year-old female client who is scheduled for abdominal surgery the following week. The client is obese and uses estrogen-based oral contraceptives. This client is at high risk for development of

○ 1. atherosclerosis.
○ 2. diabetes.
○ 3. Raynaud's disease.
○ 4. thrombophlebitis.

77. The nurse observes that an older woman has small to moderate, distended and tortuous veins running along the inner aspect of her lower legs. These are commonly called
○ 1. aneurysms.
○ 2. lipomas.
○ 3. ulcers.
○ 4. varicose veins.

78. Which of the following clients is at risk for varicose veins?
○ 1. A client who has had a cerebral vascular accident.
○ 2. A client who has had anemia.
○ 3. A client who has had thrombophlebitis.
○ 4. A client who has had transient ischemia attacks.

79. A client weighs 300 pounds and has a history of DVT and thrombophlebitis. When reviewing a teaching plan with this client, the nurse knows that the client has understood the nurse's instructions when he states he will
○ 1. avoid exercise.
○ 2. lose weight.
○ 3. perform leg lifts every 4 hours.
○ 4. wear support hose using rubber bands to hold the stockings up.

80. When an arterial embolus has been diagnosed, an emergency embolectomy may be considered if the involved extremity is viable. After an embolectomy, a *priority* goal is to
○ 1. administer pain medication.
○ 2. administer the anticoagulants as ordered.
○ 3. encourage activity within the guidelines specified by the physician.
○ 4. monitor the pulses.

The Client With an Aneurysm

81. The client comes to the emergency department complaining of severe abdominal pain. A radiograph reveals a large abdominal aortic aneurysm. The *primary* goal at this time is to
○ 1. maintain circulation.
○ 2. manage pain.
○ 3. prepare the client for emergency surgery.
○ 4. teach postoperative breathing exercises.

82. Before surgery for a known aortic aneurysm, the client's pulse pressure begins to widen, suggesting increased aortic valvular insufficiency. If the branches of the aortic arch are involved, the client will have

○ 1. loss of consciousness.
○ 2. anxiety.
○ 3. headache.
○ 4. disorientation.

83. A client complains of sudden, severe pain in his back and chest, accompanied by shortness of breath. The individual describes the pain as a "tearing" sensation. The physician suspects the man is experiencing a dissecting aortic aneurysm. Emergency equipment is brought into the room because one complication of a dissecting aneurysm is
○ 1. cardiac tamponade.
○ 2. cerebral vascular accident.
○ 3. pulmonary edema.
○ 4. myocardial infarction.

84. Which of the following increases the risk of having a large abdominal aortic aneurysm rupture?
○ 1. Anemia.
○ 2. Dehydration.
○ 3. High blood pressure.
○ 4. Hyperglycemia.

85. Which of the following represents a significant risk immediately after surgery for repair of an aortic aneurysm?
○ 1. Potential alteration in renal perfusion.
○ 2. Potential electrolyte imbalance.
○ 3. Potential ineffective coping.
○ 4. Potential wound infection.

86. When repairing an abdominal aortic aneurysm, the surgeon uses an incision that extends from the xiphoid process to the pubis. A nasogastric tube is inserted during the surgical procedure to decompress the stomach and bowel. After surgery, which of the following may contribute to development of a paralytic ileus?
○ 1. Use of cold fluids.
○ 2. Use of warming blankets.
○ 3. Insertion of a nasogastric tube.
○ 4. Use of narcotic pain medication.

87. A client is discharged after an aortic aneurysm repair. She received a synthetic graft to replace part of her aorta. Therefore, the nurse explains to the client the importance of notifying her physician before having
○ 1. blood drawn.
○ 2. an intravenous line inserted.
○ 3. major dental work.
○ 4. an x-ray examination.

88. The client with a deep vein thrombus has been receiving Coumadin for 2 months. The client reports bleeding gums, increased bruising, and dark stools. These symptoms indicate that the medication
○ 1. does not need to be changed.
○ 2. needs to be decreased.
○ 3. needs to be increased.
○ 4. is not being taken as prescribed.

The Client With a Variety of Vascular Problems

89. An older woman has a history of a left radical mastectomy and now presents with a swollen left arm. The nurse understands that it is appropriate to
○ 1. take the blood pressure only in the unaffected arm.
○ 2. start an intravenous line in the affected arm.
○ 3. encourage a dependent position of the affected arm.
○ 4. allow blood draws in the affected arm.

90. The pain associated with migraine headaches is believed to be caused by
○ 1. dilation of the cranial arteries.
○ 2. a temporary decrease in intracranial pressure.
○ 3. irritation and inflammation of the openings of the sinuses.
○ 4. sustained contraction of muscles around the scalp and face.

Correct Answers and Rationale

The letters in parentheses following the rationale identify the step of the nursing process (A, D, P, I, E) and client needs (1, 2, 3, 4, 5, 6, 7, 8, 9, 10). See the inside front cover for the key.

The Client With Peripheral Vascular Disease

1. 4. Blood flows in a unidirectional manner, and the blood flow involves the differences in pressure between the arterial and venous systems. The two variables influencing blood flow within this closed system are the pressure differences and the resistance to blood flow throughout the system. The greater the resistance, the greater the driving force needed, which results in an increase in the force of the contraction of the heart. Blood viscosity is important, and diameter influences resistance, but flow is dependent on pressure differences and resistance. (D, 4)

2. 3. The blood pressure is the highest in the aorta as the blood is being ejected out of the left ventricle into the aorta. The pressure declines as the blood flows through the arteries, capillaries, arterioles, veins, capillaries, and venules. (D, 4)

3. 2. The diameter of the vessel is the most important component in determining resistance in the systemic circulation. The length of the vessel is also a factor in determining resistance. Viscosity, whether the blood is "thin" or "thick," is less important when discussing blood flow. (D, 4)

4. 2. High serum lipids are associated with an increased incidence of PVD. High serum calcium, low serum potassium, and low serum lipids have no relation to PVD. (D, 9)

5. 4. It is the sympathetic nervous system (adrenergic) that is involved in regulating the blood flow in the peripheral blood vessels. The autonomic nervous system is divided into two branches, the sympathetic branch and the parasympathetic branch. The parasympathetic nervous system does not control peripheral blood flow. The central nervous system is composed of the brain and the spinal cord and does not have an influential effect on peripheral blood flow. (D, 4)

6. 1. *Claudication* is the term used to describe the discomfort a person experiences when oxygen demand in the leg muscles is greater than the supply. The pain is a result of tissue hypoxia in the working muscle. Symptoms include aching, cramping, and weakness. (D, 10)

7. 2. Assessing pedal pulses involves palpating both the dorsalis pedis and the posterior tibial arteries. These pulses are located on the top of the foot (ventral aspect) and the inner aspect of the ankle (medial surface of the ankle). (I, 4)

8. 2. As people age, the accumulation of collagen in the intima of the blood vessels results in the vessels' becoming stiff and less flexible. Consequently, there is an increased resistance within the aging adult's circulatory system. (D, 3)

9. 1. Decreased blood flow is a common characteristic of all PVD. When the demand for oxygen to the working muscles becomes greater than the supply, pain is the outcome. Slow blood flow throughout the circulatory system may suggest pump failure. Thrombus formation can result from stasis or damage to the intima of the vessels. (A, 9)

10. 1. A client with PVD and pump failure will experience a decreased blood flow. In this situation, low exercise tolerance (oxygen demand becomes greater than the oxygen supply) may be related to less blood being ejected from the left ventricle into the systemic circulation. Decreased blood supply to the tissues results in pain. Increased blood viscosity may be a component, but it is of much less importance than the disease processes. (D, 9)

11. 4. In PVD, a decreased blood flow can result in increased venous pressure. The increase in venous pressure results in an increase in capillary hydrostatic pressure, which causes a net filtration of fluid out of the capillaries into the interstitial space, resulting in edema. Valves often become incompetent with PVD. Blood volume is not decreased in this condition. Decreased muscular action would contribute to the formation of edema in the lower extremities. (D, 9)

12. 2. Presence or absence of a peripheral pulse is essential data when assessing peripheral pulses in clients with PVD. The quality of the pulse is the next important piece of information needed. The client's cardiac rhythm, or pattern, is not assessed by evaluating pulses in the lower extremities. The heart rate is not assessed during evaluation of the peripheral pulses. (A, 10)

13. 2. A common result of atherosclerosis is the formation of an aneurysm. Arteriosclerosis, or "hardening" of the arteries, involves the endothelial lining and results in thickened arterial walls. Varicose veins are the outcome of incompetent valves in the venous system. (D, 10)

14. 4. Yellowish, smooth, fatty streaks are associated with atherosclerosis of the arteries. Atheromas, calcium plaques, and thickening of the intima are associated with arteriosclerosis. (D, 9)

15. 2. Age is a nonmodifiable risk factor for atherosclerosis. The nurse instructs the client to manage modifiable risk factors such as comorbid diseases (eg, diabetes), activity level, and diet. Controlling serum blood glucose levels, engaging in regular aerobic activity, and choosing a diet low in saturated fats can reduce the risk of developing atherosclerosis. (I, 3)

16. 2. Reduction of blood flow to a specific area results in decreased oxygen and nutrients. As a result, the skin may appear mottled. Loss of hair and cool, dry skin are the other data that the nurse may observe in a client with PVD of the lower extremities. (A, 3)

17. 3. Generally, a 50% to 75% occlusion in the arterial lumen causes symptoms associated with intermittent claudication. When the demand for oxygen becomes greater than the supply in the working muscle, the client experience pain (aching, cramping). When the individual sits down and rests, the demand and supply of oxygen become balanced and the discomfort dissipates. Occlusion of 100% would result in ischemia and necrosis of tissue distal to the artery and would require immediate surgical intervention. (D, 9)

18. 3. When pedal pulses are not palpable, the nurse should obtain a Doppler ultrasound device. Auscultation is not likely to be helpful if the pulse isn't palpable. Inspection of the lower extremity can be done simultaneously when palpating, but the nurse should first try to locate a pulse by Doppler. Calling the physician may be necessary if there is a change in the client's condition. (I, 10)

19. 2. The sound produced by the Doppler machine reflects all of the vascular structures in the path of the sound beam; therefore, it may be hard to differentiate between arterial and venous blood flow. Capillary and arteriole blood flow cannot be auscultated with a Doppler instrument. (A, 10)

20. 3. An increased LDL cholesterol concentration has been documented as a risk factor for the development of atherosclerosis. LDL cholesterol is not broken down in the liver but is deposited into the intima of the blood vessels. Low triglyceride levels are desirable. High HDL and low LDL levels are beneficial and are known to be protective for the cardiovascular system. (D, 8)

21. 4. Coldness in the left foot and ankle is consistent with complete arterial obstruction. Other expected findings would include paralysis and pallor. Aching pain, a burning sensation, or numbness and tingling are earlier signs of tissue hypoxia and ischemia and are commonly associated within incomplete obstruction. (A, 10)

22. 1. Anxiety stimulates the sympathetic nervous system, which results in the secretion of epinephrine, angiotensin, and serum proteins that cause vasoconstriction in the arteries of the peripheral circulatory system. As a result, peripheral vascular resistance is increased. This vasoconstriction may increase the pain in the areas where the PVD is the greatest. The lymphatic system does not affect the blood supply of tissues. (P, 10)

23. 1. Activity Intolerance related to poor circulation and pain is a common problem with clients experiencing claudication. The goal would be to educate the individual to maintain his level of activity and incorporate frequent rest periods to prevent episodes of decreased blood supply. The data do not suggest that the client is not coping with his chronic pain, that he cannot perform self-care activities, or that his skin integrity is impaired. It would be appropriate to incorporate the diagnosis of Risk for Impaired Skin Integrity into the client's plan of care. (I, 3)

24. 2. Evaluation of the presence and quality of the pedal pulses in the affected extremity is essential after surgery to validate that the bypass graft is functioning. Assessing and providing the client information immediately after surgery is important but is secondary to determining the status of the circulation. (A, 10)

25. 1. Decreasing venous congestion in the extremities is a desired outcome for clients with heart failure. The nurse would elevate the client's legs above the level of the heart to achieve this goal. (I, 4)

26. 3. The term *gangrene* refers to blackened, decomposing tissue that is devoid of circulation. Chronic ischemia and death of the tissue can lead to gangrene in the affected extremity. Injury, edema, and decreased circulation lead to infection, gangrene, and tissue death. Atrophy is the shrinking of tissue, and contraction is joint stiffening secondary to disuse. The term *rubor* denotes a reddish color of the skin. (D, 10)

27. 1. The ankle-brachial index is based on the ratio of the ankle systolic blood pressure to arm systolic blood pressure. It allows one to quantify the degree of arterial stenosis. (D, 9)

28. 1. An arteriogram involves injecting a radiopaque contrast agent directly into the vascular system to visualize the vessels. It usually involves computed tomographic scanning. The velocity of the blood flow can be estimated by duplex ultrasound. The client's ankle-brachial index is determined, and then the client is requested to walk. The normal response is little or no drop in ankle systolic pressure after exercise. (D, 9)

29. 2. Clients may have immediate or delayed reaction to the radiopaque dye. The physician should be notified immediately, because the symptoms may suggest an allergic reaction. Treatment may involve administering

oxygen and epinephrine. It would not be inappropriate to ignore significant symptoms such as these or to attribute the symptoms to anxiety. The nurse must notify the physician first and would have to receive an order to administer epinephrine. (I, 10)

30. 3. The client is at greater risk for skin breakdown in the lower extremities related to the edema and to remaining in one position, which increases capillary pressure. Turning every 1 to 2 hours promotes vasodilatation and prevents vascular compression. Administering pain medication will not have an effect on skin integrity. Encouraging fluids is not a direct intervention for maintaining skin integrity, although being well hydrated is a goal for most clients. Maintaining hygiene does influence skin integrity but is secondary in this situation. (I, 10)

31. 4. The client should avoid using iodine or over-the-counter medications. Iodine is a highly toxic solution. An individual who has known PVD should be seen by a physician for treatment to avoid infection. The client with PVD should avoid heating pads and crossing the legs, and should wear leather shoes. A heating pad can cause injury, which, because of the decreased blood supply, can be difficult to heal. Crossing the legs can further impede blood flow. Leather shoes provide better protection. (E, 3)

32. 1. Maintaining circulation in the affected extremity after surgery is the focus of care. The graft can become occluded, and the client must be assessed frequently to determine whether the graft is patent. Preventing infection and relieving pain are important but are secondary to maintaining graft patency. Education should have taken placed in the preoperative phase and then continued during the recovery phase. (I, 10)

33. 4. PTA would be attempted first. If the blood flow is being diverted from the cranial circulation, other surgical procedures involving bypass grafts may be indicated. Amputation is necessary only if gangrene from complete loss of blood supply develops. Coronary artery bypass grafting is a specific procedure involving the arteries in the heart. (P, 10)

34. 4. If surgery is scheduled, the nurse should avoid venipunctures in the affected extremity. The goal would be to prevent unnecessary trauma and possible infection in the affected arm. Disruptions in skin integrity and even minor skin irritations can cause the surgery to be canceled. (P, 9)

The Client With Peripheral Vascular Disease Having an Amputation

35. 2. Slow, steady walking is a recommended activity for clients with peripheral vascular disease because it stim-

ulates the development of collateral circulation. The client with peripheral vascular disease should not remain inactive. Elevating the legs above the heart or wearing antiembolism stockings is a strategy for alleviating venous congestion and may worsen peripheral arterial disease. (E, 7)

36. 2. Encouraging the client who is undergoing amputation to verbalize feelings is the most therapeutic nursing intervention. By eliciting concerns, the nurse may be able to provide information to help the client cope. The nurse should avoid value-laden responses, such as "You'll still have one good leg," that may make the client feel guilty or hostile and block further communication. The nurse should not ignore the client's expressed concerns, nor should the nurse reinforce the client's concern about invalidism and dependency or assume that his wife is willing to care for him. (I, 5)

37. 2. The level of amputation often cannot be accurately determined until surgery, when the surgeon can directly assess the adequacy of the circulation of the residual limb. A longer residual limb facilitates prosthesis fitting, and this aspect will be considered in the final decision, but it is not the primary factor. (P, 10)

38. 1. Leg crossing is contraindicated because it causes adduction of the hips and decreases the flow of blood into the lower extremities. This may result in increased pressure in the graft in the affected leg. Elevating the legs, flexing the ankles, and extending the knees are not necessarily contraindicated. (I, 7)

39. 4. Because amputation requires severing and tying off major arteries and veins, hemorrhage, although unexpected, is a possible complication. A tourniquet should be available at the bedside during the early postoperative period to manage such a complication. Suction equipment should be available for the client who has undergone head and neck surgery. It is not likely that the client will require suctioning after an amputation. There is no reason to obtain an emergency cart or an airway for the client who has undergone an amputation. (P, 10)

40. 3. The purpose of wrapping the stump is to shape the residual limb to accept a prosthesis and bear weight. The compression bandaging should be worn at all times for many weeks after surgery and should be reapplied as needed to keep it free of wrinkles and snug. The dressing should be changed daily to allow for inspection of the stump incision. No lotions should be applied to the stump unless specifically ordered by the physician. The stump should not be elevated on pillows, because this will contribute to the formation of flexion contractures. Contractures will prevent the client from wearing a prosthesis and ambulating. (E, 10)

41. 3. Nicotine causes vasospasm and impedes blood. Stopping smoking is the most significant lifestyle change the client can make. The client should eat low-fat foods as part of a balanced diet. The legs should not be elevated above the heart, because this will impede arterial flow. The legs should be in a slightly dependent position. Jogging is not necessary and probably is not possible for many clients with arterial occlusive disease. A rehabilitation program that includes daily walking is suggested. (I, 3)

42. 4. In this case, the exercise prescription needs to be individualized because walking causes discomfort. To maintain the level of activity and decrease venous congestion, riding a stationary bike is another appropriate exercise behavior. Use of a stationary bike provides a non–weight-bearing exercise modality, which allows a longer duration of activity. Jogging and cross-country skiing are weight-bearing activities. In addition, cross-country skiing involves a cold environment, and maintaining warmth is essential in promoting arterial blood flow and preventing vasoconstriction. Jogging is a weight-bearing activity. Golfing is a good activity, but it is not typically considered an exercise that causes aerobic changes in the body. (D, 3)

43. 4. Diltiazem is a calcium-channel blocker that blocks the influx of calcium into the cell. In this situation, the primary use of diltiazem is to promote vasodilation and prevent spasms of the arteries. As a result of the vasodilation, blood, oxygen, and nutrients can reach the muscle and tissues. Diltiazem is not an antianxiety agent and does not promote sedation. It also does not cause vasoconstriction, which would be contraindicated for the client with PVD. (D, 8)

44. 3. Although pentoxifylline's precise mechanism of action is unknown, its therapeutic effect is to increase blood flow. It is commonly prescribed for clients experiencing intermittent claudication. Pentoxifylline should not be used for clients with coronary artery disease; a side effect of pentoxifylline is angina. It does not have any therapeutic effect on gastric reflux, and it is not a treatment for transient ischemic attacks. (D, 8)

45. 4. Pentoxifylline can potentiate the effects of theophylline and increase the risk of theophylline toxicity. Therefore, the nurse would monitor the client's theophylline level. Pentoxifylline does not interact with digoxin. Pentoxifylline can interact with heparin, and the client's PTT would need to be monitored closely if the client were taking heparin. It does not affect cholesterol levels. (A, 8)

46. 2. Angina is an adverse reaction to pentoxifylline, which should be used cautiously in clients with coronary artery disease. The nurse should report the client's symptoms to the physician, who may order nitroglyc-

erin and possibly discontinue the pentoxifylline. The client should rest until the chest pain subsides, and documentation is essential when a client experiences an adverse reaction with medications that have been prescribed; however, the nurse's top priority is to call the physician, report the problem, and obtain an order for nitroglycerin. The client's complaints should never be dismissed. (I, 10)

47. 1. Assessing the individual's health behavior before surgery will help the nurse and client to develop strategies to change the client's unhealthy lifestyle behaviors to healthier ones. (I, 3)

48. 4. Before beginning dietary interventions, the nurse must assess the client's pattern of food intake, life cycle, food preferences, and ethnic, cultural, and financial influences. (P, 7)

The Client With Buerger's Disease (Thromboangiitis Obliterans)

49. 1. Buerger's disease is an inflammation of the intermediate and small arteries and veins. The tibial artery and vessels of the feet are affected in about 70% of clients with this disease. The forearms and hands are affected in approximately 30% of cases. The head, neck, and lower back are not affected. (D, 10)

50. 1. Daily use of nicotine, either by smoking or by use of smokeless tobacco products, is associated with Buerger's disease. Occupational exposure to radiation and hypertension are not associated with the condition. Although this disorder is commonly observed in the male population 20 to 40 years old, smoking is the most strongly associated risk factor; the disease does not occur in nonsmokers. (D, 3)

51. 3. Because of the inflammation, a common complication of Buerger's disease is thrombus formation and potential occlusion of the vessel. Inflammation of the immediate and small arteries and veins is involved in the disease process. Embolus is a potential risk if a thrombus has developed. Fat embolus is associated with fractures of the bones. Thrombophlebitis occurs after thrombus formation. (P, 3)

52. 3. When helping a client change detrimental health behavior, it is critical to learn how the client perceives the situation or problem. The client is more likely to change detrimental health behaviors if he or she realizes that there is a problem and that these behaviors lead to the problem. (A, 3)

53. 1. Pharmacologic nicotine (eg, Nicotrol) is given in controlled and decreasing doses for the management of nicotine withdrawal symptoms as an adjunct to a smoking cessation program. Pharmacologic nicotine

can be administered by various routes: transdermal, topical, oral, or nasal sprays. The nicotine dosage is titrated in declining dosage over 4 to 6 weeks. Nitroglycerin is used for anginal symptoms, furosemide is a diuretic, and ibuprofen is an anti-inflammatory medication; these agents have no role in a smoking cessation program. (D, 8)

54. 2. Beurger's disease is characterized by inflammation and fibrosis of arteries, veins, and nerves. White blood cells infiltrate the area and become fibrotic, which results in occlusion of the vessels. Symptoms include slowly developing claudication, cyanosis, coldness, and pain at rest. Thickening of the intima and media of the artery is characteristic of atherosclerosis. Vasospasm lasting several minutes is characteristic of Raynaud's disease. Pain, pallor, and pulselessness are symptoms of acute occlusion of an artery by an embolus or other cause (eg, compartment syndrome). (E, 3)

The Client With Raynaud's Disease

55. 2. Raynaud's disease is more common in young women and is associated with collagen diseases such as rheumatoid arthritis and lupus. (D, 10)

56. 1. Raynaud's disease is characterized by vasospasms of the small cutaneous arteries involving the fingers and toes. (D, 10)

57. 3. Initially the vasoconstriction effect produces pallor or a whitish coloring, followed by cyanosis (bluish) and finally rubor (red). Gangrene is the end result of complete arterial occlusion. The skin is blackened and without a blood supply. (A, 9)

58. 4. Raynaud's disease involves the small cutaneous arteries of the fingers and toes. The nurse will be able to palpate the radial artery. If the disease process affects the lower extremities, the nurse will be able to palpate the dorsalis pedis artery during a vasospastic episode. (D, 10)

59. 3. Extreme changes in temperature can precipitate a vasospastic episode and should be avoided by clients with Raynaud's disease. The client should be encouraged to wear gloves when handling frozen foods or ice. The client should immerse the involved extremity in warm water during an episode to promote vasodilation and relaxation of the small arteries that are in spasm. The client can help prevent vasospasm brought on by temperature changes by wearing warm clothes. Living in a cold climate will exacerbate the symptoms. (I, 3)

60. 2. The data suggest a diagnosis of Anxiety related to change in health status. The client's statements support this diagnosis. The goal for the client is to learn strategies for effective coping with anxiety-producing situations. (P, 5)

61. 3. Propranolol (Inderal) is the only β-adrenergic medication listed. Tamsulosin hydrochloride (Flomax) blocks the smooth muscle α-adrenergic receptors in the prostate, leading to relaxation of the prostate and bladder. Terazosin hydrochloride (Hytrin) is classified as an α-adrenergic blocker and selectively blocks postsynaptic α-adrenergic receptors. This blocking action decreases sympathetic tone on the vasculature, dilating arterioles and veins. Labetalol hydrochloride (Trandate) competitively blocks α- and β-receptors. (D, 8)

62. 1. Beta-adrenergic medications block the β-adrenergic receptors. Therefore, the expected outcome of the medication is to decrease the influence of the sympathetic nervous system on the blood vessels in the hands. Beta-adrenergic blockers have no analgesic effects. Increasing blood supply to the affected area is an indirect effect of β-adrenergic blockers. They do not increase monoamine oxidase, which does not play a role in Raynaud's disease. (I, 8)

63. 4. Sympathectomy is scheduled only after other treatment alternatives have been explored and have failed. Medication and stress management are beneficial strategies to prevent advancement of the disease process. If the disease is controlled by medication, there is no reason for surgery. (D, 10)

The Client With Thrombophlebitis and Embolus Formation

64. 2. Performing active ankle and foot range-of-motion exercises periodically during the ride home will promote muscular contraction and provide support to the venous system. It is the muscular action that facilitates return of the blood from the lower extremities, especially when in the dependent position. (I, 9)

65. 3. Deep vein thrombosis is commonly associated with venous stasis in the legs when there is a lack of the skeletal muscle pump that enhances venous return to the heart. When a client is confined to bed rest, venous compression occurs because of the position of the lower extremities. This increased pressure causes damage to the intima lining of the veins and causes platelets to adhere to the damaged site. A deep vein thrombosis increases the risk that a displaced plaque will become a pulmonary embolus. Arteriosclerosis is hardening of the arteries; aneurysm is the abnormal dilation of a vessel; and varicose veins are swollen, tortuous veins. These are not generally considered causes of pulmonary embolism. (D, 10)

66. 3. Thrombolytic agents are used for clients with a history of thrombus formation, cerebral vascular accidents, and chronic atrial fibrillation. The thrombolytic agents act by dissolving emboli. (E, 8)

67. 4. Thrombophlebitis is an inflammation of a vein. The underlying etiology involves stasis of blood, increased blood coagulability, and vessel wall injury. The symptoms of thrombophlebitis are pain, swelling, and deep muscle tenderness. Air embolus is a result of air entering the vascular system. Fat embolus is associated with the presence of intracellular fat globules in the lung parenchyma and peripheral circulation after long-bone fractures. Stress fractures are associated with the musculoskeletal system. (D, 3)

68. 4. Current literature suggests that approximately 65% of the clients receiving IV therapy will develop superficial vein thrombophlebitis. (D, 9)

69. 3. The first action would be to discontinue the IV. The nurse should restart the IV elsewhere and then apply a warm compress to the affected area. The nurse would administer acetaminophen or an anti-inflammatory agent only if ordered by the physician. The type of infusion cannot be changed without a physician's order, and such a change would not help in this case. (I, 9)

70. 4. Three factors contribute to the formation of venous thrombus and thrombophlebitis: damage to the inner lining of the vein (prolonged pressure), hypercoagulability of the blood, and venous stasis. Bed rest and immobilization are associated with decreased blood flow and venous pooling in the lower extremities. Keeping the client in the supine position would not be appropriate. Turning the client every 1 to 2 hours, passive and active range-of-motion exercises, and use of TED hose help prevent venous stasis in the lower extremities. (A, 3)

71. 2. The client demonstrates classic symptoms of DVT. (D, 4)

72. 3. A history of recent abdominal surgery is a risk factor for developing a DVT, thrombophlebitis, or thromboembolism. Exercising on a regular basis helps prevent venous stasis and DVT. Wearing antithrombotic hose is a measure to help prevent venous stasis. Living alone has no link to development of DVT. (D, 10)

73. 4. Heparin dosage is usually determined by the doctor based on the client's aPTT and INR laboratory values. Therefore, the nurse monitors these values to prevent complications. Taking aspirin when the client is on heparin is contraindicated. Green leafy vegetables are high in vitamin K and therefore are not recommended for clients receiving heparin. Monitoring of the client's PT is done when the client is receiving warfarin sodium (Coumadin). (I, 7)

74. 4. The use of pneumatic compression stockings is an intervention used to prevent DVT. Other strategies include early ambulation, leg exercises if the client is confined to bed, adequate fluid intake, and administering anticoagulant medication as ordered. Deep breathing would be encouraged postoperatively, but it does not prevent DVT. (D, 3)

75. 4. Risk for Impaired Skin Integrity is the primary nursing diagnosis. With rubor or hyperemia, there is increased blood flow to the area, raising filtration pressure. As a result, capillary permeability is altered, causing damage to capillary walls. The increased permeability, obstruction of lymphatic drainage, elevation of venous pressure, and decrease in plasma protein osmotic force results in edema. (P, 10)

76. 4. The data suggest an increased risk for thrombophlebitis. The risk factors in this situation include abdominal surgery, obesity, and use of estrogen-based oral contraceptives. (D, 10)

77. 4. Varicose veins are tortuous, distended veins where blood has pooled. Varicose veins are commonly observed in the lower extremities. An aneurysm is a localized, abnormal dilatation of a blood vessel. A lipoma is a fatty tumor. An ulcer is an open sore or lesion of the skin or mucous membrane, accompanied by sloughing of inflamed necrotic tissue. (D, 4)

78. 3. Secondary varicosities can result from previous thrombophlebitis of the deep femoral veins, with subsequent valvular incompetence. Cerebral vascular accident, anemia, and transient ischemic attacks are not associated with an increased risk for varicose veins. (P, 3)

79. 2. The client is at risk for development of varicose veins. Therefore, prevention is key in the treatment plan. Maintaining ideal body weight is the goal. In order to achieve this, the client should consume a balanced diet and participate in a regular exercise program. Depending on the individual, leg lifts may or may not be an appropriate form of activity. Performing leg lifts provides muscular activity and should be done more often than every 4 hours. Wearing support hose is helpful. However, the client should not use rubber bands to hold the stockings up. (E, 9)

80. 4. The nurse will monitor the pulses in the affected extremity after arterial embolectomy. Monitoring peripheral pulses below the site of occlusion checks the arterial circulation in the involved extremity. (P, 10)

The Client With an Aneurysm

81. 3. The primary goal is to prepare the client for emergency surgery. The goal would be to prevent rupture of the aneurysm and potential death. Circulation is maintained, unless the aneurysm ruptures. (P, 10)

82. 1. If the aortic arch is involved there will be a decrease in the blood flow to the cerebrum. Therefore, loss of consciousness will be observed. A sudden loss of consciousness is a primary symptom of rupture and no blood flow to the brain. (A, 4)

83. 1. Cardiac tamponade is a life-threatening complication of a dissecting thoracic aneurysm. The sudden and painful "tearing" sensation is typically associated with the sudden release of blood. (P, 10)

84. 3. In the preoperative phase, the goal is to prevent rupture. The patient is placed in a semi-Fowler's position and in a quiet environment. The systolic blood pressure is maintained at the lowest level the client can tolerate. Anemia, dehydration, and hyperglycemia do not put the client at risk for rupture. (D, 3)

85. 1. There is a potential for an alteration in renal perfusion, manifested by decreased urine output. The altered renal perfusion may be related to renal artery embolism, prolonged hypotension, or prolonged aortic cross-clamping during surgery. Electrolyte imbalance, ineffective coping, and wound infection may occur after any surgery. (P, 10)

86. 4. Severe pain is associated with a major abdominal procedure. The goal is to maintain adequate pain relief. As a result, narcotics such as morphine are given. Side effects of morphine include dry mouth, nausea, and constipation. Bowel manipulation, immobility, and the use of pain medications are all factors that contribute to a postoperative ileus. Insertion of a nasogastric tube generally helps a postoperative ileus. (A, 7)

87. 3. The client with a synthetic graft may need to be treated with prophylactic antibiotics before undergoing major dental work. This reduces the danger of systemic infection caused by bacteria from the oral cavity. (D, 8)

88. 2. These symptoms suggest that the client is receiving too much Coumadin. Coumadin hinders the hepatic synthesis of vitamin K–dependent clotting factors and prolongs the clotting time. Because many factors influence the effectiveness of Coumadin, the dosage is monitored closely. Signs of blood loss include bleeding gums, petechiae, bruises, dark stools, and dark urine. (D, 8)

The Client with a Variety of Vascular Problems

89. 1. Lymphedema occurs frequently after radical mastectomy when lymph nodes are removed. Aplasia, or the absence of lymph nodes, prevents proper lymph drainage. The tissue swelling is caused by obstructed lymph flow in the extremity. The blood pressure is taken in the unaffected arm to avoid further accumulation of lymphedema. An intravenous line should not be started in the affected arm. Blood draws in the affected arm should not be allowed. The nurse would encourage the client to elevate the extremity above the level of the heart. (A, 10)

90. 1. A vascular disturbance involving branches of the carotid artery is believed to cause migraine attacks. Vasoconstriction of blood vessels apparently occurs first. The extracranial and intracranial arteries then dilate, causing the headache. A family history of migraine headaches is present in more than half of all people who experience migraines. (A, 10)

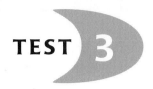

The Client With Hematologic Health Problems

▶ **The Client With Red Blood Cell Disorders**

▶ **The Client With Platelet Disorders**

▶ **The Client With White Blood Cell Disorders**

▶ **The Client With Lymphoma**

▶ **The Client Who Is in Shock**

▶ **Correct Answers and Rationale**

Select the one best answer, and indicate your choice by filling in the circle in front of the option.

The Client With Red Blood Cell Disorders

1. The nurse is preparing to teach a client with microcytic hypochromic anemia about the diet to follow after discharge. Which of the following foods should be included in the diet?
   ○ 1. Eggs.
   ○ 2. Lettuce.
   ○ 3. Citrus fruits.
   ○ 4. Cheese.

2. The nurse should instruct the client to eat which of the following foods to obtain the best supply of vitamin B_{12}?
   ○ 1. Whole grains.
   ○ 2. Green leafy vegetables.
   ○ 3. Meats and dairy products.
   ○ 4. Broccoli and brussels sprouts.

3. The nurse has just admitted a 35-year-old female client with severe arthritis and a well-controlled seizure disorder who has a serum vitamin B_{12} concentration of 800 pg/mL. Which of the following laboratory findings would cue the nurse to focus the client history on specific drug or alcohol use?
   ○ 1. Total bilirubin, 0.3 mg/dL.
   ○ 2. Serum creatinine, 0.5 mg/dL.
   ○ 3. Hemoglobin, 16 g/dL.
   ○ 4. Folate, 1.5 ng/mL.

4. The nurse understands that the client with pernicious anemia will have which distinguishing laboratory findings?
   ○ 1. Schilling's test, elevated.
   ○ 2. Intrinsic factor, absent.
   ○ 3. Sedimentation rate, 16 mm/hour.
   ○ 4. Red blood cells (RBCs), 5.0 million/μL^3.

5. The nurse devises a teaching plan for the patient with aplastic anemia. Which of the following is the most important concept to teach for health maintenance?
   ○ 1. Eat animal protein and dark green leafy vegetables every day.
   ○ 2. Avoid exposure to others with acute infections.
   ○ 3. Practice yoga and meditation to decrease stress and anxiety.
   ○ 4. Get 8 hours of sleep at night and take naps during the day.

6. A client with Crohn's disease comes to the Women's Health Clinic 3 years after a resection of the terminal ileum. She is complaining of weakness, shortness of breath, weight loss, and a sore tongue. The nurse recognizes a knowledge deficit when the client states which of the following?
   ○ 1. "I have been drinking plenty of fluids."
   ○ 2. "I have been gargling with warm salt water for my sore tongue."
   ○ 3. "I have three to four loose stools per day."
   ○ 4. "I take a vitamin B_{12} tablet every day."

7. A vegetarian who was admitted with perimenopausal bleeding, palpitations, dizziness, and profuse sweating was referred to a dietitian for nutritional counseling for anemia. Which client outcome indicates that the client does not understand the counseling? The client
   ○ 1. adds dried fruit to cereal and baked goods.
   ○ 2. cooks tomato-based foods in iron pots.
   ○ 3. drinks coffee or tea with meals.
   ○ 4. adds vitamin C to all meals.

8. A 26-year-old executive who was admitted to the hospital with iron-deficiency anemia stated that he had been experiencing gastrointestinal upset and blood-streaked vomiting. When taking his nursing

281

history, which question is most appropriate for the nurse to ask in determining the extent of the client's activity intolerance?

  ○ 1. "What daily activities were you able to do 6 months ago compared with the present?"

  ○ 2. "How long have you had this problem?"

  ○ 3. "Have you been able to keep up with all your usual activities?"

  ○ 4. "Are you more tired now than you used to be?"

9. Which position would most help to decrease a client's discomfort when the client's spouse injects vitamin B_{12} using the ventrogluteal site?

  ○ 1. Lying on the side with legs extended.

  ○ 2. Lying on the abdomen with toes pointed inward.

  ○ 3. Leaning over edge of a low table with the hips flexed.

  ○ 4. Standing upright with the feet one shoulder's-width apart.

10. The primary purpose of the Schilling test is to measure the client's ability to

  ○ 1. store vitamin B_{12}.

  ○ 2. digest vitamin B_{12}.

  ○ 3. absorb vitamin B_{12}.

  ○ 4. produce vitamin B_{12}.

11. The nurse implements which of the following for the client who is starting a Schilling test?

  ○ 1. Administering methylcellulose (Citrucel).

  ○ 2. Starting a 24- to 48-hour urine specimen collection.

  ○ 3. Maintaining NPO status.

  ○ 4. Starting a 72-hour stool specimen collection.

12. A 16-year-old boy, visiting from his Mediterranean homeland, was admitted through the emergency room with thalassemia after passing out. His laboratory tests revealed the following: blood glucose, 130 mg/dL; hemoglobin, 9.4 g/dL; hematocrit, 37%; mean corpuscular hemoglobulin concentration, 34%; and bilirubin, 2 mg/dL. The nurse assessed that the client was slightly jaundiced with pale mucous membranes, was mentally slow with a Down syndrome appearance, was 5 feet 4 inches tall, and had splenomegaly and hepatomegaly. What is the primary focus of nursing interventions for this client?

  ○ 1. Providing activities of daily living on the time schedule of his homeland.

  ○ 2. Offering foods of his preference to increase his intake of calories.

  ○ 3. Decreasing his cardiac demands by promoting a 1:3 ratio of rest to activity as tolerated.

  ○ 4. Listening to his concerns about his hospitalization.

13. A client with pernicious anemia asks why she must take vitamin B_{12} injections for the rest of her life. What is the nurse's *best* response?

  ○ 1. "The reason for your vitamin deficiency is an inability to absorb the vitamin because the stomach is not producing sufficient acid."

  ○ 2. "The reason for your vitamin deficiency is an inability to absorb the vitamin because the stomach is not producing sufficient intrinsic factor."

  ○ 3. "The reason for your vitamin deficiency is an excessive excretion of the vitamin because of kidney dysfunction."

  ○ 4. "The reason for your vitamin deficiency is an increased requirement for the vitamin because of rapid red blood cell production."

14. An African-American woman had experienced severe palpitations, weakness, and shortness of breath after taking bacitracin (Bactrim) for a urinary tract infection. As a part of the discharge planning, the nurse evaluates the client's knowledge about her

  ○ 1. increased folic acid needs.

  ○ 2. congenital enzyme deficiency.

  ○ 3. restricted activity in hot weather.

  ○ 4. need for blood transfusions.

15. The nurse is assessing a client's activity tolerance by having the client walk on a treadmill for 5 minutes. Which of the following indicates an abnormal response?

  ○ 1. Pulse rate increased by 20 bpm immediately after the activity.

  ○ 2. Respiratory rate decreased by 5 breaths/minute.

  ○ 3. Diastolic blood pressure increased by 7 mm Hg.

  ○ 4. Pulse rate within 6 bpm of resting pulse after 3 minutes of rest.

16. When comparing the hematocrit levels of a postoperative splenectomy client, the nurse notes that the hematocrit decreased from 36% to 34% on the third day even though the RBC and hemoglobin values remained stable at 4.5 million/mm³ and 11.9 g/dL, respectively. Which nursing intervention is most appropriate?

  ○ 1. Check the dressing and drains for frank bleeding.

  ○ 2. Call the physician.

  ○ 3. Continue to monitor vital signs.

  ○ 4. Start oxygen at 2 L/minute per nasal cannula.

17. The nurse administers packed red blood cells (PRBCs) to a client with pernicious anemia. Which of the following nursing actions is appropriate?

  ○ 1. Discontinue the intravenous catheter if a blood transfusion reaction occurs.

  ○ 2. Administer the PRBCs through a percutaneously inserted central catheter line with a 20-gauge needle.

  ○ 3. Flush PRBCs with 5% dextrose and 0.45% normal saline.

  ○ 4. Stay with the client during the first 15 minutes of infusion.

18. A client had received 25 mL of PRBCs when she began to experience low lack pain and mild itching. After stopping the infusion, the nurse should
    ○ 1. administer prescribed aspirin and antihistamines.
    ○ 2. collect blood and urine samples to be sent to the laboratory.
    ○ 3. administer prescribed diuretics, oxygen, and morphine.
    ○ 4. administer prescribed vasopressors.

19. A client is to receive epoetin (Epogen) injections. What laboratory value should the nurse assess before giving the injection?
    ○ 1. Hematocrit.
    ○ 2. Partial thromboplastin time.
    ○ 3. Hemoglobin concentration.
    ○ 4. Prothrombin time.

20. An elderly client states that she is afraid of receiving vitamin B_{12} injections every month because of potential toxic reactions. What is the nurse's best response to relieve these fears?
    ○ 1. "Vitamin B_{12} will cause ringing in the ears before a toxic level is reached."
    ○ 2. "Vitamin B_{12} may cause a very mild skin rash initially."
    ○ 3. "Vitamin B_{12} may cause mild nausea but nothing toxic."
    ○ 4. "Vitamin B_{12} is generally free of toxicity because it is water soluble."

21. A vegetarian with microcytic anemia is having trouble selecting food from the hospital menu. Which food is best for the nurse to suggest for satisfying the client's nutritional needs and personal preferences?
    ○ 1. Egg yolks.
    ○ 2. Brown rice.
    ○ 3. Vegetables.
    ○ 4. Tea.

22. A client with macrocytic anemia has a burn on her foot and states that she had been watching television while lying on a heating pad. What is the nurse's first response?
    ○ 1. Assess for potential abuse.
    ○ 2. Check for diminished sensations.
    ○ 3. Document the findings.
    ○ 4. Clean and dress the area.

23. Which of the following nursing assessments is a late symptom of polycythemia vera?
    ○ 1. Headache.
    ○ 2. Dizziness.
    ○ 3. Pruritus.
    ○ 4. Shortness of breath.

24. When a client is diagnosed with aplastic anemia, the nurse monitors for changes in which of the following physiologic functions?
    ○ 1. Bleeding tendencies.
    ○ 2. Intake and output.

○ 3. Peripheral sensation.
○ 4. Bowel function.

The Client With Platelet Disorders

25. Which of the following nursing interventions is appropriate for a client with a platelet count of $31,000/mm^3$?
    ○ 1. Pad sharp surfaces to avoid minor trauma when walking.
    ○ 2. Assess for spontaneous petechiae in the extremities.
    ○ 3. Keep the room darkened.
    ○ 4. Check for blood in the urine.

26. A 30-year-old woman with a history of systemic lupus erythematosus was admitted with a severe viral respiratory infection and flu. The nurse observed diffuse petechiae. Based on these data, it is most important that the nurse further evaluate the client's recent
    ○ 1. quality and quantity of food intake.
    ○ 2. type and amount of fluid intake.
    ○ 3. weakness, fatigue, and ability to get around.
    ○ 4. length and amount of menstrual flow.

27. When a client with thrombocytopenia complains of a severe headache, the nurse interprets that this may indicate which of the following?
    ○ 1. Stress of the disease.
    ○ 2. Cerebral bleeding.
    ○ 3. A migraine headache.
    ○ 4. Sinus congestion.

28. The nurse evaluates that the client correctly understands how to report signs of bleeding when she makes which of the following statements?
    ○ 1. "Petechiae are large red skin bruises."
    ○ 2. "Ecchymoses are large purple skin bruises."
    ○ 3. "Purpura is an open cut on the skin."
    ○ 4. "Abrasion is small pinpoint red dots on the skin."

29. The client states she does not understand what causes idiopathic thrombocytopenia purpura (ITTP). The nurse provides which of the following explanations?
    ○ 1. It is believed that the platelets are coated with antibodies and the spleen sees them as foreign bodies.
    ○ 2. It is believed that the liver identifies the platelets as foreign bodies.
    ○ 3. It is now believed that the syndrome is related to an underactive immune system.
    ○ 4. The cause is unknown.

30. The nurse should instruct the client with a platelet count of less than $150,000/\mu L$ to avoid which of the following activities?
    ○ 1. Ambulation.

○ 2. Valsalva's maneuver.

○ 3. Visiting with children.

○ 4. Semi-Fowler's position.

31. If a client who is taking Bufferin Arthritis Strength caplets develops prolonged bleeding from a superficial injury, the nurse recognizes that this clinical manifestation most likely reflects

    ○ 1. a prothrombin time (PT) of 10 seconds.

    ○ 2. an activated partial thromboplastin time (aPTT) of 40 seconds.

    ○ 3. a bleeding time of 8 minutes.

    ○ 4. a coagulation time (CT) of 8 minutes.

32. A client's bone marrow report reveals normal stem cells and precursors of platelets (megakaryocytes) in the presence of decreased circulating platelets. The nurse recognizes a knowledge deficit when the client makes which of the following statements?

    ○ 1. "I need to stop flossing and throw away my hard toothbrush."

    ○ 2. "I am glad that my report turned out normal."

    ○ 3. "Now I know why I have all these bruises."

    ○ 4. "I shouldn't jump off that last step anymore."

33. Which early symptom does the nurse observe in a client with thrombocytopenia who has developed a hemorrhage?

    ○ 1. Tachycardia.

    ○ 2. Bradycardia.

    ○ 3. Decreased $PaCO_2$.

    ○ 4. Narrowed pulse pressure.

34. The client with immune thrombocytopenia purpura asks the nurse why she has to take steroids. Which is the nurse's best response?

    ○ 1. Steroids destroy the antibodies covering the platelets and prolong the life of platelets.

    ○ 2. Steroids neutralize the antigens that were attacking the platelets and prolong the life of platelets.

    ○ 3. Steroids increase phagocytosis by increasing the defenses surrounding the platelets to increase the life of the platelets.

    ○ 4. Steroids alter the spleen's recognition of platelets as foreign bodies and increase the life of the platelets.

35. A client is to be discharged on prednisone. Which of the following statements indicates that the client understands important concepts about the medication therapy?

    ○ 1. "I need to take the medicine in divided doses at morning and bedtime."

    ○ 2. "I am to take 40 mg of prednisone for 2 months and then stop."

    ○ 3. "I need to wear or carry identification that I am taking prednisone."

    ○ 4. "Prednisone will give me extra protection from colds and flu."

36. When teaching the client older than 50 years of age who are receiving long-term prednisone therapy, which of the following actions does the nurse recommend?

    ○ 1. Take the prednisone with food.

    ○ 2. Take over-the-counter drugs as needed.

    ○ 3. Exercise three to four times a week.

    ○ 4. Eat foods that are low in potassium.

37. The nurse is preparing a teaching plan about increased exercise for a 51-year-old female client who is receiving long-term corticosteroid therapy for chronic immune thrombocytopenia purpura. What type of exercise is most appropriate for this client?

    ○ 1. Floor exercises.

    ○ 2. Stretching.

    ○ 3. Running.

    ○ 4. Walking.

38. A client with a history of acquired thrombocytopenia has been instructed on how to prevent and control hemorrhage. Which statement indicates that the client needs further intervention?

    ○ 1. "I can apply direct pressure over small cuts for at least 5 to 10 minutes to stop a venous bleed."

    ○ 2. "I can count the number of tissues saturated to detect blood loss during a nosebleed."

    ○ 3. "I can take hormones to decrease blood loss during menses."

    ○ 4. "I can count the number of sanitary napkins to detect excess blood loss during menses."

39. Which of the following clinical manifestations does the nurse find in the client who has systemic adverse effects from long-term corticosteroid therapy?

    ○ 1. Weight gain.

    ○ 2. High serum albumin.

    ○ 3. Low sodium.

    ○ 4. Hyperkalemia.

40. Platelets should not be administered under which of the following conditions?

    ○ 1. The platelet bag is cold.

    ○ 2. The platelets are 2 days old.

    ○ 3. The platelet bag is at room temperature.

    ○ 4. The platelets are 12 hours old.

41. The nurse is preparing to administer platelets. The nurse should

    ○ 1. check the ABO compatibility.

    ○ 2. administer the platelets slowly.

    ○ 3. gently rotate the bag.

    ○ 4. use a whole blood tubing set.

42. Which of the following indicates that a client has achieved the goal of correctly demonstrating deep breathing for an upcoming splenectomy? The client

    ○ 1. breathes in through the nose and out through the mouth.

    ○ 2. breathes in through the mouth and out through the nose.

3. uses diaphragmatic breathing in the lying, sitting, and standing positions.
4. holds a pillow to the stomach, takes a deep breath in through the nose, and blows out through pursed lips.

43. A client is scheduled for an elective splenectomy after failure to respond to conservative treatment for chronic immune thrombocytopenia purpura. Before the client goes to surgery, the nurse's final assessment is the client's
1. empty bladder.
2. signed consent.
3. vital signs.
4. name band.

44. A client with chronic immune thrombocytopenia purpura undergoes a splenectomy. Immediately after receiving the client from the postanesthesia recovery room, what should the nurse assess after first assessing the airway and vital signs?
1. Nasogastric drainage.
2. Urinary catheter.
3. Dressing.
4. Need for pain medication.

45. The client's family asks why the client has a nasogastric tube. A nasogastric tube is used to
1. move the stomach away from where the spleen was removed.
2. irrigate the operative site.
3. decrease abdominal distention.
4. assess for the gastric pH as peristalsis returns.

46. A client with chronic immune thrombocytopenia purpura who had a splenectomy is being discharged. Of the following discharge instructions, which is most specific to the client's surgical procedure?
1. Do not drive.
2. Alternate rest and activity.
3. Make an appointment for the staples to be removed.
4. Report early signs of infection.

47. What is the earliest and most obvious clinical manifestation that the nurse finds on assessment of a client with acute disseminated intravascular coagulation (DIC)?
1. Severe shortness of breath.
2. Bleeding without previous history or cause.
3. Orthopnea.
4. Hematuria.

48. Which of the following is contraindicated for a client diagnosed with DIC?
1. Treating the underlying cause.
2. Administering heparin.
3. Administering Coumadin.
4. Replacing depleted blood products.

49. A client with DIC develops clinical manifestations of microvascular thrombosis. The nurse should assess the client for
1. hemoptysis.
2. focal ischemia.
3. petechiae.
4. hematuria.

50. Recognizing early clinical manifestations of internal bleeding is an important nursing goal for a client with DIC. Which of the following is a finding associated with internal bleeding?
1. Bradycardia.
2. Hypertension.
3. Increasing abdominal girth.
4. Petechiae.

The Client With White Blood Cell Disorders

51. A client with aplastic anemia has daily white blood cell (WBC) counts. The nurse notes that his WBC level has dropped overnight from 3900 to 2900/μL. What is the appropriate nursing intervention?
1. Continue monitoring the client.
2. Call the laboratory to verify the report.
3. Document the finding.
4. Call the physician and place the client in reverse isolation.

52. A client who had an exploratory laparotomy 3 days ago has a differential with a shift to the left. The nurse instructs unlicensed personnel to report which clinical manifestation?
1. Swelling around the incision.
2. Redness around the incision.
3. Elevated temperature.
4. Purulent wound drainage.

53. What does the nurse calculate as the absolute neutrophil count (ANC) for a client with a WBC count of 1200/μL with bands, 1%; neutrophils, 34%; eosinophils, 3%; and basophils, 4%?
1. 440.
2. 420.
3. 468.
4. 456.

54. A client with neutropenia has an ANC of 900. What is the client's risk of infection?
1. Normal risk.
2. Moderate risk.
3. High risk.
4. Extremely high risk.

55. What factor besides the degree of neutropenia does the nurse assess in determining the client's risk for infection?
1. Length of time neutropenia has existed.
2. Health status before neutropenia.
3. Body build and weight.
4. Resistance to infection in childhood.

56. What nursing action is important in preventing cross-contamination?
○ 1. Change gloves immediately after use.
○ 2. Stand 2 feet from the patient.
○ 3. Speak minimally when in the room.
○ 4. Wear long-sleeved shirts.

57. The nurse should teach the neutropenic client and the family to avoid which of the following?
○ 1. Using suppositories or enemas.
○ 2. Using a high-efficiency particulate air (HEPA) filter mask.
○ 3. Performing perineal care after every bowel movement.
○ 4. Performing oral care after every meal.

58. The nurse should remind family members who are visiting a client with granulocytopenia to
○ 1. visit only if they do not have a cold.
○ 2. wash their hands.
○ 3. leave the children at home.
○ 4. avoid kissing the client on the lips.

59. The nurse should remind the unlicensed personnel that which of the following is the most important goal in the care of the neutropenic client in isolation?
○ 1. Listening to the client's feelings of concern.
○ 2. Completing the client's care in a nonhurried manner.
○ 3. Completing all of the client's care at one time.
○ 4. Instructing the client to dispose of tissue after blowing the nose.

60. The nurse's role in the consent for the bone marrow aspiration includes all of the following *except*
○ 1. witnessing the client sign the consent form for the bone marrow aspiration.
○ 2. evaluating that the client has a congruent understanding of the bone marrow aspiration procedure.
○ 3. explaining the risks of the procedure to the client.
○ 4. verifying that the client is signing the consent form by his or her free will.

61. An elderly client is about to undergo bone marrow aspiration of the sternum. The nurse understands that the client will be better prepared if the procedure and any anticipated sensations are explained. Which of the following statements will help prepare this client for the procedure?
○ 1. "You may feel a warm solution being wiped over your entire front from your neck down to your navel and out to your shoulders."
○ 2. "You will not feel the local anesthetic being applied because it will be sprayed on."
○ 3. "You will feel a pulling type of discomfort for a few seconds."
○ 4. "After the needle is removed, a bandage will be applied around your chest for the first 24 hours."

62. Twenty-four hours after a bone marrow aspiration, the nurse evaluates which of the following as an appropriate client outcome?
○ 1. The client maintains bed rest.
○ 2. There is redness and swelling at aspiration site.
○ 3. The client requests morphine sulfate 2 mg IM every 2 hours.
○ 4. There is no bleeding at aspiration site.

63. The client tells the nurse that the physician wants to do more tests to see which kind of leukemia she has. The client states, "Who cares what kind it is, I have leukemia and I'm tired of the tests. I just want to get it treated now!" What is the nurse's *best* response?
○ 1. "I'm sure you are frustrated and want to be well now."
○ 2. "Your treatment can be more effective if it is based on more specific information about your disease."
○ 3. "Now, you know the tests are necessary and that you are just upset right now."
○ 4. "I understand how you feel."

64. During the induction stage for treatment of leukemia, the nurse should remove which items that the family has brought into the room?
○ 1. A Bible.
○ 2. A picture.
○ 3. A sachet of lavender.
○ 4. A hairbrush.

65. The nurse identifies deficient knowledge when the client undergoing induction therapy for leukemia makes which of the following statements?
○ 1. "I will have to pace my activities with rest periods."
○ 2. "I can't wait to get home to my cat!"
○ 3. "I will use warm saline gargle instead of brushing my teeth."
○ 4. "I must report a temperature of 100 degrees Fahrenheit."

66. A 60-year-old client with acute myeloid leukemia (AML) states that he overheard one of the other patients say that AML had a very poor prognosis. The client explains to the nurse that he had understood his doctor to say that he had a relatively good prognosis. What is the nurse's *best* response?
○ 1. "You must have misunderstood. Whom did you hear that from?"
○ 2. "AML does have a very poor prognosis for poorly differentiated cells."
○ 3. "AML is the most common nonlymphocytic leukemia."
○ 4. "Your doctor stated your prognosis based on the differentiation of your cells."

67. The goal of nursing care for a client with acute myeloid leukemia is to prevent
○ 1. cardiac arrhythmias.

○ 2. liver failure.
○ 3. renal failure.
○ 4. hemorrhage.

68. Which of the following does the nurse observe in the client with chronic myeloid leukemia (CML)?
○ 1. Lymphadenopathy.
○ 2. Hyperplasia of the gum.
○ 3. Bone pain from expansion of marrow.
○ 4. Shortness of breath or slight confusion.

69. What is the peak age range for acquiring acute lymphocytic leukemia (ALL)?
○ 1. 4 to 12 years.
○ 2. 20 to 30 years.
○ 3. 40 to 50 years.
○ 4. 60 to 70 years.

70. The client with ALL develops nausea and a headache. These clinical manifestations may indicate all of the following *except*
○ 1. gastric distention.
○ 2. meningeal irritation.
○ 3. chemotherapy side effects.
○ 4. effects of radiation.

71. In assessing a client in the early stage of chronic lymphocytic leukemia (CLL), the nurse is aware that the client is prone to experiencing which of the following?
○ 1. Enlarged, painless lymph nodes.
○ 2. Headache.
○ 3. Hyperplasia of the gums.
○ 4. Unintentional weight loss.

72. Which does the nurse suggest as the most appropriate intervention to manage mucositis for a client with acute leukemia?
○ 1. "After each meal or every 4 hours while awake, use lemon-glycerin swabs."
○ 2. "After each meal or every 4 hours while awake, use a commercial mouthwash."
○ 3. "After each meal or every 4 hours while awake, use a saline or baking soda solution."
○ 4. "After each meal or every 4 hours while awake, use your own toothpaste and brush."

73. The client with acute leukemia and the nurse establish improved tidal volume and activity tolerance as goals of care. Progress toward these goals can be accomplished through all *except* which of the following?
○ 1. Ambulating in the hallway.
○ 2. Sitting up in a chair.
○ 3. Lying in bed and taking deep breaths.
○ 4. Using a stationary bicycle in the room.

74. The nurse is evaluating the client's learning about combination chemotherapy. Which of the following statements about reasons for using combination chemotherapy indicates the need for *further* explanation?

○ 1. "Combination chemotherapy is used to interrupt cell growth cycle at different points."
○ 2. "Combination chemotherapy is used to destroy cancer cells and treat side effects simultaneously."
○ 3. "Combination chemotherapy is used to decrease resistance."
○ 4. "Combination chemotherapy is used to minimize the toxicity from using high doses of a single agent."

75. In providing care to the client with leukemia who has developed thrombocytopenia, the nurse assesses the most common sites for bleeding. Which of the following is not a common site?
○ 1. Biliary system.
○ 2. Gastrointestinal tract.
○ 3. Brain and meninges.
○ 4. Pulmonary system.

76. The nurse's *best* explanation for why the severely neutropenic client is placed in reverse isolation is that reverse isolation helps prevent the spread of organisms
○ 1. to the client from sources outside the client's environment.
○ 2. from the client to health care personnel, visitors, and other clients.
○ 3. by using special techniques to dispose of contaminated materials.
○ 4. by using special techniques to handle the client's linens and personal items.

The Client With Lymphoma

77. Which of the following clinical manifestations does the nurse most likely observe in a client with Hodgkin's disease?
○ 1. Difficulty swallowing.
○ 2. Painless, enlarged cervical lymph nodes.
○ 3. Difficulty breathing.
○ 4. A feeling of fullness over the liver.

78. A client with Hodgkin's disease is scheduled for an excisional biopsy of an enlarged cervical lymph node under local anesthesia. What action is correct for handling the lymph node biopsy specimen for histologic examination?
○ 1. Call the laboratory and ask for specific instructions.
○ 2. Place the specimen on a sponge in gloved hand. Next, place the sponge on the gloved hand. Then, pull the glove over the specimen and take it to the laboratory.
○ 3. Place the specimen in a container and send it to the laboratory when someone is available to take it.
○ 4. Call for a laboratory technician to assist the physician.

79. The client with Hodgkin's disease undergoes an excisional cervical lymph node biopsy under local anesthesia. After the procedure, what does the nurse assess *first*?
    - ○ 1. Vital signs.
    - ○ 2. The incision.
    - ○ 3. The airway.
    - ○ 4. Neurologic signs.

80. The nurse explains to the client that a biopsy of the enlarged lymph node is important because, if Hodgkin's disease is present, the histologic examination will reveal which of the following?
    - ○ 1. Tay-Sachs cells.
    - ○ 2. Sarcoidosis cells.
    - ○ 3. Reed-Sternberg cells.
    - ○ 4. Duchenne's cells.

81. When assessing the client with Hodgkin's disease, the nurse is alert for which of the following findings?
    - ○ 1. Herpes zoster infections.
    - ○ 2. Discolored teeth.
    - ○ 3. Hemorrhage.
    - ○ 4. Hypercellular immunity.

82. The client with Hodgkin's disease develops B symptoms. These manifestations indicate which of the following?
    - ○ 1. The client has a low-grade fever (temperature lower than 100°F [37.8°C]).
    - ○ 2. The client has a weight loss of 5% or less of body weight.
    - ○ 3. The client has night sweats.
    - ○ 4. The client probably has not progressed to an advanced stage.

83. The client tells his nurse that he wants to be sure that he is receiving the latest staging technique for his lymphoma. Based on advances in technology and research, the nurse tells the client that which of the following is being used *less* often in the staging of lymphomas?
    - ○ 1. Body scans.
    - ○ 2. Radiography.
    - ○ 3. Blood studies.
    - ○ 4. Exploratory laparotomy with lymph node biopsy.

84. The client asks the nurse to explain what it means that his Hodgkin's disease is diagnosed at stage 1A. Which of the following describes the involvement of the disease?
    - ○ 1. Involvement of a single lymph node.
    - ○ 2. Involvement of two or more lymph nodes on the same side of the diaphragm.
    - ○ 3. Involvement of lymph node regions on both sides of the diaphragm.
    - ○ 4. Diffuse disease of one or more extralymphatic organs.

85. A client is undergoing a bone marrow aspiration and biopsy. What is the best way for the nurse to help the client handle her stress?
    - ○ 1. Allow the client's family to stay with her as long as possible.
    - ○ 2. Stay with the client and hold her hand without speaking.
    - ○ 3. Encourage the client to take slow, deep breaths to relax.
    - ○ 4. Allow the client time to express her feelings.

86. The nurse explains to the client with Hodgkin's disease that a bone marrow biopsy will be taken after the aspiration. What should the nurse explain about the biopsy?
    - ○ 1. "Your biopsy will be performed before the aspiration because enough tissue may be obtained so that you won't have to go through the aspiration."
    - ○ 2. "You will feel a pressure sensation when the biopsy is taken but should not feel actual pain; if you do, tell the doctor so that you can be given extra numbing medicine."
    - ○ 3. "You may hear a crunch as the needle passes through the bone, but when the biopsy is taken, you will feel a suction-type pain that will last for just a moment."
    - ○ 4. "You will be shaved and cleaned with an antiseptic agent, after which the doctor will inject a needle without making an incision to aspirate out the bone marrow."

87. A client with Hodgkin's disease that is resistant to aggressive treatment is readmitted as death is imminent. The goal of nursing care is to help relieve the client's
    - ○ 1. fear of pain.
    - ○ 2. fear of further therapy.
    - ○ 3. feelings of isolation.
    - ○ 4. feelings of social inadequacy.

88. The client is a survivor of non-Hodgkin's lymphoma. Which of the following statements indicates the client needs additional information?
    - ○ 1. "Regular screening is very important for me."
    - ○ 2. "The survivor rate is directly proportional to the incidence of second malignancy."
    - ○ 3. "The survivor rate is indirectly proportionate to the incidence of second malignancy."
    - ○ 4. "It is important for survivors to know the stage of the disease and their current treatment plan."

The Client Who Is in Shock

89. Which of the following is the most important goal of nursing care for a client who is in shock?
    - ○ 1. Manage fluid overload.

○ 2. Manage increased cardiac output.
○ 3. Manage inadequate tissue perfusion.
○ 4. Manage vasoconstriction of vascular beds.

90. Which of the following nursing assessment findings indicates hypovolemic shock in a client who has had a 15% blood loss?
○ 1. Pulse rate less than 60 bpm.
○ 2. Respiratory rate of 4 breaths/minute.
○ 3. Pupils unequally dilated.
○ 4. Systolic blood pressure less than 90 mm Hg.

91. Which of the following findings is the best indication that fluid replacement for the client in hypovolemic shock is adequate?
○ 1. Urine output greater than 30 mL/hour.
○ 2. Systolic blood pressure greater than 110 mm Hg.
○ 3. Diastolic blood pressure greater than 90 mm Hg.
○ 4. Respiratory rate of 20 breaths/minute.

92. Which of the following is a risk factor for hypovolemic shock?
○ 1. Hemorrhage.
○ 2. Antigen-antibody reaction.
○ 3. Gram-negative bacteria.
○ 4. Vasodilatation.

93. What is a priority assessment for the client in shock who is receiving an intravenous infusion of packed red blood cells and normal saline solution?
○ 1. Fluid balance.
○ 2. Anaphylactic reaction.
○ 3. Pain.
○ 4. Altered level of consciousness.

94. The client who does not respond adequately to fluid replacement has an order for an intravenous infusion of dopamine hydrochloride at 5 μg/kg per minute. The desired effect of this drug is
○ 1. increased renal and mesenteric blood flow.
○ 2. increased cardiac output.
○ 3. vasoconstriction.
○ 4. reduced preload and afterload.

95. Which of the following would be an essential nursing action for the client who is receiving dopamine hydrochloride for treatment of shock?
○ 1. Administer pain medication concurrently.

○ 2. Monitor blood pressure continuously.
○ 3. Evaluate arterial blood gases at least every 2 hours.
○ 4. Monitor for signs of infection.

96. When a client is stabilized from a blood loss of 500 mL and is awaiting surgery to control a gastric hemorrhage, the nurse keeps the client in a warm, calm, quiet, and dimly-lit environment with 1 or 2 family members present and gives simple answers to questions about the surgery. What is the primary rationale for these nursing interventions?
○ 1. To stabilize fluid and electrolyte balance.
○ 2. To minimize oxygen consumption.
○ 3. To increase client and family comfort.
○ 4. To prevent infection.

97. When assessing a client for early septic shock, the nurse observes for which of the following?
○ 1. Cool, clammy skin.
○ 2. Warm, flushed skin.
○ 3. Decreased systolic blood pressure.
○ 4. Hemorrhage.

98. A client with toxic shock has been receiving ceftriaxone sodium (Rocephin, 1 g every 12 hours). In addition to culture and sensitivity studies, what other laboratory findings does the nurse monitor?
○ 1. Serum creatinine.
○ 2. Spinal fluid analysis.
○ 3. Arterial blood gases.
○ 4. Serum osmolality.

99. What nursing intervention is *most* important in preventing septic shock?
○ 1. Administering intravenous fluid replacement therapy as ordered.
○ 2. Obtaining vital signs every 4 hours for all clients.
○ 3. Monitoring red blood cell counts for elevation.
○ 4. Maintaining asepsis of indwelling urinary catheters.

100. Which of the following is an indication of a complication of septic shock?
○ 1. Anaphylaxis.
○ 2. Acute respiratory distress syndrome.
○ 3. Chronic obstructive pulmonary disease.
○ 4. Mitral valve prolapse.

Correct Answers and Rationale

The letters in parentheses following the rationale identify the step of the nursing process (A, D, P, I, E) and client needs (1, 2, 3, 4, 5, 6, 7, 8, 9, 10). See the inside front cover for the key.

The Client With Red Blood Cell Disorders

1. 1. One of the microcytic, hypochromic anemias is iron-deficiency anemia. A rich source of iron is needed in the diet, and eggs are high in iron. Other foods high in iron include organ and muscle (dark) meats; shellfish, shrimp, and tuna; enriched, whole-grain, and fortified cereals and breads; legumes, nuts, dried fruits, and beans; oatmeal; and sweet potatoes. Dark green leafy vegetables and citrus fruits are good sources of vitamin C. Cheese is a good source of calcium. (P, 7)

2. 3. Good sources of vitamin B_{12} include meats and dairy products. Whole grains are a good source of thiamine. Green leafy vegetables are good sources of niacin, folate, and carotenoids (precursors of vitamin A). Broccoli and brussels sprouts are good sources of ascorbic acid (vitamin C). (I, 7)

3. 4. The normal range of folic acid is 1.8 to 9 ng/mL, and the normal range of vitamin B_{12} (cyanocobalamin) is 200 to 900 pg/mL. A low folic acid level in the presence of a normal vitamin B_{12} level is indicative of a primary folic acid–deficiency anemia. Factors that affect the absorption of folic acid are drugs such as methotrexate, oral contraceptives, antiseizure drugs, and alcohol. The total bilirubin, serum creatinine, and hemoglobin values are within normal limits. (D, 9)

4. 2. The defining characteristic of pernicious anemia, a megaloblastic anemia, is lack of the intrinsic factor, which results from atrophy of the stomach wall. Without the intrinsic factor, vitamin B_{12} cannot be absorbed in the small intestines, and folic acid needs vitamin B_{12} for DNA synthesis of RBCs. The gastric analysis was done to determine the primary cause of the anemia. An elevated excretion of the injected radioactive vitamin B_{12}, which is protocol for the first and second stage of the Schilling test, indicates that the client has the intrinsic factor and can absorb vitamin B_{12} into the intestinal tract. A sedimentation rate of 16 mm/hour is normal for both men and women and is a nonspecific test to detect the presence of inflammation. It is not specific to anemias. An RBC value of 5.0 million/mm³ is a normal value for both men and women and does not indicate an anemia. (A, 9)

5. 2. Clients with aplastic anemia are severely immunocompromised and at risk for infection and possible death related to bone marrow suppression and pancytopenia. Strict aseptic technique and reverse isolation are important measures to prevent infection. Although diet, reduced stress, and rest are valued in supporting health, the potentially fatal consequence of an acute infection places it as a priority for teaching the client about health maintenance. Animal meat and dark green leafy vegetables, good sources of vitamin B_{12} and folic acid, should be included in the daily diet. Yoga and meditation are good complementary therapies to reduce stress. Eight hours of rest and naps are good for spacing and pacing activity and rest. (E, 2)

6. 4. Vitamin B_{12} combines with intrinsic factor in the stomach and is then carried to the ileum, where it is absorbed into the bloodstream. In this situation, vitamin B_{12} cannot be absorbed regardless of the amount of oral intake of sources of vitamin B_{12} such as animal protein or vitamin B_{12} tablets. Vitamin B_{12} needs to be injected every month, because the ileum has been surgically removed. Replacement of fluids and electrolytes is important when the client has continuous multiple loose stools on a daily basis. Warm salt water is used to soothe sore mucous membranes. Crohn's disease and a small-bowel resection may cause several loose stools a day. (E, 4)

7. 3. Coffee and tea increase gastrointestinal motility and inhibit the absorption of nonheme iron. Clients are instructed to add dried fruits to dishes at every meal because dried fruits are a nonheme or nonanimal iron source. Cooking in iron cookware, especially acid-based foods such as tomatoes, adds iron to the diet. Clients are instructed to add a rich supply of vitamin C to every meal because the absorption of iron is increased when food with vitamin C or ascorbic acid is consumed. (E, 7)

8. 1. It is difficult to determine activity intolerance without objectively comparing activities from one time frame to another. Because iron-deficiency anemia can occur gradually and individual endurance varies, the nurse can best assess the client's activity tolerance by asking the client to compare activities 6 months ago and at present. Asking a client how long a problem has existed is a very open-ended question that allows for too much subjectivity for any definition of the client's activity tolerance. Also, the client may not even identify that a "problem" exists. Asking the client whether he is staying abreast of usual activities addresses whether the tasks were completed, not the tolerance of the client while the tasks were being completed or the

resulting condition of the client after the tasks were completed. Asking the client if he is more tired now than usual does not address his activity tolerance. Tiredness is a subjective evaluation and again can be distorted by factors such as the gradual onset of the anemia or the endurance of the individual. (E, 4)

9. 2. To promote comfort when injecting at the ventrogluteal site, the position of choice is with the client lying on the abdomen with toes pointed inward. This positioning promotes muscle relaxation, which decreases the discomfort of making an injection into a tense muscle. Lying on the side with legs extended will not provide the greatest muscle relaxation. Leaning over the edge of a table with the hips flexed and standing upright with the feet apart will increase muscular tension. (I, 8)

10. 3. Pernicious anemia is caused by the body's inability to absorb vitamin B_{12}. This results from a lack of intrinsic factor in the gastric juices. Schilling's test helps diagnose pernicious anemia by determining the client's ability to absorb vitamin B_{12}. (I, 9)

11. 2. Urinary vitamin B_{12} levels are measured after the ingestion of radioactive vitamin B_{12}. A 24- to 48-hour urine specimen is collected after administration of an oral dose of radioactively tagged vitamin B_{12} and an injection of nonradioactive vitamin B_{12}. In a healthy state of absorption, excess vitamin B_{12} is excreted in the urine; in a malabsorptive state or when the intrinsic factor is missing, vitamin B_{12} is excreted in the feces. Citrucel is a bulk-forming agent. Laxatives interfere with the absorption of vitamin B_{12}. The client is NPO 8 to 12 hours before the test but is not NPO during the test. A stool collection is not a part of the Schilling test. If stool contaminates the urine collection, the results will be altered. (I, 9)

12. 3. This client has clinical manifestations of thalassemia major, a disease found in descendants from the Mediterranean Sea area whose mother and father both possess the gene for thalassemia (ie, the client is homozygous for the gene). The severe hemolytic anemia causes sequestration of RBCs in the spleen and liver, which leads to engorgement of the organs, and chronic bone marrow hyperplasia, which leads to widening of the bones. Mental and physical growth is retarded, and the only treatment is blood transfusion, and chelation therapy if numerous transfusions have been administered. Death may result from cardiac enlargement and failure. (E, 7)

13. 2. Most clients with pernicious anemia have deficient production of intrinsic factor in the stomach. Intrinsic factor attaches to the vitamin in the stomach and forms a complex that allows the vitamin to be absorbed in the small intestine. The stomach is producing enough acid, there is not an excessive excretion of the vitamin, and there is not a rapid production of RBCs in this condition. (I, 4)

14. 2. This client presented with the typical signs of glucose-6-phospate dehydrogenase (G6PD)–deficiency anemia. Ten percent of African Americans inherit an X-linked recessive disorder of the G6PD enzyme in the RBC. When cells with decreased levels of G6PD are exposed to certain drugs, such as sulfonamides, acetylsalicylic acid, thiazide diuretics, and vitamin K, the RBC may hemolyze and anemia and jaundice may occur. The reaction is self-limited as soon as the causative agent is withheld. No further treatment is necessary except counseling to prevent acute incidence by avoiding exposure to specific drugs. There is no need for increased folic acid, restricted activity in hot weather, or blood transfusions. (E, 4)

15. 2. The normal physiologic response to activity is an increased metabolic rate over the resting basal rate. The decrease in respiratory rate indicates that the client is not strong enough to complete the mechanical cycle of respiration needed for gas exchange. The postactivity pulse is expected to increase immediately after activity but by no more than 50 bpm if it is strenuous activity. The diastolic blood pressure is expected to rise but by no more than 15 mm Hg. The pulse returns to within 6 bpm of the resting pulse after 3 minutes of rest. (E, 10)

16. 3. The nurse should continue to monitor the client, because this value reflects a normal physiologic response. The physician does not need to be called, and oxygen does not need to be started based on these laboratory findings. Immediately after surgery, the client's hematocrit reflects a falsely high value related to the body's compensatory response to the stress of sudden loss of fluids and blood. Activation of the intrinsic pathway and the renin-angiotensin cycle via antidiuretic hormone produces vasoconstriction and retention of fluid for the first 1 to 2 days postoperatively. By the second to third day, this response decreases and the client's hematocrit level is more reflective of the amount of RBCs in the plasma. Fresh bleeding is a less likely occurrence on the third postoperative day but is not impossible; however, the nurse would have expected to see a decrease in the RBC and hemoglobin values accompanying the hematocrit. (E, 4)

17. 4. The most likely time for a blood transfusion reaction to occur is during the first 15 minutes or first 50 mL of the infusion. If a blood transfusion reaction does occur, it is imperative to keep an established intravenous line so that medication can be administered to prevent or treat cardiovascular collapse in case of anaphylaxis. PRBCs should be administered through a 19-gauge or larger needle; a peripherally inserted central catheter line is not recommended, in order to avoid a slow flow. RBCs will hemolyze in dextrose or lactated Ringer's solution and should be infused with only normal saline. (I, 8)

18. 2. Low back pain occurs when the RBCs of the recipient's serum antibodies react with the donor RBC antigens. The renal tubules become obstructed with the hemoglobin freed from the hemolysis of RBCs. Hemoglobinuria can lead to acute renal failure. Freed hemoglobin in the urine and blood samples taken at the time of the reaction provide evidence of a hemolytic blood transfusion reaction. Antipyretics are administered with febrile, nonhemolytic transfusion reactions. Diuretics, oxygen, and morphine are administered with circulatory overload. Vasopressors are administered with septic transfusion reactions. (I, 8)

19. 1. Epogen is a recombinant DNA form of erythropoietin, which stimulates the production of RBCs and therefore causes the hematocrit to rise. The elevation in hematocrit causes an elevation in the blood pressure; therefore, the blood pressure is a vital sign that should be checked. The partial thromboplastin time, hemoglobin level, and prothrombin time are not monitored for this drug. (E, 8)

20. 4. Vitamin B$_{12}$ is a water-soluble vitamin. When water-soluble vitamins are taken in excess of the body's needs, they are filtered through the kidneys and excreted. Vitamin B$_{12}$ is considered to be nontoxic. Adverse reactions that have occurred are believed to be related to impurities or to the preservative in B$_{12}$ preparations. Ringing in the ears, skin rash, and nausea are not considered to be related to vitamin B$_{12}$ administration. (I, 5)

21. 2. Brown rice is a source of iron from plant sources (nonheme iron). Other sources of nonheme iron are whole-grain cereals and breads, dark green vegetables, legumes, nuts, dried fruits (apricots, raisins, dates), oatmeal, and sweet potatoes. Egg yolks have iron but it is not as well absorbed as from other sources. Vegetables are a good source of vitamins that may facilitate iron absorption. Tea contains tannin, which combines with nonheme iron, preventing its absorption. (I, 7)

22. 2. Macrocytic anemias can result from deficiencies in vitamin B$_{12}$ or ascorbic acid. Only vitamin B$_{12}$ deficiency causes diminished sensations of peripheral nerve endings. The nurse should assess for peripheral neuropathy and instruct the client in self-care activities for her diminished sensation to heat and pain (eg, using a heating pad at a lower heat setting, making frequent checks to protect against skin trauma). The burn could be related to abuse, but this conclusion would require more supporting data. The findings should be documented, but the nurse would want to address the client's sensations first. The decision of how to treat the burn should be determined by the physician. (D, 4)

23. 3. Pruritus is a late symptom that results from abnormal histamine metabolism. Headache and dizziness are early symptoms from engorged veins. Shortness of breath is an early symptom from congested mucous membrane and ineffective gas exchange. (D, 10)

24. 1. Aplastic anemia decreases the bone marrow production of RBCs, white blood cells, and platelets. The client is at risk for bruising and bleeding tendencies. A change in the client's intake and output is important, but assessment for the potential for bleeding takes priority. Change in the peripheral nervous system is a priority problem specific to clients with vitamin B$_{12}$ deficiency. Change in bowel function is not associated with aplastic anemia. (A, 9)

The Client With Platelet Disorders

25. 1. A client with a platelet count of 30,000 to 50,000/mm^3 is susceptible to bruising with minor trauma. Padding areas that the client might bump, scratch, or hit may help prevent minor trauma. A platelet count of 15,000 to 30,000/mm^3 may result in spontaneous petechiae and bruising, especially on the extremities. Safety measures to pad surfaces would still be used, but the focus would be on assessing for new spontaneous petechiae. Keeping the room dark does not help the client with a low platelet count. When the count is lower than 20,000/mm^3, the client is at risk for spontaneous bleeding from the mucous membranes (oral, nasal, urinary, and rectal) and intracranial bleeding. (I, 9)

26. 4. A recent viral infection in a female client between the ages of 20 and 30 years with a history of systemic lupus erythematosus and an insidious onset of diffuse petechiae are hallmarks of idiopathic thrombocytopenia purpura (ITTP). It is important to ask whether the client's recent menses have been lengthened or are heavier. Determining her ability to clot can help determine her risk for increased bleeding tendency until a platelet count is drawn. Petechiae are not caused by poor nutrition. Because of poor food and fluid intake or weakness and fatigue, the client may have gotten bruises from falling or bumping into things, but not petechiae. (D, 9)

27. 2. When the platelet count is very low, red blood cells leak out of the blood vessels and into the tissue. If the blood pressure is elevated and the platelet count falls to less than 15,000/mm^3, internal bleeding in the brain can occur. A severe headache occurs from meningeal irritation when blood leaks out of the cerebral vasculature. When a client has thrombocytopenia, the nurse should always assess for cerebral bleeding by checking vital signs and performing neurologic checks. (A, 9)

28. 2. Large purplish skin lesions caused by hemorrhage are called ecchymoses. Small, flat, red pinpoint lesions are petechiae. Numerous petechiae result in a reddish,

bruised appearance called purpura. An abrasion is a wound caused by scraping. (E, 9)

29. 1. Previously the cause was unknown, but recent research suggests that ITTP occurs when antibody-coated platelets are identified as foreign bodies and destroyed by macrophages in the spleen. It is not an idiosyncratic response and is not related to a depressed immune system. (I, 5)

30. 2. When the platelet count is less than 150,000/mL, prolonged bleeding can occur from trauma, injury, or straining such as with the Valsalva maneuver. Clients should avoid any activity that causes straining to evacuate the bowel. Clients can ambulate, but pointed or sharp surfaces should be padded. Clients can visit with their families but should avoid any scratches, bumps, or scraps. Clients can sit in a semi-Fowler's position but should change positions to promote circulation and check for petechiae. (I, 9)

31. 3. Bufferin contains aspirin, which is an antiplatelet agent that prevents platelet aggregation. After a 300-mg dose of aspirin, the bleeding time can be prolonged as long as 5 days. One of the best methods to check for platelet deficiency is the bleeding time test. A number of other drugs, such as alcohol, sulfonamides, and thiazide diuretics, can prolong the bleeding time. The PT evaluates the extrinsic pathway (coagulation factor VIII) and represents the time it takes to form a firm clot. The PT value is normal in severe thrombocytopenia. The aPTT evaluates the intrinsic and common coagulation pathway and represents the time it takes to form a firm clot. It is basically the same as the PTT but is considered to be more reliably reproducible and faster. The aPTT value is normal in severe thrombocytopenia. The CT or Lee-White coagulation time is normal, but it is an old and insensitive test that does not rule out a coagulation defect. (I, 8)

32. 2. The client who states that the test results are normal has only heard that the bone marrow is functioning. The etiology is in the destruction of circulating platelets. Further tests must be completed to determine the cause (eg, a coating of the platelets with antibodies that are seen as foreign bodies). The bone marrow result does rule out other potential diagnoses such as anemia, leukemia, or myeloproliferative disorders that involve bone marrow depression. The client needs to stop flossing and throw away his hard toothbrush, which can lead to bleeding of the gums. The destruction of the circulating platelets accounts for the easy bruising and the need to protect oneself from further bruising. The client should not jump or increase exertion of joints, which may lead to bleeding in the joints and joint pain. (D, 9)

33. 1. The nurse observes tachycardia in the hemorrhaging client because the heart beats faster to compensate for decreased circulating volume and decreased numbers of oxygen-carrying red blood cells. The degree of cardiopulmonary distress and anemia will be related to the amount of hemorrhage that occurred and the period of time over which it occurred. Bradycardia is a late symptom of hemorrhage; it occurs after the client is no longer able to compromise and is debilitating further into shock. If it is left untreated, the client will die from cardiovascular collapse. Decreased $PaCO_2$ is a late symptom of hemorrhage, after transport of oxygen to the tissue has been affected. A narrow pulse pressure is not an early sign of hemorrhage. (A, 10)

34. 4. Immune thrombocytopenia purpura is treated with steroids to suppress the splenic macrophages from phagocytizing the antibody-coated platelets, which are recognized as foreign bodies, so that the platelets live longer. The steroids also suppress the binding of the autoimmune antibody to the platelet surface. Steroids do not destroy the antibodies on the platelets, neutralize antigens, or increase phagocytosis. (A, 8)

35. 3. The client needs to wear information containing the name of the drug, dosage, physician and contact information, and emergency instructions, because additional corticosteroid drug therapy would be needed during emergency situations. Prednisone should be taken in the morning because it can cause insomnia and because exogenous corticosteroid suppression of the adrenal cortex is less when it is administered in the morning. Prednisone must never be stopped suddenly. It must be tapered off to allow for the adrenal cortex to recover from drug-induced atrophy so that it can resume its function. Prednisone suppresses the immune response and masks infections. It does not provide extra protection against infection. (E, 8)

36. 1. Nausea, vomiting, and peptic ulcers are gastrointestinal adverse effects of prednisone, so it is recommended that clients take the prednisone with food. In some instances, the client may be advised to take a prescribed antacid prophylactically. The client should never take over-the-counter drugs without notifying the physician who prescribed the prednisone. The client should ask the physician about the amount and kind of exercise because of the need to establish baseline physical values before starting an exercise program and because of the increased potential for comorbidity with increasing age. The client should eat foods that are high in potassium to prevent hypokalemia. (I, 8)

37. 4. The best exercise for perimenopausal and postmenopausal women who are on long-term corticosteroid therapy is a low-impact weight-bearing exercise such as walking or weight lifting. Floor exercises do not provide for the weight bearing. Stretching is appropriate but does not offer sufficient weight bearing. Running provides for weight bearing but is hard on the joints and may cause bleeding. (P, 7)

38. 2. The client needs further teaching if she thinks that the number of tissues saturated represents all of the blood lost during a nosebleed. During a nosebleed, a significant amount of blood can be swallowed and go undetected. It is important that clients with severe thrombocytopenia do not take a nosebleed lightly. Clients with thrombocytopenia can apply pressure for 5 to 10 minutes over a small, superficial cut. Clients with thrombocytopenia can take hormones to suppress menses and control menstrual blood loss. Clients can also count the number of saturated sanitary napkins to approximate blood loss during menses. Some authorities estimate that a completely soaked sanitary napkin holds 50 mL. (E, 3)

39. 1. Adverse effects of prednisone are weight gain, retention of sodium and fluids with hypertension and cushingoid features, a low serum albumin, suppressed inflammatory processes with masked symptoms, and osteoporosis. A diet high in protein, potassium, calcium, vitamin D, and vitamin C is recommended. (A, 8)

40. 1. Platelets cannot survive cold temperatures. The platelets should be stored at room temperature and last for no more than 5 days. (E, 8)

41. 3. The bag containing platelets needs to be gently rotated to prevent clumping. ABO compatibility is not a necessary requirement, but human leukocyte antigen (HLA) matching of lymphocytes may be completed to avoid development of anti-HLA antibodies when multiple platelet transfusions are necessary. Platelets should be administered as fast as can be tolerated by the client to avoid aggregation. Most institutions use tubing especially for platelets instead of tubing for blood and blood products. (I, 8)

42. 4. The correct technique for deep breathing postoperatively to avoid atelectasis and pneumonia is to take in a deep breath through the nose and hold it for 5 seconds, then blow it out through pursed lips. The goal is to fully expand and empty the lungs for pulmonary hygiene. (I, 9)

43. 3. An elective surgical procedure is scheduled in advance so that all preparations can be completed ahead of time. The vital signs are the final check that must be completed before the client leaves the room so that continuity of care and assessment is provided for. The first assessment that will be completed in the preoperative holding area or operating room will be the client's vital signs. The client should have emptied the bladder before receiving preoperative medications so that the bladder is empty when it is time for transport into the operating room. The client should have signed the consent before the transport time so that if there were any questions or concerns there was time to meet with the surgeon. Also, the consent form must be signed before any sedative medications are given. The client's name band should be placed as soon as the client arrives in the perioperative setting, and it remains in place through discharge. (A, 9)

44. 3. The client with chronic immune thrombocytopenia purpura after a splenectomy is at high risk for hypovolemia and hemorrhage. The dressing should be checked often; if drainage is present, a circle should be drawn around the drainage and the time noted to help determine how fast bleeding is occurring. The nasogastric tube should be connected, but this can wait until the dressing has been checked. A urinary catheter is not needed. The last pain medication administration and the patient's current pain level should be communicated in the exchange report. Checking for hemorrhage is a greater priority that assessing pain level. (D, 9)

45. 3. A splenectomy may involve manipulation of the upper abdominal organs such as diaphragm, stomach, liver, spleen, and small intestines. Manipulation of these organs and resulting inflammation lead to a slowed peristalsis. A nasogastric tube is placed to decrease abdominal distention in the immediate postoperative phase. The stomach does not need to be manipulated away from the spleen postoperatively, nor would a nasogastric tube accomplish this. The nasogastric tube drains gastric contents and air in the stomach; it is not in the operative site, and therefore cannot be used to irrigate it. The gastric juices are not checked as an indicator that peristalsis has returned; instead, the bowel sounds are auscultated in all four quadrants to indicate the return of peristalsis. (D, 7)

46. 4. Clients who have had a splenectomy are especially prone to infection. The reduction of immunoglobulin M leaves the client especially at risk for immunologic deficiency infections. All clients who have had major abdominal surgery usually receive discharge instructions not to drive because the stomach muscles are not strong enough to brake hard or quickly after the abdominal muscles have been separated. All clients need to pace activity and rest when going home after major surgery. Rest and sleep allow the growth hormone to repair the tissue, and activity allows the energy and strength to build endurance and muscle strength. An appointment is usually made to see the surgeon in the office 1 week after discharge for follow-up and to remove sutures or staples if this has not already been done. (I, 7)

47. 2. There is no well-defined sequence for acute DIC other than that the client starts bleeding without a previous history or cause and does not stop bleeding. Later signs may include severe shortness of breath, hypotension, pallor, petechiae, hematoma, orthopnea, hematuria, vision changes, and joint pain. (A, 10)

48. 3. DIC has not been found to respond to oral anticoagulants such as Coumadin. Treatments for DIC are controversial but include treating the underlying cause, administering heparin, and replacing depleted blood products. (I, 10)

49. 2. Clinical manifestations of microvascular thrombosis are those that represent a blockage of blood flow and oxygenation to the tissue which results in eventual death of the organ. Examples of microvascular thrombosis include acute respiratory distress syndrome (ARDS), focal ischemia, superficial gangrene, oliguria, azotemia, cortical necrosis, acute ulceration, delirium, and coma. Hemoptysis, petechiae, and hematuria are signs of hemorrhage. (A, 10)

50. 3. As blood collects in the peritoneal cavity it causes dilatation and distention, which is reflected in increased abdominal girth. The patient would be tachycardic and hypotensive. Petechiae reflect bleeding in the skin. (A, 10)

The Client With White Blood Cell Disorders

51. 4. The client will need an order to be placed in reverse (protective) isolation because his normal defenses are ineffective and place him at risk for infection (leukopenia, less than 5000/μL). The faster the decrease in WBCs, the greater the bone marrow suppression, and the more susceptible the client is to infection from not only pathogenic but nonpathogenic organisms. The client will continue to be monitored, the laboratory may be called, and the report will be placed on the chart, but protection of the client must be instituted immediately. (D, 10)

52. 3. A shift to the left means that more immature than mature WBCs are at the site of inflammation or infection. Immature WBCs are less effective at phagocytosis and do not produce classic signs of inflammation such as pus, redness, swelling, or heat. Fever is the only sign, and therefore it is a significant sign of infection in a client with immature or depressed WBCs. (I, 9)

53. 2. The ANC is calculated by multiplying the total WBC count by the sum of percentage of neutrophils and the percentage of bands and dividing by 100. In this case, $1200 \times (1 + 34) / 100 = 420$. (D, 2)

54. 2. A client is at moderate risk when the ANC is less than 1000. The ANC decreases proportionately to the increased risk of infection. The client is at normal risk of infection if the ANC is 1500 or greater. The client is at high risk of infection if the ANC is less than 500. An ANC of 100 or less is life-threatening. (A, 9)

55. 1. The one factor that may be more important than the degree of neutropenia in determining the risk for infection is the duration of the neutropenia. (A, 2)

56. 1. Bedside rails, call bells, drug-administration controls operated by the patient, and other surface areas are frequently touched by caregivers with used gloves. Changing gloves immediately after use protects the client from contamination by organisms. Cross-contamination is a break in technique of serious consequence to the severely compromised client. Standing 2 feet from the patient, speaking minimally, and wearing long-sleeved shirts are not required in standard interventions for risk of infection. (I, 2)

57. 1. The neutropenic client is at risk for infection, especially bacterial infection of the respiratory and gastrointestinal tracts. Breaks in the mucous membranes, such as those that could be caused by the insertion of a suppository or enema tube, would be a break in the first line of the body's defense and a direct port of entry for infection. The client with neutropenia is encouraged to wear a HEPA filter mask and to use an incentive spirometer for pulmonary hygiene. The client needs to know the importance of completing meticulous total body hygiene daily, including perianal care after every bowel movement, to decrease the flora at normal body orifices. The client also needs to know the importance of performing oral care after every meal and every 4 hours while the client is awake to decrease the bacterial buildup in the oropharynx. (I, 2)

58. 2. The Centers for Disease Control advises that washing hands before, during, and after care has a significant effect in reducing infections. It is advisable to avoid introducing a cold or children's germs and to avoid kissing on the lips, but the primary prevention technique is handwashing. (I, 2)

59. 4. The most common source of infection and microbial colonization in neutropenic clients is their own nonpathogenic normal flora. Attention to personal hygiene such as oral, pulmonary, urinary, and rectal care is essential. It is important to acknowledge the client's concerns and fears and to provide organized, nonhurried, caring care, but it is more important to teach the client how to prevent an infection that could be life-threatening. (I, 2)

60. 3. The nurse's role does not include explaining the risks of the procedure and giving the informed consent. This is the role of the person who is to perform the procedure, such as the doctor. One of the nurse's roles is to witness the client's signing of the consent form. The nurse also ascertains whether the client has an understanding that is consistent with the procedure listed on the form and determines that the client is signing the consent of his or her own free will. (I, 1)

61. 3. As the bone marrow is being aspirated, the client will feel a suction or pulling type of sensation or discomfort that lasts a few seconds. A systemic premedication may be given to decrease this discomfort. A small area over the sternum is cleaned with an antiseptic. It is unnecessary to paint the entire anterior chest. The local anesthetic is injected through the subcutaneous tissue to numb the tissue for the larger-bore needle that is used for aspiration and biopsy. After the needle is removed, pressure is held over the aspiration site for 5 to 10 minutes to achieve hemostasis. A small dressing is applied; a large pressure dressing, such as an Ace bandage, would restrict the expansion of the lungs and is not used. (I, 5)

62. 4. After a bone marrow aspiration, the puncture site should be checked every 10 to 15 minutes for bleeding. For a short period after the procedure, bed rest may be ordered. Signs of infection such as redness and swelling are not anticipated at the aspiration site. A mild analgesic may be ordered. If the client continues to need the morphine for longer than 24 hours, the nurse should suspect that internal bleeding or increased pressure at the puncture site may be the cause of the pain and should consult with the physician. (E, 10)

63. 2. The nurse is an advocate for the client with leukemia who can be empowered with knowledge of the treatment. Immunologic, cytogenic, morphologic, histochemical, and other means are used to identify cell subtypes and stages of leukemia cell development for very specific and optimal treatment. The nurse should not label the client's feeling such as frustration or emotional; only the client can identify her own feelings. Chastising the client is not helpful. It disavows the client's emotional state and responses to her diagnosis and involved treatment. Unless nurses have had leukemia, they cannot possibly know how the client feels even though they may be trying to offer her empathy. (I, 5)

64. 3. The induction phase of chemotherapy is an aggressive treatment to kill leukemia cells. The client is severely immunocompromised and severely at risk for infection. Flowers, herbs, and plants should be avoided during this time. The client's Bible, pictures, and other personal belongings can be cleaned before being brought into the room to prevent contact with pathogenic and nonpathogenic organisms. (I, 2)

65. 2. The nurse identifies that the client does not understand that contact with animals must be avoided because they carry infection and the induction therapy will destroy the client's WBCs. The induction therapy will cause anemia, and the client will experience fatigue and will have to pace activities with rest periods. Platelet production will be decreased, and the client will be at risk for bleeding tendencies; oral hygiene will have to be provided by using a warm saline gargle instead of brushing the teeth and gums. The client will be at risk for infection owing to the decrease in WBC production and should report a temperature of 100°F (37.8°C) or higher. (D, 10)

66. 4. The statement, "Your doctor stated your prognosis based on the differentiation of your cells" addresses the client's situation on an individual basis. The nurse is clarifying that clients have different prognoses—even though they may the same type of leukemia—because of the cell differentiation. Stating that the client misunderstood is inappropriate for an advocate of the client and serves no useful purpose. The statements are true but do not address this client's individual concern. (A, 5)

67. 4. Bleeding and infection are the major complications and causes of death for clients with AML. Bleeding is related to the degree of thrombocytopenia, and infection is related to the degree of neutropenia. Cardiac arrhythmias rarely occur as a result of AML. Liver or renal failure may occur, but these are not major causes of death in AML. (I, 9)

68. 4. Although the clinical manifestations of CML vary, clients usually have confusion and shortness of breath related to decreased capillary perfusion to the brain and lungs. Lymphadenopathy is rare in CML. Hyperplasia of the gum and bone pain are clinical manifestations of AML. (A, 10)

69. 1. The peak incidence of ALL is at 4 years of age. ALL is uncommon after 15 years of age. The median age at incidence of CML is 40 to 50 years. The peak incidence of AML occurs at 60 years of age. Two thirds of cases of chronic lymphocytic leukemia (CLL) occur in clients older than 60 years of age. (P, 3)

70. 1. ALL does not cause gastric distention. ALL does invade the central nervous system, and clients experience headaches and vomiting from meningeal irritation. Clients with ALL receive chemotherapy, which may also cause nausea and vomiting. (D, 10)

71. 4. Clients with CLL develop unintentional weight loss; fever and drenching night sweats; enlarged, painful lymph nodes, spleen, and liver; decreased reaction to skin sensitivity tests (anergy); and susceptibility to viral infections. Enlarged painless lymph nodes are a clinical manifestation of Hodgkin's lymphoma. A headache would not be one of the early signs and symptoms expected in CLL because CLL does not cross the blood-brain barrier and would not irritate the meninges. Hyperplasia of the gums is a clinical manifestation of AML. (A, 10)

72. 3. Simple rinses with saline or baking soda solution are effective and moisten the oral mucosa. Commercial mouthwashes and lemon-glycerin swabs contain glycerin and alcohol, which are drying to the mucosa and should be avoided. Brushing after each meal is recommended, but every 4 hours may be too traumatic. During acute leukemia, the neutrophil and platelet counts are often low and a soft-bristle toothbrush, instead of the client's usual brush, should be used to prevent bleeding gums. (I, 7)

73. 3. The client with acute leukemia experiences fatigue and deconditioning. Lying in bed and taking deep breaths will not help achieve the goals. The client must get out of bed to increase activity tolerance and improve tidal volume. Ambulating in the hall (using a HEPA filter mask if neutropenic) is a sensible activity and helps improve conditioning. Sitting up in a chair facilitates lung expansion. Using a stationary bicycle in the room allows the client to increase activity as tolerated. (P, 7)

74. 2. Combination chemotherapy does not mean two groups of drugs, one to kill the cancer cells and one to treat the side effects of the chemotherapy. Combination chemotherapy means that multiple drugs are given to interrupt the cell growth cycle at different points, to decrease resistance to a chemotherapy agent, and to minimize the toxicity associated with use of a high dose of a single agent (ie, by using multiple agents with different toxicities). (E, 8)

75. 1. The biliary system is not especially prone to hemorrhage. Thrombocytopenia (a low platelet count) leaves the client at risk for a potentially life-threatening spontaneous hemorrhage in the gastrointestinal, respiratory, and intracranial cavities. (A, 10)

76. 1. The primary purpose of reverse isolation is to reduce transmission of organisms to the client from sources outside the client's environment. (I, 2)

The Client With Lymphoma

77. 2. Painless and enlarged cervical lymph nodes, tachycardia, weight loss, weakness and fatigue, and night sweats are signs of Hodgkin's disease. Difficulty swallowing and breathing may occur, but only with mediastinal node involvement. Hepatomegaly is a late-stage manifestation. (A, 10)

78. 1. If the nurse is not familiar with helping with a biopsy, the nurse may need to call the laboratory for instructions in handling the specimen. In most cases, a lymph node biopsy is sent immediately to the laboratory once it is placed in a specific solution in a closed container. It is incorrect to send a biopsy in a sponge covered by a glove in an open public hallway, or to wait until someone is available to take it. The nurse is an expert in sterile technique and should assist with the

procedure because the client may be at increased risk for infection. (I, 9)

79. 3. Assessing for an open airway is always first. The procedure involves the neck; the anesthesia may have affected the swallowing reflex, or the inflammation may have closed in on the airway leading to ineffective air exchange. Once a patent airway is confirmed and an effective breathing pattern established, the circulation is checked. Vital signs and the incision are assessed as soon as possible, but only after it is established that the airway is patent and the client is breathing normally. A neurologic assessment is completed as soon as possible after other important assessments. (A, 9)

80. 3. A definitive diagnosis of Hodgkin's disease is made if Reed-Sternberg cells are found in the histologic examination of the excisional lymph node biopsy. Tay-Sachs disease is an inherited disease carried by an autosomal recessive gene. Sarcoidosis is an inflammatory granulomatous disease. Duchenne's disease is a type of muscular disorder. (I, 9)

81. 1. Herpes zoster infections are common in patients with Hodgkin's disease. Discoloring of the teeth is not related to Hodgkin's disease but rather to the ingestion of iron supplements or some antibiotics such as tetracycline. Mild anemia is common in Hodgkin's, but the platelet count is not affected until the tumor has invaded the bone marrow. A cellular immunity defect occurs in Hodgkin's disease in which there is little or no reaction to skin sensitivity tests. This is called anergy. (A, 9)

82. 3. A temperature higher than 100.4°F (38°C), profuse night sweats, and an unintentional weight loss of 10% of body weight represent the cluster of clinical manifestations known as the B symptoms. Forty percent of clients with Hodgkin's disease have B symptoms, and B symptoms are more common in advanced stages of the disease. (A, 10)

83. 4. Invasive procedures such as exploratory laparotomy and lymphangiography are being used less often because noninvasive technologies such as radiography, body scans, and blood tests provide reliable indications of lymph node and surrounding tissue or organ involvement. (P, 9)

84. 1. In the staging process, the designations A and B signify, respectively, that symptoms were or were not present when Hodgkin's disease was found. The Roman numerals I through IV indicate the extent and location of involvement of the disease. Stage I indicates involvement of a single lymph node; stage II, two or more lymph nodes on the same side of the diaphragm; stage III, lymph node regions on both sides of the diaphragm; and stage IV, diffuse disease of one or more extralymphatic organs. (D, 9)

85. 3. Encouraging the client to take slow, deep breaths during uncomfortable parts of procedures is the best method of decreasing the stress response of tightening and tensing the muscles. Slow, deep breathing affects the level of carbon dioxide in the brain to increase the client's sense of well-being. Allowing the client's family to stay with her may be appropriate if the family has a calming effect on the client. Silence can be therapeutic, but when the client is faced with a potentially life-threatening diagnosis and a new, invasive procedure, she really needs words in addition to touch unless another health care provider is talking to her. Expressing feelings is important, but the client will have to hold still for the procedure. (A, 5)

86. 2. A biopsy needle is inserted through a separate incision in the anesthetized area. The client will feel a pressure sensation when the biopsy is taken but should not feel actual pain. The client should be instructed to inform the physician if pain is felt so that more anesthetic agent can be administered to keep the client comfortable. The biopsy is performed after the aspiration and from a slightly different site so that the tissue is not disturbed by either test. The client will feel a suction-type pain for a moment when the aspiration is being performed, not the biopsy. A small incision is made for the biopsy to accommodate the larger-bore needle. This may require a stitch. (I, 9)

87. 3. Terminally ill clients most often describe feelings of isolation because they tend to be ignored; they are often left out of conversations (especially those dealing with the future); and they sense the attitudes of discomfort that many people feel in their presence. Helpful nursing measures include taking the time to be with the client; offering opportunities to talk about feelings; and answering questions honestly. (P, 5)

88. 2. It is incorrect that the survivor rate is directly proportional to the incidence of second malignancy. The survivor rate is indirectly proportional to the incidence of second malignancy, and regular screening is very important to detect a second malignancy, especially AML or myelodyplasic syndrome (MDS). Survivors should know the stage of the disease and their current treatment plan so that they can remain active participants in their health care. (E, 1)

The Client Who Is in Shock

89. 3. Nursing interventions and collaborative management are focused on correcting and maintaining adequate tissue perfusion. Inadequate tissue perfusion may be caused by hemorrhage, as in hypovolemic shock; by decreased cardiac output, as in cardiogenic shock; or by massive vasodilatation of the vascular bed, as in neurogenic, anaphylactic, and septic shock. Fluid deficit, not fluid overload, occurs in shock. (P, 10)

90. 4. Typical signs and symptoms of hypovolemic shock include systolic blood pressure less than 90 mm Hg, narrowing pulse pressure, tachycardia, tachypnea, cool and clammy skin, decreased urine output, and mental status changes such as irritability or anxiety. Unequal dilation of the pupils is related to central nervous system injury or possible to a previous history of eye injury. (D, 10)

91. 1. Urine output provides the most sensitive indication of the client's response to therapy for hypovolemic shock. Urine output should be consistently greater than 30 to 35 mL/hour. Blood pressure is a more accurate reflection of the adequacy of vasoconstriction than of tissue perfusion. Respiratory rate is not a sensitive indicator of fluid balance in the client recovering from hypovolemic shock. (E, 8)

92. 1. Causes of hypovolemic shock include external fluid loss, such as hemorrhage; internal fluid shifting, such as ascites and severe edema; and dehydration. Massive vasodilatation is the initial phase of vasogenic or distributive shock, which can be further subdivided into three types of shock: septic, neurogenic, and anaphylactic shock. A severe antigen–antibody reaction occurs in anaphylactic shock. Gram-negative bacterial infection is the most common cause of septic shock. Loss of sympathetic tone (vasodilation) occurs in neurogenic shock. (A, 10)

93. 2. The client who is receiving a blood product requires astute assessment for signs and symptoms of allergic reaction and anaphylaxis, including pruritus (itching), urticaria (hives), facial or glottal edema, and shortness of breath. If such a reaction occurs, the nurse should stop the transfusion immediately, but leave the intravenous line intact, and notify the physician. Usually, an antihistamine, such as diphenhydramine hydrochloride (Benadryl), is administered. Epinephrine and corticosteroids may be administered in severe reactions. Fluid balance is not an immediate concern during the blood administration. The administration should not cause pain unless it is extravasating out of the vein, in which case the intravenous administration should be stopped. Administration of a unit of blood should not affect the level of consciousness. (E, 8)

94. 2. At medium doses (4 to 8 µg/kg per minute), dopamine hydrochloride slightly increases the heart rate and improves contractility to increase cardiac output and improve tissue perfusion. When given at a low doses (0.5 to 3.0 µg/kg per minute), dopamine increases renal and mesenteric blood flow. At high doses (8 to 10 µg/kg per minute), dopamine produces vasoconstriction, which is an undesirable effect.

Dopamine is not given to affect the preload and afterload. (E, 8)

95. 2. The client who is receiving dopamine hydrochloride requires continuous blood pressure monitoring with an invasive or noninvasive device. The nurse may titrate the intravenous infusion to maintain a systolic blood pressure of 90 mm Hg. Administration of a pain medication concurrently with dopamine hydrochloride, which is a potent sympathomimetic with dose-related α-adrenergic agonist, β₁-selective adrenergic agonist, and dopaminergic blocking effects, is not an essential nursing action for a client who is in shock with already low hemodynamic values. Arterial blood gas concentrations should be monitored according the patient's respiratory status and acid–base balance status and are not directly related to the dopamine hydrochloride dosage. Monitoring for signs of infection is not related to the nursing action for the client receiving dopamine hydrochloride. (I, 8)

96. 2. Nursing interventions to provide warmth and rest and minimize anxiety decrease the body's need for oxygen and nutrients. This is important for a client who has lost 500 mL or a unit of blood in a short period from a gastric hemorrhage. If the client has been stabilized, the fluid and electrolyte balance has already been established for the present. The comfort of the client and family is always important and is actually accomplished while the client's oxygen consumption is being minimized, which is a priority and the primary rationale. These nursing interventions are not specific to the prevention of infection. (P, 7)

97. 2. Warm, flushed skin from a high cardiac output with vasodilatation occurs in warm shock or the hyperdynamic phase (first phase) of septic shock. Other signs and symptoms of early septic shock include fever with restlessness and confusion; decreased blood pressure with tachypnea and tachycardia; increased or normal urinary output; and nausea and vomiting or diarrhea. Cool, clammy skin occurs in the hypodynamic or cold phase (later phase). Hemorrhage is not a factor in septic shock. (A, 10)

98. 1. The nurse monitors for the blood levels of antibiotics, white blood cells, serum creatinine, and blood urea nitrogen because of the decreased perfusion to the kidneys, which are responsible for filtering out the Rocephin. It is possible that the clearance of the antibiotic has been decreased enough to cause toxicity. Increased levels of these laboratory values should be reported to the physician immediately. A spinal fluid analysis is done to examine cerebral spinal fluid, but there is no indication of central nervous system involvement in this case. Arterial blood gases are used to determine actual blood gas levels and assess acid–base balance. Serum osmolality is used to monitor fluid and electrolyte balance. (A, 8)

99. 4. Maintaining asepsis of indwelling urinary catheters is essential to prevent infection. Preventing septic shock is a major focus of nursing care, because the mortality rate for septic shock is as high as 90% in some populations. Very young and elderly clients (those younger than 2 years or older than 65 years of age) are at increased risk for septic shock. Administering intravenous fluid replacement therapy, obtaining vital signs every 4 hours on all clients, and monitoring red blood cell counts for elevation do not pertain to septic shock prevention. (I, 2)

100. 2. Acute respiratory distress syndrome (ARDS) is a complication associated with septic shock. ARDS causes respiratory failure and may lead to death, even after the client has recovered from shock. Anaphylaxis is a type of distributive or vasogenic shock. Chronic obstructive pulmonary disease is a functional category of pulmonary disease that consists of persistent obstruction of bronchial airflow and involves chronic bronchitis and chronic emphysema. Mitral valve prolapse is a condition in which the mitral valve is pushed back too far during ventricular contraction. (A, 10)

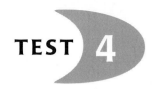
The Client With Respiratory Health Problems

Select the one best answer, and indicate your choice by filling in the circle in front of the option.

The Client With an Upper Respiratory Tract Infection

1. A client with allergic rhinitis is instructed on the correct technique for using an intranasal inhaler. Which of the following statements would demonstrate to the nurse that the client understands the instructions?
   ○ 1. "I should limit the use of the inhaler to early morning and bedtime use."
   ○ 2. "It is important to not shake the canister, because that can damage the spray device."
   ○ 3. "I should hold one nostril closed while I insert the spray into the other nostril."
   ○ 4. "The inhaler tip is inserted into the nostril and pointed toward the inside nostril wall."

2. Which of the following would be an expected outcome for a client recovering from an upper respiratory tract infection?
   ○ 1. The client maintains a fluid intake of 800 mL every 24 hours.
   ○ 2. The client experiences chills only once a day.
   ○ 3. The client coughs productively without chest discomfort.
   ○ 4. The client experiences less nasal obstruction and discharge.

3. The nurse teaches the client how to instill nasal drops. Which of the following techniques is correct?

   ○ 1. The client uses sterile technique when handling the dropper.
   ○ 2. The client blows the nose gently before instilling drops.
   ○ 3. The client uses a new dropper for each installation.
   ○ 4. The client sits in a semi-Fowler's position with the head tilted forward after administration of the drops.

4. A client with acute sinusitis is examined in an ambulatory clinic. The nurse can anticipate the use of which of the following medications in the client's treatment plan?
   ○ 1. Antibiotics.
   ○ 2. Antihistamines.
   ○ 3. Bronchodilators.
   ○ 4. Oral corticosteroids.

5. The nurse should include which of the following instructions in the teaching plan for a client with chronic sinusitis?
   ○ 1. Avoid the use of caffeinated beverages.
   ○ 2. Perform postural drainage every day.
   ○ 3. Take hot showers twice daily.
   ○ 4. Report a temperature of 102°F (38.9°C) or higher.

6. Which of the following individuals would the nurse consider to have the highest priority for receiving an influenza vaccination?

○ 1. A 60-year-old man with a hiatal hernia.

○ 2. A 36-year-old woman with three children.

○ 3. A 50-year-old woman caring for a spouse with cancer.

○ 4. A 60-year-old woman with osteoarthritis.

7. A client with allergic rhinitis asks the nurse what he should do to decrease his symptoms. Which of the following instructions would be appropriate for the nurse to give the client?

○ 1. "Use your nasal decongestant spray regularly to help clear your nasal passages."

○ 2. "Ask the doctor for antibiotics. Antibiotics will help decrease the secretion."

○ 3. "It is important to increase your activity. A daily brisk walk will help promote drainage."

○ 4. "Keep a diary of when your symptoms occur. This can help you identify what precipitates your attacks."

8. An elderly client has been ill with the flu, experiencing headache, fever, and chills. After 3 days, she develops a cough productive of yellow sputum. The nurse auscultates her lungs and hears diffuse crackles. How would the nurse best interpret these assessment findings?

○ 1. It is likely that the client is developing a secondary bacterial pneumonia.

○ 2. The assessment findings are consistent with influenza and are to be expected.

○ 3. The client is getting dehydrated and needs to increase her fluid intake to decrease secretions.

○ 4. The client has not been taking her decongestants and bronchodilators as prescribed.

9. Guaifenesin 300 mg four times a day has been ordered as an expectorant. The dosage strength of the liquid is 200 mg/5 mL. How many milliliters should the nurse administer for each dose?

○ 1. 5.0 mL.

○ 2. 7.5 mL.

○ 3. 9.5 mL.

○ 4. 10.0 mL.

10. Pseudoephedrine (Sudafed) has been ordered as a nasal decongestant. Which of the following is a possible side effect of this drug?

○ 1. Constipation.

○ 2. Bradycardia.

○ 3. Diplopia.

○ 4. Restlessness.

The Client Undergoing Nasal Surgery

11. A 27-year-old woman has had elective nasal surgery for a deviated septum. Which of the following would be an important initial clue that bleeding was occurring even if the nasal drip pad remained dry and intact?

○ 1. Complaints of nausea.

○ 2. Repeated swallowing.

○ 3. Increased respiratory rate.

○ 4. Increased pain.

12. A client who has undergone outpatient nasal surgery is ready for discharge and has nasal packing in place. Which of the following discharge instructions would be appropriate for the client?

○ 1. Avoid activities that elicit the Valsalva maneuver.

○ 2. Take aspirin to control nasal discomfort.

○ 3. Avoid brushing the teeth until the nasal packing is removed.

○ 4. Apply heat to the nasal area to control swelling.

13. Which of the following statements would indicate to the nurse that a client has understood the discharge instructions provided after her nasal surgery?

○ 1. "I should not shower until my packing is removed."

○ 2. "I will take stool softeners and modify my diet to prevent constipation."

○ 3. "Coughing every 2 hours is important to prevent respiratory complications."

○ 4. "It is important to blow my nose each day to remove the dried secretions."

14. The nurse is planning to give preoperative instructions to a client who will be undergoing rhinoplasty. Which of the following instructions should be included?

○ 1. After surgery, nasal packing will be in place for 7 to 10 days.

○ 2. Normal saline nose drops will need to be administered preoperatively.

○ 3. The results of the surgery will be immediately obvious postoperatively.

○ 4. Aspirin-containing medications should not be taken for 2 weeks before surgery.

15. Which of the following assessments would be a priority immediately after nasal surgery?

○ 1. Assessing the client's pain.

○ 2. Inspecting for periorbital ecchymosis.

○ 3. Assessing respiratory status.

○ 4. Measuring intake and output.

16. After nasal surgery, the client expresses concern about how to decrease facial pain and swelling while recovering at home. Which of the following discharge instructions would be most effective for decreasing pain and edema?

○ 1. Take analgesics every 4 hours around the clock.

○ 2. Use corticosteroid nasal spray as needed to control symptoms.

○ 3. Use a bedside humidifier while sleeping.

○ 4. Apply cold compresses to the area.

17. A client is being discharged with nasal packing in

place. He should be told to implement which of the following activities into his home care?
- ○ 1. Perform frequent mouth care.
- ○ 2. Use normal saline nose drops daily.
- ○ 3. Sneeze and cough with mouth closed.
- ○ 4. Gargle every 4 hours with salt water.

18. Which of the following activities should the nurse teach the client to implement after the removal of nasal packing on the second postoperative day?
- ○ 1. Avoid cleaning the nares until swelling has subsided.
- ○ 2. Apply water-soluble jelly to lubricate the nares.
- ○ 3. Keep a nasal drip pad in place to absorb secretions.
- ○ 4. Use a bulb syringe to gently irrigate nares.

19. The nurse is teaching a client how to manage a nosebleed. Which of the following instructions would be appropriate to give the client?
- ○ 1. "Tilt your head backward and pinch your nose."
- ○ 2. "Lie down flat and place an ice compress over the bridge of the nose."
- ○ 3. "Blow your nose gently with your neck flexed."
- ○ 4. "Sit down, lean forward, and pinch the soft portion of your nose."

20. An elderly client had posterior packing inserted to control a severe nosebleed. After insertion of the packing, the client should be closely monitored for which of the following complications?
- ○ 1. Vertigo.
- ○ 2. Bell's palsy.
- ○ 3. Hypoventilation.
- ○ 4. Loss of gag reflex.

The Client With Cancer of the Larynx

21. Which of the following is a *priority* nursing diagnosis for the client with a total laryngectomy due to cancer?
- ○ 1. Deficient Fluid Volume related to difficulty swallowing.
- ○ 2. Impaired Verbal Communication related to inability to speak.
- ○ 3. Feeding Self-care Deficit related to inability to swallow.
- ○ 4. Powerlessness related to diagnosis of cancer.

22. A client who has had a total laryngectomy appears withdrawn and depressed. He keeps the curtain drawn, refuses visitors, and indicates a desire to be left alone. Which nursing intervention would most likely be therapeutic for the client?
- ○ 1. Discussing his behavior with his wife to determine the cause.

- ○ 2. Exploring his future plans.
- ○ 3. Respecting his need for privacy.
- ○ 4. Encouraging him to express his feelings nonverbally and in writing.

23. The nurse is suctioning a client who had a laryngectomy. What is the maximum amount of time the nurse should suction the client?
- ○ 1. 10 seconds.
- ○ 2. 15 seconds.
- ○ 3. 25 seconds.
- ○ 4. 30 seconds.

24. When suctioning a tracheostomy or laryngectomy tube, the nurse should follow which of the following procedures?
- ○ 1. Use a sterile catheter each time the client is suctioned.
- ○ 2. Cleanse the catheter in sterile water after each use and reuse for no longer than 8 hours.
- ○ 3. Protect the catheter in sterile packaging between suctioning episodes.
- ○ 4. Use a clean catheter with each suctioning, and disinfect it in hydrogen peroxide between uses.

25. The client with a laryngectomy communicates to the nurse that he does not want his family to see him. He indicates that he thinks the opening in his throat is disgusting. Which of the following nursing diagnoses would be most appropriate?
- ○ 1. Deficient Knowledge about the care of a stoma.
- ○ 2. Disturbed Personal Identity related to change in appearance.
- ○ 3. Disturbed Body Image related to neck surgery.
- ○ 4. Hopelessness related to irreversible changes in body functioning.

26. The nurse is preparing a community presentation on the prevention of cancer. Which of the following should be included as a *primary* risk factor for developing laryngeal cancer?
- ○ 1. Chronic allergy.
- ○ 2. Chewing tobacco.
- ○ 3. Exposure to airborne environmental toxins.
- ○ 4. Smoking.

27. Which of the following signs and symptoms would the nurse include in a teaching plan as an early warning sign of laryngeal cancer?
- ○ 1. Dysphagia.
- ○ 2. Hoarseness.
- ○ 3. Airway obstruction.
- ○ 4. Stomatitis.

28. A client has just returned from the postanesthesia care unit (PACU) after undergoing a laryngectomy. Which of the following interventions should the nurse include in the plan of care?
- ○ 1. Maintain the head of the bed at 30 to 40 degrees.
- ○ 2. Teach the client how to use esophageal speech.

○ 3. Initiate small feedings of soft foods.

○ 4. Irrigate drainage tubes as needed.

29. Which of the following is an appropriate expected outcome for a client recovering from a total laryngectomy?

○ 1. The client will regain the ability to taste and smell food.

○ 2. The client will demonstrate appropriate care of the gastrostomy tube.

○ 3. The client will communicate feelings about body image changes.

○ 4. The client will demonstrate sterile suctioning technique for stoma care.

30. Which of the following home care instructions would be appropriate for a client with a laryngectomy?

○ 1. Perform mouth care every morning and evening.

○ 2. Provide adequate humidity in the home.

○ 3. Maintain a soft, bland diet.

○ 4. Limit physical activity to shoulder and neck exercises.

The Client With Pneumonia

31. A 79-year-old female client is admitted to the hospital with a diagnosis of bacterial pneumonia. While obtaining the client's health history, the nurse learns that the client has osteoarthritis, follows a vegetarian diet, and is very concerned with cleanliness. Which of the following would most likely be a predisposing factor for the diagnosis of pneumonia?

○ 1. Age.

○ 2. Osteoarthritis.

○ 3. Vegetarian diet.

○ 4. Daily bathing.

32. A client with bacterial pneumonia is to be started on intravenous antibiotics. Which of the following diagnostic tests must be completed before antibiotic therapy begins?

○ 1. Urinalysis.

○ 2. Sputum culture.

○ 3. Chest radiograph.

○ 4. Red blood cell count.

33. When caring for the client who is receiving an aminoglycoside antibiotic, the nurse monitors which of the following laboratory values?

○ 1. Serum sodium.

○ 2. Serum potassium.

○ 3. Serum creatinine.

○ 4. Serum calcium.

34. A client with pneumonia has a temperature of 102.6°F (39.2°C), is diaphoretic, and has a productive cough. The nurse should include which of the following measures in the plan of care?

○ 1. Position changes every 4 hours.

○ 2. Nasotracheal suctioning to clear secretions.

○ 3. Frequent linen changes.

○ 4. Frequent offering of a bedpan.

35. Bed rest is prescribed for a client with pneumonia during the acute phase of the illness. Bed rest serves which of the following purposes?

○ 1. It reduces the cellular demand for oxygen.

○ 2. It decreases the episodes of coughing.

○ 3. It promotes safety.

○ 4. It promotes clearance of secretions.

36. The cyanosis that accompanies bacterial pneumonia is primarily caused by which of the following?

○ 1. Decreased cardiac output.

○ 2. Pleural effusion.

○ 3. Inadequate peripheral circulation.

○ 4. Decreased oxygenation of the blood.

37. A client with pneumonia is experiencing pleuritic chest pain. Which of the following describes pleuritic chest pain?

○ 1. A mild but constant aching in the chest.

○ 2. Severe midsternal pain.

○ 3. Moderate pain that worsens on inspiration.

○ 4. Muscle spasm pain that accompanies coughing.

38. Which of the following measures would most likely be successful in reducing pleuritic chest pain in a client with pneumonia?

○ 1. Encourage the client to breathe shallowly.

○ 2. Have the client practice abdominal breathing.

○ 3. Offer the client incentive spirometry.

○ 4. Teach the client to splint the rib cage when coughing.

39. Aspirin is administered to clients with pneumonia because of its antipyretic and

○ 1. analgesic effects.

○ 2. anticoagulant effects.

○ 3. adrenergic effects.

○ 4. antihistamine effects.

40. Which of the following mental status changes may occur when a client with pneumonia is first experiencing hypoxia?

○ 1. Coma.

○ 2. Apathy.

○ 3. Irritability.

○ 4. Depression.

41. The client with pneumonia develops mild constipation, and the nurse administers docusate sodium (Colace) as ordered. This drug works by

○ 1. softening the stool.

○ 2. lubricating the stool.

○ 3. increasing stool bulk.

○ 4. stimulating peristalsis.

42. A client with pneumonia has a temperature ranging between 101° and 102°F (38.3° and 38.8°C) and

periods of diaphoresis. Based on this information, which of the following nursing interventions would be a priority?
- ○ 1. Maintain complete bed rest.
- ○ 2. Administer oxygen therapy.
- ○ 3. Provide frequent linen changes.
- ○ 4. Provide fluid intake of 3 L/day.

43. Which of the following would be an appropriate expected outcome for an elderly client recovering from bacterial pneumonia?
- ○ 1. A respiratory rate of 25 to 30 breaths/minute.
- ○ 2. The ability to perform activities of daily living without dyspnea.
- ○ 3. A maximum loss of 5 to 10 pounds of body weight.
- ○ 4. Chest pain that is minimized by splinting the ribcage.

The Client With Tuberculosis

44. Which of the following symptoms is common in clients with active tuberculosis?
- ○ 1. Weight loss.
- ○ 2. Increased appetite.
- ○ 3. Dyspnea on exertion.
- ○ 4. Mental status changes.

45. The nurse obtains a sputum specimen from a client with suspected tuberculosis for laboratory study. Which of the following laboratory techniques is most commonly used to identify tubercle bacilli in sputum?
- ○ 1. Acid-fast staining.
- ○ 2. Sensitivity testing.
- ○ 3. Agglutination testing.
- ○ 4. Dark-field illumination.

46. Which of the following antituberculosis drugs can cause damage to the eighth cranial nerve?
- ○ 1. Streptomycin.
- ○ 2. Isoniazid (INH).
- ○ 3. Para-aminosalicylic acid (PAS).
- ○ 4. Ethambutol hydrochloride (Myambutol).

47. The client who experiences eighth cranial nerve damage will most likely report which of the following symptoms?
- ○ 1. Vertigo.
- ○ 2. Facial paralysis.
- ○ 3. Impaired vision.
- ○ 4. Difficulty swallowing.

48. The nurse should teach clients that the most common route of transmitting tubercle bacilli from person to person is through contaminated
- ○ 1. dust particles.
- ○ 2. droplet nuclei.
- ○ 3. water.
- ○ 4. eating utensils.

49. What is the rationale that supports multidrug treatment for clients with tuberculosis?
- ○ 1. Multiple drugs potentiate the drugs' actions.
- ○ 2. Multiple drugs reduce undesirable drug side effects.
- ○ 3. Multiple drugs allow reduced drug dosages to be given.
- ○ 4. Multiple drugs reduce development of resistant strains of the bacteria.

50. The client with tuberculosis is to be discharged home with community health nursing follow-up. Of the following interventions, which would have the *highest* priority?
- ○ 1. Offering the client emotional support.
- ○ 2. Teaching the client about the disease and its treatment.
- ○ 3. Coordinating various agency services.
- ○ 4. Assessing the client's environment for sanitation.

51. Which of the following techniques for administering the Mantoux test is correct?
- ○ 1. Hold the needle and syringe almost parallel to the client's skin.
- ○ 2. Pinch the skin when inserting the needle.
- ○ 3. Aspirate before injecting the medication.
- ○ 4. Massage the site after injecting the medication.

52. Which of the following family members exposed to tuberculosis would be at highest risk for contracting the disease?
- ○ 1. 45-year-old mother.
- ○ 2. 17-year-old daughter.
- ○ 3. 8-year-old son.
- ○ 4. 76-year-old grandmother.

53. A client has a positive reaction to the Mantoux test. The nurse correctly interprets this reaction to mean that the client
- ○ 1. has active tuberculosis.
- ○ 2. has had contact with *Mycobacterium tuberculosis*.
- ○ 3. has developed a resistance to tubercle bacilli.
- ○ 4. has developed passive immunity to tuberculosis.

54. INH treatment is associated with the development of peripheral neuropathies. Which of the following interventions would the nurse teach the client to help prevent this complication?
- ○ 1. Adhere to a low-cholesterol diet.
- ○ 2. Supplement the diet with pyridoxine (vitamin B_6).
- ○ 3. Get extra rest.
- ○ 4. Avoid excessive sun exposure.

55. The nurse should caution sexually active female clients taking INH that the drug has which of the following effects?
- ○ 1. Increases the risk of vaginal infection.
- ○ 2. Has mutagenic effects on ova.
- ○ 3. Decreases the effectiveness of oral contraceptives.
- ○ 4. Inhibits ovulation.

56. Clients who have had active tuberculosis are at risk for recurrence. Which of the following conditions increases that risk?
  ○ 1. Cool and damp weather.
  ○ 2. Active exercise and exertion.
  ○ 3. Physical and emotional stress.
  ○ 4. Rest and inactivity.

57. In which areas of the United States is the incidence of tuberculosis highest?
  ○ 1. Rural farming areas.
  ○ 2. Inner-city areas.
  ○ 3. Areas where clean water standards are low.
  ○ 4. Suburban areas with significant industrial pollution.

58. The nurse should include which of the following instructions when developing a teaching plan for clients who are receiving INH and rifampin for treatment of tuberculosis?
  ○ 1. Take the medications with antacids.
  ○ 2. Double the dosage if a drug dose is forgotten.
  ○ 3. Increase intake of dairy products.
  ○ 4. Limit alcohol intake.

59. The public health nurse is providing follow-up care to a client with tuberculosis who does not regularly take his medication. Which nursing action would be most appropriate for this client?
  ○ 1. Ask the client's spouse to supervise the daily administration of the medications.
  ○ 2. Visit the client weekly to ask him whether he is taking his medications regularly.
  ○ 3. Notify the physician of the client's noncompliance and request a different prescription.
  ○ 4. Remind the client that tuberculosis can be fatal if it is not treated promptly.

The Client With Chronic Obstructive Pulmonary Disease

60. A client with chronic obstructive pulmonary disease (COPD) reports steady weight loss and being "is too tired from just breathing to eat." Which of the following nursing diagnoses would be most appropriate when planning nutritional interventions for this client?
  ○ 1. Altered Nutrition: Less Than Body Requirements related to fatigue.
  ○ 2. Activity Intolerance related to dyspnea.
  ○ 3. Weight Loss related to COPD.
  ○ 4. Ineffective Breathing Pattern related to alveolar hypoventilation.

61. When developing a discharge plan to manage the care of a client with COPD, the nurse should anticipate which of the following?
  ○ 1. The client will develop infections easily.
  ○ 2. The client will maintain current status.

  ○ 3. The client will require less supplemental oxygen.
  ○ 4. The client will show permanent improvement.

62. Which of the following outcome criteria would be appropriate for a client with COPD who has been discharged to home?
  ○ 1. The client promises to do pursed-lip breathing at home.
  ○ 2. The client states actions to reduce pain.
  ○ 3. The client states that he will use oxygen via a nasal cannula at 5 L/minute.
  ○ 4. The client agrees to call the physician if dyspnea on exertion increases.

63. Which of the following physical assessment findings would the nurse expect to find in a client with advanced COPD?
  ○ 1. Increased anteroposterior chest diameter.
  ○ 2. Underdeveloped neck muscles.
  ○ 3. Collapsed neck veins.
  ○ 4. Increased chest excursions with respiration.

64. When instructing clients on how to decrease the risk of COPD, the nurse should emphasize which of the following behaviors?
  ○ 1. Participate regularly in aerobic exercises.
  ○ 2. Maintain a high-protein diet.
  ○ 3. Avoid exposure to people with known respiratory infections.
  ○ 4. Abstain from cigarette smoking.

65. Which of the following is the primary reason to teach pursed-lip breathing to clients with emphysema?
  ○ 1. To promote oxygen intake.
  ○ 2. To strengthen the diaphragm.
  ○ 3. To strengthen the intercostal muscles.
  ○ 4. To promote carbon dioxide elimination.

66. Which of the following is a priority goal for the client with COPD?
  ○ 1. Maintaining functional ability.
  ○ 2. Minimizing chest pain.
  ○ 3. Increasing carbon dioxide levels in the blood.
  ○ 4. Treating infectious agents.

67. A client's arterial blood gas values are as follows: pH, 7.31; PaO_2, 80 mm Hg; $PaCO_2$, 65 mm Hg; HCO_3^-, 36 mEq/L. Which of the following signs or symptoms would the nurse expect?
  ○ 1. Cyanosis.
  ○ 2. Flushed skin.
  ○ 3. Irritability.
  ○ 4. Anxiety.

68. When performing postural drainage, which of the following factors promotes the movement of secretions from the lower to the upper respiratory tract?
  ○ 1. Friction between the cilia.
  ○ 2. Force of gravity.
  ○ 3. Sweeping motion of cilia.
  ○ 4. Involuntary muscle contractions.

69. When teaching a client with COPD to conserve energy, the nurse should teach the client to lift objects
    - ○ 1. while inhaling through an open mouth.
    - ○ 2. while exhaling through pursed lips.
    - ○ 3. after exhaling but before inhaling.
    - ○ 4. while taking a deep breath and holding it.

70. The nurse teaches a client with COPD to assess for signs and symptoms of right-sided heart failure. Which of the following signs and symptoms should be included in the teaching plan?
    - ○ 1. Clubbing of nail beds.
    - ○ 2. Hypertension.
    - ○ 3. Peripheral edema.
    - ○ 4. Increased appetite.

71. The nurse assesses the respiratory status of a client who is experiencing an exacerbation of COPD secondary to an upper respiratory tract infection. Which of the following findings would be expected?
    - ○ 1. Normal breath sounds.
    - ○ 2. Prolonged inspiration.
    - ○ 3. Normal chest movement.
    - ○ 4. Coarse crackles and rhonchi.

72. Which of the following blood gas abnormalities should the nurse anticipate in a client with advanced COPD?
    - ○ 1. Increased $PaCO_2$.
    - ○ 2. Increased PaO_2.
    - ○ 3. Increased pH.
    - ○ 4. Increased oxygen saturation.

73. A client with COPD is experiencing dyspnea and has a low PaO_2 level. The nurse plans to administer oxygen as ordered. Which of the following statements is true concerning oxygen administration to a client with COPD?
    - ○ 1. High oxygen concentrations will cause coughing and dyspnea.
    - ○ 2. High oxygen concentrations may inhibit the hypoxic stimulus to breathe.
    - ○ 3. Increased oxygen use will cause the client to become dependent on the oxygen.
    - ○ 4. Administration of oxygen is contraindicated in clients who are using bronchodilators.

74. Which of the following diets would be most appropriate for a client with COPD?
    - ○ 1. Low-fat, low-cholesterol diet.
    - ○ 2. Bland, soft diet.
    - ○ 3. Low-sodium diet.
    - ○ 4. High-calorie, high-protein diet.

75. The nurse administers theophylline to the client. To evaluate the effectiveness of this medication, which of the following drug actions would the nurse anticipate?
    - ○ 1. Suppression of the client's respiratory infection.
    - ○ 2. Decrease in bronchial secretions.

    - ○ 3. Relaxation of bronchial smooth muscle.
    - ○ 4. Thinning of tenacious, purulent sputum.

76. The nurse is planning to teach a client with COPD how to cough effectively. Which of the following instructions should be included?
    - ○ 1. Take a deep abdominal breath, bend forward, and cough three or four times on exhalation.
    - ○ 2. Lie flat on the back, splint the thorax, take two deep breaths, and cough.
    - ○ 3. Take several rapid, shallow breaths and then cough forcefully.
    - ○ 4. Assume a side-lying position, extend the arm over the head, and alternate deep breathing with coughing.

The Client With Asthma

77. A 34-year-old woman with a history of asthma is admitted to the emergency department. The nurse notes that the client is dyspneic, with a respiratory rate of 35 breaths/minute, nasal flaring, and use of accessory muscles. Auscultation of the lung fields reveals greatly diminished breath sounds. Based on these findings, what action should the nurse take to initiate care of the client?
    - ○ 1. Initiate oxygen therapy and reassess the client in 10 minutes.
    - ○ 2. Draw blood for an arterial blood gas analysis and send the client for a chest x-ray.
    - ○ 3. Encourage the client to relax and breathe slowly through the mouth.
    - ○ 4. Administer bronchodilators.

78. The nurse would anticipate which of the following arterial blood gas results in a client experiencing a prolonged, severe asthma attack?
    - ○ 1. Decreased $PaCO_2$, increased PaO_2, and decreased pH.
    - ○ 2. Increased $PaCO_2$, decreased PaO_2, and decreased pH.
    - ○ 3. Increased $PaCO_2$, increased PaO_2, and increased pH.
    - ○ 4. Decreased $PaCO_2$, decreased PaO_2, and increased pH.

79. A client with acute asthma is prescribed short-term corticosteroid therapy. What is the rationale for the use of steroids in clients with asthma?
    - ○ 1. Corticosteroids promote bronchodilation.
    - ○ 2. Corticosteroids act as an expectorant.
    - ○ 3. Corticosteroids have an anti-inflammatory effect.
    - ○ 4. Corticosteroids prevent development of respiratory infections.

80. A client is prescribed metaproterenol (Alupent) via a metered-dose inhaler (MDI), two puffs every 4

hours. The nurse instructs the client to report side effects. Which of the following are potential side effects of metaproterenol?
○ 1. Irregular heartbeat.
○ 2. Constipation.
○ 3. Pedal edema.
○ 4. Decreased pulse rate.

81. A client has been taking flunisolide (AeroBid), two inhalations a day, for treatment of asthma. He tells the nurse that he has painful, white patches in his mouth. Which response by the nurse would be most appropriate?
○ 1. "This is an anticipated side effect of your medication. It should go away in a couple of weeks."
○ 2. "You are using your inhaler too much and it has irritated your mouth."
○ 3. "You have developed a fungal infection from your medication. It will need to be treated with an antibiotic."
○ 4. "Be sure to brush your teeth and floss daily. Good oral hygiene will treat this problem."

82. The nurse is observing an elderly client use his MDI to administer his bronchodilator medication. Which of the following client actions should the nurse correct to improve the client's technique?
○ 1. The client shakes the inhaler immediately before use.
○ 2. The client waits 30 seconds between puffs.
○ 3. The client activates the MDI on inspiration.
○ 4. The client holds his breath for 10 seconds after inhalation.

83. Which of the following would be an appropriate expected outcome for an adult client with well-controlled asthma?
○ 1. Chest x-ray demonstrates minimal hyperinflation.
○ 2. Temperature remains lower than 100°F (37.8°C).
○ 3. Arterial blood gas analysis demonstrates a decrease in PaO_2.
○ 4. Breath sounds are clear.

84. Which of the following health promotion activities should the nurse include in the discharge teaching plan for a client with asthma?
○ 1. Incorporate physical exercise as tolerated into the daily routine.
○ 2. Monitor peak flow numbers after meals and at bedtime.
○ 3. Eliminate stressors in the work and home environment.
○ 4. Use sedatives to ensure uninterrupted sleep at night.

85. The client with asthma should be taught that which of the following is one of the most common precipitating factors of an acute asthma attack?

○ 1. Occupational exposure to toxins.
○ 2. Viral respiratory infections.
○ 3. Exposure to cigarette smoke.
○ 4. Exercising in cold temperatures.

86. Which of the following findings would most likely indicate the presence of a respiratory infection in a client with asthma?
○ 1. Cough productive of yellow sputum.
○ 2. Bilateral expiratory wheezing.
○ 3. Chest tightness.
○ 4. Respiratory rate of 30 breaths/minute.

The Client With Lung Cancer

87. A client who has been diagnosed with lung cancer is to have a left lower lobectomy. Which of the following assessment findings obtained during the nurse's admission interview would increase the client's risk of developing postoperative pulmonary complications?
○ 1. The client is 5 feet, 7 inches tall and weighs 110 pounds.
○ 2. The client tends to keep her real feelings to herself.
○ 3. The client ambulates and can climb one flight of stairs without dyspnea.
○ 4. The client is 58 years of age.

88. The nurse in the perioperative area is preparing a female client for surgery and notices that the client looks sad. The client says, "I'm scared of having cancer. It's so horrible and I brought it on myself. I should have quit smoking years ago." What would be the nurse's best response to the client?
○ 1. "It's okay to be scared. What is it about cancer that you're afraid of?"
○ 2. "It's normal to be scared. I would be, too. We'll help you through it."
○ 3. "Don't be so hard on yourself. You don't know if your smoking caused the cancer."
○ 4. "Do you feel guilty because you smoked?"

89. A client who underwent a left lower lobectomy has been out of surgery for 48 hours. She is receiving morphine sulfate via a patient-controlled analgesia (PCA) system. She complains of moderately severe pain in her left thorax that worsens when she coughs. The nurse should
○ 1. let the client rest, so that she is not stimulated to cough.
○ 2. encourage the client to take deep breaths to help control the pain.
○ 3. check that the PCA device is functioning properly, and then reassure the client that the machine is working and will relieve her pain.
○ 4. assess the pain systematically with the hospital-approved scale.

90. Which of the following areas is a priority to evaluate when completing discharge planning for a client who has had a lobectomy for treatment of lung cancer?
    ○ 1. The support available to assist the client at home.
    ○ 2. The distance the client lives from the hospital.
    ○ 3. The client's ability to do home blood pressure monitoring.
    ○ 4. The client's knowledge of the causes of lung cancer.

91. Which of the following would be a major intervention to help prevent lung cancer?
    ○ 1. Encourage cigarette smokers to have yearly chest radiographs.
    ○ 2. Instruct people about techniques for smoking cessation.
    ○ 3. Recommend that people have their houses and apartments checked for asbestos leakage.
    ○ 4. Encourage people to install central air cleaners in their homes.

92. After a thoracotomy, clients should be instructed to perform deep-breathing exercises for which of the following reasons?
    ○ 1. Deep breathing elevates the diaphragm, which enlarges the thorax and increases the lung surface available for gas exchange.
    ○ 2. Deep breathing increases blood flow to the lungs to allow them to recover from the trauma of surgery.
    ○ 3. Deep breathing controls the rate of air flow to the remaining lobe so that it will not become hyperinflated.
    ○ 4. Deep breathing expands the alveoli and increases the lung surface available for ventilation.

93. Which of the following is the most important aspect of pain management for the client after a thoracotomy?
    ○ 1. Repositioning the client immediately after administering pain medication.
    ○ 2. Reassessing the client 30 minutes after administering pain medication.
    ○ 3. Verbally reassuring the client after administering pain medication.
    ○ 4. Readjusting the pain medication dosage as needed according to the client's condition.

94. While assessing a thoracotomy incisional area from which a chest tube exits, the nurse feels a crackling sensation under the fingertips along the entire incision. Which of the following should be the nurse's first action?
    ○ 1. Lower the head of the bed and call the physician.
    ○ 2. Prepare an aspiration tray.
    ○ 3. Mark the area with a skin pencil at the outer periphery of the crackling.
    ○ 4. Turn off the suction of the chest drainage system.

95. When teaching a client to deep breathe effectively after a lobectomy, the nurse should instruct the client to do which of the following?
    ○ 1. Contract the abdominal muscles, take a slow deep breath through the nose and hold it for 3 to 5 seconds, then exhale.
    ○ 2. Contract the abdominal muscles, take a deep breath through the mouth, and exhale slowly as if trying to blow out a candle.
    ○ 3. Relax the abdominal muscles, take a slow deep breath through the nose, and hold it for 3 to 5 seconds.
    ○ 4. Relax the abdominal muscles, take a deep breath through the mouth, and exhale slowly over 10 seconds.

96. Which of the following rehabilitative measures should the nurse teach the client who has undergone chest surgery to prevent shoulder ankylosis?
    ○ 1. Turn from side to side.
    ○ 2. Raise and lower the head.
    ○ 3. Raise the arm on the affected side over the head.
    ○ 4. Flex and extend the elbow on the affected side.

97. When caring for a client with a chest tube and water-seal drainage system, the nurse should implement which of the following interventions?
    ○ 1. Verify that the air vent on the water-seal drainage system is capped when the suction is off.
    ○ 2. Strip the chest drainage tubes at least every 4 hours if excessive bleeding occurs.
    ○ 3. Ensure that the chest tube is clamped when moving the client out of the bed.
    ○ 4. Make sure that the drainage apparatus is always below the client's chest level.

98. A client has a chest tube attached to a water-seal drainage system and the nurse notes that the fluid in the chest tube and in the water-seal column has stopped fluctuating. Which of the following is the explanation?
    ○ 1. The lung has fully expanded.
    ○ 2. The lung has collapsed.
    ○ 3. The chest tube is in the pleural space.
    ○ 4. The mediastinal space has decreased.

99. The nurse observes a constant gentle bubbling in the water-seal column of a water-seal chest drainage system. This observation should prompt the nurse to do which of the following?
    ○ 1. Continue monitoring as usual; this is expected.
    ○ 2. Check the connectors between the chest and drainage tubes and where the drainage tube enters the collection bottle.
    ○ 3. Decrease the suction to −15 cm H_2O and continue observing the system for changes in bubbling during the next several hours.
    ○ 4. Drain half of the water from the water-seal chamber.

100. A client who underwent a lobectomy and has a water-seal chest drainage system is breathing with a little more effort and at a faster rate than 1 hour ago. The client's pulse rate is also increased. Which of the following actions should the nurse implement?
    ○ 1. Check the tubing to ensure that the client is not lying on it or kinking it.
    ○ 2. Increase the suction.
    ○ 3. Lower the drainage bottles 2 to 3 feet below the level of the client's chest.
    ○ 4. Ensure that the chest tube has two clamps on it to prevent air leaks.

101 The nurse is assessing a client who has chest drainage. According to Figure 1, the nurse should
    ○ 1. clamp the chest tube near the insertion site to prevent air from entering the pleural cavity.
    ○ 2. chart the amount of chest drainage.
    ○ 3. add water to maintain the water seal.
    ○ 4. change the chest drainage system.

102. Which of the following should be readily available at the bedside of a client with a chest tube in place?
    ○ 1. A tracheostomy tray.
    ○ 2. Another sterile chest tube.
    ○ 3. A bottle of sterile water.
    ○ 4. A spirometer.

The Client With Chest Trauma

103. A 21-year-old male client is transported by ambulance to the emergency department after a serious automobile accident. He complains of severe pain in his right chest where he struck the steering wheel. What is the primary client goal at this time?
    ○ 1. Reduce the client's anxiety.
    ○ 2. Maintain adequate oxygenation.

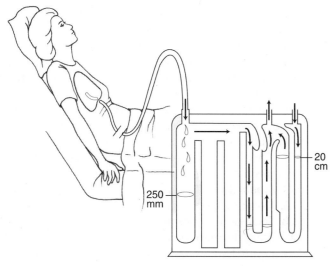

Figure 1.

○ 3. Decrease chest pain.
○ 4. Maintain adequate circulating volume.

104. A client with rib fractures and a pneumothorax has a chest tube inserted that is connected to a water-seal chest tube drainage system. The nurse notes that the fluid in the water-seal column is fluctuating with each breath that the client takes. What is the significance of this fluctuation?
    ○ 1. An obstruction is present in the chest tube.
    ○ 2. The client is developing subcutaneous emphysema.
    ○ 3. The chest tube system is functioning properly.
    ○ 4. There is a leak in the chest tube system.

105. A client who is recovering from chest trauma is to be discharged home with a chest tube drainage system intact. The nurse should instruct the client to call the physician for which of the following?
    ○ 1. Respiratory rate greater than 16 breaths/ minute.
    ○ 2. Continuous bubbling in the water-seal chamber.
    ○ 3. Fluid in the chest tube.
    ○ 4. Fluctuation of fluid in the water-seal chamber.

106. Which of the following findings would suggest pneumothorax in a trauma victim?
    ○ 1. Pronounced crackles.
    ○ 2. Inspiratory wheezing.
    ○ 3. Dullness on percussion.
    ○ 4. Absent breath sounds.

107. For a client with rib fractures and a pneumothorax, the physician prescribes morphine sulfate, 1 to 2 mg/hour, given intravenously as needed for pain. The primary objective of this order is to provide adequate pain control so that the client can breathe effectively. Which of the following outcomes would indicate successful achievement of this objective?
    ○ 1. Pain rating of 0 on a scale of 0 to 10 by the client.
    ○ 2. Decreased client anxiety.
    ○ 3. Respiratory rate of 26 breaths/minute.
    ○ 4. PaO$_2$ of 70 mm Hg.

108. A client undergoes surgery to repair lung injuries. Postoperative orders include the transfusion of one unit of packed red blood cells at a rate of 60 mL/hour. How long would this transfusion take to infuse?
    ○ 1. 2 hours.
    ○ 2. 4 hours.
    ○ 3. 6 hours.
    ○ 4. 8 hours.

109. The primary reason for infusing blood at a rate of 60 mL/hour is to help prevent which of the following complications?
    ○ 1. Emboli formation.
    ○ 2. Fluid volume overload.
    ○ 3. Red blood cell hemolysis.
    ○ 4. Allergic reaction.

110. A client's chest tube is to be removed by the physician. Which of the following items should the nurse have

ready to be placed directly over the wound when the chest tube is removed?
- ○ 1. Butterfly dressing.
- ○ 2. Montgomery strap.
- ○ 3. Fine-mesh gauze dressing.
- ○ 4. Petrolatum gauze dressing.

111. Which of the following is a sign or symptom of a moderate pneumothorax?
- ○ 1. Sudden, sharp chest pain.
- ○ 2. Wheezing breath sounds over affected side.
- ○ 3. Hemoptysis.
- ○ 4. Cyanosis.

112. A chest tube is inserted in a client with a pneumothorax for which of the following reasons?
- ○ 1. For administration of oxygen.
- ○ 2. To promote formation of lung scar tissue.
- ○ 3. To insert antibiotics into the pleural space.
- ○ 4. To remove air and fluid.

Care of the Client With Acute Respiratory Failure

113. Which of the following interventions would be most likely to prevent the development of acute respiratory distress syndrome (ARDS)?
- ○ 1. Teaching cigarette smoking cessation.
- ○ 2. Maintaining adequate serum potassium levels.
- ○ 3. Monitoring clients for signs of hypercapnia.
- ○ 4. Replacing fluids adequately during hypovolemic states.

114. Which of the following nursing diagnoses would be a priority for a client with ARDS?
- ○ 1. Ineffective Breathing Pattern.
- ○ 2. Pain.
- ○ 3. Ineffective Health Maintenance.
- ○ 4. Risk for Infection.

115. The nurse interprets which of the following as an early sign of ARDS in a client at risk?
- ○ 1. Elevated carbon dioxide level.
- ○ 2. Hypoxia not responsive to oxygen therapy.
- ○ 3. Metabolic acidosis.
- ○ 4. Severe, unexplained electrolyte imbalance.

116. A client has the following arterial blood gas values: pH, 7.52; PaO_2, 50 mm Hg; $PaCO_2$, 28 mm Hg; HCO_3^-, 24 mEq/L. From the client's $PaCO_2$ level, the nurse determines that the client is experiencing which of the following conditions?
- ○ 1. Hypoxemia.
- ○ 2. Hypoventilation.
- ○ 3. Hyperventilation.
- ○ 4. Oxygen toxicity.

117. A client has the following arterial blood gas values: pH, 7.52; PaO_2, 50 mm Hg; $PaCO_2$; 28 mm Hg; HCO_3^-, 24 mEq/L. Based upon the client's PaO_2, which of the following conclusions would be accurate?
- ○ 1. The client is severely hypoxic.
- ○ 2. The oxygen level is low but poses no risk for the client.
- ○ 3. The client's PaO_2 level is within normal range.
- ○ 4. The client requires oxygen therapy with very low oxygen concentrations.

118. A client has the following arterial blood gas values: pH, 7.52; PaO_2, 50 mm Hg; $PaCO_2$, 28 mm Hg; HCO_3^-, 24 mEq/L. The nurse determines that which of the following is a possible cause for these findings?
- ○ 1. Chronic obstructive pulmonary disease (COPD).
- ○ 2. Diabetic ketoacidosis with Kussmaul's respirations.
- ○ 3. Myocardial infarction.
- ○ 4. Pulmonary embolus.

119. Which of the following interventions should the nurse anticipate in a client who has been diagnosed with ARDS?
- ○ 1. Tracheostomy.
- ○ 2. Intermittent positive-pressure breathing.
- ○ 3. Mechanical ventilation.
- ○ 4. Insertion of a chest tube.

120. The nurse should anticipate that which of the following conditions can place a client at risk for ARDS?
- ○ 1. Septic shock.
- ○ 2. COPD.
- ○ 3. Asthma.
- ○ 4. Heart failure.

121. Which one of the following assessments would be most appropriate for determining the correct placement of an endotracheal tube in a mechanically ventilated client?
- ○ 1. Assessing the client's skin color.
- ○ 2. Monitoring the respiratory rate.
- ○ 3. Verifying the amount of cuff inflation.
- ○ 4. Auscultating lung sounds bilaterally.

122. Which of the following nursing interventions would promote effective airway clearance in a client with acute respiratory distress?
- ○ 1. Administering oxygen every 2 hours.
- ○ 2. Turning the client every 4 hours.
- ○ 3. Administering sedatives to promote rest.
- ○ 4. Suctioning if cough is ineffective.

123. Which of the following complications is associated with mechanical ventilation?
- ○ 1. Gastrointestinal hemorrhage.
- ○ 2. Immunosuppression.
- ○ 3. Increased cardiac output.
- ○ 4. Pulmonary emboli.

Correct Answers and Rationale

The letters in parentheses following the rationale identify the step of the nursing process (A, D, P, I, E) and client needs (1, 2, 3, 4, 5, 6, 7, 8, 9, 10). See the inside front cover for the key.

The Client With an Upper Respiratory Tract Infection

1. 3. When using an intranasal inhaler, it is important to close off one nostril while inhaling the spray into the other nostril to ensure the best inhalation of the spray. Use of the inhaler is not limited to mornings and bedtime. The canister should be shaken immediately before use. The inhaler tip should be inserted into the nostril and pointed toward the outside nostril wall to maximize inhalation of the medication. (E, 8)

2. 4. A client recovering from an upper respiratory tract infection should report decreasing or no nasal discharge and obstruction. Daily fluid intake should be increased to more than 1 L every 24 hours to liquefy secretions. The temperature should be below 100°F (37.8°C) with no chills or diaphoresis. A productive cough with chest pain indicates a pulmonary infection, not an upper respiratory tract infection. (E, 10)

3. 2. The client should blow the nose before instilling nose drops. Instilling nose drops is a clean technique. The dropper should be cleaned after each administration, but it does not need to be changed. The client should assume a position that will allow the medication to reach the desired area; this is usually a supine position. (E, 8)

4. 1. The plan of care for a client who has acute sinusitis includes antibiotics to treat the bacterial infection. In addition, nasal corticosteroids and decongestants are frequently ordered to decrease mucosal inflammation and edema. Nasal corticosteroids are preferred to oral corticosteroids because they do not produce systematic side effects when used as prescribed. Antihistamines can promote an increase in secretion viscosity and continued symptoms; they should be avoided. Bronchodilators are ineffective in sinusitis. (P, 8)

5. 3. The client with chronic sinusitis should be instructed to take hot showers in the morning and evening to promote drainage of secretions. There is no need to limit caffeine intake. Performing postural drainage will inhibit removal of secretions, not promote it. Clients should elevate the head of the bed to promote drainage. Clients should report all temperatures higher than 100.4°F (38°C), because a temperature that high can indicate infection. (I, 9)

6. 3. Individuals who are household members or home care providers for high-risk individuals are high-priority targeted groups for immunization against influenza to prevent transmission to those who have a decreased capacity to deal with the disease. The wife who is caring for a husband with cancer has the highest priority of the clients described, because her husband is likely to be immunocompromised and particularly susceptible to the flu. A healthy 60-year-old man or a healthy 36-year-old woman is not in a high-priority category for influenza vaccination. A 60-year-old woman with osteoporosis does not have a higher priority for influenza vaccination than a home care provider. (A, 9)

7. 4. It is important for clients with allergic rhinitis to determine the precipitating factors so that they can be avoided. Keeping a diary can help identify these triggers. Nasal decongestant sprays should not be used regularly because they can cause a rebound effect. Antibiotics are not appropriate for allergic rhinitis because an infection is not present. Increasing activity will not control the clients symptoms; in fact, walking outdoors may increase them if the client is allergic to pollen. (I, 9)

8. 1. Pneumonia is the most common complication of influenza, especially in the elderly. The development of a purulent cough and crackles may be indicative of a bacterial infection and are not consistent with a diagnosis of influenza. These findings are not indicative of dehydration. Decongestants and bronchodilators are not typically prescribed for the flu. (D, 10)

9. 2. 300 mg/x = 200 mg/5 mL; x = 7.5 mL. (I, 8)

10. 4. Side effects of pseudoephedrine are experienced primarily in the cardiovascular system and through sympathetic effects on the central nervous system (CNS). The most common CNS side effects include restlessness, dizziness, tension, anxiety, insomnia, and weakness. Common cardiovascular side effects include tachycardia, hypertension, palpitations, and arrhythmias. Constipation and diplopia are not side effects of pseudoephedrine. Tachycardia, not bradycardia, is a side effect of pseudoephedrine. (A, 8)

The Client Undergoing Nasal Surgery

11. 2. Because of the dense nasal packing, bleeding may not be apparent through the nasal drip pad. Instead, the blood may run down the throat, causing the client

to swallow frequently. The back of the throat, where the blood will be apparent, can be assessed with a flashlight. An accumulation of blood in the stomach can cause nausea and vomiting, but nausea would not be the initial indicator of bleeding. An increased respiratory rate occurs in shock but is not an early sign of bleeding in a client who has undergone nasal surgery. Increased pain warrants further assessment but is not an indicator of bleeding. (A, 11)

12. 1. The client should be instructed to avoid any activities that cause Valsalva's maneuver (eg, constipation, vigorous coughing, exercise) in order to reduce bleeding and stress on suture lines. The client should not take aspirin because of its antiplatelet properties, which may cause bleeding. Oral hygiene is important to rid the mouth of old dried blood and to enhance the client's appetite. Cool compresses, not heat, should be applied to decrease swelling and control discoloration of the area. (I, 10)

13. 2. Constipation can cause straining during defecation, which can induce bleeding. Showering is not contraindicated. The client should take measures to prevent coughing, which can cause bleeding. The client should avoid blowing her nose for 48 hours after the packing is removed. Thereafter, she should blow her nose gently, using the open-mouth technique to minimize bleeding in the surgical area. (E, 10)

14. 4. Aspirin-containing medications should be discontinued for 2 weeks before surgery to decrease the risk of bleeding. Nasal packing is usually removed the day after surgery. Normal saline nose drops are not routinely administered preoperatively. The results of the surgery will not be obvious immediately after surgery because of edema and ecchymosis. (P, 9)

15. 3. Immediately after nasal surgery, ineffective breathing patterns may develop as a result of the nasal packing and nasal edema. Nasal packing may dislodge, leading to obstruction. Assessing for airway obstruction is a priority. Assessing for pain is important, but it is not as high a priority as assessment of the airways. It is too early to detect ecchymosis. Measuring intake and output is not typically a priority nursing assessment after nasal surgery. (A, 10)

16. 4. Applying cold compresses helps to decrease facial swelling and pain from edema. Analgesics may decrease pain, but they do not decrease edema. A corticosteroid nasal spray would not be administered postoperatively because it can impair healing. Use of a bedside humidifier promotes comfort by providing moisture for nasal mucosa, but it does not decrease edema. (I, 7)

17. 1. Frequent mouth care is important to provide comfort and encourage eating. Mouth care promotes moist mucous membranes. Nose drops cannot be used with nasal packing in place. When sneezing and coughing, the client should do so with the mouth open to decrease the chance of dislodging the packing. Gargling should not be attempted with packing in place. (I, 7)

18. 2. After removal of nasal packing, the client should be instructed to apply water-soluble jelly to the nares to lubricate the nares and promote comfort. Swelling gradually subsides over several weeks; the client can gently cleanse the nares as soon as packing is removed. A nasal drip pad is not needed after removal of packing. Irrigation with a bulb syringe may interfere with healing and introduce infection. (I, 7)

19. 4. The client should assume a sitting position and lean forward. Firm pressure should be applied to the soft portion of the nose for approximately 10 minutes. Tilting the head backward can cause the client to swallow blood, which can obscure the amount of bleeding and also can lead to nausea. Ice compresses may be applied, but the client should not lie flat. Blowing the nose is to be avoided because it can increase bleeding. (I, 9)

20. 3. Posterior packing may alter the respiratory status of the client, especially in elderly clients, causing hypoventilation. Clients should be observed carefully for changes in level of consciousness, respiratory rate, and heart rate and rhythm after the insertion of the packing. Vertigo does not occur as a result of the insertion of posterior packing. Bell's palsy, a disorder of the seventh cranial nerve, is not associated with epistaxis or nasal packing. Loss of gag reflex does not occur as a result of the insertion of posterior packing. (A, 9)

The Client With Cancer of the Larynx

21. 2. The client will be unable to speak after the laryngectomy, and an alternative method of communication must be used. The method (writing or using a communication board with letters, words, or pictures as desired) should be determined and practiced preoperatively. The client with a laryngectomy is able to swallow but may have difficulty swallowing initially. Intravenous fluids will be administered to maintain an adequate fluid volume. Although Powerlessness may be an important diagnosis for clients with cancer, there are no data to support that it is indicated for this client. (D, 10)

22. 4. The client has undergone body changes and permanent loss of verbal communication. He may feel isolated and insecure. The nurse can encourage him to express his feelings and use this information to develop an appropriate care plan. Discussing the client's behavior with his wife may not reveal his feelings. Exploring future plans is not appropriate at this time because

more information about the client's behavior is needed before proceeding to this level. The nurse can respect the client's need for privacy while also encouraging him to express his feelings. (I, 5)

23. 1. A client should be suctioned for no longer than 10 seconds at a time. Suctioning for longer than 10 seconds may reduce the client's oxygen level so much that he becomes hypoxic. (I, 9)

24. 1. The recommended technique is to use a sterile catheter each time the client is suctioned. There is a danger of introducing organisms into the respiratory tract when strict aseptic technique is not used. Reusing a suction catheter is not consistent with aseptic technique. The nurse does not use a clean catheter when suctioning a tracheostomy; it is a sterile procedure. (I, 9)

25. 3. Disturbed Body Image is the most appropriate nursing diagnosis based on the client's statements at this time. Most clients are concerned about how their family members will respond to the physical changes that have occurred as a result of radical neck surgery. The nurse should allow the client to verbalize any negative feelings or concerns that exist because of the surgery. Referral to a support group for laryngectomy clients may be helpful to the client and family members in coping with the changes in their lives. The client's feelings are not related to a knowledge deficit, but rather to a permanent change in physical appearance and functioning. The diagnosis of Disturbed Personal Identity refers to a client's inability to distinguish self from nonself. Hopelessness may be an issue for the client experiencing a body image disturbance; however, there are no data to support this diagnosis at this time. (D, 5)

26. 4. The primary risk factor for laryngeal cancer is cigarette smoking. The use of alcohol, in combination with smoking, appears to increase the risk. Approximately 90% of head and neck cancers, including laryngeal cancer, develop after prolonged use of tobacco and alcohol. Chronic allergy conditions are not implicated in cancer of the larynx. The use of chewing tobacco and snuff can lead to the development of oral cancer. Exposure to noxious fumes or polluted air and voice abuse are also factors in the development of laryngeal cancer, but they are not primary factors. (P, 4)

27. 2. Early warning signs of laryngeal cancer can vary depending on tumor location. Hoarseness lasting longer than 2 weeks should be evaluated because it is one of the most common warning signs. Other early warning signs include a lump in the neck, persistent sore throat, cough, earache, or the feeling of a lump in the throat. Later signs and symptoms include dysphagia, hemoptysis, pain, and airway obstruction. Stomatitis is not a sign of laryngeal cancer. (P, 4)

28. 1. Immediately after surgery the client should be maintained in a position with the head of the bed elevated 30 to 40 degrees (semi-Fowler's position) to decrease tissue edema, facilitate breathing, and decrease pain related to edema formation. Immediately postoperatively, the client should be provided alternative means of communicating, such as a communication board. As healing progresses and edema subsides, a speech therapist should work with the client to explore various voice restoration options such as the use of a voice prosthesis, electrolarynx, artificial larynx, or esophageal speech. Food is not initiated in the immediate postoperative phase; enteral feedings are usually used to meet nutritional needs until edema subsides. Irrigation of the drainage tubes is an inappropriate action. (P, 7)

29. 3. It is important that the client be able to communicate his or her feelings about the body image changes that have occurred as a result of surgery. Open communication helps promote adjustment. The client may not regain the ability to taste and smell food because of no longer breathing through the nose or because of radiation therapy treatments, or both. A gastrostomy tube would not typically be placed after a total laryngectomy, nor would it be necessary for the client to demonstrate sterile suctioning technique for stoma care. The client would use clean technique. (E, 10)

30. 2. Adequate humidity should be provided in the home to help keep secretions moist. A bedside humidifier is recommended. A high fluid intake is also important to liquefy secretions. Mouth care is important to prevent drying of mucous membranes and should be performed frequently throughout the day, especially before and after meals, to help stimulate appetite. The client may eat any food that can be chewed and swallowed comfortably. The client may resume physical activity as tolerated. (I, 9)

The Client With Pneumonia

31. 1. The client's age is a predisposing factor for pneumonia; pneumonia is more common in elderly or debilitated clients. Other predisposing factors include smoking, upper respiratory tract infections, malnutrition, immunosuppression, and the presence of a chronic illness. Osteoarthritis, a nutritionally sound vegetarian diet, and frequent bathing are not predisposing factors for pneumonia. (A, 9)

32. 2. A sputum specimen is obtained for culture to determine the causative organism. After the organism is identified, an appropriate antibiotic can be prescribed. Beginning antibiotic therapy before obtaining the sputum specimen may alter the results of the test. Neither a urinalysis, a chest radiograph, nor a red blood cell

count needs to be obtained before initiation of antibiotic therapy for pneumonia. (I, 9)

33. 3. It is essential to monitor serum creatinine in the client receiving an aminoglycoside antibiotic because of the potential of these drugs to cause acute tubular necrosis. Aminoglycoside antibiotics do not affect serum sodium, potassium, or calcium levels. (A, 8)

34. 3. Frequent linen changes are appropriate for this client because of the diaphoresis. Diaphoresis produces general discomfort. The client should be kept dry to promote comfort. Position changes need to be done every 2 hours. Nasotracheal suctioning is not indicated with the client's productive cough. Frequent offering of a bedpan is not indicated by the data provided in this scenario. (I, 7)

35. 1. Exudate in the alveoli interferes with ventilation and the diffusion of gases in clients with pneumonia. During the acute phase of the illness, it is essential to reduce the body's need for oxygen at the cellular level; bed rest is the most effective method for doing so. Bed rest does not decrease coughing or promote clearance of secretions, and it does not necessarily provide a safe environment. (I, 10)

36. 4. A client with pneumonia has less lung surface available for the diffusion of gases because of the inflammatory pulmonary response that creates lung exudate and results in reduced oxygenation of the blood. The client becomes cyanotic because blood is not adequately oxygenated in the lungs before it enters the peripheral circulation. Decreased cardiac output may be a comorbid condition in some clients with pneumonia; however, it is not the cause of cyanosis. Pleural effusions are a potential complication of pneumonia but are not the primary cause of decreased oxygenation. Inadequate peripheral circulation is also not the cause of the cyanosis that develops with bacterial pneumonia. (A, 10)

37. 3. Chest pain in pneumonia is generally caused by friction between the pleural layers. It is more severe on inspiration than on expiration, secondary to chest wall movement. Pleuritic chest pain is usually described as sharp, not mild or aching. Pleuritic chest pain is not localized to the sternum, and it is not the result of a muscle spasm. (A, 10)

38. 4. The pleuritic pain is triggered by chest movement and is particularly severe during coughing. Splinting the chest wall will help reduce the discomfort of coughing. Deep breathing is essential to prevent further atelectasis. Incentive spirometry facilitates effective deep breathing but does not decrease pleuritic chest pain. Abdominal breathing is not as effective in decreasing pleuritic chest pain as is splinting of the rib cage. (I, 10)

39. 1. Aspirin is administered to clients with pneumonia because it is an analgesic that helps control chest discomfort and an antipyretic that helps reduce fever. It is also an anti-inflammatory agent that reduces inflammation. Aspirin has an anticoagulant effect, but that is not the reason for prescribing it for a client with pneumonia. Aspirin does not have adrenergic or antihistamine effects, and drugs with adrenergic or antihistamine effects are not used for the treatment of pneumonia. (I, 8)

40. 3. Clients who are experiencing hypoxia characteristically exhibit irritability, restlessness, or anxiety as initial mental status changes. As the hypoxia becomes more pronounced, the client may become confused and combative. Coma is a late clinical manifestation of hypoxia. Apathy and depression are not symptoms of hypoxia. (A, 10)

41. 1. Docusate sodium is a stool softener that allows fluid and fatty substances to enter the stool and soften it. Docusate sodium does not lubricate the stool, increase stool bulk, or stimulate peristalsis. (I, 8)

42. 4. A fluid intake of at least 3 L/day should be provided to replace any fluid loss occurring as a result of the fever and diaphoresis; this is a high-priority intervention. Although clients with pneumonia may be prescribed bed rest, complete bed rest is not necessary solely because of the elevated temperature. Administration of oxygen therapy also is not indicated for the purposes of treating the fever. Frequent linen changes is an appropriate intervention, but it is not of the highest priority among the options given. (I, 9)

43. 2. An expected outcome for a client recovering from pneumonia would be the ability to perform activities of daily living without experiencing dyspnea. A respiratory rate of 25 to 30 breaths/minute indicates the client is experiencing tachypnea, which would not be expected on recovery. A weight loss of 5 to 10 pounds is undesirable; the expected outcome would be to maintain normal weight. A client who is recovering from pneumonia should experience decreased or no chest pain. (E, 1)

The Client With Tuberculosis

44. 1. Tuberculosis typically produces anorexia and weight loss. Other signs and symptoms may include fatigue, low-grade fever, and night sweats. Increased appetite is not a symptom of tuberculosis; dyspnea on exertion and change in mental status are not common symptoms of tuberculosis. (A, 10)

45. 1. The most commonly used technique to identify tubercle bacilli is acid-fast staining. The bacilli have a waxy surface, which makes them difficult to stain in

the laboratory. However, once they are stained, the stain is resistant to removal, even with acids. Therefore, tubercle bacilli are often called acid-fast bacilli. Sensitivity testing, agglutination testing, and dark-field illumination are not used to identify tubercle bacilli. (A, 9)

46. 1. Streptomycin is an aminoglycoside, and eighth cranial nerve damage (ototoxicity) is a common side effect of aminoglycosides. A common side effect of INH is peripheral neuritis. A common side effect of PAS is gastrointestinal disturbance. A common side effect of ethambutol hydrochloride (Myambutol) is optic neuritis. (A, 8)

47. 1. The eighth cranial nerve is the vestibulocochlear nerve, which is responsible for hearing and equilibrium. Streptomycin can damage this nerve (ototoxicity). Symptoms of ototoxicity include vertigo, tinnitus, hearing loss, and ataxia. Facial paralysis would result from damage to the facial nerve (VII). Impaired vision would result from damage to the optic (II), oculomotor (III), or the trochlear (IV) nerves. Difficulty swallowing would result from damage to the glossopharyngeal (IX) or the vagus (X) nerve. (E, 8)

48. 2. Tubercle bacilli is spread by airborne droplet nuclei. Droplet nuclei are the residue of evaporated droplets containing the bacilli, which remain suspended and are circulated in the air. Dust particles and water do not spread tubercle bacilli. Tuberculosis is not spread by eating utensils, dishes, or other fomites. (I, 2)

49. 4. Use of a combination of antituberculosis drugs slows the rate at which organisms develop drug resistance. Combination therapy also appears to be more effective than single-drug therapy. Many drugs potentiate (or inhibit) the actions of other drugs; however, this is not the rationale for using multiple drugs to treat tuberculosis. Treatment with multiple drugs does not reduce side effects and may expose the client to more side effects. Combination therapy may allow some medications (eg, antihypertensives) to be given in reduced dosages; however, reduced dosages are not prescribed for antibiotics and antituberculosis drugs. (P, 8)

50. 2. Ensuring that the client is well educated about tuberculosis is the highest priority. Education of the client and family is essential to help the client understand the need for completing the prescribed drug therapy to cure the disease. Offering the client emotional support, coordinating various agency services, and assessing the environment may be part of the care for the client with tuberculosis; however, these interventions are of less importance than education about the disease process and its treatment. (P, 7)

51. 1. The Mantoux test is administered via intradermal injection. The appropriate technique for an intradermal

injection includes holding the needle and syringe almost parallel to the client's skin, keeping the skin slightly taut when the needle is inserted, and inserting the needle with the bevel side up. There is no need to aspirate, a technique that assesses for incorrect placement in a blood vessel, when giving an intradermal injection. The injection site is not massaged. (I, 8)

52. 4. Elderly persons are believed to be at higher risk for contracting tuberculosis because of decreased immunocompetence. Other high-risk populations in the United States include the urban poor, clients with acquired immunodeficiency syndrome (AIDS), and minority groups. (A, 2)

53. 2. A positive Mantoux skin test indicates that the client has been exposed to tubercle bacilli. Exposure does not necessarily mean that active disease exists. A positive Mantoux test does not mean that the client has developed resistance. Unless involved in treatment, the client may still develop active disease at any time. Immunity to tuberculosis is not possible. (E, 9)

54. 2. INH competes for the available vitamin B_6 in the body and leaves the client at risk for development of neuropathies related to vitamin deficiency. Supplemental vitamin B_6 is routinely prescribed. Following a low-cholesterol diet, getting extra rest, and avoiding excessive sun exposure will not prevent the development of peripheral neuropathies. (P, 8)

55. 3. INH interferes with the effectiveness of oral contraceptives, and female clients of childbearing age should be counseled to use an alternate form of birth control while taking the drug. INH does not increase the risk of vaginal infection, nor does it affect the ova or ovulation. (I, 8)

56. 3. Tuberculosis can be controlled but never completely eradicated from the body. Periods of intense physical or emotional stress increase the likelihood of recurrence. Clients should be taught to recognize the signs and symptoms of a potential recurrence. Weather and activity levels are not related to recurrences of tuberculosis. (I, 10)

57. 2. Statistics show that of the four geographic areas described, most cases of tuberculosis are found in inner-core residential areas of large cities, where health and sanitation standards tend to be low. Substandard housing, poverty, and crowded living conditions also generally characterize these city areas and contribute to the spread of the disease. Farming areas have a low incidence of tuberculosis. Variations in water standards and industrial pollution are not correlated to tuberculosis incidence. (A, 2)

58. 4. INH and rifampin are hepatotoxic drugs. Clients should be warned to limit intake of alcohol during drug therapy. Both drugs should be taken on an empty stomach. If antacids are needed for gastrointestinal dis-

tress, they should be taken 1 hour before or 2 hours after these drug are administered. Clients should not double the dosage of these drugs because of their potential toxicity. Clients taking INH should avoid foods that are rich in tyramine, such as cheese and dairy products, or they may develop hypertension. (P, 8)

59. 1. Directly observed therapy (DOT) can be implemented with clients who are not compliant with drug therapy. In DOT, a responsible person, who may be a family member or a health care provider, observes the client taking the medication. Visiting the client, changing the prescription, or threatening the client will not ensure compliance if the client will not or cannot follow the prescribed treatment. (I, 2)

The Client With Chronic Obstructive Pulmonary Disease

60. 1. The client's problem is altered nutrition—specifically, less than required. The cause, as stated by the client, is the fatigue associated with the disease process. Activity Intolerance is a likely diagnosis but is not related to the client's nutritional problems. Weight Loss is not a nursing diagnosis. Ineffective Breathing Pattern may be a problem, but this diagnosis does not specifically address the problem of weight loss described by the client. (D, 7)

61. 1. A client with COPD is at high risk for development of respiratory infections. COPD is slowly progressive; therefore, maintaining current status and establishing a goal that the client will require less supplemental oxygen are unrealistic expectations. Treatment may slow progression of the disease, but permanent improvement is highly unlikely. (P, 1)

62. 4. Increasing dyspnea on exertion indicates that the client may be experiencing complications of COPD, and therefore the physician should be notified. Extracting promises from clients is not an outcome criterion. Pain is not a common symptom of COPD. Clients with COPD use low-flow oxygen supplementation (1 to 2 L/minute) to avoid suppressing the respiratory drive, which, for these clients, is stimulated by hypoxia. (E, 7)

63. 1. Increased anteroposterior chest diameter is characteristic of advanced COPD. Air is trapped in the overextended alveoli, and the ribs are fixed in an inspiratory position. The result is the typical barrel-chested appearance. Overly developed, not underdeveloped, neck muscles are associated with COPD because of their increased use in the work of breathing. Distended, not collapsed, neck veins are associated with COPD as a symptom of the heart failure that the client may experience secondary to the increased workload on the heart to pump blood into the pulmonary vasculature.

Diminished, not increased, chest excursion is associated with COPD. (A, 10)

64. 4. Cigarette smoking is the primary cause of COPD. Other risk factors include exposure to environmental pollutants and chronic asthma. Participating in an aerobic exercise program, although beneficial, will not decrease the risk of COPD. Insufficient protein intake and exposure to people with respiratory infections do not increase the risk of COPD. (I, 4)

65. 4. Pursed-lip breathing prolongs exhalation and prevents air trapping in the alveoli, thereby promoting carbon dioxide elimination. By prolonging exhalation and helping the client relax, pursed-lip breathing helps the client learn to control the rate and depth of respiration. Pursed-lip breathing does not promote the intake of oxygen, strengthen the diaphragm, or strengthen intercostal muscles. (I, 10)

66. 1. A priority goal for the client with COPD is to manage the signs and symptoms of the disease process so as to maintain the client's functional ability. Chest pain is not a typical symptom of COPD. The carbon dioxide concentration in the blood is increased to an abnormal level in clients with COPD; it would not be a goal to increase the level further. Preventing infection would be a goal of care for the client with COPD. (P, 7)

67. 2. The high $PaCO_2$ level causes flushing due to vasodilation. The client also becomes drowsy and lethargic because carbon dioxide has a depressant effect on the central nervous system. Cyanosis is a sign of hypoxia. Irritability and anxiety are not common with a $PaCO_2$ level of 65 mm Hg but are associated with hypoxia. (A, 9)

68. 2. The principle behind using postural drainage is that gravity will help move secretions from smaller to larger airways. Postural drainage is best used after percussion has loosened secretions. Coughing or suctioning is then used to remove secretions. Movement of cilia is not sufficient to move secretions. Muscle contractions do not move secretions within the lungs. (I, 10)

69. 2. Exhaling requires less energy than inhaling. Therefore, lifting while exhaling saves energy and reduces perceived dyspnea. Pursing the lips prolongs exhalation and provides the client with more control over breathing. Lifting after exhaling but before inhaling is similar to lifting with the breath held. This should not be recommended because it is similar to the Valsalva maneuver, which can stimulate cardiac dysrhythmias. (I, 7)

70. 3. Right-sided heart failure is a complication of COPD that occurs because of pulmonary hypertension. Signs and symptoms of right-sided heart failure include peripheral edema, jugular venous distention, hepatomegaly, and weight gain due to increased fluid volume. Clubbing of nail beds is associated with conditions of chronic hypoxemia. Hypertension is associated with

left-sided heart failure. Clients with heart failure have decreased appetites. (I, 10)

71. 4. Exacerbations of COPD are frequently caused by respiratory infections. Coarse crackles and rhonchi would be auscultated as air moves through airways obstructed with secretions. In COPD, breath sounds are diminished because of an enlarged anteroposterior diameter of the chest. Expiration, not inspiration, becomes prolonged. Chest movement is decreased as lungs become overdistended. (A, 10)

72. 1. As COPD progresses, the client typically develops increased $PaCO_2$ levels and decreased PaO_2 levels. This results in decreased pH and decreased oxygen saturation. These changes are the result of air trapping and hypoventilation. (D, 9)

73. 2. Clients who have a long history of COPD may retain carbon dioxide (CO_2). Gradually the body adjusts to the higher CO_2 concentration, and the high levels of CO_2 no longer stimulate the respiratory center. The major respiratory stimulant then becomes hypoxemia. Administration of high concentrations of oxygen eliminates this respiratory stimulus and leads to hypoventilation. Oxygen can be drying if it is not humidified, but it does not cause coughing and dyspnea. Increased oxygen use will not create an oxygen dependency; clients should receive oxygen as needed. Oxygen is not contraindicated with the use of bronchodilators. (P, 7)

74. 4. The client should eat high-calorie, high-protein meals to maintain nutritional status and prevent weight loss that results from the increased work of breathing. The client should be encouraged to eat small, frequent meals. A low-fat, low-cholesterol diet is indicated for clients with coronary artery disease. The client with COPD does not necessarily need to follow a sodium-restricted diet, unless otherwise medically indicated. There is no need for the client to eat bland, soft foods. (I, 7)

75. 3. Theophylline is a bronchodilator that is administered to relax airways and decrease dyspnea. Theophylline is not used to treat infections and does not decrease or thin secretions. (E, 8)

76. 1. The goal of effective coughing is to conserve energy, facilitate removal of secretions, and minimize airway collapse. The client should assume a sitting position with feet on the floor if possible. The client should bend forward slightly and, using pursed-lip breathing, exhale. After resuming an upright position, the client should use abdominal breathing to slowly and deeply inhale. After repeating this process three or four times, the client should take a deep abdominal breath, bend forward, and cough three or four times upon exhalation ("huff" cough). Lying flat does not enhance lung expansion; sitting upright promotes full expansion of the thorax. Shallow breathing does not facilitate removal of secretions, and forceful coughing promotes collapse of airways. A side-lying position does not allow for adequate chest expansion to promote deep breathing. (P, 7)

The Client With Asthma

77. 4. In an acute asthma attack, diminished or absent breath sounds can be an ominous sign indicating lack of air movement in the lungs and impending respiratory failure. The client requires immediate intervention with inhaled bronchodilators, intravenous corticosteroids, and possibly intravenous theophylline. Administering oxygen and reassessing the client 10 minutes later would delay needed medical intervention, as would drawing blood for an arterial blood gas analysis and obtaining a chest x-ray. It would be futile to encourage the client to relax and breath slowly without providing the necessary pharmacologic intervention. (D, 1)

78. 2. As the severe asthma attack worsens, the client becomes fatigued and alveolar hypoventilation develops. This leads to carbon dioxide retention and hypoxemia. The client develops respiratory acidosis. Therefore, the $PaCO_2$ level increases, the PaO_2 level decreases, and the pH decreases, indicating acidosis. (P, 10)

79. 3. Corticosteroids have an anti-inflammatory effect and act to decrease edema in the bronchial airways and decrease mucus secretion. Corticosteroids do not have a bronchodilator effect, act as expectorants, or prevent respiratory infections. (D, 8)

80. 1. Irregular heartbeats should be reported promptly to the care provider. Metaproterenol may cause irregular heartbeat, tachycardia, or anginal pain because of its adrenergic effect on β-adrenergic receptors in the heart. It is not recommended for use in clients with known cardiac disorders. Metaproterenol does not cause constipation, pedal edema, or bradycardia. (I, 8)

81. 3. Use of oral inhalant corticosteroids, such as flunisolide, can lead to the development of oral thrush, a fungal infection. Once developed, thrush must be treated by antibiotic therapy; it will not resolve on its own. Fungal infections can develop even without overuse of the corticosteroid inhaler. Although good oral hygiene can help prevent development of a fungal infection, it cannot be used alone to treat the problem. (D, 8)

82. 2. When using inhalers, clients should wait about 1 minute between puffs to allow adequate absorption of the medication. It is correct technique to shake the inhaler immediately before use, to activate the MDI on inhalation, and to hold the breath for 10 seconds after inhalation is complete. (I, 8)

83. 4. Between attacks, breath sounds should be clear on auscultation with good air flow present throughout lung fields. Chest x-rays should be normal. The client should remain afebrile. Arterial blood gases should be normal. (E, 10)

84. 1. Physical exercise is beneficial and should be incorporated as tolerated into the client's schedule. Peak flow numbers should be monitored daily, usually in the morning (before taking medication). Peak flow does not need to be monitored after each meal. Stressors in the client's life should be modified but cannot be totally eliminated. Although adequate sleep is important, it is not recommended that sedatives be routinely taken to induce sleep. (P, 9)

85. 2. The most common precipitator of asthma attacks is viral respiratory infection. Clients with asthma should avoid people who have the flu or a cold and should get yearly flu vaccinations. Environmental exposure to toxins or heavy particulate matter can trigger asthma attacks; however, far fewer asthmatics are exposed to such toxins than are exposed to viruses. Cigarette smoke can also trigger asthma attacks, but to a lesser extent than viral respiratory infections. Some asthmatic attacks are triggered by exercising in cold weather. (I, 9)

86. 1. A cough productive of yellow sputum is the most likely indicator of a respiratory infection. The other signs and symptoms—wheezing, chest tightness, and increased respiratory rate—are all findings associated with an asthma attack and do not necessarily mean an infection is present. (A, 10)

The Client With Lung Cancer

87. 1. Risk factors for postoperative pulmonary complications include malnourishment, which is indicated by this client's height and weight. It is thought that emotional responses can affect overall health; however, not verbalizing one's feelings is not a contributing factor in postoperative pulmonary complications. The client's current activity level and age do not place her at increased risk for complications. (A, 10)

88. 1. Acknowledging the basic feeling the client expresses—fear—and asking an open-ended question allows the client to explain her fears. The other options dismiss the client's feelings and may give false reassurance or label the client's feelings. The client should be encouraged to explore her own feelings. (I, 5)

89. 4. Systematic pain assessment is necessary for adequate pain management in the postoperative client. Guidelines from the Agency for Health Care Research recommend that institutions adopt a pain assessment scale to assist in facilitating pain management. Even though the client is receiving morphine sulfate by PCA, assessment is needed if she is experiencing pain. The concern is not to eliminate coughing but to control pain adequately. Coughing is necessary to prevent postoperative atelectasis and pneumonia. Breathing exercises may help control pain in some circumstances; however, most clients with thoracic surgery require parenteral opioid analgesics in the early postoperative period. Although it is necessary that the PCA device be checked periodically to ensure that it is functioning properly, if the machine is functional and the client's pain is not relieved further intervention, beginning with a pain assessment, is indicated. (A, 7)

90. 1. Because clients are discharged as soon as possible from the hospital, it is essential to evaluate the support they have to assist them with self-care at home. The distance the client lives from the hospital is not a critical factor in discharge planning. There are no data indicating that home blood pressure monitoring is needed. Knowledge of the causes of lung cancer, although important, is not the most essential area to evaluate given the client's postoperative status. (E, 5)

91. 2. Epidermoid cancer involving the larger bronchi is almost entirely associated with heavy cigarette smoking. The American Cancer Society reports that smoking is responsible for more than 80% of lung cancers in men and women. The prevalence of lung cancer is related to the duration and intensity of the smoking, so nurses can best prevent lung cancer by persuading clients to stop smoking. Chest radiographs aid in detection of lung cancer; they do not prevent it. Exposure to asbestos has been implicated as a risk factor for lung cancer, but cigarette smoking is the major risk factor. There are no data to support the use of home air cleaners in the prevention of lung cancer. (I, 4)

92. 4. Deep breathing helps prevent microatelectasis and pneumonitis and also helps force air and fluid out of the pleural space into the chest tubes. More than half of the ventilatory process is accomplished by the rise and fall of the diaphragm. The diaphragm is the major muscle of respiration; deep breathing causes it to descend, not elevate, thereby increasing the ventilating surface. Deep breathing increases blood flow to the lungs; however, the primary reason for deep breathing is to expand alveoli and prevent atelectasis. The remaining lobe naturally hyperinflates to fill the space created by the resected lobe. This is an expected phenomenon. (I, 10)

93. 2. It is essential that the nurse evaluate the effects of pain medication after the medication has had time to act; reassessment is necessary to determine the effectiveness of the pain management plan. Although it is

prudent to check for discomfort related to positioning when assessing the client's pain, repositioning the client immediately after administering pain medication is not necessary. Verbally reassuring the client after administering pain medication may be useful to help instill confidence in the treatment plan; however, it is not as important as evaluating the effectiveness of the medication. Readjusting the pain medication dosage as needed according to the client's condition is essential, but the effectiveness of the medication must be evaluated first. (I, 10)

94. 3. This crackling sensation is subcutaneous emphysema. Subcutaneous emphysema is not an unusual finding, and it is not dangerous if confined. But progression can be serious, especially if the neck is involved; a tracheotomy may be needed. If emphysema progresses noticeably in 1 hour, the physician should be notified. Lowering the head of the bed will not arrest the progress or provide any further information. A tracheotomy tray would be useful if emphysema progresses to the neck. Emphysema may progress if the chest drainage system does not adequately remove air and fluid; therefore, the system should not be turned off. (I, 10)

95. 1. The recommended procedure for teaching clients postoperatively to deep breathe includes contracting (pulling in) the abdominal muscles and taking a slow, deep breath through the nose. This breath is held 3 to 5 seconds, which facilitates alveolar ventilation by improving the inspiratory phase of ventilation. Exhaling slowly as if trying to blow out a candle is a technique used in pursed-lip breathing to facilitate exhalation in clients with chronic obstructive pulmonary disease. It is recommended that the abdominal muscles be contracted, not relaxed, to promote deep breathing. The client should breathe through the nose. (I, 10)

96. 3. A client who has undergone chest surgery should be taught to raise the arm on the affected side over the head to help prevent shoulder ankylosis. This exercise helps restore normal shoulder movement, prevents stiffening of the shoulder joint, and improves muscle tone and power. Turning from side to side, raising and lowering the head, and flexing and extending the elbow on the affected side do not exercise the shoulder joint. (I, 7)

97. 4. The drainage apparatus is always kept *below* the client's chest level to prevent back flow of fluid into the pleural space. The air vent must always be open in the closed chest drainage system to allow air from the client to escape. Stripping a chest tube causes excessive negative intrapleural pressure and is not recommended. Clamping a chest tube when moving a client is not recommended. (I, 10)

98. 1. Cessation of fluid fluctuation in the tubing can mean one of several things: the lung has fully expanded and

negative intrapleural pressure has been re-established; the chest tube is occluded; or the chest tube is not in the pleural space. Fluid fluctuation occurs because, during inspiration, intrapleural pressure exceeds the negative pressure generated in the water-seal system. Therefore, drainage moves toward the client. During expiration, the pleural pressure exceeds that generated in the water-seal system, and fluid moves away from the client. When the lung is collapsed or the chest tube is in the pleural space, fluid fluctuation is likely to be noted. The chest tube is not inserted in the mediastinal space. (A, 10)

99. 2. There should never be constant bubbling in the water-seal bottle; normally the bubbling is intermittent. Constant bubbling in the water-seal bottle indicates an air leak, which means that less negative pressure is being exerted on the pleural space. Decreasing the suction or draining part of the water in the water-seal chamber will not reduce the leak. (I, 10)

100. 1. In this case, there may be some obstruction to the flow of air and fluid out of the pleural space, causing air and fluid to collect and build up pressure. This prevents the remaining lung from re-expanding and can cause a mediastinal shift to the opposite side. The nurse's first response is to assess the tubing for kinks or obstruction. Increasing the suction is not done without a physician's order. The normal position of the drainage bottles is 2 to 3 feet below chest level. Clamping the tubes obstructs the flow of air and fluid out of the pleural space and should not be done. (I, 10)

101. 2. The chest drainage system is set up properly. The chest tube is attached to the drainage system and does not need to be clamped; there is sufficient water to maintain the water seal; the drainage from the patient has not exceeded the capacity of the drainage system. The nurse should chart the amount and color of the drainage every 4 to 8 hours. (I, 10)

102. 3. A bottle of sterile water should be readily available and in view when a client has a chest tube so that the tube can be immediately submersed in the water if the chest tube system becomes disconnected. The chest tube should be reconnected to the water-seal system as soon as a sterile functioning system can be re-established. There is no need for a tracheostomy tray, another chest tube, or a spirometer to be placed at the bedside for emergency use. (P, 10)

The Client With Chest Trauma

103. 2. Blunt chest trauma may lead to respiratory failure, and maintenance of adequate oxygenation is the priority for the client. Decreasing the client's anxiety is related to maintaining effective respirations and oxygenation. Although pain is distressing to the client and can increase anxiety and decrease respiratory effectiveness, pain control is secondary to maintaining oxygenation. Maintaining adequate circulatory volume is also secondary to maintaining adequate oxygenation. (P, 10)

104. 3. Fluctuation of fluid in the water-seal column with respirations indicates that the system is functioning properly. If an obstruction were present in the chest tube, fluid fluctuation would be absent. Subcutaneous emphysema occurs when air pockets can be palpated beneath the client's skin around the chest tube insertion site. A leak in the system is indicated when continuous bubbling occurs in the water-seal column. (E, 10)

105. 2. Continuous bubbling in the water-seal chamber indicates a leak in the system, and the client needs to be instructed to notify the physician if continuous bubbling occurs. A respiratory rate of more than 16 breaths/minute may not be unusual and does not necessarily mean that the client should notify the physician. Fluid in the chest tube is expected, as is fluctuation of the fluid in the water-seal chamber. (I, 10)

106. 4. Pneumothorax means that the lung has collapsed and is not functioning. The nurse will hear no sounds of air movement on auscultation. Movement of air through mucus produces crackles. Wheezing occurs when airways become obstructed. Dullness on percussion indicates increased density of lung tissue, usually caused by accumulation of fluid. (A, 10)

107. 1. If the client reports no pain, then the objective of adequate pain relief has been met. Decreased anxiety is not related only to pain control; it could also be related to other factors. A respiratory rate of 26 breaths/minute is not within normal limits. A PaO_2 of 70 mm Hg is not within normal limits. (E, 10)

108. 2. One unit of packed red blood cells is about 250 mL. If the blood is delivered at a rate of 60 mL/hour, it will take about 4 hours to infuse the entire unit. The transfusion of a single unit of packed red blood cells should not exceed 4 hours to prevent the growth of bacteria and minimize the risk of septicemia. (I, 8)

109. 2. Too-rapid infusion of blood, or any intravenous fluid, can cause fluid volume overload and related problems such as pulmonary edema. Emboli formation, red blood cell hemolysis, and allergic reaction are not related to rapid infusion. (I, 8)

110. 4. Immediately after chest tube removal, a petrolatum gauze is placed over the wound and covered with a dry sterile dressing. This serves as an airtight seal to prevent air leakage or air movement in either direction. Bandages are not applied directly over wounds. Montgomery straps are used in place of adhesive when a dressing require very frequent changes and the constant removal of adhesive would damage the skin.

They are not placed over open wounds. Mesh gauze would allow air movement. (I, 10)

111. 1. Pneumothorax signs and symptoms include sudden, sharp chest pain; tachypnea; and tachycardia. Other signs and symptoms include diminished or absent breath sounds over the affected lung, anxiety, and restlessness. Breath sounds are diminished or absent over the affected side. Hemoptysis and cyanosis are not typically present with a moderate pneumothorax. (A, 10)

112. 4. A chest tube is inserted to re-expand the lung and remove air and fluid. Oxygen is not administered through a chest tube. Chest tubes are not inserted to promote scar tissue formation. Antibiotics are not used to treat a pneumothorax. (D, 7)

Care of the Client With Acute Respiratory Failure

113. 4. One of the major risk factors for development of ARDS is hypovolemic shock. Adequate fluid replacement is essential to minimize the risk of ARDS in these clients. Teaching smoking cessation does not prevent ARDS. An abnormal serum potassium level and hypercapnia are not risk factors for ARDS. (I, 10)

114. 1. Ineffective Breathing Pattern is a priority nursing diagnosis category for the client with ARDS. The massive shift of fluid from the capillaries to the alveoli, as well as the reduced surfactant, greatly increases the work of breathing. The lungs become stiff and noncompliant, and the client becomes severely hypoxic. The client with ARDS usually requires endotracheal intubation and mechanical ventilation. Pain and Ineffective Health Maintenance are not priority nursing diagnoses for a client with ARDS. Although the client may be at risk for development of an infection, a higher-priority nursing diagnosis is maintaining an airway. (D, 10)

115. 2. A hallmark of early ARDS is refractory hypoxemia. The client's PaO_2 level continues to fall, despite higher concentrations of administered oxygen. Elevated carbon dioxide and metabolic acidosis occur late in the disorder. Severe electrolyte imbalances are not indicators of ARDS. (A, 10)

116. 3. The $PaCO_2$ level of 28 mm Hg indicates that the client is hyperventilating. Normal $PaCO_2$ levels are between 35 and 45 mm Hg. In hyperventilation, carbon dioxide is excreted at an increased rate, and the $PaCO_2$ falls below 35 mm Hg. The client develops respiratory alkalosis. $PaCO_2$ levels do not measure arterial blood oxygen. Hypoventilation causes increased $PaCO_2$ levels. Oxygen toxicity does not cause decreased $PaCO_2$ levels. (D, 10)

117. 1. Normal PaO_2 level ranges between 80 and 100 mm Hg. When the PaO_2 value falls to 50 mm Hg, the nurse

should be alert for signs of hypoxia and impending respiratory failure. An oxygen level this low poses a severe risk for respiratory failure. The PaO_2 is not within normal range. The client will require oxygenation at a concentration that maintains the PaO_2 at 55 to 60 mm Hg or more. (D, 10)

118. 4. A $PaCO_2$ of 28 mm Hg and PaO_2 of 50 mm Hg are both abnormal; the PaO_2 of 50 mm Hg signifies acute respiratory failure. In evaluating possible causes for this disorder, the nurse should consider conditions that lead to hypoxia and hyperventilation, such as pulmonary embolus. COPD is typically associated with respiratory acidosis and elevated $PaCO_2$. The client with diabetic ketoacidosis most often has metabolic acidosis. A myocardial infarction does not often cause an acid-base imbalance because the primary problem is cardiac in origin. (D, 10)

119. 3. Endotracheal intubation and mechanical ventilation are required in ARDS to maintain adequate respiratory support. Endotracheal intubation, not a tracheostomy, is usually the initial method of maintaining an airway. (P, 10)

120. 1. The two risk factors most commonly associated with the development of ARDS are gram-negative septic shock and gastric content aspiration. Nurses should be particularly vigilant in assessing a client for onset of ARDS if the client has experienced direct lung trauma or a systemic inflammatory response syndrome (which can be caused by any physiologic insult that leads to widespread inflammation). (P, 9)

121. 4. Auscultation for bilateral breath sounds is the most appropriate method for determining cuff placement. The nurse should also look for the symmetric rise and fall of the chest and should note the location of the exit mark on the tube. Assessments of skin color, respiratory rate, and the amount of cuff inflation cannot validate the placement of the endotracheal tube. (I, 7)

122. 4. The nurse should suction the client if the client is not able to cough up secretions and clear the airway. Administering oxygen will not promote airway clearance. The client should be turned every 2 hours to help move secretions; every 4 hours is not often enough. Administering sedatives is contraindicated in acute respiratory distress because sedatives can depress respirations. (I, 10)

123. 1. Gastrointestinal hemorrhage occurs in about 25% of clients receiving prolonged mechanical ventilation, because of the development of stress ulcers. Clients who are receiving steroid therapy and those with a previous history of ulcers are most likely to be at risk. Other possible complications include incorrect ventilation, oxygen toxicity, fluid imbalance, decreased cardiac output, pneumothorax, infection, and atelectasis. (A, 10)

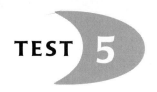

TEST 5

The Client With Upper Gastrointestinal Tract Health Problems

- ▶ **The Client With Disorders of the Oral Cavity**
- ▶ **The Client With Peptic Ulcer Disease**
- ▶ **The Client With Cancer of the Stomach**
- ▶ **The Client With Gastroesophageal Reflux Disease**
- ▶ **Correct Answers and Rationale**

Select the one best answer, and indicate your choice by filling in the circle in front of the option.

The Client With Disorders of the Oral Cavity

1. A client who has a history of a mitral valve prolapse tells the nurse during a clinic visit that she is scheduled to get her teeth cleaned. Which of the following replies by the nurse is *most* appropriate?
   - ○ 1. "The physician will need to re-evaluate the status of your heart condition before your dental appointment."
   - ◉ 2. "Be sure to remind your dentist that you have a heart condition."
   - ○ 3. "It is important for you to care for your teeth because your heart condition makes you more susceptible to developing oral infections."
   - ◉ 4. "We will prescribe a prophylactic antibiotic for you to take before getting your teeth cleaned."

2. The nurse instructs the nursing assistant on how to provide oral hygiene for a client who cannot perform this task for himself. Which of the following techniques should the nurse tell the assistant to incorporate into the client's daily care?
   - ○ 1. Assess the oral cavity each time mouth care is given and record observations.
   - ◉ 2. Use a soft toothbrush to brush the client's teeth after each meal.
   - ○ 3. Swab the client's tongue, gums, and lips with a soft foam applicator every 2 hours.
   - ○ 4. Rinse the client's mouth with mouthwash several times a day.

3. During the assessment of a client's mouth, the nurse notes the absence of saliva. The client is also complaining of pain in the area of the ear. The client has been NPO for several days because of the insertion of a nasogastric tube. Based on these findings, the

nurse suspects that the client may be developing which of the following mouth conditions?
   - ○ 1. Stomatitis.
   - ○ 2. Oral candidiasis.
   - ◉ 3. Parotitis.
   - ○ 4. Gingivitis.

4. The nurse is preparing a community presentation on oral cancer. Which of the following is a primary risk factor for oral cancer that the nurse should include in the presentation?
   - ◉ 1. Use of alcohol.
   - ○ 2. Frequent use of mouthwash.
   - ○ 3. Lack of vitamin B_{12}.
   - ○ 4. Lack of regular teeth cleaning by a dentist.

5. A client has entered a smoking cessation program to quit a two-pack-a-day cigarette habit. He tells the occupational health nurse at his place of employment that he has not smoked a cigarette for 3 weeks, but is afraid he is going to "slip up" and smoke because of current job pressures. What would be the most appropriate reply for the nurse to make in response to the client's comments?
   - ○ 1. "Don't worry about it. Everybody has difficulty quitting smoking, and you should expect to as well."
   - ○ 2. "If you increase your self-control, I am sure you will be able to avoid smoking."
   - ○ 3. "Try taking a couple of days of vacation to relieve the stress of your job."
   - ◉ 4. "It is good that you can talk about your concerns. Try calling a friend when you want to smoke."

6. A client who was in a motor vehicle accident has a fractured mandible. Surgery has been performed to

immobilize the injury by wiring the jaw. What is the nurse's priority in regard to care in the immediate postoperative phase?
- ○ 1. Prevent nausea and vomiting.
- ◉ 2. Maintain a patent airway.
- ○ 3. Provide frequent oral hygiene.
- ○ 4. Establish a way for the client to communicate.

7. A client has returned from surgery during which her jaws were wired as treatment for a fractured mandible. The client is in stable condition. The nurse is instructing the assistant on how to properly position the client. Which instructions about positioning would be appropriate for the nurse to give the assistant?
- ◉ 1. Keep the client in a side-lying position with the head slightly elevated.
- ○ 2. Do not reposition the client without the assistance of a registered nurse.
- ○ 3. The client can assume any position that is comfortable.
- ○ 4. Keep the client's head elevated on two pillows at all times.

8. A client who has had her jaws wired begins to vomit. What should be the nurse's *first* action?
- ○ 1. Insert a nasogastric tube and connect it to suction.
- ◉ 2. Use wire cutters to cut the wire.
- ◉ 3. Suction the client's airway as needed.
- ○ 4. Administer an antiemetic intravenously.

The Client With Peptic Ulcer Disease

9. A client is admitted to the hospital after vomiting bright red blood and is diagnosed with a bleeding duodenal ulcer. The client develops a sudden, sharp pain in the midepigastric region along with a rigid, boardlike abdomen. These clinical manifestations most likely indicate which of the following?
- ○ 1. An intestinal obstruction has developed.
- ○ 2. Additional ulcers have developed.
- ○ 3. The esophagus has become inflamed.
- ○ 4. The ulcer has perforated.

10. A client with peptic ulcer disease tells the nurse that he has black stools, which he has not reported to his physician. Based on this information, which nursing diagnosis would be appropriate for this client?
- ○ 1. Ineffective Coping related to fear of diagnosis of chronic illness.
- ◉ 2. Deficient Knowledge related to unfamiliarity with significant signs and symptoms.
- ○ 3. Constipation related to decreased gastric motility.
- ○ 4. Imbalanced Nutrition: Less Than Body Requirements related to gastric bleeding.

11. The client asks the nurse what causes a peptic ulcer to develop. The nurse responds that recent research indicates that many peptic ulcers are the result of which of the following?
- ○ 1. Work-related stress.
- ○ 2. *Helicobacter pylori* infection.
- ○ 3. Diets high in fat.
- ○ 4. A genetic defect in the gastric mucosa.

12. A client with a peptic ulcer reports epigastric pain that frequently awakens her during the night, a feeling of fullness in the abdomen, and a feeling of anxiety about her health. Based on this information, which nursing diagnosis would be *most* appropriate?
- ○ 1. Imbalanced Nutrition: Less than Body Requirements related to anorexia.
- ○ 2. Disturbed Sleep Pattern related to epigastric pain.
- ○ 3. Ineffective Coping related to exacerbation of duodenal ulcer.
- ○ 4. Activity Intolerance related to abdominal pain.

13. The nurse is preparing to teach a client with a peptic ulcer about the diet that should be followed after discharge. The nurse should explain that the diet will most likely consist of which of the following?
- ○ 1. Bland foods.
- ○ 2. High-protein foods.
- ○ 3. Any foods that are tolerated.
- ○ 4. Large amounts of milk.

14. The nurse finds a client who has been diagnosed with a peptic ulcer surrounded by papers from his briefcase and arguing on the telephone with a coworker. The nurse's response to observing these actions should be based on knowledge that
- ○ 1. involvement with his job will keep the client from becoming bored.
- ○ 2. a relaxed environment will promote ulcer healing.
- ○ 3. not keeping up with his job will increase the client's stress level.
- ○ 4. setting limits on the client's behavior is an important nursing responsibility.

15. A client with a peptic ulcer has been instructed to avoid intense physical activity and stress. Which activity should the client incorporate into the home care plan?
- ○ 1. Conduct physical activity in the morning so that he can rest in the afternoon.
- ○ 2. Have the family agree to perform the necessary yard work at home.
- ○ 3. Give up jogging and substitute a less demanding hobby.
- ○ 4. Incorporate periods of physical and mental rest in his daily schedule.

16. A client is to take one daily dose of ranitidine (Zantac) at home to treat her peptic ulcer. The nurse

knows that the client understands proper drug administration of ranitidine when she says that she will take the drug at which of the following times?
○ 1. Before meals.
○ 2. With meals.
○ 3. At bedtime.
○ 4. When pain occurs.

17. A client has been taking aluminum hydroxide (Amphojel) 30 mL six times per day at home to treat his peptic ulcer. He tells the nurse that he has been unable to have a bowel movement for 3 days. Based on this information, the nurse would determine that which of the following is the most likely cause of the client's constipation?
○ 1. The client has not been including enough fiber in his diet.
○ 2. The client needs to increase his daily exercise.
○ 3. The client is experiencing a side effect of the aluminum hydroxide.
○ 4. The client has developed a gastrointestinal obstruction.

18. A client is taking an antacid for treatment of a peptic ulcer. Which of the following statements best indicates that the client understands how to correctly take the antacid?
○ 1. "I should take my antacid before I take my other medications."
○ 2. "I need to decrease my intake of fluids so that I don't dilute the effects of my antacid."
○ 3. "My antacid will be most effective if I take it whenever I experience stomach pains."
○ 4. "It is best for me to take my antacid 1 to 3 hours after meals."

19. Which of the following would be an expected outcome for a client with peptic ulcer disease?
○ 1. The client will demonstrate appropriate use of analgesics to control pain.
○ 2. The client will explain the rationale for eliminating alcohol from the diet.
○ 3. The client will verbalize the importance of monitoring hemoglobin and hematocrit every 3 months.
○ 4. The client will eliminate contact sports from his or her lifestyle.

The Client With Cancer of the Stomach

20. A client with suspected gastric cancer undergoes an endoscopy of the stomach. Which of the following assessments made after the procedure would indicate the development of a potential complication?
○ 1. The client complains of a sore throat.
○ 2. The client displays signs of sedation.

○ 3. The client experiences a sudden increase in temperature.
○ 4. The client demonstrates a lack of appetite.

21. A client has been diagnosed with adenocarcinoma of the stomach and is scheduled to undergo a subtotal gastrectomy (Billroth II procedure). During preoperative teaching, the nurse is reinforcing information about the surgical procedure. Which of the following explanations is most accurate?
○ 1. The procedure will result in enlargement of the pyloric sphincter.
○ 2. The procedure will result in anastomosis of the gastric stump to the jejunum.
○ 3. The procedure will result in removal of the duodenum.
○ 4. The procedure will result in repositioning of the vagus nerve.

22. The client tells the nurse that since his diagnosis of stomach cancer, he has been having trouble sleeping and is frequently preoccupied with thoughts about how his life will change. He says, "I wish my life could stay the same." Based on this information, which one of the following nursing diagnoses would be appropriate at this time?
○ 1. Ineffective Coping related to the diagnosis of cancer.
○ 2. Disturbed Sleep Pattern related to fear of the unknown.
○ 3. Anticipatory Grieving related to the diagnosis of cancer.
○ 4. Anxiety related to the need for gastric surgery.

23. After a subtotal gastrectomy, the nurse should anticipate that nasogastric tube drainage will be what color for about 12 to 24 hours after surgery?
○ 1. Dark brown.
○ 2. Bile green.
○ 3. Bright red.
○ 4. Cloudy white.

24. After a subtotal gastrectomy, care of the client's nasogastric tube and drainage system should include which of the following nursing interventions?
○ 1. Irrigate the tube with 30 mL of sterile water every hour, if needed.
○ 2. Reposition the tube if it is not draining well.
○ 3. Monitor the client for nausea, vomiting, and abdominal distention.
○ 4. Turn the machine to high suction if the drainage is sluggish on low suction.

25. The nurse understands that the best position for the client who has undergone a gastrectomy is
○ 1. prone.
○ 2. supine.
○ 3. low Fowler's.
○ 4. right or left Sims'.

26. As part of the client's discharge planning after a subtotal gastrectomy, the nurse has identified Imbalanced Nutrition: Less Than Body Requirements as a major nursing diagnosis. To help the client meet nutritional goals at home, the nurse should develop a plan of care that includes which of the following interventions?
    - ○ 1. Instruct the client to increase the amount eaten at each meal.
    - ○ 2. Encourage the client to eat smaller amounts more frequently.
    - ○ 3. Explain that if vomiting occurs after a meal, nothing more should be eaten that day.
    - ○ 4. Inform the client that bland foods are typically less nutritional and should be used minimally.

27. As a result of a gastric resection, the client is at risk for development of dumping syndrome. The nurse would prepare a plan of care for this client based on knowledge that this problem stems primarily from which of the following gastrointestinal changes?
    - ○ 1. Excess secretion of digestive enzymes in the intestines.
    - ○ 2. Rapid emptying of stomach contents into the small intestine.
    - ○ 3. Excess glycogen production by the liver.
    - ○ 4. Loss of gastric enzymes.

28. To reduce the risk of dumping syndrome, the nurse should teach the client which of the following interventions?
    - ○ 1. Sit upright for 30 minutes after meals.
    - ○ 2. Drink liquids with meals, avoiding caffeine.
    - ○ 3. Avoid milk and other dairy products.
    - ○ 4. Decrease the carbohydrate content of meals.

29. A client who is recovering from a subtotal gastrectomy asks the nurse, "When will I be able to eat three meals a day again like I used to?" Which of the following responses by the nurse is most appropriate?
    - ○ 1. "Eating six meals a day is time-consuming, isn't it?"
    - ○ 2. "You will have to eat six small meals a day for the rest of your life."
    - ○ 3. "You will be able to tolerate three meals a day before you are discharged."
    - ○ 4. "Most clients can resume their normal meal patterns in about 6 to 12 months."

30. Which of the following symptoms would be indicative of the dumping syndrome?
    - ○ 1. Hunger.
    - ○ 2. Vomiting.
    - ○ 3. Diaphoresis.
    - ○ 4. Heartburn.

31. After surgery for gastric cancer, a client is scheduled to undergo radiation therapy. It will be most important for the nurse to include information about which of the following in the client's teaching plan?

- ○ 1. Nutritional intake.
- ○ 2. Management of alopecia.
- ○ 3. Exercise and activity levels.
- ○ 4. Access to community resources.

32. Which of the following would be an expected nutritional outcome for a client who has undergone a subtotal gastrectomy for cancer?
    - ○ 1. Regain weight loss within 1 month after surgery.
    - ○ 2. Resume normal dietary intake of three meals a day.
    - ○ 3. Control nausea and vomiting through regular use of antiemetics.
    - ○ 4. Achieve optimal nutritional status through oral or parenteral feedings.

The Client With Gastroesophageal Reflux Disease

33. The client is scheduled to have an upper gastrointestinal tract series. Which of the following treatments should the nurse anticipate after the examination?
    - ○ 1. Administering a laxative.
    - ○ 2. Placing the client on a clear liquid diet.
    - ○ 3. Giving the client a tapwater enema.
    - ○ 4. Starting an intravenous infusion.

34. A client who has been diagnosed with gastroesophageal reflux disease (GERD) complains of heartburn. To decrease the heartburn, the nurse should instruct the client to eliminate which of the following items from the diet?
    - ○ 1. Lean beef.
    - ○ 2. Air-popped popcorn.
    - ○ 3. Hot chocolate.
    - ○ 4. Raw vegetables.

35. The client with GERD complains of a chronic cough. The nurse understands that in a client with GERD this symptom may be indicative of which of the following conditions?
    - ○ 1. Development of laryngeal cancer.
    - ○ 2. Irritation of the esophagus.
    - ○ 3. Esophageal scar tissue formation.
    - ○ 4. Aspiration of gastric contents.

36. Bethanechol (Urecholine) has been ordered for a client with GERD. The nurse should evaluate the client for which of the following side effects?
    - ○ 1. Constipation.
    - ○ 2. Urinary urgency.
    - ○ 3. Hypertension.
    - ○ 4. Dry oral mucosa.

37. The client attends two sessions with the dietitian to learn about diet modifications to minimize gastroesophageal reflux. The teaching would be considered

successful if the client says that she will decrease her intake of which of the following foods?

- ○ 1. Fats.
- ○ 2. High-sodium foods.
- ○ 3. Carbohydrates.
- ○ 4. High-calcium foods.

38. Which of the following dietary measures would be useful in preventing esophageal reflux?

- ○ 1. Eating small, frequent meals.
- ○ 2. Increasing fluid intake.
- ○ 3. Avoiding air swallowing with meals.
- ○ 4. Adding a bedtime snack to the dietary plan.

39. The nurse understands that the primary symptoms of a sliding hiatal hernia are associated with reflux. Therefore, the nurse should assess the client for which of the following symptoms?

- ○ 1. Heartburn.
- ○ 2. Jaundice.
- ○ 3. Anorexia.
- ○ 4. Stomatitis.

40. Which of the following factors would most likely contribute to the development of a client's hiatal hernia?

- ○ 1. Having a sedentary desk job.
- ○ 2. Being 5 feet, 3 inches tall and weighing 190 pounds.
- ○ 3. Using laxatives frequently.
- ○ 4. Being 40 years old.

41. Which of the following nursing interventions would most likely promote self-care behaviors in the client with a hiatal hernia?

- ○ 1. Introduce the client to other people who are successfully managing their care.
- ○ 2. Include the client's daughter in the teaching so that she can help implement the plan.
- ○ 3. Ask the client to identify other situations in which he demonstrated responsibility for himself.
- ○ 4. Reassure the client that he will be able to implement all aspects of the plan successfully.

42. The client has been taking magnesium hydroxide (milk of magnesia) at home in an attempt to control hiatal hernia symptoms. The nurse should assess the client for which of the following conditions most commonly associated with the ongoing use of magnesium-based antacids?

- ○ 1. Anorexia.
- ○ 2. Weight gain.
- ○ 3. Diarrhea.
- ○ 4. Constipation.

43. Which of the following lifestyle modifications should the nurse encourage the client with a hiatal hernia to include in activities of daily living?

- ○ 1. Daily aerobic exercise.
- ○ 2. Eliminating smoking and alcohol use.
- ○ 3. Balancing activity and rest.
- ○ 4. Avoiding high-stress situations.

44. In developing a teaching plan for the client with a hiatal hernia, the nurse's assessment of which work-related factors would be most useful?

- ○ 1. Number and length of breaks.
- ○ 2. Body mechanics used in lifting.
- ○ 3. Temperature in the work area.
- ○ 4. Cleaning solvents used.

45. The nurse instructs the client on health maintenance activities to help control symptoms from her hiatal hernia. Which of the following statements would indicate that the client has understood the instructions?

- ○ 1. "I'll avoid lying down after a meal."
- ○ 2. "I can still enjoy my potato chips and cola at bedtime."
- ○ 3. "I wish I didn't have to give up swimming."
- ○ 4. "If I wear a girdle, I'll have more support for my stomach."

46. The physician prescribes metoclopramide hydrochloride (Reglan) for the client with hiatal hernia. The nurse plans to instruct the client that this drug is used in hiatal hernia therapy to accomplish which of the following objectives?

- ○ 1. Increase the resting tone of the esophageal sphincter.
- ○ 2. Neutralize gastric secretions.
- ○ 3. Delay gastric emptying.
- ○ 4. Reduce secretion of digestive juices.

47. The nurse should instruct the client to avoid which of the following drugs while taking metoclopramide hydrochloride (Reglan)?

- ○ 1. Antacids.
- ○ 2. Antihypertensives.
- ○ 3. Anticoagulants.
- ○ 4. Alcohol.

48. Cimetidine (Tagamet) may also be used to treat hiatal hernia. The nurse should understand that this drug is used to prevent which of the following?

- ○ 1. Esophageal reflux.
- ○ 2. Dysphagia.
- ○ 3. Esophagitis.
- ○ 4. Ulcer formation.

49. The client asks the nurse whether he will need surgery to correct his hiatal hernia. Which reply by the nurse would be most accurate?

- ○ 1. "Surgery is usually required, although medical treatment is attempted first."
- ○ 2. "Hiatal hernia symptoms can usually be successfully managed with diet modifications, medications, and lifestyle changes."
- ○ 3. "Surgery is not performed for this type of hernia."
- ○ 4. "A minor surgical procedure to reduce the size of the diaphragmatic opening will probably be planned."

Correct Answers and Rationale

The letters in parentheses following the rationale identify the step of the nursing process (A, D, P, I, E) and client needs (1, 2, 3, 4, 5, 6, 7, 8, 9, 10). See the inside front cover for the key.

The Client With Disorders of the Oral Cavity

1. 4. Clients who are at risk for developing infective endocarditis due to cardiac conditions such as mitral valve prolapse must take prophylactic antibiotics before any dental procedure that may cause bleeding. The client is not more susceptible to developing oral infections. Rather, the client is more susceptible to developing endocarditis that results from oral bacteria that enter the circulation during the dental procedure. The physician does not necessarily need to re-evaluate the heart condition of a client who is stable, but antibiotics must be prescribed. It is not enough to simply remind the dentist about the heart condition. (I, 9)

2. 2. A soft toothbrush should be used to brush the client's teeth after every meal and more often as needed. Mechanical cleansing is necessary to maintain oral health, stimulate gingiva, and remove plaque. Assessing the oral cavity and recording observations is the responsibility of the nurse, not the nursing assistant. Swabbing with a safe foam applicator does not provide enough friction to cleanse the mouth. Mouthwash can be a drying irritant and is not recommended for frequent use. (I, 7)

3. 3. The lack of saliva, pain near the area of the ear, and the prolonged NPO status of the client should lead the nurse to suspect the development of parotitis, or inflammation of the parotid gland. Parotitis usually develops in cases of dehydration combined with poor oral hygiene or when clients have been NPO for an extended period. Preventive measures include the use of sugarless hard candy or gum to stimulate saliva production, adequate hydration, and frequent mouth care. Stomatitis (inflammation of the mouth) produces excessive salivation and a sore mouth. Oral candidiasis (thrush) causes bluish-white mouth lesions. Gingivitis can be recognized by the inflamed gingiva and bleeding that occur during toothbrushing. (A, 7)

4. 1. Chronic and excessive use of alcohol can lead to oral cancer. Smoking and use of smokeless tobacco are other significant risk factors. Additional risk factors include chronic irritation such as a broken tooth or ill-fitting dentures, poor dental hygiene, overexposure to sun (lip cancer), and syphilis. Use of mouthwash, lack of vitamin B_{12}, and lack of regular teeth cleaning appointments have not been implicated as primary risk factors for oral cancer. (P, 4)

5. 4. It is important for individuals who are engaged in smoking cessation efforts to feel comfortable with sharing their fears of failure with others and seeking support. Although fewer than 5% of smokers successfully quit on their first attempt, it is not helpful to tell a client that he should anticipate failure. Telling the client to exercise more self-control does not provide him with support. Taking a vacation to avoid job pressures does not address the issue of fearing he will smoke a cigarette when in a stressful situation. (I, 5)

6. 2. The priority of care in the immediate postoperative phase is to maintain a patent airway. The nurse should observe the client carefully for signs of respiratory distress. If the client becomes nauseated, antiemetics should be administered to decrease the chance of vomiting with obstruction of the airway and aspiration of vomitus. Providing frequent oral hygiene and an alternative means of communication are important aspects of nursing care, but maintaining a patent airway is most important. (P, 10)

7. 1. Immediately after surgery the client should be placed on the side with the head slightly elevated. This position helps facilitate removal of secretions and decreases the likelihood of aspiration should vomiting occur. A registered nurse does not need to be present to reposition the client, unless the client's condition warrants the presence of the nurse. Although it is important to elevate the head, there is no need to keep the client's head elevated on two pillows unless that position is comfortable for the client. (I, 9)

8. 3. The nurse's first action is to clear the client's airway as necessary. Inserting a nasogastric tube or administering an antiemetic may prevent future vomiting episodes, but these procedures are not helpful when the client is actually vomiting. Cutting the wires is done only as a last resort or in case of respiratory or cardiac arrest. (I, 10)

The Client With Peptic Ulcer Disease

9. 4. The body reacts to perforation of an ulcer by immobilizing the area as much as possible. This results in boardlike abdominal rigidity, usually with extreme pain. This may occur over several hours or days. It is a medical emergency requiring immediate intervention.

An intestinal obstruction would not cause midepigastric pain. Esophageal inflammation or the development of additional ulcers would not cause a rigid, boardlike abdomen. (D, 10)

10. 2. Black, tarry stools are an important warning sign of bleeding in peptic ulcer disease. Digested blood in the stool causes it to be black. The odor of the stool is very offensive. Clients with peptic ulcer disease should be instructed to report the incidence of black stools promptly to their primary health care provider. (D, 7)

11. 2. Recent research has indicated that most peptic ulcers may be caused by *Helicobacter pylori*, which is a gram-negative bacterium. If this organism is detected through diagnostic tests, treatment of the ulcer will include the use of antibiotics and bismuth compounds such as Pepto-Bismol. It has not been proven that work-related stress or a genetic defect causes ulcers. Diets high in fat do not cause peptic ulcer disease. (I, 10)

12. 2. Based on the data provided, the most appropriate nursing diagnosis would be Disturbed Sleep Pattern. A client with a duodenal ulcer commonly awakens during the night with pain. The client's feelings of anxiety do not necessarily indicate that she is coping ineffectively. (D, 7)

13. 3. Diet therapy for ulcer disease is a controversial issue. There is no scientific evidence that diet therapy promotes healing. Most clients are instructed to follow a diet that they can tolerate. There is no need for the client to ingest only a bland or high-protein diet. Milk may be included in the diet, but it is not recommended in excessive amounts. (P, 7)

14. 2. A relaxed environment is an essential component of ulcer healing. Nurses can help clients understand the importance of relaxation and explore with them ways to balance work and family demands to promote healing. Not keeping up with his job will probably increase the client's stress level, but the nurse's response is best if it is based on the fact that a relaxed environment is an essential component of ulcer healing. Nurses cannot set limits on a client's behavior; clients must make the decision to make lifestyle changes. (P, 7)

15. 4. It would be most effective for the client to develop a health maintenance plan that incorporates regular periods of physical and mental rest in the daily schedule. Strategies should be identified to deal with the types of physical and mental stressors that the client needs to cope with in the home and work environments. Scheduling physical activity to occur only in the morning would not be restful or practical. There is no need for the client to avoid yard work or jogging if these activities are not stressful. (P, 5)

16. 3. Ranitidine blocks secretion of hydrochloric acid. Clients who take only one daily dose of ranitidine are usually advised to take it at bedtime to inhibit nocturnal secretion of acid. Clients who take the drug twice a day are advised to take it in the morning and at bedtime. (E, 8)

17. 3. It is most likely that the client is experiencing a side effect of the antacid. Antacids with aluminum salt products, such as aluminum hydroxide, form insoluble salts in the body. These precipitate and accumulate in the intestines, causing constipation. Increasing dietary fiber intake or daily exercise may be a beneficial lifestyle change for the client but is not likely to relieve the constipation caused by the aluminum hydroxide. Constipation, in isolation from other symptoms, is not a sign of a bowel obstruction. (D, 8)

18. 4. Antacids are most effective if taken 1 to 3 hours after meals and at bedtime. When an antacid is taken on an empty stomach, the duration of the drug's action is greatly decreased. Taking antacids 1 to 3 hours after a meal lengthens the duration of action, thus increasing the therapeutic action of the drug. Antacids should be administered about 2 hours after other medications to decrease the chance of drug interactions. It is not necessary to decrease fluid intake when taking antacids. If antacids are taken more frequently than recommended, the likelihood of developing side effects increases. Therefore, the client should not take antacids as often as desired to control pain. (E, 8)

19. 2. Alcohol is a gastric irritant that should be eliminated from the intake of the client with peptic ulcer disease. Analgesics are not used to control ulcer pain; many analgesics are gastric irritants. The client's hemoglobin and hematocrit typically do not need to be monitored every 3 months, unless gastrointestinal bleeding is suspected. The client can maintain an active lifestyle and does not need to eliminate contact sports as long as they are not stress-inducing. (E, 9)

The Client With Cancer of the Stomach

20. 3. The most likely complication of an endoscopic procedure is perforation. A sudden temperature spike within 1 to 2 hours after the procedure is indicative of a perforation and should be reported immediately to the physician. A sore throat is to be anticipated after an endoscopy. Clients are given sedatives during the procedure, so it is expected that they will display signs of sedation after the procedure is completed. A lack of appetite could be the result of many factors, including the disease process. (D, 9)

21. 2. A Billroth II procedure bypasses the duodenum and connects the gastric stump directly to the jejunum. The pyloric sphincter is removed, along with some of the stomach fundus. (I, 10)

22. 3. The information presented most clearly supports a nursing diagnosis of Anticipatory Grieving. The feelings expressed in this situation are more related to grieving about the changes that will occur in the client's life as a result of the diagnosis of gastric cancer than to fear of the unknown or anxiety about the surgery. There is no evidence of ineffective coping at this time. (D, 5)

23. 1. About 12 to 24 hours after a subtotal gastrectomy, gastric drainage is normally brown, which indicates digested blood. Bile green or cloudy white drainage is not expected during the first 12 to 24 hours after a subtotal gastrectomy. Drainage during the first 6 to 12 hours contains some bright red blood, but large amounts of blood or excessive bloody drainage should be reported to the physician promptly. (E, 9)

24. 3. Nausea, vomiting, or abdominal distention indicates that gas and secretions are accumulating within the gastric pouch due to impaired peristalsis or edema at the operative site and may indicate that the drainage system is not working properly. Saline solution is used to irrigate nasogastric tubes. Hypotonic solutions such as water increase electrolyte loss. In addition, a physician's order is needed to irrigate the nasogastric tube, because this procedure could disrupt the suture line. After gastric surgery, only the surgeon repositions the nasogastric tube because of the danger of rupturing or dislodging the suture line. The amount of suction varies with the type of tube used and is ordered by the physician. High suction may create too much tension on the gastric suture line. (I, 9)

25. 3. A client who has had abdominal surgery is best placed in a low Fowler's position postoperatively. This positioning relaxes abdominal muscles and provides for maximum respiratory and cardiovascular function. The prone, supine, or Sims position would not be tolerated by a client who has had abdominal surgery, nor do those positions support respiratory or cardiovascular functioning. (I, 10)

26. 2. Because of the client's reduced stomach capacity, frequent small feedings are recommended. Early satiety can result, and large quantities of food are not well tolerated. Each client should progress at his or her own pace, gradually increasing the amount of food eaten. The goal is three meals daily if possible, but this can take 6 months or longer to achieve. Nausea can be episodic and can result from eating too fast or eating too much at one time. Eating less and eating more slowly, rather than not eating at all, can be a solution. Bland foods are recommended as starting foods because they are easily digested and are less irritating to the healing mucosa. Bland foods are not less nutritional. (P, 7)

27. 2. After a gastric resection, ingested food moves rapidly from the remaining stomach into the duodenum or jejunum. The food has not undergone adequate preliminary digestion in the stomach. It is concentrated (hypertonic), distends the intestine, and stimulates significant secretion of insulin by the pancreas, as well as a shift of fluid into the bowel. The dumping syndrome results from these factors, which are initiated by the rapid movement of food out of the stomach. (P, 9)

28. 4. Carbohydrates are restricted, but protein, including meat and dairy products, is recommended because it is digested more slowly. Lying down for 30 minutes after a meal is encouraged to slow movement of the food bolus. Fluids are restricted to reduce the bulk of food. There is no need to avoid caffeine. (I, 7)

29. 4. The symptoms related to dumping syndrome that occur after a gastrectomy usually disappear by 6 to 12 months after surgery. Most clients can begin to resume normal meal patterns after signs of the dumping syndrome have stopped. Acknowledging that eating six meals a day is time-consuming does not address the client's question and makes an assumption about the client's concerns. It is not necessarily true that a six-meal-a-day dietary pattern will be required for the rest of the client's life. Clients will not be able to eat three meals a day before hospital discharge. (I, 10)

30. 3. Symptoms of the dumping syndrome usually begin 15 to 30 minutes after eating and include weakness, dizziness, diaphoresis, palpitations, a sense of fullness, abdominal cramps, and diarrhea. These symptoms result when a large bolus of hypertonic fluid enters the small intestine and causes a sudden decrease in plasma volume as fluid is shifted into the bowel. Heartburn is the result of gastric reflex, not the dumping syndrome. (A, 10)

31. 1. Clients who have had gastric surgery are prone to postoperative complications such as dumping syndrome and postprandial hypoglycemia that can affect nutritional intake. Vitamin absorption can also be an issue, depending on the extent of the gastric surgery. Radiation therapy to the upper gastrointestinal area also can affect nutritional intake by causing anorexia, nausea, and esophagitis. The client would not be expected to develop alopecia. Exercise and activity levels as well as access to community resources are important teaching areas, but nutritional intake is a priority need. (P, 9)

32. 4. An appropriate expected outcome is for the client to achieve optimal nutritional status through the use of oral feedings or total parenteral nutrition (TPN). TPN may be used to supplement oral intake, or it may be used alone if the client cannot tolerate oral feedings. The client would not be expected to regain lost weight within 1 month after surgery or to tolerate a normal dietary intake of three meals a day. Nausea and vomiting would not be considered an expected outcome of gastric surgery, and regular use of antiemetics would not be anticipated. (E, 10)

The Client With Gastroesophageal Reflux Disease

33. 1. A laxative is administered after an upper gastrointestinal series to stimulate a bowel movement. This examination involves the administration of barium, which must be promptly eliminated from the body because it may harden and cause an obstruction. A clear liquid diet or an intravenous infusion would have no effect on stimulating removal of the barium. An enema would be ineffective because the barium is too high in the gastrointestinal tract. (P, 9)

34. 3. With GERD, eating substances that decrease lower esophageal sphincter pressure causes heartburn. A decrease in the lower esophageal sphincter pressure allows gastric contents to reflux into the lower end of the esophagus. Foods that can cause a decrease in esophageal sphincter pressure include fatty foods, chocolate, caffeinated beverages, peppermint, and alcohol. A diet high in protein and low in fat is recommended for clients with GERD. Lean beef, popcorn, and raw vegetables would be acceptable. (I, 10)

35. 4. Clients with GERD can develop pulmonary symptoms such as coughing, wheezing, and dyspnea that are caused by the aspiration of gastric contents. GERD does not predispose the client to the development of laryngeal cancer. Irritation of the esophagus and esophageal scar tissue formation can develop as a result of GERD. However, GERD is more likely to cause painful and difficult swallowing. (D, 10)

36. 2. Bethanechol (Urecholine), a cholinergic drug, may be used in GERD to increase lower esophageal sphincter pressure and facilitate gastric emptying. Cholinergic side effects may include urinary urgency, diarrhea, abdominal cramping, hypotension, and increased salivation. To avoid these side effects, the client should be closely monitored to establish the minimum effective dose. (E, 8)

37. 1. Fats are associated with decreased esophageal sphincter tone, which increases reflux. Obesity contributes to the development of hiatal hernia, and a low-fat diet might also aid in weight loss. Carbohydrates and foods high in sodium or calcium do not affect gastroesophageal reflux. (E, 7)

38. 1. Esophageal reflux worsens when the stomach is overdistended with food. Therefore, an important measure is to eat small, frequent meals. Fluid intake should be decreased during meals to reduce abdominal

distention. Avoiding air swallowing does not prevent esophageal reflux. Food intake in the evening should be strictly limited to reduce the incidence of nighttime reflux, so bedtime snacks are not recommended. (I, 7)

39. 1. Heartburn, the most common symptom of a sliding hiatal hernia, results from reflux of gastric secretions into the esophagus. Regurgitation of gastric contents and dysphagia are other common symptoms. Jaundice, which results from a high concentration of bilirubin in the blood, is not associated with hiatal hernia. Anorexia is not a typical symptom of hiatal hernia. Stomatitis is inflammation of the mouth. (A, 10)

40. 2. Any factor that increases intra-abdominal pressure, such as obesity, can contribute to the development of hiatal hernia. Other factors include abdominal straining, frequent heavy lifting, and pregnancy. Hiatal hernia is also associated with older age and occurs in women more frequently than in men. Having a sedentary desk job, using laxatives frequently, or being 40 years old is not likely to be a contributing factor in development of a hiatal hernia. (A, 9)

41. 3. Self-responsibility is the key to individual health maintenance. Using examples of situations in which the client has demonstrated self-responsibility can be reinforcing and supporting. The client has ultimate responsibility for his personal health habits. Meeting other people who are managing their care and involving family members can be helpful, but individual motivation is more important. Reassurance can be helpful but is less important than individualization of care. (I, 7)

42. 3. The magnesium salts in magnesium hydroxide are related to those found in laxatives and may cause diarrhea. Aluminum salt products can cause constipation. Many clients find that a combination product is required to maintain normal bowel elimination. The use of magnesium hydroxide does not cause anorexia or weight gain. (P, 8)

43. 2. Smoking and alcohol use both reduce esophageal sphincter tone and can result in reflux. They therefore should be avoided by clients with hiatal hernia. Daily aerobic exercise, balancing activity and rest, and avoiding high-stress situations may increase the client's general health and well-being, but they not directly associated with hiatal hernia. (P, 4)

44. 2. Bending, especially after eating, can cause gastroesophageal reflux. Lifting heavy objects increases intra-abdominal pressure. Assessing the client's lifting techniques enables the nurse to evaluate the client's knowledge of factors contributing to hiatal hernia and how to prevent complications. The other work-related factors are not directly related to treatment of hiatal hernia. Number and length of breaks, temperature in the work area, and cleaning solvents used are not directly related to treatment of hiatal hernia. (A, 7)

45. 1. A client with a hiatal hernia should avoid the recumbent position immediately after meals to minimize gastric reflux. Bedtime snacks, as well as high-fat foods and carbonated beverages, should be avoided. Excessive vigorous exercise also should be avoided, especially after meals, but there is no reason why the client must give up swimming. Wearing tight constrictive clothing, such as a girdle, can increase intra-abdominal pressure and thus lead to reflux of gastric juices. (E, 7)

46. 1. Metoclopramide hydrochloride increases sphincter tone and facilitates gastric emptying; both actions reduce the incidence of reflux. Other drugs, such as antacids or histamine receptor antagonists, may also be prescribed to help control reflux and esophagitis and to decrease or neutralize gastric secretions. Reglan is not effective in decreasing or neutralizing gastric secretions. (P, 8)

47. 4. Metoclopramide hydrochloride can cause sedation. Alcohol and other central nervous system depressants add to this sedation. A client who is taking this drug should be cautioned to avoid driving or performing other hazardous activities for a few hours after taking the drug. Clients may take antacids, antihypertensives, and anticoagulants while on metoclopramide. (I, 8)

48. 3. Cimetidine is a histamine receptor antagonist that decreases the quantity of gastric secretions. It may be used in hiatal hernia therapy to prevent or treat the esophagitis and heartburn associated with reflux. Cimetidine is not used to prevent reflux, dysphagia, or ulcer development. (P, 8)

49. 2. Most clients can be treated successfully with a combination of diet restrictions, medications, weight control, and lifestyle modifications. Surgery to correct a hiatal hernia, which commonly produces complications, is performed only when medical therapy fails to control the symptoms. (I, 9)

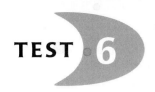

The Client With Lower Gastrointestinal Tract Health Problems

Select the one best answer, and indicate your choice by filling in the circle in front of the option.

The Client With Cancer of the Colon

1. Which of the following has been identified as a potential risk factor for the development of colon cancer?
   ○ 1. Chronic constipation.
   ○ 2. Long-term use of laxatives.
   ○ 3. History of smoking.
   ○ 4. History of inflammatory bowel disease.

2. The nurse is preparing a teaching plan for a community presentation on the prevention and early detection of colon cancer. Which of the following would the nurse identify to the audience as the most common symptom of colon cancer?
   ○ 1. Abdominal pain.
   ○ 2. Diarrhea.
   ○ 3. Rectal bleeding.
   ○ 4. Abdominal distention.

3. When teaching a client with signs and symptoms of colon cancer about the diagnostic workup, the nurse instructs the client to take which of the following types of medication after a barium enema?
   ○ 1. Laxative.
   ○ 2. Anticholinergic.
   ○ 3. Antacid.
   ○ 4. Demulcent.

4. The client with colon cancer has an abdominal–perineal resection with a colostomy. Which of the following nursing interventions is most appropriate for this client in the postoperative period?
   ○ 1. Maintain the client in a semi-Fowler's position.
   ○ 2. Assist the client with warm sitz baths.
   ○ 3. Administer 30 mL of milk of magnesia to stimulate colostomy activity.
   ○ 4. Remove the ostomy pouch as needed so the stoma can be assessed.

5. The nurse evaluates the client's stoma during the initial postoperative period. Which of the following observations should be reported immediately to the physician?
   ○ 1. The stoma is slightly edematous.
   ○ 2. The stoma is dark red to purple.
   ○ 3. The stoma oozes a small amount of blood.
   ○ 4. The stoma does not expel stool.

6. While changing the client's colostomy bag and dressing, the nurse assesses that the client is ready to participate in her care by noting which of the following?
   ○ 1. The client asks what time the doctor will visit that day.
   ○ 2. The client asks about the supplies used during the dressing change.
   ○ 3. The client talks about something she read in the morning newspaper.
   ○ 4. The client complains about the way the night nurse changed the dressing.

7. Which of the following skin preparations would be best to apply around the client's colostomy?
   ○ 1. Karaya.
   ○ 2. Petrolatum.
   ○ 3. Cornstarch.
   ○ 4. Antiseptic cream.

8. A client is recovering from an abdominal–perineal resection. Which of the following measures would most effectively promote wound healing after the perineal drains have been removed?
   ○ 1. Taking sitz baths.
   ○ 2. Taking daily showers.
   ○ 3. Applying warm, moist dressings to the area.
   ○ 4. Applying a protected heating pad to the area.

9. When planning diet teaching for the client with a colostomy, the nurse would develop a plan that emphasizes which of the following dietary instructions?
   ○ 1. Foods containing roughage should not be eaten.
   ○ 2. Liquids are best limited to prevent diarrhea.
   ○ 3. Clients should experiment to find the diet that is best for them.
   ○ 4. A high-fiber diet will produce a regular passage of stool.

10. Which of the following would be an expected outcome for a client who is recovering from an abdominal–perineal resection with a colostomy?
    ○ 1. The client will maintain a fluid intake of 3000 mL/day.
    ○ 2. The client will eliminate fiber from the diet.
    ○ 3. The client will limit physical activity to light exercise.
    ○ 4. The client will accept that sexual activity will be diminished.

The Client With Hemorrhoids

11. A 36-year-old female client has been diagnosed with hemorrhoids. Which of the following factors in the client's history would most likely be a primary cause of her hemorrhoids?
    ○ 1. Her age.
    ○ 2. Three vaginal delivery pregnancies.
    ○ 3. Her job as a schoolteacher.
    ○ 4. Varicosities in her legs.

12. Which position would be ideal for the client in the early postoperative period after a hemorrhoidectomy?
    ○ 1. High Fowler's.
    ○ 2. Supine.
    ○ 3. Side-lying.
    ○ 4. Trendelenburg's.

13. The nurse instructs the client who has had a hemorrhoidectomy not to use sitz baths until at least 12 hours postoperatively to avoid inducing which of the following complications?
    ○ 1. Hemorrhage.
    ○ 2. Rectal spasm.
    ○ 3. Urinary retention.
    ○ 4. Constipation.

14. The nurse teaches the client who has had rectal surgery the proper timing for sitz baths. The nurse knows that the client has understood the teaching when the client states that it is most important to take a sitz bath
    ○ 1. first thing each morning.
    ○ 2. as needed for discomfort.
    ○ 3. after a bowel movement.
    ○ 4. at bedtime.

The Client With Inflammatory Bowel Disease

15. A client who had ulcerative colitis for the past 5 years is admitted to the hospital with an exacerbation of the disease. Which of the following factors was most likely of greatest significance in causing an exacerbation of ulcerative colitis?
    ○ 1. A demanding and stressful job.
    ○ 2. Changing to a modified vegetarian diet.
    ○ 3. Beginning a weight-training program.
    ○ 4. Walking 2 miles every day.

16. Which goal for the client's care should take priority during the first days of hospitalization for an exacerbation of ulcerative colitis?
    ○ 1. Promoting self-care and independence.
    ○ 2. Managing diarrhea.
    ○ 3. Maintaining adequate nutrition.
    ○ 4. Promoting rest and comfort.

17. The client with ulcerative colitis is following orders for bed rest with bathroom privileges. What would be the primary rationale for this activity restriction?
    ○ 1. To conserve energy.
    ○ 2. To reduce intestinal peristalsis.
    ○ 3. To promote rest and comfort.
    ○ 4. To prevent injury.

18. A client's ulcerative colitis symptoms have been present for longer than 1 week. The nurse recognizes that the client should be assessed carefully for signs of which of the following complications?
    ○ 1. Heart failure.
    ○ 2. Deep vein thrombosis.
    ○ 3. Hypokalemia.
    ○ 4. Hypocalcemia.

19. A client who has ulcerative colitis says to the nurse, "I can't take this anymore! I'm constantly in pain, and I can't leave my room because I need to stay by the toilet. I don't know how to deal with this."

Based on these comments, an appropriate nursing diagnosis for this client would be
- 1. Impaired Physical Mobility related to fatigue.
- 2. Disturbed Thought Processes related to pain.
- 3. Social Isolation related to chronic fatigue.
- 4. Ineffective Coping related to chronic abdominal pain.

20. A client newly diagnosed with ulcerative colitis has been placed on steroids. He states that he has heard that taking steroids can be dangerous and asks the nurse why steroids are prescribed. Which of the following statements by the nurse provides the client with accurate information about the use of steroid therapy in the treatment of ulcerative colitis?
- 1. "Ulcerative colitis can be cured by the use of steroids."
- 2. "Steroids are used in severe flare-ups because they can decrease the incidence of bleeding."
- 3. "Long-term use of steroids will prolong periods of remission."
- 4. "The side effects of steroids outweigh their benefit to clients with ulcerative colitis."

21. A client who has ulcerative colitis has persistent diarrhea. He is thin and has lost 12 pounds since the exacerbation of his ulcerative colitis. The nurse should anticipate that the physician will order which of the following treatment approaches to help the client meet his nutritional needs?
- 1. Initiate continuous enteral feedings.
- 2. Encourage a high-calorie, high-protein diet.
- 3. Implement total parenteral nutrition.
- 4. Provide six small meals a day.

22. The physician prescribes sulfasalazine (Azulfidine) for the client with ulcerative colitis to continue taking at home. What instructions should the nurse give the client about taking this medication?
- 1. Avoid taking it with food.
- 2. Take the total dose at bedtime.
- 3. Take it with a full glass (240 mL) of water.
- 4. Stop taking it if urine turns orange-yellow.

23. A client with ulcerative colitis expresses serious concerns about her career as an attorney because of the effects of stress on ulcerative colitis. Which of the following nursing interventions will be most helpful to the client?
- 1. Review her current coping mechanisms and develop alternatives, if needed.
- 2. Suggest a less stressful career in which she would still use her education and experience.
- 3. Suggest that she ask her colleagues to help decrease her stress by giving her the easier cases.
- 4. Prepare family members for the fact that she will have to work part-time.

24. Which of the following diets would be most appropriate for the client with ulcerative colitis?
- 1. High calorie, low protein.
- 2. High protein, low residue.
- 3. Low fat, high fiber.
- 4. Low sodium, high carbohydrate.

25. A client who has a history of Crohn's disease is admitted to the hospital with fever, diarrhea, cramping, abdominal pain, and weight loss. Which of the following laboratory findings would be anticipated for the client?
- 1. Hyperalbuminemia.
- 2. Thrombocytopenia.
- 3. Hypokalemia.
- 4. Hypercalcemia.

26. A client with Crohn's disease experiences rectal bleeding along with 15 to 20 watery stools per day. Which of the following signs would be indicative of dehydration?
- 1. Sunken eyeballs.
- 2. Decreased pulse rate.
- 3. Moist skin.
- 4. Pitting edema.

27. Which of the following would be a priority focus of care for a client experiencing an exacerbation of his Crohn's disease?
- 1. Encouraging regular ambulation.
- 2. Promoting bowel rest.
- 3. Maintaining current weight.
- 4. Decreasing episodes of rectal bleeding.

The Client With an Intestinal Obstruction

28. A client is admitted to the hospital complaining of nausea, vomiting, and abdominal pain. Bowel obstruction is suspected. During the initial assessment, the nurse hears high-pitched tinkling bowel sounds on auscultation and flat sounds on percussion. The flat sounds are caused by
- 1. hyperactive peristalsis.
- 2. excessive gas trapped in the intestine.
- 3. the presence of a mass or tumor in the bowel.
- 4. fluid trapped in the intestine.

29. The physician orders intestinal decompression with a Cantor tube for the client. The primary purpose of a nasoenteric tube such as a Cantor tube is
- 1. to remove fluid and gas from the intestine.
- 2. to prevent fluid accumulation in the stomach.
- 3. to break up the obstruction.
- 4. to provide an alternative route for drug administration.

30. After insertion of a nasoenteric tube, the nurse should place the client in which position?
- 1. Supine.
- 2. Right side-lying.
- 3. Semi-Fowler's.
- 4. Upright in a bedside chair.

31. Which of the following statements about nasoenteric tubes is correct?
    - ○ 1. The tube cannot be attached to suction.
    - ○ 2. The tube contains a soft rubber bag filled with mercury.
    - ○ 3. The tube is taped securely to the client's cheek after insertion.
    - ○ 4. The tube can have its placement determined only by auscultation.

32. Which of the following nursing diagnoses would be most appropriate for a client with an intestinal obstruction?
    - ○ 1. Impaired Swallowing related to NPO status.
    - ○ 2. Urinary Retention related to deficient fluid volume.
    - ○ 3. Deficient Fluid Volume related to nausea and vomiting.
    - ○ 4. Chronic Pain related to abdominal distention.

33. The client with an intestinal obstruction continues to have acute pain even though the nasoenteric tube is patent and draining. Which action by the nurse would be most appropriate?
    - ○ 1. Reassure the client that the nasoenteric tube is functioning.
    - ○ 2. Assess the client for a rigid abdomen.
    - ○ 3. Administer narcotic as ordered.
    - ○ 4. Reposition the client on the left side.

34. Before abdominal surgery for an intestinal obstruction, the nurse monitors the client's urine output and finds that the total output for the past 2 hours was 35 mL. The nurse then assesses the client's total intake and output over the last 24 hours and notes that he had 2000 mL of intravenous fluid for intake, 500 mL of drainage from the nasogastric tube, and 700 mL of urine for a total output of 1200 mL. This would indicate which of the following?
    - ○ 1. Decreased renal functioning.
    - ○ 2. Inadequate pain relief.
    - ○ 3. Extension of the obstruction.
    - ○ 4. Inadequate fluid replacement.

The Client With an Ileostomy

35. A client is scheduled for an ileostomy. Which of the following interventions would be most helpful in preparing the client psychologically for the surgery?
    - ○ 1. Include family members in preoperative teaching sessions.
    - ○ 2. Encourage the client to ask questions about managing an ileostomy.
    - ○ 3. Provide a brief, thorough explanation of all preoperative and postoperative procedures.
    - ○ 4. Invite a member of the ostomy association to visit the client.

36. A client who is scheduled for an ileostomy has an order for oral neomycin to be administered before surgery. The nurse understands that the rationale for administering oral neomycin before surgery is to
    - ○ 1. prevent postoperative bladder infection.
    - ○ 2. reduce the number of intestinal bacteria.
    - ○ 3. decrease the potential for postoperative hypostatic pneumonia.
    - ○ 4. increase the body's immunologic response to the stressors of surgery.

37. Of the following goals for client care after an ileostomy, which has the *highest* priority?
    - ○ 1. To provide relief from constipation.
    - ○ 2. To assist the client with self-care activities.
    - ○ 3. To maintain fluid and electrolyte balance.
    - ○ 4. To minimize odor formation.

38. The client asks the nurse, "Is it really possible to lead a normal life with an ileostomy?" Which action by the nurse would be the most effective to address this question?
    - ○ 1. Have the client talk with a member of the clergy about these concerns.
    - ○ 2. Tell the client to worry about those concerns after surgery.
    - ○ 3. Arrange for a person with an ostomy to visit the client preoperatively.
    - ○ 4. Notify the surgeon of the client's question.

39. The nurse explains to the client that some form of skin barrier must be used around the stoma at all times. The primary function of a skin barrier is to
    - ○ 1. help prevent the formation of odor.
    - ○ 2. help maintain an accurate output record.
    - ○ 3. protect against irritation from ileostomy effluent.
    - ○ 4. allow the client to keep the ostomy pouch on longer.

40. The nurse should instruct the client with an ileostomy to report which of the following symptoms immediately?
    - ○ 1. Passage of liquid stool from the stoma.
    - ○ 2. Occasional presence of undigested food in the effluent.
    - ○ 3. Absence of drainage from the ileostomy for 6 or more hours.
    - ○ 4. Temperature of 99.8°F (37.7°C).

41. The nurse finds the client crying. The client explains to the nurse, "I'm upset because I know I won't be able to have children now that I have an ileostomy." Which of the following would be the best response for the nurse?
    - ○ 1. "Many women with ileostomies decide to adopt. Why don't you consider that option?"
    - ○ 2. "Having an ileostomy does not necessarily mean that you can't bear children. Let's talk

about your concerns."
- 3. "I can understand your reasons for being upset. Having children must be important to you."
- 4. "I'm sure you will adjust to this situation with time. Try not to be too upset."

42. The nurse evaluates the client's understanding of ileostomy care. Which of the following statements indicates that discharge teaching has been effective?
- 1. "I should be able to resume weight lifting in 2 weeks."
- 2. "I can return to work in 2 weeks."
- 3. "I need to drink at least 3000 mL a day of fluid."
- 4. "I will need to avoid getting my stoma wet while bathing."

43. A client calls the nurse at a clinic to report the sudden onset of abdominal cramps, vomiting, and watery discharge from his ileostomy. How should the nurse respond to this client?
- 1. Tell the client to come into the clinic for an examination if the symptoms persist for longer than 24 hours.
- 2. Encourage the client to increase fluid intake to 3 L/day to replace fluid lost through vomiting.
- 3. Instruct the client to take 30 mL of milk of magnesia to stimulate a bowel movement.
- 4. Tell the client that he needs to be examined immediately by the physician.

The Client Receiving Total Parenteral Nutrition

44. A client with inflammatory bowel disease is receiving total parenteral nutrition (TPN). The basic component of the client's TPN solution is most likely to be
- 1. an isotonic dextrose solution.
- 2. a hypertonic dextrose solution.
- 3. a hypotonic dextrose solution.
- 4. a colloidal dextrose solution.

45. TPN is ordered for a client with Crohn's disease. While administering the TPN solution, it is important for the nurse to remember that total parental solutions are used to
- 1. increase cell nutrition.
- 2. treat metabolic acidosis.
- 3. provide hydration.
- 4. reverse a positive nitrogen balance.

46. The nurse would regularly assess a client's ability to metabolize the TPN solution adequately by monitoring the client for which of the following signs?
- 1. Tachycardia.
- 2. Hypertension.
- 3. Elevated blood urea nitrogen concentration.
- 4. Hyperglycemia.

47. Which of the following interventions should the nurse include in the client's care plan to prevent complications associated with TPN administered through a central line?
- 1. Use a clean technique for all dressing changes.
- 2. Tape all connections of the system.
- 3. Encourage bed rest.
- 4. Cover the insertion site with a moisture-proof dressing.

48. When developing a care plan for a client who is receiving TPN, which one of the following potential nursing diagnoses would be most appropriate?
- 1. Impaired Swallowing.
- 2. Impaired Gas Exchange.
- 3. Risk for Fluid Volume Excess.
- 4. Ineffective Tissue Perfusion.

49. A client's TPN fluid is being administered through central intravenous tubing. Which complication can occur if the tubing becomes disconnected?
- 1. Phlebitis.
- 2. Pneumothorax.
- 3. Hemorrhage.
- 4. Air embolus.

50. The nurse discovers that a client's TPN solution was running at an incorrect rate and is now 2 hours behind schedule. Which action is most appropriate for the nurse to take to correct the problem?
- 1. Readjust the solution to infuse the desired amount.
- 2. Continue the infusion at the current rate, but run the next bottle at an increased rate.
- 3. Double the infusion rate for 2 hours.
- 4. Notify the physician.

51. The purpose of administering fat emulsion solution during TPN is
- 1. to provide essential fatty acids.
- 2. to provide extra carbohydrates.
- 3. to promote effective metabolism of glucose.
- 4. to maintain a normal body weight.

52. Which of the following should the nurse interpret as an indication of a complication after the first few days of TPN therapy?
- 1. Glycosuria.
- 2. A 1- to 2-lb weight gain.
- 3. Decreased appetite.
- 4. Elevated temperature.

53. Which of the following side effects would the nurse expect the client to exhibit in the event of too rapid an infusion of TPN solution?
- 1. Negative nitrogen balance.
- 2. Circulatory overload.
- 3. Hypoglycemia.
- 4. Hypokalemia.

The Client With Diverticular Disease

54. Which of the following laboratory findings would the nurse expect to find in a client with diverticulitis?
    - ○ 1. Elevated red blood cell count.
    - ○ 2. Decreased platelet count.
    - ○ 3. Elevated white blood cell count.
    - ○ 4. Elevated serum blood urea nitrogen concentration.

55. The nurse is aware that the diagnostic tests typically ordered for acute diverticulitis do not include a barium enema. The reason for this is that a barium enema
    - ○ 1. can perforate an intestinal abscess.
    - ○ 2. would greatly increase the client's pain.
    - ○ 3. is of minimal diagnostic value in diverticulitis.
    - ○ 4. is too lengthy a procedure for the client to tolerate.

56. Which of the following measures should the client with diverticulitis be taught to integrate into his daily routine at home?
    - ○ 1. Using enemas to relieve constipation.
    - ○ 2. Decreasing fluid intake to increase the formed consistency of the stool.
    - ○ 3. Eating a high-fiber diet when symptomatic with diverticulitis.
    - ○ 4. Refraining from straining and lifting activities.

57. Which of the following medications would the nurse anticipate administering to a client with diverticular disease?
    - ○ 1. Psyllium hydrophilic mucilloid (Metamucil).
    - ○ 2. Diphenoxylate with atropine sulfate (Lomotil).
    - ○ 3. Diazepam (Valium).
    - ○ 4. Aluminum hydroxide (Amphojel).

58. Which of the following signs would be indicative of peritonitis in a client with diverticulitis?
    - ○ 1. Hyperactive bowel sounds.
    - ○ 2. Rigid abdominal wall.
    - ○ 3. Explosive diarrhea.
    - ○ 4. Excessive flatulence.

The Client With Appendicitis

59. In a client with acute appendicitis, the nurse should anticipate which of the following treatments?
    - ○ 1. Administration of enemas to cleanse bowel.
    - ○ 2. Insertion of a nasogastric tube.
    - ○ 3. Placement of client on NPO status.
    - ○ 4. Administration of heat to the abdomen.

60. A client with acute appendicitis develops a fever, tachycardia, and hypotension. Based on these assessment findings, the nurse suspects which of the following complications?
    - ○ 1. Deficient fluid volume.
    - ○ 2. Intestinal obstruction.
    - ○ 3. Bowel ischemia.
    - ○ 4. Peritonitis.

61. Postoperative nursing care for a client after an appendectomy would include which of the following interventions?
    - ○ 1. Administering sitz baths four times a day.
    - ○ 2. Noting the first bowel movement after surgery.
    - ○ 3. Limiting the client's activity to bathroom privileges.
    - ○ 4. Measuring abdominal girth every 2 hours.

62. A client who had an appendectomy for a perforated appendix returns from surgery with a drain inserted in the incisional site. The nurse understands that the purpose of the drain is to accomplish which of the following?
    - ○ 1. Provide access for wound irrigation.
    - ○ 2. Promote drainage of wound exudate.
    - ○ 3. Minimize development of scar tissue.
    - ○ 4. Decrease postoperative discomfort.

The Client With an Inguinal Hernia

63. A client who has a history of an inguinal hernia is admitted to the hospital with complaints of sudden, severe abdominal pain; vomiting; and abdominal distention. Based on these assessment findings, the nurse suspects that which of the following complications has developed?
    - ○ 1. Peritonitis.
    - ○ 2. Incarcerated hernia.
    - ○ 3. Strangulated hernia.
    - ○ 4. Intestinal perforation.

64. A client has just had an inguinal herniorrhaphy. Which of the following nursing interventions would be appropriate for his care?
    - ○ 1. Help the client to turn, cough, and deep-breathe every 2 hours.
    - ○ 2. Apply an ice bag to the scrotum.
    - ○ 3. Apply a truss before the client ambulates.
    - ○ 4. Maintain the client in a high Fowler's position while in bed.

65. After an inguinal herniorrhaphy, the nurse should evaluate the client carefully for which of the following likely complications?
    - ○ 1. Hypostatic pneumonia.
    - ○ 2. Deep vein thrombosis.
    - ○ 3. Paralytic ileus.
    - ○ 4. Urinary retention.

Correct Answers and Rationale

The letters in parentheses following the rationale identify the step of the nursing process (A, D, P, I, E) and client needs (1, 2, 3, 4, 5, 6, 7, 8, 9, 10). See the inside front cover for the key.

The Client With Cancer of the Colon

1. 4. A history of inflammatory bowel disease is a risk factor for colon cancer. Other risk factors include age (older than 40 years), history of familial polyposis, colorectal polyps, and high-fat and/or low-fiber diet. (A, 9)

2. 3. Rectal bleeding is the most common symptom of colon cancer. Other commonly seen symptoms include alternating constipation and diarrhea, narrowing of stool caliber, and a sense of incomplete evacuation. Iron-deficiency anemia and occult bleeding may also be present. Colon cancer may be asymptomatic in early stages. Abdominal pain and distention are not necessarily present in the early stages of colon cancer. (P, 9)

3. 1. After a barium enema, a laxative is ordinarily prescribed. This is done to promote elimination of the barium. Retained barium predisposes the client to constipation and fecal impaction. Anticholinergic drugs decrease gastrointestinal motility. Antacids decrease gastric acid secretion. Demulcents soothe mucous membranes of the gastrointestinal tract and are used to treat diarrhea. (P, 9)

4. 2. Appropriate nursing interventions after an abdominal–perineal resection with a colostomy include assisting the client with warm sitz baths three to four times a day to cleanse the perineal incision. The client will be more comfortable assuming a side-lying position because of the perineal incision. It would be inappropriate to administer milk of magnesia to stimulate colostomy activity. Stool passage will begin as peristalsis returns. It is not necessary or desirable to change the ostomy pouch daily to assess the stoma. The ostomy pouch should be transparent to allow easy observation of the stoma and drainage. (I, 10)

5. 2. A dark red to purple stoma indicates inadequate blood supply. Mild edema and slight oozing of blood are normal in the early postoperative period. The colostomy would typically not begin functioning until 2 to 4 days after surgery. (E, 10)

6. 2. A client who displays interest in the procedure and asks about supplies used for dressings may be ready to participate in self-care. Inquiring about the physician's visit, discussing news events, and complaining about a

dressing change are behaviors that avoid the subject of the colostomy. (E, 5)

7. 1. Karaya and Stomahesive are both effective agents for protecting the skin around a colostomy. They keep the skin healthy and prevent skin irritation from stoma drainage. Petrolatum, cornstarch, and antiseptic creams do not protect the skin adequately and may prevent an adequate seal between the skin and the colostomy bag. (I, 7)

8. 1. Sitz baths are an effective way to cleanse the operative area after an abdominal–perineal resection. Sitz baths bring warmth to the area, improve circulation, and promote healing and cleanliness. Most clients find them comfortable and relaxing. Between sitz baths, the area should be kept clean and dry. A shower will not adequately cleanse the perineal area. Moist dressings may promote wound contamination and delay healing. A heating pad applied to the area for longer than 20 minutes may cause excessive vasodilation, leading to congestion and discomfort. (I, 10)

9. 3. It is best to adjust the diet of a client with a colostomy in a manner that suits the client rather than trying special diets. Severe restriction of roughage is not recommended. The client is encouraged to drink 2 to 3 L of fluid per day. A high-fiber diet may produce loose stools. (P, 7)

10. 1. An expected outcome is that the client will maintain an intake of 3000 mL/day unless contraindicated. There is no need to eliminate fiber from the diet; the client can eat whatever foods are desires, avoiding those that are bothersome. Physical activity does not need to be limited to light exercise. The client can resume normal activities as tolerated, usually within 6 to 8 weeks. The client's sexual activity may be affected, but it does not need to be diminished. (E, 10)

The Client With Hemorrhoids

11. 2. Hemorrhoids are associated with prolonged sitting or standing, portal hypertension, chronic constipation, and prolonged increased intra-abdominal pressure, as associated with pregnancy and the strain of vaginal delivery. Her job as a schoolteacher does not require prolonged sitting or standing. Age and leg varicosities are not related to the development of hemorrhoids. (A, 9)

12. 3. Positioning in the early postoperative phase should avoid stress and pressure on the operative site. The prone and side-lying positions are ideal from a comfort perspective. A high Fowler's or supine position will

place pressure on the operative site and is not recommended. There is no need for Trendelenburg's position. (I, 10)

13. 1. Applying heat during the immediate postoperative period may cause hemorrhage at the surgical site. Moist heat may relieve rectal spasms after bowel movements. Urinary retention caused by reflex spasm may also be relieved by moist heat. Increasing fiber and fluid in the diet can help prevent constipation. (I, 10)

14. 3. Adequate cleansing of the anal area is difficult but essential. After rectal surgery, sitz baths assist in this process, so the client should take a sitz bath after a bowel movement. Other times are dictated by client comfort. (E, 9)

The Client With Inflammatory Bowel Disease

15. 1. Stressful and emotional events have been clearly linked to exacerbations of ulcerative colitis, although their role in the etiology of the disease has been disproved. A modified vegetarian diet or an exercise program is an unlikely cause of the exacerbation. (A, 10)

16. 2. Diarrhea is the primary symptom in an exacerbation of ulcerative colitis, and decreasing the frequency of stools is the first goal of treatment. The other goals are ongoing and will be best achieved by halting the exacerbation. The client may receive antidiarrheal agents, antispasmodic agents, bulk hydrophilic agents, or anti-inflammatory drugs. (P, 10)

17. 2. Although modified bed rest does help conserve energy and promotes comfort, its primary purpose in this case is to help reduce the hypermotility of the colon. Preventing injury is accomplished by other means, such as providing assistance, education, and monitoring of clients at risk for injury. (P, 10)

18. 3. Excessive diarrhea causes significant depletion of the body's stores of sodium and potassium as well as fluid. The client should be closely monitored for hypokalemia and hyponatremia. Ulcerative colitis does not place the client at risk for heart failure, deep vein thrombosis, or hypocalcemia. (A, 9)

19. 4. It is not uncommon for clients with ulcerative colitis to become apprehensive and upset about the frequency of stools and the presence of abdominal cramping. During these acute exacerbations, clients need emotional support and encouragement to verbalize their feelings about their chronic health concerns and assistance in developing effective coping methods. The client has not expressed feelings of fatigue or isolation or demonstrated disturbed thought processes. (D, 5)

20. 2. Steroids are effective in management of the acute symptoms of ulcerative colitis. Steroids do not cure ulcerative colitis, which is a chronic disease. Long-term use is not effective in prolonging the remission and is not advocated. Clients should be assessed carefully for side effects related to steroid therapy, but the benefits of short-term steroid therapy usually outweigh the potential side effects. (P, 8)

21. 3. Food will be withheld from the client with severe symptoms of ulcerative colitis to rest the bowel. To maintain the client's nutritional status, the client will be started on total parenteral nutrition. Enteral feedings or dividing the diet into six small meals does not allow the bowel to rest. A high-calorie, high-protein diet will worsen the client's symptoms. (P, 10)

22. 3. Adequate fluid intake of at least 8 glasses a day prevents crystalluria and stone formation during sulfasalazine therapy. Sulfasalazine can cause gastrointestinal distress and is best taken after meals and in equally divided doses. Sulfasalazine gives alkaline urine an orange-yellow color, but it is not necessary to stop the drug when this occurs. (I, 8)

23. 1. A client with ulcerative colitis need not curtail career goals. Self-care is the cornerstone of long-term management, and learning to cope with and modify stressors will enable the client to live with the disease. Giving up a desired career could discourage and even depress the client. Placing the responsibility for minimizing stressors at work in the hands of others leads to a feeling of loss of control and decreases the sense of responsibility needed for sound self-care. Working part-time rather than full-time is unnecessary. (I, 5)

24. 2. Clients with ulcerative colitis should follow a well-balanced high-protein, high-calorie, low-residue diet, avoiding such high-residue foods as whole-wheat grains, nuts, and raw fruits and vegetables. Clients with ulcerative colitis need more protein for tissue healing and should avoid excess roughage. There is no need for clients with ulcerative colitis to follow low-sodium diets. (I, 7)

25. 3. Hypokalemia is the most expected laboratory finding owing to the diarrhea. Hypoalbuminemia can also occur in Crohn's disease; however, the client's potassium level is of greater importance at this time because a low potassium can cause cardiac arrest. Anemia is an expected development, but thrombocytopenia is not. Calcium levels are not affected. (A, 10)

26. 1. Signs and symptoms of dehydration include sunken eyeballs, postural hypotension, increased pulse rate, dry skin, weight loss, thirst, dry oral mucosa, and restlessness. Pitting edema is an indication of fluid excess. (A, 10)

27. 2. A priority goal of care during an acute exacerbation of Crohn's disease is to promote bowel rest. This is accomplished through decreasing activity, encouraging rest, and initially placing client on NPO status while maintaining nutritional needs parenterally. Regular ambulation is important, but the priority is bowel rest. The client will probably lose some weight during the acute phase of the illness. Diarrhea is nonbloody in Crohn's disease, and episodes of rectal bleeding are not expected. (P, 10)

The Client With an Intestinal Obstruction

28. 4. On percussion, air or gas produces a resonant sound, and fluid produces a flat sound. An intestinal obstruction traps large amounts of fluid in the intestine. Hyperactive peristalsis resulting in the frequent high-pitched tinkling sounds would be apparent on auscultation above the area of obstruction. Masses cause a dull sound when percussed. (A, 4)

29. 1. Intestinal decompression is accomplished with a Cantor, Harris, or Miller-Abbott tube. These 6- to 10-foot tubes are passed into the small intestine to the obstruction. They remove accumulated fluid and gas, relieving the pressure. Obstructions are not "broken up" but resolve with decompression or surgical intervention. A nasogastric tube is used to remove fluid from the stomach. The length of the nasoenteric tubes prohibits its use as an alternative route for medication administration. (I, 9)

30. 2. The client is placed in a right side-lying position to facilitate movement of the mercury-weighted tube through the pyloric sphincter. After the tube is in the intestine, the client is turned from side to side or encouraged to ambulate to facilitate tube movement through the intestinal loops. Placing the client in the supine position, in a semi-Fowler's position, or sitting out of bed in a chair will not facilitate tube progression. (I, 9)

31. 2. A nasoenteric tube does have a small balloon at its tip that is weighted with mercury. The weight of the mercury helps advance the tube by gravity through the intestine. A nasoenteric tube is not taped in position until it has reached the obstruction. Nasoenteric tubes are attached to suction. Because the tube has a radiopaque strip, its progress through the intestinal tract can be followed by fluoroscopy. (I, 9)

32. 3. A client with an intestinal obstruction is particularly susceptible to deficient fluid volume and electrolyte imbalances. NPO status does not impair swallowing. Urinary retention is not caused by deficient fluid volume. The client's pain is acute in nature, not chronic. (D, 10)

33. 2. The client's pain may be indicative of peritonitis, and the nurse should assess for signs such as a rigid abdomen, elevated temperature, and increasing pain. Reassuring the client is important, but accurate assess-

ment of the client is essential. The full assessment should occur before pain relief measures are employed. Repositioning the client to the left side will not resolve the pain. (I, 8)

34. 4. Considering that there is usually 1 L of insensible fluid loss, this client's output exceeds his intake (intake, 2000 mL; output, 2200 mL), indicating deficient fluid volume. The kidneys are concentrating urine in response to low circulating volume, as evidenced by a urine output of less than 30 mL/hour. This indicates that increased fluid replacement is needed. Decreasing urine output can be a sign of decreased renal functioning, but the data provided suggest that the client is dehydrated. Pain does not affect urine output. There are no data to suggest that the obstruction has worsened. (E, 9)

The Client With an Ileostomy

35. 3. Providing explanations of preoperative and postoperative procedures helps the client prepare and understand what to expect. It also provides an opportunity for the client to share concerns. Including family members in the teaching sessions is beneficial but does not focus on the client's psychological preparation. Encouraging the client to ask questions about managing the ileostomy may be rushing the client psychologically into accepting the change in body image and function. The client may need time to first handle the stress of surgery and then observe the care of the ileostomy by others before it is appropriate to begin discussing self-management. The nurse should gently explore whether the client is ready to ask questions about management throughout the hospitalization. The client should have the opportunity to express concerns and to agree to an ostomy association visitor before an invitation is extended. (I, 5)

36. 2. The rationale for the administration of oral neomycin is to decrease intestinal bacteria and thereby decrease the potential for peritonitis and wound infection postoperatively. Neomycin will not alter the client's potential for developing a urinary or respiratory infection. Neomycin does not affect the body's immune system. (P, 8)

37. 3. A high-priority goal after ileostomy surgery is the maintenance of fluid and electrolyte balance. The client will experience continuous liquid to semiliquid stools. The client should be engaged in self-care activities, and minimizing odor formation is important; however, these goals do not take priority over maintaining fluid and electrolyte balance. (P, 10)

38. 3. If the client agrees, having a visit by a person who has successfully adjusted to living with an ileostomy would be the most helpful measure. This would let the client actually see that typical activities of daily living can be pursued postoperatively. Someone who has felt some of the same concerns can answer the client's questions. A visit from the clergy may be helpful to some clients but would not provide this client with the information sought. Disregarding the client's concerns is not helpful. Although the physician should know about the client's concerns, this in itself will not reassure the client about life after an ileostomy. (I, 5)

39. 3. Because of high concentrations of digestive enzymes, ileostomy effluent is irritating to skin and can cause excoriation and ulceration. Some form of protection must be used to keep the effluent from contacting the skin. A skin barrier does not decrease odor formation; odor is controlled by diet. The barrier does not affect the accuracy of output records. Pouches are usually worn for 4 to 7 days before being changed. (I, 7)

40. 3. Any sudden decrease in drainage or onset of severe abdominal pain should be reported to the physician immediately because it could mean that an obstruction has developed. The ileostomy drains liquid stool at frequent intervals throughout the day. Undigested food may be present at times. A temperature of 99.8°F is not necessarily abnormal or a cause for concern. (A, 9)

41. 2. The fact that the client has an ileostomy does not necessarily mean that she cannot get pregnant and bear children. It may be recommended, however, that the number of pregnancies be limited. Women of childbearing age should be encouraged to discuss their concerns with their physician. Discussing their concerns about sexual functioning and pregnancy will help decrease fears and anxiety. Empathizing or telling the woman that she can adopt does not address her concerns. Her current fears may be based on erroneous understanding. Telling the client that she will adjust to the situation ignores her concerns. (I, 5)

42. 3. To maintain an adequate fluid balance, the client needs to drink at least 3000 mL/day. Heavy lifting should be avoided; the physician will indicate when the client can participate in sports again. The client will not resume working as soon as 2 weeks after surgery. Water does not harm the stoma, so the client does not have to worry about getting it wet. (E, 10)

43. 4. Sudden onset of abdominal cramps, vomiting, and watery discharge with no stool from an ileostomy are likely indications of an obstruction. It is imperative that the client be examined immediately. If an obstruction is present, ingesting fluids or taking milk of magnesia will increase the severity of symptoms. Oral intake is avoided when a bowel obstruction is suspected. In addition, the client is vomiting and, although he may very well need fluid replacement, he will not be able to

tolerate oral fluids. Laxatives are contraindicated in cases of suspected bowel obstruction. (I, 9)

The Client Receiving Total Parenteral Nutrition

44. 2. The TPN solution is usually a hypertonic glucose solution. The greater the concentration of dextrose in solution, the greater the tonicity. Hypertonic glucose solutions are used to meet the body's calorie demands in a volume of fluid that will not overload the cardiovascular system. An isotonic dextrose solution (eg, 5% dextrose in water) or a hypotonic dextrose solution will not provide enough calories to meet metabolic needs. Colloids are plasma expanders and blood products and are not used in TPN. (I, 8)

45. 1. The goal of TPN is to meet the client's nutritional needs. TPN is not used to treat metabolic acidosis; ketoacidosis can actually develop as a result of administering TPN. TPN is a hypertonic solution containing carbohydrates, amino acids, electrolytes, trace elements, and vitamins. It is not used to meet the hydration needs of clients. TPN is administered to provide a positive nitrogen balance. (P, 8)

46. 4. During TPN administration, the client should be monitored regularly for hyperglycemia. The client may require small amounts of insulin to improve glucose metabolism. The client should also be observed for signs of hypoglycemia, which may occur if the body overproduces insulin in response to a high glucose intake or if too much insulin is administered to help improve glucose metabolism. Tachycardia or hypertension is not indicative of the client's ability to metabolize the solution. An elevated blood urea nitrogen concentration is indicative of renal status and fluid balance. (A, 8)

47. 2. Complications associated with administration of TPN through a central line include infection and air embolism. To prevent these complications, strict aseptic technique is used for all dressing changes, the insertion site is covered with an air-occlusive dressing, and all connections of the system are taped. Ambulation and activities of daily living are encouraged and not limited during the administration of TPN. (I, 8)

48. 3. The most appropriate nursing diagnosis is Risk for Excess Fluid Volume. Clients receiving TPN are at high risk for development of fluid overload. To prevent fluid imbalances, the nurse must carefully monitor the rate of the infusion and the client's response to the infusion. The diagnoses of Impaired Swallowing, Impaired Gas Exchange, and Ineffective Tissue Perfusion have no application to clients specifically related to administration of TPN. (D, 8)

49. 4. An air embolus can occur if the intravenous tubing becomes disconnected. The tubing connection should be carefully secured to prevent separation of tubing. The client should be instructed to take a deep breath and hold it when changing tubing to prevent an air embolus. Phlebitis can occur as a result of irritation from the hypertonic infusion. Pneumothorax and hemorrhage are complications of catheter placement. (P, 9)

50. 4. When TPN fluids are infused too rapidly or too slowly, the physician should be notified. TPN solutions must be carefully and accurately infused. Rate adjustments should not be made without a written order from the physician. Significant alterations in rate (10% increase or decrease) can result in fluctuations of blood glucose levels. Speeding up the solution can result in too much glucose entering the system. (I, 8)

51. 1. The administration of fatty acids provides additional calories and essential fatty acids to meet the body's energy needs. Fatty acids are lipids, not carbohydrates. Fatty acids do not aid in the metabolism of glucose. Although they are necessary for meeting the complete nutritional needs of the client, fatty acids do not necessarily help a client maintain normal body weight. (P, 8)

52. 4. An elevated temperature can be an indication of an infection at the insertion site or in the catheter. Vital signs should be taken every 2 to 4 hours after initiation of TPN therapy to detect early signs of complications. Glycosuria is to be expected during the first few days of therapy until the pancreas adjusts by secreting more insulin. A gradual weight gain is to be expected as the client's nutritional status improves. Some clients experience a decreased appetite during TPN therapy. (D, 9)

53. 2. Too rapid infusion of a TPN solution can lead to circulatory overload. The client should be assessed carefully for indications of excessive fluid volume. A negative nitrogen balance occurs in nutritionally depleted individuals, not when TPN fluids are administered in excess. When TPN is administered too rapidly the client is at risk for receiving an excess of dextrose and electrolytes. Therefore, the client is at risk for hyperglycemia and hyperkalemia. (A, 8)

The Client With Diverticular Disease

54. 3. Because of the inflammatory nature of diverticulitis, the nurse would anticipate an elevated white blood cell count. The remaining laboratory findings are not associated with diverticulitis. Elevated red blood cell counts occur in clients with polycythemia vera or fluid volume deficit. Decreased platelet counts can occur as a result of aplastic anemias or malignant blood disorders, as a side effect of some drugs, and as a result of some heritable conditions. Elevated serum blood urea nitrogen is usually associated with renal conditions. (A, 9)

55. 1. Barium enemas and colonoscopies are contraindicated in clients with acute diverticulitis because they can lead to perforation of the colon and peritonitis. A barium enema may be ordered after the client has been treated with antibiotic therapy and the inflammation has subsided. A barium enema is diagnostic in diverticulitis. (A, 9)

56. 4. Clients with diverticular disease should refrain from any activities, such as lifting, straining, or coughing, that increase intra-abdominal pressure and may precipitate an attack. Enemas are contraindicated because they increase intestinal pressure. Fluid intake should be increased, rather than decreased, to promote soft, formed stools. A low-fiber diet is used when inflammation is present. (I, 1)

57. 1. Diverticular disease is treated with a high-fiber diet and bulk laxatives such as psyllium hydrophilic mucilloid (Metamucil). Fiber decreases the intraluminal pressure and makes it easier for stool to pass through the colon. Antidiarrheals such as Lomotil and tranquilizers such as Valium are not used to treat diverticular disease. Antacids are used to decrease gastric acidity and are not useful for treating diverticular disease. (P, 8)

58. 2. Diverticular rupture causes peritonitis from the release of intestinal contents (chemicals and bacteria) into the peritoneal cavity. The inflammatory response of the peritoneal tissue produces severe abdominal rigidity and pain, diminished intestinal motility, and retention of intestinal contents (air, fluid, and stool). Because of decreased intestinal motility, bowel sounds will be hypoactive or absent and the client will not experience bowel movements or flatulence. (A, 10)

The Client With Appendicitis

59. 3. A client who is diagnosed with acute appendicitis is placed on NPO status in anticipation of surgery. Enemas are not administered because they can lead to perforation and peritonitis. A nasogastric tube is not usually inserted, unless the client has suffered a perforation. Heat is contraindicated because it may lead to perforation of the appendix. (P, 9)

60. 4. Complications of acute appendicitis are perforation, peritonitis, and abscess development. Signs of the development of peritonitis include abdominal pain and distention, tachycardia, tachypnea, nausea, vomiting, and fever. Because peritonitis can cause hypovolemic shock, hypotension can develop. Deficient fluid volume would not cause a fever. Intestinal obstruction would cause abdominal distention, diminished or absent bowel sounds, and abdominal pain. Bowel ischemia has signs and symptoms similar to those found with intestinal obstruction. (A, 10)

61. 2. Noting the client's first bowel movement after surgery is important because this indicates that normal peristalsis has returned. Sitz baths are used after rectal surgery, not appendectomy. Ambulation is started the day of surgery and is not confined to bathroom privileges. The abdomen should be auscultated for bowel sounds and palpated for softness, but there is no need to measure the girth every 2 hours. (I, 10)

62. 2. Drains are inserted postoperatively in appendectomies when an abscess was present or the appendix was perforated. The purpose is to promote drainage of exudate from the wound and facilitate healing. A drain is not used for irrigation of the wound. The drain will not minimize scar tissue development or decrease postoperative discomfort. (I, 7)

The Client With an Inguinal Hernia

63. 3. The symptoms are indicative of a strangulated hernia. In a strangulated hernia, the hernia cannot be reduced back into the abdominal cavity. The intestinal lumen and the blood supply to the intestine are obstructed, causing an acute intestinal obstruction. Without immediate intervention, necrosis and gangrene may develop. Surgery is required to release the strangulation. Although many of these signs and symptoms are present with peritonitis or perforated bowel, abdominal rigidity, a cardinal sign of peritonitis and perforated bowel, is not mentioned. Therefore, the nurse would not immediately suspect these conditions. An incarcerated hernia refers to a hernia that is irreducible but has not necessarily resulted in an obstruction. (D, 10)

64. 2. After inguinal herniorrhaphy repair, an ice bag to the scrotum will help decrease pain and edema. The client is encouraged to turn and deep-breathe, but coughing is not encouraged, to decrease straining on the surgical area. A truss is not needed for support after surgery. While resting, the client may be most comfortable in a semi-Fowler's position, but there is no need to maintain a high Fowler's position. (I, 10)

65. 4. The most common complication after an inguinal hernia repair is the inability to void, especially in men. The nurse should evaluate the client carefully for urinary retention. Hypostatic pneumonia, deep vein thrombosis, and paralytic ileus are potential postoperative problem with any surgical client but are not as likely to occur after an inguinal hernia repair as is urinary retention. (E, 9)

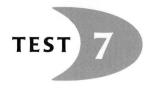

The Client With Biliary Tract Disorders

▶ **The Client With Cholecystitis**

▶ **The Client With Pancreatitis**

▶ **The Client With Viral Hepatitis**

▶ **The Client With Cirrhosis**

▶ **Correct Answers and Rationale**

Select the one best answer, and indicate your choice by filling in the circle in front of the option.

The Client With Cholecystitis

1. A client is admitted to the hospital with a diagnosis of cholecystitis from cholelithiasis. The client is complaining of severe abdominal pain and extreme nausea and has vomited several times. Based on this data, which nursing diagnosis would have the *highest* priority for intervention at this time?
   ○ 1. Anxiety related to severe abdominal discomfort.
   ○ 2. Deficient Fluid Volume related to vomiting.
   ○ 3. Pain related to gallbladder inflammation.
   ○ 4. Imbalanced Nutrition: Less Than Body Requirements related to vomiting.

2. If a gallstone becomes lodged in the common bile duct, the nurse should anticipate that the client's stools would most likely become what color?
   ○ 1. Green.
   ○ 2. Gray.
   ○ 3. Black.
   ○ 4. Brown.

3. When the client's common bile duct is obstructed, the nurse should evaluate the client for signs of which of the following complications?
   ○ 1. Respiratory distress.
   ○ 2. Circulatory overload.
   ○ 3. Urinary tract infection.
   ○ 4. Prolonged bleeding time.

4. A client who has been scheduled to have a choledocholithotomy expresses anxiety about having surgery. Which of the following nursing interventions would help achieve the goal of reducing the client's anxiety?
   ○ 1. Provide the client with information about what to expect postoperatively.
   ○ 2. Tell the client it is normal to be afraid.
   ○ 3. Reassure the client by telling her that surgery is a common procedure.
   ○ 4. Stress the importance of following the physician's instructions after surgery.

5. A client undergoes a traditional cholecystectomy and choledochotomy and returns from surgery with a T-tube. To evaluate the effectiveness of the T-tube, the nurse should understand that the primary reason for the T-tube is to accomplish which of the following goals?
   ○ 1. Promote wound drainage.
   ○ 2. Provide a way to irrigate the biliary tract.
   ○ 3. Minimize the passage of bile into the duodenum.
   ○ 4. Prevent bile from entering the peritoneal cavity.

6. How much bile would the nurse expect the T-tube to drain during the first 24 hours after a choledocholithotomy?
   ○ 1. 50 to 100 mL.
   ○ 2. 150 to 250 mL.
   ○ 3. 300 to 500 mL.
   ○ 4. 550 to 700 mL.

7. The nurse measures the amount of bile drainage from a T-tube and records it by which one of the following methods?
   ○ 1. Adding it to the client's urine output.
   ○ 2. Charting it separately on the output record.
   ○ 3. Adding it to the amount of wound drainage.
   ○ 4. Subtracting it from the total intake for each day.

8. After a cholecystectomy it is recommended that the client follow a low-fat diet at home. Which of the following foods would be most appropriate to include in a low-fat diet?
   ○ 1. Cheese omelet.
   ○ 2. Peanut butter.
   ○ 3. Ham salad sandwich.
   ○ 4. Roast beef.

9. A client with cholecystitis is complaining of severe right upper quadrant pain. Which of the following medications would the nurse anticipate administering to relieve the client's pain?
   ○ 1. Meperidine (Demerol).

    ○ 2. Acetaminophen with codeine.

    ○ 3. Promethazine (Phenergan).

    ○ 4. Morphine sulfate.

10. A client undergoes a laparoscopic cholecystectomy. Which of the following dietary instructions would the nurse give the client immediately after surgery?

    ○ 1. "You cannot eat or drink anything for 24 hours."

    ○ 2. "You may resume your normal diet the day after your surgery."

    ○ 3. "Drink liquids today and eat lightly for a few days."

    ○ 4. "You can progress from a liquid to a bland diet as tolerated."

11. Which of the following discharge instructions would be appropriate for a client who has had a laparoscopic cholecystectomy?

    ○ 1. Avoid showering for 48 hours after surgery.

    ○ 2. Return to work within 1 week.

    ○ 3. Change the dressing daily until incision heals.

    ○ 4. Use acetaminophen (Tylenol) to control any fever.

The Client With Pancreatitis

12. The initial diagnosis of pancreatitis is confirmed if the client's blood work shows a significant elevation in which of the following serum values?

    ○ 1. Amylase.

    ○ 2. Glucose.

    ○ 3. Potassium.

    ○ 4. Trypsin.

13. The client who has been hospitalized with pancreatitis does not drink alcohol because of her religious convictions. She becomes upset when the physician persists in asking her about alcohol intake. The nurse should explain that the reason for these questions is that

    ○ 1. there is a strong link between alcohol use and acute pancreatitis.

    ○ 2. alcohol intake can interfere with the tests used to diagnose pancreatitis.

    ○ 3. alcoholism is a major health problem, and all clients are questioned about alcohol intake.

    ○ 4. the physician must obtain the pertinent facts, regardless of religious beliefs.

14. The nurse monitors the client with pancreatitis for early signs of shock. Which of the following conditions is primarily responsible for making it difficult to manage shock in pancreatitis?

    ○ 1. Severity of intestinal hemorrhage.

    ○ 2. Vasodilating effects of kinin peptides.

    ○ 3. Tendency toward congestive heart failure.

    ○ 4. Frequent incidence of acute tubular necrosis.

15. Which of the following signs and symptoms would the nurse expect to see in a client with acute pancreatitis?

    ○ 1. Diarrhea.

    ○ 2. Jaundice.

    ○ 3. Hypertension.

    ○ 4. Ascites.

16. The nurse evaluates the client's most recent laboratory data. Which laboratory finding would be consistent with a diagnosis of acute pancreatitis?

    ○ 1. Hyperglycemia.

    ○ 2. Leukopenia.

    ○ 3. Thrombocytopenia.

    ○ 4. Hyperkalemia.

17. The initial treatment plan for a client with pancreatitis most likely would focus on which of the following objectives as a priority?

    ○ 1. Resting the gastrointestinal tract.

    ○ 2. Ensuring adequate nutrition.

    ○ 3. Maintaining fluid and electrolyte balance.

    ○ 4. Preventing the development of an infection.

18. When providing care for a client with acute pancreatitis, the nurse would anticipate which of the following orders?

    ○ 1. Increase oral intake to 3000 mL every 24 hours.

    ○ 2. Insert a nasogastric tube and connect it to low suction.

    ○ 3. Place the client in the reverse Trendelenburg position.

    ○ 4. Place the client on enteric precautions.

19. The nurse carefully monitors the client with acute pancreatitis for which of the following complications?

    ○ 1. Congestive heart failure.

    ○ 2. Duodenal ulcer.

    ○ 3. Cirrhosis.

    ○ 4. Pneumonia.

20. The nurse notes that a client with acute pancreatitis occasionally experiences muscle twitching and jerking. How should the nurse interpret the significance of these symptoms?

    ○ 1. The client may be developing hypocalcemia.

    ○ 2. The client is experiencing a reaction to meperidine (Demerol).

    ○ 3. The client has a nutritional imbalance.

    ○ 4. The client needs a muscle relaxant to help him rest.

21. Which of the following medications would most likely be given to the client with acute pancreatitis to augment pain control?

    ○ 1. Ibuprofen (Motrin).

    ○ 2. Magnesium hydroxide (Maalox).

    ○ 3. Propantheline bromide (Pro-Banthine).

    ○ 4. Propranolol (Inderal).

22. Which of the following would most likely be a

major nursing diagnosis for a client with acute pancreatitis?

- ○ 1. Ineffective Airway Clearance.
- ○ 2. Excess Fluid Volume.
- ○ 3. Impaired Swallowing.
- ○ 4. Imbalanced Nutrition: Less Than Body Requirements.

23. Which of the following dietary instructions would be appropriate for the nurse to give a client who is recovering from acute pancreatitis?
- ○ 1. Avoid crash dieting.
- ○ 2. Restrict carbohydrate intake.
- ○ 3. Eat six small meals a day.
- ○ 4. Decrease sodium in diet.

24. Pancreatic enzyme replacements are ordered for the client with chronic pancreatitis. When should the nurse instruct the client to take them to obtain the most therapeutic effect?
- ○ 1. Three times daily between meals.
- ○ 2. With each meal and snack.
- ○ 3. In the morning and at bedtime.
- ○ 4. Every 4 hours, at specified times.

25. The nurse should teach the client with chronic pancreatitis to monitor the effectiveness of pancreatic enzyme replacement therapy by doing which of the following?
- ○ 1. Monitoring fluid intake.
- ○ 2. Performing regular glucose fingerstick tests.
- ○ 3. Observing stools for steatorrhea.
- ○ 4. Testing urine for ketones.

26. The client with chronic pancreatitis should be monitored closely for the development of which of the following disorders?
- ○ 1. Cholelithiasis.
- ○ 2. Hepatitis.
- ○ 3. Irritable bowel syndrome.
- ○ 4. Diabetes mellitus.

The Client With Viral Hepatitis

27. The nurse is planning a community education program on how to prevent the transmission of viral hepatitis. Which of the following types of hepatitis is considered to be primarily a sexually transmitted disease?
- ○ 1. Hepatitis A.
- ○ 2. Hepatitis B.
- ○ 3. Hepatitis C.
- ○ 4. Hepatitis D.

28. The nurse would expect the client to exhibit which of the following symptoms during the icteric phase of viral hepatitis?
- ○ 1. Tarry stools.
- ○ 2. Yellowed sclera.
- ○ 3. Shortness of breath.
- ○ 4. Light, frothy urine.

29. The nurse plans care for the client with hepatitis A with the understanding that the causative virus will be excreted from the client's body primarily through the
- ○ 1. skin.
- ○ 2. feces.
- ○ 3. urine.
- ○ 4. blood.

30. The nurse is planning a staff development program for health care staff on how to care for clients with hepatitis A. Which of the following precautions would the nurse indicate as essential when caring for clients with hepatitis A?
- ○ 1. Gowning when entering a client's room.
- ○ 2. Wearing a mask when providing care.
- ○ 3. Assigning the client to a private room.
- ○ 4. Wearing gloves when giving direct care.

31. A client who is recovering from hepatitis A continues to complain of fatigue and malaise. The client asks the nurse, "When will my strength return?" Which of the following responses by the nurse is most appropriate?
- ○ 1. "Your fatigue should be gone by now. We will evaluate you for a secondary infection."
- ○ 2. "Your fatigue is a side effect of your drug therapy. It will disappear when your treatment regimen is complete."
- ○ 3. "It is important for you to increase your activity level. That will help decrease your fatigue."
- ○ 4. "It is normal for you to feel fatigued. The fatigue should go away in the next 2 to 4 months."

32. When developing a plan of care for the client with viral hepatitis, the nurse should incorporate nursing orders that reflect the primary treatment. Emphasis will be on ensuring that the client receives which of the following?
- ○ 1. Adequate bed rest.
- ○ 2. Generous fluid intake.
- ○ 3. Regular antibiotic therapy.
- ○ 4. Daily intravenous electrolyte therapy.

33. Which of the following test results would the nurse use to assess the liver function of a client with viral hepatitis?
- ○ 1. Glucose tolerance.
- ○ 2. Creatinine clearance.
- ○ 3. Serum transaminase.
- ○ 4. Serum electrolytes.

34. In a client with viral hepatitis, the nurse would closely assess for indications of which of the following abnormal laboratory values?
- ○ 1. Prolonged prothrombin time.
- ○ 2. Decreased blood glucose levels.

○ 3. Elevated serum potassium.
○ 4. Decreased serum calcium.

35. Which of the following diets would most likely be prescribed for a client with viral hepatitis?
    ○ 1. High fat, low protein.
    ○ 2. High protein, low carbohydrate.
    ○ 3. High carbohydrate, high calorie.
    ○ 4. Low sodium, low fat.

36. The nurse develops a teaching plan for the client about how to prevent the transmission of hepatitis A. Which of the following discharge instructions is appropriate for the client?
    ○ 1. Spray the house to eliminate infected insects.
    ○ 2. Tell family members to try to stay away from the client.
    ○ 3. Tell family members to wash their hands frequently.
    ○ 4. Disinfect all clothing and eating utensils.

37. The nurse assesses that the client with hepatitis is experiencing fatigue, weakness, and a general feeling of malaise. The client tires rapidly during morning care. Based on this information, which of the following would be an appropriate nursing diagnosis?
    ○ 1. Impaired Physical Mobility related to malaise.
    ○ 2. Self-Care Deficit related to fatigue.
    ○ 3. Ineffective Coping related to long-term illness.
    ○ 4. Activity Intolerance related to fatigue.

38. A client has been admitted to the hospital with a diagnosis of hepatitis B. The client tells the nurse, "I feel so isolated from my friends and family. Nobody wants to be around me." What would be the most appropriate nursing diagnosis for this client?
    ○ 1. Anxiety related to feelings of isolation.
    ○ 2. Social Isolation related to significant others' fear of contracting disease.
    ○ 3. Powerlessness related to lack of social support.
    ○ 4. Low Self-Esteem related to feelings of rejection.

39. What would be the nurse's *best* response to the client's expressed feelings of isolation as a result of having hepatitis?
    ○ 1. "Don't worry. It's normal to feel that way."
    ○ 2. "Your friends are probably afraid of contracting hepatitis from you."
    ○ 3. "I'm sure you're imagining that!"
    ○ 4. "Tell me more about your feelings of isolation."

40. Which of the following measures would prevent transmission of the hepatitis C virus to health care personnel?
    ○ 1. Administer hepatitis C vaccine to all health care personnel.
    ○ 2. Decrease contact with blood and blood-contaminated fluids.
    ○ 3. Wear gloves when emptying the bedpan.
    ○ 4. Wear a gown and mask when providing direct care.

41. Interferon alfa-2b has been prescribed to treat a client with chronic hepatitis B. Which side effects are most commonly associated with the administration of interferon alfa-2b?
    ○ 1. Retinopathy.
    ○ 2. Constipation.
    ○ 3. Flulike symptoms.
    ○ 4. Hypoglycemia.

42. The nurse is preparing a community education program about preventing hepatitis B infection. Which of the following would be appropriate to incorporate into the teaching plan?
    ○ 1. Hepatitis B is relatively uncommon among college students.
    ○ 2. Frequent ingestion of alcohol can predispose an individual to development of hepatitis B.
    ○ 3. Good personal hygiene habits are most effective to preventing the spread of hepatitis B.
    ○ 4. The use of a condom is advised for sexual intercourse.

43. Which of the following expected outcomes would be appropriate for a client with viral hepatitis?
    ○ 1. The client will demonstrate a decrease in fluid retention related to ascites.
    ○ 2. The client will verbalize the importance of reporting bleeding gums or bloody stools.
    ○ 3. The client will limit use of alcohol to 2 to 3 drinks per week.
    ○ 4. The client will restrict activity to within the home to prevent disease transmission.

The Client With Cirrhosis

44. The nurse is assessing a client who is in the early stages of cirrhosis of the liver. Which sign would the nurse anticipate finding?
    ○ 1. Peripheral edema.
    ○ 2. Ascites.
    ○ 3. Anorexia.
    ○ 4. Jaundice.

45. A client with cirrhosis begins to develop ascites. Spironolactone (Aldactone) is prescribed to treat the ascites. The nurse should monitor the client closely for which of the following drug-related side effects?
    ○ 1. Constipation.
    ○ 2. Hyperkalemia.
    ○ 3. Irregular pulse.
    ○ 4. Dysuria.

46. What diet should be implemented for a client who is in the early stages of cirrhosis?
    ○ 1. High calorie, high carbohydrate.
    ○ 2. High protein, low fat.
    ○ 3. Low fat, low protein.
    ○ 4. High carbohydrate, low sodium.

47. A client with cirrhosis complains that his skin always feels itchy and that he "scratches himself raw" while he sleeps. The nurse should recognize that the itching is the result of which abnormality associated with cirrhosis?
    ○ 1. Folic acid deficiency.
    ○ 2. Prolonged prothrombin time.
    ○ 3. Increased bilirubin levels.
    ○ 4. Hypokalemia.

48. Which one of the following health promotion activities would be appropriate for the nurse to suggest that the client with cirrhosis add to the daily routine at home?
    ○ 1. Supplement the diet with daily multivitamins.
    ○ 2. Limit daily alcohol intake.
    ○ 3. Take a sleeping pill at bedtime.
    ○ 4. Limit contact with other people whenever possible.

49. The client with cirrhosis has developed ascites. The nurse should recognize that the pathologic basis for the development of ascites in clients with cirrhosis is portal hypertension and
    ○ 1. an excess serum sodium level.
    ○ 2. an increased metabolism of aldosterone.
    ○ 3. a decreased flow of hepatic lymph.
    ○ 4. a decreased serum albumin level.

50. Which of the following positions would be appropriate for a client with severe ascites?
    ○ 1. Fowler's.
    ○ 2. Side-lying.
    ○ 3. Reverse Trendelenburg.
    ○ 4. Sims'.

51. The client with cirrhosis receives 100 mL of 25% serum albumin intravenously. Which finding would best indicate that the albumin is having its desired effect?
    ○ 1. Increased urine output.
    ○ 2. Increased serum albumin level.
    ○ 3. Decreased anorexia.
    ○ 4. Increased ease of breathing.

52. A client with cirrhosis vomits bright red blood and the physician suspects bleeding esophageal varices. The physician decides to insert a Sengstaken-Blakemore tube. The nurse should explain to the client that the tube acts by
    ○ 1. providing a large diameter for effective gastric lavage.
    ○ 2. applying direct pressure to gastric bleeding sites.
    ○ 3. blocking blood flow to the stomach and esophagus.
    ○ 4. applying direct pressure to the esophagus.

53. About 30 minutes after a Sengstaken-Blakemore tube is inserted, the nurse observes that the client appears to be having difficulty breathing. The nurse's first action should be to

○ 1. remove the tube.
○ 2. deflate the esophageal portion of the tube.
○ 3. determine whether the tube is obstructing the airway.
○ 4. increase the oxygen flow rate.

54. The physician orders oral neomycin as well as a neomycin enema for a client with cirrhosis. The nurse understands that the purpose of this therapy is to
    ○ 1. reduce abdominal pressure.
    ○ 2. prevent straining during defecation.
    ○ 3. block ammonia formation.
    ○ 4. reduce bleeding within the intestine.

55. The nurse monitors a client with cirrhosis for the development of hepatic encephalopathy. Which of the following would be an indication that hepatic encephalopathy is developing?
    ○ 1. Decreased mental status.
    ○ 2. Elevated blood pressure.
    ○ 3. Decreased urinary output.
    ○ 4. Labored respirations.

56. A client's serum ammonia level is elevated, and the physician orders 30 mL of lactulose (Cephulac). Which of the following side effects of this drug would the nurse expect to see?
    ○ 1. Increased urine output.
    ○ 2. Improved level of consciousness.
    ○ 3. Increased bowel movements.
    ○ 4. Nausea and vomiting.

57. A client is to be discharged with a prescription for lactulose (Cephulac). The nurse teaches the client and the client's spouse how to administer this medication. Which of the following statements would indicate that the client has understood the information?
    ○ 1. "I'll take it with Maalox."
    ○ 2. "I'll mix it with apple juice."
    ○ 3. "I'll take it with a laxative."
    ○ 4. "I'll mix the crushed tablets in some gelatin."

58. The nurse is providing discharge instructions for a client with cirrhosis. Which of the following statements best indicates that the client has understood the teaching?
    ○ 1. "I should eat a high-protein, high-carbohydrate diet to provide energy."
    ○ 2. "It is safer for me to take acetaminophen (Tylenol) for pain instead of aspirin."
    ○ 3. "I should avoid constipation to decrease chances of bleeding."
    ○ 4. "If I get enough rest and follow my diet, it is possible for my cirrhosis to be cured."

59. The nurse is preparing a client for a paracentesis. Which of the following activities would be appropriate before the procedure?
    ○ 1. Have the client void immediately before the procedure.

  ○ 2. Place the client in a side-lying position.

  ○ 3. Initiate an intravenous line to administer sedatives.

  ○ 4. Place client on NPO status 6 hours before the procedure.

60. Which of the following interventions would the nurse anticipate incorporating into the client's plan of care when hepatic encephalopathy initially develops?

  ○ 1. Inserting a nasogastric tube.

  ○ 2. Restricting fluids to 1000 mL/day.

  ○ 3. Administering intravenous salt-poor albumin.

  ○ 4. Implementing a low-protein diet.

61. A client with ascites and peripheral edema is at risk for impaired skin integrity. Which of the following interventions would be implemented to prevent skin breakdown?

  ○ 1. Range-of-motion exercise every 4 hours.

  ○ 2. Massage of the abdomen once a shift.

  ○ 3. Use of alternating air pressure mattress.

  ○ 4. Elevation of the lower extremities.

Correct Answers and Rationale

The letters in parentheses following the rationale identify the step of the nursing process (A, D, P, I, E) and client needs (1, 2, 3, 4, 5, 6, 7, 8, 9, 10). See the inside front cover for the key.

The Client With Cholecystitis

1. 3. The primary goal of nursing care at this time is to decrease the client's severe abdominal pain. The pain, which is frequently accompanied by nausea and vomiting, is caused by biliary spasm. Narcotic analgesics are given to relieve the severe pain and spasm of cholecystitis. Relief of pain may decrease nausea and vomiting and thereby decrease the client's likelihood of developing further complications, such as deficient fluid volume and imbalanced nutrition. (D, 10)

2. 2. When bile is not reaching the intestine, the feces do not contain bile pigments. The stool then becomes gray, claylike, or putty-like in color. Dark green color in the stool is the result of bile pigment. Black stool can be caused by upper gastrointestinal bleeding and by certain medications, such as iron supplements. Brown stool is normal. (A, 10)

3. 4. A client with an obstructed common bile duct should be monitored for prolonged bleeding time. Such an obstruction prevents bile from entering the intestinal tract, thus decreasing the absorption of fat-soluble vitamins A, D, E, and K. Vitamin K is necessary for prothrombin formation. Prothrombin deficiency causes delayed blood clotting, which results in prolonged bleeding time. An obstructed bile duct does not cause respiratory distress, circulatory overload, or urinary tract infection. (E, 10)

4. 1. Providing information can help to answer the client's questions and decrease anxiety. Fear of the unknown can increase anxiety. Telling the client not to be afraid, that the procedure is a common one, or to follow her physician's orders will not necessarily decrease anxiety. (I, 5)

5. 4. A T-tube is used after exploration of the common duct to help prevent bile from spilling into the peritoneal cavity. The tube also helps maintain patency of the common bile duct and helps ensure bile drainage out of the body, until the edema in the common bile duct subsides. After this occurs, bile can drain into the duodenum. (E, 9)

6. 3. The T-tube usually drains 300 to 500 mL in the first 24 hours after a choledocholithotomy. After 3 to 4 days, as the edema subsides in the common bile duct, the amount decreases to less than 200 mL per 24 hours. (A, 9)

7. 2. T-tube bile drainage is recorded separately on the output record. Adding the T-tube drainage to the urine output or wound drainage makes it difficult to accurately determine the amounts of bile, urine, or drainage. The client's total intake will be incorrect if drainage is subtracted from it. (I, 9)

8. 4. Lean meats such as beef, lamb, veal, and well-trimmed lean ham and pork are low in fat. Rice, pasta, and vegetables are low in fat when not served with butter, cream, or sauces. Fruits are low in fat. The amount of fat allowed in a client's diet after a cholecystectomy will depend on the client's ability to tolerate fat. Typically, the client does not require a special diet but is encouraged to avoid excessive fat intake. A cheese omelet and peanut butter have high fat content. Ham salad is high in fat from the fat in salad dressing. (P, 7)

9. 1. Meperidine (Demerol) would be the narcotic analgesic of choice for a client with cholecystitis. Acetaminophen with codeine would not be appropriate to administer, because the codeine could cause biliary duct spasm and increase pain, as could opiates such as morphine sulfate. Promethazine (Phenergan) is an antiemetic. (P, 8)

10. 3. Immediately after surgery, the client will drink liquids. A light diet can be resumed the day after surgery. There is no need for the client to remain NPO after surgery, because peristaltic bowel activity should not be affected. The client will probably not be able to tolerate a full meal comfortably the day after surgery. There is no need for the client to stay on a bland diet after a laparoscopic cholecystectomy. The client should, however, avoid excessive fats. (I, 10)

11. 2. After a laparoscopic cholecystectomy, clients can return to work within 1 week. The client can remove dressings from the puncture site and shower the day after surgery. The site does not need to be rebandaged but should be left open to air. The client should report any fever, which could be an indication of a complication. (I, 9)

The Client With Pancreatitis

12. 1. The primary diagnostic tests for pancreatitis are serum amylase, serum lipase, and urine amylase. All three laboratory results are typically elevated. Serum

amylase is the most common test; the result is usually higher than 200 units/dL. Serum glucose may be elevated in pancreatitis because of beta-cell damage, but this is not used to diagnose pancreatitis. Serum potassium and trypsin levels are not affected in pancreatitis. (A, 9)

13. 1. Alcoholism is a major cause of acute pancreatitis in the United States. Because some clients are reluctant to discuss alcohol use, staff may inquire about it in several ways. All clients are asked about alcohol and drug use on hospital admission, but this information is especially pertinent for clients with pancreatitis. Physicians do need to seek facts, but this can be done while respecting the client's religious beliefs. Respecting religious beliefs is important in providing holistic client care. Generally, alcohol intake does not interfere with the tests used to diagnose pancreatitis. Recent ingestion of large amounts of alcohol, however, may cause an increased serum amylase level. Large amounts of ethyl and methyl alcohol may produce an elevated urinary amylase concentration. (I, 4)

14. 2. Life-threatening shock is a potential complication of pancreatitis. Kinin peptides activated by the trapped trypsin cause vasodilation and increased capillary permeability. These effects exacerbate shock and are not easily reversed with pharmacologic agents such as vasopressors. Hemorrhage may occur into the pancreas, but not in the intestines. Systemic complications include pulmonary complications, but not congestive heart failure or acute tubular necrosis. (A, 10)

15. 2. Jaundice may be present in acute pancreatitis owing to obstruction of the biliary tract. Bowel sounds may be decreased or absent, so diarrhea would not be expected. Hypotension is likely to develop because of pancreatic hemorrhage or toxemia. Ascites develops as a result of portal hypertension and is common in liver disease, but not in pancreatitis. (A, 10)

16. 1. Pancreatitis interferes with beta-cell functioning, and clients must be monitored carefully for hyperglycemia. The client may also develop hypocalcemia and hyperlipidemia. Pancreatitis does not decrease blood cell counts or affect platelet production or potassium levels. (E, 9)

17. 1. There is little definitive treatment for pancreatitis. As a primary objective, it is important to decrease pancreatic enzymes to reduce stimulation of the pancreas. This is done by keeping the client NPO to rest the gastrointestinal tract and thereby suppress pancreatic enzyme secretion. Ensuring adequate nutrition, maintaining fluid and electrolyte balance, and preventing the development of an infection are issues for the client with pancreatitis but are not the primary focus of treatment. (P, 10)

18. 2. Nasogastric suction is frequently used in the treatment of pancreatitis to decrease pancreatic secretions and gastric distention. Foods and fluids are withheld during the acute phase of pancreatitis to rest the pancreas. Intravenous fluids are administered to provide hydration. Placing the client in the reverse Trendelenburg position is not appropriate. Most clients will be more comfortable if they are placed in a side-lying position with the head of the bed elevated to relieve abdominal tension. There is no need to place the client on enteric precautions. (P, 9)

19. 4. The client with acute pancreatitis is prone to complications associated with the respiratory system. Pneumonia, atelectasis, and pleural effusion are examples of respiratory complications that can develop as a result of pancreatic enzyme exudate. Pancreatitis does not cause congestive heart failure, ulcer formation, or cirrhosis. (A, 9)

20. 1. Hypocalcemia develops in severe cases of acute pancreatitis. The exact cause is unknown. Signs and symptoms of hypocalcemia include jerking and muscle twitching, numbness of fingers and lips, and irritability. Meperidine may cause tremors or convulsions as an adverse effect, but not muscle twitching. (E, 9)

21. 3. Antispasmodic drugs such as propantheline bromide may be administered along with narcotics to deal with the intense pain associated with pancreatitis. Antispasmodics relax smooth muscle and decrease gastric motility and pancreatic enzyme secretion, thereby decreasing pain. Ibuprofen does not have an antispasmodic effect and would not be as effective in relieving pain. Propranolol (Inderal) and magnesium hydroxide do not have antispasmodic effects and would not be effective in relieving pain. Antacids may be given to neutralize gastric secretions. (I, 8)

22. 4. Imbalanced Nutrition: Less Than Body Requirements is likely to be a priority nursing diagnosis because the abdominal pain, nausea, and vomiting that are typical of pancreatitis can affect the client's food and fluid intake. Treatment of pancreatitis also frequently involves stopping all oral intake until the inflammation is resolved. Clients with pancreatitis are at risk for development of malnutrition. Intravenous therapy is used for fluid replacement, and total parenteral nutrition may be ordered to prevent malnourishment. Clients with pancreatitis do not have airway clearance or swallowing difficulties. Clients with pancreatitis are more likely to develop deficient fluid volume and to require fluid replacement. (D, 10)

23. 1. Crash dieting or bingeing may cause an acute attack of pancreatitis and should be avoided. Carbohydrate intake should be increased, because carbohydrates are less stimulating to the pancreas. There is no need to

maintain a dietary pattern of six meals a day; the client can eat whenever desired. There is no need to place the client on a sodium-restricted diet, because pancreatitis does not promote fluid retention. (I, 10)

24. 2. In chronic pancreatitis, destruction of pancreatic tissue requires pancreatic enzyme replacement. Pancreatic enzymes are prescribed to facilitate the digestion of proteins and fats and should be taken in conjunction with every meal and snack. Specified hours or limited times for administration are ineffective because the enzymes must be taken in conjunction with food ingestion. (I, 8)

25. 3. If the dosage and administration of pancreatic enzymes are adequate, the client's stool will be relatively normal. Any increase in odor or fat content would indicate the need for dosage adjustment. Stable body weight would be another indirect indicator. Fluid intake does not affect enzyme replacement therapy. If diabetes has developed, the client will need to monitor glucose levels. However, glucose and ketone levels are not affected by pancreatic enzyme therapy and would not indicate effectiveness of the therapy. (E, 8)

26. 4. Clients with chronic pancreatitis are likely to develop diabetes as a result of the pancreatic fibrosis that occurs. The pancreas becomes unable to secrete insulin. Cholelithiasis, hepatitis, and irritable bowel syndrome are not caused by chronic pancreatitis. (A, 9)

The Client With Viral Hepatitis

27. 2. Hepatitis B is considered to be a sexually transmitted disease. It can also be transmitted by percutaneous exposure to infected blood. Hepatitis A is transmitted via the fecal–oral route. Hepatitis C is primarily transmitted percutaneously and, less frequently, sexually. Hepatitis D is transmitted percutaneously. (P, 2)

28. 2. Liver inflammation and obstruction block the normal flow of bile. Excess bilirubin turns the skin and sclera yellow and the urine dark and frothy. Profound anorexia is also common. Tarry stools are indicative of gastrointestinal bleeding and would not be expected in hepatitis. Light- or clay-colored stools may occur in hepatitis owing to bile duct obstruction. The urine is dark and frothy. Shortness of breath would be unexpected. (A, 10)

29. 2. The organism causing hepatitis A is transmitted primarily through feces. Viral hepatitis is not transmitted via the skin or urine. Hepatitis B, C, and D are transmitted through exposure to blood, but hepatitis A is not. (P, 2)

30. 4. Contact precautions are recommended for clients with hepatitis A. This includes wearing gloves for direct care. These recommendations are made by the Centers for Disease Control and Prevention. A gown is not required unless substantial contact with the client is anticipated. It is not necessary to wear a mask. The client does not need a private room unless incontinent of stool. (P, 2)

31. 4. During the convalescent or posticteric stage of hepatitis, fatigue and malaise are the most common complaints. These symptoms usually disappear within 2 to 4 months. Fatigue and malaise are not evidence of a secondary infection. Hepatitis A is not treated by drug therapy. It is important that the client continue to balance activity with periods of rest. (I, 9)

32. 1. Treatment of hepatitis consists primarily of bed rest with bathroom privileges. Bed rest is maintained during the acute phase to reduce metabolic demands on the liver, thus increasing its blood supply and promoting liver cell regeneration. When activity is gradually resumed, the client should be taught to rest before becoming overly tired. Although adequate fluid intake is important, it is not necessary to force fluids to treat hepatitis. Antibiotics are not used to treat hepatitis. Electrolyte imbalances are not typical of hepatitis. (I, 7)

33. 3. Serum levels of bilirubin and liver enzymes, such as alanine aminotransferase (ALT [formerly SGPT]) and aspartate aminotransferase (AST [formerly SGOT]), are carefully monitored during hepatitis. They provide important data about liver function. Blood glucose levels, the creatinine clearance, and serum electrolyte levels provide no information about liver function. (A, 9)

34. 1. The prothrombin time may be prolonged because of decreased absorption of vitamin K and decreased production of prothrombin by the liver. The client should be assessed carefully for bleeding tendencies. Blood glucose and serum potassium and calcium levels are not affected by hepatitis. (A, 9)

35. 3. Unlike the cirrhosis of alcoholism, viral forms of hepatitis are not usually associated with nutritional depletion. A well-balanced diet is advocated. It is a challenge to ensure that clients with hepatitis ingest a balanced diet with sufficient carbohydrates and calories, because these clients are generally anorexic and have little interest in eating. Low-fat, high-protein foods are encouraged with hepatitis clients. There is no need to restrict sodium intake. (P, 7)

36. 3. The hepatitis A virus is transmitted via the fecal–oral route. The virus is spread through contaminated hands, water, and food, especially shellfish growing in contaminated water. Certain animal handlers are at risk for hepatitis A, particularly those handling primates. Frequent handwashing is probably the single most important preventive action. Insects do not transmit hepatitis A. Family members do not need to stay

away from the client with hepatitis. It is not necessary to disinfect food and clothing. (I, 2)

37. 4. The most appropriate diagnosis for this client is Activity Intolerance related to fatigue. The major goal of care for the client with hepatitis is to increase activity gradually as tolerated. Periods of alternating rest and activity should be included in the plan of care. There is no evidence that the client is physically immobile, unable to provide self-care, or coping ineffectively. (D, 7)

38. 2. The client expresses feelings of isolation. The most appropriate nursing diagnosis for this client is Social Isolation. Clients with hepatitis frequently feel guilty about possibly exposing others to the disease. Family and friends may experience fear of contracting the disease. The data provided do not indicate that the client is necessarily anxious, feeling powerless, or experiencing low self-esteem. (D, 5)

39. 4. The nurse should encourage the client to further verbalize feelings of isolation. Instead of dismissing these feelings or making assumptions about the cause of isolation, the nurse should allow clients to verbalize their fears and provide education on how to prevent infection transmission. (I, 5)

40. 2. Hepatitis C is usually transmitted through blood exposure or needlesticks. A hepatitis C vaccine is currently under development, but it is not available for use. The first line of defense against hepatitis B is the hepatitis B vaccine. Hepatitis C is not transmitted through feces or urine. Wearing a gown and mask will not prevent transmission of the hepatitis C vaccine if the caregiver comes in contact with infected blood or needles. (P, 2)

41. 3. Interferon alfa-2b most commonly causes flulike side effects such as myalgia, arthralgia, headache, nausea, fever, and fatigue. Retinopathy is a potential side effect, but not a common one. Diarrhea may develop as a side effect. Clients are advised to administer the drug at bedtime and get adequate rest. Medications may be prescribed to treat the symptoms. The drug may also cause hematologic changes; therefore laboratory tests such as a complete blood count and differential should be conducted monthly during the drug therapy. Blood glucose laboratory values should be monitored for the development of hyperglycemia. (A, 8)

42. 4. Hepatitis B is spread through exposure to blood or blood products and through high-risk sexual activity. Hepatitis B is considered to be a sexually transmitted disease. High-risk sexual activities include sex with multiple partners, unprotected sex with an infected individual, male homosexual activity, and sexual activity with intravenous drug users. The Centers for Disease Control and Prevention recommend immuniza-

tion of all newborns and adolescents. College students are at high risk for development of hepatitis B and are encouraged to be immunized. Alcohol intake by itself does not predispose an individual to hepatitis B, but it can lead to high-risk behaviors such as unprotected sex. Good personal hygiene alone will not prevent the transmission of hepatitis B. (P, 2)

43. 2. The client should be able to verbalize the importance of reporting any bleeding tendencies that could be the result of a prolonged prothrombin time. Ascites is not typically a clinical manifestation of hepatitis; it is associated with cirrhosis. Alcohol use should be eliminated for at least 1 year after the diagnosis of hepatitis to allow the liver time to fully recover. There is no need for a client to be restricted to the home, because hepatitis is not spread through casual contact between individuals. (E, 10)

The Client With Cirrhosis

44. 3. Early clinical manifestations of cirrhosis are subtle and usually include gastrointestinal symptoms such as anorexia, nausea, vomiting, and changes in bowel patterns. These changes are caused by the liver's altered ability to metabolize carbohydrates, proteins, and fats. Peripheral edema, ascites, and jaundice are later signs of liver failure and portal hypertension. (A, 10)

45. 2. Spironolactone (Aldactone) is a potassium-sparing diuretic; therefore, clients should be monitored closely for hyperkalemia. Other common side effects include abdominal cramping, diarrhea, dizziness, headache, and rash. Constipation and dysuria are not common side effects of spironolactone. An irregular pulse is not a side effect of spironolactone but could develop if serum potassium levels are not closely monitored. (A, 8)

46. 1. For clients who have cirrhosis without complications, a high-calorie, high-carbohydrate diet is preferred to provide an adequate supply of nutrients. In the early stages of cirrhosis, there is no need to restrict fat, protein, or sodium. (I, 10)

47. 3. Excess retained bilirubin produces an irritating effect on the peripheral nerves, causing intense itching. Folic acid deficiency causes varied symptoms, but not itching. Itching is not a symptom of a prolonged prothrombin time or of hypokalemia. (E, 9)

48. 1. General health promotion measures include maintaining good nutrition, avoiding infection, and abstaining from alcohol. Rest and sleep are essential, but an impaired liver may not be able to detoxify sedatives and barbiturates. Such drugs must be used cautiously, if at all, by clients with cirrhosis. The client does not need to limit contact with others but should exercise caution to stay away from ill people. (I, 7)

49. 4. Ascites results from increased pressure in the venous system caused by a low level of serum albumin (which contributes to decreased colloid osmotic pressure) and sodium retention. The serum sodium level is not increased. There is a decreased aldosterone clearance and an increased flow of hepatic lymph. (A, 10)

50. 1. Ascites can compromise the action of the diaphragm and increase the client's risk of respiratory problems. Ascites also greatly increases the risk of skin breakdown. Frequent position changes are important, but the preferred position is Fowler's. Placing the client in Fowler's position helps facilitate the client's breathing by relieving pressure on the diaphragm. The other positions do not relieve pressure on the diaphragm. (I, 7)

51. 1. Normal serum albumin is administered to reduce ascites. Hypoalbuminemia, a mechanism underlying ascites formation, results in decreased colloid osmotic pressure. Administering serum albumin increases the plasma colloid osmotic pressure, which causes fluid to flow from the tissue space into the plasma. Increased urine output is the best indication that the albumin is having the desired effect. An increased serum albumin level and increased ease of breathing may indirectly imply that the administration of albumin is effective in relieving the ascites. However, it is not as direct an indicator as increased urinary output. Anorexia is not affected by the administration of albumin. (E, 8)

52. 4. The Sengstaken-Blakemore tube has a small gastric balloon that anchors the tube and applies pressure to the area of the cardiac sphincter. The large esophageal balloon applies direct pressure on the bleeding sites in the esophagus. A tube passing through the balloons allows for aspiration and irrigation. The Sengstaken-Blakemore tube is not used for gastric lavage. It would not be desirable to block blood flow to the stomach and esophageal tissue. (P, 9)

53. 3. If the gastric balloon should rupture or deflate, the esophageal balloon can move and partially or totally obstruct the airway, causing respiratory distress. The client must be observed closely. No direct action should be taken until the condition is accurately diagnosed. (I, 9)

54. 3. Neomycin is administered to decrease the bacterial action on protein in the intestines, which results in ammonia production. This ammonia, if not detoxified by the liver, can result in hepatic encephalopathy and coma. The antibiotic does not reduce abdominal pressure, prevent straining during defecation, or decrease hemorrhaging within the intestine. (P, 8)

55. 1. The client should be monitored closely for changes in mental status. Ammonia has a toxic effect on central nervous system tissue and produces an altered level of consciousness, marked by drowsiness and irritability. If this process is unchecked, the client may lapse into coma. Increasing ammonia levels are not detected by changes in blood pressure, urinary output, or respirations. (A, 10)

56. 3. Lactulose increases intestinal motility, thereby trapping and expelling ammonia in the feces. An increase in the number of bowel movements is expected as a side effect. Lactulose does not affect urine output. Any improvements in mental status would be the result of increased ammonia elimination, not a side effect of the drug. Nausea and vomiting are not common side effects of lactulose. (P, 8)

57. 2. The taste of lactulose is a problem for some clients. Mixing it with fruit juice, water, or milk can make it more palatable. Lactulose should not be given with antacids, which may inhibit its action. Lactulose comes in the form of syrup for oral or rectal administration. (E, 8)

58. 3. Clients with cirrhosis should be instructed to avoid constipation and straining at stool to prevent hemorrhage. The client with cirrhosis has bleeding tendencies because of the liver's inability to produce clotting factors. A low-protein and high-carbohydrate diet is recommended. Clients with cirrhosis should not take acetaminophen, which is potentially hepatotoxic. Aspirin also should be avoided if esophageal varices are present. Cirrhosis is a chronic disease. (E, 9)

59. 1. Immediately before a paracentesis, the client should empty the bladder to prevent perforation. The client will be placed in a high Fowler's position or seated on the side of the bed for the procedure. Intravenous sedatives are not usually administered. The client does not need to be NPO. (I, 9)

60. 4. When hepatic encephalopathy develops, measures are taken to reduce ammonia formation. Protein is restricted in the diet. A nasogastric tube is not inserted initially but may be necessary as the disease progresses. Fluid restriction and salt-poor albumin are incorporated into the treatment of ascites, but not hepatic encephalopathy. (I, 10)

61. 3. Edematous tissue is easily traumatized and must receive meticulous care. An alternating air pressure mattress will help decrease pressure on the edematous tissue. Range-of-motion exercises are important to maintain joint function, but they do not necessarily prevent skin breakdown. When abdominal skin is stretched taut due to ascites, it must be cleansed very carefully. The abdomen should not be massaged. Elevation of the lower extremities promotes venous return and decreases swelling. (I, 9)

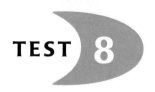

The Client With Endocrine Health Problems

Select the one best answer, and indicate your choice by filling in the circle in front of the option.

The Client With Thyrotoxicosis

1. The nurse is completing a health assessment of a 42-year-old woman with suspected Graves' disease. The nurse should assess this client for
   ○ 1. anorexia.
   ○ 2. tachycardia.
   ○ 3. weight gain.
   ○ 4. cold skin.

2. A female client with thyrotoxicosis would probably report which changes related to the menstrual cycle during initial assessment?
   ○ 1. Dysmenorrhea.
   ○ 2. Metrorrhagia.
   ○ 3. Oligomenorrhea.
   ○ 4. Menorrhagia.

3. Propylthiouracil (PTU) is prescribed for a client with Graves' disease to decrease circulating thyroid hormone. The nurse should teach the client to immediately report which of the following signs and symptoms?
   ○ 1. Sore throat.
   ○ 2. Painful, excessive menstruation.
   ○ 3. Constipation.
   ○ 4. Increased urine output.

4. A client with thyrotoxicosis says to the nurse, "I am so irritable. I am having problems at work because I lose my temper very easily." Which of the following responses by the nurse would give the client the most accurate explanation of her behavior?
   ○ 1. "Your behavior is caused by temporary confusion brought on by your illness."

   ○ 2. "Your behavior is caused by the excess thyroid hormone in your system."
   ○ 3. "Your behavior is caused by your worrying about the seriousness of your illness."
   ○ 4. "Your behavior is caused by the stress of trying to manage a career and cope with illness."

5. Serum concentrations of thyroid hormones and thyroid-stimulating hormone (TSH) are tests ordered for the client with thyrotoxicosis. Which of the following laboratory values are indicative of thyrotoxicosis?
   ○ 1. Elevated thyroid hormone concentrations and normal TSH.
   ○ 2. Elevated TSH and normal thyroid hormone concentrations.
   ○ 3. Decreased thyroid hormone concentrations and elevated TSH.
   ○ 4. Elevated thyroid hormone concentrations and decreased TSH.

6. The nurse should teach the client to prevent corneal irritation from mild exophthalmos by
   ○ 1. massaging the eyes at regular intervals.
   ○ 2. instilling an ophthalmic anesthetic as ordered.
   ○ 3. wearing dark-colored glasses.
   ○ 4. covering both eyes with moistened gauze pads.

7. A client with Graves' disease is treated with radioactive iodine (RAI) in the form of sodium iodide ^{131}I. Which of the following statements by the nurse will explain to the client how the drug works?
   ○ 1. "The radioactive iodine stabilizes the thyroid hormone levels before a thyroidectomy."
   ○ 2. "The radioactive iodine reduces uptake of thyroxine and thereby improves your condition."

○ 3. "The radioactive iodine lowers the levels of thyroid hormones by slowing your body's production of them."

○ 4. "The radioactive iodine destroys thyroid tissue so that thyroid hormones are no longer produced."

8. Which of the following nursing diagnoses would most likely be appropriate for a client with Graves' disease performing self-care after treatment with RAI in the form of sodium iodide ^{131}I?

○ 1. Risk for Injury related to altered level of consciousness.

○ 2. Ineffective Breathing Pattern related to effects of radioactive iodine.

○ 3. Total Self-Care Deficit related to the need for immobilization after RAI therapy.

○ 4. Risk for Ineffective Therapeutic Regimen related to lack of knowledge about disease management.

9. After treatment with RAI in the form of sodium iodide ^{131}I, the nurse teaches the client to

○ 1. monitor for signs and symptoms of hyperthyroidism.

○ 2. rest for 1 week to prevent complications of the medication.

○ 3. take thyroxine replacement for the remainder of the client's life.

○ 4. assess for hypertension and tachycardia resulting from altered thyroid activity.

10. A client with a large goiter is scheduled for a subtotal thyroidectomy to treat thyrotoxicosis. Saturated solution of potassium iodide (SSKI) is prescribed preoperatively for the client. The primary reason for using this drug is that it helps

○ 1. slow progression of exophthalmos.

○ 2. reduce the vascularity of the thyroid gland.

○ 3. decrease the body's ability to store thyroxine.

○ 4. increase the body's ability to excrete thyroxine.

11. Which of the following measures is most often recommended when preparing SSKI for administration?

○ 1. Pour the solution over ice chips.

○ 2. Mix the solution with an antacid.

○ 3. Dilute the solution with water, milk, or fruit juice and have the client drink it with a straw.

○ 4. Disguise the solution in a pureed fruit or vegetable.

12. The nurse asks the client to state her name as soon as she regains consciousness postoperatively after a subtotal thyroidectomy and at each assessment. The nurse does this primarily to monitor for signs of which of the following?

○ 1. Internal hemorrhage.

○ 2. Decreasing level of consciousness.

○ 3. Laryngeal nerve damage.

○ 4. Upper airway obstruction.

13. A client who has undergone a subtotal thyroidectomy is subject to complications in the first 48 hours after surgery. The nurse should obtain and keep at the bedside equipment to

○ 1. begin total parenteral nutrition.

○ 2. start a cutdown infusion.

○ 3. administer tube feedings.

○ 4. perform a tracheostomy.

14. Which of the following symptoms might indicate that a client was developing tetany after a subtotal thyroidectomy?

○ 1. Pains in the joints of the hands and feet.

○ 2. Tingling in the fingers.

○ 3. Bleeding on the back of the dressing.

○ 4. Tension on the suture line.

15. Which of the following medications should be available to provide emergency treatment if a client develops tetany after a subtotal thyroidectomy?

○ 1. Sodium phosphate.

○ 2. Calcium gluconate.

○ 3. Echothiophate iodide.

○ 4. Sodium bicarbonate.

16. A 60-year-old woman is diagnosed with hypothyroidism. Signs and symptoms of hypothyroidism include

○ 1. tachycardia.

○ 2. weight gain.

○ 3. diarrhea.

○ 4. anorexia.

17. Appropriate nursing diagnoses for a client with hypothyroidism would probably include which of the following?

○ 1. Risk for Injury (corneal abrasion) related to incomplete closure of eyelid.

○ 2. Imbalanced Nutrition: Less Than Body Requirements related to hypermetabolism.

○ 3. Deficient Fluid Volume related to diarrhea.

○ 4. Activity Intolerance related to fatigue associated with the disorder.

18. When discussing recent onset of feelings of sadness and depression in a client with hypothyroidism, the nurse should inform the client that these feelings are

○ 1. the effects of thyroid hormone replacement therapy and will diminish over time.

○ 2. related to the thyroid hormone replacement therapy and will not diminish over time.

○ 3. a normal part of having a chronic illness.

○ 4. most likely related to low thyroid hormone levels and will improve with treatment.

The Client With Diabetes Mellitus

19. A 55-year-old male client has recently been diagnosed with type 2 diabetes mellitus (DM) and is pre-

scribed the sulfonylurea compound tolbutamide (Orinase). He is concerned about the diagnosis and says he knows nothing about diabetes. The nurse determines that the client needs teaching and support. The nurse explains that tolbutamide is believed to lower the blood glucose level by which of the following actions?
○ 1. Potentiating the action of insulin.
○ 2. Lowering the renal threshold of glucose.
○ 3. Stimulating insulin release from functioning beta cells in the pancreas.
○ 4. Combining with glucose to render it inert.

20. When teaching the diabetic client about foot care, the nurse should instruct the client to do which of the following
○ 1. Avoid going barefoot.
○ 2. Buy shoes a half size larger.
○ 3. Cut toenails at angles.
○ 4. Use heating pads for sore feet.

21. A client with DM asks the nurse to recommend something to remove corns from his toes. The nurse should advise him to
○ 1. apply a high-quality corn plaster to the area.
○ 2. consult his physician or podiatrist about removing the corns.
○ 3. apply iodine to the corns before peeling them off.
○ 4. soak his feet in borax solution to peel off the corns.

22. A client with DM presents to the clinic for a regular 3-month follow-up appointment. The nurse notes several small bandages covering cuts on the client's hands. The client says, "I'm so clumsy. I'm always cutting my finger cooking or burning myself on the iron." Which of the following responses by the nurse would be most appropriate?
○ 1. "Wash all wounds in isopropyl alcohol."
○ 2. "Keep all cuts clean and covered."
○ 3. "Why don't you have your children to do the cooking and ironing?"
○ 4. "You really should be fine as long as you take your daily medication."

23. The client with DM says, "If I could just avoid what you call carbohydrates in my diet, I guess I would be okay." The nurse should base the response to this comment on the knowledge that diabetes affects metabolism of which of the following?
○ 1. Carbohydrates only.
○ 2. Fats and carbohydrates only.
○ 3. Protein and carbohydrates only.
○ 4. Proteins, fats, and carbohydrates.

24. A client with type 1 DM is admitted to the emergency department. Which of the following respiratory patterns requires immediate action?
○ 1. Deep, rapid respirations with long expirations.

○ 2. Shallow respirations alternating with long expirations.
○ 3. Regular depth of respirations with frequent pauses.
○ 4. Short expirations and inspirations.

25. The nurse should caution the client with DM who is taking a sulfonylurea medication that alcoholic beverages should be avoided while taking these drugs because they can cause which of the following?
○ 1. Hypokalemia.
○ 2. Hyperkalemia.
○ 3. Hypocalcemia.
○ 4. Disulfiram (Antabuse)–like symptoms.

26. Which of the following conditions is the most significant risk factor for the development of type 2 DM?
○ 1. Cigarette smoking.
○ 2. High-cholesterol diet.
○ 3. Obesity.
○ 4. Hypertension.

27. Which of the following indicates a potential complication of DM?
○ 1. Inflamed, painful joints.
○ 2. Blood pressure of 160/100 mm Hg.
○ 3. Stooped appearance.
○ 4. Hemoglobin of 9 g/dL.

28. The nurse is teaching the client about home blood glucose monitoring. Which of the following blood glucose measurements indicates impending hypoglycemia?
○ 1. 59 mg/dL.
○ 2. 75 mg/dL.
○ 3. 108 mg/dL.
○ 4. 119 mg/dL.

29. Assessment of the diabetic client for common complications should always include examination of the
○ 1. abdomen.
○ 2. lymph glands.
○ 3. pharynx.
○ 4. eyes.

30. The client with type 1 DM is taught to take isophane insulin suspension NPH (Humulin N) at 5 PM each day. The client should be instructed that the greatest risk for hypoglycemia will occur at about what time?
○ 1. 11 AM, shortly before lunch.
○ 2. 1 PM, shortly after lunch.
○ 3. 6 PM, shortly after dinner.
○ 4. 1 AM, while sleeping.

31. A client with type 1 DM who jogs daily is given the following education regarding the preferred sites for insulin absorption.
○ 1. The preferred sites are the arms.
○ 2. The legs are the preferred sites of injection since the client is a jogger.

○ 3. The abdomen would provide a consistent and effective absorption site.

○ 4. Jogging does not cause altered insulin absorption, and the client does not have to be concerned about preferred sites.

32. The diabetic client who is taking insulin lispro (Humalog) injections would be advised to eat
    ○ 1. within 10 to 15 minutes after the injection.
    ○ 2. 1 hour after the injection.
    ○ 3. at any time, because timing of meals with Humalog injections is unnecessary.
    ○ 4. 2 hours before the injection.

33. The best indicator that allows the nurse to judge that the client has learned how to give an insulin self-injection correctly is when the client can do which of the following?
    ○ 1. Perform the procedure safely and correctly.
    ○ 2. Critique the nurse's performance of the procedure.
    ○ 3. Explain all steps of the procedure correctly.
    ○ 4. Correctly answer a post-test about the procedure.

34. Angiotensin-converting enzyme (ACE) inhibitors may be prescribed for the client with DM to reduce vascular changes and possibly prevent or delay development of
    ○ 1. chronic obstructive pulmonary disease.
    ○ 2. pancreatic cancer.
    ○ 3. renal failure.
    ○ 4. cerebral vascular accident.

35. The nurse should teach the diabetic client that which of the following is the most common symptom of hypoglycemia?
    ○ 1. Nervousness.
    ○ 2. Anorexia.
    ○ 3. Kussmaul's respirations.
    ○ 4. Bradycardia.

36. The nurse is assessing the client's use of medications. Which of the following medications may cause a complication with the treatment plan of a client with diabetes?
    ○ 1. Aspirin.
    ○ 2. Steroids.
    ○ 3. Sulfonylureas.
    ○ 4. ACE inhibitors.

37. A female client with type 1 DM is experiencing minor illness with the flu. The nurse should instruct the client
    ○ 1. to increase the frequency of self-monitoring (blood glucose testing).
    ○ 2. that she should try to reduce food intake to diminish nausea.
    ○ 3. that she does not need to take the insulin if she cannot eat.
    ○ 4. to take half of the normal dose of insulin.

38. Which of the following is a priority nursing diagnosis for the diabetic client who is taking insulin and has nausea and vomiting from a viral illness or influenza?
    ○ 1. Imbalanced Nutrition: Less than Body Requirements.
    ○ 2. Impaired Health Maintenance related to ineffective coping skills.
    ○ 3. Risk for Activity Intolerance.
    ○ 4. Activity Intolerance.

39. During a home visit, a diabetic client begins to cry and says, "I just cannot stand the thought of having to give myself a shot every day." Which of the following would be the best response by the nurse?
    ○ 1. "If you do not give yourself your insulin shots, you will die."
    ○ 2. "We can teach your daughter to give the shots so you will not have to do it."
    ○ 3. "I can arrange to have a home care nurse give you the shots every day."
    ○ 4. "What is it about giving yourself the insulin shots that bothers you?"

40. A client presents to the emergency room with diabetic ketoacidosis. The nurse would identify which of the following nursing diagnoses as a *priority* problem?
    ○ 1. Disturbed Sleep Pattern.
    ○ 2. Impaired Health Maintenance.
    ○ 3. Imbalanced Nutrition: Less than Body Requirements.
    ○ 4. Deficient Fluid Volume.

The Client With Pituitary Adenoma

41. Galactorrhea is caused by overproduction of which hormone?
    ○ 1. Prolactin.
    ○ 2. Adrenocorticotropic hormone (ACTH).
    ○ 3. Growth hormone (GH).
    ○ 4. Thyroid-stimulating hormone (TSH).

42. Which of the following symptoms are common in male clients with prolactin-secreting tumors?
    ○ 1. Severe lethargy and fatigue.
    ○ 2. Decreased libido and impotence.
    ○ 3. Bony proliferation of the hands, jaw, and feet.
    ○ 4. Deepening or coarsening of the voice.

43. Surgical management for large, invasive pituitary tumors is a transsphenoidal hypophysectomy. The nurse would explain that the surgery will be performed through an incision in the
    ○ 1. back of the mouth.
    ○ 2. nose.
    ○ 3. sinus channel below the right eye.
    ○ 4. upper gingival mucosa in the space between the upper gums and lip.

44. To help minimize the risk of postoperative respiratory complications after a hypophysectomy, the nurse would focus the client's preoperative teaching on the importance of
   ○ 1. using blow bottles.
   ○ 2. making frequent position changes.
   ○ 3. deep breathing.
   ○ 4. coughing.

45. Which of the following monitoring activities would be a major focus when planning nursing care for a client who has undergone transsphenoidal hypophysectomy?
   ○ 1. Monitoring for cerebrospinal fluid (CSF) leak.
   ○ 2. Monitoring for fluctuating blood glucose levels.
   ○ 3. Monitoring for Cushing's syndrome.
   ○ 4. Monitoring for cardiac arrest.

46. A client expresses concern about how a hypophysectomy will affect his sexual function. Which of the following statements provides the most accurate information about the physiologic effects of hypophysectomy?
   ○ 1. Removing the source of excess hormone should restore the client's libido, erectile function, and fertility.
   ○ 2. Potency will be restored, but the client will remain infertile.
   ○ 3. Fertility will be restored, but impotence and decreased libido will persist.
   ○ 4. Exogenous hormones will be needed to restore erectile function after the adenoma is removed.

47. Before undergoing a transsphenoidal hypophysectomy for pituitary adenoma, the client asks the nurse how the surgeon will close the incision made in the dura. The nurse would respond based on the knowledge that
   ○ 1. dissolvable sutures are used to close the dura.
   ○ 2. nasal packing provides pressure until normal wound healing occurs.
   ○ 3. a patch is made with a piece of fascia.
   ○ 4. a synthetic mesh is placed to facilitate healing.

48. Initial treatment for a CSF leak after transsphenoidal hypophysectomy would most likely involve
   ○ 1. repacking the nose.
   ○ 2. returning the client to surgery.
   ○ 3. enforcing bed rest with the head of the bed elevated.
   ○ 4. administering high-dose corticosteroid therapy.

49. Oral hygiene for a client recovering from transsphenoidal hypophysectomy would include which of the following?
   ○ 1. Rinsing the mouth with saline solution.
   ○ 2. Performing frequent toothbrushing.
   ○ 3. Cleaning the teeth with an electric toothbrush.
   ○ 4. Vigorous flossing.

50. The nurse teaches the client to monitor for signs and symptoms of which potential complication after hypophysectomy?
   ○ 1. Acromegaly.
   ○ 2. Cushing's disease.
   ○ 3. Diabetes mellitus.
   ○ 4. Hypopituitarism.

51. After pituitary surgery the nurse should assess the client for which of the following?
   ○ 1. Urine specific gravity less than 1.010.
   ○ 2. Urine output between 1 and 2 L/day.
   ○ 3. Blood glucose level higher than 300 mg/100 mL.
   ○ 4. Urine negative for glucose and ketones.

52. Vasopressin is administered to the client with diabetes insipidus (DI) because it
   ○ 1. decreases blood pressure.
   ○ 2. increases tubular reabsorption of water.
   ○ 3. increases release of insulin from the pancreas.
   ○ 4. decreases glucose production within the liver.

53. Which of the following constitutes a *priority* outcome criterion for the client with DI?
   ○ 1. Maintains normal fluid and electrolyte balance.
   ○ 2. Selects American Diabetes Association diet correctly.
   ○ 3. States dietary restrictions.
   ○ 4. Exhibits serum glucose level within normal range.

The Client With Addison's Disease

54. Which of the following is the *priority* goal for a client in addisonian crisis?
   ○ 1. Controlling hypertension.
   ○ 2. Preventing irreversible shock.
   ○ 3. Preventing infection.
   ○ 4. Relieving anxiety.

55. Which of the following would be an expected finding in a client with adrenal crisis (addisonian crisis)?
   ○ 1. Fluid retention.
   ○ 2. Pain.
   ○ 3. Peripheral edema.
   ○ 4. Hunger.

56. The client is receiving an intravenous infusion of 5% dextrose in normal saline running at 125 mL/hour. When hanging a new bag of fluid, the nurse notes swelling and hardness at the infusion site. Which immediate action would be indicated?
   ○ 1. Discontinue the infusion.
   ○ 2. Apply a warm soak to the site.
   ○ 3. Stop the flow of solution temporarily.
   ○ 4. Irrigate the needle with normal saline.

57. The client's wife asks the nurse whether the intravenous infusion is meeting her husband's nutri-

tional needs because he has vomited several times. The nurse's response should be based on the knowledge that 1 L of 5% dextrose in normal saline delivers

○ 1. 170 calories.

○ 2. 250 calories.

○ 3. 340 calories.

○ 4. 500 calories.

58. A client with Addison's disease is admitted to the medical unit. The nurse diagnoses the client with Deficient Fluid Volume related to inadequate fluid intake and to fluid loss secondary to inadequate adrenal hormone secretion. As the client's oral intake increases, which of the following fluids would be most appropriate?

○ 1. Milk and diet soda.

○ 2. Water and eggnog.

○ 3. Bouillon and juice.

○ 4. Coffee and milkshakes.

59. After stabilization of Addison's disease, a client attends a stress management class because stress can precipitate addisonian crisis. Which of the following actions taught by the nurse in the class is based on principles of stress management?

○ 1. Remove all sources of stress from your life.

○ 2. Use relaxation techniques such as music.

○ 3. Take antianxiety drugs daily.

○ 4. Avoid discussing stressful experiences.

60. When teaching a client newly diagnosed with primary Addison's disease, the nurse should explain that the disease results from

○ 1. insufficient secretion of growth hormone (GH).

○ 2. dysfunction of the hypothalamic pituitary.

○ 3. idiopathic atrophy of the adrenal gland.

○ 4. oversecretion of the adrenal medulla.

61. The nurse would expect the client with Addison's disease to exhibit which of the following signs and symptoms?

○ 1. Weight gain.

○ 2. Hunger.

○ 3. Lethargy.

○ 4. Muscle spasms.

62. Which of the following findings would be typical of Addison's disease?

○ 1. Hypokalemia.

○ 2. Hypernatremia.

○ 3. Hypoglycemia.

○ 4. Decreased blood urea nitrogen (BUN) level.

63. The client with Addison's disease is taking glucocorticoids at home. Which of the following statements correctly reflects the principle governing administration and dosage of glucocorticoids?

○ 1. Various circumstances increase the need for glucocorticoids, so dosage adjustments will be needed.

○ 2. The need for glucocorticoids stabilizes, and a predetermined dose is taken once a day.

○ 3. Glucocorticoids are cumulative, so a dose is taken every third day.

○ 4. A dose is taken every 6 hours to ensure consistent blood levels of glucocorticoids.

64. Cortisone acetate (Cortone Acetate) and fludrocortisone acetate (Florinef Acetate) are prescribed as replacement therapy for a client with Addison's disease. What administration schedule should be followed for this therapy?

○ 1. Take both drugs three times a day.

○ 2. Take the entire dose of both drugs first thing in the morning.

○ 3. Take all the fludrocortisone acetate and two thirds of the cortisone acetate in the morning, and take the remaining cortisone acetate in the afternoon.

○ 4. Take half of each drug in the morning and the remaining half of each drug at bedtime.

65. Which statement should the nurse make when teaching the client about taking oral glucocorticoids?

○ 1. "Take your medication with a full glass of water."

○ 2. "Take your medication on an empty stomach."

○ 3. "Take your medication at bedtime to increase absorption."

○ 4. "Take your medication with meals or with an antacid."

66. Which of the following is the best indicator for determining whether a client with Addison's disease is receiving the correct amount of glucocorticoid replacement?

○ 1. Skin turgor.

○ 2. Temperature.

○ 3. Thirst.

○ 4. Daily weight.

67. Which of the following signs and symptoms would probably indicate that the client with Addison's disease is receiving too much glucocorticoid replacement?

○ 1. Anorexia.

○ 2. Dizziness.

○ 3. Rapid weight gain.

○ 4. Poor skin turgor.

68. Which of the following is a *priority* goal for the client with Addison's disease?

○ 1. Maintain medication compliance.

○ 2. Avoid normal activities with stress.

○ 3. Follow a 2-g sodium diet.

○ 4. Prevent hypertensive episodes.

69. The client with Addison's disease should anticipate the need for increased glucocorticoid supplementation in which of the following situations?

○ 1. Returning to work after a weekend.

○ 2. Going on vacation.

○ 3. Having oral surgery.

○ 4. Having a routine medical checkup.

70. The nurse should teach the client with Addison's disease that the side effect of bronze-colored skin is thought to be caused by which of the following?

○ 1. Hypersensitivity to sun exposure.

○ 2. Increased serum bilirubin level.

○ 3. Side effects of the glucocorticoid therapy.

○ 4. Increased secretion of adrenocorticotropic hormone (ACTH).

71. Which of the following would most likely be a *priority* nursing diagnosis for the client experiencing addisonian crisis?

○ 1. Total Self-Care Deficit (Level I) related to weakness and fatigue.

○ 2. Imbalanced Nutrition: More Than Body Requirements related to increased appetite.

○ 3. Imbalanced Nutrition: More Than Body Requirements related to decreased exercise.

○ 4. Excess Fluid Volume related to reduced urinary excretion of fluid.

The Client With Cushing's Disease

72. A 42-year-old female client reports that she has gained weight and that her face and body are "rounder," while her legs and arms have become thinner. A tentative diagnosis of Cushing's disease is made. When examining this client, the nurse would expect to find

○ 1. orthostatic hypotension.

○ 2. muscle hypertrophy in the extremities.

○ 3. bruised areas on the skin.

○ 4. decreased body hair.

73. Signs and symptoms of Cushing's disease include

○ 1. weight loss.

○ 2. thin, fragile skin.

○ 3. hypotension.

○ 4. abdominal pain.

74. Cushing's disease is manifested by the excessive secretion of corticosteroids. The hormones involved are

○ 1. glucocorticoids and aldosterone.

○ 2. adrenocorticotropic hormone (ACTH).

○ 3. glucocorticoids, aldosterone, and androgens.

○ 4. catecholamines.

75. Which of the following test results would be consistent with a diagnosis of Cushing's disease?

○ 1. Postprandial hypoglycemia.

○ 2. Hypokalemia.

○ 3. Hyponatremia.

○ 4. Decreased urinary calcium level.

76. A client with Cushing's disease tells the nurse that the physician said her morning serum cortisol level was within normal limits. She asks, "How can that be? I'm not imagining all these symptoms!" The nurse's response will be based on which of the following concepts?

○ 1. Some clients are very sensitive to the effects of cortisol and develop symptoms even with normal levels.

○ 2. A single random blood test cannot provide reliable information about endocrine levels.

○ 3. The excessive cortisol levels seen in Cushing's disease commonly result from loss of the normal diurnal secretion pattern.

○ 4. Tumors tend to secrete hormones irregularly, and the hormones are often not present in the blood.

77. The client with Cushing's disease needs to modify dietary intake to control symptoms. In addition to increasing protein, which strategy would be most appropriate?

○ 1. Increase calories.

○ 2. Restrict sodium.

○ 3. Restrict potassium.

○ 4. Reduce fat to 10%.

78. Bone resorption is a possible complication of Cushing's disease. Which of the following interventions should the nurse recommend to help the client prevent this complication?

○ 1. Increase the amount of potassium in the diet.

○ 2. Maintain a regular program of weight-bearing exercise.

○ 3. Limit dietary vitamin D intake.

○ 4. Perform isometric exercises.

79. A client has been found to have an adrenal tumor and is scheduled for a bilateral adrenalectomy. The nurse begins preoperative teaching, which includes the importance of deep breathing. Which of the following would be the most accurate instructions?

○ 1. "Sit in an upright position and take a deep breath."

○ 2. "Hold your abdomen firmly with a pillow and take several deep breaths."

○ 3. "Tighten your stomach muscles as you inhale and breathe normally."

○ 4. "Raise your shoulders to expand your chest."

80. A priority goal in the first 24 hours after a bilateral adrenalectomy is to

○ 1. begin oral nutrition.

○ 2. promote self-care activities.

○ 3. prevent adrenal crisis.

○ 4. ambulate in the hallway.

81. A client undergoing a bilateral adrenalectomy has postoperative orders for hydromorphone hydrochloride (Dilaudid) 2 mg to be given subcutaneously every 4 hours PRN for pain. This drug is administered in relatively small doses primarily because it is

○ 1. less likely to cause dependency in small doses.

○ 2. less irritating to subcutaneous tissues in small doses.

○ 3. as potent as most other analgesics in larger doses.

○ 4. excreted before accumulating in toxic amounts in the body.

82. Adrenal function is affected by the drug ketoconazole (Nizoral), an antifungal agent used to treat severe fungal infections. How is this effect manifested?

○ 1. Ketoconazole suppresses adrenal steroid secretion.

○ 2. Ketoconazole destroys adrenocortical cells, resulting in a "medical" adrenalectomy.

○ 3. Ketoconazole increases ACTH-induced corticosteroid serum levels.

○ 4. Ketoconazole decreases duration of adrenal suppression when administered with corticosteroids.

83. In the early postoperative period after a bilateral adrenalectomy, the nurse should recognize that the most probable cause of temperature elevation is

○ 1. dehydration.

○ 2. poor lung expansion.

○ 3. wound infection.

○ 4. urinary tract infection.

84. A client who is recovering from a bilateral adrenalectomy has a patient-controlled analgesia (PCA) system with morphine sulfate. Which of the following actions is a *priority* nursing intervention for the client?

○ 1. Observing the client at regular intervals for narcotic addiction.

○ 2. Encouraging the client to reduce analgesic use and tolerate the pain.

○ 3. Evaluating pain control at least every 2 hours.

○ 4. Increasing the amount of morphine if the client does not administer the medication.

85. After surgery for bilateral adrenalectomy, the client is kept on bed rest for several days to stabilize the body's need for steroids postoperatively. Which of the following exercises has been found to be especially helpful in preparing a client for ambulation after a period of bed rest?

○ 1. Alternately flexing and extending the knees.

○ 2. Alternately abducting and adducting the legs.

○ 3. Alternately stretching the Achilles tendons.

○ 4. Alternately flexing and relaxing the quadriceps femoris muscles.

86. As the nurse helps the postoperative client out of bed, the client complains of gas pains in her abdomen. Which of the following is the most effective nursing intervention to relieve this discomfort?

○ 1. Encourage the client to ambulate.

○ 2. Insert a rectal tube.

○ 3. Insert a nasogastric tube.

○ 4. Encourage the client to drink carbonated liquids.

87. Because of steroid excess, the client who has undergone a bilateral adrenalectomy is at an increased risk for

○ 1. postoperative confusion.

○ 2. delayed wound healing.

○ 3. emboli.

○ 4. malnutrition.

88. The client who has undergone a bilateral adrenalectomy is ready to return home. She tells the nurse that she is concerned about persistent body changes and the fact that her moods are still so unpredictable. She says, "I thought surgery was supposed to fix all that." The nurse should base her teaching about recovery on which of the following concepts?

○ 1. The body changes are permanent and she will not be the same as before this condition.

○ 2. The body and mood will gradually return to normal.

○ 3. The physical changes are permanent, but the mood swings will disappear.

○ 4. The physical changes are temporary, but the mood swings are permanent.

89. After bilateral adrenalectomy for Cushing's disease, the client is told by her physician that she needs periodic testosterone injections. She asks the nurse, "What is that for? Did he forget I'm a woman?" What would be the nurse's *best* response?

○ 1. "Testosterone is needed to balance the reproductive cycle."

○ 2. "Testosterone is needed to restore the body's sodium and potassium balance."

○ 3. "Testosterone is given to stimulate protein anabolism."

○ 4. "Testosterone is given to stabilize mood swings."

90. Which of the following should the nurse include in the teaching plan of a female client with bilateral adrenalectomy?

○ 1. Emphasizing that the client will need steroid replacement for the rest of her life.

○ 2. Instructing the client about the importance of tapering steroid medication carefully to prevent crisis.

○ 3. Informing the client that steroids will be required only until her body can manufacture sufficient quantities.

○ 4. Emphasizing that the client will need to take steroids whenever her life involves physical or emotional stress.

The Female Client With Perimenopausal or Menopausal Syndrome

91. The client with perimenopause or menopause syndrome is primarily experiencing a deficiency of the hormone
    ○ 1. progesterone.
    ○ 2. estrogen.
    ○ 3. prolactin.
    ○ 4. oxytocin.

92. A woman with perimenopausal syndrome asks the nurse why she is having irregular periods. The nurse explains that she has a deficiency of estrogen caused by decreased function of the
    ○ 1. ovarian follicle.
    ○ 2. pituitary gland.
    ○ 3. adrenal cortex.
    ○ 4. thyroid.

93. A menopausal woman with an intact uterus is taking a combined estrogen and progesterone replacement medication, Prempro 0.625 mg / 2.5 mg. Combined hormonal therapy is given because estrogen alone
    ○ 1. would not be effective for hot flashes.
    ○ 2. could be a risk factor for endometrial cancer.
    ○ 3. would not be sufficient to maintain libido.
    ○ 4. could be a risk factor for ovarian cancer.

94. A woman in menopause is a good candidate for hormone replacement therapy (HRT) if she
    ○ 1. has a family history of breast cancer.
    ○ 2. had breast cancer a year ago.
    ○ 3. has a family history of heart disease.
    ○ 4. had an estrogen-dependent dysplasia.

95. The nurse teaches the client prescribed HRT to contact her health care provider immediately if she experiences which of the following?
    ○ 1. Hot flashes.
    ○ 2. Irregular vaginal bleeding.
    ○ 3. Breast tenderness.
    ○ 4. Vaginal pH changes.

The Client With Pheochromocytoma

96. A client is admitted with pheochromocytoma. The nurse assesses the client's blood pressure frequently. This is based on the knowledge that pheochromocytoma of the adrenal medulla releases excessive amounts of
    ○ 1. renin.
    ○ 2. aldosterone.
    ○ 3. catecholamines.
    ○ 4. glucocorticoids.

97. The primary feature of pheochromocytoma's effect on blood pressure is
    ○ 1. systolic hypertension.
    ○ 2. diastolic hypertension.
    ○ 3. hypertension that is resistant to treatment with drugs.
    ○ 4. widening pulse pressure.

98. The client with pheochromocytoma is scheduled for surgical resection of the tumor in the adrenal medulla. The nurse monitors the client postoperatively for which of the following potential complications?
    ○ 1. Orthostatic hypotension.
    ○ 2. Hemorrhage.
    ○ 3. Hypoglycemia.
    ○ 4. Hypertensive crisis.

99. The client with pheochromocytoma should be instructed to avoid activities that precipitate hypertensive crises or paroxysms, such as
    ○ 1. jogging.
    ○ 2. the Valsalva maneuver.
    ○ 3. anxiety.
    ○ 4. hypoglycemia.

100. Which of the following therapeutic classes of drugs is used to treat tachycardia and angina in a client with pheochromocytoma?
    ○ 1. Angiotensin-converting enzyme (ACE) inhibitors.
    ○ 2. Calcium channel blockers.
    ○ 3. β-blockers.
    ○ 4. Diuretics.

Correct Answers and Rationale

The letters in parentheses following the rationale identify the step of the nursing process (A, D, P, I, E) and client needs (1, 2, 3, 4, 5, 6, 7, 8, 9, 10). See the inside front cover for the key.

The Client With Thyrotoxicosis

1. 2. Graves' disease, the most common type of thyrotoxicosis, is a state of hypermetabolism. The increased metabolic rate generates heat and produces tachycardia and fine muscle tremors. Anorexia is associated with hypothyroidism. Loss of weight, despite a good appetite and adequate caloric intake, is a common feature of hyperthyroidism. Cold skin is associated with hypothyroidism. (A, 10)

2. 3. A change in the menstrual interval, diminished menstrual flow (oligomenorrhea), or even the absence of menstruation (amenorrhea) may result from the hormonal imbalances of thyrotoxicosis. Oligomenorrhea in women and decreased libido and impotence in men are common features of thyrotoxicosis. Dysmenorrhea is painful menstruation. Metrorrhagia, blood loss between menstrual periods, is a symptom of hypothyroidism. Menorrhagia, excessive bleeding during menstrual periods, is a symptom of hypothyroidism. (A, 10)

3. 1. The most serious side effects of PTU are leukopenia and agranulocytosis, which usually occur within the first 3 months of treatment. The client should be taught to promptly report to the health care provider any signs and symptoms of infection, such as a sore throat and fever. Any client complaining of a sore throat and fever should have an immediate white blood cell count and differential performed, and the drug must be held until the results are obtained. Painful menstruation, constipation, and increased urine output are not associated with PTU therapy. (I, 8)

4. 2. A typical sign of thyrotoxicosis is irritability caused by the high levels of circulating thyroid hormones in the body. This symptom decreases as the client responds to therapy. Thyrotoxicosis does not cause confusion. The client may be worried about her illness, and stress may influence her mood; however, irritability is a common symptom of thyrotoxicosis and the client should be informed of that fact rather than blamed. (I, 5)

5. 4. Elevated serum concentrations of thyroid hormones and suppressed serum TSH are the features of thyrotoxicosis. Decreased or absent serum TSH is a very accurate indicator of thyrotoxicosis. Increased levels of circulating thyroid hormones cause the feedback mechanism to the brain to suppress TSH secretion. (A, 10)

6. 3. Treatment of mild ophthalmopathy that may accompany thyrotoxicosis includes measures such as wearing sunglasses to protect the eye from corneal irritation. Treatment of ophthalmopathy should be performed in consultation with an ophthalmologist. Massaging the eyes will not help to protect the cornea. An ophthalmic anesthetic is used to examine and possibly treat a painful eye, not protect the cornea. Covering the eyes with moist gauze pads is not a satisfactory nursing measure to protect the eyes of a client with exophthalmos, because treatment is not focused on moisture to the eye but rather on protecting the cornea and optic nerve. In exophthalmos, the retrobulbar connective tissues and extraocular muscle volume are expanded because of fluid retention. The pressure is also increased. (I, 9)

7. 4. Sodium iodide ^{131}I destroys the thyroid follicular cells, and thyroid hormones are no longer produced. Use of RAI is often recommended for many clients with Graves' disease, especially the elderly. The treatment results in a "medical thyroidectomy." RAI is given in lieu of surgery, not before surgery. RAI does not reduce uptake of thyroxine. The outcome of giving the RAI is the destruction of the thyroid follicular cells. It is possible to slow the production of thyroid hormones with RAI. (I, 8)

8. 4. Management of the disease process is a priority for the client who has undergone RAI therapy with sodium iodide ^{131}I. Signs of hyperthyroidism usually persist for 1 to 2 months and may be still present for up to 1 year until thyroid hormone production stops. Permanent hypothyroidism is the major complication of radioactive ^{131}I treatment. At that time, the client will need to be able to recognize symptoms of hypothyroidism. Changes in level of consciousness or breathing pattern are not expected. The client does not need to be immobilized after RAI treatment. (D, 8)

9. 3. The client needs to be educated about the need for lifelong thyroid hormone replacement. Permanent hypothyroidism is the major complication of RAI ^{131}I treatment. Lifelong medical follow-up and thyroid replacement are warranted. The client needs to monitor for signs and symptoms of hypothyroidism, not hyperthyroidism. Resting for 1 week is not necessary. Hypertension and tachycardia are signs of hyperthyroidism, not hypothyroidism. (I, 8)

10. 2. SSKI is frequently administered before a thyroidectomy because it helps decrease the vascularity of the

thyroid gland. A highly vascular thyroid gland is very friable, a condition that presents a hazard during surgery. Preparation of the client for surgery includes depleting the gland of thyroid hormone and decreasing vascularity. SSKI does not decrease the progression of exophthalmos, and it does not decrease the body's ability to store thyroxine or increase the body's ability to excrete thyroxine. (P, 8)

11. 3. SSKI should be diluted well in milk, water, juice, or a carbonated beverage before administration to help disguise the strong, bitter taste. Also, this drug is irritating to mucosa if taken undiluted. The client should sip the diluted preparation through a drinking straw to help prevent staining of the teeth. Pouring the solution over ice chips will not sufficiently dilute the SSKI or cover the taste. Antacids are not used to dilute or cover the taste of SSKI. Mixing in a puree would put the SSKI in contact with the teeth. (I, 8)

12. 3. Laryngeal nerve damage is a potential complication of thyroid surgery because of the proximity of the thyroid gland to the recurrent laryngeal nerve. Asking the client to speak helps assess for signs of laryngeal nerve damage. Persistent or worsening hoarseness and weak voice are signs of laryngeal nerve damage and should be reported to the physician immediately. Internal hemorrhage is detected by changes in vital signs. The client's level of consciousness can be partially assessed by asking her to speak, but that is not the primary reason for doing so in this situation. Upper airway obstruction is detected by color and respiratory rate and pattern. (I, 9)

13. 4. Equipment for an emergency tracheostomy should be kept in the room, in case tracheal edema and airway occlusion occur. Laryngeal nerve damage can result in vocal cord spasm and respiratory obstruction. A tracheostomy set, oxygen and suction equipment, and a suture removal set (for respiratory distress from hemorrhage) make up the emergency equipment that should be readily available. Total parenteral nutrition is not anticipated for the client undergoing thyroidectomy. Intravenous infusion via a cutdown is not an expected possible treatment after thyroidectomy. Tube feedings are not anticipated emergency care. (P, 10)

14. 2. Tetany may occur after thyroidectomy if the parathyroid glands are accidentally injured or removed during surgery. This would cause a disturbance in serum calcium levels. An early sign of tetany is numbness and tingling of the fingers or toes and in the circumoral region. Tetany may occur from 1 to 7 days postoperatively. Late signs of tetany include seizures, contraction of the glottis, and respiratory obstruction. Pains in the joints of the hands and feet are not early symptoms of tetany. Bleeding on the back of the dressing is related to possible incisional complications. Ten-

sion on the suture line may indicate swelling, infection, or internal bleeding, but it is not related to tetany. (A, 10)

15. 2. The client with tetany is suffering from hypocalcemia, which is treated by administering an intravenous preparation of calcium, such as calcium gluconate or calcium chloride. Oral calcium is then necessary until normal parathyroid function returns. Sodium phosphate is a laxative. Echothiophate iodide is an eye preparation used as a miotic for an antiglaucoma effect. Sodium bicarbonate is a potent systemic antacid. (I, 8)

16. 2. Typical symptoms of hypothyroidism include weight gain, fatigue, decreased energy, apathy, brittle nails, dry skin, cold intolerance, hair loss, constipation, and numbness and tingling in the fingers. Tachycardia is a sign of hyperthyroidism, not hypothyroidism. Diarrhea and anorexia are not symptoms of hypothyroidism. (A, 10)

17. 4. A major problem for the person with hypothyroidism is fatigue. Other signs and symptoms include lethargy, personality changes, generalized edema, impaired memory, slowed speech, cold intolerance, dry skin, muscle weakness, constipation, weight gain, and hair loss. Incomplete closure of the eyelids, hypermetabolism, and diarrhea are associated with hyperthyroidism. (D, 7)

18. 4. Hypothyroidism may contribute to sadness and depression. It is good practice for clients with newly diagnosed depression to be monitored for hypothyroidism by checking the serum thyroid hormone and TSH levels. This client needs to know that these feelings may be related to her low thyroid hormone levels and may improve with treatment. Replacement therapy does not cause depression. Depression may accompany chronic illness, but it is not "normal." (I, 10)

The Client With Diabetes Mellitus

19. 3. Oral hypoglycemic agents of the sulfonylurea group, such as tolbutamide (Orinase), lower the blood glucose level by stimulating functioning beta cells in the pancreas to release insulin. These agents also increase insulin's ability to bind to the body's cells. They may also act to increase the number of insulin receptors in the body. Tolbutamide does not potentiate the action of insulin. Tolbutamide does not lower the renal threshold of glucose, which would not be a factor in the treatment of diabetes in any case. Tolbutamide does not combine with glucose to render it inert. (P, 8)

20. 1. The client with diabetes is prone to serious foot injuries secondary to peripheral neuropathy and decreased circulation. The client should be taught to

avoid going barefoot to prevent injury. Shoes that do not fit properly should not be worn, because they will cause blisters that can become nonhealing, serious wounds for the diabetic client. Toenails should be cut straight across. A heating pad should not be used because of the risk for burns due to insensitivity to temperature. (I, 9)

21. 2. A client with diabetes should be advised to consult a physician or podiatrist for corn removal because of the danger of traumatizing the foot tissue and potential development of ulcers. The diabetic client should never self-treat foot problems but should consult a physician or podiatrist. (I, 9)

22. 2. Proper and careful first-aid treatment is important when a client with diabetes has a skin cut or laceration. The skin should be kept supple and as free of organisms as possible. Washing and bandaging the cut will accomplish this. Washing wounds with alcohol is too caustic and drying to the skin. Having the children help is an unrealistic suggestion and does not educate the client about proper care of wounds. Tight control of blood glucose levels through adherence to the medication regimen is vitally important; however, it does not mean that careful attention to cuts can be ignored. (I, 9)

23. 4. DM is a multifactorial, systemic disease associated with problems in the metabolism of all food types. The client's diet should contain appropriate amounts of all three nutrients, plus adequate minerals and vitamins. (I, 7)

24. 1. Deep, rapid respirations with long expirations is indicative of Kussmaul's respiration, which occurs in metabolic acidosis. The respirations increase in rate and depth, and the breath has a "fruity" or acetone-like odor. This breathing pattern is the body's attempt to blow off carbon dioxide and acetone, thus compensating for the acidosis. The other breathing patterns listed are not related to ketoacidosis and would not compensate for the acidosis. (A, 10)

25. 4. A client with diabetes who takes any first- or second-generation sulfonylurea should be advised to avoid alcohol intake. Sulfonylureas in combination with alcohol can cause serious reactions of disulfiram (Antabuse)–like reactions including flushing, angina, palpitations, and vertigo. Serious reactions such as seizures and possibly death may also occur. Hypokalemia, hyperkalemia, and hypocalcemia do not result from taking sulfonylureas in combination with alcohol. (I, 8)

26. 3. The most important factor predisposing to the development of type 2 DM is obesity. Insulin resistance increases with obesity. Cigarette smoking is not a predisposing factor, but it is a risk factor that increases complications of DM. A high-cholesterol diet does not necessarily predispose to DM, but it may contribute to obesity and hyperlipidemia. Hypertension is not a predisposing factor, but it is a risk factor for developing complications of DM. (A, 4)

27. 2. The client with DM is especially prone to hypertension due to atherosclerotic changes, which leads to problems of the microvascular and macrovascular systems. This can result in complications in the heart, brain, and kidneys. Heart disease and stroke are twice as common among people with DM than among people without the disease. Painful, inflamed joints accompany rheumatoid arthritis. A stooped appearance accompanies osteoporosis with narrowing of the vertebral column. A low hemoglobin concentration accompanies anemia, especially iron-deficiency anemia and anemia of chronic disease. (A, 4)

28. 1. Although some individual variation exists, when the blood sugar decreases to less than 60 mg/dL the client experiences or is at risk for hypoglycemia. Hypoglycemia can occur in both type 1 and type 2 DM, although it is more common when the client is taking insulin. The nurse should instruct the client on the prevention, detection, and treatment of hypoglycemia. (A, 10)

29. 4. Diabetic retinopathy, cataracts, and glaucoma are common complications in diabetics, necessitating eye assessment and examination. The feet should also be examined at each client encounter, monitoring for thickening, fissures, or breaks in the skin; ulcers; and thickened nails. Although assessments of the abdomen, pharynx, and lymph glands are included in a thorough examination, they are not pertinent to common diabetic complications. (D, 9)

30. 4. The client with DM who is taking NPH (Humulin N) insulin in the evening is most likely to become hypoglycemic shortly after midnight because this insulin peaks in 6 to 12 hours. The client needs to eat a bedtime snack to help prevent hypoglycemia while sleeping. (I, 8)

31. 3. If the client engages in an activity or exercise that focuses on one area of the body, that area may cause inconsistent absorption of insulin. A good regimen for a jogger is to inject the abdomen for 3 weeks and then rotate to the buttock. A jogger may have inconsistent absorption in the legs or arms with strenuous running. (I, 8)

32. 1. Insulin lispro (Humalog) begins to act within 10 to 15 minutes and lasts approximately 4 hours. A major advantage of Humalog is that the client can eat almost immediately after the insulin is administered. The client needs to be instructed regarding the onset, peak, and duration of all insulin, as meals need to be timed with these parameters. Waiting 1 hour to eat may pre-

cipitate hypoglycemia. Eating 2 hours before the insulin lispro could cause hyperglycemia if the client does not have circulating insulin to metabolize the carbohydrate. (I, 8)

33. 1. The nurse would judge that learning has occurred from evidence of a change in the client's behavior. A client who performs a procedure safely and correctly demonstrates that he or she has acquired a skill. Evaluation of this skill acquisition requires performance of that skill by the client with observation by the nurse. The client must also demonstrate cognitive understanding, as shown by the ability to critique the nurse's performance. Explaining the steps demonstrates acquisition of knowledge at the cognitive level only. A posttest would not indicate the degree to which the client has learned a psychomotor skill. (E, 8)

34. 3. Renal failure frequently results from the vascular changes associated with DM. ACE inhibitors increase renal blood flow and are effective in decreasing diabetic nephropathy. Obstructive pulmonary disease is not a complication of diabetes, nor is it prevented by ACE inhibitors. Pancreatic cancer is neither prevented by ACE inhibitors nor considered a complication of diabetes. Cerebral vascular accident is not directly prevented by ACE inhibitors, although management of hypertension will decrease vascular disease. (I, 8)

35. 1. The four most commonly reported signs and symptoms of hypoglycemia are nervousness, weakness, perspiration, and confusion. Other signs and symptoms include hunger, incoherent speech, tachycardia, and blurred vision. Anorexia and Kussmaul's respirations are clinical manifestations of hyperglycemia or ketoacidosis. Bradycardia is not associated with hypoglycemia; tachycardia is. (I, 9)

36. 2. Steroids can cause hyperglycemia because of their effects on carbohydrate metabolism, making diabetic control more difficult. Aspirin is not known to affect glucose metabolism. Sulfonylureas are oral hypoglycemic agents used in the treatment of DM. ACE inhibitors are not known to affect glucose metabolism. (I, 8)

37. 1. Colds and influenza present special challenges to the client with DM because the body's need for insulin increases during illness. Therefore, the client must take the prescribed insulin dose, increase the frequency of blood testing, and maintain an adequate fluid intake to counteract the dehydrating effect of hyperglycemia. Clear fluids, juices, and Gatorade are encouraged. Not taking insulin when sick, or taking half the normal dose, may cause the client to develop ketoacidosis. (I, 9)

38. 1. Imbalanced Nutrition: Less than Body Requirements is a priority diagnosis for the client with DM who is experiencing vomiting with influenza. The diabetic client should eat small, frequent meals of 50 g of carbohydrate or food equal to 200 calories every 3 to 4 hours. If the client cannot eat the carbohydrates or any fluids, the physician or nurse should be called or the client should go to the emergency room. The diabetic client is in danger of complications with dehydration, electrolyte imbalance, and ketoacidosis. Increasing the client's coping skills is important to lifestyle behaviors, but it is not a priority during this acute illness of influenza. Comfort is a need for this client, but it is not the first priority; neither is altered activity. (D, 7)

39. 4. The best response would be to allow the client to verbalize her fears about giving herself a shot each day. Tactics that increase fear are not effective in changing behavior. If possible, the client needs to be responsible for his or her own care, including giving self-injections. It is unlikely that the client's insurance company will pay for such a service if the client is capable of self-administration. (I, 5)

40. 4. Deficient Fluid Volume, causing dehydration and possible hypovolemic shock, is the main problem in diabetic ketoacidosis because increased osmolarity from the glucose leads to a fluid shift from the intracellular to the extracellular space. The fluid shift leads to increased renal excretion of glucose and fluid. Severe dehydration, electrolyte imbalance, and possible hypovolemic shock is a medical emergency requiring immediate administration of insulin and intravenous fluid and electrolytes. Disturbed Sleep Pattern is not a priority nursing diagnosis for the critically ill client. It is possible that the client's condition has resulted from Impaired Health Maintenance; however, physiologic problems and diagnoses take priority over psychosocial problems and diagnoses. There are no data to support the diagnosis of Imbalanced Nutrition. (D, 10)

The Client With Pituitary Adenoma

41. 1. Galactorrhea, or abnormal flow of breast milk, results from overproduction of prolactin. Pituitary tumors are almost always secreting tumors, and they are classified by the specific hormone secreted. Pituitary tumors can cause oversecretion of ACTH, GH, or TSH. Overproduction of ACTH results in Cushing's disease. Overproduction of GH results in gigantism. Overproduction of TSH results in hypothyroidism. (I, 10)

42. 2. Excessive prolactin secretion in men results in decreased libido and impotence; these are often the only significant symptoms until the tumor becomes large. Symptoms of pituitary tumors result from both the presence of a space-occupying mass in the cranium and the excess secretion of hormones. Lethargy and fatigue are associated with hypothyroidism or addis-

onian crisis. Bony proliferation and voice changes are associated with excessive GH. (A, 10)

43. 4. With transsphenoidal hypophysectomy, the sella turcica is entered from below, through the sphenoid sinus. There is no external incision; the incision is made between the upper lip and gums. (P, 9)

44. 3. Deep breathing is the best choice for helping prevent atelectasis. The client should be placed in the semi-Fowler's position (or as ordered) and taught deep breathing, sighing, mouth breathing, and how to avoid coughing. Blow bottles are not effective in preventing atelectasis because they do not promote sustained alveolar inflation to maximal lung capacity. Frequent position changes help loosen lung secretions, but deep breathing is most important in preventing atelectasis. Coughing is contraindicated because it increases intracranial pressure and can cause cerebrospinal fluid (CSF) to leak from the point at which the sella turcica was entered. (I, 10)

45. 1. A major focus of nursing care after transsphenoidal hypophysectomy is prevention of and monitoring for a CSF leak. CSF leakage can occur if the patch or incision is disrupted. The nurse should monitor for signs of infection, including elevated temperature, increased white blood cell count, rhinorrhea, nuchal rigidity, and persistent headache. Hypoglycemia and adrenocortical insufficiency may occur. Monitoring for fluctuating blood glucose levels is not related specifically to transsphenoidal hypophysectomy. The client will be given intravenous fluids postoperatively to supply carbohydrates. Cushing's disease results from adrenocortical excess, not insufficiency. Monitoring for postoperative complications contributing to possible cardiac arrest is always important, but it is not related specifically to transsphenoidal hypophysectomy. (P, 10)

46. 1. The client's sexual problems are directly related to the excessive prolactin level. Removing the source of excessive hormone secretion should allow the client to return gradually to a normal physiologic pattern. Fertility will return, and erectile function and sexual desire will return to baseline as hormone levels return to normal. (I, 10)

47. 3. The dural opening is typically repaired with a patch of muscle or fascia taken from the abdomen or thigh. The client should be prepared preoperatively for the presence of this additional incision in the abdomen or thigh. The client will need the patch of muscle or fascia to replace the dura. Disposable sutures alone will not provide an intact suture line. Nasal packing will not provide closure for the dural opening. A synthetic mesh is not the tissue of choice for surgical repair of the dura. (I, 9)

48. 3. If CSF leakage is suspected or confirmed, the client is treated initially with bed rest with the head of the bed elevated to decrease pressure on the graft site. Most leaks heal spontaneously, but occasionally surgical repair of the site in the sella turcica is needed. Repacking the nose will not heal the leak at the graft site in the dura. The client will not be returned to surgery immediately, because most leaks heal spontaneously. High-dose corticosteroid therapy is not effective in healing a CSF leak. (I, 10)

49. 1. After transsphenoidal surgery, the client must be careful not to disturb the suture line while healing occurs. Frequent oral care should be provided with rinses of saline, and the teeth may be gently cleaned with Toothettes. Frequent or vigorous toothbrushing or flossing is contraindicated because it may disturb or cause tension on the suture line. (P, 10)

50. 4. Most clients who undergo adenoma removal experience a gradual return of normal pituitary secretion and do not experience complications. However, hypopituitarism can cause deficits of GH, gonadotropins, TSH, and ACTH. The client should be taught to monitor for change in mental status, energy level, muscle strength, and cognitive function. In adults, changes in sexual function, impotence, or decreased libido should be reported. Acromegaly and Cushing's disease are conditions of hypersecretion. Diabetes mellitus is related to the function of the pancreas and is not directly related to the function of the pituitary. (I, 9)

51. 1. Pituitary diabetes insipidus (DI) is a potential complication after pituitary surgery because of possible interference with the production of antidiuretic hormone (ADH). One major manifestation of DI is polyuria, because lack of ADH results in insufficient water reabsorption by the kidneys. The polyuria leads to a decreased urine specific gravity (between 1.001 and 1.010). The client may drink and excrete 5 to 40 L of fluid daily. DI does not affect metabolism. A blood glucose level higher than 300 mg/100 mL is associated with impaired glucose metabolism or diabetes mellitus. Urine negative for sugar and ketones is normal. (A, 9)

52. 2. The major characteristic of DI is decreased tubular reabsorption of water due to insufficient amounts of ADH. Vasopressin is administered to the client with DI because it has pressor and ADH activities. Vasopressin (Pitressin) works to increase the concentration of the urine by increasing tubular reabsorption, thus preserving up to 90% water. Vasopressin is administered to the client with DI because it is a synthetic ADH. The administration of vasopressin results in increased tubular reabsorption of water, and it is effective for emergency treatment or daily maintenance of mild DI. Vasopressin does not decrease blood pressure or affect insulin production or glucose metabolism, nor is insulin production a factor in DI. (P, 8)

53. 1. Because DI involves excretion of large amounts of fluid, maintaining normal fluid and electrolyte balance is a priority for this client. Special dietary programs or restrictions are not indicated in treatment of DI. Serum glucose levels are priorities in diabetes mellitus but not in DI. (E, 10)

The Client With Addison's Disease

54. 2. Addison's disease is caused by a deficiency of adrenal corticosteroids and can result in severe hypotension and shock because of uncontrolled loss of sodium in the urine and impaired mineralocorticoid function. This results in loss of extracellular fluid and dangerously low blood volume. Glucocorticoids must be administered to reverse hypotension. Preventing infection is not an appropriate goal of care in this life-threatening situation. Relieving anxiety is appropriate when the client's condition is stabilized, but the calm, competent demeanor of the emergency department staff will be initially reassuring. (P, 10)

55. 2. Adrenal hormone deficiency can cause profound physiologic changes. The client may experience severe pain (headache, abdominal pain, back pain, or pain in the extremities). Inhibited gluconeogenesis commonly produces hypoglycemia, and impaired sodium retention causes decreased, not increased, fluid volume. Edema would not be expected. Gastrointestinal disturbances including nausea and vomiting are expected findings in Addison's disease, not hunger. (A, 10)

56. 1. Signs of infiltration include slowing of the infusion and swelling, pain, hardness, pallor, and coolness of the skin at the site. If these signs occur, the intravenous (IV) line should be discontinued and restarted at another infusion site. The new anatomic site, time, and type of cannula used should be documented. The nurse may apply a warm soak to the site, but only after the IV line is discontinued. Parenteral administration of fluids should not be stopped intermittently. Stopping the flow does not treat the problem, nor does it address the client's needs for fluid replacement. Infiltrated IV sites should not be irrigated; doing so will only causing more swelling and pain. (I, 8)

57. 1. Each liter of 5% dextrose in normal saline solution contains 170 calories. The nurse should consult with the physician and dietitian when a client is on intravenous therapy or is NPO for any extended period, because further electrolyte supplementation or alimentation therapy may be needed. (I, 8)

58. 3. Electrolyte imbalances associated with Addison's disease include hypoglycemia, hyponatremia, and hyperkalemia. Salted bouillon and fruit juices provide glucose and sodium to replenish these deficits. Diet soda does not contain sugar. Water could cause further sodium dilution. Coffee's diuretic effect would aggravate the fluid deficit. Milk contains potassium and sodium. (I, 7)

59. 2. Finding alternative methods of dealing with stress, such as relaxation techniques, is a cornerstone of stress management. Removing all sources of stress from one's life is not possible. Antianxiety drugs are prescribed by physicians for temporary management during periods of major stress, and they are not an intervention in stress management classes. Avoiding discussion of stressful situations will not necessarily reduce stress. (I, 5)

60. 3. Primary Addison's disease refers to a problem in the gland itself. Primary Addison's disease occurs from idiopathic atrophy of the glands. The process is believed to be autoimmune in nature. The most common causes of primary adrenocortical insufficiency are autoimmune destruction (70%) and tuberculosis (20%). Hyposecretion of glucocorticoids, aldosterone, and androgens occur with Addison's disease. Insufficient secretion of GH causes dwarfism or growth delay. Pituitary dysfunction can cause Addison's disease, but this is not a primary disease process. Oversecretion of the adrenal medulla causes pheochromocytoma. (I, 10)

61. 3. Although many of the disease symptoms are vague and nonspecific, most clients experience lethargy and depression as early symptoms. Other early symptoms include mood changes, emotional lability, irritability, weight loss, muscle weakness, fatigue, nausea, and vomiting. Most clients experience a loss of appetite. Muscles become weak, not spastic, because of adrenocortical insufficiency. (A, 10)

62. 3. Decreased hepatic gluconeogenesis and increased tissue glucose uptake cause hypoglycemia, not hyperglycemia. Elevated glucose is associated with cortisol excess, as in Cushing's disease. Hyperkalemia and hyponatremia are characteristic of Addison's disease. There is decreased renal perfusion and excretion of waste products, which causes an elevated BUN level. (A, 9)

63. 1. The need for glucocorticoids changes with circumstances. The basal dose is established when the client is discharged, but this dose covers only normal daily needs and does not provide for additional stressors. As the manager of the medication schedule, the client needs to know signs of excessive and insufficient dosages. Glucocorticoid needs fluctuate. Glucocorticoids are not cumulative and must be taken daily. They must never be discontinued suddenly; in the absence of endogenous production, addisonian crisis could result. Two thirds of the daily dose should be taken at about 8 AM and the remainder at about 4 PM. This schedule approximates the diurnal pattern of normal secretion, with highest levels between 4 AM and 6 AM and lowest levels in the evening. (I, 8)

64. 3. Fludrocortisone acetate can be administered once a day, but cortisone acetate administration should follow the body's natural diurnal pattern of secretion. Greater amounts of cortisol are secreted during the day to meet increased demand of the body. Typically, baseline administration of cortisone acetate is 25 mg in the morning and 12.5 mg in the afternoon. Taking it three times a day would result in an excessive dose. Taking the drug only in the morning would not meet the needs of the body later in the day and evening. (I, 8)

65. 4. Oral steroids can cause gastric irritation and ulcers and should be administered with meals, if possible, or otherwise with an antacid. Only instructing the client to take the medication with a full glass of water will not help prevent gastric complications from steroids. Steroids should never be taken on an empty stomach. Glucocorticoids should be taken in the morning, not at bedtime. (I, 8)

66. 4. Measuring daily weight is a reliable, objective way to monitor fluid balance. Rapid variations in weight reflect changes in fluid volume, which suggests insufficient control of the disease and the need for more glucocorticoids in the client with Addison's disease. Nurses should instruct clients taking oral steroids to weigh themselves daily and to report any unusual weight loss or gain. Skin turgor testing does supply information about fluid status, but daily weight monitoring is more reliable. Temperature is not a direct measurement of fluid balance. Thirst is a nonspecific and very late sign of weight loss. (E, 8)

67. 3. Rapid weight gain, because it reflects excess fluids, is a warning sign that the client is receiving too much hormone replacement. It may be difficult to individualize the correct dosage for a client taking glucocorticoids, and the therapeutic range between underdosage and overdosage is narrow. Maintaining the client on the lowest dose that provides satisfactory clinical response is always the goal of pharmacotherapeutics. Fluid balance is an important indicator of the adequacy of hormone replacement. Anorexia is not present with glucocorticoid therapy, because these drugs increase the appetite. Dizziness is not specific to the effects of glucocorticoid therapy. Poor skin turgor is a late sign of fluid volume deficit. (E, 8)

68. 1. Medication compliance is an essential part of the self-care required to manage Addison's disease. The client must learn to adjust the glucocorticoid dose in response to the normal and unexpected stresses of daily living. The nurse should instruct the client never to stop taking the drug without consulting the health care provider to avoid an addisonian crisis. Regularity in daily habits makes adjustment easier, but the client should not be encouraged to withdraw from normal activities to avoid stress. The client does not need to restrict sodium. The client is at risk for hyponatremia. Hypotension, not hypertension, is more common with Addison's disease. (P, 8)

69. 3. Illness or surgery places tremendous stress on the body, necessitating increased glucocorticoid dosage. Extreme emotional or psychological stress also necessitates dosage adjustment. Increased dosages are needed in times of stress to prevent drug-induced adrenal insufficiency. Returning to work after the weekend, going on a vacation, or having a routine checkup usually will not alter glucocorticoid dosage needs. (P, 9)

70. 4. Bronzing, or general deepening of skin pigmentation, is a classic sign of Addison's disease and is caused by melanocyte-stimulating hormone produced in response to increased ACTH secretion. The hyperpigmentation is typically found in the distal portion of extremities and in areas exposed to sun. Additionally, areas that may not be exposed to sun, such as the nipples, genitalia, tongue, and knuckles, become bronze-colored. Treatment of Addison's disease usually reverses the hyperpigmentation. Bilirubin level is not related to the pathophysiology of Addison's disease. Hyperpigmentation is not related to the effects of the glucocorticoid therapy. (I, 10)

71. 1. Weakness, fatigue, lethargy, and inability to perform usual activities are major problems for the client experiencing addisonian crisis. A client in crisis requires bed rest until the crisis has been resolved and hormone levels return to normal. A client with addisonian crisis experiences nausea, not increased appetite, and Imbalanced Nutrition: Less Than Body Requirements. Fluid volume deficit, not excess, is another priority diagnosis. (D, 10)

The Client With Cushing's Disease

72. 3. Skin bruising from increased skin and blood vessel fragility is a classic sign of Cushing's disease. Hyperpigmentation and bruising are caused by the hypersecretion of glucocorticoids. Fluid retention causes hypertension, not hypotension. Muscle wasting occurs in the extremities. Hair on the head thins, while body hair increases. (A, 10)

73. 2. In Cushing's disease, excessive cortisol secretion causes rapid protein catabolism, depleting the collagen support of the skin. The skin becomes thin and fragile and susceptible to easy bruising. The typical "cushingoid" appearance of the client includes a moon face, buffalo hump, central obesity, and thin musculature.

Weight gain, mood swings, and slow wound healing are other symptoms of Cushing's disease. Hypertension, not hypotension, is a sign of Cushing's disease. Abdominal pain is not a symptom of Cushing's disease. (A, 10)

74. 3. Excessive levels of glucocorticoids, aldosterone, and androgens secreted from the adrenal cortex result in the constellation of symptoms known as Cushing's disease. Cushing's disease can be caused by a tumor, overstimulation from the pituitary, or the use of prescription steroid drugs. Androgens are also secreted in excess. ACTH is only one hormone that is abnormal in Cushing's disease. Excessive secretion of catecholamines accompanies pheochromocytoma, a disease of the adrenal medulla. (A, 10)

75. 2. Sodium retention is typically accompanied by potassium depletion. Hypertension, hypokalemia, edema, and congestive heart failure may result from the hypersecretion of aldosterone. The client with Cushing's disease exhibits postprandial or persistent hyperglycemia. Clients with Cushing's disease have hypernatremia, not hyponatremia. Bone resorption of calcium increases the urine calcium level. (A, 9)

76. 3. Cushing's disease is often caused by loss of the diurnal cortisol secretion pattern. The client's random morning cortisol level may be within normal limits, but secretion continues at that level throughout the entire day. Cortisol levels should normally decrease after the morning peak. Analysis of a 24-hour urine specimen is often useful in identifying the cumulative excess. Clients will not have symptoms with normal cortisol levels. Hormones are present in the blood. (I, 9)

77. 2. A primary dietary intervention is to restrict sodium, thereby reducing fluid retention. Increased protein catabolism results in loss of muscle mass and necessitates supplemental protein intake. The client may be asked to restrict total calories to reduce weight. The client should be encouraged to eat potassium-rich foods because serum levels are typically depleted. Although reducing fat intake as part of an overall plan to restrict calories is appropriate, fat intake of less than 20% of total calories is not recommended. (P, 7)

78. 2. Osteoporosis is a serious outcome of prolonged cortisol excess because calcium is resorbed out of the bone. Regular daily weight-bearing exercise (eg, brisk walking) is an effective way to drive calcium back into the bones. The client should also be instructed to have a dietary and/or supplemental intake of calcium of 1500 mg daily. Potassium levels are not relevant to prevention of bone resorption. Vitamin D is needed to aid in the absorption of calcium. Isometric exercises condition muscle tone but do not build bones. (I, 9)

79. 2. Effective splinting for a high incision reduces stress on the incision line, decreases pain, and increases the client's ability to deep breathe effectively. Deep breathing should be done hourly by the client after surgery. Sitting upright ignores the need to splint the incision to prevent pain. Tightening the stomach muscles is not an effective strategy for promoting deep breathing. Raising the shoulders is not a feature of deep breathing exercises. (I, 10)

80. 3. The primary goal in the first 24 hours after adrenalectomy is to identify and prevent adrenal crisis. Monitoring of vital signs is the most important evaluation measure. Hypotension, tachycardia, postural hypotension, and dysrhythmias can be indicators of pending vascular collapse and hypovolemic shock that can occur with adrenal crisis. Beginning oral nutrition is important, but not necessarily in the first 24 hours after surgery, and it is not more important than preventing adrenal crisis. Promoting self-care activities is not as important as preventing adrenal crisis. Ambulating in the hallway is not a priority in the first 24 hours after adrenalectomy. (P, 10)

81. 3. Hydromorphone hydrochloride is about five times more potent than morphine sulfate, from which it is prepared. Therefore, it is administered only in small doses. Hydromorphone hydrochloride can cause dependency in any dose; however, fear of dependency developing in the postoperative period is unwarranted. The dose is determined by the client's need for pain relief. Hydromorphone hydrochloride is not irritating to subcutaneous tissues. As with opioid analgesics, excretion depends on normal liver function. (I, 8)

82. 1. Ketoconazole suppresses adrenal steroid secretion and may cause acute hypoadrenalism. The adverse effect should reverse when the drug is discontinued. Ketoconazole does not destroy adrenal cells. Mitotane (Lysodren) is the drug that destroys the cells and may be used to obtain a medical adrenalectomy. Ketoconazole decreases, not increases, ACTH-induced serum corticosteroid levels. It increases the duration of adrenal suppression when given with steroids. (I, 8)

83. 2. Poor lung expansion from bed rest, pain, and retained anesthesia is a common cause of slight postoperative temperature elevation. Nursing care includes turning, coughing, and deep breathing the client every 1 to 2 hours, or more frequently as ordered. The client will have postoperative intravenous fluid replacement ordered to prevent dehydration. Wound infections typically appear 4 to 7 days after surgery. Urinary tract infections would not be typical with this surgery. (A, 10)

84. 3. Pain control should be evaluated at least every 2 hours for the client with a PCA system. Addiction is not

a common problem for the postoperative client. A client should not be encouraged to tolerate pain; in fact, other nursing actions besides PCA should be implemented to enhance the action of narcotics. One of the purposes of PCA is for the client to determine frequency of administering the medication; the nurse should not interfere unless the client is not obtaining pain relief. The nurse should ensure that the client is instructed on the use of the PCA control button and that the button is always within reach. (I, 8)

85. 4. Alternately flexing and relaxing the quadriceps muscles helps prepare the client for ambulation. This exercise helps maintain the strength in the quadriceps, which is the major muscle group used when walking. The other exercises listed do not increase a client's readiness for walking. (I, 7)

86. 1. Decreased mobility is one of the most common causes of abdominal distention related to retained gas in the intestines. Peristalsis has been inhibited by the general anesthesia, analgesics, and inactivity during the immediate postoperative period. Ambulation increases peristaltic activity and helps move gas. Walking can prevent the need for a rectal tube, which is a more invasive procedure. A nasogastric tube is also a more invasive procedure and requires a doctor's order. It is not a preferred treatment for gas postoperatively. Walking should prevent the need for further interventions. Carbonated liquids can increase gas formation. (I, 9)

87. 2. Persistent cortisol excess undermines the collagen matrix of the skin, impairing wound healing. It also carries an increased risk of infection and of bleeding. The wound should be observed and documentation performed regarding the status of healing. Confusion and emboli are not expected complications after adrenalectomy. Malnutrition also is not an expected complication after adrenalectomy. Nutritional status should be regained postoperatively. (I, 9)

88. 2. As the body readjusts to normal cortisol levels, mood and physical changes will gradually return to a normal state. (I, 10)

89. 3. Testosterone is an androgen hormone that is responsible for protein metabolism as well as maintenance of secondary sexual characteristics. Therefore, it is needed by both males and females. Removal of both adrenal glands necessitates replacement of glucocorticoids and androgens. (I, 10)

90. 1. Bilateral adrenalectomy requires lifelong adrenal hormone replacement therapy. If unilateral surgery is performed, most clients gradually reestablish a normal secretion pattern. The client and family will require extensive teaching and support to maintain self-care management at home. Information on dosing, side effects, what to do if a dose is missed, and follow-up examinations is needed in the teaching plan. Although steroids are tapered when given for an intermittent or one-time problem, they are not discontinued when given to clients who have undergone bilateral adrenalectomy, because they will not regain the ability to manufacture steroids. Steroids must be taken on a daily basis, not just during periods of physical or emotional stress. (P, 10)

The Female Client With Perimenopausal or Menopausal Syndrome

91. 2. Deficiency of estrogen causes the major characteristics of perimenopause/menopause. As estrogen decreases, many physiologic changes occur with perimenopause. Although many of the changes occur in the female reproductive system, other organs and systems are affected as well. Progesterone is the hormone responsible for maintaining pregnancy. Prolactin is one of the hormones responsible for lactation. Oxytocin is secreted by the posterior pituitary and is responsible for labor. (A, 10)

92. 1. As the ovarian follicle ceases to produce estrogen, menopause occurs. The endocrine changes that occur in menopause due to cessation of the ovarian follicle include hot flashes, headaches, and mood changes with irritability and anxiety (A, 10)

93. 2. Unopposed estrogen in a woman with an intact uterus can cause overgrowth of the endometrium, or endometrial hyperplasia. This hyperplasia can be a precursor to endometrial cancer. Estrogen is effective to control hot flashes. If libido is a major problem, testosterone is usually deficient. Hormone replacement therapy (HRT) is not known to be related to the incidence of ovarian cancer. (I, 8)

94. 3. A woman with a family history of heart disease or with actual heart disease is a good candidate for HRT. Estrogen has a protective effect against heart disease, the leading cause of death in aging women. The incidence of cardiovascular disease rises markedly in women after menopause. A family or personal history of breast cancer or a history of any estrogen-dependent dysplasia is an absolute contraindication for HRT. (P, 8)

95. 2. Endometrial cancer is a potential complication for postmenopausal women on HRT. Unfortunately, no symptoms except irregular vaginal bleeding are evident in endometrial cancer. Any menopausal or postmenopausal woman with irregular bleeding requires a biopsy to rule out endometrial cancer. Hot flashes may occur during perimenopause even if the client is on HRT; however, they are a benign symptom. Breast tenderness is a possible side effect of HRT, but it is not nec-

essary to report it immediately to the health care provider. Changes in vaginal pH may occur but need not be reported. (P, 9)

The Client With Pheochromocytoma

96. 3. Pheochromocytomas release catecholamines, both epinephrine and norepinephrine. The excessive hormone secretion can be constant or episodic, producing constant or episodic severe hypertension. (A, 10)

97. 3. The release of catecholamines, epinephrine and norepinephrine, causes hypertension that is resistant to treatment. Although pheochromocytoma accounts for fewer than 1% of the cases of hypertension, it is important to diagnose so the client may be correctly treated. The hypertension occurs with both systolic and diastolic pressures, and the pressures may be very labile. Widening pulse pressure is not related to pheochromocytoma. (D, 9)

98. 4. Postoperative management is directed at maintaining a normal blood pressure, because the client may be hypertensive immediately after surgery. The nurse must monitor blood pressure frequently and report abnormalities. Clients in hypertensive crisis should be in an intensive care unit for cardiac, blood pressure, and neurologic monitoring. Orthostatic hypotension may be a concern for clients on prolonged bed rest or with fluid deficits. Although hemorrhage may accompany any surgery, it is unlikely with this surgery. Elevated blood glucose concentrations, not hypoglycemia, occur with pheochromocytoma. (I, 9)

99. 2. Bending, lifting, and the Valsalva maneuver can precipitate hypertensive crises or paroxysms. These activities increase transabdominal pressure and may cause cardiac-stimulating effects. The blood pressure is very labile with these activities, and paroxysms may be accompanied by tachycardia, palpitations, angina, or electrocardiographic changes. (A, 1)

100. 3. A β-blocker such as propranolol is administered to block the cardiac-stimulating effects of epinephrine. ACE inhibitors and calcium channel blockers do not block sympathetic activity as β-blockers do. Diuretics decrease fluid volume and peripheral resistance, but they do not block sympathetic activity. (I, 8)

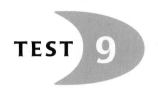

The Client With Urinary Tract Health Problems

Select the one best answer, and indicate your choice by filling in the circle in front of the option.

The Client With Cancer of the Bladder

1. Which of the following symptoms is the most common clinical finding associated with bladder cancer?
   ○ 1. Suprapubic pain.
   ○ 2. Dysuria.
   ○ 3. Painless hematuria.
   ○ 4. Urinary retention.

2. A client is to have a cystoscopy to rule out cancer of the bladder. Which of the following symptoms would indicate that the client has developed a complication after the cystoscopy?
   ○ 1. Dizziness.
   ○ 2. Chills.
   ○ 3. Pink-tinged urine.
   ○ 4. Bladder spasms.

3. If the client develops lower abdominal pain after a cystoscopy, the nurse should instruct the client to do which of the following?
   ○ 1. Apply an ice pack to pubic area.
   ○ 2. Massage the abdomen gently.
   ○ 3. Ambulate as much as possible.
   ○ 4. Sit in a tub of warm water.

4. A client who has been diagnosed with bladder cancer is scheduled for an ileal conduit. Preoperatively, the nurse reinforces the client's understanding of the surgical procedure by explaining that an ileal conduit
   ○ 1. is a temporary procedure that can be reversed later.
   ○ 2. diverts urine into the sigmoid colon, where it is expelled through the rectum.
   ○ 3. conveys urine from the ureters to a stoma opening on the abdomen.
   ○ 4. creates an opening in the bladder that allows urine to drain into an external pouch.

5. After surgery for an ileal conduit, the nurse should closely evaluate the client for the occurrence of which of the following complications related to pelvic surgery?
   ○ 1. Peritonitis.
   ○ 2. Thrombophlebitis.
   ○ 3. Ascites.
   ○ 4. Inguinal hernia.

6. The nurse is assessing the urine of a client who has had an ileal conduit and notes that the urine is yellow with a moderate amount of mucus. Based on the data, which of the following nursing interventions would be most appropriate at this time?
   ○ 1. Change the appliance bag.
   ○ 2. Notify the physician.
   ○ 3. Obtain a urine specimen for culture.
   ○ 4. Encourage a high fluid intake.

7. When teaching the client to care for an ileal conduit, the nurse instructs the client to empty the appliance frequently, primarily to help prevent which of the following problems?
   ○ 1. Rupture of the ileal conduit.
   ○ 2. Interruption of urine production.
   ○ 3. Development of odor.
   ○ 4. Separation of the appliance from the skin.

8. The nurse should teach the client with an ileal conduit to prevent urine leakage when changing the appliance by using which of the following procedures?

○ 1. Insert a gauze wick into the stoma.

○ 2. Close the opening temporarily with a cellophane seal.

○ 3. Suction the stoma before changing the appliance.

○ 4. Avoid oral fluids for several hours before changing the appliance.

9. The client with an ileal conduit will be using a reusable appliance at home. The nurse should teach the client to clean the appliance routinely with which product?

○ 1. Baking soda.

○ 2. Soap.

○ 3. Hydrogen peroxide.

○ 4. Alcohol.

10. Which of the following solutions will be useful to help control odor in the urine collecting bag after it has been cleaned?

○ 1. Salt water.

○ 2. Vinegar.

○ 3. Ammonia.

○ 4. Bleach.

11. A female client who has a urinary diversion tells the nurse, "This urinary pouch is embarrassing. Everyone will know that I'm not normal. I don't see how I can go out in public anymore." The most appropriate nursing diagnosis for this client is

○ 1. Anxiety related to the presence of urinary diversion.

○ 2. Deficient Knowledge about how to care for the urinary diversion.

○ 3. Low Self-Esteem related to feelings of worthlessness.

○ 4. Disturbed Body Image related to creation of a urinary diversion.

12. The nurse teaches the client with a urinary diversion to attach the appliance to a standard urine collection bag at night. The most important reason for doing this is to prevent

○ 1. urine reflux into the stoma.

○ 2. appliance separation.

○ 3. urine leakage.

○ 4. the need to restrict fluids.

13. The nurse teaches the client with an ileal conduit measures to prevent a urinary tract infection. Which of the following measures would be most effective?

○ 1. Avoid people with respiratory tract infections.

○ 2. Maintain a daily fluid intake of 2000 to 3000 mL.

○ 3. Use sterile technique to change the appliance.

○ 4. Irrigate the stoma daily.

14. The nurse evaluates the effectiveness of the client's postoperative plan of care. Which of the following would be an expected outcome for a client with an ileal conduit?

○ 1. The client verbalizes the understanding that his physical activity must be curtailed.

○ 2. The client states that he will place an aspirin in the drainage pouch to help control odor.

○ 3. The client demonstrates how to catheterize the stoma.

○ 4. The client states that he will empty the drainage pouch frequently throughout the day.

The Client With Renal Calculi

15. A client is admitted to the hospital with a diagnosis of renal calculi. She is experiencing severe flank pain and complains of nausea. Her temperature is 100.6°F (38.1°C). Which of the following would be a *priority* outcome for this client?

○ 1. Prevention of urinary tract complications.

○ 2. Alleviation of nausea.

○ 3. Alleviation of pain.

○ 4. Maintenance of fluid and electrolyte balance.

16. The client is scheduled to have a kidney, ureter, and bladder (KUB) radiograph. Which of the following would be ordered to prepare the client for this radiograph?

○ 1. Fluid and food will be withheld the morning of the examination.

○ 2. A tranquilizer will be given before the examination.

○ 3. An enema will be given before the examination.

○ 4. No special preparation is required for the examination.

17. In addition to nausea and severe flank pain, a female client with renal calculi complains of pain in the groin and bladder. The nurse would determine that these symptoms most likely result from which of the following?

○ 1. Nephritis.

○ 2. Referred pain.

○ 3. Urine retention.

○ 4. Additional stone formation.

18. Which of the following nursing interventions is likely to provide the most relief from the pain associated with renal colic?

○ 1. Applying moist heat to the flank area.

○ 2. Administering meperidine (Demerol).

○ 3. Encouraging high fluid intake.

○ 4. Maintaining complete bed rest.

19. A client who has been diagnosed with renal calculi reports that the pain is intermittent and less colicky. Which of the following nursing actions is most important at this time?

○ 1. Report hematuria to the physician.

○ 2. Strain the urine carefully.

○ 3. Administer meperidine (Demerol) every 3 hours.

○ 4. Apply warm compresses to the flank area.

20. The client is scheduled for an intravenous pyelogram (IVP) to determine the location of the renal calculi. Which of the following measures would be most important for the nurse to include in pretest preparation?
○ 1. Ensuring adequate fluid intake on the day of the test.
○ 2. Preparing the client for the possibility of bladder spasms during the test.
○ 3. Checking the client's history for allergy to iodine.
○ 4. Determining when the client last had a bowel movement.

21. After an IVP, the nurse should anticipate incorporating which of the following measures into the client's plan of care?
○ 1. Maintaining bed rest.
○ 2. Encouraging adequate fluid intake.
○ 3. Assessing for hematuria.
○ 4. Administering a laxative.

22. The nurse finds a container with the client's urine specimen sitting on a counter in the bathroom. The client states that the specimen has been sitting in the bathroom for at least 2 hours. What would be the nurse's most appropriate action?
○ 1. Discard the urine and obtain a new specimen.
○ 2. Send the urine to the laboratory as quickly as possible.
○ 3. Add fresh urine to the collected specimen and send the specimen to the laboratory.
○ 4. Refrigerate the specimen until it can be transported to the laboratory.

23. A client has a ureteral catheter in place after renal surgery. A priority nursing action for care of the ureteral catheter would be to
○ 1. irrigate the catheter with 30 mL of normal saline every 8 hours.
○ 2. ensure that the catheter is draining freely.
○ 3. clamp the catheter every 2 hours for 30 minutes.
○ 4. ensure that the catheter drains at least 30 mL/hour.

24. Which of the following interventions would be the most appropriate for preventing the development of a paralytic ileus in a client who has undergone renal surgery?
○ 1. Encourage the client to ambulate every 2 to 4 hours.
○ 2. Offer 3 to 4 ounces of a carbonated beverage periodically.
○ 3. Encourage use of the incentive spirometer every 2 hours.
○ 4. Continue intravenous fluid therapy.

25. The nurse is conducting a postoperative assessment of a client on the first day after renal surgery. Which of the following findings would be most important for the nurse to report to the physician?
○ 1. Temperature, 99.8°F (37.7°C).
○ 2. Urine output, 20 mL/hour.
○ 3. Absence of bowel sounds.
○ 4. A 2×2-inch area of serous sanguineous drainage on the flank dressing.

26. A client with a history of renal calculi formation is being discharged after surgery to remove the calculus. What instructions should the nurse include in the client's discharge teaching plan?
○ 1. Increase daily fluid intake to at least 2 to 3 L.
○ 2. Strain urine at home regularly.
○ 3. Eliminate dairy products from the diet.
○ 4. Follow measures to alkalinize the urine.

27. Because a client's renal stone was found to be composed of uric acid, a low-purine, alkaline-ash diet was ordered. Incorporation of which of the following food items into the home diet would indicate that the client understands the necessary diet modifications?
○ 1. Milk, apples, tomatoes, and corn.
○ 2. Eggs, spinach, dried peas, and gravy.
○ 3. Salmon, chicken, caviar, and asparagus.
○ 4. Grapes, corn, cereals, and liver.

28. Allopurinol (Zyloprim), 200 mg/day, is prescribed for the client with renal calculi to take at home. The nurse should teach the client about which of the following side effects of this medication?
○ 1. Retinopathy.
○ 2. Maculopapular rash.
○ 3. Nasal congestion.
○ 4. Dizziness.

29. The client has a clinic appointment scheduled for 10 days after discharge. Which laboratory finding at that time would indicate that allopurinol (Zyloprim) has had a therapeutic effect?
○ 1. Decreased urinary alkaline phosphatase level.
○ 2. Increased urinary calcium excretion.
○ 3. Increased serum calcium level.
○ 4. Decreased serum uric acid level.

The Client With Acute Renal Failure

30. Which of the following urinary symptoms is the most common initial manifestation of acute renal failure?
○ 1. Dysuria.
○ 2. Anuria.
○ 3. Hematuria.
○ 4. Oliguria.

31. A client developed shock after a severe myocardial infarction and has now developed acute renal failure. The client's family asks the nurse why the client

has developed acute renal failure. The nurse should base the response on the knowledge that there was
○ 1. a decrease in the blood flow through the kidneys.
○ 2. an obstruction of urine flow from the kidneys.
○ 3. a blood clot formed in the kidneys.
○ 4. structural damage to the kidney resulting in acute tubular necrosis.

32. The client's blood urea nitrogen (BUN) concentration is elevated in acute renal failure. What is the likely cause of this finding?
○ 1. Fluid retention.
○ 2. Hemolysis of red blood cells.
○ 3. Below-normal metabolic rate.
○ 4. Reduced renal blood flow.

33. The client's serum potassium is elevated in acute renal failure, and the nurse administers sodium polystyrene sulfonate (Kayexalate). This drug acts to
○ 1. increase potassium excretion from the colon.
○ 2. release hydrogen ions for sodium ions.
○ 3. increase calcium absorption in the colon.
○ 4. exchange sodium for potassium ions in the colon.

34. If the client's serum potassium continues to rise in acute renal failure, the nurse should be prepared for which of the following emergency situations?
○ 1. Cardiac arrest.
○ 2. Pulmonary edema.
○ 3. Circulatory collapse.
○ 4. Hemorrhage.

35. A high-carbohydrate, low-protein diet is prescribed for the client with acute renal failure. The rationale for the high-carbohydrate diet is that carbohydrates will
○ 1. act as a diuretic.
○ 2. reduce demands on the liver.
○ 3. help maintain urine acidity.
○ 4. prevent the development of ketosis.

36. The client with acute renal failure asks the nurse for a snack. Because the client's potassium level is elevated, which of the following snacks would be most appropriate?
○ 1. A gelatin dessert.
○ 2. Yogurt.
○ 3. An orange.
○ 4. Peanuts.

37. In the oliguric phase of acute renal failure, the nurse should anticipate the development of which of the following complications?
○ 1. Pulmonary edema.
○ 2. Metabolic alkalosis.
○ 3. Hypotension.
○ 4. Hypokalemia.

38. The client in acute renal failure has an external cannula inserted in the forearm for hemodialysis. Which of the following nursing measures is appropriate for the care of this client?

○ 1. Use the unaffected arm for blood pressure measurements.
○ 2. Draw blood from the cannula for routine laboratory work.
○ 3. Percuss the cannula for bruits each shift.
○ 4. Inject heparin into the cannula each shift.

39. The nurse initiates the client's first hemodialysis treatment. The client develops a headache, confusion, and nausea. These symptoms indicate which of the following potential complications?
○ 1. Disequilibrium syndrome.
○ 2. Myocardial infarction.
○ 3. Air embolism.
○ 4. Peritonitis.

40. If disequilibrium syndrome occurs during dialysis, which of the following would be the *priority* nursing action?
○ 1. Administer oxygen per nasal cannula.
○ 2. Slow the rate of dialysis.
○ 3. Reassure the client that the symptoms are normal.
○ 4. Place the client in Trendelenburg's position.

41. The client receives heparin while on hemodialysis. The nurse explains the rationale supporting anticoagulation by making which of the following statements?
○ 1. "Regional anticoagulation is achieved by putting heparin in the dialysis machine and protamine sulfate, which reverses the anticoagulation, in the client."
○ 2. "You will receive warfarin sodium (Coumadin) to maintain anticoagulation between treatments."
○ 3. "Heparin does not enter the body, so there is no risk of bleeding."
○ 4. "Clotting time is seriously prolonged for several hours after each treatment."

42. Which of the following abnormal blood values would not be improved by dialysis treatment?
○ 1. Elevated serum creatinine.
○ 2. Hyperkalemia.
○ 3. Decreased hemoglobin.
○ 4. Hypernatremia.

43. The nurse teaches the client how to recognize signs of infection in the shunt by telling the client to assess the shunt each day for
○ 1. absence of a bruit.
○ 2. sluggish capillary refill time.
○ 3. coolness of the involved extremity.
○ 4. swelling at the shunt site.

44. The client with acute renal failure is recovering and asks the nurse, "Will my kidneys ever function normally again?" The nurse's response is based on knowledge that the client's renal status will most likely

○ 1. continue to improve over a period of weeks.
○ 2. result in the need for permanent hemodialysis.
○ 3. improve only if the client receives a renal transplant.
○ 4. result in end-stage renal failure.

The Client With Urinary Tract Infection

45. A 24-year-old female client comes to an ambulatory care clinic in moderate distress with a probable diagnosis of acute cystitis. Which of the following symptoms would the nurse most likely expect the client to report during the assessment?
    ○ 1. Fever and chills.
    ○ 2. Frequency and burning on urination.
    ○ 3. Flank pain and nausea.
    ○ 4. Hematuria.

46. The client asks the nurse, "How did I get this urinary tract infection?" The nurse should explain that in most instances, cystitis is caused by
    ○ 1. congenital strictures in the urethra.
    ○ 2. an infection elsewhere in the body.
    ○ 3. urine stasis in the urinary bladder.
    ○ 4. an ascending infection from the urethra.

47. The nurse is instructing the unlicensed assistant on the correct technique for obtaining a clean-catch urine culture from a female client. Which of the following statements indicates that the assistant has understood the instructions?
    ○ 1. "I will have the client completely empty her bladder into the specimen cup."
    ○ 2. "I will need to catheterize the client to get the urine specimen."
    ○ 3. "I will ask the client to cleanse her labia, void into the toilet, and then into the specimen cup."
    ○ 4. "I will obtain the specimen in the afternoon after the client has had plenty of fluids."

48. The client, who is a newlywed, is afraid to discuss her diagnosis of cystitis with her husband. Which would be the nurse's best approach?
    ○ 1. Arrange a meeting with the client, her husband, the doctor, and the nurse.
    ○ 2. Insist that the client talk with her husband because good communication is necessary for a successful marriage.
    ○ 3. Talk first with the husband alone and then with both of them together to share the husband's reactions.
    ○ 4. Spend time with the client addressing her concerns and then stay with her while she talks with her husband.

49. The nurse teaches a client who has cystitis methods to relieve her discomfort until the antibiotic takes effect. Which of the following responses by the

client would indicate that she understands the nurse's instructions?
    ○ 1. "I will place ice packs on my perineum."
    ○ 2. "I will take hot tub baths."
    ○ 3. "I will drink a cup of warm tea every hour."
    ○ 4. "I will void every 5 to 6 hours."

50. The client with cystitis is also given a prescription for phenazopyridine hydrochloride (Pyridium). The nurse should teach the client that this drug is used to treat urinary tract infections by
    ○ 1. releasing formaldehyde and providing bacteriostatic action.
    ○ 2. potentiating the action of the antibiotic.
    ○ 3. providing an analgesic effect on the bladder mucosa.
    ○ 4. preventing the crystallization that can occur with sulfa drugs.

51. Before the client starts taking phenazopyridine hydrochloride (Pyridium), she should be taught about which of the drug's side effects?
    ○ 1. Bright orange-red urine.
    ○ 2. Incontinence.
    ○ 3. Constipation.
    ○ 4. Slight drowsiness.

52. Which of the following statements by the client would indicate that she is at high risk for a recurrence of cystitis?
    ○ 1. "I can usually go 8 to 10 hours without needing to empty my bladder."
    ○ 2. "I take a tub bath every evening."
    ○ 3. "I wipe from front to back after voiding."
    ○ 4. "I drink a lot of water during the day."

53. To prevent recurrence of cystitis, the nurse should plan to encourage the client to include which of the following measures in her daily routine?
    ○ 1. Wearing cotton underpants.
    ○ 2. Increasing citrus juice intake.
    ○ 3. Douching regularly with 0.25% acetic acid.
    ○ 4. Using vaginal sprays.

54. The nurse explains to the client the importance of drinking large quantities of fluid to prevent cystitis. To help her understand, the nurse should tell her to drink
    ○ 1. twice as much fluid as she usually drinks.
    ○ 2. at least 1 quart more than she usually drinks.
    ○ 3. a lot of water, juice, and other fluids throughout the day.
    ○ 4. at least 3000 mL of fluids daily.

The Client With Pyelonephritis

55. Which of the following symptoms would most likely indicate pyelonephritis?
    ○ 1. Ascites.

○ 2. Costovertebral angle (CVA) tenderness.

○ 3. Polyuria.

○ 4. Nausea and vomiting.

56. Which of the following factors would put the client at increased risk for pyelonephritis?
    ○ 1. History of hypertension.
    ○ 2. Intake of large quantities of cranberry juice.
    ○ 3. Fluid intake of 2000 mL/day.
    ○ 4. History of diabetes mellitus.

57. Which of the following groups of laboratory tests is most important for assessing the client's renal status?
    ○ 1. Serum sodium and potassium levels.
    ○ 2. Arterial blood gases and hemoglobin.
    ○ 3. Serum blood urea nitrogen (BUN) and creatinine levels.
    ○ 4. Urinalysis and urine culture.

58. The client with pyelonephritis asks the nurse, "How will I know whether the antibiotics are effectively treating my infection?" The nurse's most appropriate response would be which of the following?
    ○ 1. "After you take the antibiotics for 2 weeks, you'll be cured."
    ○ 2. "The doctor can tell by the color and odor of your urine."
    ○ 3. "The doctor can determine your progress through urine cultures."
    ○ 4. "When your symptoms disappear, you'll know that your infection is gone."

59. The client with acute pyelonephritis wants to know the possibility of developing chronic pyelonephritis. The nurse's response is based on knowledge that which of the following disorders most commonly leads to chronic pyelonephritis?
    ○ 1. Acute pyelonephritis.
    ○ 2. Recurrent urinary tract infections.
    ○ 3. Acute renal failure.
    ○ 4. Glomerulonephritis.

The Client With Chronic Renal Failure

60. The nurse assesses the client who has chronic renal failure and notes the following: crackles in the lung bases, elevated blood pressure, and weight gain of 2 pounds in 1 day. Based on these data, which of the following nursing diagnoses is appropriate?
    ○ 1. Excess Fluid Volume related to the kidney's inability to maintain fluid balance.
    ○ 2. Increased Cardiac Output related to fluid overload.
    ○ 3. Ineffective Tissue Perfusion related to interrupted arterial blood flow.
    ○ 4. Ineffective Therapeutic Regimen Management related to lack of knowledge about therapy.

61. What is the primary disadvantage of using peritoneal dialysis for long-term management of chronic renal failure?
    ○ 1. The danger of hemorrhage is high.
    ○ 2. It cannot correct severe imbalances.
    ○ 3. It is a time-consuming method of treatment.
    ○ 4. The risk of contracting hepatitis is high.

62. The client with chronic renal failure complains of feeling nauseated at least part of every day. The nurse should explain that the nausea is the result of
    ○ 1. acidosis caused by the medications.
    ○ 2. accumulation of waste products in the blood.
    ○ 3. chronic anemia and fatigue.
    ○ 4. excess fluid load.

63. The dialysis solution is warmed before use in peritoneal dialysis primarily to
    ○ 1. encourage the removal of serum urea.
    ○ 2. force potassium back into the cells.
    ○ 3. add extra warmth to the body.
    ○ 4. promote abdominal muscle relaxation.

64. Which of the following assessments would be most appropriate for the nurse to make while the dialysis solution is dwelling within the client's abdomen?
    ○ 1. Assess for urticaria.
    ○ 2. Observe respiratory status.
    ○ 3. Check capillary refill time.
    ○ 4. Monitor electrolyte status.

65. During the client's dialysis, the nurse observes that the solution draining from the abdomen is consistently blood-tinged. The client has a permanent peritoneal catheter in place. Which interpretation of this observation would be correct?
    ○ 1. Bleeding is expected with a permanent peritoneal catheter.
    ○ 2. Bleeding indicates abdominal blood vessel damage.
    ○ 3. Bleeding can indicate kidney damage.
    ○ 4. Bleeding is caused by too-rapid infusion of the dialysate.

66. During dialysis, the nurse observes that the flow of dialysate stops before all the solution has drained out. The nurse should
    ○ 1. have the client sit in a chair.
    ○ 2. turn the client from side to side.
    ○ 3. reposition the peritoneal catheter.
    ○ 4. have the client walk.

67. Which of the following nursing interventions should be included in the client's care plan during dialysis therapy?
    ○ 1. Limit the client's visitors.
    ○ 2. Monitor client's blood pressure.
    ○ 3. Pad the side rails of the bed.
    ○ 4. Keep the client NPO.

68. What is the most potentially dangerous complication of peritoneal dialysis?
    ○ 1. Abdominal pain.
    ○ 2. Gastrointestinal bleeding.
    ○ 3. Peritonitis.
    ○ 4. Muscle cramps.

69. After completion of peritoneal dialysis, the nurse would expect the client to exhibit which of the following characteristics?
    ○ 1. Hematuria.
    ○ 2. Weight loss.
    ○ 3. Hypertension.
    ○ 4. Increased urine output.

70. Aluminum hydroxide gel (Amphojel) is prescribed for the client with chronic renal failure to take at home. What is the purpose of giving this drug to a client with chronic renal failure?
    ○ 1. To relieve the pain of gastric hyperacidity.
    ○ 2. To prevent Curling's stress ulcers.
    ○ 3. To bind phosphate in the intestine.
    ○ 4. To reverse metabolic acidosis.

71. The nurse teaches the client with chronic renal failure when to take the aluminum hydroxide gel. Which of the following statements would indicate that the client understands the teaching?
    ○ 1. "I'll take it every 4 hours around the clock."
    ○ 2. "I'll take it between meals and at bedtime."
    ○ 3. "I'll take it when I have a sour stomach."
    ○ 4. "I'll take it with meals and bedtime snacks."

72. The client with chronic renal failure tells the nurse he takes magnesium hydroxide (milk of magnesia) at home for constipation. The nurse suggests that the client switch to psyllium hydrophilic mucilloid (Metamucil) because
    ○ 1. Milk of magnesia can cause magnesium intoxication.
    ○ 2. Milk of magnesia is too harsh on the bowel.
    ○ 3. Metamucil is more palatable.
    ○ 4. Milk of magnesia is high in sodium.

73. In planning teaching strategies for the client with chronic renal failure, the nurse must keep in mind the neurologic impact of uremia. Which teaching strategy would be most appropriate?
    ○ 1. Providing all needed teaching in one extended session.
    ○ 2. Validating frequently the client's understanding of the material.
    ○ 3. Conducting a one-on-one session with the client.
    ○ 4. Using videotapes to reinforce the material as needed.

74. The nurse helps the client with chronic renal failure develop a home diet plan with the goal of helping the client maintain adequate nutritional intake. Which of the following diets would be most appropriate for a client with chronic renal failure?

○ 1. High carbohydrate, high protein.
○ 2. High calcium, high potassium, high protein.
○ 3. Low protein, low sodium, low potassium.
○ 4. Low protein, high potassium.

75. Sexual problems can be troublesome to clients with chronic renal failure. Which one of the following strategies would be most useful in helping a client cope with such a problem?
    ○ 1. Help the client to accept that sexual activity will be decreased.
    ○ 2. Suggest using alternative forms of sexual expression and intimacy.
    ○ 3. Tell the client to plan rest periods after sexual activity.
    ○ 4. Suggest that the client avoid sexual activity to prevent embarrassment.

77. A client with chronic renal failure has asked to be evaluated for a home continuous ambulatory peritoneal dialysis (CAPD) program. The nurse should explain that the major advantage of this approach is that it
    ○ 1. is relatively low in cost.
    ○ 2. allows the client to be more independent.
    ○ 3. is faster and more efficient than standard peritoneal dialysis.
    ○ 4. has fewer potential complications than standard peritoneal dialysis.

77. The client asks whether her diet would change on CAPD. Which of the following would be the nurse's best response?
    ○ 1. "Diet restrictions are more rigid with CAPD because standard peritoneal dialysis is a more effective technique."
    ○ 2. "Diet restrictions are the same for both CAPD and standard peritoneal dialysis."
    ○ 3. "Diet restrictions with CAPD are fewer than with standard peritoneal dialysis because dialysis is constant."
    ○ 4. "Diet restrictions with CAPD are fewer than with standard peritoneal dialysis because CAPD works more quickly."

78. Which of the following is the most significant sign of peritoneal infection?
    ○ 1. Cloudy dialysate fluid.
    ○ 2. Swelling in the legs.
    ○ 3. Poor drainage of the dialysate fluid.
    ○ 4. Redness at the catheter insertion site.

The Client With Urinary Incontinence

79. When developing a plan of care for the client with stress incontinence, the nurse should take into consideration that stress incontinence is best defined as the involuntary loss of urine associated with

○ 1. a strong urge to urinate.
○ 2. overdistention of the bladder.
○ 3. activities that increase abdominal pressure.
○ 4. obstruction of the urethra.

80. Which of the following assessment data would most likely be related to a client's current complaint of stress incontinence?
   ○ 1. The client's intake of 2 to 3 L of fluid per day.
   ○ 2. The client's history of three full-term pregnancies.
   ○ 3. The client's age of 45 years.
   ○ 4. The client's history of competitive swimming.

81. The primary goal of nursing care for a client with stress incontinence is to
   ○ 1. help the client adjust to the frequent episodes of incontinence.
   ○ 2. eliminate all episodes of incontinence.
   ○ 3. prevent the development of urinary tract infections.
   ○ 4. decrease the number of incontinence episodes.

82. The nurse is developing a teaching plan for a client with stress incontinence. Which of the following instructions should be included?
   ○ 1. Avoid activities that are stressful and upsetting.
   ○ 2. Avoid caffeine and alcohol.
   ○ 3. Do not wear a girdle.
   ○ 4. Limit physical exertion.

83. A client has urge incontinence. Which of the following signs and symptoms would the nurse expect to find in this client?
   ○ 1. Inability to empty the bladder.
   ○ 2. Loss of urine when coughing.
   ○ 3. Involuntary urination with minimal warning.
   ○ 4. Frequent dribbling of urine.

84. Which of the following interventions would be most appropriate for a client who has urge incontinence?
   ○ 1. Have the client urinate on a timed schedule.
   ○ 2. Provide a bedside commode.
   ○ 3. Administer prophylactic antibiotics.
   ○ 4. Teach the client intermittent self-catheterization technique.

Correct Answers and Rationale

The letters in parentheses following the rationale identify the step of the nursing process (A, D, P, I, E) and client needs (1, 2, 3, 4, 5, 6, 7, 8, 9, 10). See the inside front cover for the key.

The Client With Cancer of the Bladder

1. 3. Painless hematuria is the most common clinical finding in bladder cancer. Other symptoms include frequency, dysuria, and urgency, but these are not as common as the hematuria. Suprapubic pain and urinary retention do not occur in bladder cancer. (A, 10)

2. 2. Chills could indicate the onset of acute infection that can progress to septic shock. Dizziness would not be an anticipated symptom after a cystoscopy. Pink-tinged urine and bladder spasms are common after cystoscopy. (E, 9)

3. 4. Lower abdominal pain after a cystoscopy is frequently caused by bladder spasms. Warm water can help relax muscles. Ice is not effective in relieving spasms. Massage and ambulation may increase bladder irritability. (I, 7)

4. 3. An ileal conduit is a permanent urinary diversion in which a portion of the ileum is surgically resected and one end of the segment is closed. The ureters are surgically attached to this segment of the ileum, and the open end of the ileum is brought to the skin surface on the abdomen to form the stoma. The client must wear a pouch to collect the urine that continually flows through the conduit. The bladder is removed during the surgical procedure and the ileal conduit is not reversible. Diversion of urine to the sigmoid colon is called a *ureteroileosigmoidostomy*. An opening in the bladder that allows urine to drain externally is called a *cystostomy*. (I, 9)

5. 2. After pelvic surgery, there is an increased chance of thrombophlebitis owing to the pelvic manipulation that can interfere with circulation and promote venous stasis. Peritonitis is a potential complication of any abdominal surgery, not just pelvic surgery. Ascites is most frequently an indication of liver disease. Inguinal hernia may be caused by an increase in intra-abdominal pressure or a congenital weakness of the abdominal wall; ventral hernia occurs at the site of a previous abdominal incision. (E, 9)

6. 4. Mucus is secreted by the intestinal segment used to create the conduit and is a normal occurrence. The client should be encouraged to maintain a large fluid intake to help flush the mucus out of the conduit. Because mucus in the urine is expected, it is not necessary to change the appliance bag or to notify the physician. The mucus is not an indication of an infection, so a urine culture is not necessary. (D, 9)

7. 4. If the appliance becomes too full, it is likely to pull away from the skin completely or to leak urine onto the skin. A full appliance will not rupture the ileal conduit or interrupt urine production. Odor formation has numerous causes. (I, 10)

8. 1. Inserting a gauze wick into the stoma helps prevent urine leakage when changing the appliance. The stoma should not be sealed or suctioned. Oral fluids do not need to be avoided. (I, 10)

9. 2. A reusable appliance should be routinely cleaned with soap and water. (I, 10)

10. 2. A distilled vinegar solution acts as a good deodorizing agent after an appliance has been cleaned well with soap and water. If the client prefers, a commercial deodorizer may be used. Salt solution does not deodorize. Ammonia and bleaching agents may damage the appliance. (I, 7)

11. 4. It is normal for clients to express fears and concerns about the body changes associated with a urinary diversion. Allowing the client time to verbalize concerns in a supportive environment and suggesting that she discuss these concerns with people who have successfully adjusted to ostomy surgery can help her begin coping with these changes in a positive manner. Although the client may be anxious about this situation and self-esteem may be diminished, the underlying problem is a disturbance in body image. There are no data to support a diagnosis of Deficient Knowledge. (D, 5)

12. 1. The most important reason for attaching the appliance to a standard urine collection bag at night is to prevent urine reflux into the stoma and ureters, which can result in infection. Use of a standard collection bag also keeps the appliance from separating from the skin and helps prevent urine leakage from an overly full bag, but the primary purpose is to prevent reflux of urine. A client with a urinary diversion should drink 2000 to 3000 mL of fluid each day; it would be inappropriate to suggest decreasing fluid intake. (I, 10)

13. 2. Maintaining a fluid intake of 2000 to 3000 mL/ likely to be most effective in preventing urin infection. A high fluid intake results in hig put, which prevents urinary stasis growth. Avoiding people with respi

tions will not prevent urinary tract infections. Clean, not sterile, technique is used to change the appliance. An ileal conduit stoma is not irrigated. (I, 10)

14. 4. It is important that the client empty the drainage pouch throughout the day to decrease the risk of leakage. The client does not normally need to curtail physical activity. Aspirin should never be placed in a pouch because aspirin can irritate or ulcerate the stoma. The client does not catheterize an ileal conduit stoma. (E, 10)

The Client With Renal Calculi

15. 3. The priority nursing goal for this client is to alleviate the pain, which can be excruciating. Prevention of urinary tract complications and alleviation of nausea are appropriate throughout the client's hospitalization, but relief of the severe pain is a priority. The client is at little risk of fluid and electrolyte imbalance. (P, 10)

16. 4. A KUB radiographic examination ordinarily requires no preparation. It is usually done while the client lies supine and does not involve the use of radiopaque substances. (P, 9)

17. 2. The pain associated with renal colic due to calculi is often referred to the groin and bladder in female clients and to the testicles in male clients. Nausea, vomiting, abdominal cramping, and diarrhea may also be present. Nephritis or urinary retention is an unlikely cause of the referred pain. The type of pain described in this situation is unlikely to be caused by additional stone formation. (D, 10)

18. 2. During episodes of renal colic, the pain is excruciating. It is necessary to administer narcotic analgesics to control the pain. Application of heat, encouraging high fluid intake, and limitation of activity are important interventions, but they will not relieve the renal colic pain. (I, 9)

19. 2. Intermittent pain that is less colicky indicates that the calculi may be moving along the urinary tract. Fluids should be encouraged to promote movement, and the urine should be strained to detect passage of the stone. Hematuria is to be expected from the irritation of the stone. Analgesics should be administered when the client needs them, not routinely. Moist heat to the flank area is helpful when renal colic occurs, but it is less necessary as pain is lessened. (I, 10)

20. 3. A client scheduled for an IVP should be assessed for allergies to iodine and shellfish. Clients with such allergies may be allergic to the IVP dye and be at risk for an anaphylactic reaction. Adequate fluid intake is important after the examination. Bowel preparation is important before an IVP to allow visualization of the ureters and bladder, but checking for allergies is most important. (I, 9)

21. 2. After an IVP, the nurse should encourage fluids to decrease the risk of renal complications caused by the contrast agent. There is no need to place the client on bed rest or administer a laxative. An IVP would not cause hematuria. (P, 9)

22. 1. The appropriate action would be to discard the specimen and obtain a new one. Urine that is allowed to stand at room temperature will become alkaline, with multiplying bacteria. The specimen should be examined within 1 hour after urination. (I, 9)

23. 2. The ureteral catheter should drain freely without bleeding at the site. The catheter is rarely irrigated, and any irrigation would be done by the physician. The catheter is never clamped. The client's total urine output (ureteral catheter plus voiding or Foley catheter output) should be 30 mL/hour. (I, 9)

24. 1. Ambulation stimulates peristalsis. A client with paralytic ileus is kept NPO until peristalsis returns. Incentive spirometry and intravenous fluid infusion are routine postoperative orders that do not have any effect on preventing paralytic ileus. Incentive spirometry is used to prevent respiratory complications. (I, 10)

25. 2. The decrease in urine output may reflect inadequate renal perfusion and should be reported immediately. Urine output of 30 mL/hour or greater is considered acceptable. A slight elevation in temperature is expected after surgery. Peristalsis returns gradually, usually the second or third day after surgery. Bowel sounds will be absent until then. A small amount of serous sanguineous drainage is to be expected. (E, 10)

26. 1. A high daily fluid intake is essential for all clients who are at risk for calculi formation because it prevents urinary stasis and concentration, which can cause crystallization. Depending on the composition of the stone, the client also may be instructed to institute specific dietary measures aimed at preventing stone formation. Clients may need to limit purine, calcium, or oxalate. Urine may need to be either alkaline or acid. There is no need to strain urine regularly. (P, 7)

27. 1. Because a high-purine diet contributes to the formation of uric acid, a low-purine diet is advocated. An alkaline-ash diet is also advocated, because uric acid crystals are more likely to develop in acid urine. Foods that may be eaten as desired in a low-purine diet include milk, all fruits, tomatoes, cereals, and corn. Foods allowed on an alkaline-ash diet include milk, fruits (except cranberries, plums, and prunes), and vegetables (especially legumes and green vegetables). Gravy, chicken, and liver are high in purine. (E, 7)

28. 2. Allopurinol is used to treat renal calculi composed of uric acid. Side effects of allopurinol include drowsiness, maculopapular rash, anemia, abdominal pain, nausea, vomiting, and bone marrow depression. Clients should

be instructed to report skin rashes and any unusual bleeding or bruising. Retinopathy, nasal congestion, and dizziness are not side effects of allopurinol. (I, 8)

29. 4. By inhibiting uric acid synthesis, allopurinol decreases its excretion. The drug's effectiveness is assessed by evaluating for a decreased serum uric acid concentration. Allopurinol does not alter the level of alkaline phosphatase, nor does it affect urinary calcium excretion or the serum calcium level. (E, 8)

The Client With Acute Renal Failure

30. 4. Oliguria is the most common initial symptom of acute renal failure. Anuria is rarely the initial symptom. Dysuria and hematuria are not associated with acute renal failure. (A, 10)

31. 1. There are three categories of acute renal failure: prerenal, intrarenal, and postrenal. Causes of prerenal failure occur outside the kidney and include poor perfusion and a decrease in circulating volume resulting from such factors as trauma, septic shock, impaired cardiac function, and dehydration. In this case of severe myocardial infarction, there was a decrease in perfusion of the kidneys caused by impaired cardiac function. An obstruction within the urinary tract, such as results from kidney stones, tumors, or benign prostatic hypertrophy, is called postrenal failure. Structural damage to the kidney resulting from acute tubular necrosis is called intrarenal failure. It is caused by conditions such as hypersensitivity (allergic disorders), renal vessel obstruction, and nephrotoxic agents. (P, 10)

32. 4. Urea, an end product of protein metabolism, is excreted by the kidneys. Impairment in renal function caused by reduced renal blood flow results in an increase in the plasma urea level. Fluid retention, hemolysis of red blood cells, and lowered metabolic rate do not cause an elevated BUN value. (A, 9)

33. 4. Polystyrene sulfonate, a cation-exchange resin, causes the body to excrete potassium through the gastrointestinal tract. In the intestines, particularly the colon, the sodium of the resin is partially replaced by potassium. The potassium is then eliminated when the resin is eliminated with feces. Although the result is to increase potassium excretion, the specific method of action is the exchange of sodium ions for potassium ions. Polystyrene sulfonate does not release hydrogen ions or increase calcium absorption. (I, 8)

34. 1. Hyperkalemia places the client at risk for serious cardiac dysrhythmias and cardiac arrest. Therefore, the nurse should carefully monitor the client for cardiac dysrhythmias and be prepared to treat cardiac arrest when caring for a client with hyperkalemia. Increased

potassium levels do not result in pulmonary edema, circulatory collapse, or hemorrhage. (P, 8)

35. 4. High-carbohydrate foods meet the body's caloric needs during acute renal failure. Protein is limited because its breakdown may result in accumulation of toxic waste products. The main goal of nutritional therapy in acute renal failure is to decrease protein catabolism. Protein catabolism causes increased levels of urea, phosphate, and potassium. Carbohydrates provide energy and decrease the need for protein breakdown. They do not have a diuretic effect. Some specific carbohydrates influence urinary pH, but this is not the reason for encouraging a high-carbohydrate, low-protein diet. There is no need to reduce demands on the liver through dietary manipulation in acute renal failure. (I, 7)

36. 1. Gelatin desserts contain little or no potassium and can be served to a client on a potassium-restricted diet. Foods high in potassium include bran and whole grains; most dried, raw, and frozen fruits and vegetables; most milk and milk products; chocolate, nuts, raisins, coconut, and strong brewed coffee. (I, 7)

37. 1. Pulmonary edema can develop during the oliguric phase of acute renal failure because of decreased urinary output and fluid retention. Metabolic acidosis develops because the kidneys cannot excrete hydrogen ions, and bicarbonate is used to buffer the hydrogen. Hypertension may develop as a result of fluid retention. Hyperkalemia develops as the kidneys lose the ability to excrete potassium. (P, 10)

38. 1. The unaffected arm should be used for blood pressure measurement. The external cannula must be handled carefully and protected from damage and disruption. In addition, a tourniquet or clamps should be kept at the bedside, because dislodgment of the cannula would cause arterial hemorrhage. The arm with the cannula is not used for blood pressure measurement, intravenous therapy, or venipuncture. Patency is assessed by auscultating for bruits every shift. Heparin is not injected into the cannula to maintain patency. Because it is part of the general circulation, the cannula cannot be heparinized. (I, 9)

39. 1. Common symptoms of disequilibrium syndrome include headache, nausea and vomiting, confusion, and even seizures. Disequilibrium syndrome typically occurs near the end or after the completion of hemodialysis treatment. It is the result of rapid changes in solute composition and osmolality of the extracellular fluid. These symptoms are not related to cardiac function, air embolism, or peritonitis. (D, 9)

40. 2. If disequilibrium syndrome occurs during dialysis, the most appropriate intervention is to slow the rate of dialysis. The syndrome is believed to result from too-

rapid removal of urea and excess electrolytes from the blood; this causes transient cerebral edema, which produces the symptoms. Administration of oxygen and position changes do not affect the symptoms. It would not be appropriate to reassure the client that the symptoms are normal. (I, 9)

41. 1. Regional anticoagulation can be achieved by infusing heparin in the dialyzer and protamine sulfate, its antagonist, in the client. Warfarin sodium is not used in dialysis treatment. There is some risk of bleeding; however, clotting time is monitored carefully. The client's clotting time will not be seriously affected, although some rebound effect may occur. (I, 8)

42. 3. Dialysis has no effect on anemia. Because some red blood cells are injured during the procedure, dialysis aggravates a low hemoglobin concentration. Dialysis will clear metabolic waste products from the body and correct electrolyte imbalances. (E, 9)

43. 4. Signs of an external access shunt infection include redness, tenderness, swelling, and drainage from around the shunt site. The absence of a bruit indicates closing of the shunt. Sluggish capillary refill time and coolness of the extremity indicates decreased blood flow to the extremity. (A, 9)

44. 1. The kidneys have a remarkable ability to recover from serious insult. Recovery may take 3 to 12 months. The client should be taught how to recognize the symptoms of decreasing renal function and to notify the physician if such problems occur. In a client who is recovering from acute renal failure, there is no need for renal transplantation or permanent hemodialysis. Chronic renal failure develops before end-stage renal failure. (P, 10)

The Client With Urinary Tract Infection

45. 2. The classic symptoms of cystitis are severe burning, urgency, and frequent urination. Systemic symptoms, such as fever and nausea and vomiting, are more likely to accompany pyelonephritis than cystitis. Hematuria may occur, but it is not as common as frequency and burning. (A, 10)

46. 4. Although various conditions may result in cystitis, the most common cause is an ascending infection from the urethra. Strictures and urinary retention can lead to infections, but these are not the most common cause. Systemic infections are rarely causes of cystitis. (I, 10)

47. 3. The correct technique for a clean-catch urine culture specimen is to have the female client cleanse the labia from front to back, void into the toilet, and then void into the cup. The client does not need to fully empty her bladder into the cup. It is not necessary to catheterize the client to obtain the specimen. The first voided specimen of the day has the highest bacterial counts. (I, 7)

48. 4. As newlyweds, the client and her husband need to develop a strong communication base. The nurse can facilitate communication by preparing and supporting the client. Given the situation, an interdisciplinary conference is inappropriate and would not promote intimacy for the client and her husband. Insisting that the client talk with her husband is not addressing her fears. Being present allows the nurse to facilitate the discussion of a difficult topic. Having the nurse speak first with the husband alone shifts responsibility away from the couple. (I, 5)

49. 2. Hot tub baths promote relaxation and help relieve urgency, discomfort, and spasm. Applying heat to the perineum is more helpful than cold because heat reduces inflammation. Although liberal fluid intake should be encouraged, caffeinated beverages such as tea, coffee, and cola can be irritating to the bladder and should be avoided. Voiding at least every 2 to 3 hours should be encouraged because it reduces urinary stasis. (E, 7)

50. 3. Phenazopyridine hydrochloride is a urinary analgesic that works directly on the bladder mucosa to relieve the distressing symptoms of dysuria. Phenazopyridine hydrochloride does not have a bacteriostatic effect. It does not potentiate antibiotics or prevent crystallization. (I, 8)

51. 1. The client should be told that phenazopyridine hydrochloride turns the urine a bright orange-red, which may stain underwear. It can be frightening for a client to see orange-red urine without having been forewarned. Other common side effects associated with phenazopyridine include headaches, gastrointestinal disturbances, and rash. Phenazopyridine hydrochloride does not cause incontinence, constipation, or drowsiness. (I, 8)

52. 1. Stasis of urine in the bladder is one of the chief causes of bladder infection, and a client who voids infrequently is at greater risk of reinfection. A tub bath does not promote urinary tract infections as long as the client avoids harsh soaps and bubble baths. Scrupulous hygiene and liberal fluid intake (unless contraindicated) are excellent preventive measures, but the client also should be taught to void every 2 to 3 hours during the day. (E, 9)

53. 1. A woman can adopt several health-promotion measures to prevent the recurrence of cystitis, including avoiding too-tight pants, noncotton underpants, and irritating substances such as bubble baths and vaginal soaps and sprays. Increasing citrus juice intake can be a bladder irritant. Regular douching is not recommended; it can alter the pH of the vagina, increasing the risk of infection. (P, 7)

54. 4. Instructions should be as specific as possible, and the nurse should avoid general statements such as "a lot." A specific goal is most useful. A mix of fluids will increase the likelihood of client compliance. It may not be sufficient to tell the client to drink twice as much as or 1 quart more than she usually drinks if her intake was inadequate to begin with. (I, 7)

The Client With Pyelonephritis

55. 2. Common symptoms of pyelonephritis include CVA tenderness, burning, urinary urgency or frequency, chills, fever, and fatigue. Ascites, polyuria, and nausea and vomiting are not indicative of pyelonephritis. (A, 10)

56. 4. A client with a history of diabetes mellitus, urinary tract infections, or renal calculi is at increased risk for pyelonephritis. Others at high risk include pregnant women and people with structural alterations of the urinary tract. A history of hypertension may put the client at risk for kidney damage, but not kidney infection. Intake of large quantities of cranberry juice and a fluid intake of 2000 mL/day are not risk factors for pyelonephritis. (A, 9)

57. 3. Serum BUN and creatinine are the tests most commonly used to assess renal function, with creatinine being the most reliable indicator. Nonrenal factors may affect BUN levels as well as serum sodium and potassium levels. Arterial blood gases and hemoglobin are not used to assess renal status. Urinalysis is a general screening test, and a urine culture is used to detect urinary tract infections. (A, 10)

58. 3. Antibiotics are usually prescribed for a 2- to 4-week period. A urine culture is needed to evaluate the effectiveness of antibiotic therapy. Urine must be examined microscopically to adequately determine the presence of bacteria. Symptoms usually disappear 48 to 72 hours after antibiotic therapy is started, but antibiotics need to continue for up to 4 weeks. (I, 8)

59. 2. Chronic pyelonephritis is most commonly the result of recurrent urinary tract infections. Chronic pyelonephritis can lead to chronic renal failure. Single cases of acute pyelonephritis rarely cause chronic pyelonephritis. Acute renal failure is not a cause of chronic pyelonephritis. Glomerulonephritis is an immunologic disorder, not an infectious disorder. (P, 10)

The Client With Chronic Renal Failure

60. 1. Crackles in the lungs, weight gain, and elevated blood pressure are indicators of excess fluid volume, a common complication in chronic renal failure. The client's fluid status should be monitored carefully for imbalances on an ongoing basis. (D, 10)

61. 3. A disadvantage of peritoneal dialysis in long-term management of chronic renal failure is that it requires large blocks of time. The risk of hemorrhage or hepatitis is not high with peritoneal dialysis. Peritoneal dialysis is effective in maintaining a client's fluid and electrolyte balance. (E, 9)

62. 2. Nausea typically results from the chronic presence of retained waste products in the body. The client can control nausea most effectively by following the diet regimen strictly to avoid wide variations in blood values between treatments. Metabolic acidosis results from impaired excretion, not medications. Chronic anemia and fatigue as well as excess fluid are potential problems but do not cause nausea. (I, 10)

63. 1. The main reason for warming the peritoneal dialysis solution is that the warm solution helps dilate peritoneal vessels, which increases urea clearance. Warmed dialyzing solution also contributes to client comfort by preventing chilly sensations, but this is a secondary reason for warming the solution. The warmed solution does not force potassium into the cells or promote abdominal muscle relaxation. (I, 9)

64. 2. During dwell time, the dialysis solution is allowed to remain in the peritoneal cavity for the time ordered by the physician (usually 20 to 45 minutes). During this time, the nurse should monitor the client's respiratory status, because the pressure of the dialysis solution on the diaphragm can create respiratory distress. The dialysis solution would not cause urticaria or affect circulation to the fingers. The client's laboratory values are obtained before beginning treatment and are monitored every 4 to 8 hours during the treatment, not just during the dwell time. (A, 9)

65. 2. Because the client has a permanent catheter in place, blood-tinged drainage should not occur. Persistent blood-tinged drainage could indicate damage to the abdominal vessels, and the physician should be notified. The bleeding is originating in the peritoneal cavity, not the kidneys. Too-rapid infusion of the dialysate can cause pain. (A, 9)

66. 2. Fluid return with peritoneal dialysis is accomplished by gravity flow. Actions that enhance gravity flow include turning the client from side to side, raising the head of the bed, and gently massaging the abdomen. The client is usually confined to a recumbent position during the dialysis. The nurse should not attempt to reposition the catheter. (I, 9)

67. 2. Because hypotension is a complication associated with peritoneal dialysis, the nurse records intake and output, monitors vital signs, and observes the client's behavior. The nurse also encourages visiting and other diversional activities. A client on peritoneal dialysis need not need to be placed in a bed with padded side rails or kept NPO. (I, 9)

68. 3. Peritonitis is a serious risk associated with peritoneal dialysis. Aseptic technique should be maintained during the procedure. Minor abdominal cramping may occur with dialysis. Gastrointestinal bleeding is an extremely rare complication. Muscle cramps are not an anticipated complication of peritoneal dialysis but may be a complication of hemodialysis. (E, 9)

69. 2. Weight loss is expected because of the removal of fluid. The client's weight before and after dialysis is one measure of the effectiveness of treatment. Blood pressure usually decreases because of the removal of fluid. Hematuria would not occur after completion of peritoneal dialysis. Dialysis only minimally affects the damaged kidneys' ability to manufacture urine. (A, 9)

70. 3. A client in renal failure develops hyperphosphatemia that causes a corresponding excretion of the body's calcium stores, leading to renal osteodystrophy. To decrease this loss, aluminum hydroxide gel is prescribed to bind phosphates in the intestine and facilitate their excretion. Gastric hyperacidity is not necessarily a problem associated with chronic renal failure. Antacids will not prevent Curling's stress ulcers and do not affect metabolic acidosis. (P, 8)

71. 4. Aluminum hydroxide gel is administered to bind the phosphates in ingested foods and must be given with or immediately after meals and snacks. There is no need for the client to take it on a 24-hour schedule. It is not administered to treat hyperacidity in clients with chronic renal failure and therefore is not prescribed between meals. (E, 8)

72. 1. Magnesium is normally excreted by the kidneys. When the kidneys fail, magnesium can accumulate and cause severe neurologic problems. Milk of magnesia is harsher than Metamucil, but magnesium toxicity is a more serious problem. A client may find both milk of magnesia and Metamucil unpalatable. Milk of magnesia is not high in sodium. (I, 8)

73. 2. Uremia can cause decreased alertness, so the nurse needs to validate the client's comprehension frequently. Because the client's ability to concentrate is limited, short lessons are most effective. If family members are present at the sessions, they can reinforce the material. Written materials that the client can review are superior to videotapes, because clients may not be able to maintain alertness during the viewing of the videotape. (P, 10)

74. 3. Dietary management for clients with chronic renal failure is usually designed to restrict protein, sodium, and potassium intake. Protein intake is reduced because the kidney can no longer excrete the byproducts of protein metabolism. The degree of dietary restriction depends on the degree of renal impairment. The client should also receive a high-carbohydrate diet along with appropriate vitamin and mineral supplements. Calcium requirements remain 1000 to 2000 mg/day. (P, 7)

75. 2. Altered sexual functioning commonly occurs in chronic renal failure and can stress marriages and relationships. Altered sexual functioning can be caused by decreased hormone levels, anemia, peripheral neuropathy, or medication. The client should not decrease or avoid sexual activity but instead should modify it. The client should rest before sexual activity. (I, 5)

76. 2. The major benefit of CAPD is that it frees the client from daily dependence on dialysis centers, health care personnel, and machines for life-sustaining treatment. This independence is a valuable outcome for some people. CAPD is costly and must be done daily. Side effects and complications are similar to those of standard peritoneal dialysis. (I, 9)

77. 3. Dietary restrictions with CAPD are fewer than those with standard peritoneal dialysis because dialysis is constant, not intermittent. The constant slow diffusion of CAPD helps prevent accumulation of toxins and allows for a more liberal diet. CAPD does not work more quickly, but more consistently. Both types of peritoneal dialysis are effective. (I, 7)

78. 1. Cloudy drainage indicates bacterial activity in the peritoneum. Other signs and symptoms of infection are fever, hyperactive bowel sounds, and abdominal pain. Swollen legs may be indicative of congestive heart failure. Poor drainage of dialysate fluid is probably the result of a kinked catheter. Redness at the insertion site indicates local infection, not peritonitis. However, a local infection that is left untreated can progress to the peritoneum. (A, 9)

The Client With Urinary Incontinence

79. 3. Stress incontinence is the involuntary loss of urine during such activities as coughing, sneezing, laughing, or physical exertion. These activities increase abdominal and detrusor pressure. A strong urge to urinate is associated with urge incontinence. Overdistention of the bladder can lead to overflow incontinence. Obstruction of the urethra can lead to urinary retention. (P, 10)

80. 2. The history of three pregnancies is most likely the cause of the client's current episodes of stress incontinence. The client's fluid intake, age, or history of swimming would not create an increase in intra-abdominal pressure. (A, 4)

81. 4. The primary goal of nursing care is to decrease the number of incontinence episodes and the amount of urine expressed in an episode. Behavioral interventions (eg, diet and exercise) and medications are the nonsurgi-

cal management methods used to treat stress incontinence. Without surgical intervention, it may not be possible to eliminate all episodes of incontinence. Helping the client adjust to the incontinence is not treating the problem. Clients with stress incontinence are not prone to the development of urinary tract infection. (P, 10)

82. 2. Clients with stress incontinence are encouraged to avoid substances such as caffeine and alcohol which are bladder irritants. Emotional stressors do not cause stress incontinence. It is caused most commonly by relaxed pelvic musculature. Wearing girdles is not contraindicated. Although clients may be inclined to limit physical exertion to avoid incontinence episodes, they should be encouraged to seek treatment instead of limiting their activities. (P, 9)

83. 3. A characteristic of urge incontinence is involuntary urination with little or no warning. The inability to empty the bladder is urinary retention. Loss of urine when coughing occurs with stress incontinence. Frequent dribbling of urine is common in male clients after some types of prostate surgery or may occur in women after the development of a vesicovaginal or urethrovaginal fistula. (A, 10)

84. 1. Instructing the client to void at regularly scheduled intervals can help decrease the frequency of incontinence episodes. Providing a bedside commode does not decrease the number of incontinence episodes and does not help the client who leads an active lifestyle. Infections are not a common cause of urge incontinence, so antibiotics would not be an appropriate treatment. Intermittent self-catheterization is appropriate for overflow or reflux incontinence, but not urge incontinence, because it does not treat the underlying cause. (I, 10)

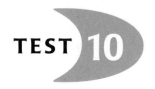
The Client With Reproductive Health Problems

Select the one best answer, and indicate your choice by filling in the circle in front of the option.

The Client With Uterine Fibroids

1. A 39-year-old female client has been experiencing intermittent vaginal bleeding for several months. Her physician tells her that she has uterine fibroids and recommends an abdominal hysterectomy. The nurse is completing the routine admission assessment when the client expresses fear about the surgery. Which of the following statements offers the best guide for the nurse's response? The nurse should
   ○ 1. reassure the client of her physician's competence.
   ○ 2. give the client opportunities to express her fears.
   ○ 3. teach the client that fear impedes recovery.
   ○ 4. change the subject of conversation to pleasantries when the client appears fearful.

2. The client having an abdominal hysterectomy is admitted the morning of surgery. Essential information the client needs before admission includes which of the following?
   ○ 1. What to wear to the hospital.
   ○ 2. What she can eat and drink before admission.
   ○ 3. The type of pain medication that will be prescribed postoperatively.
   ○ 4. Preoperative teaching about exercises at home.

3. The nurse is witnessing the client's signature on the informed surgical consent for an abdominal hysterectomy. It is important to ascertain that the client understands that with this surgical procedure she will have

○ 1. deceased libido.
○ 2. infertility.
○ 3. depression.
○ 4. weight gain.

4. During the immediate postoperative period after an abdominal hysterectomy, the client requires catheterization because she is unable to void. When preparing to insert the catheter into the urinary meatus, the nurse locates the anatomic structures between the labia minora. Starting from the area nearer the pubic bone and moving downward toward the anus, in which of the following order do the clitoris, vaginal opening, and urinary meatus lie?
   ○ 1. Clitoris, vaginal opening, urinary meatus.
   ○ 2. Urinary meatus, vaginal opening, clitoris.
   ○ 3. Vaginal opening, clitoris, urinary meatus.
   ○ 4. Clitoris, urinary meatus, vaginal opening.

5. The nurse is assigning tasks to the unlicensed assistive personnel (UAP) for a client with an abdominal hysterectomy on the first postoperative day. Which of the following cannot be delegated to the UAP?
   ○ 1. Taking vital signs.
   ○ 2. Recording intake and output.
   ○ 3. Giving perineal care.
   ○ 4. Assessing the incision site.

6. Which of the following physical sensations will the client who has had an abdominal hysterectomy most likely experience if she hyperventilates while performing deep breathing exercises?
   ○ 1. Dyspnea.
   ○ 2. Dizziness.

○ 3. Blurred vision.

○ 4. Mental confusion.

7. The UAP reports to the nurse that the client with an abdominal hysterectomy who returned from the recovery room 1 hour earlier has saturated the blue pad with bright red blood. The nurse should
   ○ 1. call the surgeon to report the bleeding.
   ○ 2. ask the UAP to obtain vital signs while the nurse calls the surgeon.
   ○ 3. ask the UAP to increase the flow of intravenous (IV) fluids to prevent shock.
   ○ 4. assess the client again in 15 minutes before the nurse takes any further action.

8. Which nursing measure would most likely relieve postoperative gas pains after abdominal hysterectomy?
   ○ 1. Offering the client a hot beverage.
   ○ 2. Providing extra warmth.
   ○ 3. Applying a snugly fitting abdominal binder.
   ○ 4. Helping the client walk.

9. On the second postoperative day after an abdominal hysterectomy, the client develops a temperature of 100.4°F (38°C). The nurse's first action should be to
   ○ 1. increase the number of wound changes to minimize infection.
   ○ 2. obtain a culture and sensitivity study of the urine to determine the source of infection.
   ○ 3. ensure that the client takes at least 10 deep breaths every hour.
   ○ 4. change the site of the client's IV fluid catheter to reduce the risk of infection.

10. The nurse in a rural hospital has just been notified that a client is being admitted from the emergency room with a nursing home–acquired pneumonia. The unit has four empty beds in semiprivate rooms. The room that would be most suitable for this client is the one with
    ○ 1. a 60-year-old client admitted for investigation of transient ischemic attacks.
    ○ 2. a 45-year-old client with an abdominal hysterectomy.
    ○ 3. a 24-year-old client with non-Hodgkin's lymphoma.
    ○ 4. a 55-year-old client with alcoholic cirrhosis.

11. The nurse is changing the dressing of a client after an abdominal hysterectomy. Which of the following nursing measures would be most appropriate if the dressing adheres to the client's incisional area?
    ○ 1. Pull off the dressing quickly and then apply slight pressure over the area.
    ○ 2. Lift an easily moved portion of the dressing and then remove it slowly.
    ○ 3. Moisten the dressing with sterile normal saline solution and then remove it.
    ○ 4. Remove part of the dressing and then remove

the remainder gradually over a period of several minutes.

12. A priority nursing diagnosis for the postoperative client who experiences wound dehiscence after an abdominal hysterectomy would be
    ○ 1. Risk for Infection.
    ○ 2. Excess Fluid Volume.
    ○ 3. Ineffective Airway Clearance.
    ○ 4. Imbalanced Nutrition: Less Than Body Requirements.

13. The client with an abdominal hysterectomy is being prepared for discharge in the morning. The nurse knows from the admission psychosocial assessment that the client has a mentally retarded adult son whom she cares for at home. The nurse would discuss with the physician the need for referral to which of the following departments?
    ○ 1. Home health care.
    ○ 2. Social work.
    ○ 3. Pastoral care.
    ○ 4. Volunteer services.

14. Which of the following hormones is likely to be prescribed for the client after an abdominal hysterectomy and removal of the ovaries and fallopian tubes?
    ○ 1. Estrogen.
    ○ 2. Thyroxine.
    ○ 3. Prolactin.
    ○ 4. Testosterone.

15. Which of the following nursing diagnoses would be most appropriate for the client being discharged from the hospital 3 days after an abdominal hysterectomy?
    ○ 1. Imbalanced Nutrition: Less Than Body Requirements related to nausea and vomiting.
    ○ 2. Excess Fluid Volume related to surgery.
    ○ 3. Ineffective Breathing Pattern related to postoperative pneumonia.
    ○ 4. Ineffective Coping related to body image disturbance.

16. When preparing discharge instructions for a client after an abdominal hysterectomy, the nurse should *first*
    ○ 1. have the client watch an educational video.
    ○ 2. assess the client's available social supports.
    ○ 3. call the social worker to evaluate the client.
    ○ 4. read the discharge instructions to the client.

The Client With Breast Disease

17. A postmenopausal woman is worried about pain in the upper outer quadrant of her left breast. The nurse's first course of action is to
    ○ 1. do a breast examination and report the results to the physician.

○ 2. explain that pain is caused by hormonal fluctuations.

○ 3. reassure the client that pain is not a symptom of breast cancer.

○ 4. teach the client the correct procedure for breast self-examination (BSE).

18. The nurse teaches a female client that the best time in the menstrual cycle to examine the breasts is during the

○ 1. week that ovulation occurs.

○ 2. week that menstruation occurs.

○ 3. first week after menstruation.

○ 4. week before menstruation occurs.

19. A woman with bilateral breast implants asks if she still needs to do breast examinations because she does not know what to feel for. Which of the following is the nurse's best response?

○ 1. "Have your partner assess your breasts on a regular basis."

○ 2. "I will show you the correct technique as I do the breast examination."

○ 3. "A breast examination is very difficult when you have had implant surgery."

○ 4. "You need to have a mammogram instead."

20. The client states that she has noticed that her bra fits more snugly at certain times of the month. She asks the nurse if this is a sign of breast disease. The nurse should base the reply to this client on the knowledge that

○ 1. benign cysts tend to cause the breasts to vary in size.

○ 2. it is normal for the breasts to increase in size before menstruation begins.

○ 3. a change in breast size warrants further investigation.

○ 4. differences in breast size are related to normal growth and development.

21. A 76-year-old client tells the nurse that she has lived long and does not need mammograms. Which of the following represents the nurse's best response?

○ 1. "You are not as at risk as a premenopausal woman."

○ 2. "The incidence of breast cancer increases with age."

○ 3. "We need to consider your family history of breast cancer first."

○ 4. "It will be sufficient if you perform breast examinations monthly."

22. After the surgeon's meeting with a client to obtain the client's informed consent for a modified radical mastectomy, the client asks the nurse many questions about breast reconstruction that the nurse finds difficult to answer. The nurse should

○ 1. inform the surgeon that the client has questions about reconstruction before she signs the consent.

○ 2. inform the client that she should concentrate on recovering from the mastectomy first.

○ 3. inform the client that she can have a consultation with the plastic surgeon in a few weeks.

○ 4. inform the client she can ask the surgeon these questions later when the surgeon makes rounds.

23. During the admission workup for a modified radical mastectomy, the client is extremely anxious and asks many questions. Which of the following statements would offer the best guide for the nurse to answer questions raised by this apprehensive preoperative client? It is usually best to

○ 1. tell the client as much as she wants to know and is able to understand.

○ 2. delay discussing the client's questions with her until she is convalescing.

○ 3. delay discussing the client's questions with her until her apprehension subsides.

○ 4. explain to the client that she should discuss her questions first with the physician.

24. A client asks the nurse, "Where is cancer usually found in the breast?" On a diagram of a left breast, the nurse would indicate that most malignant tumors occur in which quadrant of the breast?

○ 1. Upper outer quadrant.

○ 2. Upper inner quadrant.

○ 3. Lower outer quadrant.

○ 4. Lower inner quadrant.

25. Atropine sulfate is included in the preoperative orders for a client undergoing a modified radical mastectomy. The primary reason for giving this drug preoperatively is that it

○ 1. helps to promote general muscular relaxation.

○ 2. helps to decrease pulse and respiratory rates.

○ 3. helps to decrease nausea.

○ 4. helps to inhibit oral and respiratory secretions.

26. During the postoperative period after a modified radical mastectomy, the client confides in the nurse that she thinks she got breast cancer because she had an abortion and she did not tell her husband. The best response of the nurse is which of the following?

○ 1. "Cancer is not a punishment; it is a disease."

○ 2. "You might feel better if you confided in your husband."

○ 3. "Tell me more about your feelings on this."

○ 4. "I can have the social worker talk to you if you would like."

27. Postoperatively after a modified radical mastectomy, a client has an incisional drainage tube attached to Hemovac suction. The primary purpose of this tube is to

○ 1. decrease intrathoracic pressure and facilitate breathing.

○ 2. increase collateral lymphatic flow toward the operative area.

○ 3. remove accumulated serum and blood in the operative area.

○ 4. prevent formation of adhesions between the skin and chest wall in the operative area.

28. Which of the following positions would be best for a client's right arm when she returns to her room after a right modified radical mastectomy?

○ 1. Across her chest wall.

○ 2. At her side at the same level as her body.

○ 3. In the position that affords her the greatest comfort without placing pressure on the incision.

○ 4. On pillows, with her hand higher than her elbow and her elbow higher than her shoulder.

29. The client with breast cancer is prescribed tamoxifen (Nolvadex) 20 mg daily. The client states she does not like taking medicine and asks the nurse if the tamoxifen is really worth taking. The nurse's best response is which of the following?

○ 1. "This drug is part of your chemotherapy program."

○ 2. "This drug has been found to decrease metastatic breast cancer."

○ 3. "This drug will act as an estrogen in your breast tissue."

○ 4. "This drug will prevent hot flashes since you can not take hormone replacement."

30. A client undergoing chemotherapy after a modified radical mastectomy asks the nurse questions about a breast prosthesis and wigs. After answering the questions directly, the nurse would also

○ 1. provide a list of resources including the local breast cancer support group.

○ 2. offer a referral to the social worker.

○ 3. call the home health care agency.

○ 4. contact the plastic surgeon.

31. A client is to have radiation therapy after a modified radical mastectomy. The client should be taught to care for the skin at the site of therapy by

○ 1. washing the area with water.

○ 2. exposing the area to dry heat.

○ 3. applying an ointment to the area.

○ 4. using talcum powder on the area.

32. The nurse would teach a client that a normal local tissue response to radiation is

○ 1. atrophy of the skin.

○ 2. scattered pustule formation.

○ 3. redness of the surface tissue.

○ 4. sloughing of two layers of skin.

33. The nurse refers a client who had a mastectomy to "Reach to Recovery." The primary purpose of the American Cancer Society's Reach to Recovery program is to

○ 1. foster rehabilitation in women who have had mastectomies.

○ 2. raise funds to support early breast cancer detection programs.

○ 3. provide free dressings for women who have had radical mastectomies.

○ 4. collect statistics for research from women who have had mastectomies.

The Client With Benign Prostatic Hypertrophy

34. A 72-year-old male client is brought to the emergency department by his son. The client is extremely uncomfortable and has been unable to void for the past 12 hours. He has known for some time that he has an enlarged prostate but has wanted to avoid surgery. The best method for the nurse to use when assessing for bladder distention in a male client is to check for

○ 1. a rounded swelling above the pubis.

○ 2. dullness in the lower left quadrant.

○ 3. rebound tenderness below the symphysis.

○ 4. urine discharge from the urethral meatus.

35. During a client's urinary bladder catheterization, the bladder is emptied gradually. The best rationale for the nurse's action is that completely emptying an overdistended bladder at one time tends to cause

○ 1. renal failure.

○ 2. abdominal cramping.

○ 3. possible shock.

○ 4. atrophy of bladder musculature.

36. The primary reason for lubricating the urinary catheter generously before inserting it into a male client is that this technique helps reduce

○ 1. spasms at the orifice of the bladder.

○ 2. friction along the urethra when the catheter is being inserted.

○ 3. the number of organisms gaining entrance to the bladder.

○ 4. the formation of encrustations that may occur at the end of the catheter.

37. The primary reason for taping an indwelling catheter laterally to the thigh of a male client is to

○ 1. eliminate pressure at the penoscrotal angle.

○ 2. prevent the catheter from kinking in the urethra.

○ 3. prevent accidental catheter removal.

○ 4. allow the client to turn without kinking the catheter.

38. The primary function of the prostate gland is

○ 1. to store underdeveloped sperm before ejaculation.

○ 2. to regulate the acidity and alkalinity of the environment for proper sperm development.

3. to produce a secretion that aids the nourishment and passage of sperm.

4. to secrete a hormone that stimulates the production and maturation of sperm.

39. Many older men with prostatic hypertrophy do not seek medical attention until urinary obstruction is almost complete. Investigations have found that the primary reason for this delay in seeking attention is that these men
    1. feel too self-conscious to seek help when reproductive organs are involved.
    2. expect that it is normal to have to live with some urinary problems as they grow older.
    3. fear that sexual indiscretions in earlier life may be the cause of their problem.
    4. have little discomfort in relation to the amount of pathology because responses to pain stimuli fade with age.

40. The nurse anticipates that a client with prostatic hypertrophy will most likely report having experienced which of the following symptoms?
    1. Voiding at less frequent intervals.
    2. Difficulty starting the flow of urine.
    3. Painful urination.
    4. Increased force of the urine stream.

41. The nurse is reviewing the medication history of a client with benign prostatic hypertrophy (BPH). Which medication should be recognized as likely to aggravate BPH?
    1. Metformin (Glucophage).
    2. Buspirone (BuSpar).
    3. Inhaled ipratropium (Atrovent).
    4. Ophthalmic timolol (Timoptic).

42. A client is scheduled to undergo a transurethral resection of the prostate gland (TURP). The procedure is to be done under spinal anesthesia. Postoperatively, the nurse should be particularly alert for early signs of
    1. convulsions.
    2. cardiac arrest.
    3. renal shutdown.
    4. respiratory paralysis.

43. A common nursing diagnosis for a client in the immediate postoperative phase after a TURP is
    1. Ineffective Peripheral Tissue Perfusion related to deep vein thrombosis.
    2. Altered Comfort related to pain of bladder spasms.
    3. Disturbed Body Image related to disfiguring surgery.
    4. Imbalanced Nutrition: Less Than Body Requirements.

44. A client with BPH is being treated with terazosin (Hytrin) 2 mg at bedtime. The nurse should monitor the client's

1. urinary nitrites.
2. white blood cell count.
3. blood pressure.
4. pulse.

45. A client underwent a TURP, and a large three-way Foley catheter was inserted in the bladder with continuous bladder irrigation. In which of the following circumstances would the nurse increase the flow rate of the continuous bladder irrigation?
    1. When the drainage is continuous but slow.
    2. When the drainage appears cloudy and dark yellow.
    3. When the drainage becomes bright red.
    4. When there is no drainage of urine and irrigating solution.

46. A client is to receive belladonna and opium suppositories, as needed, postoperatively after a TURP. The nurse should give the client this drug when he demonstrates signs of
    1. a urinary tract infection.
    2. urinary retention.
    3. frequent urination.
    4. pain from bladder spasms.

47. A nursing assistant tells the nurse, "I think the client is confused. He keeps telling me he has to void, but that isn't possible because he has a catheter in place that is draining well." Which of the following responses would be most appropriate for the nurse to make?
    1. "His catheter is probably plugged. I'll irrigate it in a few minutes."
    2. "That's a common complaint after prostate surgery. The client only imagines the urge to void."
    3. "The urge to void is usually created by the large catheter, and he may be having some bladder spasms."
    4. "I think he may be somewhat confused."

48. A report on a urine culture indicates numerous white and red blood cells and a moderate amount of bacterial growth. The nurse evaluating these findings would deduce that the client most likely has
    1. a urethral stricture.
    2. a decreased renal filtration rate.
    3. a urinary tract infection.
    4. a prostate gland malignancy.

49. In discussing home care with a client after a TURP, the nurse should teach the male client that dribbling of urine
    1. can be a chronic problem.
    2. can persist for several months.
    3. is an abnormal sign that requires intervention.
    4. is a sign of healing within the prostate.

50. A priority nursing diagnosis for the client who is being discharged to home 3 days after a TURP would be

397

○ 1. Deficient Fluid Volume.
○ 2. Imbalanced Nutrition: Less Than Body Requirements.
○ 3. Impaired Tissue Integrity.
○ 4. Ineffective Airway Clearance.

51. If a client's prostate enlargement is caused by a malignancy, which of the following blood examinations should the nurse anticipate to assess whether metastasis has occurred?
○ 1. Serum creatinine level.
○ 2. Serum acid phosphatase level.
○ 3. Total nonprotein nitrogen level.
○ 4. Endogenous creatinine clearance time.

The Client With a Sexually Transmitted Disease

52. A home care nurse begins caring for a 25-year-old female client who has just been diagnosed with human immunodeficiency virus (HIV) infection. The client asks the nurse, "How could this have happened?" The nurse responds to the question based on the most frequent mode of HIV transmission, which is
○ 1. hugging an HIV-positive sexual partner without using barrier precautions.
○ 2. inhaling cocaine.
○ 3. sharing food utensils with an HIV-positive person without proper cleansing of the utensils.
○ 4. having sexual intercourse with an HIV-positive person without using a condom.

53. A client with HIV is taking zidovudine (AZT). AZT is a drug that acts to
○ 1. destroy the virus.
○ 2. enhance the body's antibody production.
○ 3. slow replication of the virus.
○ 4. neutralize toxins produced by the virus.

54. Women who have herpes genitalis are at risk for development of
○ 1. sterility.
○ 2. cervical cancer.
○ 3. uterine fibroid tumors.
○ 4. irregular menses.

55. Which of the following nursing diagnoses would most likely be a priority for a client with herpes genitalis?
○ 1. Disturbed Sleep Pattern.
○ 2. Imbalanced Nutrition: Less Than Body Requirements.
○ 3. Pain.
○ 4. Ineffective Breathing Pattern.

56. The primary reason that a herpes simplex virus (HSV) infection is a serious concern to a client with HIV infection is that it
○ 1. is an acquired immunodeficiency virus (AIDS)–defining illness.
○ 2. is curable only after 1 year of antiviral therapy.

○ 3. leads to cervical cancer.
○ 4. causes severe electrolyte imbalances.

57. In educating a client about HIV, the nurse should take into account the fact that the most effective method known to control the spread of HIV infection is
○ 1. premarital serologic screening.
○ 2. prophylactic treatment of exposed people.
○ 3. laboratory screening of pregnant women.
○ 4. ongoing sex education about preventive behaviors.

58. A male client with HIV infection becomes depressed and tells the nurse "I have nothing worth living for now." Which of the following statements would be the best response by the nurse?
○ 1. "You are a young person and have a great deal to live for."
○ 2. "You should not be too depressed; we are close to finding a cure for AIDS."
○ 3. "You are right; it is very depressing to have HIV."
○ 4. "Tell me more about how you are feeling about being HIV positive."

59. The organism responsible for causing syphilis is classified as a
○ 1. virus.
○ 2. fungus.
○ 3. rickettsia.
○ 4. spirochete.

60. The typical chancre of syphilis appears as
○ 1. a grouping of small, tender pimples.
○ 2. an elevated wart.
○ 3. a painless, moist ulcer.
○ 4. an itching, crusted area.

61. When interviewing a client with newly diagnosed syphilis, the public health nurse should be aware that the spread of the disease can be controlled by
○ 1. motivating the client to undergo treatment.
○ 2. obtaining a list of the client's sexual contacts.
○ 3. increasing the client's knowledge of the disease.
○ 4. reassuring the client that records are confidential.

62. Benzathine penicillin G, 2.4 million units IM, is prescribed as treatment for an adult client with primary syphilis. The intramuscular injection is administered in
○ 1. the deltoid.
○ 2. the upper outer quadrant of the buttock.
○ 3. the quadriceps lateralis of the thigh.
○ 4. the midlateral aspect of the thigh.

63. A priority nursing diagnosis for a client with primary syphilis is
○ 1. Deficient Knowledge related to lack of exposure to information about mode of transmission.
○ 2. Pain related to cutaneous skin lesions on palms and soles.

○ 3. Ineffective Tissue Perfusion related to a bleeding chancre.

○ 4. Disturbed Body Image related to alopecia.

64. An 18-year-old female college student is seen at the university health center. She undergoes a pelvic examination and is diagnosed with gonorrhea. Which of the following responses by the nurse would be best when the client says that she is nervous about the upcoming pelvic examination?
○ 1. "Can you tell me more about how you're feeling?"
○ 2. "You're not alone. Most women feel uncomfortable about this examination."
○ 3. "Do not worry about Dr. Smith. He's a specialist in female problems."
○ 4. "We'll do everything we can to avoid embarrassing you."

65. When educating a female client with gonorrhea, the nurse should emphasize that for women gonorrhea
○ 1. is often marked by symptoms of dysuria or vaginal bleeding.
○ 2. does not lead to serious complications.
○ 3. can be treated but not cured.
○ 4. may not cause symptoms until serious complications occur.

66. Which of the following groups has experienced the greatest rise in the incidence of STDs over the past two decades?
○ 1. Teenagers.
○ 2. Divorced people.
○ 3. Young married couples.
○ 4. Older adults.

67. A female client with gonorrhea informs the nurse that she has had sexual intercourse with her boyfriend and asks the nurse, "Would he have any symptoms?" The nurse responds that in men the symptoms of gonorrhea include
○ 1. impotence.
○ 2. scrotal swelling.
○ 3. urinary retention.
○ 4. dysuria.

68. The nurse assesses the mouth and oral cavity of a client with HIV because the most common opportunistic infection initially presents as
○ 1. HSV lesions on the lips.
○ 2. oral candidiasis.
○ 3. cytomegalovirus (CMV) infection.
○ 4. aphthae on the gingiva.

The Client With Cancer of the Cervix

69. A 45-year-old female client makes a clinic appointment for a routine gynecologic examination. The position of choice for a client undergoing a vaginal examination is the

○ 1. Sims' position.
○ 2. lithotomy position.
○ 3. genupectoral position.
○ 4. dorsal recumbent position.

70. A client asks the nurse to explain the meaning of her abnormal Pap smear result. Which of the following concepts should the nurse include in the response?
○ 1. An atypical Pap smear means that abnormal viral cells were found in the smear.
○ 2. An atypical Pap smear means that cancer cells were found in the smear.
○ 3. A positive Pap smear alone is not very important diagnostically because there are many false-positive results.
○ 4. Abnormal cells in a Pap smear may be caused by various conditions other than cancer.

71. Which of the following is a risk factor for cervical cancer?
○ 1. Sexual experiences with one partner.
○ 2. Sedentary lifestyle.
○ 3. Obesity.
○ 4. Adolescent pregnancy.

72. The American Cancer Society recommends that adult women follow which schedule for Pap smear screening?
○ 1. Annually for women in the high-risk category.
○ 2. Annually if sexually active; every 5 years if sexually abstinent.
○ 3. Every 3 years after one initial negative test.
○ 4. Every 3 years until age 40 and annually thereafter.

73. A woman tells the nurse that she is always nervous about the pelvic examination and Pap smear because "there's been a lot of cancer in my family." The nurse should be aware that an early sign of cervical cancer is
○ 1. pain.
○ 2. leg edema.
○ 3. urinary and rectal symptoms.
○ 4. light bleeding or watery vaginal discharge.

74. A 30-year-old female client asks the nurse about douching. What information would the nurse include in the teaching plan?
○ 1. Douching during menstruation is safe.
○ 2. Daily douching will decrease any vaginal odor.
○ 3. Perfumed douches are recommended to decrease odors.
○ 4. Douching removes natural mucus and changes the balance of normal vaginal flora.

75. The husband of a client with cervical cancer says to the nurse, "The doctor told my wife that her cancer is curable. Is he just trying to make us feel better?" Which would be the nurse's most accurate response?
○ 1. "When cervical cancer is detected early and treated aggressively, the cure rate is almost 100%."

○ 2. "The 5-year survival rate is about 75%, which makes the odds pretty good."

○ 3. "Saying a cancer is curable means that 50% of all women with the cancer survive at least 5 years."

○ 4. "Cancers of the female reproductive tract tend to be slow growing and respond well to treatment."

76. A client with suspected cervical cancer is undergoing a colposcopy with conization. The nurse gives instructions to the client about her menstrual periods, emphasizing that
○ 1. her periods will return to normal.
○ 2. her next two or three periods may be heavier and more prolonged than usual.
○ 3. her next two or three periods will be lighter than normal.
○ 4. she may skip her next two periods.

77. A client with cervical cancer is undergoing internal radium implant therapy. A lead-lined container and a pair of long forceps are kept in the client's hospital room for
○ 1. disposal of emesis or other bodily secretions.
○ 2. handling of the dislodged radiation source.
○ 3. disposal of the client's eating utensils.
○ 4. storage of the radiation dose.

78. The mother of a client who has a radium implant asks why so many nurses are involved in her daughter's care. She states, "The doctor said I can be in the room for up to 2 hours each day, but the nurses say they're restricted to 30 minutes." The nurse explains that this variation is based on the fact that nurses
○ 1. touch the client, which increases their exposure to radiation.
○ 2. work with many clients and could carry infection to a client receiving radiation therapy, if exposure is prolonged.
○ 3. work with radiation on an ongoing basis, while visitors have infrequent exposure to radiation.
○ 4. are at greater risk from the radiation because they are younger than the mother.

79. A priority nursing diagnosis for a client with cervical cancer who has an internal radium implant would be
○ 1. Pain related to cervical tumor.
○ 2. Anxiety related to self-care deficit from imposed immobility during radiation.
○ 3. Impaired Health Maintenance related to surgery.
○ 4. Disturbed Sleep Pattern related to interruptions by health care personnel.

80. A client with condylomata acuminata (genital warts) is being treated by a colposcopy. The client asks the nurse if this procedure is really necessary.

The nurse explains that the procedure to treat the warts is important because warts can lead to
○ 1. infertility.
○ 2. cervical cancer.
○ 3. pelvic inflammatory disease.
○ 4. rectal cancer.

81. Which of the following would be standard nursing care for a client with cervical cancer who has an internal radium implant in place?
○ 1. Offer the bedpan every 2 hours.
○ 2. Provide perineal care twice daily.
○ 3. Check the position of the applicator hourly.
○ 4. Offer a low-residue diet.

82. The nurse should carefully observe a client with internal radium implants for typical side effects associated with radiation therapy to the cervix. These effects include
○ 1. severe vaginal itching.
○ 2. confusion.
○ 3. high fever in the afternoon or evening.
○ 4. nausea and a foul vaginal discharge.

The Client With Testicular Disease

83. A 28-year-old male client is diagnosed with acute epididymitis. The nurse would expect to find that the symptoms that caused the client to seek medical care are
○ 1. burning and pain on urination.
○ 2. severe tenderness and swelling in the scrotum.
○ 3. foul-smelling ejaculate.
○ 4. foul-smelling urine.

84. A 20-year-old client is being treated for epididymitis. Teaching for this client should include the fact that epididymitis is often a result of a
○ 1. virus.
○ 2. parasite.
○ 3. sexually transmitted infection.
○ 4. protozoa.

85. When teaching a client to perform testicular self-examination, the nurse explains that the examination should be performed
○ 1. after intercourse.
○ 2. at the end of the day.
○ 3. after a warm bath or shower.
○ 4. after exercise.

86. The normal testis can be described as
○ 1. soft.
○ 2. egg shaped.
○ 3. spongy.
○ 4. lumpy.

87. A client has a testicular nodule that is highly suspicious for testicular cancer. A laboratory test that supports this diagnosis is
○ 1. decreased α-fetoprotein (AFP).

2. decreased β-human chorionic gonadotropin (hCG).

3. increased testosterone.

4. increased AFP.

88. Although the cause of testicular cancer is unknown, it is associated with a history of

1. undescended testes.

2. sexual relations at an early age.

3. seminal vesiculitis.

4. epididymitis.

89. Risk factors associated with testicular malignancies include

1. African-American race.

2. residing in a rural area.

3. lower socioeconomic status.

4. age older than 40 years.

90. A client with a testicular malignancy undergoes a radical orchiectomy. A priority problem in the immediate postoperative period is

1. bladder spasms.

2. urinary elimination.

3. pain.

4. nausea.

91. A right orchiectomy is performed on a client with a testicular malignancy. The client expresses concerns regarding his sexuality. The nurse should base the response on the knowledge that

1. the client is not a candidate for sperm banking.

2. the client should retain normal sexual drive and function.

3. the client will be impotent.

4. the client will have a change in secondary sexual characteristics.

92. A client diagnosed with seminomatous testicular cancer expresses fear and questions the nurse about his prognosis. The nurse should base the response on the knowledge that

1. testicular cancer is almost always fatal.

2. testicular cancer has a cure rate of 90% when diagnosed early.

3. surgery is the treatment of choice for testicular cancer.

4. testicular cancer has a 50% cure rate when diagnosed early.

The Client With Cancer of the Prostate

93. A client asks the nurse why the prostate specific antigen (PSA) level is determined before the digital rectal examination. The nurse's best response is which of the following?

1. "It is easier for the client."

2. "A prostate examination can possibly decrease the PSA."

3. "A prostate examination can possibly increase the PSA."

4. "If the PSA is normal, the client will not have to undergo the rectal examination."

94. During a digital rectal examination, a key sign for prostate cancer is

1. a hard prostate, localized or diffuse.

2. abdominal pain.

3. a boggy, tender prostate.

4. a nonindurated prostate.

95. A client is undergoing a total prostatectomy for prostate cancer. The client asks questions about his sexual function. The best response of the nurse is which of the following?

1. "Loss of the prostate gland means that you will be impotent."

2. "Loss of the prostate gland means that you will be infertile and there will be no ejaculation. You can still experience the sensations of orgasm."

3. "Loss of the prostate gland means that you will have no loss of sexual function and drive."

4. "Loss of the prostate gland means that your erectile capability will return immediately after surgery."

96. A 65-year-old client has been told by the physician that his prostate cancer was graded at stage IIB. The client inquires if this means he is going to die soon. The best response of the nurse is which of the following?

1. "Prostate cancer at this stage is very slow growing."

2. "Prostate cancer at this stage is very fast growing."

3. "Prostate cancer at this stage has spread to the bone."

4. "Prostate cancer at this stage is difficult to predict."

97. A client with prostate cancer is treated with hormone therapy consisting of diethylstilbestrol (DES; Stilphostrol), 2 mg daily. The nurse should instruct the client that the medication can cause

1. tenderness of the scrotum.

2. tenderness of the breasts.

3. loss of pubic hair.

4. decreased blood pressure.

The Client With Erectile Dysfunction

98. A male client complains of impotence. The nurse examines the client's medication regimen and is aware that a contributing factor to impotence could be

1. aspirin.

2. antihypertensives.

3. nonsteroidal anti-inflammatory drugs.

4. anticoagulants.

99. A 65-year-old male client with erectile dysfunction

(ED) asks the nurse, "Is all this just in my head? Am I crazy?" The best response of the nurse is based on the knowledge that

○ 1. ED is believed to be psychogenic in most cases.

○ 2. more than 50% of the cases are attributed to organic causes.

○ 3. evaluation of nocturnal erections is not helpful in the differentiation of psychogenic or organic causes.

○ 4. ED is an uncommon problem among men older than 65 years of age.

100. The nurse should teach the client with ED to alter his lifestyle to

○ 1. avoid alcohol.

○ 2. follow a low-salt diet.

○ 3. decrease smoking.

○ 4. increase attempts at sexual intercourse.

Correct Answers and Rationale

The letters in parentheses following the rationale identify the step of the nursing process (A, D, P, I, E) and client needs (1, 2, 3, 4, 5, 6, 7, 8, 9, 10). See the inside front cover for the key.

The Client With Uterine Fibroids

1. 2. The best approach for a client who is fearful about having surgery is to allow the client opportunities to express her fears. Open-ended questions should elicit the client's individual and specific fears. This then gives the nurse the opportunity to provide clarification, information, and support and possibly to offer other resources. The other actions are not supportive and deny the client the opportunity to express her feelings. (I, 5)

2. 2. It is a priority that the client knows she will not be able to eat or drink for 8 hours before admission. A client who consumes food and fluid before a general anesthetic is at risk for aspiration, which can lead to aspiration pneumonia, respiratory arrest, and even death. The clothing she should wear to the hospital and the type of medication she will receive are important, but not the priority. Information on exercise and resumption of normal activities can be included in the discharge teaching. (I, 7)

3. 2. The client needs to understand that with removal of the uterus she will no longer be able to bear children or have menstrual periods. The surgical procedure should not change the woman's libido or sexual functioning. Research does not support the idea that hysterectomy contributes to depression or weight gain. Research demonstrates that women who have managed health problems for some time before the hysterectomy may actually have a more positive effect, with less worry about their health condition and about contraception or pregnancy. (P, 1)

4. 4. Starting from the area nearer the pubic bone and moving toward the anus, the anatomic order is clitoris, urinary meatus, and vaginal opening. (I, 9)

5. 4. The registered nurse is responsible to monitor the surgical site for condition of the dressing, status of the incision, and any signs of complications. UAP who have been trained to report abnormalities to the registered nurse supervising the care may take vital signs, record intake and output, and give perineal care. (P, 1)

6. 2. Hyperventilation occurs when the client breathes so rapidly and deeply that she exhales excessive amounts of carbon dioxide. A characteristic symptom of hyperventilation is dizziness. To avoid hyperventilation, the nurse should assist the client in the practice of slow, deep breathing in a regular breathing pattern. Dyspnea, blurred vision, and mental confusion are not associated with hyperventilation. (A, 10)

7. 2. The surgeon should be notified when a client who has had an abdominal hysterectomy develops vaginal bleeding that saturates a blue pad in 1 hour, and care should be managed so that other personnel can obtain vital signs while the nurse contacts the surgeon. The client may need to have IV fluids increased, but the surgeon needs to be notified first. Waiting 15 minutes while the client is having bright red bleeding is an unsafe nursing action; the client will probably lose a large amount of blood. (I, 1)

8. 4. The discomfort associated with gas pains is likely to be relieved when the client ambulates. The gas will be more easily expelled with exercise. The anesthesia, analgesics, and immobility have altered normal peristalsis. Peristalsis will be stimulated by exercise. Offering a hot beverage, providing extra warmth, and applying an abdominal binder are not recommended and could aggravate the discomfort of postoperative gas pains. (I, 10)

9. 3. Elevated temperature on the second postoperative day is suggestive of a respiratory tract infection. Respiratory infections most often occur during the first 48 hours after surgery. The client's vital signs should be monitored closely, and abnormalities should be reported to the surgeon. Signs of infection, if present in the wound or urinary tract, are likely to occur later in the postoperative period. There is no indication that the IV catheter is the source of infection. (I, 10)

10. 1. The client with a possible transient ischemic attack is the only client who has not had surgery and is not immunocompromised. The client with a recent surgery and incision should not be exposed to a client with infection. Clients with cancer or alcoholic cirrhosis are very susceptible to infection, and it would not be safe to expose them to a client with a respiratory infection. (P, 1)

11. 3. When a dressing sticks to a wound, it is best to moisten the dressing with sterile normal saline solution and then remove it carefully. Trying to remove a dry dressing is likely to irritate the skin and wound. This may contribute to tension or tearing along the suture line. (I, 1)

12. 1. Dehiscence, the opening of a wound, places the client at an immediate increased risk for infection. The wound should be covered with sterile saline and reported to the surgeon immediately. The fluid and caloric needs of the client should be maintained by IV replacement. Ineffective airway clearance or imbalanced nutrition could be an applicable diagnosis but not a priority diagnosis in this situation. Excess Fluid Volume is not an applicable diagnosis. (D, 10)

13. 2. The social worker will be able to coordinate respite care for the son and other community resources for this family. Home health care would provide care for the client herself, but respite care for the son is the priority need for this family. Pastoral care provides spiritual care. The volunteer department would not be responsible for coordination of care at the client's home. (P, 1)

14. 1. The primary ovarian hormone is estrogen. It may be prescribed for a woman whose ovaries, fallopian tubes, and uterus have been surgically removed, creating a "surgical menopause." Thyroxine is synthesized by the thyroid gland and is unaffected by a hysterectomy. Prolactin is the hormone involved in the production of breast milk. Testosterone is the male hormone. (I, 8)

15. 4. Body image disturbance related to loss of female reproductive organs may lead to ineffective coping in some women. Therefore, interventions to address this problem should be incorporated into discharge planning. The nurse should address any concerns regarding image, sexuality, and loss of fertility with the client. The other diagnoses are not expected problems 3 days after a hysterectomy. (D, 5)

16. 2. Assessment is the first step in planning client education. Assessing social support resources is a key aspect of discharge planning that begins when the client is admitted to the hospital. It is imperative to know what assistance and support the client has at home. Assessment includes obtaining data about any family or home responsibilities the client is concerned with during the recovery period. (I, 5)

The Client With Breast Disease

17. 1. This complaint warrants the nurse's performing an examination and reporting the results to the physician. Hormone fluctuations do cause breast discomfort, but an examination must be done at this time to assess the breast. Although pain is not common with breast cancer, it can be a symptom. Teaching the client to perform BSE is important, but it is not the priority action in this case. (I, 10)

18. 3. It is generally recommended that the breasts be examined during the first week after menstruation. During this time, the breasts are least likely to be tender or swollen because estrogen is at its lowest level. Therefore, the examination will be more comfortable for the client. The examination may also be more accurate, because the client is more likely to notice an actual change in her breast that is not simply related to hormonal changes. (I, 4)

19. 2. The client needs to become more confident and knowledgeable about the normal feel of the implants and her breast tissue. The best technique is for the nurse to demonstrate BSE to the client as the nurse conducts the clinical breast examination. Implant surgery does not exclude the need for monthly BSE. A mammogram is not a substitute for monthly BSE. (I, 4)

20. 2. The breasts may vary in size before menstruation because of breast engorgement caused by hormonal changes. A woman may then note that her bra fits more tightly than usual. Benign cysts do not cause variation in breast size. A change in breast size that does not follow hormonal changes could warrant further assessment. The breasts normally are about the same size, although some women have one breast slightly larger than the other. (I, 4)

21. 2. Advancing age in postmenopausal women has been identified as a risk factor for breast cancer. A 76-year-old client needs monthly BSE and a yearly clinical breast examination and mammogram to comply with the screening schedule. Family history is important, but only about 5% of breast cancers are genetic. (A, 4)

22. 1. If a client has questions the nurse cannot answer, it is best to delay the signing of the consent until the questions are clarified for the client. The surgeon should be notified, and the appropriate information or collaboration should be provided for the client before she signs the surgical consent. Telling her she should concentrate on recovery first ignores the client's questions and concerns. Frequently the plastic surgeon needs to be consulted at the beginning of the treatment, because various surgical decisions depend on the future plans for breast reconstruction. (I, 1)

23. 1. An important nursing responsibility is preoperative teaching, and the most frequently recommended guide for teaching is to tell the client as much as she wants to know and is able to understand. Delaying discussion of issues about which the client has concerns is likely to aggravate the situation and cause the client to feel distrust. As a general guide, the client would not ask the question if she were not ready to discuss her situation. The nurse is available to answer the client's questions and concerns and should not delay discussing these with the client. (I, 5)

24. 1. About half of malignant breast tumors occur in the upper outer quadrant of the breast. For no known reason, cancer appears in the left breast more often than in the right breast. The upper outer quadrants of the breast, and especially the axillary area, should be covered thoroughly in the clinical breast examination and BSE. (A, 10)

25. 4. Atropine sulfate, a cholinergic blocking agent, is given preoperatively to reduce secretions in the mouth and respiratory tract. This assists in maintaining the integrity of the respiratory system during general anesthesia. Atropine is not used to promote muscle relaxation, decrease nausea and vomiting, or decrease pulse and respiratory rates. It causes the pulse to increase. (I, 8)

26. 3. The nurse should respond with an open-ended statement that elicits further exploration of the client's feelings. Women with cancer may feel guilt or shame. Previous life decisions, sexuality, and religious beliefs may influence a client's adjustment to a diagnosis of cancer. The nurse should not contradict her feelings of punishment or offer advice such as confiding in the husband. A social worker referral may be beneficial in the future, but is not the first response needed to elicit exploration of the client's feelings. (I, 5)

27. 3. A drainage tube is placed in the wound after a modified radical mastectomy to help remove accumulated blood and fluid in the area. Removal of the drainage fluids assists in wound healing and is intended to decrease the incidence of hematoma or abscess formation and decrease the incidence of infection. Drainage tubes placed in a wound do not decrease intrathoracic pressure, increase collateral lymphatic flow, or prevent adhesion formation. (I, 9)

28. 4. Lymph nodes are ordinarily removed from the axillary area when a modified radical mastectomy is done, and each of the nodes is biopsied. To facilitate drainage from the arm on the affected side, the client's arm should be elevated on pillows with her hand higher than her elbow and her elbow higher than her shoulder. (I, 10)

29. 2. Tamoxifen is an antiestrogen drug that has been found to be effective against metastatic breast cancer and to improve the survival rate. The drug causes hot flashes as a side effect. (I, 8)

30. 1. Giving the client a list of community resources that could provide support and guidance assists the client to maintain her self-image and independence. The support group will include other women who have undergone similar therapies and can offer suggestions for breast products and wigs. (I, 1)

31. 1. A client receiving radiation therapy should avoid lotions, ointments, and anything that may cause irritation to the skin, such as exposure to sunlight, heat, or talcum powder. The area may safely be washed with water if it is done gently and if care is taken not to injure the skin. (I, 9)

32. 3. The most common reaction of the skin to radiation therapy is redness of the surface tissues. Dryness, tanning, and capillary dilation are also common. Atrophy of the skin, pustules, and sloughing of two layers would not be expected and should be reported to the radiologist. (I, 9)

33. 1. The American Cancer Society's Reach to Recovery is a rehabilitation program for women who have had breast surgery. It is designed to meet their physical, psychological, and emotional needs. The Reach to Recovery program is implemented by women who have had breast cancer themselves. Many women benefit from this peer information and support. (I, 5)

The Client With Benign Prostatic Hypertrophy

34. 1. The best way to assess for a distended bladder in either a male or female client is to check for a rounded swelling above the pubis. This swelling represents the distended bladder rising above the pubis into the abdominal cavity. Dullness does not indicate a distended bladder. The client might experience tenderness or pressure above the symphysis. No urine discharge is expected; the urine flow is blocked by the enlarged prostate.

35. 3. Rapid emptying of an overdistended bladder may cause hypotension and shock due to the sudden change of pressure within the abdominal viscera. Previously, removing no more than 1000 mL at one time was the standard of practice, but this is no longer thought to be necessary so long as the overdistended bladder is emptied slowly. (I, 9)

36. 2. Liberal lubrication of the catheter before catheterization of a male decreases friction along the urethra and reduces irritation and trauma to urethral tissues. Because the male urethra is tortuous, a liberal amount of lubrication is advised to ease catheter passage. The female urethra is not tortuous, and, although the catheter should be lubricated before insertion, less lubricant is necessary. (I, 9)

37. 1. The primary reason for taping an indwelling catheter to a male client so that the penis is held in a lateral position is to prevent pressure at the penoscrotal angle. Prolonged pressure at the penoscrotal angle can cause a ureterocutaneous fistula. (I, 9)

38. 3. The prostate gland is located below the bladder and surrounds the urethra. It serves one primary purpose: to produce a secretion that aids the nourishment and passage of sperm. (A, 10)

39. 2. Research shows that older men tend to believe it is normal to live with some urinary problems. As a result, these men often overlook symptoms and simply attribute them to aging. As part of preventive care for men older than 40 years of age, the yearly physical examination should include palpation of the prostate via rectal examination. The nurse should teach male clients the value of early detection and adequate follow-up for the prostate. (E, 5)

40. 2. Signs and symptoms of prostatic hypertrophy include difficulty starting the flow of urine, urinary frequency and hesitancy, decreased force of the urine stream, interruptions in the urine stream when voiding, and nocturia. The prostate gland surrounds the urethra, and these symptoms are all attributed to obstruction of the urethra resulting from prostatic hypertrophy. Nocturia from incomplete emptying of the bladder is common. Straining and urinary retention are often the symptoms that influence the client to seek care. Painful urination is generally not a symptom of prostatic hypertrophy. (A, 10)

41. 3. Atrovent is a bronchodilator, and its anticholinergic effects can aggravate urinary retention. Glucophage and BuSpar do not affect the urinary system; timolol does not have a systemic effect. (I, 8)

42. 4. If paralysis of vasomotor nerves in the upper spinal cord occurs when spinal anesthesia is used, the client is likely to develop respiratory paralysis. Artificial ventilation is required until the effects of the anesthesia subside. Convulsions, cardiac arrest, and renal shutdown are not likely results of spinal anesthesia. (A, 10)

43. 2. The pain of bladder spasms frequently necessitates pharmacologic intervention, as ordered by the surgeon. Deep vein thrombosis is not common after a TURP. The surgery is not disfiguring because no incision is made; the surgical entry is via the urethral meatus. The client resumes dietary intake shortly after the procedure, because a general anesthetic was not administered. (D, 10)

44. 3. Terazosin (Hytrin) is an antihypertensive drug that is also used in the treatment of BPH. Blood pressure must be monitored to ensure that the client does not develop hypotension, syncope, or orthostatic hypotension. The client should be instructed to change positions slowly. Urinary nitrates, white blood cell count, and pulse rate are not affected by terazosin. (I, 8)

45. 3. The decision by the surgeon to insert a catheter after a TURP or prostatectomy depends on the amount of bleeding that is expected after the procedure. During continuous bladder irrigation after a TURP or prostatectomy, the rate at which the solution enters the bladder should be increased when the drainage becomes brighter red. The color indicates the presence of blood. Increasing the flow of irrigating solution helps flush the catheter well so that clots do not plug it. There would be no reason to increase the flow rate when the return is continuous or when the return appears cloudy and dark yellow. Increasing the flow would be contraindicated when there is no return of urine and irrigating solution. (I, 8)

46. 4. Belladonna and opium suppositories are prescribed and administered to reduce bladder spasms that cause pain after a TURP. Bladder spasms frequently accompany any urologic procedure. Antispasmodics offer relief by eliminating or reducing the spasms. (I, 8)

47. 3. The Foley catheter creates the urge to void and can also cause bladder spasms. The nurse should ensure adequate bladder emptying by monitoring urine output and characteristics. Urine output should be at least 50 mL/hour. A plugged catheter, imagining the urge to void, and confusion are less likely reasons for the client's complaint. (I, 9)

48. 3. The presence of red and white blood cells and moderate bacteria in the urine is most typical of a urinary tract infection (UTI). Positive leukocyte esterase and nitrites are also significant for UTI. The pH increases with UTI, becoming more alkaline. A urethral stricture, decreased renal filtration rate, or prostate malignancy would not be evident in the urinalysis. (E, 9)

49. 2. Dribbling of urine can occur for several months after a TURP, and the client needs to be informed that this is expected. The nurse should teach the client perineal exercises to strengthen sphincter tone. The client may need to use pads for temporary incontinence. The client should be reassured that continence will return in a few months. (I, 7)

50. 1. Deficient Fluid Volume is a priority diagnosis, because the client needs to drink a large amount of fluids to keep the urine clear. The urine should be almost without color. About 2 weeks after a TURP, when desiccated tissue is sloughed out, a secondary hemorrhage could occur. The client should be instructed to call the surgeon or go to the emergency department if at any time the urine turns bright red. The client is not specifically at risk for nutritional problems after a TURP. The client is not specifically at risk for impaired tissue integrity because there is no external incision, and the client is not specifically at risk for airway problems because the procedure is done under spinal anesthesia. (D, 7)

51. 2. The most specific examination to determine whether a malignancy extends outside of the prostatic capsule is a study of the serum acid phosphatase level. The level increases when a malignancy has metastasized. A prostate specific antigen (PSA) determination and a digital rectal examination are done when screening for prostate cancer. Serum creatinine level, total nonprotein nitrogen level, and endogenous creatinine clearance time give information about kidney functioning, not prostate malignancy. (A, 9)

The Client With a Sexually Transmitted Disease

52. 4. HIV infection is transmitted through blood and body fluids, particularly vaginal and seminal fluids. A blood transfusion is one way the disease can be contracted. Other modes of transmission are sexual intercourse with an infected partner and sharing needles for intravenous drug injections with an infected person. Women now have the highest rate of newly diagnosed HIV infection. Many of these women have contracted the HIV virus from unprotected sex with male partners. HIV cannot be transmitted by hugging, inhaling cocaine, or sharing food utensils. (A, 2)

53. 3. Zidovudine (AZT) interferes with replication of HIV and thereby slows progression of HIV infection to acquired immunodeficiency syndrome (AIDS). There is no known cure for HIV infection. Today, clients are not treated with monotherapy but are usually on triple therapy due to a much-improved clinical response. Decreased viral loads with the drug combinations have improved the longevity and quality of life in clients with HIV/AIDS. AZT does not destroy the virus, enhance the body's antibody production, or neutralize toxins produced by the virus. (I, 8)

54. 2. Women who have herpes genitalis are more likely to develop cervical cancer than women who have never had the disease. Cervical cancer is now considered a sexually transmitted disease (STD). Regular examinations, including Pap tests, are recommended to detect and treat cervical cancer at an early stage. Herpes genitalis does not cause sterility, uterine fibroid tumors, or irregular menses. (A, 10)

55. 3. Pain is a common problem in women with herpes genitalis. Analgesia may be prescribed for the pain. Clients frequently describe the pain as an intense burning. Urination can be very painful because of the burning sensation from herpes lesions in the perineal area. Sleep disturbances, nutritional deficits, and ineffective breathing patterns are not frequently associated with herpes genitalis. (D, 10)

56. 1. HSV infection is one of a group of disorders that, when diagnosed in the presence of HIV infection, are considered to be diagnostic for AIDS. Other AIDS-defining illnesses include Kaposi's sarcoma; cytomegalovirus of the liver, spleen, or lymph nodes; and *Pneumocystis carinii* pneumonia. HSV infection is not curable and does not cause severe electrolyte imbalances. Herpes genitalis can lead to cervical cancer. (A, 10)

57. 4. Education to prevent behaviors that cause HIV transmission is the primary method of controlling HIV infection. Behaviors that place people at risk for HIV infection include unprotected sexual intercourse and sharing of needles for intravenous drug injection. Educating clients about using condoms during sexual relations is a priority in controlling HIV transmission. (I, 4)

58. 4. The nurse should respond with a statement that allows the client to express his thoughts and feelings. After sharing feelings about their diagnosis, clients will need information, support, and community resources. Statements of encouragement or agreement do not provide an opportunity for the client to express himself. (I, 5)

59. 4. *Treponema pallidum*, the organism that causes syphilis, is classified as a spirochete because of its corkscrew appearance. There are more than 100 different types of STD caused by various types of organisms. Viruses and bacteria are responsible for many common STDs. Fungi and rickettsia do not cause STDs. (A, 9)

60. 3. The chancre of syphilis is characteristically a painless, moist ulcer. The serous discharge is very infectious. Because the chancre is usually painless and disappears, the client may not be aware of it or may not seek care. (A, 10)

61. 2. An important aspect of controlling the spread of STDs is obtaining a list of the sexual contacts of an infected client. These contacts, in turn, should be encouraged to obtain immediate care. Many people with STDs are reluctant to reveal their sexual contacts, which makes controlling STDs difficult. Increasing clients' knowledge of the disease and reassuring clients that their records are confidential can motivate them to seek treatment, which does help to control the spread of the disease, but it is not as critical as information about the client's sexual contacts. (P, 10)

62. 2. Because of the large dose, the upper outer quadrant of the buttocks is the recommended site. The Centers for Disease Control and Prevention (CDC) recommends Benzathine penicillin G 2.4 million units IM in a single dose for adults with primary or secondary syphilis who are not allergic to penicillin. The deltoid and the quadriceps lateralis of the thigh are not large enough for the recommended dose. In infants and small children, the midlateral aspect of the thigh may be preferred. (I, 8)

63. 1. A client with primary syphilis is at risk of transmitting the disease to sexual partners if he or she is not knowledgeable about how the disease is spread. Cutaneous lesions on the palms and soles and alopecia are signs of secondary syphilis. Chancres do not bleed sufficiently to alter tissue perfusion. Chancres often disappear even without treatment. (D, 10)

64. 1. Asking the client to describe her nervousness gives her the opportunity to express her concerns. It also allows the nurse to understand her better and gives the nurse a base to respond to the client's stated fears, questions, or need for further information. Responses that make assumptions about the source of the concern or offer reinforcement are not supportive and block successful communication. (I, 5)

65. 4. Many women do not seek treatment because they are unaware that they have gonorrhea. They may be symptom free or have only very mild symptoms until the disease progresses to pelvic inflammatory disease (PID). Dysuria and vaginal bleeding are not present in gonorrhea. Gonorrhea can lead to very serious complications. It can be cured with the proper treatment. (I, 10)

66. 1. Statistics reveal that the incidence of STDs is rising more rapidly among teenagers than among any other age group. Many reasons have been given for this trend, including a change in societal mores and increasing sexual activity among teenagers. During this developmental stage, teenagers may engage in high-risk sexual behaviors because they often are living in the present and feel that it won't happen to them. (E, 4)

67. 4. Dysuria and a mucopurulent urethral discharge characterize gonorrhea in men. Gonococcal symptoms are so painful and bothersome for men that they usually seek treatment with the onset of symptoms. Impotence, scrotal swelling, and urinary retention are not associated with gonorrhea. (I, 10)

68. 2. The most common opportunistic infection in HIV initially presents as oral candidiasis, or thrush. The client with HIV should always have an oral assessment. HSV and CMV are opportunistic infections that present later in AIDS. Aphthous stomatitis, or recurrent canker sores, is not an opportunistic infection, although the sores are thought to occur more often when the client is under stress. (A, 4)

The Client With Cancer of the Cervix

69. 2. Although other positions may be used, the preferred position for a vaginal examination is the lithotomy position. This position offers the best visualization. If the client is elderly and frail, staff members may need to support the client's flexed legs while the examiner conducts the examination and obtains the Pap smear. (I, 4)

70. 4. The Pap smear identifies atypical cervical cells that may be present for various reasons. Cancer is the most common possible cause, but not the only one. The Pap smear does not show abnormal viral cells. An adequate smear provides accurate diagnostic data; the false-positive rate is only about 5%. (I, 9)

71. 4. Young age at first pregnancy is a risk factor for cervical cancer. Other risk factors include a family history of the disease, sexual experience with multiple partners, and a history of sexually transmitted disease (eg, syphilis, human papillomavirus, gonorrhea, herpes genitalis). Cigarette smoking, promiscuous male partner, human immunodeficiency virus infection or other immunosuppression, and low socioeconomic status are other risk factors. Sexual relations with one partner, sedentary lifestyle, and obesity are not risk factors. (A, 4)

72. 1. Annual screening is recommended for any woman in the high-risk category. When detected early, cervical cancer has an excellent prognosis. Most women who die of cervical cancer have never had a Pap test or have not had one in the last 5 years. Current American Cancer Society guidelines advocate Pap smears every 3 years after a pattern of three initial negative annual tests is established and the woman is deemed to be at low risk for development of cervical cancer. Sexual activity is not related to frequency of Pap tests. (P, 9)

73. 4. In its early stages, cancer of the cervix is usually asymptomatic, which underscores the importance of regular Pap smears. A light bleeding or serosanguineous discharge may be apparent as the first noticeable symptom. Pain, leg edema, urinary and rectal symptoms, and weight loss are late signs of cervical cancer. (A, 4)

74. 4. The vagina naturally cleanses itself, and douching is not recommended unless it is prescribed by a health care provider for a medical condition. Daily douching could destroy normal flora. Perfumed douches could trigger allergenic responses. Douching should be avoided during menses. (I, 9)

75. 1. When cervical cancer is detected early and treated aggressively, the cure rate approaches 100%. The incidence of cervical cancer has increased among African Americans, Native Americans, and Latinas, and these women often have a poorer prognosis because the cancer is not identified early. Pap smears and colposcopy have the potential to decrease mortality from invasive carcinoma when these screening and treatment programs are utilized by women. (I, 10)

76. 2. The client should be informed that her next two or three periods could be heavy and prolonged. The client is instructed to report any excessive bleeding. The nurse should reinforce the necessity for the follow-up check and the review of the biopsy results with the client. The client's periods will not be normal for 2 to 3 months. (A, 4)

77. 2. Dislodged radioactive materials should not be touched with bare or gloved hands. Forceps are used to place the material in the lead-lined container, which shields the radiation. Exposure to radiation can occur only by direct exposure to the encased radioactive substance; it cannot result from contact with emesis or urine or from touching the client. Disposal of eating utensils cannot lead to radiation exposure. Radioactive dose materials are kept only in the radiation department. (I, 9)

78. 3. The three factors related to radiation safety are time, distance, and shielding. Nurses on radiation oncology units work with radiation frequently and so must limit their contact. Nurses are physically closer to clients than are visitors, who are often asked to sit 6 feet away from the client. Touching the client does not increase the amount of radiation exposure. Aseptic technique and isolation prevent the spread of infection. Age is a risk factor for people in their reproductive years. (I, 9)

79. 2. A client can experience anxiety because she is immobilized on strict bed rest and is unable to care for herself while the implant is in place. During an intracavity implant, the woman is kept flat in bed to prevent dislodgement of the radioactive substance. The implant may be left in place for 24 to 72 hours. Usually, the tumor is removed before implant insertion. Impaired Health Maintenance and Disturbed Sleep Pattern are not priorities. (D, 5)

80. 2. Genital warts can lead to dysplastic changes of the cervix, referred to as cervical intraepithelial neoplasia (CIN). The development of cervical cancer remains the largest threat of all condyloma-associated neoplasias. Infertility, pelvic inflammatory disease, and rectal cancer are not complications of genital warts. (I, 4)

81. 4. Bowel movements can be difficult with the radium applicator in place. The purpose of the low-residue diet is to decrease bowel movements. The bowel is cleansed before therapy, and the woman is maintained on a low-residue diet during treatment to prevent bowel distention and defecation. To prevent dislodgement of the applicator, the client is maintained on strict bed rest and allowed only to turn from side to side. Perineal care is omitted during radium implant therapy, although any vaginal discharge should be reported to the doctor. It is rare for the applicator to extrude, so this does not need to be checked every hour. (I, 9)

82. 4. Nausea, vomiting, and a foul vaginal discharge are common side effects of internal radiation therapy for cervical cancer. A foul-smelling discharge may develop from the destruction and sloughing of cells. Vaginal discharge may persist for some time. General symptoms of radiation syndrome include nausea, vomiting, anorexia, and malaise. Vaginal itching, confusion, and high fever are not typical side effects of radiation therapy for cervical cancer. (A, 9)

The Client With Testicular Disease

83. 2. Epididymitis causes acute tenderness and pronounced swelling of the scrotum. Gradual onset of unilateral scrotal pain, urethral discharge, and fever are other key signs. It is occasionally, but not routinely, associated with urinary tract infection. Burning and pain on urination and foul-smelling ejaculate or urine are not classic symptoms of epididymitis. (A, 10)

84. 3. Among men younger than 35 years of age, epididymitis is most frequently caused by a sexually transmitted infection. Causative organisms are usually chlamydia or *Neisseria gonorrhea*. The other major form of epididymitis is bacterial, caused by the *Escherichia coli* or *Pseudomonas*. The nurse should always include safe sex teaching for a client with epididymitis. The client should also be advised against anogenital intercourse, because this is a mode of transmission of gram-negative rods to the epididymis. (P, 4)

85. 3. After a warm bath or shower, the testes hang lower and are both relaxed and in the ideal position for manual evaluation and palpation. (I, 4)

86. 2. Normal testes feel smooth, egg-shaped, and firm to the touch, without lumps. The surface should feel smooth and rubbery. The testes should not be soft or spongy to the touch. Testicular malignancies are usually nontender, nonpainful hard lumps. Any lumps, swelling, nodules, or signs of inflammation should be reported to the physician. (A, 4)

87. 4. AFP and hCG are considered markers that indicate the presence of testicular disease. Elevated AFP and hCG and decreased testosterone are markers for testicular disease. Measurements of AFP, HCG, and testosterone are also obtained throughout the course of therapy to help measure the effectiveness of treatment. (A, 10)

88. 1. Cryptorchidism (undescended testis) carries a greatly increased risk for testicular cancer. Undescended testes occurs in about 3% of male infants, with an increased incidence in premature infants. Other possible causes of malignancy include chemical carcinogens, trauma, orchitis, and environmental factors. Testicular cancer is not associated with early sexual relations in men, even though cervical cancer is associated with early sexual relations in women. Testicular cancer is not associated with seminal vesiculitis or epididymitis. (A, 4)

89. 2. The incidence of testicular cancer is higher in men who live in rural rather than suburban areas. Testicular cancer is more common in white than in black men. Men with higher socioeconomic status seem to have a greater incidence of testicular cancer. The exact cause of testicular cancer is unknown. Cancer of the testes is the leading cause of death from cancer in the 15- to 35-year-old age group. (A, 4)

90. 3. Because of the location of the incision in the high inguinal area, pain is a major problem during the immediate postoperative period. The incisional area and discomfort caused by movement contribute to increased pain. Bladder spasms and elimination problems are more commonly associated with prostate surgery. Nausea is not a priority problem. (D, 10)

91. 2. Unilateral orchiectomy alone does not result in impotence if the other testis is normal. The other testis should produce enough testosterone to maintain normal sexual drive, functioning, and characteristics. Sperm banking before treatment is often recommended, because radiation or chemotherapy can affect fertility. (I, 8)

92. 2. When diagnosed early and treated aggressively, testicular cancer has a cure rate of about 90%. Treatment of testicular cancer is based on tumor type, and seminoma cancer has the best prognosis. Modes of treatment include combinations of orchiectomy, radiation therapy, and chemotherapy. The chemotherapeutic regimen used currently is responsible for the successful treatment of testicular cancer. (P, 10)

The Client With Cancer of the Prostate

93. 3. Manipulation of the prostate during the digital rectal examination may falsely increase the PSA levels. The PSA determination and the digital rectal examination are both necessary as screening tools for prostate cancer, and both are recommended for all men older than 50 years of age. Prostate cancer is the most common cancer in men and the second leading killer from cancer among men in the United States. Incidence increases sharply with age, and the disease is predominant in the 60- to 70-year-old age group. (A, 4)

94. 1. On digital rectal examination, key signs of prostate cancer are a hard prostate, induration of the prostate, and an irregular, hard nodule. Accompanying symptoms of prostate cancer can include constipation, weight loss, and lymphadenopathy. Abdominal pain usually does not accompany prostate cancer. A boggy, tender prostate is found with infection (eg, acute or chronic prostatitis). (A, 4)

95. 2. Loss of the prostate gland interrupts the flow of semen, so there will be no ejaculation fluid. The sensations of orgasm remain intact. The client needs to be advised that return of erectile capability is often disrupted after surgery, but within 1 year 95% of men have returned to normal erectile function with sexual intercourse. (I, 10)

96. 1. Clients who have stage IA or IIB prostate cancer have an excellent survival rate. Prostate cancer is usually slow growing, and many men who have prostate cancer do not die from it. A stage I or II tumor is confined to the prostate gland and has not spread to the extrapelvic region or bone. (I, 10)

97. 2. Diethylstilbestrol causes engorgement and tenderness of the breasts (gynecomastia). Stilbestrol is prescribed as palliative therapy for men with androgen-dependent prostatic carcinoma. An increase in blood pressure can occur. Tenderness of the scrotum and dramatic changes in secondary sexual characteristics should not occur. (I, 8)

The Client With Erectile Dysfunction

98. 2. Antihypertensive drugs, especially β-blockers such as propanolol (Inderal), can cause impotence. When a male client complains of impotence, the nurse should always examine the client's medication regimen as a potential contributing factor. Aspirin, nonsteroidal anti-inflammatory drugs, and anticoagulants do not cause erectile dysfunction. (I, 8)

99. 2. ED is multifactorial in origin, and more than 50% of the cases can be attributed to organic causes. Causes include alteration in vascular supply, hormonal changes, neurologic dysfunction, medications, and associated systemic diseases such as diabetes mellitus or alcoholism. The presence of nocturnal erections is the first evaluation to differentiate between organic and psychogenic causes. ED is a common problem among men older than 65 years of age. (I, 5)

100. 1. Avoidance of alcohol can improve the outcome of therapy. Alcohol and smoking can affect a man's ability to have and maintain an erection. The client should be encouraged to follow a healthy diet, but no specific diet is associated with improvement of sexual function. The client should cease smoking, not just decrease smoking. Increasing attempts at intercourse without treatment will not facilitate improvement. The client should be reassured that ED is a common problem and that help is available.

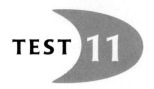

The Client With Neurologic Health Problems

▶ **The Client With a Head Injury**

▶ **The Client With Seizures**

▶ **The Client With a Cerebrovascular Accident**

▶ **The Client With Parkinson's Disease**

▶ **The Client With Multiple Sclerosis**

▶ **The Unconscious Client**

▶ **The Client in Pain**

▶ **Correct Answers and Rationale**

Select the one best answer, and indicate your choice by filling in the circle in front of the option.

The Client With a Head Injury

1. When an unconscious client with multiple injuries arrives in the emergency room, which nursing intervention receives the *highest* priority?
   - ○ 1. Establishing an airway.
   - ○ 2. Replacing blood loss.
   - ○ 3. Stopping bleeding from open wounds.
   - ○ 4. Checking for a neck fracture.

2. The nurse monitors the client who is at risk for increased intracranial pressure (ICP) for
   - ○ 1. unequal pupil size.
   - ○ 2. decreasing systolic blood pressure.
   - ○ 3. tachycardia.
   - ○ 4. decreasing body temperature.

3. What is the correct nursing intervention when a client with a head injury begins to have clear drainage from his nose?
   - ○ 1. Compress the nares.
   - ○ 2. Tilt the head back.
   - ○ 3. Give the client a white pad to collect the fluid.
   - ○ 4. Administer an antihistamine for postnasal drip.

4. Which of the following respiratory patterns indicate increasing ICP in the brain stem?
   - ○ 1. Slow, irregular respirations.
   - ○ 2. Rapid, shallow respirations.
   - ○ 3. Asymmetric chest excursion.
   - ○ 4. Nasal flaring.

5. Which of the following nursing interventions is appropriate for a client with an ICP of 20 mm Hg?
   - ○ 1. Give the client a warming blanket.
   - ○ 2. Administer low-dose barbiturates.
   - ○ 3. Encourage the client to hyperventilate.
   - ○ 4. Restrict fluids.

6. A client has signs of increased ICP. Which of the following is an early indicator of deterioration in the client's condition?
   - ○ 1. Widening pulse pressure.
   - ○ 2. Decrease in the pulse rate.
   - ○ 3. Dilated, fixed pupil.
   - ○ 4. Decrease in level of consciousness.

7. A nurse obtains a specimen of clear nasal drainage from a client with a head injury. Which of the following tests differentiates mucus from cerebrospinal fluid (CSF)?
   - ○ 1. pH.
   - ○ 2. Specific gravity.
   - ○ 3. Glucose.
   - ○ 4. Microorganisms.

8. The client has a sustained ICP of 20 mm Hg. The nurse should position the client
   - ○ 1. with the head of the bed elevated 30 to 45 degrees.
   - ○ 2. in Trendelenburg's position.
   - ○ 3. in left Simm's position.
   - ○ 4. with the head elevated on two pillows.

9. The nurse administers mannitol (Osmitrol) to the client with increased ICP and closely monitors
   - ○ 1. muscle relaxation.
   - ○ 2. intake and output.
   - ○ 3. widening of the pulse pressure.
   - ○ 4. pupil dilation.

10. A male client with a head injury regains consciousness after several days. Which of the following nursing statements is most appropriate as the client awakens?

○ 1. "I'll get your family."
○ 2. "Can you tell me your name and where you live?"
○ 3. "I'll bet you're a little confused right now."
○ 4. "You are in the hospital. You were in an accident and unconscious."

11. A client who is regaining consciousness after a craniotomy becomes restless and attempts to pull out her intravenous line. Which nursing intervention protects the client without increasing her ICP?
○ 1. Place her in a jacket restraint.
○ 2. Wrap her hands in soft "mitten" restraints.
○ 3. Tuck her arms and hands under the draw sheet.
○ 4. Apply a wrist restraint to each arm.

12. Which postoperative activity does the nurse encourage the client to avoid when there is a risk for increased ICP?
○ 1. Deep breathing.
○ 2. Turning.
○ 3. Coughing.
○ 4. Passive range-of-motion exercises.

13. Which of the following is *most* effective in assessing the client with a head injury for the development of diabetes insipidus?
○ 1. Taking vital signs every 2 hours.
○ 2. Measuring urine output hourly.
○ 3. Assessing arterial blood gas values every other day.
○ 4. Checking blood glucose.

14. After 4 weeks of hospitalization, a client who had a serious head injury with increased ICP is to be discharged to a rehabilitation facility to continue his recovery. Which of the following expected outcomes would be appropriate for the client at this stage of rehabilitation?
○ 1. The client will exhibit no further episodes of short-term memory loss.
○ 2. The client will be able to return to his construction job in 3 weeks.
○ 3. The client will actively participate in the rehabilitation process as appropriate.
○ 4. The client will be emotionally stable and display personality traits that were present before injury.

15. Which of the following describes decerebrate posturing?
○ 1. Internal rotation and adduction of arms with flexion of elbows, wrists, and fingers.
○ 2. Back hunched over, rigid flexion of all four extremities with supination of arms and plantar flexion of feet.
○ 3. Supination of arms, dorsiflexion of the feet.
○ 4. Back arched, rigid extension of all four extremities.

16. When noting cluster breathing in a client who is on a ventilator in the vent-assisted mode after a craniotomy for an intracranial bleed in the occipital lobe, the nurse should
○ 1. count the rate to be sure that ventilations are deep enough to be sufficient.
○ 2. call the physician while another nurse checks the vital signs and ascertains the patient's Glasgow Coma Scale score.
○ 3. call the physician to adjust the ventilator settings.
○ 4. check deep tendon reflexes to determine the best motor response.

17. In planning the care for a client who has had a posterior fossa (infratentorial) craniotomy, the nurse understands that, when positioning the client, which of the following is contraindicated?
○ 1. Keeping the client flat on one side or the other.
○ 2. Elevating the head of the bed to 30 degrees.
○ 3. Log rolling or turning as a unit when turning.
○ 4. Keeping the neck in a neutral position.

The Client With Seizures

18. Which of the following is contraindicated for a client with seizure precautions?
○ 1. Encouraging him to perform his own personal hygiene.
○ 2. Allowing him to wear his own clothing.
○ 3. Assessing oral temperature with a glass thermometer.
○ 4. Encouraging him to be out of bed.

19. Which of the following will the nurse observe in the client in the ictal phase of a generalized grand mal (tonic-clonic) seizure?
○ 1. Jerking in one extremity that spreads gradually to adjacent areas.
○ 2. Vacant staring and an abrupt cessation of all activity.
○ 3. Facial grimaces, patting motions, and lip smacking.
○ 4. Loss of consciousness, body stiffening, and violent muscle contractions.

20. Which statement best prepares the client for a computed tomographic (CT) scan of the head without contrast to be completed the next morning?
○ 1. "You must shampoo your hair tonight to remove all oil and dirt."
○ 2. "You may drink fluids until midnight; but after that drink nothing until the scan is completed."
○ 3. "You will have some hair shaved to attach the small electrode to your scalp."
○ 4. "You will need to hold your head very still during the examination."

21. An electroencephalogram (EEG) is ordered for the client. What nursing intervention does the nurse take when the client is served a breakfast consisting of a soft-boiled egg, toast with butter and marmalade, orange juice, and coffee on the morning of the EEG?
    - ○ 1. Remove all the food.
    - ○ 2. Remove the coffee.
    - ○ 3. Remove the toast, butter, and marmalade only.
    - ○ 4. Substitute vegetable juice for the orange juice.

22. The client asks the nurse, "What caused me to have a seizure? I've never had one before." The primary cause of tonic-clonic seizures in adults older than 20 years is
    - ○ 1. head trauma.
    - ○ 2. electrolyte imbalance.
    - ○ 3. a congenital defect.
    - ○ 4. epilepsy.

23. What does the nurse include in the teaching plan for a client with seizures who is going home with a prescription for gabapentin (Neurontin)?
    - ○ 1. Take all the medication until it is gone.
    - ○ 2. Notify the physician if vision changes occur.
    - ○ 3. Store gabapentin in the refrigerator.
    - ○ 4. Take gabapentin with an antacid to protect against ulcers.

24. What is the *priority* nursing intervention in the postictal phase of a seizure?
    - ○ 1. Reorient the client to time, person, and place.
    - ○ 2. Determine the client's level of sleepiness.
    - ○ 3. Assess the client's breathing pattern.
    - ○ 4. Position the client comfortably.

25. Which intervention is most effective in minimizing the risk of seizure activity in a client who is undergoing diagnostic studies after having experienced several episodes of seizures?
    - ○ 1. Maintain the client on bed rest.
    - ○ 2. Administer butabarbital sodium (phenobarbital) 30 mg orally, three times per day.
    - ○ 3. Close the door to the room to minimize stimulation.
    - ○ 4. Administer carbamazepine (Tegretol) 200 mg orally, twice per day.

26. What nursing assessments should be documented at the beginning of the ictal phase of a seizure?
    - ○ 1. Heart rate, respirations, pulse oximeter, and blood pressure.
    - ○ 2. Last dose of anticonvulsant and circumstances at the time.
    - ○ 3. Type of visual, auditory, and olfactory aura the client experienced.
    - ○ 4. Movement of the head, eyes, and muscle rigidity.

27. Which clinical manifestation does the nurse expect in the client in the postictal phase of grand mal seizure?
    - ○ 1. Drowsiness.
    - ○ 2. Inability to move.
    - ○ 3. Paresthesia.
    - ○ 4. Hypotension.

28. A client with seizures asks the nurse how phenytoin sodium (Dilantin) will help. Based on knowledge of the drug's action, what is the nurse's best response? The drug is thought to act by
    - ○ 1. correcting the abnormal synthesis of norepinephrine in the body.
    - ○ 2. depressing transmission of abnormal impulses in the spinal cord.
    - ○ 3. reducing the responsiveness of neurons in the brain to abnormal impulses.
    - ○ 4. interrupting the flow of abnormal impulses from peripheral neurons in the viscera to the brain.

29. The nurse is preparing to teach a client about phenytoin sodium (Dilantin) therapy. It is most important for the nurse to include the fact that Dilantin should not be stopped suddenly because
    - ○ 1. physical dependency on the drug develops over time.
    - ○ 2. status epilepticus may develop.
    - ○ 3. a hypoglycemic reaction develops.
    - ○ 4. heart block is likely to develop.

30. A client states that she is afraid she will not be able to drive again because of her seizures. The nurse's best response should indicate that driving will depend on local laws, but that most laws require
    - ○ 1. that a person with a history of seizures drive only during daytime hours.
    - ○ 2. evidence that the seizures are under medical control.
    - ○ 3. evidence that seizures occur no more often than every 12 months.
    - ○ 4. that a person with a history of seizures carry a medical identification card when driving.

31. A client tells the nurse that he is unclear about what an aura is. The nurse's response should indicate that an aura is
    - ○ 1. a postictal state of amnesia.
    - ○ 2. an hallucination that occurs during a seizure.
    - ○ 3. a symptom that occurs just before a seizure.
    - ○ 4. a feeling of relaxation as the seizure begins to subside.

32. Which of the following statements by a client with a seizure disorder who is taking topiramate (Topamax) indicates the client has understood the nurses' instruction?
    - ○ 1. "I will take the medicine before going to bed."
    - ○ 2. "I will drink 6 to 8 glasses of water a day."
    - ○ 3. "I will eat plenty of fresh fruits."
    - ○ 4. "I will take the medicine with a meal or snack."

33. Which clinical manifestation in a client does the

nurse assess as a typical reaction to long-term phenytoin sodium (Dilantin) therapy?
- ○ 1. Weight gain.
- ○ 2. Insomnia.
- ○ 3. Excessive growth of gum tissue.
- ○ 4. Deteriorating eyesight.

The Client With a Cerebrovascular Accident

34. Regular oral hygiene is an essential intervention for the client who has had a cerebrovascular accident (CVA). Which of the following nursing measures is inappropriate when providing oral hygiene?
- ○ 1. Placing the client on the back with a small pillow under the head.
- ○ 2. Keeping portable suctioning equipment at the bedside.
- ○ 3. Opening the client's mouth with a padded tongue blade.
- ○ 4. Cleansing the client's mouth and teeth with a toothbrush.

35. When a client arrives in the emergency department with an ischemic CVA, what is the priority for the nurse to assess in relation to the treatment of tissue plasminogen activator (t-PA) administration?
- ○ 1. Current medications.
- ○ 2. Complete physical and history.
- ○ 3. Time of onset of current CVA.
- ○ 4. Upcoming surgical procedures.

36. During the first 24 hours after thrombolytic treatment for an ischemic CVA, the primary goal is to control the client's
- ○ 1. pulse.
- ○ 2. respirations.
- ○ 3. blood pressure.
- ○ 4. temperature.

37. What is a priority nursing assessment in the first 24 hours after admission for the client with a thrombotic CVA?
- ○ 1. Cholesterol level.
- ○ 2. Pupil size and pupillary response.
- ○ 3. Bowel sounds.
- ○ 4. Echocardiogram.

38. What is a priority nursing intervention when suctioning an unconscious client to maintain cerebral perfusion?
- ○ 1. Hyperoxygenate before and after suctioning.
- ○ 2. Administer analgesics.
- ○ 3. Provide oral hygiene.
- ○ 4. Administer diuretics.

39. The nursing assessment of a client's functional status before and after a CVA is essential. Why is it so important?
- ○ 1. The rehabilitation plan will be guided by it.
- ○ 2. Functional status before the CVA will help predict outcomes.
- ○ 3. It will help the client recognize his physical limitations.
- ○ 4. The client can be expected to regain much of his functioning.

40. Which of the following techniques does the nurse avoid when changing a client's position in bed if the client has hemiparalysis?
- ○ 1. Rolling the client onto her side.
- ○ 2. Sliding the client to move her up in bed.
- ○ 3. Lifting the client when moving her up in bed.
- ○ 4. Having the client help lift herself off the bed using a trapeze.

41. Which nursing intervention has been found to be the *most* effective means of preventing plantar flexion in a client who has had a CVA with residual paralysis?
- ○ 1. Place the client's feet against a firm footboard.
- ○ 2. Reposition the client every 2 hours.
- ○ 3. Have the client wear ankle-high tennis shoes at intervals throughout the day.
- ○ 4. Massage the client's feet and ankles regularly.

42. The nurse is planning the care of a hemiplegic client to prevent joint deformities of the arm. What position is *not* appropriate?
- ○ 1. Placing a pillow in the axilla so that the arm is away from the body.
- ○ 2. Placing a pillow under the slightly flexed arm so that the hand is higher than the elbow.
- ○ 3. Positioning the hands in a slightly pronated position.
- ○ 4. Positioning a roll in the hand so that the fingers are barely flexed.

43. For the client who is experiencing expressive aphasia, which nursing intervention is *most* helpful in promoting communication?
- ○ 1. Speaking loudly.
- ○ 2. Using a picture board.
- ○ 3. Writing directions so client can read them.
- ○ 4. Speaking in short sentences.

44. The nurse is teaching the family of a client with dysphagia about decreasing the risk of aspiration while eating. Which of the following strategies is inappropriate?
- ○ 1. Maintaining an upright position.
- ○ 2. Restricting the diet to liquids until swallowing improves.
- ○ 3. Introducing foods on the unaffected side of the mouth.
- ○ 4. Keeping distractions to a minimum.

45. Which food-related behaviors would the nurse observe in a client who has had a CVA that has left him with homonymous hemianopia?
- ○ 1. Increased preference for foods high in salt.

○ 2. Eating food on only half of the plate.

○ 3. Forgetting the names of foods.

○ 4. Inability to swallow liquids.

46. The nurse is teaching the client about ways to adapt to a visual disability. Which does the nurse identify as the primary safety precaution to use?
○ 1. Wear a patch over one eye.
○ 2. Place personal items on the sighted side.
○ 3. Lie in bed with the unaffected side toward the door.
○ 4. Turn the head from side to side when walking.

47. A client is experiencing mood swings after a CVA and often has episodes of tearfulness that are distressing to the family. Which is the best technique for the nurse to instruct family members to try when the client experiences a crying episode?
○ 1. Sit quietly with the client until the episode is over.
○ 2. Ignore the behavior.
○ 3. Attempt to divert the client's attention.
○ 4. Tell the client that this behavior is unacceptable.

48. The client who has had a CVA with residual physical handicaps becomes discouraged by his physical appearance. What attitude is best for the nurse to display to help the client overcome his negative self-concept?
○ 1. Helpfulness and sympathy.
○ 2. Concern and charity.
○ 3. Directives and firmness.
○ 4. Encouragement and patience.

49. When communicating with a client who has aphasia, which of the following nursing interventions is inappropriate?
○ 1. Present one thought at a time.
○ 2. Encourage the client not to write messages.
○ 3. Speak with normal volume.
○ 4. Make use of gestures.

50. Based on the nurse's knowledge of thrombolytic therapy, what is the expected outcome of this drug therapy?
○ 1. Increased vascular permeability.
○ 2. Vasoconstriction.
○ 3. Dissolved emboli.
○ 4. Prevention of hemorrhage.

The Client With Parkinson's Disease

51. Which of the following is an initial sign of Parkinson's disease?
1. Rigidity.
2. Tremor.
3. Bradykinesia.
4. Akinesia.

52. The nurse develops a teaching plan for a client newly diagnosed with Parkinson's disease. Which of the following topics that the nurse plans to discuss is the *most* important?
○ 1. Maintaining a balanced nutritional diet.
○ 2. Enhancing the immune system.
○ 3. Maintaining a safe environment.
○ 4. Engaging in diversional activity.

53. The nurse observes that a client's upper arm tremors disappear as he unbuttons his shirt. Which statement best guides the nurse's analysis of these observations about the client's tremors?
○ 1. The tremors are probably psychological and can be controlled at will.
○ 2. The tremors sometimes disappear with purposeful and voluntary movements.
○ 3. The tremors disappear when the client's attention is diverted by some activity.
○ 4. There is no explanation for the observation; it is probably a chance occurrence.

54. When does the nurse encourage a client with Parkinson's disease to schedule the most demanding physical activities to minimize the effects of hypokinesia?
○ 1. Early in the morning, when the client's energy level is high.
○ 2. To coincide with the peak action of drug therapy.
○ 3. Immediately after a rest period.
○ 4. When family members will be available.

55. Which goal is the most realistic and appropriate for a client diagnosed with Parkinson's disease?
○ 1. To cure the disease.
○ 2. To stop progression of the disease.
○ 3. To begin preparations for terminal care.
○ 4. To maintain optimal body function.

56. What is the primary goal collaboratively established by the nurse, the physical therapist, and the client with Parkinson's disease?
○ 1. To maintain joint flexibility.
○ 2. To build muscle strength.
○ 3. To improve muscle endurance.
○ 4. To reduce ataxia.

57. A client with Parkinson's disease is prescribed levodopa (L-dopa) therapy. The nurse determines that the drug is effective when the client experiences an improvement in which of the following?
○ 1. Mood.
○ 2. Muscle rigidity.
○ 3. Appetite.
○ 4. Alertness.

58. A client is being switched from levodopa to carbidopa-levodopa (Sinemet). The nurse should monitor for which of the following possible complications that can occur during the period of medication change and dosage adjustment?

○ 1. Euphoria.
○ 2. Jaundice.
○ 3. Vital sign fluctuation.
○ 4. Symptoms of diabetes.

59. When administering a new medication regimen to a client with Parkinson's disease, the nurse makes certain that the medication is taken
○ 1. at bedtime.
○ 2. all at one time.
○ 3. 2 hours before mealtime.
○ 4. at the time scheduled.

60. A client with Parkinson's disease needs a long time to complete her morning hygiene, but she becomes annoyed when the nurse offers assistance and refuses all help. Which statement is the nurse's best initial response in this situation?
○ 1. Tell the client firmly that she needs assistance and help her with her care.
○ 2. Praise the client for her desire to be independent and give her extra time and encouragement.
○ 3. Tell the client that she is being unrealistic about her abilities and must accept the fact that she needs help.
○ 4. Suggest to the client that if she insists on self-care, she should at least modify her routine.

61. A client with Parkinson's disease asks the nurse to explain to his nephew "what the doctor said the pallidotomy would do." What is the nurse's best response? The main goal for the client after pallidotomy is improved
○ 1. functional ability.
○ 2. emotional stress.
○ 3. alertness.
○ 4. appetite.

The Client With Multiple Sclerosis

62. Which of the following is not a typical clinical manifestation of multiple sclerosis (MS)?
○ 1. Double vision.
○ 2. Sudden bursts of energy.
○ 3. Weakness in the extremities.
○ 4. Muscle tremors.

63. The nurse determines that baclofen (Lioresal) is accomplishing its intended purpose for a client with MS when it achieves which of the following?
○ 1. Induces sleep.
○ 2. Stimulates the client's appetite.
○ 3. Relieves muscular spasticity.
○ 4. Reduces the urine bacterial count.

64. A client has had MS for 15 years and has received various drug therapies. What is the primary reason why the nurse has found it difficult to evaluate the effectiveness of the drugs that the client has used? Clients with MS

○ 1. exhibit intolerance to many drugs.
○ 2. experience spontaneous remissions from time to time.
○ 3. require multiple drugs simultaneously.
○ 4. endure long periods of exacerbation before the illness responds to a particular drug.

65. When the nurse talks with a client with MS who has slurred speech, which nursing intervention is contraindicated?
○ 1. Encouraging the client to speak slowly.
○ 2. Encouraging the client to speak distinctly.
○ 3. Asking the client to repeat indistinguishable words.
○ 4. Asking the client to speak louder when tired.

66. The right hand of a client with MS trembles severely whenever she attempts a voluntary action. She spills her coffee twice at lunch and cannot get her dress fastened securely. Which is the best legal documentation in nursing notes of the chart for this client assessment?
○ 1. "Has an intention tremor of the right hand."
○ 2. "Right-hand tremor worsens with purposeful acts."
○ 3. "Needs assistance with dressing and eating due to severe trembling and clumsiness."
○ 4. "Slight shaking of right hand increases to severe tremor when client tries to button her clothes or drink from a cup."

67. A client with MS is experiencing bowel incontinence and is starting a bowel retraining program. Which strategy is inappropriate?
○ 1. Eating a diet high in fiber.
○ 2. Setting a regular time for elimination.
○ 3. Using an elevated toilet seat.
○ 4. Limiting fluid intake to 1000 mL/day.

68. Which of the following is an inappropriate goal to establish with a client who has MS?
○ 1. The client will develop joint mobility.
○ 2. The client will develop muscle strength.
○ 3. The client will develop cognition.
○ 4. The client will develop mood elevation.

69. The nurse is preparing a client with MS for discharge from the hospital to home. Which of the following instructions is appropriate?
○ 1. "You will need to accept the necessity for a quiet and inactive lifestyle."
○ 2. "Keep active, use stress reduction strategies, and avoid fatigue."
○ 3. "Follow good health habits to change the course of the disease."
○ 4. "Practice using the mechanical aids that you will need when future disabilities arise."

70. Which of the following is inappropriate for the nurse to include in the discharge plan for a client with MS who has an impaired peripheral sensation?

○ 1. Carefully test the temperature of bath water.
○ 2. Avoid kitchen activities because of the risk of injury.
○ 3. Avoid hot water bottles and heating pads.
○ 4. Inspect the skin daily for injury or pressure points.

71. Which intervention should the nurse suggest to help a client with MS avoid episodes of urinary incontinence?
○ 1. Limit fluid intake to 1000 mL/day.
○ 2. Insert an indwelling urinary catheter.
○ 3. Establish a regular voiding schedule.
○ 4. Administer prophylactic antibiotics, as ordered.

72. A client with MS lives with her daughter and 3-year-old granddaughter. The daughter asks the nurse what she can do at home to help her mother. The nurse explains that the client would benefit most by which of the following measures?
○ 1. Psychotherapy.
○ 2. Regular exercise.
○ 3. Day care for the granddaughter.
○ 4. Weekly visits by another person with MS.

The Unconscious Client

73. A client is brought to the emergency department unconscious. An empty bottle of aspirin was found in his car, and a drug overdose is suspected. In anticipation of further emergency treatment for the client, which of the following medications should the nurse have available?
○ 1. Vitamin K.
○ 2. Dextrose 50%.
○ 3. Activated charcoal powder.
○ 4. Sodium thiosulfate.

74. The wife and sister of a client who had attempted suicide with an overdose are distraught about his comatose condition and the possibility that he took an intentional drug overdose. Which of the following would be an appropriate initial nursing intervention with this family?
○ 1. Explain that because the client was found on hospital property, he was probably asking for help and did not intentionally overdose.
○ 2. Give the wife and sister a big hug and assure them that the client is in good hands.
○ 3. Encourage the wife and sister to express their feelings and concerns, and listen carefully.
○ 4. Allow the wife and sister to help care for the client by rubbing his back when he is turned.

75. Which of the following is a *priority* goal during the first 24 hours of hospitalization for a comatose client with suspected drug overdose?

○ 1. Educate regarding drug abuse.
○ 2. Minimize pain.
○ 3. Maintain intact skin.
○ 4. Increase caloric intake.

76. It is essential for the nurse to complete which of the following interventions on an unconscious intubated client, if not contraindicated because of increased intracranial pressure?
○ 1. Monitor the oral temperature, keep the room temperature at 70°F (21.1°C), and place the client on a cooling blanket if the client's temperature is higher than 101°F (38.3°C).
○ 2. Clean the mouth carefully, apply a thin coat of petroleum jelly, and move the endotracheal tube to the opposite side daily.
○ 3. Position the client in the supine position with the head to the side and slightly elevated on two pillows.
○ 4. Turn the client with a draw sheet and place a pillow behind the back and one between the legs.

77. An unconscious client has been positioned on one side. The nurse anticipates that which of the following anatomic areas is a pressure point in this position?
○ 1. Sacrum.
○ 2. Occiput.
○ 3. Ankles.
○ 4. Heels.

78. The client is placed in a right side-lying position. Which of the following positions is incorrect?
○ 1. The head is placed on a small pillow.
○ 2. The right leg is extended without pillow support.
○ 3. The left arm is rested on the mattress with the elbow flexed.
○ 4. The left leg is supported on a pillow with the knee flexed.

79. What is the intended outcome for the nursing intervention of performing passive range-of-motion exercises on an unconscious client?
○ 1. Preservation of muscle mass.
○ 2. Prevention of bone demineralization.
○ 3. Increase in muscle tone.
○ 4. Maintenance of joint mobility.

80. When the nurse performs oral hygiene for an unconscious client, which nursing intervention is the *priority*?
○ 1. Keep a suction machine available.
○ 2. Place the client in a prone position.
○ 3. Wear sterile gloves while brushing the client's teeth.
○ 4. Use gauze wrapped around the fingers to cleanse the client's gums.

81. The nurse observes that the client's right eye does

not close totally. Based on this finding, which nursing intervention is *most* appropriate?
- ○ 1. Make sure the client wears eyeglasses at all times.
- ○ 2. Place an eye patch over the completely closed right eye.
- ○ 3. Instill artificial tears once every shift.
- ○ 4. Cleanse the eyelid with a clean washcloth every shift.

82. Which symptom is an early indicator of hypoxia in the unconscious client?
- ○ 1. Cyanosis.
- ○ 2. Decreased respirations.
- ○ 3. Restlessness.
- ○ 4. Hypotension.

83. When administering intermittent enteral feeding to an unconscious client, the nurse should
- ○ 1. heat the formula in a microwave.
- ○ 2. place the client in a semi-Fowler's position.
- ○ 3. obtain a sterile gavage bag and tubing.
- ○ 4. weigh the client before administering the feeding.

84. The client is to receive 200 mL of tube feeding every 4 hours. When the nurse checks for the client's gastric residual before administering the next scheduled feeding and obtains 40 mL of gastric residual, what is the appropriate intervention?
- ○ 1. Withhold the tube feeding and notify the physician.
- ○ 2. Dispose of the residual and continue with the feeding.
- ○ 3. Delay feeding the client for 1 hour and then recheck the residual.
- ○ 4. Readminister the residual to the client and continue with the feeding.

85. Of the following nursing interventions for catheter care, which should have the *highest* priority?
- ○ 1. Cleansing the area around the urethral meatus.
- ○ 2. Clamping the catheter periodically to maintain muscle tone.
- ○ 3. Irrigating the catheter with several ounces of normal saline solution.
- ○ 4. Changing the location where the catheter is taped to the client's leg.

The Client in Pain

86. A 34-year-old Chinese man is admitted with multiple injuries from a motor vehicle accident. He complains of severe pain and requests frequent medication. The assistive nursing personnel express surprise, saying, "I thought Asian people were very stoic about pain." Which is the nurse's best response about pain?
- ○ 1. Expression and perception of pain vary widely from person to person.
- ○ 2. Tolerance of pain is about the same in all people.
- ○ 3. Tolerance of pain is determined by a person's genetic makeup.
- ○ 4. Pain perception is about the same in all people.

87. The nurse finds it difficult to relieve a client's pain satisfactorily. Which of the following measures should the nurse take into consideration when continuing efforts to promote comfort?
- ○ 1. Improve the nurse–client relationship.
- ○ 2. Enlist the help of the client's family.
- ○ 3. Allow the client additional time to work through his or her own responses to pain.
- ○ 4. Arrange to have the client share a room with a client who has little pain.

88. A client from China tells the nurse, "If I could be among my people, I could receive acupuncture for this pain." The nurse should understand that acupuncture in the Asian culture is based on the theory that it
- ○ 1. eliminates evil spirits.
- ○ 2. promotes tranquility with a higher being.
- ○ 3. restores the balance of energy.
- ○ 4. blocks nerve pathways to the brain.

89. The client's physician decides to change the analgesia medication from meperidine hydrochloride (Demerol) 75 mg intramuscularly every 4 hours as needed to meperidine hydrochloride by the oral route. What dosage of oral meperidine hydrochloride is required to provide an equivalent analgesic dose?
- ○ 1. 25 to 50 mg.
- ○ 2. 75 to 100 mg.
- ○ 3. 125 to 150 mg.
- ○ 4. 250 to 300 mg.

90. When the nurse administers meperidine hydrochloride, its effectiveness as an analgesic is related to its ability to
- ○ 1. reduce the perception of pain.
- ○ 2. decrease the sensitivity of pain receptors.
- ○ 3. interfere with pain impulses traveling along sensory nerve fibers.
- ○ 4. block the conduction of pain impulses along the central nervous system.

91. The nurse bases interventions to reduce pain on the gate-control theory of pain. This theory holds that a regulatory process controls impulses reaching the brain. This regulatory process is believed to be located in the
- ○ 1. brain stem.
- ○ 2. cerebellum.
- ○ 3. spinal cord.
- ○ 4. hypothalamus.

92. A client is arousing from a coma and keeps saying, "Just stop the pain." The nurse understands that the human body typically and automatically responds to pain first with attempts to
    ○ 1. tolerate the pain.
    ○ 2. decrease the perception of pain.
    ○ 3. escape the source of pain.
    ○ 4. divert attention from the source of pain.

93. Ergotamine tartrate (Gynergen) is prescribed for a client's migraine headaches. The nurse would judge correctly that the drug is effective when the client reports that
    ○ 1. the migraine is aborted.
    ○ 2. the severity of the migraine is reduced.
    ○ 3. the sleeplessness experienced in the past after a migraine is relieved.
    ○ 4. the visual problems experienced in the past after a migraine are relieved.

94. The client asks the nurse why she has migraine headaches. What is the nurse's best response?
    ○ 1. Migraine headaches are believed to be caused by dilation of the cranial arteries.
    ○ 2. Migraine headaches are believed to be caused by a temporary decrease in intracranial pressure.
    ○ 3. Migraine headaches are believed to be caused by irritation and inflammation of the openings of the sinuses.
    ○ 4. Migraine headaches are believed to be caused by sustained contraction of muscles around the scalp and face.

95. The nurse explains to the client with pain that the purpose of biofeedback is to enable him to exert control over his physiologic processes by
    ○ 1. regulating the body processes through electrical control.
    ○ 2. shocking himself when an undesirable response is elicited.
    ○ 3. monitoring the body processes for the therapist to interpret.
    ○ 4. translating the signals of his body processes into observable forms.

96. The nurse explains to the client that the main reason a back rub is used as therapy to relieve pain is because the massage
    ○ 1. blocks pain impulses from the spinal cord to the brain.
    ○ 2. blocks pain impulses from the brain to the spinal cord.
    ○ 3. stimulates the release of endorphins.
    ○ 4. distracts the client's focus on the source of the pain.

97. Nursing responsibilities for the client with a patient-controlled analgesia (PCA) system would include
    ○ 1. reassuring the client that pain will be relieved.
    ○ 2. documenting the client's response to pain medication on a routine basis.
    ○ 3. instructing the client to continue pressing the system's button whenever pain occurs.
    ○ 4. titrating of the client's pain medication until the client is free of pain.

98. When locating the ventrogluteal site before giving an intramuscular injection, the nurse should place the palm on the client's
    ○ 1. iliac crest.
    ○ 2. greater trochanter.
    ○ 3. anterior superior iliac spine.
    ○ 4. posterior superior iliac spine.

99. The nurse using healing touch affects a client's pain primarily through
    ○ 1. energy fields.
    ○ 2. touch therapy.
    ○ 3. massage.
    ○ 4. hypnosis.

100. A client asks why the nurse does not give a 1.5-mL intramuscular injection into the upper arm. The nurse should explain that the deltoid muscle is not used because the muscle
    ○ 1. is small.
    ○ 2. is difficult to locate.
    ○ 3. has many pain receptors.
    ○ 4. has a poor blood supply.

Correct Answers and Rationale

The letters in parentheses following the rationale identify the step of the nursing process (A, D, P, I, E) and client needs (1, 2, 3, 4, 5, 6, 7, 8, 9, 10). See the inside front cover for the key.

The Client With a Head Injury

1. 1. The highest priority for a client with multiple injuries is to establish an open airway for effective ventilation and oxygenation. Unless the client has a patent airway, other care measures will be futile. Replacing blood loss, stopping bleeding from open wounds, and checking for a neck fracture are important nursing interventions to be completed after the airway and ventilation are established. (D, 4)

2. 1. Increasing ICP causes unequal pupils as a result of pressure on the third cranial nerve. Increasing ICP causes an increase in the systolic pressure, which reflects the additional pressure needed to perfuse the brain. It increases the pressure on the vagus nerve, which produces bradycardia, and it causes an increase in body temperature from hypothalamic damage. (A, 9)

3. 3. The clear drainage must be analyzed to determine whether it is nasal drainage or cerebrospinal fluid (CSF). The nurse would not place tissues at the bedside because it is important to know how much leakage of CSF is occurring. Compressing the nares will obstruct the drainage flow. It is inappropriate to tilt the head back, which would allow the fluid to drain down the throat and not be collected for a sample. It is inappropriate to administer an antihistamine because the drainage may not be from postnasal drip. (I, 4)

4. 1. Neural control of respiration takes place in the brain stem. Deterioration and pressure produce irregular respiratory patterns. Rapid, shallow respirations, asymmetric chest movements, and nasal flaring are more characteristic of respiratory distress or hypoxia. (A, 10)

5. 3. Normal ICP is 15 mm Hg or less for 15 to 30 seconds or longer. Hyperventilation causes vasoconstriction, which reduces CSF and blood volume, two important factors for reducing a sustained ICP of 20 mm Hg. A cooling blanket is used to control the elevation of temperature because a fever increases the metabolic rate, which in turn increases ICP. High doses of barbiturates may be used to reduce the increased cellular metabolic demands. Fluid volume and inotropic drugs are used to maintain cerebral perfusion by supporting the cardiac output and keeping the cerebral perfusion pressure greater than 80 mm Hg. (I, 10)

6. 4. A decrease in the client's level of consciousness is an early indicator of deterioration of the client's neurologic status. Changes in level of consciousness, such as restlessness and irritability, may be subtle. Widening of the pulse pressure, decrease in the pulse rate, and dilated, fixed pupils occur later if the increased ICP is not treated. (A, 10)

7. 3. The constituents of CSF are similar to those of blood plasma. An examination for glucose content is done to determine whether body fluid is mucus or CSF. CSF contains glucose; mucus does not. (I, 9)

8. 1. The client's ICP is elevated, and the client should be positioned to avoid extreme neck flexion or extension. The head of the bed is usually elevated 30 to 45 degrees to drain the venous sinuses and thus decrease the ICP. Trendelenburg's position places the client's head lower than the body, which would increase ICP. The Simm's position (side lying) and elevating the head on two pillows may extend or flex the neck, which increases ICP. (I, 9)

9. 2. After administering mannitol (Osmitrol), the nurse closely monitors intake and output, because mannitol promotes diuresis and is given primarily to pull water from the extracellular fluid of the edematous brain. Mannitol can cause hypokalemia and may lead to muscle contractions, not muscle relaxation. Signs such as widening of the pulse pressure and pupil dilation should not occur, because the mannitol serves to decrease ICP. (A, 8)

10. 4. It is important to first explain where a client is to orient him to time, person, and place. Offering to get his family and asking him questions to determine whether he is oriented are important, but the first comments should let the client know where he is and what happened to him. It is useful to be empathetic to the client, but making a comment such as "I'll bet you're a little confused" when he first awakens is not helpful and may cause him anxiety. (I, 5)

11. 2. It is best for the client to wear mitts, because restraining her movements will cause agitation and lead to an increase of the ICP. (I, 10)

12. 3. Coughing is contraindicated for a client at risk for increased ICP because coughing increases ICP. Deep breathing can be continued. Turning and passive range-of-motion exercises can be continued with care not to extend or flex the neck. (I, 4)

13. 2. Diabetes insipidus results from deficiency of antidiuretic hormone (ADH). The condition may occur in

conjunction with head injuries as well as with other disorders. In ADH deficiency, the client is extremely thirsty and excretes large amounts of highly diluted urine. Measuring the urine output to detect excess amount and checking the specific gravity of urine samples to determine urine concentration are appropriate measures to determine the onset of diabetes insipidus. The patient may be tachycardic and hypotensive from fluid deficit; however, altered vital signs in a patient with a head injury may occur for other reasons as well. Blood gas analysis and blood glucose levels will not reveal diabetes insipidus. (A, 10)

14. 3. Recovery from a serious head injury is a long-term process that may continue for months or years. Depending on the extent of the injury, clients who are transferred to rehabilitation facilities most likely will continue to exhibit cognitive and mobility impairments as well as behavior and personality changes. The client would be expected to participate in the rehabilitation efforts to the extent he is capable. Family members and significant others will need long-term support to help them cope with the changes that have occurred in the client. (P, 7)

15. 4. Decerebrate posturing occurs in patients with damage to the upper brain stem, midbrain, or pons and is demonstrated clinically by arching of the back, rigid extension of the extremities, pronation of the arms, and plantar flexion of the feet. Internal rotation and adduction of arms with flexion of elbows, wrists, and fingers describes decorticate posturing, which indicates damage to corticospinal tracts and cerebral hemispheres. (A, 10)

16. 2. Cluster breathing consists of clusters of irregular breaths followed by periods of apnea on an irregular basis. A lesion in the upper medulla or lower pons is usually the cause of cluster breathing. Because the client had a bleed in the occipital lobe, which is just superior and posterior to the pons and medulla, clinical manifestations that indicate a new lesion are monitored very closely in case another bleed ensues. The physician is notified immediately so that treatment can begin before respirations cease. Another nurse needs to assess vital signs and score the client according to the Glasgow Coma Scale, but time is also of the essence. Checking deep tendon reflexes is one part of the Glasgow Coma Scale analysis. (A, 10)

17. 2. Elevating the head of the bed to 30 degrees is contraindicated for infratentorial craniotomies because it could cause herniation of the brain down onto the brain stem and spinal cord, resulting in sudden death. Elevation of the head of the bed to 30 degrees with the head turned to the side opposite the incision, if not contraindicated by the ICP, is used for *supratentorial* craniotomies. (P, 9)

The Client With Seizures

18. 3. Temperatures are not assessed orally with a glass thermometer because the thermometer could break and cause injury if a seizure occurred. The client can perform personal hygiene. There is no clinical reason to discourage the client from wearing his own clothes. As long as there are no other limitations, the client should be encouraged to be out of bed. (I, 10)

19. 4. A grand mal seizure involves both a tonic phase and a clonic phase. The tonic phase consists of loss of consciousness, dilated pupils, and muscular stiffening or contraction, which lasts about 20 to 30 seconds. The clonic phase involves repetitive movements. The grand mal seizure ends with confusion, drowsiness, and resumption of respiration. A partial seizure starts in one region of the cortex and may stay focused or spread (eg, jerking in the extremity spreading to other areas of the body). A petit mal seizure usually occurs in children and involves a vacant stare with a brief loss of consciousness that often goes unnoticed. A complex partial seizure involves facial grimacing with patting and smacking. (A, 10)

20. 4. The client will be asked to hold the head very still during the examination, which lasts about 30 to 60 minutes. In some instances, food and fluids may be withheld for 4 to 6 hours before the procedure if a contrast medium is used, because the radiopaque substance sometimes causes nausea. There is no special preparation for a CT scan, so a shampoo the night before is not required. The client may drink fluids until 4 hours before the scan is scheduled. Electrodes are not used for a CT scan, nor is the head shaved. (I, 9)

21. 2. Beverages containing caffeine, such as coffee, tea, and cola drinks, are withheld before an EEG because of the stimulating effects of the caffeine on the brain waves. A meal should not be omitted before an EEG, because low blood sugar could alter brain wave patterns. (I, 9)

22. 1. Trauma is one of the primary causes of brain damage and seizure activity in adults. Other common causes of seizure activity in adults include neoplasms, withdrawal from drugs and alcohol, and vascular disease. (I, 10)

23. 2. Gabapentin may impair vision. Changes in vision, concentration, or coordination should be reported to the physician. Gabapentin should not be stopped abruptly because of the potential for status epilepticus; this is a medication that must be tapered off. Gabapentin is to be stored at room temperature and out of direct light. It should not be taken with antacids. (P, 8)

24. 3. A priority goal for the client in the postictal phase (after a seizure) is to assess the client's breathing pattern for effective rate, rhythm, and depth. The nurse should apply oxygen and ventilation to the client as appropriate. Other interventions, to be completed after the airway has been established, include reorientation of the client to time, person, and place. Determining the client's level of sleepiness is useful, but it is not a priority. Positioning the client comfortably promotes rest but is of less importance than ascertaining that the airway is patent. (I, 9)

25. 4. Carbamazepine (Tegretol) is an anticonvulsant that helps prevent further seizures. Bed rest, sedation (phenobarbital), and providing privacy do not minimize the risk of seizures. (I, 9)

26. 4. During a seizure, the nurse should note movement of the client's head, eyes, and muscle rigidity, especially when the seizure first begins, to obtain clues about the location of the trigger focus in the brain. Other important assessments would include noting the progression and duration of the seizure, respiratory status, loss of consciousness, pupil size, and incontinence of urine and stool. It is typically not possible to assess the client's pulse and blood pressure during a tonic-clonic seizure because the muscle contractions make assessment difficult to impossible. The last dose of anticonvulsant medication can be evaluated later. The nurse should focus on maintaining an open airway, preventing injury to the client, and assessing the onset and progression of the seizure to determine the type of brain activity involved. The type of aura should assessed in the preictal phase of the seizure. (A, 10)

27. 1. The nurse would expect a client to experience drowsiness to somnolence in the postictal phase, because exhaustion results from the abnormal spontaneous neuron firing and tonic-clonic motor response. An inability to move a muscle part is not expected after a tonic-clonic or grand mal seizure, because a lack of motor function would be related to a complication such as a lesion, tumor, or cerebrovascular accident in the correlating brain tissue. A change in sensation would not be expected, because this would indicate a complication such as an injury to the peripheral nerve pathway to the corresponding part from the central nervous system. Hypotension is not typically a problem after a seizure. (A, 10)

28. 3. Exactly how phenytoin sodium helps control seizures is unclear. The most common theory is that it reduces the responsiveness of neurons in the brain to abnormal impulses—that is, it depresses neural activity. Dilantin does not influence norepinephrine or transmission of impulses in the spinal cord, nor does it interrupt the flow of abnormal impulses from peripheral neurons in the viscera to the brain. (A, 8)

29. 2. Anticonvulsant drug therapy should never be stopped suddenly; doing so can lead to the life-threat-

ening status epilepticus. Phenytoin sodium does not carry a risk of physical dependency or lead to hypoglycemia. Phenytoin sodium has antiarrhythmic properties, and discontinuation does not cause heart block. (P, 8)

30. 2. Specific motor vehicle regulations and restrictions for people who experience seizures vary locally. Most commonly, evidence that the seizures are under medical control is required before the person is given permission to drive. Time of day is not a consideration when determining driving restrictions related to seizures. The amount of time a person has been seizure free is a consideration for lifting driving restrictions; however, the time frame is usually 2 years. It is recommended, not required, that a person who is subject to seizures carry a card or wear an identification bracelet describing the illness to facilitate quick identification in the event of an emergency. (P, 1)

31. 3. An aura is a premonition of an impending seizure. Auras usually are of a sensory nature (ie, an olfactory, visual, gustatory, or auditory sensation); some may be of a psychic nature. Evaluating an aura may help identify the area of the brain from which the seizure originates. (I, 10)

32. 2. Toxic effects of topiramate are nephrolithiasis, and clients are encouraged to drink 6 to 8 glasses of water a day to dilute the urine and flush the renal tubules to avoid stone formation. Topamax is taken in divided doses because it produces drowsiness. Although eating fresh fruits is desirable from a nutritional standpoint, this is not related to the topiramate. The drug does not have to be taken with meals. (E, 8)

33. 3. A common side effect of long-term phenytoin therapy is an overgrowth of gingival tissues. Problems may be minimized with good oral hygiene, but in some cases, overgrown tissues must be removed surgically. (A, 8)

The Client With a Cerebrovascular Accident

34. 1. A helpless client should be positioned on the side, not on the back, with the head on a small pillow. A lateral position helps secretions escape from the throat and mouth, minimizing the risk of aspiration. (I, 7)

35. 3. Studies show that clients who receive recombinant t-PA treatment within 3 hours after the onset of a CVA have better outcomes. The time from the onset of stroke to t-PA treatment is a priority assessment. A complete physical and history is not possible when a client is receiving emergency care. Upcoming surgical procedures may need to be delayed because of the administration of t-PA administration, which is a priority in the immediate treatment of the current CVA. (A, 10)

36. 3. Control of blood pressure is critical during the first 24 hours after treatment because an intracerebral hemorrhage is the major side effect of thrombolytic therapy. Vital signs are monitored, and the blood pressure is maintained as identified by the physician and specific to the client's ischemic tissue needs and risk of bleeding from treatment. (P, 10)

37. 2. It is crucial to monitor the pupil size and pupillary response to indicate changes around the cranial nerves. The cholesterol level is not a priority assessment, although it may be an assessment to be addressed for long-term healthy lifestyle rehabilitation. Bowel sounds need to be assessed because an ileus or constipation can develop, but this is not a priority in the first 24 hours, when the primary concerns are cerebral hemorrhage and increased intracranial pressure. An echocardiogram is not needed for the client with a thrombotic CVA without heart problems. (A, 10)

38. 1. It is a priority to hyperoxygenate the client before and after suctioning to prevent hypoxia and to maintain cerebral perfusion. Analgesics are administered to provide pain relief. Oral hygiene provides asepsis and comfort. Diuretics assist in reducing the intracranial pressure. (D, 9)

39. 1. The primary reason for the nursing assessment of a client's functional status before and after a CVA is to guide the plan. The assessment does not help to predict how far the rehabilitation team can help the client to recover from the residual effects of the CVA, only what plans can help a client who has moved from one functional level to another. The nursing assessment of the client's functional status is not a motivating factor. (A, 7)

40. 2. Sliding a client on a sheet causes friction and is to be avoided. Friction injures skin and predisposes to pressure ulcer formation. Rolling the client is an acceptable method to use when changing positions as long as the client is maintained in anatomically neutral positions and her limbs are properly supported. The client may be lifted as long as the nurse has assistance and uses proper body mechanics to avoid injury to the himself or herself or the client. Having the client help lift herself off the bed with a trapeze is an acceptable means to move a client without causing friction burns or skin breakdown. (I, 7)

41. 3. The use of ankle-high tennis shoes has been found to be most effective in preventing plantar flexion (foot drop) because they add support to the foot and keep it in the correct anatomic position. Footboards stimulate spasms and are not routinely recommended. Regular repositioning and range-of-motion exercises are important interventions, but the client's foot needs to be left in correct anatomic position to prevent overextension of the muscle and tendon of the foot. (I, 7)

42. 3. When voluntary muscle control is lost, the flexor muscles, which are stronger, exert control over the extensor muscles. Folding the arms over the chest allows the flexor muscles to flex and exert control over the already weaker extensor muscles. It is better to extend the arms of the client to allow the extensor muscles to exert control over the flexor muscles and prevent contractures. Placing a pillow in the axilla so that the arm is away from the body keeps the arm abducted and prevents skin from touching skin, which leads to skin breakdown. Placing a pillow under the slightly flexed arm so that the hand is higher than the elbow prevents edema. Positioning a roll in the hand so that the fingers are barely flexed prevents the flexor muscles from overtaking the extensors. (P, 7)

43. 2. Expressive aphasia is a condition in which the client understands what is heard or written but cannot say what he or she wants to say. A communication or picture board helps the client communicate with others in that the client can point to objects or activities that he or she desires. (I, 5)

44. 2. A client with dysphagia (difficulty swallowing) frequently has the most difficulty ingesting thin liquids, which are easily aspirated. Liquids should be thickened to avoid aspiration. Maintaining an upright position while eating is appropriate because it minimizes the risk of aspiration. Introducing foods on the unaffected side allows the client to have better control over the food bolus. The client should concentrate on chewing and swallowing; therefore, distractions should be avoided. (I, 2)

45. 2. Homonymous hemianopia is blindness in half of the visual field; therefore, the client would see only half of his plate. Eating only the food on half of the plate results from an inability to coordinate visual images and spatial relationships. There may be an increased preference for foods high in salt after a CVA, but this would not be related to homonymous hemianopia. Forgetting the names of foods would be aphasia, which involves a cerebral cortex lesion. Being unable to swallow liquids is dysphagia, which involves motor pathways of cranial nerves IX and X, including the lower brain stem. (E, 10)

46. 4. To expand the visual field, the partially sighted client should be taught to turn the head from side to side when walking. Neglecting to do so may result in accidents. This technique helps maximize the use of remaining sight. (I, 2)

47. 3. A client who has brain damage may be emotionally labile and may cry or laugh for no explainable reason. Crying episodes are best dealt with by attempting to divert the client's attention. Ignoring the behavior will not affect the mood swing or the crying and may

increase the client's sense of isolation. Telling the client to stop is inappropriate. (I, 5)

48. 4. When offering emotional support to a client who is discouraged and has a negative self-concept because of physical handicaps, the nurse should display encouragement and patience. The client should be praised when he shows progress in his efforts to overcome handicaps. An attitude of helpfulness and sympathy allows the client to assume a role of someone not ordinary, someone who is not like others. Regardless of the handicap, the client still feels the same on the inside and has the same innate needs for his growth and developmental age group. An attitude of concern and charity tends to make the client feel like a "charity case" or like someone who is given something free because of his "condition." The client feels unequal to his peers or unable to fulfill the role relationships that were obtained before the CVA. An attitude of directives and firmness is inappropriate because it implies that the client can do better if he just tries harder and leaves no room for softness in the approach to overcoming a negative self-concept. (I, 5)

49. 2. The nurse should encourage the client to write messages or use alternative forms of communication to avoid frustration. Presenting one thought at a time decreases stimuli that may distract the client, as does speaking in a normal volume and tone. The nurse should ask the client to "show me" and should encourage the use of gestures to assist in getting the message across with minimal frustration and exhaustion for the client. (I, 5)

50. 3. Thrombolytic enzyme agents are used for clients with a thrombotic CVA to dissolve emboli, thus reestablishing cerebral perfusion. They do not increase vascular permeability, cause vasoconstriction, or prevent further hemorrhage. (E, 8)

The Client With Parkinson's Disease

51. 2. The first sign of Parkinson's disease is usually tremors. The client often is the first to notice this sign, because the tremors may be minimal at first. Rigidity is the second sign, and bradykinesia is the third sign. Akinesia is a later stage of bradykinesia. (A, 10)

52. 3. The primary focus is on maintaining a safe environment, because the client with Parkinson's disease often has a propulsive gait, characterized by a tendency to take increasingly quicker steps while walking. This type of gait often causes the client to fall or to have trouble stopping. (P, 7)

53. 2. Voluntary and purposeful movements often temporarily decrease or stop the tremors associated with Parkinson's disease. In some clients, however, tremors

may increase with voluntary effort. Tremors associated with Parkinson's disease are not psychogenic but are related to an imbalance between dopamine and acetylcholine. (E, 10)

54. 2. Demanding physical activity should be performed during the peak action of drug therapy. Clients should be encouraged to maintain independence in self-care activities to the greatest extent possible. (I, 7)

55. 4. The most appropriate and realistic goal is to help the client function at his or her best. There is no known cure for Parkinson's disease. Parkinson's disease progresses in severity, and there is no known way to stop its progression. Many clients live for years with the disease, however, and it would not be appropriate to start planning terminal care at this time. (P, 7)

56. 1. The primary goal of physical therapy and nursing interventions is to maintain joint flexibility and muscle strength. Parkinson's disease involves a degeneration of dopamine-producing neurons; therefore, it would be an unrealistic goal to attempt to build muscles or increase endurance. The decrease in dopamine neurotransmitters results in ataxia secondary to extrapyramidal motor system effects. Attempts to reduce ataxia through physical therapy would not be effective. (P, 7)

57. 2. Levodopa is prescribed to decrease severe muscle rigidity. (E, 8)

58. 3. Vital signs should be monitored, especially during periods of adjustment. Changes such as orthostatic hypotension, cardiac irregularities, palpitations, and lightheadedness should be reported immediately. The client may actually experience suicidal or paranoid ideation instead of euphoria. The nurse should monitor the client for elevated liver enzymes such as lactate dehydrogenase, aspartate aminotransferase, alanine aminotransferase, blood urea nitrogen, and alkaline phosphatase, but the client should not be jaundiced. The client should not experience symptoms of diabetes or a low serum glucose, but the nurse should check the hemoglobin and hematocrit levels. (E, 8)

59. 4. While the client is hospitalized for adjustment of medication, it is essential that the medications be administered exactly at the scheduled time, for accurate evaluation of effectiveness. For example, Sinemet is taken in divided doses over the day, not all at one time, for optimum effectiveness. (I, 8)

60. 2. Ongoing self-care is a major goal for clients with Parkinson's disease. The client should be given additional time as needed and praised for her efforts to remain independent. Firmly telling the client that she needs assistance will undermine her self-esteem and defeat her efforts to be independent. Telling the client that her perception is unrealistic does not foster hope in her ability to care for herself. Suggesting that the client modify her routine seems to put the hospital or the nurse's time schedule before the patient's needs. This will only decrease the client's self-esteem and her desire to try to continue self-care, which is obviously important to her. (I, 6)

61. 1. The goal of a pallidotomy is to improve functional ability for the client with Parkinson's disease. This is a priority. The pallidotomy creates lesions in the globus pallidus to control extrapyramidal disorders that affect control of movement and gait. If functional ability is improved by the pallidotomy, the client may experience a secondary response of an improved emotional response, but this is not the primary goal of the surgical procedure. (P, 9)

The Client With Multiple Sclerosis

62. 2. With MS, hyperexcitability and euphoria may occur, but because of muscle weakness sudden bursts of energy are unlikely. Visual disturbances, weakness in the extremities, and loss of muscle tone and tremors are common symptoms of MS. (A, 10)

63. 3. Baclofen is a centrally acting skeletal muscle relaxant that helps relieve the muscle spasms common in MS. Drowsiness is a side effect, and driving should be avoided if the medication produces a sedative effect. Baclofen does not stimulate the appetite or reduce bacteria in the urine. (E, 8)

64. 2. Evaluating drug effectiveness is difficult because a high percentage of clients with MS exhibit unpredictable episodes of remission, exacerbation, and steady progress without apparent cause. Clients with MS do not necessarily have increased intolerance to drugs, nor do they endure long periods of exacerbation before the illness responds to a particular drug. Multiple drug use is not what makes evaluation of drug effectiveness difficult. (E, 8)

65. 4. Asking a client to speak louder even when tired may aggravate the problem. (I, 6)

66. 4. The nurse's notes should be concise, objective, clearly stated, and relevant. This client trembles when she attempts voluntary actions such as drinking a beverage or fastening clothing. This activity should be described exactly as it occurs so that others reading the note will have no doubt about the nurse's observation of the client's behavior. Identifying the "intentional" activity of daily living will help the interdisciplinary team individualize the client's plan of care. Clarifying what is meant by "worsening" with a purposeful act will facilitate the inter-rater reliability of the team. It is better to state what the client did than to give vague nursing orders in the nursing notes. (I, 1)

67. 4. Limiting fluid intake is likely to aggravate rather than relieve symptoms when a bowel-training program is being implemented. Furthermore, water imbalance, as well as electrolyte imbalance, tends to aggravate symptoms of MS. A diet high in fiber helps keep bowel movements regular. Setting a regular time each day for elimination helps train the body to maintain a schedule. Using an elevated toilet seat facilitates transfer of the client from the wheelchair to the toilet or from a standing to a sitting position. (I, 7)

68. 3. MS is a progressive, chronic neurologic disease characterized by patchy demyelination throughout the central nervous system. This interferes with the transmission of electrical impulses from one nerve cell to the next. MS affects speech, coordination, and vision, but not cognition. Care for the client with MS is directed toward maintaining joint mobility, preventing deformities, maintaining muscle strength, rehabilitation, preventing and treating depression, and providing client motivation. (P, 7)

69. 2. The nurse's most positive approach is to encourage a client with MS to keep active, use stress reduction strategies, and avoid fatigue because it is important to support the immune system while remaining active. A quiet, inactive lifestyle is not necessarily indicated. Good health habits are not likely to alter the course of the disease, although they may help minimize complications. Practicing using aids that will be needed for future disabilities may be helpful but also can be discouraging. (I, 7)

70. 2. The client should not be instructed to avoid kitchen activities out of fear of injury; independence and self-care are also important. However, the client should meet with an occupational therapist to learn about assistive devices and techniques that can reduce injuries, such as burns and cuts, that are common in kitchen activities. A client with impaired peripheral sensation does not feel pain as readily as someone whose sensation is unimpaired; therefore, water temperatures should be tested carefully. The client should be advised to avoid using hot water bottles or heating pads. Because the client cannot relay on minor pain to alert him to damaged skin or sore spots, he should carefully inspect the skin daily to visualize any injuries that he cannot feel. (P, 2)

71. 3. Maintaining a regular voiding pattern is the most appropriate measure to help the client avoid urinary incontinence. Fluid intake is not related to incontinence. Incontinence is related to the strength of the detrusor and urethral sphincter muscles. Inserting an indwelling catheter would be a treatment of last resort because of the increased risk for infection. If catheterization is required, intermittent self-catheterization is preferred because of its lower risk of infection. Antibiotics do not influence urinary incontinence. (P, 7)

72. 2. An individualized regular exercise program benefits the client to relieve muscle spasms. The client can be trained to use unaffected muscles to promote coordination because MS is a progressive debilitating condition. (I, 7)

The Unconscious Client

73. 3. Activated charcoal powder is administered to absorb remaining particles of salicylate. Vitamin K is an antidote for warfarin sodium. Dextrose 50% is used to treat hypoglycemia. Sodium thiosulfate is an antidote for cyanide. (P, 8)

74. 3. The initial response to crisis is high anxiety. Anxiety must dissipate before a person can deal with the actual situation. Allowing family members to ventilate their feelings can help diffuse their anxiety. The reasons for the client's actions are unknown; assumptions must be validated before they become facts. Touch can be appropriate, but not when it is used as false reassurance. Helping with the client's care is appropriate at a later time. (I, 5)

75. 3. Maintaining intact skin is a priority goal for the unconscious client. Unconscious clients need to be turned every hour to prevent complications of immobility, which include pressure ulcers and stasis pneumonia. The unconscious client cannot be educated at this time. Pain is not a concern. During the first 24 hours, the unconscious client will mostly likely be NPO. (P, 9)

76. 2. The nurse must clean the unconscious client's mouth carefully, apply a thin coat of petroleum jelly, and move the endotracheal tube to the opposite side daily to prevent dryness, crusting, inflammation, and parotiditis. The unconscious client's temperature should be monitored by a route other than the oral route (eg, rectal, tympanic), because oral temperatures will be inaccurate. The client should be positioned in a lateral or semiprone position, not a supine position, to allow for drainage of secretions and for the jaw and tongue to fall forward. The client should be not be dragged when turned, as may happen when a draw sheet is used. Care should be take to lift the client's heels, buttocks, arms, and head off of the sheets when turning. Trochanter rolls, splints, foam boot aids, specialty beds, and so on—not just two pillows—should be used to keep the client in correct body position and to decrease pressure on bony prominences. (I, 9)

77. 3. Pressure points in the side-lying position include the ears, shoulders, ribs, greater trochanter, medial or lateral condyles, and ankles. The sacrum, occiput, and heels are pressure points in the supine position. (D, 10)

78. 3. The client is not in proper body alignment if, when in the right side-lying position, the client's left arm rests on the mattress with the elbow flexed. This positioning of the arm pulls the left shoulder out of good alignment, restricting respiratory movements. The arm should be supported on a pillow. The client's head also should be placed on a small pillow to keep it in alignment with the body. The right leg should be extended on the mattress without a pillow to avoid hyperrotation of the hip. A pillow should be placed between the left and right legs with the left knee flexed so that on no parts of the legs is skin touching skin. (I, 10)

79. 4. The goal of performing passive range-of-motion exercises is to maintain joint mobility. Active exercise is needed to preserve bone and muscle mass. Passive range-of-motion movements do not prevent bone demineralization or have a positive effect on the client's muscle tone. (P, 10)

80. 1. Maintaining a patent airway is the priority. Therefore, the nurse should keep suction equipment available to remove secretions. The client should be placed in a side-lying position, not prone. Performing oral hygiene is a clean procedure; therefore, the nurse wears clean gloves, not sterile gloves. The nurse should never place any fingers in an unconscious client's mouth; the client may bite down. Padded tongue blades, swabs, or a toothbrush should be used instead; but maintaining the airway is the priority. (I, 10)

81. 2. When the blink reflex is absent or the eyes do not close completely, the cornea may become dry and irritated. Placing a patch over the completely closed eye is the most appropriate intervention to prevent eye injury. Having the client wear eyeglasses or cleaning the eyelid with a washcloth will not protect the cornea from dryness or irritation. Instilling artificial tears may be ordered to help prevent dryness and irritation; however, administration of artificial tears once per shift would be too infrequent to be of benefit. (I, 10)

82. 3. Restlessness is an early indicator of hypoxia. The nurse should suspect hypoxia in the unconscious client who becomes restless. The most accurate method for determining the presence of hypoxia is to evaluate the pulse oximeter value and/or arterial blood gas values. Cyanosis and decreased respirations are late indicators of hypoxia. Hypertension, not hypotension, is a sign of hypoxia. (A, 10)

83. 2. The client should be placed in a semi-Fowler's position to reduce the risk of aspiration. The formula should be at room temperature, not heated. Administering enteral tube feedings is a clean procedure, not a sterile one; therefore, sterile supplies are not required. Clients receiving enteral feedings should be weighed regularly, but not necessarily before each feeding. (I, 9)

84. 4. Gastric residuals are checked before administration of enteral feedings to determine whether gastric emptying is delayed. A residual of less than 50% of the previous feeding volume is usually considered acceptable. In this case, the amount is not excessive and the nurse should re-instill the aspirate through the tube and then administer the feeding. If the amount of gastric residual is excessive, the nurse should notify the physician and withhold the feeding. Disposing of the residual can cause electrolyte and fluid losses. (I, 9)

85. 1. Good catheter care, including meticulous cleansing of the area around the urethral meatus, is the highest priority for the client with an indwelling catheter. Clamping an indwelling catheter is not recommended. Irrigation of the catheter, which requires breaking the closed system, is not recommended. Manipulation of the catheter taped to the client's leg causes trauma to the urethral meatus, which can predispose the client to an infection and is also not recommended. (I, 9)

The Client in Pain

86. 1. Pain perception is an individual experience. Research indicates that pain tolerance and perception vary widely among individuals, even within cultures. (P, 5)

87. 1. Experience has demonstrated that clients who feel confidence in the persons who are caring for them do not require as much therapy for pain relief as those who have less confidence do. Without the client's confidence, developed in an effective nurse–client relationship, other interventions may be less effective. Arranging for the client to share a room with another client who has little pain may have negative effects on the client who has pain that is difficult to relieve. (P, 7)

88. 3. Acupuncture, like acupressure and acumassage, is performed in certain Asian cultures to help restore the energy balance within the body. Pressure, massage, and fine needles are applied to "energy pathways" to help restore the body's balance. In the Western world, many researchers think that the gate-control theory of pain may be applicable to acupuncture, acumassage, and acupressure. The concept of evil spirits is not appropriate or relevant to the practice of acupuncture. Promoting tranquility with a higher being is not the purpose of acupuncture. Acupuncture does not block nerve pathways to the brain. (P, 9)

89. 4. Although meperidine hydrochloride can be given orally, it is more effective when given intramuscularly. The equianalgesic dose of oral meperidine hydrochloride is up to four times the intramuscular dose ($75 \times 4 = 300$). (I, 8)

90. 1. Opioid analgesics relieve pain by reducing or altering the perception of pain. Meperidine hydrochloride does not decrease the sensitivity of pain receptors, interfere with pain impulses traveling along sensory nerve fibers, or block the conduction of pain impulses in the central nervous system. (P, 8)

91. 3. According to the gate-control theory, the regulatory process that controls pain impulses reaching the brain most probably occurs in the spinal cord. (P, 10)

92. 3. The client's innate responses to pain are directed initially toward escaping from the source of pain. Variations in individuals' tolerance and perception of pain are apparent only in conscious clients, and only conscious clients are able to employ distraction to help relieve pain. (A, 10)

93. 1. Ergotamine tartrate is used to help abort a migraine attack. It should be taken as soon as prodromal symptoms of migraine appear. (A, 8)

94. 1. Migraine headaches are believed to be caused by a vascular disturbance involving branches of the carotid artery, where vasoconstriction of blood vessels apparently occurs first. The extracranial and intracranial arteries then dilate, causing the headache. There is no temporary decrease in intracranial pressure. Sinusitis is not the cause of migraine headaches. Muscle contractions of the head and neck are often caused by stress and result in a tension headache. (A, 10)

95. 4. Biofeedback translates body processes into observable signs so that the client can develop some control over certain body processes. Biofeedback does not involve any electrical stimulation. Use of unpleasant stimuli such as electrical shock is a form of aversion therapy. Biofeedback does not involve monitoring body processes for the therapist to interpret; rather, it is a self-directed, self-care activity that reinforces learning because the client can see the results of his actions. (P, 9)

96. 1. A back rub stimulates the large-diameter cutaneous fibers, which block transmission of pain impulses from the spinal cord to the brain. It does not block the transmission of pain impulses or stimulate the release of endorphins. A back rub may distract the client, but the physiologic process of fiber stimulation is the main reason a back rub is used as therapy for pain relief. (A, 7)

97. 2. It is essential that the nurse document the client's response to pain medication on a routine, systematic basis. Reassuring the client that pain will be relieved is often not realistic. A client who continually presses the PCA button may not be getting adequate pain relief, but through careful assessment and documentation, the effectiveness of pain relief interventions can be evaluated and modified. Pain medication is not titrated until the client is free from pain but rather until an acceptable level of pain management is reached. (I, 8)

98. 2. To locate the ventrogluteal site, the nurse places the palm on the client's greater trochanter for careful and correct identification to avoid tissue or nerve damage. The middle finger slides on the skin along the iliac crest while the palm is on the greater trochanter. The nurse places the index finger on the anterosuperior iliac spine. The posterior iliac spine is a landmark for locating the dorsogluteal site. (I, 8)

99. 1. The nurse using healing touch affects a client's pain primarily through assessing and directing the flow of energy fields. Healing touch can involve touching, but it does not have to involve body contact. Massage and hypnosis are not parts of healing touch. (I, 9)

100. 1. The deltoid muscle is small and is not used for injections greater than 1 mL. The muscle is easy to locate. It does not have excessive pain receptors. The deltoid muscle does have a good blood supply, just as the other muscles in the body have. (I, 8)

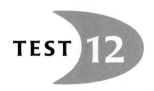

TEST 12

The Client With Musculoskeletal Health Problems

▶ The Client With Rheumatoid Arthritis

▶ The Client With Osteoarthritis

▶ The Client With a Hip Fracture

▶ The Client With a Herniated Disk

▶ The Client With an Amputation due to Peripheral Vascular Disease

▶ The Client With Fractures

▶ The Client With a Femoral Fracture

▶ The Client With a Spinal Cord Injury

▶ Correct Answers and Rationale

Select the one best answer, and indicate your choice by filling in the circle in front of the option.

The Client With Rheumatoid Arthritis

1. On a visit to the clinic, a client reports the onset of early symptoms of rheumatoid arthritis. Which of the following would the nurse *most* likely assess?
   ○ 1. Limited motion of joints.
   ○ 2. Deformed joints of the hands.
   ○ 3. Early morning stiffness.
   ○ 4. Rheumatoid nodules.

2. A client being evaluated for rheumatoid arthritis tells the nurse, "I can't seem to do my household chores anymore without becoming tired. My knees hurt whenever I walk; it's difficult for me to get around my house and yard." Based on these data, which nursing diagnosis would be the *most* appropriate for the client at this time?
   ○ 1. Activity Intolerance related to fatigue and pain.
   ○ 2. Self-Care Deficit Level II related to increasing joint pain.
   ○ 3. Ineffective Coping related to chronic pain.
   ○ 4. Disturbed Body Image related to fatigue and joint pain.

3. After teaching the client about risk factors for rheumatoid arthritis, which of the following, if stated by the client as a risk factor, would indicate to the nurse that the client needs additional teaching?
   ○ 1. History of Epstein-Barr virus infection.
   ○ 2. Female gender.
   ○ 3. Adults between the ages of 60 to 75 years.
   ○ 4. Positive testing for human leukocyte antigen (HLA) DR4 allele.

4. When developing the plan of care for a client during the acute phase of rheumatoid arthritis, which of the following would the nurse identify as the *lowest* priority?
   ○ 1. Relieving pain.
   ○ 2. Preserving joint function.
   ○ 3. Maintaining usual ways of accomplishing tasks.
   ○ 4. Preventing joint deformity.

5. After the nurse teaches a client about heat and cold treatments to manage arthritis pain, which of the following client statements indicates that the client still has a knowledge deficit?
   ○ 1. "I can use heat and cold as often as I want."
   ○ 2. "With heat, I should apply it for no longer than 20 minutes at a time."
   ○ 3. "Heat-producing liniments can be used with other heat devices."
   ○ 4. "Ten to 15 minutes per application is the maximum time for cold applications."

6. The client with rheumatoid arthritis tells the nurse, "I have a friend who took gold shots and had a wonderful response. Why didn't my doctor let me try that?" Which of the following responses by the nurse would be *most* appropriate?
   ○ 1. "It's the doctor's prerogative to decide how to treat you. The doctor has chosen what is best for your situation."
   ○ 2. "Tell me more about your friend's arthritic condition. Maybe I can answer that question for you."

○ 3. "That drug is used for cases that are worse than yours. It wouldn't help you, so don't worry about it."

○ 4. "Every person is different. What works for one patient may not always be effective for another."

7. When developing the teaching plan for the client with rheumatoid arthritis to promote rest, which of the following would the nurse expect to instruct the client to *avoid* during rest periods?

○ 1. Proper body alignment.

○ 2. Elevating the part.

○ 3. Prone lying positions.

○ 4. Positions of flexion.

8. After teaching the client with rheumatoid arthritis about measures to conserve energy in his activities of daily living specifically involving the small joints, which of the following, if stated by the client, would indicate the need for additional teaching?

○ 1. Pushing with palms when rising from a chair.

○ 2. Holding packages close to the body.

○ 3. Sliding objects.

○ 4. Carrying a laundry basket with clinched fingers and fists.

9. After teaching the client with severe rheumatoid arthritis about the newly prescribed medication methotrexate (Rheumatrex), which of the following statements indicates the need for *further* teaching?

○ 1. "I will take my vitamins while I'm on this drug."

○ 2. "I must not drink any alcohol while I'm taking this drug."

○ 3. "I should brush my teeth after every meal."

○ 4. "I will continue taking my birth control pills."

10. A 25-year-old client taking hydroxychloroquine (Plaquenil) for rheumatoid arthritis reports difficulty seeing out of her left eye. The nurse interprets this assessment finding as indicating which of the following?

○ 1. Development of a cataract.

○ 2. Possible retinal degeneration.

○ 3. Part of the disease process.

○ 4. A coincidental occurrence.

11. A client with a history of severe rheumatoid arthritis undergoes surgery. Postoperatively, the client's right leg is placed in a continuous passive motion (CPM) device. Which of the following would the nurse perform when caring for a client receiving CPM therapy?

○ 1. Adjusting the settings as needed to prevent client discomfort.

○ 2. Increasing the range-of-motion settings at least every 8 hours.

○ 3. Maintaining proper positioning of the joint on the CPM machine.

○ 4. Discontinuing the CPM therapy when range of motion increases to 90 degrees.

12. A client with rheumatoid arthritis tells the nurse, "I know it is important to exercise my joints so that I won't lose mobility, but my joints are so stiff and painful that exercising is difficult." Which of the following responses by the nurse would be *most* appropriate?

○ 1. "You are probably exercising too much. Decrease your exercise to every other day."

○ 2. "Tell the doctor about your symptoms. Maybe your analgesic medication can be increased."

○ 3. "Stiffness and pain are part of the disease. Learn to cope by focusing on activities you enjoy."

○ 4. "Take a warm tub bath or shower before exercising. This may help with your discomfort."

The Client With Osteoarthritis

13. When completing the history and physical examination of a client diagnosed with osteoarthritis, which of the following would the nurse assess?

○ 1. Anemia.

○ 2. Osteoporosis.

○ 3. Weight loss.

○ 4. Local joint pain.

14. Which of the following statements indicates that the client with osteoarthritis understands the effects of capsaicin (Zostrix) cream?

○ 1. "I always wash my hands right after I apply the cream."

○ 2. "After I apply the cream, I wrap my knee with an ace bandage."

○ 3. "I keep the cream in the cabinet above the stove in the kitchen."

○ 4. "I also use the same cream when I get a cut or a burn."

15. At which of the following times would the nurse instruct the client to take ibuprofen (Motrin), prescribed for left hip pain secondary to osteoarthritis, to minimize gastric mucosal irritation?

○ 1. At bedtime.

○ 2. On arising.

○ 3. Immediately after a meal.

○ 4. On an empty stomach.

16. When preparing a teaching plan for the client with osteoarthritis who is taking celecoxib (Celebrex), the nurse expects to explain that the major advantage of celecoxib over diclofenac (Voltaren) is that celecoxib is less likely to produce which of the following?

○ 1. Hepatotoxicity.

○ 2. Renal toxicity.

○ 3. Gastrointestinal (GI) bleeding.

○ 4. Nausea and vomiting.

17. The client diagnosed with osteoarthritis states, "My friend takes steroid pills for her rheumatoid arthritis. Why don't I take steroids for my osteoarthritis?" The nurse's response to the client is based on an understanding of which of the following?

○ 1. Intra-articular corticosteroid injections are used to treat osteoarthritis.

○ 2. Oral corticosteroids can be used in osteoarthritis.

○ 3. A systemic effect is needed in osteoarthritis.

○ 4. Rheumatoid arthritis and osteoarthritis are two similar diseases.

18. In preparation for total knee surgery, a 200-pound client with osteoarthritis is being discharged from the hospital to lose weight to reduce the risks of anesthesia. In conjunction with a weight loss program, which of the following exercises would the nurse recommend as *best* if the client has no contraindications?

○ 1. Weight lifting.

○ 2. Walking.

○ 3. Aquatic exercise.

○ 4. Tai chi exercise.

19. The physician recommends a total hip replacement for a client with osteoporosis who reports increasingly severe pain in the left hip. The nurse would initiate the preoperative teaching plan for the client, beginning with which of the following?

○ 1. Teaching how to prevent hip flexion.

○ 2. Demonstrating coughing and deep breathing techniques.

○ 3. Showing the client what an actual hip prosthesis looks like.

○ 4. Assessing the client's fears about the procedure.

20. After the client undergoes a total knee replacement for severe osteoarthritis, which of the following assessment findings would lead the nurse to suspect possible nerve damage?

○ 1. Numbness.

○ 2. Bleeding.

○ 3. Dislocation.

○ 4. Pinkness.

21. After surgery and insertion of a total joint prosthesis, a client develops severe sudden pain and an inability to move the extremity. The nurse interprets these findings as indicating which of the following?

○ 1. A developing infection.

○ 2. Bleeding in the operative site.

○ 3. Joint dislocation.

○ 4. Glue seepage into soft tissue.

The Client With a Hip Fracture

22. Which of the following would the nurse assess in a client with an intracapsular hip fracture?

○ 1. Internal rotation.

○ 2. Muscle flaccidity.

○ 3. Shortening of affected leg.

○ 4. Absence of pain in the fracture area.

23. When developing the plan of care for an older adult client with a hip fracture, which of the following

chronic health problems would the nurse be *least* likely to assess in the client?

○ 1. Hypertension.

○ 2. Cardiac decompensation.

○ 3. Pulmonary disease.

○ 4. Multiple sclerosis.

24. When teaching a client with an extracapsular hip fracture scheduled for surgical internal fixation with the insertion of a pin, the nurse bases the teaching on the understanding that this surgical repair is the treatment of choice for which of the following reasons?

○ 1. Hemorrhage at the fracture site is prevented.

○ 2. Neurovascular impairment risk is decreased.

○ 3. The risk for infection at the site is lessened.

○ 4. The client is able to be mobilized sooner.

25. A client with an extracapsular hip fracture returns to the nursing unit after internal fixation and pin insertion with a drainage tube at the incision site. Her husband asks, "Why does she have this tube inserted in her hip?" Which of the following responses by the nurse demonstrates understanding of the primary purpose for this drainage tube?

○ 1. "The tube helps us to detect a wound infection early on."

○ 2. "This way we won't have to irrigate the wound."

○ 3. "Fluid won't be allowed to accumulate at the site."

○ 4. "We have a way to administer antibiotics into the wound."

26. When assessing a client who has just received a femoral head prosthesis, which of the following would alert the nurse to the possibility of neurologic impairment in the affected extremity?

○ 1. Decreased distal pulse.

○ 2. Inability to move.

○ 3. Diminished capillary refill.

○ 4. Coolness to the touch.

27. A client with a hip fracture has undergone surgery for insertion of a femoral head prosthesis. Which of the following activities would the nurse instruct the client to avoid?

○ 1. Crossing the legs while sitting down.

○ 2. Sitting on a raised commode seat.

○ 3. Using an abductor splint while lying on the side.

○ 4. Rising straight from a chair to a standing position.

28. The nurse encourages the client who has had a femoral head prosthesis placement to use which of the following types of chairs to sit in during the first 6 to 8 weeks after surgery?

○ 1. A desk-type swivel chair.

○ 2. A padded upholstered chair.

○ 3. A high-backed chair with armrests.

○ 4. A recliner with an attached footrest.

29. While assessing the home environment of an elderly client who is using crutches during the postoperative recovery phase after hip pinning, which of the following would pose the greatest hazard to the client as a risk for falling at home?
    ○ 1. A 4-year-old cocker spaniel.
    ○ 2. Scatter rugs.
    ○ 3. Snack tables.
    ○ 4. Rocking chairs.

The Client With a Herniated Disk

30. The nurse is observing a client who is recovering from back strain lift a box as shown in Figure 1. According to the figure, the nurse should
    ○ 1. praise the client for using correct body mechanics.
    ○ 2. suggest to the client that she put both knees on the floor before attempting to lift the box.
    ○ 3. advise the client to bend from the waist rather than stretching her back in this position.
    ○ 4. inform the client that it will be better for her to keep her back straight by squatting with both knees parallel.
31. Which of the following activities would the nurse instruct the client with low back pain to *avoid*?
    ○ 1. Keeping light objects below the level of the elbows when lifting.
    ○ 2. Leaning forward while bending the knees.
    ○ 3. Exceeding prescribed exercise program.
    ○ 4. Sleeping on the side with legs flexed.
32. A client was brought to the hospital because he could not get out of bed because of low back pain radiating down to his right heel and lateral foot. When developing the client's plan of care, which of the following categories of medication would the nurse anticipate the physician's ordering?
    ○ 1. Angiotensin-converting enzyme (ACE) inhibitors.

○ 2. β-Adrenergic blocking agents.
○ 3. Nonsteroidal anti-inflammatory drugs (NSAIDs).
○ 4. Barbiturates.

33. A client with a ruptured intervertebral disc at L4–5 stands with a flattened spine slightly tilted forward and slightly flexed to the affected side. The nurse interprets this finding as indicating which of the following?
    ○ 1. Motor changes.
    ○ 2. Postural deformity.
    ○ 3. Alteration of reflexes.
    ○ 4. Sensory changes.
34. Which of the following positions would be most comfortable for a client with a ruptured disc at L5–S1 right?
    ○ 1. Prone.
    ○ 2. Supine with the legs flexed.
    ○ 3. High Fowler's.
    ○ 4. Right Sims'.
35. The client with a herniated intervertebral disc scheduled for a myelogram asks the nurse about the procedure. The nurse explains that radiographs will be taken of the client's spine after an injection of which of the following?
    ○ 1. Sterile water.
    ○ 2. Normal saline solution.
    ○ 3. Liquid nitrogen.
    ○ 4. Radiopaque dye.
36. Which of the following would be inappropriate to include when preparing a client for magnetic resonance imaging (MRI) to evaluate a ruptured disc?
    ○ 1. Informing the client that the procedure is painless.
    ○ 2. Taking a thorough history of past surgeries.
    ○ 3. Checking for previous complaints of claustrophobia.
    ○ 4. Starting an intravenous line at keep-open rate.
37. A client complaining of numbness from the back of his left buttock to the dorsum of his foot and big toe is scheduled to undergo a laminectomy. The operative consent form states, "a left lumbar laminectomy of L3–4." Based on the nurse's understanding of the client's complaints and intended surgical procedure, which of the following would the nurse do next?
    ○ 1. Have the client sign the consent form.
    ○ 2. Call the surgeon.
    ○ 3. Change the consent form.
    ○ 4. Review the client's history.
38. After a bilateral lumbar laminectomy at L5–S1, which of the following is a priority nursing diagnosis for the client in the immediate postoperative phase?
    ○ 1. Impaired Physical Mobility related to back pain.
    ○ 2. Imbalanced Nutrition: Less Than Body Requirements related to postoperative status.

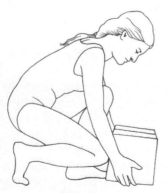

Figure 1.

3. Bowel Incontinence related to decreased physical activity.
4. Disturbed Body Image related to fear of disfiguring surgical scar.

39. Immediately after the lumbar laminectomy, the nurse administers ondansetron hydrochloride (Zofran) to the client as ordered. The nurse determines that the drug is effective when which of the following is controlled?
   ○ 1. Muscle spasms.
   ○ 2. Nausea.
   ○ 3. Shivering.
   ○ 4. Dry mouth.

40. After a laminectomy, the client states, "The doctor said that I can do anything I want to." Which of the following activities, if stated by the client, indicates the need for *further* teaching?
   ○ 1. Drying the dishes.
   ○ 2. Sitting outside on firm cushions.
   ○ 3. Making the bed walking from side to side.
   ○ 4. Sweeping the front porch.

41. When developing the discharge teaching plan for a client who has undergone a lumbar laminectomy L4–5 left and will be returning to work in 6 weeks, which of the following actions would the nurse encourage the client to *avoid*?
   ○ 1. Placing one foot on a stepstool during prolonged standing.
   ○ 2. Sleeping on the back with support under the knees.
   ○ 3. Maintaining average body weight for height.
   ○ 4. Sitting whenever possible.

42. A male client, who had normal preoperative baseline data except for dysfunction associated with his operative diagnosis, underwent a spinal fusion yesterday. Which of the following nursing assessments would alert the nurse to the development of a possible complication?
   ○ 1. Lateral rotation of the head and neck.
   ○ 2. Clear yellowish fluid on the dressing.
   ○ 3. Use of the standing position to void.
   ○ 4. Nonproductive cough.

43. After a spinal fusion, a client is required to wear a back brace. Which of the following would the nurse expect to do before applying the brace?
   ○ 1. Have the client in bed lying on the side.
   ○ 2. Verify with the physician the position to use.
   ○ 3. Ask the client to stand with arms held out to the side.
   ○ 4. Encourage the client to sit in a straight chair.

44. After teaching a client required to wear a back brace after a spinal fusion, which of the following client statements indicates effective teaching about skin protection measures with the brace?
   ○ 1. "I will apply lotion before putting on the brace."

2. "I will be sure to pad the area around my iliac crest."
3. "I can use baby powder under the brace to absorb perspiration."
4. "I should wear a thin cotton undershirt under the brace."

45. When developing the teaching plan for a client scheduled for a spinal fusion, which of the following would the nurse expect to include?
   ○ 1. The client typically experiences more pain at the donor site than at the fusion site.
   ○ 2. The surgeon will apply a simple gauze dressing to the donor site.
   ○ 3. Neurovascular checks are unnecessary if the fibula is the donor site.
   ○ 4. The client's level of activity restriction is determined by the amount of pain.

46. The nurse determines that the client who has had a lumbar laminectomy with a spinal fusion understands his postoperative instructions when he places his feet in which of the following positions when sitting in a chair?
   ○ 1. On the floor with the feet flat.
   ○ 2. On a low footstool.
   ○ 3. In any comfortable position with legs uncrossed.
   ○ 4. On a high footstool so the feet are level with the chair seat.

47. When developing the plan of care for a client undergoing a lumbar laminectomy, which of the following activities would be contraindicated during the initial postoperative period?
   ○ 1. Assisting with her daily hygiene activities.
   ○ 2. Lying flat in bed.
   ○ 3. Walking in the hall.
   ○ 4. Sitting all afternoon in her room.

48. Which of the following exercises would the nurse advise the client to avoid after a lumbar laminectomy?
   ○ 1. Knee-to-chest lifts.
   ○ 2. Hip tilts.
   ○ 3. Sit-ups.
   ○ 4. Pelvic tilts.

The Client With an Amputation due to Peripheral Vascular Disease

49. When obtaining the history of a client with peripheral vascular disease who requires an amputation, which of the following would the nurse identify as the *least* likely factor contributing to the client's peripheral vascular disease?
   ○ 1. Uncontrolled diabetes mellitus for 15 years.
   ○ 2. A 20-pack-year history of cigarette smoking.
   ○ 3. Current age of 39 years.

○ 4. A serum cholesterol concentration of 275 mg/dL.

50. When assessing the client with severe arterial occlusive disease and gangrene of the left great toe, which of the following findings would the nurse observe in the client's left leg and foot?
○ 1. Edema around the ankle.
○ 2. Loss of hair on the lower leg.
○ 3. Thin, soft toenails.
○ 4. Warmth in the foot.

51. A client with absent peripheral pulses and pain at rest is scheduled for an arterial Doppler study of the affected extremity. Which of the following would the nurse include when preparing the client for this test?
○ 1. Have the client sign a consent form for the procedure.
○ 2. Administer a pretest sedative as appropriate.
○ 3. Keep the client tobacco-free for 30 minutes before the test.
○ 4. Wrap the client's affected foot with a blanket.

52. The client with peripheral arterial disease says, "I've really tried to manage my condition well." Which of the following, if reported by the client during the history, would the nurse determine as appropriate for this client?
○ 1. Resting with the legs elevated above the level of the heart.
○ 2. Walking slowly but steadily for 30 minutes twice a day.
○ 3. Minimizing activity as much and as often as possible.
○ 4. Wearing antiembolism stockings at all times when out of bed.

53. Which of the following would the nurse include in the teaching plan for a client with arterial insufficiency to the feet who is being managed conservatively?
○ 1. Daily lubrication of the feet.
○ 2. Soaking the feet in warm water.
○ 3. Applying antiembolism stockings.
○ 4. Wearing firm, supportive leather shoes.

54. While the nurse is providing preoperative teaching, the client says, "I hate the idea of being an invalid after they cut off my leg." Which of the following would be the nurse's *most* therapeutic response?
○ 1. "At least you will still have one good leg to use."
○ 2. "Tell me more about how you're feeling."
○ 3. "Let's finish the preoperative teaching."
○ 4. "You're lucky to have a wife to care for you."

55. The client asks the nurse, "Why can't the doctor tell me exactly how much of my leg he's going to take off? Don't you think I should know that?" The nurse responds based on the understanding that the final decision about the level of amputation required depends primarily on which of the following?
○ 1. The need to remove as much of the leg as possible.
○ 2. The adequacy of the blood supply to the tissues.
○ 3. The ease with which a prosthesis can be fitted.
○ 4. The client's ability to walk with a prosthesis.

56. Which of the following actions would be the priority for a client who has been in the postanesthesia care unit (PACU) for 45 minutes after an above-the-knee amputation and develops a dime-size bright red spot on the ace bandage above the amputation site?
○ 1. Elevating the stump.
○ 2. Reinforcing the dressing.
○ 3. Calling the surgeon.
○ 4. Drawing a mark around the site.

57. A client in the PACU with a left below-the-knee amputation complains of pain in her left big toe. Which of the following would the nurse do *first*?
○ 1. Tell the client it is impossible to feel the pain.
○ 2. Show the client that the toes are not there.
○ 3. Explain to the client that her pain is real.
○ 4. Give the client the prescribed narcotic analgesic.

58. The client with an above-the-knee amputation is to use crutches while his prosthesis is being adjusted. In which of the following exercises would the nurse instruct the client to best prepare him for using crutches?
○ 1. Abdominal exercises.
○ 2. Isometric shoulder exercises.
○ 3. Quadriceps setting exercises.
○ 4. Triceps stretching exercises.

59. A client who has an above-the-knee amputation is to use crutches until the prosthesis is properly fitted. When teaching the client about using the crutches, the nurse instructs the client to support her weight primarily on which of the following body areas?
○ 1. Axillae.
○ 2. Elbows.
○ 3. Upper arms.
○ 4. Hands.

60. The client requiring a left above-the-knee amputation due to arterial occlusive peripheral vascular disease is to be discharged on a low-fat, low-cholesterol, low-sodium diet. Which of the following would be the nurse's *first* step in planning the dietary instructions?
○ 1. Determining the client's knowledge level about cholesterol.
○ 2. Asking the client to name foods that are high in fat, cholesterol, and salt.

3. Explaining the importance of complying with the diet.
4. Assessing the client's and family's typical food preferences.

The Client With Fractures

61. Three hours ago a client was thrown from a car into a ditch, and he is now admitted to the emergency department in a stable condition with vital signs within normal limits, alert and oriented with good coloring and an open fracture of the right tibia. When assessing the client, the nurse would be especially alert for signs and symptoms of which of the following?
   - 1. Hemorrhage.
   - 2. Infection.
   - 3. Deformity.
   - 4. Shock.

62. The client with a fractured tibia has been taking methocarbamol (Robaxin). When teaching the client about this drug, which of the following would the nurse include as the drug's primary effect?
   - 1. Killing of microorganisms.
   - 2. Reduction in itching.
   - 3. Relief of muscle spasms.
   - 4. Decrease in nervousness.

63. A client who has been taking carisoprodol (Soma) at home for a fractured arm is admitted with a blood pressure of 80/50 mg Hg, a pulse rate of 115 bpm, and respirations of 8 breaths/minute and shallow. The nurse interprets these findings as indicating which of the following?
   - 1. Expected common side effects.
   - 2. Hypersensitivity reaction.
   - 3. Possible habituating effect.
   - 4. Hemorrhage from gastrointestinal irritation.

64. When admitting a client with a fractured extremity, the nurse would focus the assessment on which of the following *first*?
   - 1. The area proximal to the fracture.
   - 2. The actual fracture site.
   - 3. The area distal to the fracture.
   - 4. The opposite extremity for baseline comparison.

65. Regardless of the type of cast material used, the nurse identifies a knowledge deficit when the client makes which of the following statements about the care of his cast?
   - 1. "I'll elevate the cast above my heart initially."
   - 2. "I'll exercise my joints above and below the cast."
   - 3. "I can pull out cast padding to scratch inside the cast."

4. "I'll apply ice for 10 minutes to control edema for the first 24 hours."

66. Which of the following interventions would be *least* appropriate for a client who is in a double hip spica cast?
   - 1. Encouraging the intake of cranberry juice.
   - 2. Advising the client to eat large amounts of cheese.
   - 3. Establishing regular times for elimination.
   - 4. Having the client dangle at the bedside.

67. When preparing the teaching plan for a client about crutch walking using a two-point gait pattern, which of the following would the nurse include?
   - 1. Advance a crutch on one side and then advance the opposite foot; repeat on the opposite side.
   - 2. Advance a crutch on one side and simultaneously advance and bear weight on the opposite foot; repeat on the opposite side.
   - 3. Advance both crutches together and then follow by lifting both lower extremities to the level of the crutches.
   - 4. Advance both crutches together and then follow by lifting both lower extremities past the level of the crutches.

68. The client returns from surgery after debridement of an open fracture of the tibia. The wound was left open, and a three-way drainage system was left in place. Which of the following would the nurse expect to assess?
   - 1. Results of culture and sensitivity testing of the wound.
   - 2. Presence of a pressure dressing over the wound.
   - 3. Complaints of increased pain from exposed nerve endings.
   - 4. Hypotension resulting from additional vessel bleeding.

69. A client who crashed her motorcycle suffered a tibial fracture that required casting. Approximately 5 hours later, the client begins to complain of increasing pain distal to the left tibial fracture despite the morphine injection administered 30 minutes previously. The nurse's *next* action should be to assess for which of the following?
   - 1. Presence of a distal pulse.
   - 2. Pain with a pain rating scale.
   - 3. Vital sign changes.
   - 4. Potential for drug tolerance.

70. A client with a fracture develops compartment syndrome. When caring for the client, the nurse would be alert for which of the following signs of possible organ failure?
   - 1. Rales.
   - 2. Jaundice.

○ 3. Generalized edema.
○ 4. Dark, scanty urine.

The Client With a Femoral Fracture

71. After determining that a client with a fractured right femur has not had any immunizations since childhood, which of the following biologic products would the nurse administer to provide the client with passive immunity for tetanus?
    ○ 1. Tetanus toxoid.
    ○ 2. Tetanus antigen.
    ○ 3. Tetanus vaccine.
    ○ 4. Tetanus antitoxin.

72. After teaching the client with a femoral fracture about treatment with skeletal traction, which of the following, if stated by the client as a purpose, would indicate the need for additional teaching?
    ○ 1. To align injured bones.
    ○ 2. To provide long-term pull.
    ○ 3. To apply 25 pounds of traction.
    ○ 4. To pull weight with a boot.

73. The nurse is planning care for the client with a femoral fracture who is in balanced suspension traction. Which of the following would the nurse be *least* likely to include in the plan of care?
    ○ 1. Use of a fraction bedpan.
    ○ 2. Checks for redness over the ischial tuberosity.
    ○ 3. Elevation of the head of bed no more than 25 degrees.
    ○ 4. Personal hygiene with a complete bedbath.

74. Which of the following nursing assessments for a client in balanced suspension traction using a half-ring Thomas splint with a Pearson attachment that suspends the lower extremity and applies direct skeletal traction for a hip fracture would be *inappropriate*?
    ○ 1. Greater trochanter skin checks.
    ○ 2. Pin site inspection.
    ○ 3. Neurovascular checks proximal to the splint.
    ○ 4. Foot movement evaluation.

75. The client in balanced suspension traction is transported to surgery for closed reduction and internal fixation of his fractured femur. When transporting the client to the operating room, which of the following would the nurse do?
    ○ 1. Transfer the client to a cart with manually suspended traction.
    ○ 2. Call the surgeon to request an order for temporarily removing the traction.
    ○ 3. Send the client on his bed with extra help to stabilize the traction.
    ○ 4. Remove the traction and send the client on a cart.

76. When caring for the client with a Pearson attachment on the traction setup, the nurse understands that the purpose of this attachment is to accomplish which of the following?
    ○ 1. Support the lower portion of the leg.
    ○ 2. Support the thigh and upper leg.
    ○ 3. Allow attachment of the skeletal pin.
    ○ 4. Prevent flexion deformities in the ankle and foot.

77. Which of the following would lead the nurse to suspect that a client with a fracture of the right femur may be developing a fat embolus?
    ○ 1. Acute respiratory distress syndrome.
    ○ 2. Migraine-like headaches.
    ○ 3. Numbness in the right leg.
    ○ 4. Muscle spasms in the right thigh.

78. The client with a fractured femur is upset and agitated about her injury and its treatment. She says, "How can I stay like this for weeks? I can't even move!" Based on these data, the nurse would identify which of the following as the *most* appropriate nursing diagnosis?
    ○ 1. Impaired Physical Mobility related to traction.
    ○ 2. Ineffective Coping related to prolonged immobility.
    ○ 3. Deficient Diversional Activity related to prolonged hospitalization.
    ○ 4. Activity Intolerance related to impaired mobility.

79. The client asks the nurse what his activity limitations are while he is in Buck's traction. Which of the following responses by the nurse would be *most* appropriate?
    ○ 1. "You can sit up whenever you want."
    ○ 2. "You must lie flat on your back most of the time."
    ○ 3. "You can turn your body."
    ○ 4. "You must lie on your stomach."

80. Because a client has a Thomas splint, the nurse would need to assess the client regularly for which of the following?
    ○ 1. Signs of skin pressure in the groin area.
    ○ 2. Evidence of decreased breath sounds.
    ○ 3. Skin breakdown behind the heel.
    ○ 4. Urinary retention.

81. The client has a nursing diagnosis of Self-Care Deficit Level II related to the confinement of traction. Which of the following would indicate a successful outcome for this diagnosis?
    ○ 1. The client assists as much as possible in his care, demonstrating increased participation over time.
    ○ 2. The client allows the nurse to complete his care in an efficient manner without interfering.
    ○ 3. The client allows his wife to assume total responsibility for his care.

○ 4. The client allows his wife to complete his care to promote feelings of usefulness.

82. The client who had an open femoral fracture was discharged to her home, where she developed fever, night sweats, chills, restlessness, and restrictive movement of the fractured leg. The nurse interprets these findings as indicating which of the following?
○ 1. Pulmonary emboli.
○ 2. Osteomyelitis.
○ 3. Fat emboli.
○ 4. Urinary tract infection.

83. When antibiotics are not producing the desired outcome for a client with osteomyelitis, the nurse interprets this as suggesting the occurrence of which of the following as *most* likely?
○ 1. Formation of scar tissue interfering with absorption.
○ 2. Development of pus leading to ischemia.
○ 3. Production of bacterial growth by avascular tissue.
○ 4. Antibiotics' not being instilled directly into the bone.

The Client With a Spinal Cord Injury

84. A client who fell during a rock-climbing trip is alert and conscious but unable to move her arms or legs on command. When planning to move a person with a possible spinal cord injury, which of the following would be the *priority* concern?
○ 1. Wrapping and supporting the extremities, which can be easily injured.
○ 2. Moving the person gently to help reduce pain.
○ 3. Immobilizing the head and neck to prevent further injury.
○ 4. Cushioning the back with pillows to ensure comfort.

85. The nurse is taking care of a client with a spinal cord injury. The extent of the client's injury is shown in Figure 2. Which of the following findings is expected when assessing this client?
○ 1. Inability to move his arms.
○ 2. Loss of sensation in his hands and fingers.
○ 3. Dysfunction of bowel and bladder.
○ 4. Difficulty breathing.

86. When the client has a cord transection at T4, which of the following is the *primary* focus of the nursing assessment?
○ 1. Renal status.
○ 2. Vascular status.
○ 3. Gastrointestinal function.
○ 4. Biliary function.

87. When assessing the client with a cord transection above T5 for possible complications, which of the

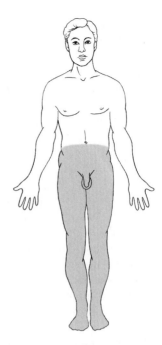

Figure 2.

following would the nurse expect as *least* likely to occur?
○ 1. Diarrhea.
○ 2. Paralytic ileus.
○ 3. Stress ulcers.
○ 4. Intra-abdominal bleeding.

88. The nurse is planning to teach the client with spinal cord injury and intermittent nasogastric suctioning about interventions to protect her integumentary system. Which of the following would the nurse include?
○ 1. Eat enough calories to maintain desired weight.
○ 2. Stay in cool environments to avoid sweating.
○ 3. Stay in warm environments to avoid chilling.
○ 4. Eat low-sodium foods to avoid edema.

89. Which of the following would the nurse use as the *best* method to assess for the development of deep vein thrombosis in a client with a spinal cord injury?
○ 1. Homan's sign.
○ 2. Pain.
○ 3. Tenderness.
○ 4. Leg girth.

90. During the period of spinal shock, the nurse would expect the client's bladder function to be which of the following?
○ 1. Spastic.
○ 2. Normal.
○ 3. Atonic.
○ 4. Uncontrolled.

91. After a month of therapy, the client in spinal shock begins to experience muscle spasms in his legs. He calls the nurse in excitement to report the leg move-

ment. Which of the following responses by the nurse would be the *most* accurate?

○ 1. "These movements indicate that the damaged nerves are healing."

○ 2. "This is a good sign. Keep trying to move all the affected muscles."

○ 3. "The return of movement means that eventually you should be able to walk again."

○ 4. "The movements occur from muscle reflexes that can't be initiated or controlled by the brain."

92. The client with a spinal cord injury asks the nurse why the dietitian has recommended that she decrease her total daily intake of calcium. Which of the following responses by the nurse would provide the *most* accurate information?

○ 1. "Excessive intake of dairy products makes constipation more common."

○ 2. "Immobility increases calcium absorption from the intestine."

○ 3. "Lack of weight bearing causes demineralization of the long bones."

○ 4. "Dairy products likely will contribute to weight gain."

93. As a first step in teaching a woman with a spinal cord injury and quadriplegia about her sexual health, the nurse assesses her understanding of her current sexual functioning. Which of the following statements by the client indicates a good understanding of her sexual functioning?

○ 1. "I won't be able to have sexual intercourse until the urinary catheter is removed."

○ 2. "I can participate in sexual activity but might not experience orgasm."

○ 3. "I can't have sexual intercourse because it causes hypertension, but other sexual activity is okay."

○ 4. "I should be able to participate in sexual activity, but I will be infertile."

94. A client with a spinal cord injury who has been active in sports and outdoor activities talks almost obsessively about his past activities. In tears, one day he asks the nurse, "Why can't I stop talking about these things? I know those days are gone forever." Which of the following responses by the nurse conveys the *best* understanding of the client's behavior?

○ 1. "Be patient. It takes time to adjust to such a massive loss."

○ 2. "Talking about the past is a form of denial. We have to help you focus on today."

○ 3. "Reviewing your losses is a way to help you work through your grief and loss."

○ 4. "It's a simple escape mechanism to go back and live again in happier times."

Correct Answers and Rationale

The letters in parentheses following the rationale identify the step of the nursing process (A, D, P, I, E) and client needs (1, 2, 3, 4, 5, 6, 7, 8, 9, 10). See the inside front cover for the key.

The Client With Rheumatoid Arthritis

1. 3. Initially, most clients with early symptoms of rheumatoid arthritis complain of early morning stiffness or stiffness after sitting still for a while. Later symptoms of rheumatoid arthritis include limited joint range of motion; deformed joints, especially of the hand; and rheumatoid nodules. (A, 10)

2. 1. Based on the client's complaints, the most appropriate nursing diagnosis would be Activity Intolerance related to fatigue and pain. Nursing interventions would focus on helping the client conserve energy and decrease episodes of fatigue. Although the client may develop a self-care deficit related to the activity intolerance and increasing joint pain, the client is voicing concerns about household chores and difficulty around the house and yard, not self-care issues. Over time, the client may develop ineffective coping or body image disturbance as the disorder becomes chronic with increasing pain and fatigue. (D, 7)

3. 3. Rheumatoid arthritis is a disorder of adults between the ages of 20 to 55 years of age, not 60 to 75 years. Research has found that rheumatoid arthritis occurs in clients who have had infectious disease such as the Epstein-Barr virus. Female gender is a risk factor, because rheumatoid arthritis occurs three times more often in women than in men. The genetic link, specifically HLA-DR4, has been found in 65% of clients with rheumatoid arthritis. (E, 9)

4. 3. Maintaining usual ways of accomplishing tasks would be the lowest priority during the acute phase. Rather, the focus is on developing less stressful ways of accomplishing routine tasks. Pain relief is a high priority during the acute phase because pain is typically severe and interferes with the client's ability to function. Preserving joint function and preventing joint deformity are high priorities during the acute phase to promote an optimal level of functioning and reduce the risk of contractures. (P, 10)

5. 3. Heat-producing liniment can produce a burn if used with other heat devices that could intensify the heat reaction. Heat and cold can be used as often as the client desires. However, each application of heat should not exceed 20 minutes, and each application of cold should not exceed 10 to 15 minutes. Application for longer periods results in the opposite of the intended effect: vasoconstriction instead of vasodilation with heat, and vasodilation instead of vasoconstriction with cold. (E, 9)

6. 4. The nurse's most appropriate response is one that is therapeutic. The basic principle of therapeutic communication and a therapeutic relationship is honesty. Therefore, the nurse needs to explain truthfully that each client is different and that there are various forms of arthritis and arthritis treatment. To state that it is the doctor's prerogative to decide how to treat the client implies that the client is not a member of his or her own health care team and is not a participant in his or her care. The statement also is defensive, which serves to block any further communication or questions from the client about the doctor. Asking the client to tell more about the friend presumes that the client knows correct and complete information, which is not a valid assumption to make. The nurse does not know about the client's friend and should not make statements about another client's condition. Stating that the drug is for cases that are worse than the patient's demonstrates that the nurse is making assumptions that are not necessarily valid or appropriate. Also, telling the client not to worry ignores the underlying emotions associated with the question, totally discounting the client's feelings. (I, 5)

7. 4. Positions of flexion should be avoided to prevent loss of functional ability of affected joints. Proper body alignment during rest periods is encouraged to maintain correct muscle and joint placement. Lying in the prone position is encouraged to avoid further curvature of the spine and internal rotation of the shoulders (P, 10)

8. 4. Carrying a laundry basket with clinched fingers and fists is not an example of conserving energy of small joints. The laundry basket should be held with both hands opened as wide as possible and with outstretched arms so that pressure is not placed on the small joints of the fingers. When rising from a chair, the palms should be used instead of the fingers so as to distribute weight over the larger area of the palms. Holding packages close to the body provides greater support to the shoulder, elbow, and wrist joints because muscles of the arms and hands are used to stabilize the weight against the body. This decreases the stress and weight or pull on small joints such as the fingers. Objects can be slid with the palm of the hand, which distributes weight over the larger area of the palms instead of stressing the small joints of the fin-

gers to pick up the weight of the object to move it to another place (E, 7)

9. 1. Because some over-the-counter vitamin supplements contain folic acid, the client should avoid self-medication with vitamins while taking methotrexate, a folic acid antagonist. Because methotrexate is hepatoxic, the client should avoid the intake of alcohol, which could increase the risk for hepatotoxicity. Methotrexate can cause bone marrow depression, placing the client at risk for infection. Therefore, meticulous mouth care is essential to minimize the risk for infection. Contraception should be used during methotrexate therapy and for 8 weeks after the therapy has been discontinued because of its effect on mitosis. Methotrexate is considered teratogenic. (E, 8)

10. 2. Difficulty seeing out of one eye, when evaluated in conjunction with the client's medication therapy regimen, leads to the suspicion of possible retinal degeneration. The possibility of an irreversible retinal degeneration caused by deposits of hydroxychloroquine (Plaquenil) in the layers of the retina requires an ophthalmologic examination before therapy is begun and at 6-month intervals. Although cataracts may develop in young adults, they are less likely, and damage from the hydroxychloroquine is the most obvious at risk factor. Eyesight is not affected by the disease process of rheumatoid arthritis. (D, 8)

11. 3. The nurse must frequently evaluate the positioning of the client's leg to prevent misalignment and development of possible contractures. Initially the client may experience some discomfort when using a CPM machine. If the client cannot tolerate the discomfort, the physician should be notified to obtain an order to adjust the settings. The settings for the machine are determined by the physician and cannot be changed without an order. Although the optimal degree of flexion is 90 degrees, therapy will continue until the individual regains the maximal degree flexion in the knee as determined by the doctor. (I, 9)

12. 4. Superficial heat applications such as tub baths, showers, and warm compresses can be helpful in relieving pain and stiffness. Exercises can be performed more comfortably and more effectively after heat applications. Typically, large doses of analgesics, which can lead to hepatotoxic effects, are not necessary. Learning to cope with the pain by refocusing is inappropriate. The client with rheumatoid arthritis must balance rest with exercise every day, not every other day. (I, 7)

The Client With Osteoarthritis

13. 4. Osteoarthritis is a degenerative joint disease with local manifestations such as local joint pain, unlike rheumatoid arthritis, which has systemic manifestation such as anemia and osteoporosis. Weight loss occurs in rheumatoid arthritis, whereas most clients with osteoarthritis are overweight. (A, 10)

14. 1. Capsaicin cream, which produces analgesia by preventing the reaccumulation of substance P in the peripheral sensory neurons, is made from the active ingredients of hot peppers. Therefore, clients should wash their hands immediately after applying capsaicin cream if they do not wear gloves, to avoid possible contact between the cream and mucous membranes. Clients are instructed to avoid wearing tight bandages over areas where capsaicin cream has been applied, because swelling may occur from inflammation of the arthritis in the joint and lead to constriction on the peripheral neurovascular system. Capsaicin cream should be stored in areas between 59°F and 86°F (between 15°C and 30°C). The cabinet over the stove in the kitchen would be too warm. Capsaicin cream should be not come in contact with irritated and broken skin, mucous membranes, or eyes. Therefore it should not be used on cuts or burns. (E, 8)

15. 3. Drugs that cause gastric irritation, such as ibuprofen (Motrin), are best taken after or with a meal, when stomach contents help minimize the local irritation. Taking the medication on an empty stomach at any time during the day will lead to gastric irritation. Taking the drug at bedtime with food may cause the client to gain weight, possibly aggravating the osteoarthritis. When the client arises, he is stiff from immobility and should use warmth and stretching until he gets food in his stomach. (I, 8)

16. 3. The major advantage of celecoxib (Celebrex), the new generation of cyclooxygenase-2 (COX-2) inhibitors, over diclofenac (Voltaren), a COX-1 inhibitor, is that celecoxib is less likely to produce GI problems such as ulcers and bleeding. There is no evidence of less hepatotoxicity, renal toxicity, or nausea and vomiting with COX-2 inhibitors. (P, 8)

17. 1. Rheumatoid arthritis and osteoarthritis are two different diseases. Corticosteroids are used for clients with osteoarthritis to obtain a local effect. Therefore, they are given only via intra-articular injection. Oral corticosteroids are avoided because they can cause an acceleration of osteoarthritis. (D, 8)

18. 3. When combined with a weight loss program, aquatic exercise would be best because it cushions the joints and allows the client to burn off calories. Aquatic exercise promotes circulation, muscle toning, and lung expansion, which promote healthy preoperative conditioning. Weight lifting and walking are too stressful to the joints, possibly exacerbating the client's osteoarthritis. Although tai chi exercise is designed for stretching and coordination, it would not be the best exercise for this client to help with weight loss. (I, 10)

19. 4. Before implementing a teaching plan, the nurse should determine the client's fears about the procedure. Only then can the client begin to hear what the nurse has to share about the individualized teaching plan designed to meet the client's needs. In the preoperative period, the client needs to learn how to correctly prevent hip flexion and to demonstrate coughing and deep breathing. However, this teaching can be effective only after the client's fears have been assessed and addressed. Although the client may appreciate seeing what a hip prosthesis looks like, so as to understand the new body part, this is not a necessity. (I, 5)

20. 1. The nurse would suspect nerve damage if numbness is present. However, whether the damage is short-term and related to edema or long-term and related to permanent nerve damage would not be clear at this point. The nurse needs to continue to assess the client's neurovascular status, including pain, pallor, pulselessness, paresthesia, and paralysis (the five P's). Bleeding would suggest vascular damage or hemorrhage. Dislocation would suggest malalignment. Pink color would suggest adequate circulation to the area. Numbness would suggest neurologic damage. (A, 9)

21. 3. The joint has dislocated when the client with a total joint prosthesis develops severe sudden pain and an inability to move the extremity. Clinical manifestations of an infection would include inflammation, redness, erythema, and possibly drainage and separation of the wound. Bleeding could be external (eg, blood visible from the wound or on the dressing) or internal and manifested by signs of shock (eg, pallor, coolness, hypotension, tachycardia). The seepage of glue into soft tissue would have occurred in the operating room, when the glue is still in the liquid form. The glue dries into the hard fixed form before the wound is closed. (D, 9)

The Client With a Hip Fracture

22. 3. With an intracapsular hip fracture, the affected leg is shorter than the unaffected leg because of the muscle spasms and external rotation. The client also experiences severe pain in the region of the fracture. (A, 10)

23. 4. Multiple sclerosis would be the least likely chronic health problem for an older adult with a hip fracture. Typically, multiple sclerosis is considered a severe crippling disorder of young adults. Hypertension is a common chronic health problem in older adults. Cardiac decompensation is common in older adults; it arises from cardiac musculature changes and age-related changes in the heart. This comorbid condition can complicate the treatment and care when the older adult experiences a hip fracture. Pulmonary disease commonly arises from age-related changes in the respiratory system. These comorbid conditions can complicate the treatment and care when the older adult experiences a hip fracture. (P, 9)

24. 4. Insertion of a pin for the internal fixation of a extracapsular fractured hip provides good fixation of the fracture. The fracture site is stabilized and fractured bone ends are well approximated. As a result, the client is able to be mobilized sooner, thus reducing the risks of complications related to immobility. Internal fixation with a pin insertion does not prevent hemorrhage or decrease the risk for neurovascular impairment, potential complications associated with any joint or bone surgery. It does not lessen the client's risk for infection at the site. (I, 9)

25. 3. The primary purpose of the drainage tube is to prevent fluid accumulation in the wound. Fluid when it accumulates creates dead space. Elimination of the dead space by keeping the wound free of fluid greatly enhances wound healing and helps prevent abscess formation. Although the characteristics of the drainage from the tube, such as a change in color or appearance, may suggest a possible infection, this is not the tube's primary purpose. The drainage tube does not eliminate the need for wound irrigation or provide a way to instill antibiotics into the wound. (I, 9)

26. 2. Being unable to move the affected leg suggests neurologic impairment. A decrease in the distal pulse, diminished capillary refill, and coolness to touch of the affected extremity suggest vascular compromise. (A, 9)

27. 1. Any activity or position that causes flexion, adduction, or internal rotation of greater than 90 degrees should be avoided until the soft tissue surrounding the prosthesis has stabilized, at approximately 6 weeks. Crossing the feet while sitting down can lead to dislocation of the femoral head from the hip socket. Sitting on a raised commode seat prevents hip flexion and adduction. Using an abductor splint while side-lying keeps the hip joint in abduction, thus preventing adduction and possible dislocation. Rising straight from a chair to a standing position is acceptable for this client because this action avoids hip flexion, adduction, and internal rotation of greater than 90 degrees. (I, 9)

28. 3. A high-backed straight chair with armrests is recommended to help keep the client in the best possible alignment after surgery for a femoral head prosthesis placement. Use of this type of chair helps to prevent dislocation of the prosthesis from the socket. A desk-type swivel chair, padded upholstered chair, or recliner should be avoided because it does not provide for good body alignment and can cause the overly flexed femoral head to dislocate. (I, 9)

29. 2. Although pets and furniture such as snack tables and rocking chairs may pose a problem, scatter rugs are the single greatest hazard in the home, especially for

elderly people who are unsure and unsteady with walking. Falls have been found to account for almost half the accidental deaths that occur in the home. The risk for falls is further compounded by the client's need for crutches. (A, 2)

The Client With a Herniated Disk

30. 1. The client is using correct body mechanics for lifting because she is keeping her back as straight as possible and is holding the box close to her body. She is using her large leg muscles to lift the box. She is using a broad base of support by placing her feet as wide apart as possible. The other suggestions would cause the client to put a strain on her back. (E, 9)

31. 3. The client with low back pain should not exceed prescribed exercises even though they may think, "If this will make me well, double will make me well quicker." When exceeding prescribed exercise programs, the client's muscle may be unconditioned and easily tired, leading to injury and increased pain. To use proper body mechanics when lifting light objects, the client should bring the item close to the center of gravity, which occurs when the object is kept below the level of the elbows. Leaning forward while bending the knees allows for the muscles of the thigh to be used instead of those of the lower back. Sleeping on the side with the legs flexed is appropriate because the spine is kept in a neutral position without twisting or pulling on muscles. (I, 9)

32. 3. For the client who has back pain radiating down to his right heel and lateral foot, suggesting radiculopathy of a herniated disc at L5–S1, typically the physician would order NSAIDs, oral analgesics, and muscle relaxants. ACE inhibitors are indicated for clients with hypertension and those with heart failure unresponsive to conventional therapy. β-Blockers are indicated for clients with cardiovascular disorders, such as hypertension and angina, and also for migraine prophylaxis. Barbiturates are central nervous system depressants; they are indicated for clients with seizures or insomnia and for those being prepared for surgery. (P, 8)

33. 2. Standing with a flattened spine slightly tilted forward and slightly flexed to the affected side indicates a postural deformity. Motor changes would include findings such as hypotonia or muscle weakness. Absent or diminished reflexes related to the level of herniation would indicate alteration in reflexes. Sensory changes would include findings such as paresthesia and numbness related to the specific tract of the herniation. (D, 10)

34. 2. A supine position with the client's legs flexed is the most comfortable position because it allows for the disc to recess off of the nerve, thus alleviating the pressure and pain. The prone position causes hyperextension of the spine and increased pressure of the disc on the nerve root on the right. A ruptured disc at L5–S1 right is a term commonly used in the analysis of a history and physical examination, magnetic resonance image, or myelogram to identify a ruptured disc compressing the right nerve root exiting the L5–S1 spinous process, as opposed to the central area or the left nerve root of that spinous process. If the ruptured area of the disc were in the central area of the spinous process, the prone position and hyperextension might relieve the disc pressure on the nerve. A high Fowler's or sitting position increases the pressure of the disc on the nerve root because of gravity, as does a right Sims' position. (I, 10)

35. 4. Myelography, used to determine the exact location of a herniated disk, involves the use of a radiopaque dye (usually an iodized oil, but in some instances a water-soluble compound). In some instances, air is used for an air-contrast study. (I, 9)

36. 4. An intravenous line is not required for an MRI. If a client has an intravenous line, it is usually converted to an intermittent infusion device, such as a heparin lock, to avoid infiltration during transport of the client and completion of the procedure. When a contrast agent is used, the client is moved out of the cylinder, the contrast material is injected, and the client is moved back in. An MRI scan is painless. Typically the staff positions the client with pillows, blankets, ear plugs, and music, to ensure client comfort, before the procedure is started. A history of past surgeries is important, especially if the surgery involved implantation of any metallic devices (eg, implants, clips, pacemakers). Additionally, the nurse needs to assess for any hearing aids, electronic devices, shrapnel, bra hooks, necklaces, jewelry, credit cards, zippers, or any type of metal that the magnet of the MRI unit would attract. Although open MRI units are now available, they are not in widespread use. Therefore, the nurse needs to check determine whether the client is claustrophobic because the unit is a closed cylinder in which the client hears pops of noise. A number of clients develop claustrophobia that causes the procedure to be cancelled. If the client is claustrophobic, the procedure may need to be rescheduled after an open MRI unit is located or made available. (I, 9)

37. 2. Based on the client's complaints, the nurse should call the surgeon to verify the location of the surgery. The client's complaints indicate radiculopathy of L4–5, but the consent form states L3–4. Radiculopathy of L3–4 involves pain radiating from the back to the buttocks to the posterior thigh to the inner calf. The nurse must act as a client advocate and not ask the client to sign the consent until the correct procedure is identified and confirmed on the consent. The nurse has no legal authority or responsibility to change the consent. The history is a source of information, but when the client is coherent and the history is contradictory, the physician should be contacted to clarify the situation. Ultimately, it is the surgeon's responsibility to identify the site of surgery specified on the surgical consent form. (D, 1)

38. 1. Impaired Physical Mobility related to back pain, muscle spasms, and tissue manipulation is a priority after a laminectomy, because based on individual factors such as the length of time of the disease and previous scarring or injury to the muscles or nerves before the surgery, spasms and pain can be quite severe. Imbalanced Nutrition: Less Than Body Requirements related to inability to eat in the supine position is not a priority problem because the client is encouraged to take fluids as soon as the gag reflex returns, no nausea is present, and bowel sounds begin to return. Bowel Incontinence related to decreased physical activity is not a priority problem because the client is encouraged to sit up and to ambulate to the bathroom with assistance as soon as the anesthesia wears off. Disturbed Body Image related to fear of disfiguring surgical scar should also not be a priority problem because the laminectomy incision is commonly small, possibly as small as 1 inch for a lumbar laminectomy L5–S1 bilateral. (D, 10)

39. 2. Ondansetron hydrochloride (Zofran) is a selective serotonin receptor antagonist that acts centrally to control the client's nausea in the postoperative phase. It does not control muscle spasms, shivering, or dry mouth. (E, 8)

40. 4. Sweeping causes a twisting motion, which should be avoided because twisting can cause undue stress on the recently ruptured disc site, muscle spasms, and a potential recurrent disc rupture. Although the client should not bend at the waist, such as when washing dishes at the sink, the client can dry dishes because no bending is necessary. The client can sit in a firm chair that keeps the back anatomically aligned. The client should not twist and pull, so when making the bed, the client should pull the covers up on one side and then walk around to the other side before trying to pull the covers up there. (E, 10)

41. 4. After a lumbar laminectomy L4–5 left, a client who is returning to work should avoid sitting whenever possible. If the client must sit, he or she should sit only in chairs that allow the knees to be higher than the hips and support the arms to maintain correct body alignment and reduce undue stress on the spine. Maintaining good body postures is most important after a lumbar laminectomy L4–5 left. By 6 weeks after the surgery, the client should have regained stamina. To maintain correct body posture, the client should also place one foot on a stepstool during prolonged standing. Sleeping on the back with a support under the knees is effective in maintaining correct body posture. Maintaining an average weight for height is important in maintaining a healthy back because carrying extra weight caused undue stress on back muscles. (P, 10)

42. 2. Clear yellowish fluid on the dressing may be cerebral spinal fluid. This fluid must be tested for glucose to determine whether it is cerebral spinal fluid. If so, the client is at great risk for an infection of the central nervous system, which has a high mortality rate. The patient should be able to laterally rotate the head and neck, which is above the surgical site in the spinal column. During the nursing postoperative neuromuscular–vascular assessment of movement of the head and neck, the nurse should find results consistent with the preoperative baseline status. Using the standing position to void is normal for a male client. Coughing is the body's defense mechanism to help clear the lungs of the anesthetic agents and to ventilate the lungs in response to a sustained deep inspiration for ventilation of the lower lobes of the lungs. A frequent cough could place a strain on the incision site and should be avoided. Also, a productive cough of thick yellow sputum would indicate the complication of a respiratory infection. (D, 9)

43. 2. The nurse should verify with the surgeon the preferred position to use before applying the brace. Traditionally, the client who had a spinal fusion was asked to lie on the side and log roll onto the brace. Now doctors also have clients stand and sit for the brace application. Therefore, the nurse needs to verify the surgeon's preference. (P, 9)

44. 4. The client should wear a thin cotton undershirt under the brace to prevent the brace from abrading directly against the skin. The cotton material also aids in absorbing any moisture, such as perspiration, which could lead to skin irritation and breakdown. Applying lotion is not recommended before applying the brace because further skin breakdown can result (related to the collection of moisture where microorganisms can grow) and irritants from the lotion can cause further irritation. Applying extra padding (eg, to the iliac crests) is not recommended because the padding can become wrinkled, producing more pressure sites and skin breakdown. Use of baby or talcum powder is not recommended because the irritation from the talcum also can cause irritation and skin breakdown. (E, 9)

45. 1. Typically, the donor site causes more pain than the fused site does because inflammation, swelling, and venous oozing around the nerve endings in the donor site, where the subcuticular tissue was removed, occurs during the first 24 to 48 hours postoperatively. After surgery, the surgeon applies a pressure dressing to the donor site to compress the veins that were transected for the removal of subcutaneous tissue but that did not stop oozing blood after surgical cauterization during the surgical procedure. Pressure on a transected vein, which is low pressure, stops the oozing and loss of blood from the venous site. When the donor site is the fibula, neurovascular checks must be performed every hour to ensure adequate neurologic function of and circulation to the area. The surgeon, not the degree or amount of pain, specifies activity restrictions. (P, 10)

46. 1. A client who has had back surgery should place his feet flat on the floor to avoid strain on the incision. Placing the feet on a low or high footstool or in any other position of comfort with the legs uncrossed increases the pressure on the suture line and increases the inflammation around the involved nerve root, thereby increasing the risk for possible rerupture of the disc site. (E, 9)

47. 4. After a lumbar laminectomy, a client should not sit for prolonged periods in a chair because of the increased pressure against the nerve root and incision site. Assisting with daily hygiene is an appropriate activity during the initial postoperative period because, as with any surgical procedure, the patient needs to return to her optimal level of functioning as soon as possible. There is no limitation on the patient's participation in daily hygiene activities except for her individual response of pain, nausea, vomiting, or weakness. Lying flat in bed is appropriate because it does not cause stress on the spinal column where the laminectomy was performed and the disc tissue was removed. Positions that should be avoided are those that would cause twisting and flexion of the spine. Walking in the hall is an acceptable activity. It promotes good postoperative ventilation, circulation, and return of peristalsis, which are needed for all surgical patients. In addition, walking provides the postoperative lumbar laminectomy patient an opportunity to build up endurance and muscle strength and to promote circulation to the operative and incision sites for healing without twisting or stressing them. (P, 10)

48. 3. Sit-ups are not recommended for the client who has had a lumbar laminectomy, because these exercises place too great a stress on the back. Knee-to-chest lifts, hip tilts, and pelvic tilt exercises are recommended to strengthen back and abdominal muscles. (I, 9)

The Client With an Amputation due to Peripheral Vascular Disease

49. 3. Typically, peripheral vascular disease is considered to be a disorder affecting older adults. Therefore, an age of 39 years would not be considered as a risk factor contributing to the development of peripheral vascular disease. Uncontrolled diabetes mellitus is considered a risk factor for peripheral vascular disease because of the macroangiopathic and microangiopathic changes that result from poor blood glucose control. Cigarette smoking is a known risk factor for peripheral vascular disease. Nicotine is a potent vasoconstrictor. Serum cholesterol levels greater than 200 mg/dL are considered a risk factor for peripheral vascular disease. (D, 4)

50. 2. The client with severe arterial occlusive disease and gangrene of the left great toe would have lost the hair on the leg due to decreased circulation to the skin. Edema around the ankle and lower leg would indicate venous insufficiency of the lower extremity. Thin, soft toenails (ie, not thickened and brittle) are a normal finding. Warmth in the foot indicates adequate circulation to the extremity. Typically the foot would be cool to cold if a severe arterial occlusion were present. (A, 10)

51. 3. The client should be tobacco-free for 30 minutes before the test to avoid false readings related to the vasoconstrictive effects of smoking on the arteries. Because this test is noninvasive, the client does not need to sign a consent form. The client should receive a narcotic analgesic, not a sedative, to control the pain as the blood pressure cuffs are inflated during the Doppler studies to determine the ankle-to-brachial pressure index. The client's ankle should not be covered with a blanket, because the weight of the blanket on the ischemic foot will cause pain. A bed cradle should be used to keep even the weight of a sheet off the affected foot. (I, 9)

52. 2. Slow, steady walking is a recommended activity for the client with peripheral arterial disease because it stimulates the development of collateral circulation needed to ensure adequate tissue oxygenation. The client with peripheral arterial disease should not minimize activity. Activity is necessary to foster the development of collateral circulation. Elevating the legs above the heart is an appropriate strategy for reducing venous congestion. Wearing antiembolism stockings promotes the return of venous circulation, which is important for clients with venous insufficiency. However, their use in clients with peripheral arterial disease may cause the disease to worsen. (D, 10)

53. 1. Daily lubrication, inspection, cleansing, and patting dry of the feet should be performed to prevent cracking of the skin and possible infection. Soaking the feet in warm water should be avoided, because soaking can lead to maceration and subsequent skin breakdown. Additionally, the client with arterial insufficiency typically experiences sensory changes, so the client may be unable to detect water that is too warm, thus placing the client at risk for burns. Antiembolism stockings, appropriate for clients with venous insufficiency, are inappropriate for clients for with arterial insufficiency and could lead to a worsening of the condition. Footwear should be roomy, soft, and protective and allow air to circulate. Therefore, firm, supportive leather shoes would be inappropriate. (I, 9)

54. 2. Encouraging the client who will be undergoing amputation to verbalize his feelings is the most therapeutic response. Asking the client to tell more about how he is feeling helps to elicit information, providing insight into his view of the situation and also providing the nurse with ideas to help him cope. The nurse should avoid value-laden responses, such as, "At least you will still have one good leg to use," that may make the client feel guilty or hostile, thereby blocking further communication. Furthermore, stating that the client still has one good leg ignores his expressed concerns. The client has verbalized feelings of helplessness by using the term "invalid." The nurse needs to focus on this concern and not try to complete the teaching first before discussing what is on the client's mind. The client's needs, not the nurse's needs, must be met first. It is inappropriate for the nurse to assume to know the relationship between the client and his wife or the roles they now must assume as dependent client and caregiver. Additionally, the response about the client's wife caring for him may reinforce the client's feelings of helplessness as an invalid. (I, 5)

55. 2. The level of amputation often cannot be accurately determined until during surgery, when the surgeon can directly assess the adequacy of the circulation of the residual limb. From a moral, ethical, and legal viewpoint, the surgeon attempts to remove as little of the leg as possible. Although a longer residual limb facilitates prosthesis fitting, unless the stump is receiving a good blood supply the prosthesis will not function properly because tissue necrosis will occur. Although the client's ability to walk with a prosthesis is important, it is not a determining factor in the decision about the level of amputation required. Blood supply to the tissue is the primary determinant. (I, 10)

56. 4. The priority action is to draw a mark around the site of bleeding to determine the rate of bleeding. Once the area is marked, the nurse can determine whether the bleeding is increasing or decreasing by the size of the area marked. Because the spot is bright red, the bleeding is most likely arterial in origin. Once the rate and source of bleeding are identified, the surgeon should be notified. The stump is not elevated because adhesions may occur, interfering with the ability to fit a prosthesis. The dressing would be reinforced if the bleeding is determined to be of venous origin, characterized by slow oozing of darker blood that ceases with the application of a pressure dressing. Typically, operative dressings are not changed for 24 hours. Therefore, the dressing is reinforced to prevent organisms from penetrating through the blood-soaked areas of the initial postoperative dressing. (I, 10)

57. 4. The nurse's first action would be to administer the prescribed narcotic analgesic to the client, because this phenomenon is phantom sensation and interventions should be provided to relieve it. Pain relief is the priority. Phantom sensation is a real sensation. It is incorrect and inappropriate to tell a client that it is impossible to feel the pain. Although it does relieve the client's apprehensions to be told that phantom sensations are a real phenomenon, the client needs prompt treatment to relieve the pain sensation. Usually phantom sensation will go away. However, showing the client that the toes are not there does nothing to provide the client with relief. (I, 10)

58. 4. Use of crutches requires significant strength from the triceps muscles. Therefore, efforts are focused on strengthening these muscles in anticipation of crutch walking. Bed and wheelchair push-ups are excellent exercises targeted at the triceps muscles. Abdominal exercises, range-of-motion and isometric exercises of the shoulders, and quadriceps and gluteal setting exercises are not helpful in preparing for crutch walking. (I, 9)

59. 4. When using crutches, the client is taught to support her weight primarily on the hands. Supporting body weight on the axillae, elbows, or upper arms must be avoided to prevent nerve damage from excessive pressure. (I, 9)

60. 4. Before beginning dietary instructions and interventions, the nurse must first assess the client's and family's food preferences, such as pattern of food intake, life cycle, food preferences, and ethnic, cultural, and financial influences. Once this information is obtained, the nurse can begin teaching based on the client's current knowledge level and then building on this knowledge base. (P, 10)

The Client With Fractures

61. 2. Because of the degree of contamination of the open fracture and the time that has passed since the accident, the risk for infection is very high. Therefore, the nurse would be especially alert for signs and symptoms of possible existing infection or early signs of infection, such as debris in the wound site, temperature abnormalities, results of laboratory studies such as complete blood count and wound culture and sensitivities, or heat or redness around or in the wound. Because the client's vital signs and cardiovascular status are stable at this time, hemorrhage is not the primary concern. The client is talking coherently at this point, so his mentation does not suggest that he is in shock. However, assessment for signs and symptoms of hemorrhage and shock would certainly be ongoing. The fracture would be corrected by surgery as soon as possible, thereby minimizing the risk for deformity. (A, 10)

62. 3. Methocarbamol (Robaxin) is a muscle relaxant and acts primarily to relieve muscle spasms. It has no effect on microorganisms, does not reduce itching, and has no effect on decreasing nervousness. (I, 8)

63. 3. Hypotension, tachycardia, and depressed respirations are signs of high levels of ingestion of muscle relaxants, and the client may be developing a habit of taking this drug for a prolonged period. The potential for abuse should be considered when large doses of a muscle relaxant such as Soma are taken for prolonged periods. Expected common side effects would include drowsiness, fatigue, lassitude, blurred vision, headache, ataxia, weakness, and gastrointestinal (GI) upset. Hemorrhage from GI irritation is not associated with this drug. Hypersensitivity reactions would be manifested by pruritus and skin rashes. (D, 8)

64. 3. The nursing assessment is first focused on the region distal to the fracture for neurovascular injury or compromise. When a nerve or blood vessel is severed or obstructed at the actual fracture site, innervation to the nerve or blood flow to the vessel is disrupted below the site; therefore, the area distal to the fracture site is the area of compromised neurologic input or vascular flow and return, not the area above the fracture site or the fracture site itself. The nurse may assess the opposite extremity at the area proximal to the fracture site for a baseline comparison of pulse quality, color, temperature, size, and so on, but the comparison would be made after the initial neurovascular assessment. (A, 10)

65. 3. Clients should not pull out cast padding to scratch inside the cast because of the hazard of skin breakdown and subsequent potential for infection. Clients are encouraged to elevate the casted extremity above the level of the heart to reduce edema and to exercise or move the joints above and below the cast to promote and maintain flexibility and muscle strength. Applying ice for 10 minutes during the first 24 hours helps to reduce edema. (E, 9)

66. 2. The client in a double hip spica cast should avoid eating foods that can be constipating, such as cheese. Rather, fresh fruits and vegetables should be encouraged and the client should be encouraged to drink at least 2500 mL/day. Drinking cranberry juice or foods high in ascorbic acid, which helps to keep urine acidic and thereby avoids the development of renal calculi, is encouraged. The client should be encouraged to establish regular times for elimination to promote regularity in bowel and bladder habits. The client will develop orthostatic hypotension unless the circulatory system is

reconditioned slowly through dangling and standing exercises. (I, 10)

67. 2. A two-point gait involves partial weight bearing on each foot, with each crutch advancing simultaneously with the opposing leg. Advancing a crutch on one side and then advancing the opposite foot, and repeating on the opposite side, illustrates the four-point gait. When the client advances both crutches together and follows by lifting both lower extremities to the same level as the crutches, the gait is called a "swing to" gait. When the client advances both crutches together and follows by lifting both lower extremities to past the level of the crutches, the gait is called a "swing through" gait. The "swing through" gait is often used by paraplegic clients because it allows them to place weight on their legs while the crutches are moved one stride ahead. (P, 9)

68. 1. The wound was left open with a three-way drainage system in place to irrigate the debrided would with normal saline or an antibiotic. Before the debridement, a sample of the would would be taken for culture and sensitivity testing so that an organism-specific antibiotic could be administered to prevent possible serious sequelae of osteomyelitis. Therefore, the nurse would assess the results of the culture and sensitivity report. A pressure dressing would not be applied to an open wound. Rather, a wet-to-dry dressing most likely would be used. There should not be increased pain related to the exposure of nerve endings in the subcutaneous tissue of the wound that was left open to the environment. The bleeding of vessels should be controlled as it would have been if the wound had been closed. Therefore, additional vessel bleeding should not be a problem. (A, 10)

69. 1. The nurse should assess the client's ability to move her toes and for the presence of distal pulses, including a neurovascular assessment of the area below the cast. Increasing pain unrelieved by usual analgesics and occurring 4 to 12 hours after the onset of casting or trauma may be the first sign of compartment syndrome, which can lead to permanent damage to nerves and muscles. Although the nurse can use a pain rating scale or assess for changes in vital signs to objectively assess the client's pain, the client's complaints suggest early and important signs of compartment syndrome requiring immediate intervention. The nurse should not confuse these signs with the potential for drug tolerance. This assessment might be appropriate once the suspicion of compartment syndrome has been ruled out. (I, 10)

70. 4. The client with compartment syndrome may release myoglobin from damaged muscle cell into the circulation. This becomes trapped in the renal tubules, resulting in dark, scanty urine, possibly leading to acute renal failure. Rales may suggest respiratory complications; jaundice suggests liver failure; and generalized edema may suggest heart failure. However, these are not associated with compartment syndrome. (A, 9)

The Client With a Femoral Fracture

71. 4. Passive immunity for tetanus is provided in the form of tetanus antitoxin or tetanus immune globulin. An antitoxin is an antibody to the toxin of an organism. Administering tetanus toxoid, antigen, or vaccine would provide active immunity by stimulating the body to produce its own antibodies. (I, 8)

72. 4. Skeletal traction is not used to pull weight with a boot. Skeletal traction involves the insertion of a wire or a pin into the bone to maintain a pull of 5 to 45 pounds on the area, promoting proper alignment of the fractured bones over a long term. (E, 9)

73. 4. The client with a femoral fracture in balanced suspension traction should not be given a complete bed-bath. Rather, the client is encouraged to participate in self-care and movement in bed, such as with a trapeze triangle. Use of a fracture bedpan is appropriate. A fraction bedpan is lower, and it is easier for the client to move on and off the bedpan without altering the line of traction. Checking for areas of redness or pressure over all areas in contact with the traction or bed, including the ischial tuberosity, is important to prevent possible skin breakdown. The client should be positioned so that the feet do not press against the footboard. Therefore, elevating the head of the bed no more than 25 degrees is recommended to keep the client from moving down in the bed. (P, 9)

74. 3. Neurovascular checks should be performed distal or past the site of the splint, not proximal or above the site of the splint, at least every 4 hours. An injury or compromise to the peripheral nervous innervation or blood flow will reflect a change on the site of the splint after the pathway from the heart and brain. Checking the skin over the greater trochanter is appropriate because the half-ring of the Thompson splint can slide around the greater trochanter area where the traction is applied; it should be checked routinely along with other areas at high risk for pressure necrosis, such as the fibial head, ischial tuberosity, malleoli, and hamstring tendons. Inspecting the pin site is appropriate because any drainage or redness might indicate an infection in the bone in which the pin is inserted. Immediate treatment is imperative to avoid osteomyelitis and possible loss of the limb. Evaluation of the foot for movement is important to obtain neuromuscular–vascular data for assessment in comparison with the baseline data of the affected extremity and with the opposite extremity to detect any compromise of the client's condition. (A, 9)

75. 3. The nurse should send the client to the operating room on his bed with extra help to keep the traction from moving to maintain the femur in the proper alignment before surgery. Transferring the client to a cart with manually suspended traction is inappropriate because doing so places the client at risk for additional trauma to the surrounding neurovascular and soft tissues, as would removing the traction. The surgeon need not be called, because the decision about transferring the client is an independent nursing action. (I, 9)

76. 1. The Pearson attachment supports the lower leg and provides increased stability in the overall traction setup. It also makes it easier to maintain correct alignment. It does not support the thigh and upper leg or prevent flexion deformities in the ankle and foot. It is not attached to the skeletal pin. (I, 9)

77. 1. Fat emboli usually result in symptoms of acute respiratory distress syndrome, such as apprehension, chest pain, cyanosis, dyspnea, tachypnea, tachycardia, and decreased partial pressure of arterial oxygen resulting from poor oxygen exchange. Migraine-like headaches are not a symptom of a fat embolism, but mental confusion, memory loss, and a headache from poor oxygen exchange may be seen with central nervous system involvement. Numbness in the right leg is a peripheral neurovascular response that most likely is related to the femoral fracture. Muscle spasms in the right thigh are a symptom of a neuromuscular response affecting the local muscle around the femoral fracture site. (D, 9)

78. 2. Based on the client's statements, Ineffective Coping is the most appropriate nursing diagnosis, because the client is voicing frustration about the current situation and her inability to move. The nurse should seek ways to help the client adjust to and cope with her present state of immobility. Emphasis should be placed on what the client can do to care for herself, such as participating in her daily care and exercises to maintain muscle strength, to help her maintain some control over her situation. (D, 5)

79. 1. The client can sit up in bed, remaining in the supine position so that an even, sustained amount traction is maintained under the bandage used in the Buck's traction. Maintenance of even, sustained traction decreases the chance that the bandage or traction strap might slip and cause compression or stress on the nerves or vascular tracts, resulting in permanent damage. The client does not have to remain flat but may adjust the head of the bed to varying degrees of elevation while remaining in the supine position. The client should not turn his body to another position, because the bandage may slip. (I, 9)

80. 1. The nurse should assess for signs of skin pressure in the groin area because the Thomas splint, which is a

half-ring that slips over the thigh and suspends the lower extremity in direct skeletal traction, may cause discomfort, pressure, or skin irritation in the groin. The nurse always assesses respirations as part of routine vital signs, but assessing for evidence of decreased breath sounds is not a routine assessment related directly to the Thomas splint. The head of the bed can be elevated to facilitate breathing, but not more than 25 degrees, to avoid continually moving the client toward the foot of the bed from the weight of the traction. The nurse always assesses for pressure areas on dependent parts, but assessing for skin breakdown behind the heel is not a routine assessment related directly to the Thomas splint, in which the heel is free of any contact with padding or metal parts of the Pearson attachment for the balanced suspension traction. The client who is in a Thomas splint is able to use a bedpan, especially the fracture bedpan for a female client and the urinal for a male to urinate. Urinary incontinence should not be a special assessment directly related to the Thomas splint, but it may be a client-specific assessment. (A, 9)

81. 1. The client's assisting as much as possible in his care and increasing participation over time indicate that the client has accomplished self-care by gaining a sense of control. If the client lets the nurse complete his care without interfering, his behavior would indicate passivity, possibly from denial or depression. If the client allows his wife to assume total responsibility for his care or to complete his care, he still has a self-care deficit and a successful outcome has not been reached. (E, 7)

82. 2. Fever, night sweats, chills, restlessness, and restrictive movement of the fractured leg are clinical manifestations of osteomyelitis, which is a pyogenic bone infection caused by bacteria, usually staphylococcus, a virus, or a fungus. The bone is inaccessible to macrophages and antibodies for protection against infections, so an infection in this site can become serious quickly. The client with a pulmonary or fat embolus would develop symptoms of pulmonary compromise, such as shortness of breath, chest pain, angina, and mental confusion. Symptoms of urinary tract infection would include pain over the suprapubic, groin, or back region with fever and chills, with no restrictive movement of the leg. (D, 9)

83. 1. With osteomyelitis, scar tissue forms because of the continuing presence of the infecting organism, usually *Staphylococcus aureus*. Subsequently, pus and bacteria collect to form avascular tissue. This scar tissue does not absorb the antibiotics. The scar tissue or devitalized (dead) tissue must be scraped from the bone so that antibiotic irrigation can be instituted to clear up the chronic osteomyelitis. (D, 10)

The Client With a Spinal Cord Injury

84. 3. The priority concern is to immobilize the head and neck to prevent further trauma when a fractured vertebra is unstable and easily displaced. Although wrapping and supporting the extremities is important, it does not take priority over immobilizing the head and neck. Pain usually is not a significant consideration with this type of injury. Cushioning is contraindicated. The neck should be kept in a neutral position and immobilized. Flexion of the neck is avoided. (P, 2)

85. 3. This client has a spinal cord injury of the sacral region of the spinal cord and will have bladder and bowel dysfunction, as well as loss of sensation and muscle control below the injury. The other options are true of a client who has quadriplegia. (A, 10)

86. 2. Although assessment of renal status, gastrointestinal function, and biliary function is important, with the spinal cord transection at T4 the client's vascular status is the primary focus of the nursing assessment, because the sympathetic feedback system is lost and the client is at risk for hypotension and bradycardia. (A, 10)

87. 1. The client with a spinal cord transection above T5 is least likely to develop diarrhea. Rather, constipation due to atonia would be possible. The client with a spinal cord transection above T5 is at risk for development of a paralytic ileus because the sympathetic nerve innervation to the vagus nerve, which dominates of all the vessels and organs below T5 (eg, the intestinal tract), has been disrupted and therefore so has movement or peristalsis. The client is at risk for development of stress ulcers because the sympathetic nerve innervation to the stomach has been disrupted, which results in an excessive release of hydrochloric acid in the stomach, allowing contact of hydrochloric acid with the stomach mucosa. The client does not feel subjective signs of stress ulcers (eg, pain, guarding, tenderness) and therefore is at increased risk for bleeding because complications of an ulcer can develop before early diagnosis. (A, 9)

88. 1. The client should eat enough calories to maintain her desired weight, a positive nitrogen balance, and enough protein to help decrease the rate of muscle atrophy and prevent skin breakdown and infection. The client with a spinal cord injury does not have poikilothermism, the ability to adjust body temperature to the environmental temperature. The client should add additional clothes or coverage below the level of transection in cool environments. The client does not sweat below the level of transection and should be sensitive to the possibility of overheating in extremely hot climates and the need for sprinkling or moving into an air-conditioned environment. The client with intermittent nasogastric suctioning is at risk for development of

a metabolic alkalosis and electrolyte imbalance that leads to decreased tissue perfusion; therefore, the client needs to increase the sodium and potassium in her diet, not decrease the sodium. (P, 9)

89. 4. Measuring the leg girth is the most appropriate method, because the usual signs, such as a positive Homan's sign, pain, and tenderness, are not present. Other means of assessing for a deep vein thrombosis in a client with a spinal cord injury are through a Doppler examination and impedance plethysmography. (A, 9)

90. 3. During the period of spinal shock, the bladder is completely atonic and will continue to fill passively unless the client is catheterized. (A, 9)

91. 4. The movements occur from muscle reflexes and cannot be initiated or controlled by the brain. After the period of spinal shock, the muscles gradually become spastic owing to an increased sensitivity of the lower motor neurons. It is an expected occurrence and does not indicate that healing is taking place or that the client will walk again. The movement is not voluntary and cannot be brought under voluntary control. (I, 10)

92. 3. Long-bone demineralization is a serious consequence of the loss of weight bearing. An excessive calcium load is brought to the kidneys, and precipitation may occur, predisposing to stone formation. Excessive intake of dairy products does not make constipation more common. Immobility does not increase calcium absorption from the intestine. Dairy products do not necessarily contribute to weight gain. (I, 7)

93. 2. The woman with spinal cord injury can participate in sexual activity but might not experience orgasm. Cessation in the nerve pathway may occur in spinal cord injury, but this does not negate the client's mental and emotional needs to creatively participate with her partner in a sexual relationship and to reach orgasm. An indwelling urinary (Foley) catheter may be left in place during intercourse and need not be removed because the Foley catheter is placed in the urethra, which is not the channel used for sexual intercourse. There are no contraindications, such as hypertension, to sexual activity in a woman with spinal cord injury. Sexual intercourse is allowed, and hypertension should be manageable. Because a spinal cord injury does not affect fertility, the client should have access to family planning information so that an unplanned pregnancy can be avoided. (E, 7)

94. 3. Spinal cord injury represents a physical loss; grief is the normal response to this loss. Working through grief entails reviewing memories and eventually letting go of them. The process may take as long as 2 years. Telling the client to be patient and that adjustment takes time is a clichéd type of response, one that is not empathetic or responsive to the client's needs. Telling the client to focus on today does not allow time for the grief process, which is necessary for the client to work through and adjust to the loss. The client is not escaping but is reminiscing on what is lost, to work through the grieving process. (I, 5)

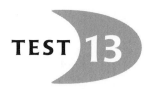
The Client With Cancer

Select the one best answer, and indicate your choice by filling in the circle in front of the option.

The Client at Risk for Cancer

1. Which of the following would be considered an iatrogenic cause of cancer?
   ○ 1. Ionizing radiation from radon.
   ○ 2. Ionizing radiation from uranium ore.
   ○ 3. X-rays used to treat a tumor.
   ○ 4. Ultraviolet radiation from the sun.

2. An epidemiologic study or investigation is to be conducted on workers in uranium mines who are currently free of any cancer. Subjects are to be monitored over a 5-year period, and the incidence rates of certain types of cancers are to be determined. This study design illustrates what kind of research study?
   ○ 1. Prospective study.
   ○ 2. Historical retrospective study.
   ○ 3. Retrospective study.
   ○ 4. Historical prospective study.

3. Carcingogenesis is irreversible in which of the following stages?
   ○ 1. Progression stage.
   ○ 2. Promotion stage.
   ○ 3. Initiation stage.
   ○ 4. Regression stage.

4. Cancer prevalence is defined as
   ○ 1. the likelihood cancer will occur in a lifetime.
   ○ 2. the number of persons with cancer at a given point in time.
   ○ 3. the number of new cancers in a year.
   ○ 4. all cancer cases more than 5 years old.

5. Which of the following groups would benefit most from education regarding potential risk factors for melanoma?
   ○ 1. Adults older than 35 years of age.
   ○ 2. Senior citizens who have been repeatedly exposed to the effects of ultraviolet A and ultraviolet B rays.

○ 3. Parents with children.
○ 4. Employees of a chemical factory.

6. A nurse is providing education in a community setting about general measures to avoid excessive sun exposure. Which of the following recommendations is appropriate?
   ○ 1. Reapply sunscreen only if you go into the water.
   ○ 2. Avoid peak exposure hours from 9 AM to 1 PM.
   ○ 3. Wear loosely woven clothing for added ventilation.
   ○ 4. Apply sunscreen with a sun protection factor (SPF) of 15 or more before sun exposure.

7. A 29-year-old woman is concerned about her personal risk factors for malignant melanoma. She is upset because her 49-year-old sister was recently diagnosed with the disease. After gathering information about the client's history of sun exposure, the nurse's best response would be to explain that
   ○ 1. some melanomas have a familial component and she should seek medical advice.
   ○ 2. her personal risk is low because most melanomas occur at age 60 or later.
   ○ 3. her personal risk is low because melanoma does not have a familial component.
   ○ 4. she should not worry because she did not experience severe sunburn as a child.

8. The nurse is palpating a female client's breast while assessing for breast disease. In Figure 1, the area of the breast in which tumors are most commonly found is
   ○ 1. Area 1.
   ○ 2. Area 2.
   ○ 3. Area 3.
   ○ 4. Area 4.

9. While being educated by the nurse about breast self-examination, a client asks what the rationale is for

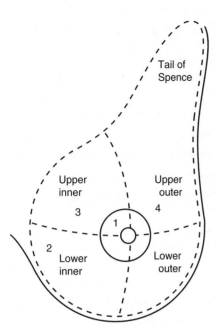

Figure 1.

moving her arms in different positions while standing in front of a mirror. The nurse explains that these positions are used to

○ 1. increase the examiner's comfort during procedure.

○ 2. more easily diagnose any masses.

○ 3. determine whether there is any nipple discharge with movement.

○ 4. emphasize any change in shape or contour of the breast.

10. A 17-year-old, sexually active female client is seen in the family planning clinic and requests oral contraceptives. Before examination, the nurse should explain the importance of regular Pap smears. This recommendation is based on the current screening guidelines of the American Cancer Society (ACS) for Pap smears, which state that

○ 1. Pap smears are recommended every other year.

○ 2. if four consecutive annual Pap smears are negative, the client should schedule repeat Pap smears every 3 years.

○ 3. the initial Pap smear should be done at age 18, or earlier if the woman is sexually active.

○ 4. if four consecutive smears are negative, the client should request a colposcopy.

11. A client with a family history of cancer asks the nurse what the single most important risk factor for cancer is. Which of the following risk factors should the nurse discuss?

○ 1. Family history.

○ 2. Lifestyle choices.

○ 3. Age.

○ 4. Menopause or hormonal events.

12. According to experimental and epidemiologic evidence, it is suggested that a high-fat diet increases the risk of several cancers. Which of the following cancers is linked to a high-fat diet?

○ 1. Ovarian.

○ 2. Lung.

○ 3. Colon.

○ 4. Liver.

13. A 42-year-old female highway construction worker is concerned about her cancer risks. She reveals that she has been married for 18 years, has two children, smokes one pack of cigarettes per day, and drinks one to two beers with her husband after work almost every day. She is 30 pounds overweight, eats fast food often, and eats fresh fruits and vegetables rarely. Her mother was diagnosed with breast cancer 2 years ago. Her father and an aunt both died of lung cancer. She had a basal cell carcinoma removed from her cheek 3 years earlier. What behavioral changes should the nurse instruct this client to make first?

○ 1. Decrease fat in the diet, decrease alcohol consumption, and use sunscreen every day.

○ 2. Decrease intake of salt-cured food, lose weight, and stop smoking.

○ 3. Stop drinking beer, decrease fiber in the diet, and use sun protection.

○ 4. Stop smoking, use sun protection, and lose weight.

14. A nurse who is teaching smoking cessation programs to healthy adult smokers is participating in what type of prevention activity?

○ 1. Primary.

○ 2. Secondary.

○ 3. Tertiary.

○ 4. Nonspecific.

15. The incidence and risk of cancer increase when smoking is combined with

○ 1. asbestos exposure and alcohol consumption.

○ 2. ultraviolet radiation exposure and alcohol consumption.

○ 3. asbestos exposure and ultraviolet radiation exposure.

○ 4. alcohol consumption and a diet high in nitrite-cured foods.

16. A 60-year-old man comes to the clinic with complaints of hoarseness. What information will be helpful in determining his risk for head and neck cancer?

○ 1. Patterns of medication use and history of alcohol consumption.

○ 2. Exposure to sun and family history of head and neck cancers.

○ 3. Exposure to wood dust and a high-fat diet.

○ 4. History of tobacco use and history of alcohol consumption.

17. A 42-year-old woman is interested in making dietary changes to reduce her risk of colon cancer. What dietary selections would the nurse suggest?
   ○ 1. Croissant, granola and peanut butter squares, whole milk.
   ○ 2. Bran muffin, skim milk, stir-fried broccoli.
   ○ 3. Granola, bagel with cream cheese, cauliflower salad.
   ○ 4. Oatmeal, raisin cookies, baked potato with sour cream, turkey sandwich.

18. Which of the following is an environmental factor that increases the risk of cancer?
   ○ 1. Gender.
   ○ 2. Nutrition.
   ○ 3. Immunologic status.
   ○ 4. Age.

19. A client at risk for lung cancer asks why he is scheduled for a computed tomography (CT) scan as part of his initial workup. The nurse's best response is which of the following?
   ○ 1. "The CT is far superior to magnetic resonance imaging for evaluating lymph node metastasis."
   ○ 2. "The CT is noninvasive and readily available."
   ○ 3. "The CT is useful for distinguishing small differences in tissue density and detecting nodal involvement."
   ○ 4. "The CT can distinguish a malignant from a non-malignant adenopathy."

20. Lifestyle influences that are considered risk factors for colorectal cancer include
   ○ 1. a diet low in vitamin C.
   ○ 2. a high dietary intake of artificial sweeteners (Aspartame).
   ○ 3. a high-fat, low-fiber diet.
   ○ 4. multiple sex partners.

21. The development of a culturally sensitive health education program for the socioeconomically disadvantaged requires the nurse to
   ○ 1. locate the program at an existing government facility.
   ○ 2. integrate folk beliefs and traditions into the content.
   ○ 3. prepare materials in the primary language of the program sponsor.
   ○ 4. exclude community leaders from initial planning efforts.

The Client With Pain

22. A 62-year-old woman is taking long-acting morphine 120 mg every 12 hours for pain from metastatic breast cancer. She can have 20 mg of immediate-release morphine every 3 to 4 hours as needed for breakthrough pain. The physician should be notified if the client uses more than how many breakthrough doses of morphine in 24 hours?
   ○ 1. Seven.
   ○ 2. Four.
   ○ 3. Two.
   ○ 4. One.

23. In addition to acetaminophen, which drugs are recommended from Step 1 of the World Health Organization (WHO) analgesic ladder for the treatment of mild to moderate cancer-related pain?
   ○ 1. Oxycodone.
   ○ 2. Nonsteroidal anti-inflammatory drugs (NSAIDs).
   ○ 3. Codeine.
   ○ 4. Propoxyphene.

24. Assessment of a client taking an NSAID for pain management should include specific questions regarding which of the following systems?
   ○ 1. Gastrointestinal.
   ○ 2. Renal.
   ○ 3. Pulmonary.
   ○ 4. Cardiac.

25. Which of the following best describes a client's response to chronic pain?
   ○ 1. Elevated vital signs, physical inactivity, facial grimacing, and periods of anxiety.
   ○ 2. Normal vital signs, physical inactivity, and normal facial expressions.
   ○ 3. Normal vital signs, normal facial expressions, and moaning.
   ○ 4. Elevated vital signs, grimacing, and depression.

26. Which of the following terms describes the condition of a client who requires an increase in dosage to maintain adequate analgesia?
   ○ 1. Pseudoaddiction.
   ○ 2. Physical dependence.
   ○ 3. Psychological dependence.
   ○ 4. Drug tolerance.

27. A client is experiencing severe pain from advanced cancer disease. The client's son is concerned about the drugs the client has taken and wonders which are the best. The nurse tells him that, overall, the drug of choice to treat advanced cancer pain is
   ○ 1. methadone (Dolophine).
   ○ 2. oxycodone.
   ○ 3. morphine sulfate.
   ○ 4. hydromorphone (Dilaudid).

28. A 52-year-old man was discharged from the hospital for cancer-related pain. His pain appeared to be well controlled on the intravenous (IV) morphine. He was switched to oral morphine when discharged 2 days ago. He now reports his pain as an 8 on a 10-point scale and wants the IV morphine. Which of the

following represents the most likely explanation for the patient's reports of inadequate pain control?
- ○ 1. He is addicted to the IV morphine.
- ○ 2. He is going through withdrawal from the IV opioid.
- ○ 3. He is physically dependent on the IV morphine.
- ○ 4. He is undermedicated on the oral opioid.

29. Which of the following components of a thorough pain assessment is most significant?
- ○ 1. Intensity.
- ○ 2. Cause.
- ○ 3. Aggravating factors.
- ○ 4. Location.

30. A 48-year-old client with cancer has been receiving 10 mg of IV morphine while hospitalized. In order to give an equivalent dose of oral morphine, the nurse should be sure the physician has ordered which of the following doses?
- ○ 1. 25 mg.
- ○ 2. 30 mg.
- ○ 3. 40 mg.
- ○ 4. 10 mg.

31. Which of the following reasons explains why meperidine (Demerol) is not recommended for chronic cancer-related pain?
- ○ 1. It has a high potential for abuse.
- ○ 2. It has agonist–antagonist properties.
- ○ 3. It must be given intramuscularly to be effective.
- ○ 4. It contains a metabolite that causes seizures.

32. A 60-year-old woman with chronic cancer pain has been receiving opiates for 4 months. She rated her pain as an 8 on a 10-point scale before starting the opioid medication. She has just had a thorough examination with no new evidence of increased disease, yet her pain is close to 8 again. The most likely explanation for her increasing pain is
- ○ 1. development of an addiction to the opioids.
- ○ 2. tolerance to the opioid.
- ○ 3. withdrawal from the opioid.
- ○ 4. placebo effect has decreased.

33. The nurse teaches the client with chronic cancer pain about optimal pain control. Which of the following recommendations is most effective for pain control?
- ○ 1. Get used to some pain and use a little less medication than needed to keep from being addicted.
- ○ 2. Take prescribed analgesics on an around-the-clock schedule to prevent recurrent pain.
- ○ 3. Take analgesics only when pain returns.
- ○ 4. Take enough analgesics around the clock so that you can sleep 12 to 16 hours a day to block the pain.

The Client Who Requires Symptom Management

34. Which of the following nursing interventions would be most helpful in making the respiratory effort of a client with metastatic lung cancer more efficient?
- ○ 1. Teaching the client diaphragmatic breathing techniques.
- ○ 2. Administering cough suppressants as ordered.
- ○ 3. Teaching and encouraging pursed-lip breathing.
- ○ 4. Placing the client in a low semi-Fowler's position.

35. When assessing the client with lung cancer who is dyspneic, the nurse observes which of the following behaviors?
- ○ 1. Euphoria.
- ○ 2. Anger.
- ○ 3. Anxiety.
- ○ 4. Laziness.

36. The nurse is teaching a 17-year-old client and the client's family about what to expect with high-dose chemotherapy and the effects of neutropenia. What should the nurse teach as the most reliable early indicator of infection in a neutropenic client?
- ○ 1. Fever.
- ○ 2. Chills.
- ○ 3. Tachycardia.
- ○ 4. Dyspnea.

37. A 28-year-old client with cancer is afraid of experiencing a febrile reaction associated with blood transfusions. He asks the nurse if this will happen to him. The nurse's best response is which of the following?
- ○ 1. "Febrile reactions are caused when antibodies on the surface of blood cells in the transfusion are directed against antigens of the recipient."
- ○ 2. "Febrile reactions can usually be prevented by administering antipyretics and antihistamines before the start of the transfusion."
- ○ 3. "Febrile reactions are rarely immune-mediated reactions and can be a sign of hemolytic transfusion."
- ○ 4. "Febrile reactions primarily occur within 15 minutes after initiation of the transfusion and occur during the blood transfusion."

38. A 56-year-old male client is admitted to the oncology unit for dyspnea. He recently had a pneumonectomy for treatment of lung cancer. The client has not had any other cancer treatment therapies. The increased dyspnea is most likely caused by
- ○ 1. fibrotic changes in lung parenchyma.
- ○ 2. pneumonia or bronchitis.
- ○ 3. anemia related to myelosuppression.
- ○ 4. pericardial effusion.

39. Which of the following has been associated with fatigue from cancer chemotherapy?
○ 1. Decreased quality of life.
○ 2. Increased risk of infection.
○ 3. Improved disease prognosis.
○ 4. Increased pain.

40. When the nurse is teaching the client and family how to manage possible nausea and vomiting at home, which of the following should be discussed?
○ 1. Eating frequent, small meals throughout the day.
○ 2. Eating three normal meals a day.
○ 3. Eating only cold foods with no odor.
○ 4. Limiting the amount of fluid intake.

41. A client informs the nurse that she is using an herbal therapy while receiving chemotherapy. Which of the following actions should the nurse take?
○ 1. Determine what substances the client is using and make sure that the physician is aware of all therapies the client is using.
○ 2. Guide the client in the decision-making process to select either Western or alternative medicine.
○ 3. Encourage the client to seek alternative modalities that do not require the ingestion of substances.
○ 4. Recommend that the client stop using the alternative medicines immediately.

42. A terminally ill 82-year-old client in hospice care is experiencing nausea and vomiting because of a partial bowel obstruction. Conservative management of the nausea and vomiting may be achieved with the use of
○ 1. a nasogastric suction tube.
○ 2. intravenous antiemetics.
○ 3. osmotic laxatives.
○ 4. a clear liquid diet.

43. A 62-year-old man is dying from metastatic lung cancer, and all treatments have been discontinued. The client's breathing pattern is labored with gurgling sounds. The client's wife asks the nurse, "Can't you do something to help with his breathing?" Which of the following is the nurse's best response in this situation?
○ 1. Direct the unlicensed personnel to assess the client's vital signs and provide oral care.
○ 2. Suction the client so that the client's wife knows all interventions were performed.
○ 3. Reposition the client, elevate the head of the bed, and provide a cool compress.
○ 4. Explain to the wife that dying clients do not need suctioning.

44. A 40-year-old woman is losing most of her hair as a result of chemotherapy. Which of the following statements best explains chemotherapy-induced alopecia?
○ 1. "The new growth of hair will be gray."

○ 2. "The hair loss is temporary."
○ 3. "New hair growth will always be same texture and color as it was before chemotherapy."
○ 4. "The client should avoid use of wigs when possible."

45. A 58-year-old man is going to have chemotherapy for lung cancer. He asks the nurse how the chemotherapeutic drugs will work. The most accurate explanation the nurse can give is which of the following?
○ 1. "Chemotherapy affects all rapidly dividing cells."
○ 2. "The molecular structure of the DNA is altered."
○ 3. "Cancer cells are susceptible to drug toxins."
○ 4. "Chemotherapy encourages cancer cells to divide."

46. A 62-year-old man with a history of chronic obstructive pulmonary disease (COPD) and metastatic carcinoma of the lung has not responded to radiation therapy and is being admitted to the hospice program. Initial client assessment will most likely reveal that the client has
○ 1. ascites.
○ 2. pleural friction rub.
○ 3. dyspnea.
○ 4. peripheral edema.

47. The nurse is working with a client who has cancer to improve the client's independence in activities of daily living after radiation therapy. Which of the following is an appropriate nursing intervention?
○ 1. Refer the client to a community support group after discharge from the rehabilitation unit.
○ 2. Make certain that a family member is present for the rehabilitation sessions.
○ 3. Provide positive reinforcement for skills achieved.
○ 4. Inform the client of rehabilitation plans made by the rehabilitation team.

48. When teaching about prevention of infection to a client with a long-term venous catheter, the nurse can document that the client has understood discharge instructions when the client states which of the following?
○ 1. "I will not remove the dressing until I return to the clinic next week."
○ 2. "My husband or I will do the dressing changes three times per week, exactly the way you showed us."
○ 3. "I will monitor my temperature once each weekday."
○ 4. "I know it is very important to wash my hands after irrigating the catheter."

49. A 58-year-old client with pancreatic cancer, who has been bed-bound for 3 weeks, has just returned from having a left subclavian, long-term, tunneled catheter inserted for administration of analgesics. The nurse has not yet received radiographic results for confirmation of placement. The client becomes restless and dyspneic and complains of chest pain radiating to the middle of his back. Physical assessment reveals tachycardia and absent breath sounds in the left lung. The nurse suspects that the client is experiencing

○ 1. an air embolus.

○ 2. a pneumothorax.

○ 3. a pulmonary embolus.

○ 4. a myocardial infarction.

50. In setting goals for a client with advanced liver cancer who has poor nutrition, the nurse determines that which of the following is a realistic desired outcome for the client?

○ 1. Normalize albumin levels.

○ 2. Return to ideal body weight.

○ 3. Gain 1 pound every 2 weeks.

○ 4. Maintain current weight.

51. The nurse administers a bolus tube feeding to a client with cancer. Which of the following nursing interventions is most appropriate to decrease the risk for aspiration?

○ 1. Place the client on bed rest with the head of the bed elevated to 60 degrees for 2 hours.

○ 2. Place the client on the left side with the head of the bed at 45 degrees for 15 minutes.

○ 3. Assist the client out of bed to sit upright in a chair for 1 hour.

○ 4. Ask the client to rest in bed with the head of the bed elevated to 30 degrees for 20 minutes.

52. A client with colon cancer had a left hemiolectomy 3 weeks previously. The client is still having difficulty maintaining an adequate oral intake to meet metabolic needs for optimal healing. Which of the following nutritional support methods would the nurse anticipate for the client?

○ 1. Total parenteral nutrition through a central catheter.

○ 2. Intravenous infusion of dextrose.

○ 3. Nasogastric feeding tube with protein supplement.

○ 4. Jejunostomy for high caloric feedings.

53. A client with stomach cancer is admitted to the oncology unit after vomiting for 3 days. Physical assessment findings include irregular pulse, muscle twitching, and complaints of prickling sensations in the fingers and hands. Laboratory results include a potassium level of 2.9 mEq/L, a pH of 7.46, and a bicarbonate level of 29 mEq/L. The client is experiencing

○ 1. respiratory alkalosis.

○ 2. respiratory acidosis.

○ 3. metabolic alkalosis.

○ 4. metabolic acidosis.

54. A 32-year-old woman meets with the nurse on her first office visit since undergoing a left mastectomy. When asked how she is doing, the woman says her appetite is still not good, she is not getting much sleep because she doesn't go to bed until her husband is asleep, and she is really anxious to get back to work. Which of the following nursing interventions should the nurse explore to support the client's current needs?

○ 1. Call the physician to discuss allowing the client to return to work earlier.

○ 2. Suggest that the client learn relaxation techniques for help with her insomnia.

○ 3. Perform a nutritional assessment to assess for anorexia.

○ 4. Ask open-ended questions about sexuality issues related to her mastectomy.

55. Which of the following client situations would require the most intensive nursing interventions for immobility?

○ 1. A 38-year-old woman receiving internal radiation therapy for cervical cancer.

○ 2. A 7-year-old boy with leukemia hospitalized for induction of high-dose chemotherapy.

○ 3. A 75-year-old man with metastatic prostate cancer hospitalized for a pathologic fracture of the femur.

○ 4. A 6-month-old undergoing surgery for placement of a central venous catheter.

56. Immobility affects several body systems because of a reduction in the amount of weight bearing and physical activity. Which of the following is most indicative of the changes that can occur with immobility?

○ 1. Cardiovascular workload increases, lung expansion increases.

○ 2. Cardiovascular workload decreases, lung expansion increases.

○ 3. Cardiovascular workload increases, metabolism decreases.

○ 4. Metabolism increases, lung expansion decreases.

57. A 56-year-old client is receiving chemotherapy that has the potential to cause pulmonary toxicity. Which of the following symptoms indicates a toxic response to the chemotherapy?

○ 1. Decrease in appetite.

○ 2. Drowsiness.

○ 3. Spasms of the diaphragm.

○ 4. Cough and shortness of breath.

58. A 52-year-old client with lung cancer is calling the outpatient center with complaints of a low-grade fever of 100.6°F (38.1°C), nonproductive cough, and increasing fatigue. He completed the radiation ther-

apy to the mass in his right lung and mediastinum 10 weeks ago and has a follow-up appointment to see the physician in 2 weeks. What is most the appropriate response for the telephone triage nurse?

○ 1. Advise the client to take two acetaminophen tablets every 4 to 6 hours for 2 days and call back if his temperature increases to 101.0°F (38.3°C) or greater.

○ 2. Advise the client that this is an expected side effect of the radiation therapy and to keep his appointment in 2 weeks.

○ 3. Advise the client to come to the office to be examined today.

○ 4. Advise the client to go to the nearest emergency room.

59. A 52-year-old African American woman has a history of breast cancer. She has developed recurrent pleural effusions. Before a scheduled thoracentesis for palliation of symptoms, the nurse should anticipate which of the following orders?

○ 1. Arterial blood gases.

○ 2. Electrocardiogram.

○ 3. White blood cell (WBC) count with differential.

○ 4. Posterior and lateral view (radiographs) of chest.

60. Impaired Spontaneous Ventilation is a nursing diagnosis most likely applicable to which of the following patient populations?

○ 1. Clients with lymphatic malignancies who are undergoing chemotherapy.

○ 2. Clients with hematopoietic malignancies who are undergoing chemotherapy.

○ 3. Clients with head and neck malignancies who are undergoing surgery.

○ 4. Clients with brain tumors who are undergoing radiation.

61. A 58-year-old man has just had a sclerosing agent instilled after chest tube drainage of a pleural effusion. The nurse should instruct the client to

○ 1. lie still to prevent a pneumothorax.

○ 2. sit upright with arms on an overhead table to promote lung expansion.

○ 3. change position frequently to distribute the agent.

○ 4. lie on the side where the thoracentesis was done to hold pressure on the chest tube site.

62. After surgery for head and neck cancer, a 67-year-old man has a permanent tracheostomy. One of the most important long-term interventions the nurse can teach the client and his family is to emphasize the importance of

○ 1. providing tracheostomy site care.

○ 2. addressing the psychosocial issues related to tracheostomy.

○ 3. observing for early signs and symptoms of skin breakdown around the tracheostomy site.

○ 4. using humidifiers to prevent thick, tenacious secretions.

63. Which of the following signs and symptoms would the nurse expect to find in a client with malignant pleural effusions?

○ 1. Hiccups, anxiety.

○ 2. Cough, weight gain.

○ 3. Peripheral edema, temperature of 99°F (37.2°C).

○ 4. Chest pain, dyspnea.

64. A 56-year-old woman is undergoing a thoracentesis. Which of the following outcomes of the procedure is *least* likely?

○ 1. Treatment of recurrent malignant effusion.

○ 2. Diagnosis of underlying disease.

○ 3. Palliation of symptoms.

○ 4. Relief of acute respiratory distress.

65. Which of the following symptoms is associated with anemia?

○ 1. Decreased salivation.

○ 2. Bradycardia.

○ 3. Cold intolerance.

○ 4. Nausea.

66. The nurse is assisting the physician with a thoracentesis for a client with suspected lung cancer. If the client has a malignant effusion, the nurse would expect the fluid to be

○ 1. milky white.

○ 2. straw-colored.

○ 3. turbid.

○ 4. bloody.

67. Many oncology clients are at risk for development of a hypercoagulable state and thrombosis. Laboratory tests to monitor for these complications include

○ 1. carcinoembryonic antigen (CEA).

○ 2. α-fetoprotein (AFP).

○ 3. prothrombin time (PT) and partial thromboplastin time (PTT).

○ 4. Complete blood count (CBC) with differential.

68. One of the most serious blood coagulation complications for individuals with cancer and for those undergoing cancer treatments is disseminated intravascular coagulation (DIC). The most common cause of this bleeding disorder is

○ 1. underlying liver disease.

○ 2. brain metastasis.

○ 3. intravenous heparin therapy.

○ 4. sepsis.

69. A 42-year-old client has a platelet count of 22,000 cells/mm^3 and has petechiae on the lower extremities. Petechiae are

○ 1. blackish colored moles arising from the nevi.

○ 2. purplish tiny nodules usually appearing over the feet and legs.

○ 3. dime-sized, dry, scaly lesions.

○ 4. tiny purplish red spots visible under the skin.

70. A 62-year-old woman has had a left modified radical mastectomy with axillary node dissection. The nurse is aware that lymphedema is a common complication that can occur

○ 1. with right-sided radical mastectomies.

○ 2. in older women.

○ 3. 7 to 10 days after surgery or not at all.

○ 4. from 6 weeks to 20 years after surgery.

71. Formation of blood clots or thrombi is a complication that can occur in clients with long-term vascular access devices (VADs). To prevent or minimize the risk of thrombus formation, prophylactic administration of daily medication appears to be helpful. What medication would the nurse expect to be ordered?

○ 1. Urokinase.

○ 2. Vitamin B_{12}.

○ 3. Warfarin (Coumadin).

○ 4. Acetaminophen (Tylenol).

72. The client with lymphedema has an increased risk of cellulitis and lymphangitis because of

○ 1. fragility of the capillaries.

○ 2. myelosuppression of the bone marrow.

○ 3. stagnation of accumulated fluid.

○ 4. increased use of extremity.

73. A 38-year-old female client with a history of breast-conserving surgery, axillary node dissection, and radiation therapy calls the clinic to report that her arm is red, warm to touch, and slightly swollen. Which of the following actions should the nurse suggest?

○ 1. Apply warm compresses to the affected arm.

○ 2. Elevate the arm on two pillows.

○ 3. See the physician immediately.

○ 4. Schedule an appointment within 2 to 3 weeks.

74. The nurse is assessing a 42-year-old client with cancer. He has lost 1 pound in 4 weeks. He is taking Compazine for nausea. He has a temperature of 101°F (38.3°C). The fever is indicative of

○ 1. inadequate nutrition.

○ 2. new resistance to current antiemetic therapy.

○ 3. expected response to chemotherapy treatment.

○ 4. infection.

75. A pneumonectomy is a surgical procedure sometimes indicated for treatment of non–small-cell lung cancer. A pneumonectomy involves removal of

○ 1. an entire lung field.

○ 2. a small, wedge-shaped lung surface.

○ 3. one lobe of a lung.

○ 4. one or more segments of a lung lobe.

76. Many biologic response modifiers (BRMs) have expected side effects of fever and chills or a flu-like syndrome. These side effects typically

○ 1. are controlled with antipyretics.

○ 2. last 24 to 72 hours.

○ 3. increase in intensity with continued therapy.

○ 4. have a biphasic pattern.

77. A 36-year-old man with lymphoma presents with signs of impending septic shock 9 days after chemotherapy. The nurse could expect which of the following to be present?

○ 1. Flushing, decreased oxygen saturation, mild hypotension.

○ 2. Low-grade fever, chills, tachycardia.

○ 3. Elevated temperature, oliguria, hypotension.

○ 4. High-grade fever, normal blood pressure, increased respirations.

78. An appropriate nursing intervention for clients with fatigue related to cancer treatment includes teaching the client to

○ 1. increase fluid intake.

○ 2. minimize naps or periods of rest during day.

○ 3. conserve energy by prioritizing activities.

○ 4. limit dietary intake of high-fiber foods.

79. The nurse is aware that the most common issue associated with sleep disturbances in the hospitalized client with cancer is

○ 1. social.

○ 2. nutritional.

○ 3. cultural.

○ 4. psychological.

80. Which of the following represents the most appropriate nursing intervention for a client with pruritus caused by cancer or the treatments?

○ 1. Administration of antihistamines.

○ 2. Steroids.

○ 3. Silk sheets.

○ 4. Medicated cool baths.

81. The nurse is caring for a client with cancer who has intractable dyspnea. The nurse is aware that the physician may order which of the following types of drugs to relieve the dyspnea?

○ 1. Mucolytic agents.

○ 2. Antidepressants.

○ 3. Narcotics.

○ 4. Diuretics.

82. A 62-year-old woman has experienced a flare-up of pruritus. Which of the client's actions could be the cause of the flare-up?

○ 1. Wearing clothes made from 100% cotton.

○ 2. Sleeping in a cool, humidified room.

○ 3. Increasing fluid intake to at least 3000 mL per day.

○ 4. Daily baths with a deodorant soap.

83. Which of the following variables is *most* important to assess when determining the impact of the cancer diagnosis and treatment modalities on a long-term survivor's quality of life?
    ○ 1. Occupation and employability.
    ○ 2. Functional status.
    ○ 3. Evidence of disease.
    ○ 4. Individual values and beliefs.

84. A 56-year-old woman is currently receiving radiation therapy to the chest wall for recurrent breast cancer. She calls her health care provider to report that she has pain while swallowing and burning and tightness in her chest. Which of the following complications of radiation therapy is most likely responsible for her symptoms?
    ○ 1. Hiatal hernia.
    ○ 2. Stomatitis.
    ○ 3. Radiation enteritis.
    ○ 4. Esophagitis.

85. A 48-year-old woman is receiving radiation therapy for treatment of breast cancer. She reports to the clinic today complaining of apathy, impaired concentration, and feeling tired all the time even though she is sleeping more and more. These complaints suggest symptoms of
    ○ 1. advanced breast cancer.
    ○ 2. fatigue.
    ○ 3. hypocalcemia.
    ○ 4. radiation pneumonitis.

86. A 68-year-old woman with breast cancer complains of abdominal bloating and cramping with no bowel movement for 5 days. She says she usually has a bowel movement every day after her morning coffee. Bowel sounds are present in all four quadrants. She received 80 mg of Adriamycin 10 days ago. The nurse can expect to administer which of the following interventions?
    ○ 1. A Fleet enema to stimulate peristalsis.
    ○ 2. A soapsuds enema until clear.
    ○ 3. An oral cathartic until the client has a bowel movement, then evaluate need for daily stool softeners.
    ○ 4. A daily stool softener for constipation and a mild narcotic for abdominal discomfort.

87. An 82-year-old elderly, alert, and oriented woman with metastatic lung cancer is admitted to the medical-surgical unit for treatment of heart failure. She was given 80 mg of furosemide (Lasix) in the emergency department. Although the client is ambulatory, the unlicensed assistive personnel are concerned about urinary incontinence because the client is frail and in a strange environment. The nurse would instruct the unlicensed personnel to assist with implementing the nursing plan of care by

○ 1. ordering adult diapers for the client so she will not have to worry about incontinence.
○ 2. requesting a Foley catheter to avoid incontinence.
○ 3. padding the bed with extra absorbent linens.
○ 4. placing a commode at the bedside and instructing the client in its use.

88. A 36-year-old woman is scheduled to receive external radiation therapy and a cesium implant for cancer of the cervix. Which of the following statements would be most accurate to include in the teaching plan about the potential effects of radiation therapy on sexuality?
    ○ 1. "You should avoid all sexual intercourse during treatment."
    ○ 2. "You may notice some vaginal dryness after treatment is completed."
    ○ 3. "You may notice some vaginal relaxation after treatment is completed."
    ○ 4. "You will continue to have normal menstrual periods during treatment."

89. A cancer patient has diarrhea and a nursing diagnosis of Impaired Skin Integrity related to the frequent diarrhea. Which of the following nursing interventions is appropriate for this diagnosis?
    ○ 1. Discourage sitz baths, because they promote bacterial growth.
    ○ 2. Apply zinc oxide ointment to the rectal area after each bowel movement to protect the skin.
    ○ 3. Apply skin-barrier dressing daily to the rectal area to form a protective barrier.
    ○ 4. Cleanse the rectal area with unscented soap and water after each bowel movement, rinse well, and pat dry.

90. Which of the following statements is most accurate regarding the long-term toxic effects of cancer treatments on the immune system?
    ○ 1. Clients with persistent immunologic abnormalities after treatment are at a much greater risk for infection than clients with a history of splenectomy.
    ○ 2. The use of radiation and combination chemotherapy can result in more frequent and more severe immune system impairment.
    ○ 3. Long-term immunologic effects have been studied only in patients with breast and lung cancer.
    ○ 4. The T-helper cells recover more rapidly than the T-supressor cells, which results in positive helper cell balance that can last 5 years.

91. The nurse caring for a client who is receiving external beam radiation therapy for treatment of lung cancer should anticipate that the client will have which of the following?

○ 1. Diarrhea.
○ 2. Improved energy level.
○ 3. Dysphagia.
○ 4. Normal white blood cell count.

92. The nurse would expect single-donor platelets to be ordered for which of the following clients?
    ○ 1. A client who is receiving multiple platelet transfusions.
    ○ 2. A client who is deficient in coagulation factors.
    ○ 3. A client whose platelet count is greater than 50,000/mm³.
    ○ 4. A client who is refractory to random-donor platelets.

The Client Who Is Coping With Loss, Grief, Bereavement, and Spiritual Distress

93. A client is newly diagnosed with cancer and is beginning a treatment plan. Which of the following nursing interventions will be most effective in helping the client cope?
    ○ 1. Assume decision making for the client.
    ○ 2. Encourage strict compliance with all treatment regimens.
    ○ 3. Inform the client of all possible adverse treatment effects.
    ○ 4. Identify available resources.

94. A daughter is concerned that her mother is in denial when discussing her diagnosis of breast cancer because she sometimes says that breast cancer isn't that serious and changes the subject. The nurse informs the daughter that denial can be a healthy defense mechanism if it is used
    ○ 1. to permit her mother to seek unconventional treatments.
    ○ 2. when making decisions about her care.
    ○ 3. alone and not in combination with other defense mechanisms.
    ○ 4. to allow her mother to continue in her role as a mother.

95. A 45-year-old single mother of three teenaged boys has metastatic breast cancer. Her parents live 750 miles away and have only been able to visit twice since her initial diagnosis 14 months ago. The progression of her disease has forced the client to consider high-dose chemotherapy with an autologous bone marrow transplant. She is concerned about her children's welfare during the intensive treatment. When assessing the client's present support systems, the nurse will be most concerned about the potential problems with
    ○ 1. denial as a primary coping mechanism.
    ○ 2. support systems and coping strategies.
    ○ 3. decision-making abilities.
    ○ 4. transportation and money for the boys.

96. Which of the following characteristics displayed by the wife of a 36-year-old man with pancreatic cancer suggests that she may be at risk for negative bereavement outcomes?
    ○ 1. She is preparing for her husband's death.
    ○ 2. Her high socioeconomic status.
    ○ 3. Her strong family support.
    ○ 4. She blames herself for her husband's cancer.

97. Which of the following factors places a person at high risk for negative bereavement outcomes?
    ○ 1. Young age.
    ○ 2. History of anxiety.
    ○ 3. Distant relationship to the deceased.
    ○ 4. Higher socioeconomic status.

98. Which of the following nursing interventions will be *most* effective when caring for a client who is experiencing powerlessness?
    ○ 1. Make certain that all staff members focus only on the client's capabilities.
    ○ 2. Encourage family members to become more responsible for the client's care.
    ○ 3. Request a referral to a psychologist.
    ○ 4. Include the client in decision making whenever possible.

99. During the initial stage of adaptation to the diagnosis of cancer and its treatment, the nurse can facilitate the client's adaptation by
    ○ 1. encouraging the client to maintain her usual role.
    ○ 2. facilitating family-related disagreements and conflicts.
    ○ 3. supporting the client in her use of denial as a coping strategy.
    ○ 4. arranging transportation and child care on treatment days.

100. The son of a 78-year-old client with metastatic prostate cancer is asking the nurse about the purpose of hospice care. Which of the following statements by the nurse best describes hospice care?
    ○ 1. "Hospice care uses a team approach to direct hospice activity."
    ○ 2. "Clients and their families are the focus of care."
    ○ 3. "The client's physician coordinates all the care."
    ○ 4. "All hospice clients will die at home."

101. A client's husband expresses concern that his dying wife keeps saying, "I have to go to the store." Which of the following statements by the nurse will be most effective in assisting the husband to understand the dying process?
    ○ 1. "Many dying patients are restless and can be treated with sedatives."
    ○ 2. "The client may be fighting death and you should leave her alone."

3. "Comments related to going somewhere or leaving on a trip are common in dying clients."
4. "Decreased circulation and lack of oxygen to the brain often causes delirium."

102. The wife of a terminally ill client asks the nurse, "Why is he having frequent bowel movements if he is not eating?" Which of the following response by the nurse informs the wife about the client's condition?
    1. "I know he is having frequent loose stools and it is distressing for you, but that's just the way it is."
    2. "I don't know when the bowels will shut down, but they will eventually."
    3. "The pain medication will eventually help to slow the process of bowel function."
    4. "The intestines still produce some waste products even when a person is not eating."

103. The nurse formulates a nursing diagnosis of Spiritual Distress related to advanced cancer disease. An appropriate goal for the client would be to
    1. start attending church or chapel services once a week.
    2. call a chaplain and set up an appointment for spiritual guidance.
    3. reflect on past accomplishments.
    4. participate in spiritual activities of the client's choice.

104. A 72-year-old woman with cancer needs assistance with her financial concerns. The nurse would suggest that which of the following persons see the client?
    1. Bank representative.
    2. Social worker.
    3. Oncology nurse.
    4. Representative of the hospital billing department.

105. The family members caring for a 72-year-old man who is near death from colon cancer are concerned about dehydration. What should the nurse tell them about dehydration at end of life?
    1. The physician will make the decision regarding hydration therapy.
    2. Dehydration may prolong the dying process.
    3. Hydration is used only in extreme situations of dehydration.
    4. Dehydration is expected during the dying process.

106. Which of the following actions should the nurse plan to do *first* when caring for a client who is experiencing spiritual distress?
    1. Make a referral to a member of the clergy.
    2. Explain the major beliefs of different religions.
    3. Suggest reading material.
    4. Help the client explore his or her own values and beliefs.

107. Clients who are newly diagnosed with cancer have many fears and concerns. Which of the following issues is of primary concern?
    1. Ability to perform in usual roles.
    2. Cost of treatments.
    3. Prognosis.
    4. Pain.

108. The most effective resource for support for clients with cancer who are grieving is
    1. health care professionals.
    2. family.
    3. clergy.
    4. community support groups.

109. A 42-year-old client with breast cancer is concerned that her husband is depressed by her diagnosis. Which of the following changes in her husband's behavior may confirm her fears?
    1. Increased decisiveness.
    2. Problem-focused coping style.
    3. Increase in social interactions.
    4. Disturbance in his sleep patterns.

110. The most appropriate advice for the hospice nurse to give a woman whose husband died 3 months ago and her three young children would be to
    1. seek group counseling support for the three children.
    2. request individual counseling and medication to manage depression.
    3. remind her gently that bereavement care before death minimizes grieving.
    4. continue her bereavement support through hospice.

111. Which of the following interventions will be *most* effective in improving transcultural communications with oncology clients and their families?
    1. Use touch to show concern and caring for the client.
    2. Focus attention on verbal communication skills only.
    3. Establish a rapport and listen to their concerns.
    4. Maintain eye contact at all times.

112. A client with cancer verbalizes that he is afraid he won't be able to cope with all the issues that will arise. The nurse can best support the coping behaviors of a client with cancer by
    1. helping the client identify available resources.
    2. encouraging compliance with treatment regimens.
    3. relieving the client of decision making as much as possible.
    4. assisting the client to prepare for adverse treatment effects.

113. The "I Can Cope," "CanSurmount," and "Reach to Recovery" programs are all designed to help cancer clients

○ 1. choose treatment centers.
○ 2. find financial help.
○ 3. obtain home health care.
○ 4. cope with cancer.

114. A 56-year-old cancer survivor feels guilty at the "I Can Cope" meetings. The nurse can help him manage his feelings of guilt by pointing out that
    ○ 1. he is really angry at the terminally ill clients in the group.
    ○ 2. he is experiencing very volatile emotions.
    ○ 3. this is a spiritual response to his illness.
    ○ 4. this is a normal reaction when surviving a life-threatening experience.

115. A 68-year-old client with colon cancer experiences an increase in his feelings of anxiety and depression and has suicidal ideation. He appears to be in great distress. The nurse realizes that he is at which stage in his disease?
    ○ 1. Initiation of definitive treatment.
    ○ 2. End of his first course of treatment.
    ○ 3. End stage of his disease.
    ○ 4. Recurrence of the disease.

116. A 57-year-old woman has difficulty with mobility after her cancer treatment therapies and states, "Why should I bother trying to get better? It doesn't seem to make any difference what I do." The nurse responds by helping the client establish reasonable activity goals, choose her own foods from the menu, and make choices about her daily activities. These interventions represent the nurse's attempt to address which of the following nursing diagnoses?
    ○ 1. Ineffective Coping.
    ○ 2. Powerlessness.
    ○ 3. Impaired Adjustment.
    ○ 4. Dysfunctional Grieving.

117. The nurse is aware that a 65-year-old widower whose only son is 500 miles away is at higher risk for psychosocial distress because he
    ○ 1. has been successful in dealing with stress all his life.
    ○ 2. does not have to deal with other stressors right now.
    ○ 3. is able to use denial as a coping mechanism.
    ○ 4. perceives he has minimal social support.

118. A client with a diagnosis of cancer is frequently disruptive and challenges the nurse. This behavior is probably caused by
    ○ 1. uncertainty and an underlying fear of recurrence.
    ○ 2. the usual trajectory of a short-term illness.
    ○ 3. a history of the behavioral illness.
    ○ 4. the one-time crisis from learning of the diagnosis.

119. A 42-year-old husband and father of a 7-year-old girl and a 10-year-old boy is concerned about what he should tell his children regarding his wife's impending death from aggressive breast cancer. The nurse should
    ○ 1. refer the family to pastoral care services.
    ○ 2. encourage the husband to come to terms with his own grief first.
    ○ 3. suggest that the children be told nothing until after death occurs.
    ○ 4. begin education about strategies for communication with his children.

120. While talking to her husband, who is caring for their children, a 52-year-old woman slams the phone down. She begins to cry and states that she is feeling guilty for being hospitalized. Which of the following interventions will best support the client emotionally?
    ○ 1. Call the physician and ask for a psychiatry consultation.
    ○ 2. Call the physician and request an antidepressant medication.
    ○ 3. Sit with the client and help her acknowledge and discuss her feelings.
    ○ 4. Sit with the client and encourage her to see the good side of the situation.

121. A 56-year-old woman who is receiving radiation therapy tells the nurse that she feels inadequate as a wife and mother because she can no longer carry out her usual duties with the same energy as before. What recommendations should the nurse make to help her cope with this situation?
    ○ 1. Suggest that she reassign all household chores to other members of the family.
    ○ 2. Suggest that she prioritize her activities and ask for help from friends and family.
    ○ 3. Suggest that she ignore the household chores during the crisis period.
    ○ 4. Tell her not to worry so much because everyone gets a little tired at this phase of the therapy.

122. A 66-year-old woman who is usually meticulous about her appearance and dress arrives today for her 23rd day of radiation therapy. She appears disheveled and emotionally labile, and her responses to the usual questions are a little inappropriate. Her heart rate is 124 bpm, her respirations are 32 breaths/minute, and her skin is cold and clammy. These findings would suggest that the client has early signs of which of the following conditions?
    ○ 1. Schizophrenia.
    ○ 2. Panic disorder.
    ○ 3. Depression.
    ○ 4. Delirium.

123. A client has undergone surgical resection for lung cancer. Which of the following nursing interventions will promote adaptation and rehabilitation?
    ○ 1. Arranging a visit from a member of the Ameri-

can Cancer Society Lost Chord Club.
  ○ 2. Planning a progressive activity regimen with the client.
  ○ 3. Teaching tracheostomy care.
  ○ 4. Planning a vigorous exercise program.

124. Which of the following activities indicates that the client with cancer is adapting well to body image changes?
  ○ 1. The client names his brother as the person to call if he is experiencing suicidal ideation.
  ○ 2. The client discusses changes in body structure and function.
  ○ 3. The client discusses the date of his return to work.
  ○ 4. The client serves as a volunteer in a client-to-client visitation program.

The Client Who Is Experiencing Problems With Sexuality

125. A 36-year-old woman is complaining of increased vaginal dryness during sexual intercourse. She has received chemotherapy in the past and has menopausal symptoms due to ovarian suppression. An appropriate nursing intervention would be to instruct the client on the use of
  ○ 1. vaginal dilators.
  ○ 2. nightly douches.
  ○ 3. water-soluble vaginal lubricants.
  ○ 4. relaxation techniques.

126. A 49-year-old man with a tracheostomy tube confides to the nurse during a clinic visit that he is beginning to avoid sexual activity because of the increased tracheostomy secretions. Which of the following statements by the nurse will be *most* helpful to the client?
  ○ 1. "Use a scopolamine patch to decrease secretions."
  ○ 2. "Avoid fluid intake 2 hours before sexual activity."
  ○ 3. "Place a thin piece of gauze over the tracheostomy."
  ○ 4. "Wash the tracheostomy area with deodorizing antibacterial soap before sexual activity."

127. A 52-year-old client is scheduled for a total abdominal hysterectomy for cervical cancer. Discussion regarding the client's feelings and the potential impact of this procedure on her sexuality should include which of the following questions?
  ○ 1. "All women experience sexual problems with this surgical procedure. Do you have any questions?"
  ○ 2. "When can I schedule an appointment with you and your partner to discuss any issues either of you may have regarding sexuality?"

  ○ 3. "Do you anticipate any problems with sex related to your scheduled hysterectomy?"
  ○ 4. "Most women have concerns about their sexuality after this type of surgery. Do you have any concerns or questions?"

128. A young man with early-stage testicular cancer is scheduled for a unilateral orchiectomy. The client confides to the nurse that he is concerned about what effects the surgery will have on his sexual performance. Which of the following responses by the nurse provides accurate information about sexual performance after an orchiectomy?
  ○ 1. "Most impotence resolves in a couple of months."
  ○ 2. "You could have early ejaculation with this type of surgery."
  ○ 3. "We will refer you to a sex therapist, because you will probably notice erectile dysfunction."
  ○ 4. "Because your surgery does not involve other organs or tissues, you will most likely not notice any change in your sexual performance."

129. A young female client is receiving chemotherapy and mentions to the nurse that she and her husband are using a diaphragm for birth control. Which of the following is most important for the nurse to discuss?
  ○ 1. Inconvenience of the diaphragm.
  ○ 2. Transmission of sexually transmitted diseases.
  ○ 3. Body changes related to hormones.
  ○ 4. Infection control.

130. To promote comfort and optimal respiratory expansion for a client with chronic obstructive pulmonary disease (COPD) during sexual intimacy, the nurse can suggest that the couple
  ○ 1. use a waterbed.
  ○ 2. use pillows to raise the affected partner's head and upper torso.
  ○ 3. have the affected partner assume a dependent position.
  ○ 4. limit the duration of the sexual activity.

Ethical and Legal Issues Related to Clients With Cancer and End-of-Life Care

131. In an attempt to call public attention to the cancer survivor's needs, a bill of rights was put forth by the
  ○ 1. American Cancer Society.
  ○ 2. National Coalition of Cancer Survivors.
  ○ 3. National Cancer Institute.
  ○ 4. National Hospice Organization.

132. A 32-year-old teacher is concerned that she will lose her job if she requests a leave of absence to care for her father who is getting daily treatment for colon

cancer in a city 300 miles away. Which legislative measure will likely protect her job during an extended illness?
- ○ 1. Family Leave Act of 1993.
- ○ 2. Americans With Disabilities Act of 1990.
- ○ 3. Medicare Coverage for Catastrophic Illness Act of 1988.
- ○ 4. Rehabilitation Act of 1973.

133. A 62-year-old woman thinks her husband's rehabilitation needs have been unmet by his employer after his diagnosis and treatment of colon cancer. The nurse should give her information about
- ○ 1. The Americans With Disabilities Act (1990).
- ○ 2. Title V Rehabilitation Act (1973).
- ○ 3. The Civil Rights Act (1964).
- ○ 4. The Patient Self-Determination Act (1991).

134. Which of the following statements best exemplifies the concept of autonomy?
- ○ 1. The professional staff of physicians defines the client's best interest.
- ○ 2. The nurse provides the client with the facts and then allows the client to reach an unassisted decision.
- ○ 3. The nurse respects a client's choice not to know particular information.
- ○ 4. The health care team makes health and treatment decisions.

135. The nurse can be an important advocate for the client who is considering an alternative method of cancer treatment. Which of the following statements best demonstrates the nurse as client advocate?
- ○ 1. The nurse will provide the information about standard therapies.
- ○ 2. The nurse will monitor blood tests as indicated by the alternative therapy.
- ○ 3. The nurse will document the client's desire to try an alternative therapy.
- ○ 4. The nurse will allow the client to make health care choices on her own but will assist in ensuring the client is fully informed when making those decisions.

136. When a 62-year-old client and his family receive the initial diagnosis of colon cancer, the nurse can act as an advocate by
- ○ 1. helping them maintain a sense of optimism and hopefulness.
- ○ 2. determining their understanding of the results of the diagnostic testing.
- ○ 3. listening carefully to their perceptions of what their needs are.
- ○ 4. providing them with written materials about the cancer site and its treatment.

Correct Answers and Rationale

The letters in parentheses following the rationale identify the step of the nursing process (A, D, P, I, E) and client needs (1, 2, 3, 4, 5, 6, 7, 8, 9, 10). See the inside front cover for the key.

The Client at Risk for Cancer

1. 3. Only treatment-related x-rays are iatrogenic. The others are agents that occur in the physical environment naturally. (A, 4)

2. 1. Prospective studies begin with an examination of presumed causes and go forward in time to observe presumed effects. Data about miners with exposure to uranium (the presumed cause) is collected over time to evaluate the incidence of cancer (the presumed effect). This is representative of a prospective study. Historical studies critically evaluate existing data to test hypotheses or answer questions about the causes or effects of past events. Retrospective studies begin with the effect (eg, cancer) and then attempt to link the effect to a presumed cause that occurred in the past. (A, 4)

3. 1. Progression is the change in a tumor from the preneoplastic state or low degree of malignancy to a rapidly growing tumor; it cannot be reversed. Promotion is reversible. Initiation is at first reversible (through repair of damaged DNA) and later irreversible. Regression is not a recognized stage of carcinogenesis. (A, 4)

4. 2. The word *prevalence* in a statistical setting is defined as the number of cases of a disease present in a specified population at a given time. (A, 4)

5. 3. Sun damage is a cumulative process. Parents should be taught to apply sunscreen and teach their children to use sunscreen at an early age. Although preventive education is always valuable, serious sunburns in childhood are associated with an increased risk of melanoma. Exposure to chemicals is not a risk factor for melanoma. (A, 4)

6. 4. The sunscreen SPF number for each person varies, but 15 is considered basic for most people. Sunscreen needs to be applied every 2 to 4 hours, especially if the person perspires heavily, as well as after swimming. Peak sun exposure usually occurs from 10 AM to 2 PM. Tightly woven clothing, protective hats, and sunglasses are recommended to decrease sun exposure. (A, 4)

7. 1. Malignant melanoma may have a familial basis, especially in families with dysplastic nevi syndrome. First-degree relatives should be monitored closely.

Malignant melanoma occurs most often in the 20- to 45-year-old age group. Severe sunburn as a child does increase the risk; however, this client is at increased risk because of her family history. (A, 4)

8. 4. The upper outer quadrant is the area of the breast in which most breast tumors are found. This area should be palpated thoroughly. Although breast tumors can be found in any area of the breast, including the nipple, the tumors are most often in the upper outer quadrant. (A, 4)

9. 4. All arm positions, except when the arms are relaxed by the sides, will accentuate skin changes. When the arms are raised over the head, visualization of the underside of the breasts is easier. When the hands are placed on the hips and arms are pressed forward, the breast tissue is pushed outward, which accentuates dimpling and puckering. Breast self-examination is not an uncomfortable procedure. Although masses may be seen on inspection, palpation is a more important maneuver for detecting masses. Nipple discharge is assessed by gently squeezing the nipples. (D, 4)

10. 3. The American Cancer Society guidelines state that a Pap smear and pelvic examination should be done annually for women who have been sexually active or who have reached the age of 18 years. Annual Pap smears are recommended only for clients at risk and not for the general female population. After three or more consecutive annual examinations with normal findings, the Pap smear may be performed less frequently at the discretion of the physician. Colposcopy is indicated for an abnormal Pap smear, not a negative Pap smear. (I, 4)

11. 3. Because more than 50% of the cancers occur in people who are older than 65 years of age, the single most important factor in determining risk would be age. (D, 4)

12. 3. Evidence suggests that a high-fat diet increases the risk of several cancers, including breast, colon, and prostate cancers. Ovarian, lung, and liver cancers have not been linked to a high-fat diet. (D, 4)

13. 4. The client is at increased risk for development of lung, skin, or breast cancer. Consequently, the most urgent changes in behavior should include smoking cessation, protection from the sun, and weight loss. Decreasing alcohol consumption is certainly desirable, as is improving overall nutritional intake (eg, eating low-fat foods, increasing fiber). (D, 4)

14. 1. Primary cancer prevention targets healthy individuals and includes steps to avoid factors that might lead to the development of disease. Secondary prevention

includes identification of high-risk groups with precursor states of disease. Early detection, screening, and treatment of early stages of disease are included in this category. Tertiary cancer prevention focuses on rehabilitation to assist individuals in achieving an optimal level of functioning. It includes minimizing the effect of cancer and preventing complications. "Nonspecific" is not a category of prevention activities. (A, 4)

15. 1. Asbestos and alcohol, when combined with smoking, produce a synergistic effect and result in increased cancer risk and incidence. (A, 4)

16. 4. Although exposure to the sun increases the risk of skin cancers and family history is significant in the development of some types of cancer, heavy tobacco use and alcohol intake have a synergistic effect and increase the risk and incidence of head and neck cancers. Patterns of medication use, exposure to wood dust, and a high-fat diet are not associated with an increased risk and incidence of head and neck cancers. (P, 4)

17. 2. High-fiber, low-fat diets are recommended to reduce risk of colon cancer. Stir-frying, poaching, steaming, and broiling are all low-fat methods to prepare foods. Croissants are made of refined flour. They are also high in fat, as are peanut butter squares and whole milk, granola, cream cheese, and sour cream. (P, 4)

18. 2. Environmental factors include place of residence, nutrition, occupation, personal habits, iatrogenic factors, and physical environment. Gender, immunologic status, and age are individual factors. (A, 4)

19. 3. CT scanning is the standard noninvasive method used in a workup for lung cancer because it can distinguish small differences in tissue density and in detecting nodal involvement. CT is comparable to magnetic resonance imaging in evaluating lymph node metastasis. CT is noninvasive and usually available, but these are not the main reasons for its use. The CT can distinguish malignancy in some situations only. (D, 10)

20. 3. A high-fat, low-fiber diet is a risk factor for colorectal cancer. A diet low in vitamin C, use of artificial sweeteners, and multiple sex partners are not considered risk factors for colorectal cancer. (P, 3)

21. 2. Strategies to reach the socioeconomically disadvantaged would include incorporating the folk beliefs and traditions of the target population into the program. Identification of a centrally located building with available access by the target population, use of materials in the native or primary language of the target population, and involvement by the community leaders will also help the program succeed. (P, 4)

The Client With Pain

22. 1. Use of more than three to five doses of breakthrough morphine means that the client is taking pain medications more than six times per day. This defeats the purpose of the long-acting morphine. (I, 7)

23. 2. Step 1 includes nonopioids, such as acetaminophen or NSAIDs. Opioid analgesics are not part of Step 1 of the WHO ladder. Mild opioids, such as oxycodone, codeine, and propoxyphene, and adjuvant therapy are included in Step 2. (D, 7)

24. 1. The most common toxicities from NSAIDs are gastrointestinal disorders (nausea, epigastric pain, ulcers, bleeding, diarrhea, and constipation). Renal dysfunction, pulmonary complications, and cardiovascular complications from NSAIDs are much less common. (A, 9)

25. 2. In the client with chronic pain, physiologic adaptation results in minimal changes in behavior and vital signs. Elevated vital signs, grimacing, and moaning are characteristic responses to acute pain. (A, 7)

26. 4. *Tolerance* is a reduced responsiveness to the effect of any drug, which necessitates larger doses to achieve an equivalent effect of the initial dose. *Pseudoaddiction* is a term used to describe the iatrogenic syndrome of drug-seeking behavior that develops as a direct consequence of inadequate pain management. *Physical dependence* refers to the state in which an individual must take the substance to feel physically normal; not taking the drug results in withdrawal symptoms. *Psychological dependence* refers to an individual's need to derive an alteration in mood from a substance. (D, 7)

27. 3. Morphine sulfate is the drug of choice to treat severe cancer pain. Methadone (Dolophine), oxycodone, and hydromorphone (Dilaudid) are not as effective as morphine in controlling severe cancer pain. (A, 7)

28. 4. Most cancer clients with inadequate pain control while taking an oral opioid after being switched from IV administration have been undermedicated. Equianalgesic conversions should be made to provide estimates of the equivalent does needed for same level of relief as provided by the IV dose. There is research to suggest that cancer clients do not become addicted to opioids when dosed adequately. There is no evidence to suggest that the client is physically addicted or is having withdrawal symptoms. (P, 7)

29. 1. Intensity is indicative of the severity of pain and is important for evaluating the efficacy of treatment modalities. (A, 7)

30. 2. There is a 1:3 ratio with equianalgesic dosing of IV to oral morphine; therefore, the physician should order three times the intravenous dose. (P, 7)

31. 4. Normeperidine is a potent long-acting metabolite, which can cause central nervous system (CNS) stimulation and seizures. Normeperidine is a short-acting drug and must be given in more frequent intervals and may require increased dosages for effectiveness. Mixed agonist—antagonists act competitively at different pain receptor sites. It is generally accepted by cancer pain experts that opioid agonist-antagonist drugs have very limited usefulness in cancer pain management because of their tendency to induce opioid withdrawal and cause severe CNS side effects. (D, 7)

32. 2. Tolerance to an opioid occurs when a larger dose of the analgesic is needed to provide the same level of pain control. The risk of addiction is low with opioids to treat cancer pain. There are no data to support that this client is experiencing withdrawal. Although the client may have experienced a placebo effect at one time, placebo effects tend to diminish over time, especially in regard to chronic cancer pain. (E, 8)

33. 2. The regular administration of analgesics provides a consistent serum level of medication, which can help prevent breakthrough pain. Therefore, taking the prescribed analgesics on a regular schedule is the best way to manage chronic cancer-related pain. There is little risk for the client with cancer-related pain to become addicted. Sleeping 12 to 16 hours a day would not allow the client to participate in usual daily activities or preferred activities. (I, 7)

The Client Who Requires Symptom Management

34. 3. For clients with obstructive versus restrictive disorders, extending exhalation through pursed-lip breathing will make the respiratory effort more efficient. The usual position of choice for this client is the upright position, leaning slightly forward to allow greater lung expansion. Teaching diaphragmatic breathing techniques will be more helpful to the client with a restrictive disorder. Administering cough suppressants will not help respiratory effort. A low semi-Fowler's position does not encourage lung expansion. Lung expansion is enhanced in the upright position. (I, 7)

35. 3. Anxiety is a common response in the dyspneic client and may be intensified with a diagnosis of cancer. The anxiety is usually caused by fear of choking or cessation of breathing. Labored respirations and lack of energy are not associated with euphoria, and they usually prevent angry behavior. Lack of energy associated with the disease should not be mistaken for laziness. (A, 10)

36. 1. Fever is an early sign requiring clinical intervention to identify potential causes. Chills and dyspnea may or may not be observed. Tachycardia can be an indicator in a variety of clinical situations when associated with infection; it usually occurs in response to an elevated temperature or change in cardiac function. (I, 9)

37. 2. The administration of antipyretics and antihistamines before initiation of the transfusion in the frequently transfused client can decrease the incidence of febrile reactions. Febrile reactions are immune-mediated and are caused by antibodies in the recipient that are directed against antigens present on the granulocytes, platelets, and lymphocytes in the transfused component. They are the most common transfusion reactions and may occur with onset, during transfusion, or hours after transfusion is completed. (P, 8)

38. 2. After surgical resection, functional lung tissue is lost, resulting in chronic difficulty meeting the body's demand for oxygen, and thus the dyspnea. Increased dyspnea may indicate an additional respiratory stress such as pneumonia or bronchitis. Fibrotic changes usually are a result of radiation therapy. There is no indication that the client has received myelosuppressive therapy to cause anemia. Pericardial effusions would be more likely to result from chemotherapy or radiation. (D, 10)

39. 1. Negative outcomes due to fatigue may include diminished quality of life, loss of self-esteem, depression, caregiver strain and fatigue, social isolation, decreased functional status, and poor disease prognosis. Increased risk for infection is not related to fatigue but is related to immunosuppression secondary to chemotherapy. Fatigue does not indicate an improved prognosis. It does not cause increased pain. Cancer pain is caused by many factors, including bone metastasis, nerve compression, infiltration of tumor into normal structures, and ischemia. (E, 5)

40. 1. Dietary suggestions to reduce side effects of cancer and cancer therapies include a soft, bland diet low in fat and sugar. Frequent, small meals are usually better tolerated. Fluid intake should be encouraged to avoid dehydration. It is not necessary to restrict the diet to cold foods. (I, 7)

41. 1. The role of the nurse is to assess what substances or medications the client is using and to document and inform other members of the health care team. It is very important to encourage the client to keep the physician informed of all therapeutic agents, medications, and supplements she is using, to avoid adverse interactions. It is not appropriate for the nurse to suggest that the client choose either Western or alternative therapies or to discourage the client's use of alternative therapies. The nurse should remain objective about the client's treatment choices and respect her autonomy. (I, 9)

42. 4. The use of diet modification is a conservative approach to treat the terminally ill or hospice clients who have nausea and vomiting related to bowel obstruction. Osmotic laxatives would be harder for the client to tolerate. A nasogastric tube is more aggressive and invasive. Intravenous antiemetics are also invasive. The hospice philosophy involves comfort and palliative care for the terminally ill. (D, 7)

43. 3. Repositioning the client, elevating the head of the bed, and providing a cool compress are comfort interventions consistent with the concept of palliative care of the dying. Directing the unlicensed personnel to assess vital signs focuses on the dying process, not the client. Suctioning may not benefit the client and is considered invasive and uncomfortable. Telling the wife an intervention is not needed discounts her judgment and concerns. (I, 5)

44. 2. Alopecia from chemotherapy is temporary. The new hair will not be necessarily gray, but the texture and color of new hair growth may be different. Clients who will be receiving chemotherapy should be encouraged to purchase a wig while they still have hair so that they can match the color and texture of their hair. Loss of hair or alopecia is a serious threat to self-esteem and should be addressed quickly before treatment. (D, 9)

45. 1. There are many mechanisms of action for chemotherapeutic agents, but most affect the rapidly dividing cells—both cancerous and noncancerous. Cancer cells are characterized by rapid cell division. Chemotherapy slows cell division. Not all chemotherapeutic agents affect molecular structure. All cells are susceptible to drug toxins, but not all chemotherapeutic agents are toxins. (I, 8)

46. 3. Dyspnea is a distressing symptom in clients with advanced cancer including metastatic carcinoma of the lung, previous radiation therapy, and coexisting COPD. Ascites does occur in clients with metastatic carcinoma; however, in the client with COPD and lung cancer, dyspnea is a more common finding. A pleural friction rub is usually associated with pneumonia, pleurisy, or pulmonary infarct. (A, 10)

47. 3. The positive reinforcement builds confidence and facilitates achievement of rehabilitation goals. Community support may or may not be applicable after discharge. Although family support is an important component of rehabilitation, reinforcing the skills the client has acquired is of greater importance when regaining independence. Rehabilitation plans should include the client, family, or both. (I, 5)

48. 2. The most important intervention for infection control is to continue meticulous catheter site care. Dress-

ings are to be changed two to three times per week depending on institutional policies. Temperature should be monitored at least once a day in someone with a vascular access device. Handwashing before and after irrigation or any manipulation of the site is a must for infection prevention. (E, 1)

49. 2. The client is exhibiting signs and symptoms of a pneumothorax from the insertion of the subclavian venous catheter. Although it is possible that the client suffered an air embolus during the procedure, and the client is at risk for pulmonary emboli because of his immobility, absent breath sounds immediately after insertion of a subclavian line are strongly suggestive of a pneumothorax. Unilateral absent breath sounds are not associated with a myocardial infarction. (D, 10)

50. 4. An appropriate and realistic outcome would be for the client to maintain current weight or not lose weight. It is unrealistic to expect that the client with advanced liver cancer will have normal albumin levels or will be able to gain weight. (P, 7)

51. 3. As long as the client is able to get out of bed, the preferred position and time frame for preventing aspiration after a bolus tube feeding is sitting upright out of bed in a chair for 30 to 60 minutes. Placing the client on the right, not the left, side may facilitate gastric emptying, but this is not the preferred position. Elevating the bed 30 degrees decreases the risk of aspiration, but this elevation must be maintained for at least 45 to 60 minutes. (I, 7)

52. 1. Total parenteral nutrition solutions supply the body with sufficient amounts of dextrose, amino acids, fats, vitamins, and minerals to meet metabolic needs. Clients who are unable to tolerate adequate quantities of foods and fluids and those who have had extensive bowel surgery may not be candidates for enteral feedings. The nurse would anticipate total parenteral nutrition via central catheter to promote wound healing. Intravenous dextrose does not supply all the nutrients required to promote wound healing. (P, 7)

53. 3. The client is experiencing metabolic alkalosis caused by loss of hydrogen and chloride ions from excessive vomiting. A normal or low bicarbonate level characterizes respiratory alkalosis, which results from hyperventilation. Respiratory acidosis is characterized by a decreased pH, which is a result of carbon dioxide retention. A decreased bicarbonate level and a decreased pH characterize metabolic acidosis, which can result from various pathophysiologic states. (D, 10)

54. 4. The content of the client's comments suggests that she is avoiding intimacy with her husband by waiting until he is asleep before going to bed. Addressing sexuality issues is appropriate for a client who has undergone a mastectomy. Rushing her return to work may debilitate her and add to her exhaustion. Suggesting that she learn relaxation techniques for help with her insomnia is appropriate; however, the nurse must first address the psychosocial and sexual issues that are contributing to her sleeping difficulties. A nutritional assessment may be useful, but there is no indication that she has anorexia. (E, 5)

55. 3. Although each client listed is at some risk of complication secondary to immobility, the 75-year-old man is in need of intensive interventions. Contributing factors include his age, pain management, extended bed rest, and the potential for preexisting nutritional deficits. (I, 2)

56. 3. Immobility sets up the tissue to atrophy and protein catabolism to increase, which results in a decreased metabolic rate. Cardiovascular workload increases because of venous stasis. Lung expansion decreases because there is less gas exchange. (D, 9)

57. 4. Cough and shortness of breath are significant symptoms because they may indicate decreasing pulmonary function secondary to drug toxicity. Decrease in appetite, spasms of the diaphragm, and difficulty in thinking clearly may occur as a result of chemotherapy; however, they are not indicative of pulmonary toxicity. (E, 10)

58. 3. The client is exhibiting early symptoms of pulmonary toxicity as a result of the radiation therapy. These are not expected side effects of radiation. He needs to be examined to differentiate between an infection and radiation pneumonitis. Suggesting that the client take acetaminophen and call back in 2 days is inappropriate. These symptoms are not indicative of a true emergency, but the client should be seen before his next scheduled office visit. (I, 9)

59. 4. Orders should include x-ray films to see whether the fluid moves freely and is amenable to removal by thoracentesis. Fluid loculation is a risk of repeated thoracentesis. A platelet count may be necessary if client is at risk for bleeding tendencies. Arterial blood gases or an electrocardiogram is not required before a thoracentesis. An abnormal WBC count may not necessarily preclude the procedure and is not required before thoracentesis. (P, 9)

60. 3. Surgery for head and neck malignancies often causes edema of the upper airway that can result in difficulty breathing and the need for a tracheostomy. (A, 3)

61. 3. Changing positions frequently aids in distributing the agent to the pleura for sealing. The majority of the pleural fluid is drained, and lung should already be re-expanded before instillation of the sclerosing agent. A pressure dressing is applied to the chest tube exit site,

and it is not necessary to lie on that side to hold pressure on the area. (P, 8)

62. 4. Providing adequate humidification for the client with a tracheostomy is essential. The client no longer has the functions of the nose for warming, moistening, or filtering the air when breathing through tracheostomy site. Providing tracheostomy site care, addressing the psychosocial issues, and observing for early signs and symptoms of skin breakdown around the tracheostomy site are also important; however, using humidifiers to prevent thick, tenacious secretions is the most important recommendation for long-term management and the prevention of pulmonary infection. (P, 7)

63. 4. A malignant pleural effusion is an accumulation of excessive fluid within the pleural space that occurs when cancer cells irritate the pleural membrane. Dyspnea can result from the increased pressure that may contribute to increased anxiety and fear of suffocation. Pain is a consequence of the pleural irritation. Cough is related to the atelectasis of the bronchi and inability to clear the airways. Hiccups are usually associated with pericardial effusions. Weight gain and peripheral edema may occur with peritoneal effusion. (D, 10)

64. 1. The thoracentesis is less likely to be successful as a treatment for recurrent pleural effusion because the fluid accumulates rapidly. Thoracentesis is usually successful for diagnosis of underlying disease, palliation of symptoms, and acute respiratory distress. Alleviation of the symptoms and distress is usually short-term in recurrent effusions. (D, 10)

65. 3. Cold intolerance may be associated with anemia because of the diminished oxygen supply to the peripheral circulation. Decreased salivation is not necessarily associated with anemia. Tachycardia may be expected in severe anemia. (A, 10)

66. 4. A bloody effusion is strong indication of a malignancy. Milky fluid suggests a chylous process from lymphatic obstruction. Straw-colored fluid is considered normal. Turbid fluid may indicate an infection. (A, 10)

67. 3. The PT and PTT are blood tests that measure factors involved in the clotting process and can give a fair indication if there is a clotting deficit. CEA and AFP are tumor markers associated with malignancies and are not used to evaluate a hypercoagulable state. A platelet count may be used in the evaluation of a hypercoagulable state, but it is not always included in the CBC and would need to be ordered separately. (A, 9)

68. 4. Bacterial endotoxins released from gram-negative bacteria activate the Hageman factor or coagulation factor XII. This factor inhibits coagulation via the intrinsic pathway of homeostasis, as well as stimulating fibrinoly-

sis. Liver disease can cause multiple bleeding abnormalities resulting in chronic, subclinical DIC; however, sepsis is the most common cause. Brain metastasis is not related to DIC. Intravenous heparin therapy is sometimes used to treat clients with DIC, but this treatment is controversial. It does not cause DIC but can result in bleeding tendencies if the therapeutic dose is exceeded. (D, 10)

69. 4. Petechiae are tiny purplish, hemorrhagic spots visible under the skin. Petechiae usually appear when platelets are depleted. Bleeding gums or oozing of blood may accompany the petechiae, and the client should seek medical assistance immediately. (D, 10)

70. 4. Chronic lymphedema is a late postoperative complication that can occur anywhere from 6 weeks to 20 years or more after surgery on either side. For most women, the affected arm becomes enlarged within the first year after mastectomy. The unpredictable and often delayed nature of lymphedema is assumed to result from a smoldering infection associated with subclinical lymphangitis, but may also be caused by venous obstruction, damage to lymphatic vessels, and/or dissection of lymph nodes. (D, 8)

71. 3. Low-dose administration of warfarin prophylactically appears to prevent or decrease the incidence of thrombus formation because of a mild anticoagulation effect. Urokinase is not used prophylactically but is used to treat massive pulmonary emboli, vascular thromboses, or occluded intravenous catheters. Vitamin B$_{12}$ is used to treat pernicious anemia, and neither it nor acetaminophen affects thrombus formation. (D, 8)

72. 3. Infection may occur in a client with lymphedema because of the stagnant accumulated fluid, which becomes an excellent medium for bacteria growth. Capillary permeability, not fragility, increases fluid in lymphedema. Myelosuppression is not related to the lymphedema, only to a neoplastic disease or sequela to treatment of neoplastic disease. Increased use of the extremity may also cause increased accumulation of fluid, but it is not a direct cause of cellulitis and lymphangitis. (D, 8)

73. 3. Redness, warmth, and swelling are all signs of infection. Treatment with antibiotics is usually indicated. Infection usually increases fluid accumulation and could worsen the lymphedema. Warm compresses could also increase fluid accumulation. Elevation will not treat the infection. It is critical that the client not delay treatment. (D, 10)

74. 4. Fever is most commonly related to infection. In a neutropenic client, fever frequently occurs in the absence of the usual clinical signs and symptoms of infection. Inadequate nutrition or antiemetic therapy resistance would

not result in fever. Fever is not usually expected with most chemotherapy drugs. (A, 8)

75. 1. A pneumonectomy is the removal of an entire lung field. A wedge resection refers to removal of a wedge-shaped section of lung tissue. A lobectomy is the removal of one lobe. Removal of one or more segments of a lung lobe is called a partial lobectomy. (D, 9)

76. 1. The fever and chills associated with the administration of BRMs tend to be predictable and usually respond very well to antipyretics. They usually diminish in 8 to 12 hours after each administration. The symptoms tend to decrease in intensity with continued therapy. There is no biphasic pattern associated with these side effects. (P, 7)

77. 2. Nine days after chemotherapy, one would expect the client to be immunocompromised. The clinical signs of shock reflect changes in cardiac function, vascular resistance, cellular metabolism, and capillary permeability. Low-grade fever, tachycardia, and flushing may be early signs of shock. The client with signs of impending septic shock may not have decreased oxygen saturation levels. Oliguria and hypotension are late signs of shock. Urine output can be initially normal or increased. (D, 8)

78. 3. Prioritizing physical activities helps to conserve energy, which promotes adaptation to fatigue. The client should learn to take short naps or short rest periods during the day for additional energy conversation. Increased fluid intake is important but may interrupt rest periods by causing frequent urination. Limiting intake of high-fiber foods can add to constipation, which may be a problem because of inactivity in fatigued clients. (I, 7)

79. 4. Most hospitalized persons are at risk for sleep disturbances. Psychological reasons (eg, anxiety and depression) and pain are related to sleep deprivation. Social, nutritional, and cultural issues are not necessarily associated with sleep disturbances. (D, 7)

80. 4. Nursing interventions to decrease the discomfort of pruritus include those that prevent vasodilation, decrease anxiety, and maintain skin integrity and hydration. Medicated baths with alicylic acid or colloidal oatmeal can be soothing as a temporary relief. The use of antihistamines or topical steroids depends on the cause of the pruritus, and these agents should be used with caution. Using silk sheets is not a practical intervention for the hospitalized client with pruritus. (A, 8)

81. 3. Narcotics can be effective in controlling intractable dyspnea and are considered safe, even though a side effect may be decreased respiratory rate. Mucolytic agents, antidepressants, and diuretics do not affect dyspnea. (P, 10)

82. 4. Use of deodorant or fragrant soaps is drying to the skin. Cotton clothing gives the least irritation to skin. A cool, humidified environment adds to the client's comfort as well as providing hydration for skin comfort.

Fluid intake of 3000 mL per day is recommended for adequate hydration. (A, 8)

83. 4. Individuals with cancer have various cultural values and beliefs that help them cope with the cancer experience. Quality of life cannot be evaluated solely by quantifiable factors such as employability, functional status, or evidence of disease. It must be evaluated by the survivors within the context of their subjective and individual values and beliefs. (A, 5)

84. 4. Difficulty in swallowing, pain, and tightness in the chest are signs of esophagitis, which is a common complication of radiation therapy of the chest wall. Hiatal hernia is a herniation of a portion of the stomach into the esophagus. The client could experience burning and tightness in the chest secondary to a hiatal hernia, but not pain when swallowing. Also, hiatal hernia is not a complication of radiation therapy. Stomatitis is an inflammation of the oral cavity characterized by pain, burning, and ulcerations. The client with stomatitis may experience pain with swallowing, but not burning and tightness in the chest. Radiation enteritis is a disorder of the large and small bowel that occurs during or after radiation therapy to the abdomen, pelvis, or rectum. Nausea, vomiting, abdominal cramping, the frequent urge to have a bowel movement, and watery diarrhea are the signs and symptoms. (D, 10)

85. 2. Impaired concentration, apathy, and feelings of tiredness despite more sleep all suggest fatigue. Fatigue is a common complaint of individuals receiving radiation therapy. There are no data to suggest advanced breast cancer, hypocalcemia, or radiation pneumonitis. (A, 10)

86. 3. Constipation lasting 3 days or longer is unusual in this client and warrants immediate action. However, because the client had chemotherapy with Adriamycin 10 days ago, she is susceptible to infection and should avoid rectal medications and treatments. Abdominal discomfort secondary to constipation will be relieved after the client has a bowel movement; a narcotic would contribute to the constipation. (I, 7)

87. 4. A bedside commode should be near the client for easy, safe access. Measurement of urine output is also important in a client with heart failure. Putting diapers on an alert and oriented individual would be demeaning and inappropriate. Indwelling catheters are associated with increased risk of infection and are not a solution to possible incontinence. There is no reason to think that the client would not be able to use the bedside commode. (P, 2)

88. 2. Radiation fields that include the ovaries usually result in premature menopause. Vaginal dryness will occur without estrogen replacement. There should be no sexual intercourse while the implant is in place.

Cesium is a radioactive isotope used for therapeutic irradiation of cancerous tissue. There is no documentation to support vaginal relaxation after treatment. (D, 10)

89. 4. The rectal area needs to be cleansed and gently dried after each bowel movement to prevent skin breakdown and inhibit growth of bacteria. Sitz baths are appropriate, because they promote comfort. Zinc oxide ointment does form a protective skin barrier, but it makes it difficult to thoroughly cleanse the perirectal area of feces and increases the risk of infection, as do skin barrier dressings. (P, 2)

90. 2. Studies of long-term immunologic effects in clients treated for leukemia, Hodgkin's disease, and breast cancer reveal that combination treatments of chemotherapy and radiation can cause overall bone marrow suppression, decreased leukocytes numbers, and profound immunosuppression. Persistent and severe immunologic impairment may follow radiation and chemotherapy (especially multiagent therapy). There is no evidence of greater risk of infection in clients with persistent immunologic abnormalities. Suppressor T-cells recover more rapidly than the helper T-cells. (D, 10)

91. 3. Radiation-induced esophagitis with dysphagia is particularly common in clients who receive radiation to the chest. The anatomic location of the esophagus is posterior to the mediastinum and is within the field of primary treatment. Diarrhea may occur with radiation to the abdomen. Decreased energy level and decreased white blood cell count are potential complications of radiation therapy. (D, 10)

92. 1. Clients who receive multiple platelet transfusions may form antibodies against many foreign antigens, thereby decreasing platelet response. Single-donor platelets are drawn from a single donor, decreasing the number of possible foreign antigens and increasing platelet response for long-term therapy. Platelets do not contain coagulation factors in clinically significant amounts. Clients with a platelet count greater than $50,000/mm^3$ are not at risk for bleeding. Human leukocyte antigen–matched platelets are used when clients become refractory to single-donor and random-donor platelets. (D, 8)

The Client Who Is Coping With Loss, Grief, Bereavement, and Spiritual Distress

93. 4. Identifying available resources for the client and family represents a respectful effort to make options available and encourages the client to become involved in treatment decisions. Assuming decision making for the client may foster dependence. Encouraging strict

compliance with all treatment regimens may increase anxiety and limit the client's options and treatment choices. Informing the client of all possible adverse treatment effects may increase anxiety and fear by focusing on adverse outcomes too soon. (I, 5)

94. 4. Denial is a defense mechanism used to shut out a situation that is too frightening or threatening to tolerate. In this case, denial allows the client to vacillate between acceptance of the illness and its treatment and denial of the actual or potential seriousness of the disease. This may allow the client more psychological freedom to maintain her current roles in the family and elsewhere. Denial can be harmful if the client ignores standard medical therapies in favor of unconventional treatments. Denial is not helpful when it interferes with a client's willingness to seek treatment or make decisions about care. Using any one defense mechanism exclusively usually reflects maladaptive coping. Other defense mechanisms that may be used include regression, humor, and sublimation. (D, 5)

95. 2. The client's resources for coping with the emotional and practical needs of herself and her family need to be assessed, because usual coping strategies and support systems are often inadequate in especially stressful situations. The nurse may be concerned with the client's use of denial, decision-making abilities, and ability to pay for transportation; however, the client's support systems will be of more importance in this situation. (P, 5)

96. 4. Variables that are most predictive of negative bereavement outcomes include anger and self-reproach, low socioeconomic status, lack of preparation for death, and lack of family support. Making preparations suggests that she is coping with her husband's approaching death. (D, 5)

97. 1. Younger people are at higher risk for negative bereavement outcomes. Having a history of depressive illness or a close relationship to the deceased is a risk factor for negative bereavement outcomes. People with a lower socioeconomic status are at higher risk for negative bereavement outcomes. (D, 5)

98. 4. Focusing on the client's physical capabilities is important, but powerlessness reflects a perceived lack of control over the current situation and the belief that one's actions will not affect the outcome. Participation in decision making is key to getting the client involved and feeling more in control of his own care. Apathy and dependence on others are characteristics of powerlessness. Encouraging others to take responsibility for the client's care will increase his feelings of powerlessness. A referral to a psychologist is not necessarily indicated. The nurse should implement strategies to involve the client in decisions about his

care and evaluate the response to this intervention before suggesting a referral. (I, 5)

99. 1. Maintaining role function has been found to be a supportive source of normalcy and positive self-esteem for the client and family during the cancer experience. Facilitating family-related disagreements and conflicts is not the nurse's role. Supporting the client in her use of denial as a coping strategy will not help facilitate the client's adaptation to the diagnosis. Arranging transportation and child care on treatment days may be helpful but does not necessarily facilitate adaptation to the diagnosis. (P, 5)

100. 2. The most important central component of hospice care is focus of care on the client as well as the family or significant other. The team approach and the physician's coordination of the hospice team are important, but they are not the focus. Not all hospice clients want to die at home. (A, 5)

101. 3. Mental changes and decreased level of consciousness are common in the dying process. Comments that allude to travel, trips, or going somewhere are also common. Suggesting that the client be sedated ignores the husband's question about what his wife is experiencing. Suggesting that the client is fighting death and that the husband should leave her alone is inappropriate and denies the husband time to spend with his wife. Although decreased circulation and lack of oxygen may cause delirium, delirium is not the norm in the dying process. (D, 5)

102. 4. It is important to give factual information to answer a loved one's questions and concerns. Stating, "That's just the way it is," is unprofessional and uncaring. Saying, "I don't know when the bowels will shut down, but they will eventually," projects an uncaring attitude and does not address the wife's concern for her husband or her need for information. Although it may be true that the pain medication will slow bowel function, this does not provide the wife with the information she is seeking. (I, 7)

103. 4. It is important to allow the client to choose his or her own form of spiritual support. The dying client who is weakened by disease may not be able to attend services. The client must be consulted before referral to a chaplain is made. Reflection on past accomplishments may be comforting to the client, but it does not directly address spiritual concerns. (P, 5)

104. 2. A social worker can provide information for supportive services and can help the patient with financial concerns. A bank representative or someone from the hospital billing department may be needed; however, it is most appropriate for the social worker to first assess the client's needs. (I, 5)

105. 4. Dehydration is an expected event within the dying process. Hydration may be used in any situation of

dehydration as long as it is within the client and family's wishes. Rehydrating the client may actually prolong the dying process. Decisions about treatment are made with the family. (D, 7)

106. 4. The nurse must first allow the patient to explore his or her own beliefs and values before making referrals, explaining various religious beliefs, or suggesting appropriate reading material. (P, 5)

107. 3. Immediately after the disclosure of a cancer diagnosis, each person sets out on a unique path characterized by highly individual physical and psychosocial responses to a situation marked by uncertainty. Most want to know, "How long do I have to live?" Ability to perform in usual roles, cost of treatments, and pain are concerns of many clients diagnosed with cancer; however, the primary concern typically is remaining life span. (A, 5)

108. 2. Family and friends have been found to constitute the largest portion of the network of social support. Clergy, community support groups, and health care professionals usually have a temporary role in providing social support. (P, 5)

109. 4. Depression can be a mixture of affective responses (feelings of worthlessness, hopelessness, sadness), behavioral responses (appetite changes, withdrawal, sleep disturbances, lethargy), and cognitive responses (decreased ability to concentrate, indecisiveness, suicidal ideation). Increased decisiveness, problem-solving ability, and increased social interactions are reflective of adaptive coping. (A, 5)

110. 4. Bereavement support after death usually continues for about 1 year or as needed at little or no cost to the remaining family. Mutual support groups by nonprofessionals are usually free or inexpensive but are not necessarily appropriate for young children. Professional individual counseling and medication are expensive, and medication may not be appropriate for young children. To remind someone of what she should have done before the death is not helpful at this time. (P, 5)

111. 3. It is important to establish rapport with the client and family by listening to verbal and nonverbal concern and showing respect for cultural differences. The use of touch or eye contact is culture specific and cannot be generalized as an intervention for all individuals with cancer. Miscommunication between individuals of different cultures is often caused by language differences, rules of communication, age, and gender. (I, 5)

112. 1. Helping the client to identify available resources allows the client respect and time to make informed decisions and encourages him to become actively involved with treatment options. Encouraging compliance with treatment regimens discourages the client

from becoming actively involved in his treatment and diminishes coping ability. Relieving the client of decision making as much as possible is not appropriate and encourages feelings of helplessness and powerlessness. Assisting the client to prepare for adverse treatment effects may foster hopelessness and increase anxiety by focusing on adverse outcomes too soon. (P, 5)

113. 4. These American Cancer Society–sponsored groups are designed to educate clients and their families experiencing cancer about the disease and methods of coping positively with it. These are self-help and support groups monitored by professionals and cancer survivors who have undergone a training course that helps them to facilitate small groups. (P, 5)

114. 4. Many cancer survivors question why they are doing so well and others are not. Often they express feeling guilty when they hear that others are not doing well. Suggesting that the client does not know how to describe his own emotions is inappropriate and may discourage him from expressing his feelings. Although the client may be experiencing volatile emotions, this is not the likely source of his feelings of guilt. Guilt about doing well after cancer treatment is not a spiritual response to illness. (I, 5)

115. 4. The recurrence of the disease is found to be the most distressing time, and clients may experience anxiety, depression, and suicidal ideation. Clients may feel a decrease in their anxiety and depression with the initiation of definitive treatment or at the end of their first courses of treatment. Clients in the end stage of the disease may feel all of these emotions; however, when clients have been free from cancer for some time and learn that there is a recurrence, they often experience a sharp increase in their feelings of distress. (D, 5)

116. 2. Powerlessness is a subjective experience of helplessness and apathy that can be threatening to one's competency and result in increased dependence on others. Effective nursing interventions will provide opportunities for the client to be involved in decision making and to regain a sense of control. Ineffective Coping may also be a response to altered mobility, but the nursing interventions would be directed toward enhancing coping skills. Impaired Adjustment is characterized by statements or actions suggesting that the client has not accepted the change in her health status. Dysfunctional grieving is characterized by sadness, reliving past experiences, and expressions of distress about the loss. (D, 5)

117. 4. The person who has minimal social support, has not been successful in dealing with stressors, and has multiple other stressors is at greater risk for psychosocial distress. Being successful in dealing with stress all his life would decrease the client's risk for psychosocial distress. Not having to deal with other stressors would be helpful in managing the current stressful situation. The denial coping mechanism, if used for short periods, can decrease the risk for psychosocial distress. (D, 5)

118. 1. Cancer clients report that the lifelong fear of recurrence is one of the most disruptive aspects of the disease. The trajectory of the disease is unpredictable and can be intertwined with many short- and long-term illnesses related to cancer and the treatment modalities. A diagnosis of cancer challenges the individual and the family with a series of crises rather than a time-limited episode. There are no data to indicate that the client has an underlying behavioral disorder. (D, 5)

119. 4. Without clear, consistent communication, the parent–child relationship may become strained during the illness and subsequent death of a parent. A great number of parents do not know how to communicate with their children, especially about difficult emotional topics at a time when they are also under great emotional stress. The nurse should begin by providing information and developmentally appropriate books about the grieving process for children. Referral to pastoral care services may be appropriate; however, the nurse's direct intervention of beginning education about strategies for communication will be of immediate and long-term benefit. The grieving process cannot be rushed for the husband, nor should an opportunity for the father and children to communicate and grieve together be delayed. Excluding children from participating in the grieving ritual is not shielding them from the sorrow and sadness. (I, 5)

120. 3. Acknowledgment and discussion of the client's feelings begins the establishment of a therapeutic relationship between nurse and client. It also acknowledges the seriousness of the current situation and validates the client's feelings. Psychiatric help and antidepressant medication may be options if the depression is severe and prolonged. Encouraging a client to see the good or positive side of a situation minimizes the client's feelings. (I, 5)

121. 2. Individuals who are experiencing fatigue need to prioritize their activities and ask for assistance from others. It is best not to take away all of the client's activities, because her role as wife and mother is obviously important to her and to her sense of self-worth. Suggesting that she ignore the household chores or telling her not to worry because everyone gets tired disregards the client's feelings and is not appropriate. (I, 10)

122. 4. Tachycardia, tachypnea, moist or clammy skin, and disorientation are classic symptoms of delirium. Clients with panic disorder do not exhibit disorientation. Clients with depression exhibit a flat affect, apathy, and sleep disturbances. (A, 10)

123. 2. A progressive activity regimen may be prescribed to increase pulmonary function after surgical lung resec-

tion. Rehabilitation should include walking and some stair climbing as tolerated. Vigorous exercise is usually not recommended initially. Joining the Lost Chord Club and learning tracheostomy care are appropriate for the client who has undergone a laryngectomy. (I, 4)

124. 4. Serving as a volunteer in a client-to-client program represents reintegration with constructive channeling of energies, which indicates a higher level of adaptation than attention to safety, knowledge, or planned activity. (E, 5)

The Client Who Is Experiencing Problems With Sexuality

125. 3. Water-soluble lubricants used during sexual intercourse can augment reduced natural vaginal lubrication caused by ovarian dysfunction and decreased circulating estrogen related to chemotherapy. The use of vaginal dilators, relaxation techniques, or nightly douches would not increase vaginal lubrication. Frequent douching can disrupt the normal vaginal environment. (I, 3)

126. 3. Placing a thin piece of gauze over the tracheostomy during sexual activity will help to contain the secretions and yet allow ventilation. Although a scopolamine patch may depress the salivary and bronchial secretions, it is not recommended for long-term use and would not be indicated in this situation. Avoiding fluids before sexual activity is not recommended to decrease secretions. Washing the tracheostomy area with any deodorizing soap may cause skin irritation and place the client at risk for infection. (P, 3)

127. 4. This question introduces some basic information and allows for support for the client who may be experiencing some sexuality concerns. Not all women experience sexual problems after undergoing a hysterectomy. Assuming that the client will want to schedule an appointment with her partner is inappropriate and may embarrass her. Simply asking the client whether she expects to have problems with sex is too abrupt and does not provide any information. (A, 5)

128. 4. There is usually no change in sexual function with a simple, unilateral surgical procedure to remove one testicle. (I, 5)

129. 4. The risk of becoming neutropenic during chemotherapy is very high. Therefore, an inserted foreign object such as a diaphragm may be a nidus for infection. Although the nurse may wish to inform the client about the ease with which various contraceptive modalities may be used, the focus of this discussion should be on preventing an infection, which can be fatal for the neutropenic client. There are no data to

suggest the client is at risk for acquiring a sexually transmitted disease. (D, 1)

130. 2. Raising the upper torso for the affected partner facilitates respiratory function. The use of a waterbed may be helpful for the sensation of movement. A dependent position may compromise respiratory expansion, even though energy may be conserved. Duration of sexual activity is not necessarily related to exertion. (I, 7)

Ethical and Legal Issues Related to Clients With Cancer and End-of-Life Care

131. 1. The American Cancer Society wrote *The Cancer Survivors' Bill of Rights*. These rights address medical care, personal life adjustment, job opportunities, and insurance coverage. (A, 5)

132. 1. The Family Leave Act of 1993 ensures that family caregivers who must take a leave of absence or decrease their hours during the treatment or recovery phase of an illness will not lose their jobs. The Americans with Disabilities Act of 1990 prohibits employment discrimination against person with disabilities or those who are perceived to have disabilities; it has an indirect economic impact for cancer victims and their families. The Medicare Coverage for Catastrophic Illness Act of 1988 provided increased coverage for clients with a catastrophic illness. The Rehabilitation Act of 1973 prohibited discrimination on the basis of handicap under any program or activity receiving federal financial as- sistance. (D, 1)

133. 1. The Americans with Disabilities Act of 1990 requires equal opportunity in selection, testing, and hiring of qualified applicants with disabilities. Under this act, anyone who has had cancer is considered disabled. This law prohibits discrimination against workers with disabilities and is similar to the Civil Rights Act of 1964 and Title V of the Rehabilitation Act of 1973. The Patient Self-Determination Act addresses the rights of clients in regard to making health care decisions and the use of advance directives. (I, 1)

134. 3. It is appropriate and ethical to respect the client's truly autonomous choice not to know particular information. The client's best interests should be determined by the client after he or she receives all the necessary information and in conjunction with other people of the client's choice, including family, physicians, and other health care personnel. In consumerism, the client is provided the facts and then left unassisted to make a decision. With paternalism, decisions are made by the health care team without determining or respecting the client's wishes. (D, 1)

135. 4. The advocacy role of the nurse implies that the nurse will ensure that the client's wishes are being respected and that she is making informed decisions. Therefore, the nurse will assist in ensuring that the client is fully informed. The other interventions are appropriate for the nurse but are not related to client advocacy. The client may not understand or have all the necessary information for standard therapy. A client who is taking an alternative therapy should be monitored for adverse effects. If a client is taking an alternative therapy, it is essential for the physician to know so that the therapy can be incorporated into the client's treatment plan and to ensure that there are no incompatibilities with other therapies or medications. (I, 1)

136. 3. The best nursing advocacy intervention is listening carefully to the client and family's perceptions of their needs. Studies have demonstrated that these needs are not necessarily what the nurse thinks they are. Intervening without listening carefully may result in a lack of responsiveness to the real needs. Helping the client and family maintain a sense of optimism and hopefulness is appropriate but is not necessarily advocacy. Determining the client's and family's understanding of the results of the diagnostic testing and providing written materials about the cancer site and its treatment are examples of the nurse's role as educator. (I, 1)

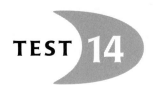

TEST 14

The Client Having Surgery

▶ The Client Who Is Preparing for Surgery

▶ The Client Who Is Receiving or Recovering From Anesthesia

▶ The Client Who Has Had Surgery

▶ Legal and Ethical Issues Associated With Surgery

▶ Correct Answers and Rationale

Select the one best answer, and indicate your choice by filling in the circle in front of the option.

The Client Who Is Preparing for Surgery

1. The nurse is reviewing the chart of a 55-year-old male client who is scheduled for a lumbar laminectomy. The nurse should notify the surgeon of which nursing assessment finding?
   ○ 1. Pimple on the lower back.
   ○ 2. Abnormal electrocardiogram (ECG).
   ○ 3. Hearing aid.
   ○ 4. Allergy to iodine.

2. The client tells the nurse on the preoperative unit that she is concerned because she cannot hear without her hearing aid and asks if she can keep it during surgery. What is the nurse's *best* response?
   ○ 1. Explain to the client that it is policy not to take personal items to surgery because they may be lost or broken.
   ○ 2. Tell the client that she will bring the hearing aid to the postanesthesia care unit so that she can have it as soon as she wakes up.
   ○ 3. Explain to the client that she will have a pre-medication that will make her sleepy before she goes to surgery and she won't need to hear.
   ○ 4. Call the surgery unit to explain the client's concern and ask if she can wear her hearing aid to surgery.

3. The client is to take clear liquids after midnight and nothing by mouth after 4 AM. The nurse recognizes that the client has deficient knowledge when he states that he
   ○ 1. ate jello at 3:30 AM.
   ○ 2. brushed his teeth at 4:00 AM but did not swallow.
   ○ 3. used a cold washcloth to hold against his lips.
   ○ 4. smoked a cigarette at 6:00 AM.

4. When a client states that she is allergic to shellfish, the nurse should suspect that she is also allergic to
   ○ 1. all other seafood.
   ○ 2. iodine skin preparations.
   ○ 3. caffeine.
   ○ 4. alcohol-based skin preparations.

5. The surgeon orders cefazolin (Ancef) 1 g to be given intravenously at 7:30 AM when the client's surgery is scheduled at 8:00 AM. The nurse understands that the primary reason to start the antibiotic exactly at 7:30 AM is
   ○ 1. that legally the medication has to be given at the ordered time.
   ○ 2. that the antibiotic is most effective in preventing infection if it is given 30 to 60 minutes before the operative incision is made.
   ○ 3. that the postoperative dose of Ancef needs to be started exactly 8 hours after the preoperative dose of Ancef.
   ○ 4. because of the peak and titer levels needed for antibiotic therapy.

6. Which of the following is the best way for the nurse to begin the preoperative interview of a client who is being admitted on the day of surgery?
   ○ 1. Walk in and ask, "Are you Mrs. Smith?"
   ○ 2. Walk in, sit down, and take the client's blood pressure.
   ○ 3. Walk in, sit down, maintain eye contact, and introduce yourself.
   ○ 4. Walk in and ask the client her name.

7. The nurse receives the laboratory results for a client who is scheduled for general anesthesia. The client has a serum potassium level of 5.8 mEq/L. What should be the nurse's *first* response?
   ○ 1. Call the surgeon.
   ○ 2. Send the client to surgery.
   ○ 3. Make a note on the front of the chart.
   ○ 4. Notify the anesthesiologist.

8. Before surgery, the preoperative nurse asks the client whether he has any allergies. The client responds, "Doesn't anyone communicate with anyone? I have been asked that question over and over!" What is the nurse's *best* response?
   ○ 1. "I'm sorry! I just have to ask that question for the record."

○ 2. "It's an important question and we just have to check."

○ 3. "You will hear it again and again as you go through surgery."

○ 4. "This question is asked for verification and safety with each new phase of treatment."

9. On the day of surgery, a diabetic client who takes insulin on a sliding scale is ordered to have nothing by mouth and all medications withheld. Her 6 AM glucose level is 300 mg/dL. What is the correct initial nursing intervention regarding the client's high blood glucose level?

○ 1. Withhold all medications as ordered.

○ 2. Administer the insulin dose dictated by the sliding scale.

○ 3. Call the physician for specific orders based on the glucose.

○ 4. Notify the surgery department.

10. The nurse is preparing a preoperative teaching plan for a client who is undergoing a bilateral breast reduction. On which component of the care plan should the nurse expect to spend the most time?

○ 1. Reduction of risk potential.

○ 2. Physiologic adaptation.

○ 3. Psychosocial integrity.

○ 4. Health promotion and maintenance.

11. A client is scheduled to have an elective mandibular osteotomy to correct a mandibular fracture sustained in an accident 6 months earlier. Which statement by the client indicates to the nurse maladaptive coping?

○ 1. "I will be glad to have my jaw fixed because my wife thinks I do not look like myself."

○ 2. "I am somewhat afraid to have the surgery but feel OK about it."

○ 3. "My wife will help me, but I don't think I will need that much help."

○ 4. "I am ready to get this over with."

12. The nurse is assessing a client's nutritional status preoperatively. Which of the following observations would indicate poor nutrition in a 5-foot 7-inch female client who is 21 years of age?

○ 1. Poor posture.

○ 2. Brittle nails.

○ 3. Dull expression.

○ 4. Weight of 128 pounds.

13. A 92-year-old male client who lives alone is admitted on the day of surgery for an inguinal hernia repair. He is very independent and states that the doctor says he will go home the day of surgery or the next morning. The preoperative nurse is planning his postoperative and discharge instructions. Which teaching method is the best approach for this client?

○ 1. Explain all the instructions to him.

○ 2. Demonstrate the instructions to him.

○ 3. Explain all the instructions to a family member.

○ 4. Write the instructions down for him.

14. A client is admitted for an arthroscopy of the right shoulder through same-day surgery. Which nurse is responsible for starting the client's discharge planning?

○ 1. The preadmission nurse.

○ 2. The preoperative nurse.

○ 3. The intraoperative nurse.

○ 4. The postoperative nurse.

15. The nurse is preparing to administer a premedication. Which of the following actions should the nurse take *first*?

○ 1. Have the family present.

○ 2. Ensure that the preoperative shave is completed.

○ 3. Have the client empty his bladder.

○ 4. Make sure the client is covered with a warm blanket.

16. While the nurse is interviewing the preoperative client, the client states that she is afraid of surgery because she had a cousin who died in surgery when she had her tonsils removed. What is the nurse's *best* response?

○ 1. Reassure the client that technology has changed over the last 10 years.

○ 2. Encourage the client to further express her concerns.

○ 3. Explain to the client that it is normal to be afraid.

○ 4. Ask the client if anyone else in her family has had trouble when they had surgery.

17. The preoperative nurse is assessing the client for risk for latex allergies. Clients are at risk for latex allergies if they are allergic to all the following *except*

○ 1. avocados.

○ 2. apples.

○ 3. kiwi.

○ 4. peaches.

18. The nurse would evaluate that which of the following clients is more at risk for latex allergies?

○ 1. A woman who is admitted for her seventh surgery.

○ 2. A man who works as a sales clerk.

○ 3. A man with well-controlled type 2 diabetes.

○ 4. A woman who is having laser surgery.

19. The nurse applies gloves, cleans the client's arm with alcohol, and begins to insert an intravenous catheter. The client begins to scratch her eyes and wipe her nose, which has begun to drain. The nurse should

○ 1. distract the client's attention.

○ 2. assess the client for pain.

○ 3. remove the catheter and assess the client's vital signs.

○ 4. increase the rate of administration of the intravenous fluids.

20. Which of the following questions would the nurse ask the client when evaluating his preoperative cognitive-perceptual pattern?
    ○ 1. "Do you have difficulty swallowing?"
    ○ 2. "Do you need special equipment to walk?"
    ○ 3. "Do you smoke?"
    ○ 4. "Do you wear glasses?"

21. The nurse is assessing a client who is scheduled for general anesthesia. When attempting to check the client's pupils, the nurse notices that the client has trouble tilting his head back. The client states that he has arthritis in his neck. Which of the following does the nurse recognize as the *primary* concern related to this finding?
    ○ 1. The client has limited movement of his neck.
    ○ 2. The client is at risk for postoperative neck pain.
    ○ 3. The client is at risk for difficult intubation.
    ○ 4. The ability to assess his pupils is limited.

22. The nurse receives the preoperative blood work report for a client who is scheduled to undergo surgery. Which of the following laboratory findings should be reported to the surgeon?
    ○ 1. Red blood cells, 4.5 million/mm³.
    ○ 2. Creatinine, 2.6 mg/dL.
    ○ 3. Hemoglobin, 12.2 g/dL.
    ○ 4. Blood urea nitrogen, 15 mg/dL.

23. A client scheduled for outpatient surgery will receive intravenous midazolam hydrochloride (Versed) for premedication. The nurse should prepare a teaching plan for the client that indicates the medication is intended to produce which of the following effects?
    ○ 1. Amnesia.
    ○ 2. Nausea.
    ○ 3. Mild agitation.
    ○ 4. Blurred vision.

24. Which nursing intervention is *most* essential when administering intravenous midazolam hydrochloride (Versed) for a premedication?
    ○ 1. Assessing the blood pressure.
    ○ 2. Monitoring the pulse oximeter.
    ○ 3. Encouraging slow, deep breaths.
    ○ 4. Explaining relaxation techniques.

25. When the nurse administers intravenous midazolam hydrochloride (Versed), the client demonstrates signs of an overdose. Which of the following interventions should the nurse be prepared to implement *first*?
    ○ 1. Ventilate with an oxygenated Ambu bag.
    ○ 2. Shock with ECG paddles.
    ○ 3. Administer 0.5 mL 1:1000 epinephrine.
    ○ 4. Titrate flumazenil (Romazicon).

26. The nurse recognizes that metoclopramide (Reglan) is ordered as a premedication for a gastroduodenoscopy primarily because of its ability to

○ 1. increase gastric pH.
○ 2. increase gastric emptying.
○ 3. reduce anxiety.
○ 4. inhibit respiratory secretions.

27. What therapeutic outcome does the nurse expect for a client who has received a premedication of glycopyrrolate (Robinul)?
    ○ 1. Increased heart rate.
    ○ 2. Increased respiratory rate.
    ○ 3. Decreased secretions.
    ○ 4. Decreased amnesia.

28. Atropine sulfate (Atropine) is contraindicated in all but which one of the following clients?
    ○ 1. A client with diabetes.
    ○ 2. A client with glaucoma.
    ○ 3. A client with urinary retention.
    ○ 4. A client with bowel obstructions.

29. After the nurse has administered droperidol (Inapsine) as a premedication, the *primary* reason that care is taken to move the client slowly in the transfer to the operating room is because of droperidol's effect on the
    ○ 1. central nervous system.
    ○ 2. respiratory system.
    ○ 3. cardiovascular system.
    ○ 4. psychoneurologic system.

30. A client has been ordered to receive enoxaparin (Lovenox) 6 hours before the scheduled time of her laparoscopic vaginal assisted hysterectomy (LAVH). Which of the following effects does the nurse recognize as being the intended therapeutic action of the enoxaparin?
    ○ 1. Increase in red blood cell production.
    ○ 2. Reduction of postoperative thrombi.
    ○ 3. Decrease in postoperative bleeding.
    ○ 4. Promotion of tissue healing.

31. During the interview the nurse obtains information about the client's medication history. It is *not* necessary for the nurse to record information about the client's
    ○ 1. current use of medications, herbs, and vitamins.
    ○ 2. over-the-counter medication use in the last 6 weeks.
    ○ 3. steroid use in the last year.
    ○ 4. use of all drugs taken in the last 18 months.

32. When the nurse is conducting a preoperative interview with a client who is having a vaginal hysterectomy, the client states that she forgot to tell her doctor that she had a total hip replacement 3 years ago. The nurse understands the importance of communicating this information to the perioperative nurse because
    ○ 1. the prosthesis may cause a problem with the electrosurgical unit used to control bleeding.

2. the client should not have her hip externally rotated when she is positioned for the procedure.

3. the perioperative nurse can inform the rest of the team about the total hip replacement.

4. there is not enough time to notify the surgeon and note this finding on the history and physical before the procedure.

33. The nurse learns that a client who is scheduled for a tonsillectomy has been taking 40 mg of oral prednisone daily for the last week for poison ivy on his leg. What is the nurse's *best* action?
   1. Document the prednisone with current medications.
   2. Notify the surgeon of the poison ivy.
   3. Notify the anesthesiologist of the prednisone administration.
   4. Send the client to surgery.

34. A client who is scheduled for an open cholecystectomy has a 20-pack-year history of smoking. The nurse understands that the client is most at risk for which of the postoperative complications?
   1. Deep vein thrombosis.
   2. Atelectasis and pneumonia.
   3. Delayed wound healing.
   4. Prolonged immobility.

35. In planning the preoperative and postoperative care for the client who is having surgery, the nurse understands that the circulating nurse
   1. passes instruments to the surgeon.
   2. answers the phone in surgery.
   3. provides the nursing process during surgery.
   4. ensures sterility of supplies.

36. The nurse explains to the family that they cannot go with the client past the doors that separate the public from the restricted area of the operating room suite because traffic control measures are designed to
   1. protect the privacy of clients.
   2. prevent any electrical sparks that could ignite the anesthetic gases.
   3. separate the family from the surgical team while they are working on the client.
   4. provide for an aseptic environment to prevent infection.

37. Which of the following clients is most at risk for potential hazards from the surgical experience?
   1. A 68-year-old client.
   2. A 50-year-old client.
   3. A 30-year-old client.
   4. A 13-year-old client.

38. The nurse recognizes that which of the following pediatric surgery clients should not play with a balloon?
   1. A child having her 15th laser surgery for a hemangioma.
   2. A child having a tonsillectomy.
   3. A child having an inguinal hernia repair.
   4. A child having an orchiopexy.

39. In which of the following clients is an autotransfusion possible?
   1. The client who has cancer.
   2. The client who is in danger of cardiac arrest.
   3. The client with a contaminated wound.
   4. The client with a ruptured bowel.

40. The nurse prepares a client who is to undergo cystoscopy by telling her that she will feel the urge to void when the procedure is over and to
   1. ignore the urge to void.
   2. force fluids.
   3. ask for the bedpan.
   4. ring for assistance to the bathroom.

41. Which of the following nursing interventions is *most* important in preventing postoperative complications?
   1. Progressive diet planning.
   2. Pain management.
   3. Bowel and elimination monitoring.
   4. Early ambulation.

The Client Who Is Receiving or Recovering From Anesthesia

42. A client arrives from surgery to the postanesthesia care unit. The nurse should complete which of the following respiratory assessments *first*?
   1. Oxygen saturation.
   2. Respiratory rate.
   3. Breath sounds.
   4. Airway flow.

43. A client who has had epidural anesthesia returns to the adult care unit. After assessing vital signs, the nurse should assess for which of the following next?
   1. Bladder distention.
   2. Headache.
   3. Postoperative pain.
   4. Ability to move the legs.

44. The nurse in the postanesthesia care unit notes that one of the client's pupils is larger than the other. Which of the following actions should the nurse perform next?
   1. Rate the client on the Glasgow scale.
   2. Administer oxygen.
   3. Check the client's baseline data.
   4. Call the surgeon.

45. A client returns to the surgical floor from the postanesthesia care unit after undergoing liposuction of the abdomen and thighs. After assessing the client's vital signs and establishing that the airway is patent, what is the nurse's next action?

○ 1. Check the dressing for signs of bleeding.

○ 2. Empty any peri-incisional drains.

○ 3. Assess the client's pain level.

○ 4. Assess the client's bladder.

46. Which is the best explanation for the nurse to give a client about general anesthesia induction?

○ 1. "Your premedication will put you to sleep."

○ 2. "You will breathe in an inhalant anesthetic mixed with oxygen through a facial mask and receive intravenous medication to make you sleepy."

○ 3. "You will receive intravenous medication to make you sleepy."

○ 4. "You will breathe in medication through a facial mask to make you sleepy."

47. Which is the best explanation for the nurse to give a child about general anesthesia induction?

○ 1. "You will be given an injection before you go to surgery to make you sleepy."

○ 2. "You will breathe in oxygen through a facial mask and receive intravenous medication to make you sleepy."

○ 3. "You will receive intravenous medication to make you sleepy."

○ 4. "You will breathe in medication through a facial mask to make you sleepy."

48. The nurse understands that the client with impaired cardiac functioning is at risk during anesthesia induction with sodium pentothal because this drug causes

○ 1. bradycardia.

○ 2. complete muscle relaxation.

○ 3. hypotension.

○ 4. tachypnea.

49. The nurse should anticipate that a client who has received propofol (Diprivan) as the induction and maintenance agent for general anesthesia will most likely experience

○ 1. minimal nausea and vomiting.

○ 2. hypotension.

○ 3. slow induction of anesthesia.

○ 4. small tremors of the skeletal muscles.

50. The nurse notices that surgical clients who go home the day of surgery receive desflurane (Suprane) or sevoflurane (Ultane) as the volatile liquid anesthesia agent. After obtaining information about these anesthetics, the nurse determines the main reason they are used is that they are

○ 1. better tolerated.

○ 2. predictable in their cardiovascular effects.

○ 3. nonirritating to the respiratory tract.

○ 4. rapidly eliminated.

51. The postanesthesia care nurse is assessing a 250-pound male client who has just returned from an arthroscopy of his right knee. His vital signs are as follows: pulse, 150 bpm; blood pressure, 90/50 mm

Hg; respiratory rate, 28 breaths/minute; and tympanic temperature, 99.8°F (37.7°C). The nurse notes that the client's muscles feel rigid. The nurse determines that the client

○ 1. is recovering as expected from the anesthesia and continues monitoring him.

○ 2. is exhibiting the effects of excessive blood loss experienced in the operating room and increases the rate of his intravenous infusion.

○ 3. is in the early stages of malignant hypothermia and obtains emergency medications and notifies the anesthesiologist.

○ 4. is in pain and offers him pain medication.

52. The nurse is assessing a client recovering from anesthesia. Which of the following signs or symptoms are the earliest indicators of hypoxemia?

○ 1. Somnolence.

○ 2. Restlessness.

○ 3. Chills.

○ 4. Urgency.

53. A nurse is planning the care for an 80-year-old client who has had spinal anesthesia with intravenous conscious sedation for a transurethral resection of the prostate (TURP). The procedure lasted 1.5 hours. The client was in the lithotomy position during the procedure and received 4000 mL of room temperature isotonic bladder irrigation. He now has continuous irrigation through a three-way Foley catheter. Which postoperative nursing intervention, after the airway and vital signs have been established, is *most* important when receiving this client from the operating room?

○ 1. Empty the catheter drainage bag.

○ 2. Cover the client with warm blankets.

○ 3. Hang new bags of irrigation.

○ 4. Turn the client.

54. Based on the nurse's knowledge of absorption and elimination of general anesthetics, which of the following clients is expected to retain the anesthesia agents longest?

○ 1. A client who is 6 feet 2 inches tall and weighs 250 pounds.

○ 2. A client who is 5 feet 4 inches tall and weighs 110 pounds.

○ 3. A client who is 5 feet 1 inch tall and weighs 200 pounds.

○ 4. A client who is 5 feet 7 inches tall and weighs 145 pounds.

55. The nurse receives a postoperative client who is awake and has received an intravenous regional nerve block (Bier block) for repair of a tendon in the wrist. The arm is bandaged, casted, and elevated on a pillow. What action should the nurse encourage the client to avoid until the intravenous regional anesthesia wears off?

○ 1. Holding the operated arm close to the face.
○ 2. Holding the operated arm with the unoperated arm.
○ 3. Using the unoperated arm.
○ 4. Using pain medication.

56. A client was given 10 mg of morphine sulfate intramuscularly for pain on return to the unit after surgery to repair a hiatal hernia. The nurse notes that the client's respirations are now 4 per minute and, after notifying the physician, prepares to administer intravenous naloxone (Narcan) to reverse the respiratory depression. The nurse plans to implement which of the following interventions after administration of the naloxone?
   ○ 1. Check respirations in 5 minutes, because naloxone is immediately effective in relieving respiratory depression.
   ○ 2. Check respirations in 30 minutes, because the effects of morphine will have worn off by then.
   ○ 3. Monitor respirations frequently for 4 to 6 hours, because the client may need repeated doses of naloxone.
   ○ 4. Monitor respirations each time the client receives morphine sulfate 10 mg intramuscularly.

57. The nurse monitors the surgical client closely for which clinical manifestation with the administration of naloxone (Narcan)?
   ○ 1. Dizziness.
   ○ 2. Biliary colic.
   ○ 3. Bleeding.
   ○ 4. Urinary retention.

58. The nurse anticipates that the client who has received epidural anesthesia is at decreased risk for a headache because
   ○ 1. a 17-gauge needle is used.
   ○ 2. a subarachnoid injection is made.
   ○ 3. a noncutting needle is used.
   ○ 4. a faster onset occurs.

59. Spinal anesthesia affects all of the following systems *except*
   ○ 1. the sympathetic nervous system.
   ○ 2. the sensory system.
   ○ 3. the parasympathetic nervous system.
   ○ 4. the motor system.

60. The nurse is to administer midazolam (Versed) 2.5 mg by slow intravenous push (IVP) over 2 minutes to a 45-year-old male client undergoing an endoscopy. This medication is available in a 5 mg/mL vial. What amount should the nurse administer?
   ○ 1. 0.5 mL.
   ○ 2. 0.25 mL.
   ○ 3. 0.45 mL.
   ○ 4. 0.75 mL.

61. When a client in the postanesthesia care unit is being actively rewarmed with an external warming device, the nurse should monitor the client's body temperature every
   ○ 1. 5 minutes.
   ○ 2. 10 minutes.
   ○ 3. 15 minutes.
   ○ 4. 20 minutes.

The Client Who Has Had Surgery

62. When transferring a very elderly, drowsy client with fragile skin from the surgery cart to the bed, how should the nurse plan to assist the client in the transfer to prevent skin shearing?
   ○ 1. With two people at each side using a draw sheet.
   ○ 2. With two people, one at each side using a draw sheet, and one person at the head.
   ○ 3. With two people using a roller and a draw sheet.
   ○ 4. With two people, one at each side using a draw sheet, one person at the head, and one person at the feet.

63. Nursing assessment of a client's ability to swallow fluids before providing any oral fluids is an important nursing action in the immediate postoperative or postprocedural period. Which of the following clients would *not* require such an assessment?
   ○ 1. The client who has undergone a bronchoscopy under local anesthesia.
   ○ 2. The client who has undergone a transurethral resection of a bladder tumor under general anesthesia.
   ○ 3. The client who has undergone a repair of carpal tunnel syndrome under local anesthesia.
   ○ 4. The client who has undergone an inguinal herniorrhaphy with spinal and intravenous conscious sedation.

64. A client is admitted to the surgical floor after having bowel surgery. The nurse observes that the client's urinary output has decreased from 50 to 20 mL/hour. The nurse considers which of the following as the most likely cause?
   ○ 1. Bowel obstruction.
   ○ 2. Side effect of opioid analgesics.
   ○ 3. Hemorrhage.
   ○ 4. Hypertension.

65. Clients are at risk for injury secondary to perioperative positioning. Which of the following would indicate that the client who has had a left thoracoscopy may have sustained such an injury?
   ○ 1. Foot drop.
   ○ 2. Knee swelling and pain.

○ 3. Tingling in the arm.

○ 4. Absence of the Achilles reflex.

66. Of the following surgeries, which is most likely to cause the client to experience postoperative nausea and vomiting?

○ 1. Total hip replacement.

○ 2. Mitral valve repair.

○ 3. Abdominal hysterectomy.

○ 4. Mastectomy of left breast.

67. The nurse is planning to teach incisional care to a client before discharge. Which of the following instructions should be included?

○ 1. Do not touch your incision before your next appointment.

○ 2. Clean your incision three times a day with hydrogen peroxide and water.

○ 3. Do not be concerned about uneven lumps under the suture lines.

○ 4. If the staples don't come out by themselves before your next appointment, the surgeon will remove them.

68. The nurse is removing the client's staples from an abdominal incision when the client sneezes and the incision splits open, exposing the intestines. Which of the following actions should the nurse take next?

○ 1. Press the emergency alarm to call the resuscitation team.

○ 2. Cover the abdominal organs with sterile dressings moistened with sterile normal saline.

○ 3. Have all visitors and family leave the room.

○ 4. Call the surgeon to come to the client's room immediately.

69. After the nurse empties a Jackson-Pratt drainage bulb, which of the following nursing interventions will ensure correct functioning of the drain?

○ 1. Irrigating it with normal saline.

○ 2. Connecting it to low intermittent suction.

○ 3. Compressing it and then plugging it to establish suction.

○ 4. Connecting it to a drainage bag and clamping it off.

70. Which of the following interventions should the nurse implement to help prevent postoperative pulmonary emboli?

○ 1. Have the client perform leg exercises every hour while awake.

○ 2. Encourage the client to cough and deep-breathe.

○ 3. Massage the calves of the client's legs.

○ 4. Have the client wear antiembolic stockings when out of bed.

71. The nurse assesses a client who has just received morphine sulfate. The client's blood pressure is 90/50 mm Hg; pulse, 58 bpm; respirations, 4 breaths/minute. What drug should the nurse prepare to administer?

○ 1. Flumazenil (Romazicon).

○ 2. Naloxone hydrochloride (Narcan).

○ 3. Doxacurium (Nuromax).

○ 4. Remifentanil (Ultiva).

72. Which of the following statements indicates to the nurse that a client who is being discharged from same-day surgery has deficient knowledge?

○ 1. "My husband is taking the day off from work to drive me home."

○ 2. "I can drive myself home after surgery."

○ 3. "I am taking a taxi home and my daughter will meet me at home."

○ 4. "My son will be here at noon to take me home."

73. The nurse is teaching a client who has had a laparoscopic cholecystectomy about postoperative pain management. Which of the following statements indicates that the client has deficient knowledge?

○ 1. "My pain is related to the gas used to distend my abdominal cavity."

○ 2. "My diet should include eating bland foods until the gas clears up."

○ 3. "My pain is related to the large incision and manipulation."

○ 4. "My pain should be relieved by walking to eliminate the gas."

74. A client undergoes an arthroscopy of the knee. Once the initial postoperative assessment is completed, the nurse does *not* need to assess which of the following parameters every 15 minutes during the first postoperative hour?

○ 1. Vital signs including pulse oximeter.

○ 2. Pain rating of the operative site.

○ 3. Urinary output.

○ 4. Neurovascular check distal to the operative site.

75. After surgery, a client was treated for postoperative nausea and vomiting and now is experiencing hypotension and tachycardia. The nurse understands that these side effects are most frequently associated with the administration of

○ 1. ondansetron hydrochloride (Zofran).

○ 2. droperidol (Inapsine).

○ 3. prochlorperazine (Compazine).

○ 4. promethazine (Phenergan).

76. When an epidural catheter is used for postoperative pain management, the nurse should

○ 1. assess but not disturb the epidural dressing.

○ 2. change the epidural dressing daily.

○ 3. change the epidural dressing daily only if it is wet.

○ 4. use strict aseptic technique when handling the epidural catheter.

77. The nurse understands that the client who has epidural pain management postoperatively can ambulate

○ 1. because the epidural catheter is in place for occasional use only.

○ 2. because a low concentration of local anesthesia with analgesia is used.

○ 3. because only analgesia is used.

○ 4. because of a low pain threshold.

78. A surgical client develops pruritus and urticaria during the administration of an intravenous antibiotic. These clinical manifestations most likely indicate that the client is having which of the following types of reactions?

○ 1. Type I—anaphylactic reaction.

○ 2. Type II—cytotoxic and cytolytic reaction.

○ 3. Type III—immune-complex reaction.

○ 4. Type IV—delayed hypersensitivity reaction.

79. A postoperative client who is coughing and short of breath complains of a feeling of doom. Her blood pressure is 80/60 mm Hg; pulse, 120 bpm; and respirations, 24 breaths/minute. These are clinical manifestations of

○ 1. malignant hyperthermia.

○ 2. anaphylaxis.

○ 3. contact dermatitis.

○ 4. cell-mediated response.

80. A 34-year-old male client who had a lumbar fusion 3 days earlier continues to take hydrocodone 7.5 mg and acetaminophen 500 mg (Lortab 7.5/500). Before administering the pain medication, the nurse should ask the client,

○ 1. "Where is your pain located?"

○ 2. "Have you emptied your bladder?"

○ 3. "How long has it been since your last dose?"

○ 4. "Is your pain better than before you had surgery?"

81. When a client wakes up in the postanesthesia care unit, she sees that she has a drain with bright red fluid in it exiting from her total hip incision. She asks the nurse, "Is this the way it is supposed to be?" Which of the following represents the nurse's best response?

○ 1. "The drainage is blood and fluid that must be drained out for healing."

○ 2. "Don't worry about it, I will explain it when you are more awake."

○ 3. "This blood is being kept sterile and will be given back to you."

○ 4. "I will give you something to make you sleep, so you will not worry."

82. A client who in the first day after surgical repair of a ruptured diverticulum has a Jackson-Pratt drainage tube in place. The client asks the nurse the purpose of the drain. What is the nurse's best response?

○ 1. "The drainage tube is used to prevent infection in the peritoneal cavity."

○ 2. "The drainage tube is used to prevent bleeding into the peritoneal cavity."

○ 3. "The drainage tube is used to prevent pressure on the bladder."

○ 4. "The drainage tube is used to prevent pressure on the gallbladder."

83. A client has had a cholecystectomy and has a biliary drainage tube in place. The client asks the nurse what the drainage should look like. The nurse informs the client that normal drainage will have which of the following qualities?

○ 1. Thin and pinkish red.

○ 2. Dark yellow-orange.

○ 3. Clear and thick.

○ 4. Green and thick.

84. A client is to be discharged from same-day surgery after his inguinal hernia repair. It has been 7 hours since his surgery. Which of the following indicates this client is ready to be discharged?

○ 1. The client voids 500 mL of urine.

○ 2. The client tolerates eating a hamburger.

○ 3. The client is pain free.

○ 4. The client walks in the hallway unassisted.

85. A client is eligible for patient-controlled analgesia (PCA) when

○ 1. a family member is able to assist with self-dosing.

○ 2. there is a court-appointed advocate to assist with self-dosing.

○ 3. the client has the ability to self-dose.

○ 4. there is a nurse to assist with self-dosing.

86. How often should the postoperative client's temperature be assessed during the first 24 hours after surgery?

○ 1. Every 2 hours.

○ 2. Every 4 hours.

○ 3. Every 6 hours.

○ 4. Every 8 hours.

87. After the first 24 hours, how often should the postsurgical client's temperature be assessed?

○ 1. Every 6 hours.

○ 2. Every 8 hours.

○ 3. Every 12 hours.

○ 4. Every 24 hours.

88. The client who has been positioned in the lithotomy position under general anesthesia for a pelvic procedure may experience postoperative discomfort in which anatomic area?

○ 1. Shoulders.

○ 2. Thighs.

○ 3. Legs.

○ 4. Feet.

89. Which of the following nursing interventions does *not* aid in meeting the goal of clear breath sounds?

○ 1. Offering pain relief before having the client cough.

○ 2. Providing a minimum of 1500 mL fluid per day.

○ 3. Monitoring breath sounds.

○ 4. Assisting with early ambulation.

90. Which of the following is *not* a sign of thromboembolism?

○ 1. Redness.

○ 2. Swelling.

○ 3. Coolness.

○ 4. Edema.

91. The nurse is teaching the client about deep-breathing techniques. The nurse determines that the client needs additional education when he makes which of the following statements?

○ 1. "I will use my incentive spirometer every hour while I'm awake."

○ 2. "I should place my hands lightly over my lower ribs and upper abdomen."

○ 3. "I should get into a comfortable position before doing my breathing exercises."

○ 4. "I should take four deep breaths and then cough deeply from the lungs."

92. A client has had a nasogastric tube connected to low intermittent suction. This intervention places the client at risk for which of the following complications?

○ 1. Confusion.

○ 2. Muscle cramping.

○ 3. Edema.

○ 4. Tremors.

93. A client returned from surgery is unable to void after 8 hours. Her bladder is distended. Which of the following interventions is contraindicated?

○ 1. Facilitate voiding by normal position.

○ 2. Pour running water over perineum.

○ 3. Insert an indwelling Foley catheter.

○ 4. Insert a straight catheter every 4 hours.

Legal and Ethical Issues Associated With Surgery

94. On admission to same-day surgery, the nurse reviews the chart to verify the client's identification documentation. Which of the following is *most* important?

○ 1. Admitting record.

○ 2. Addressograph labels.

○ 3. Identification bracelet.

○ 4. Location of family.

95. Which of the following items of documentation is *not* required for the nurse to have on the chart before the client is transported to the operating suite?

○ 1. Operative consent.

○ 2. History and physical information.

○ 3. Laboratory test results.

○ 4. Anesthesia note.

96. A 15-year-old client needs life-saving emergency surgery, but his relatives live an hour away from the hospital and cannot sign the consent form. What is the nurse's *best* response?

○ 1. Send the client to surgery without the consent.

○ 2. Call the family for a consent over the telephone and have another nurse listen as a witness.

○ 3. No action is necessary in this case because consent is not needed.

○ 4. Have the family sign the consent form as soon as they arrive.

97. A client is being prepared to have a craniotomy for a brain tumor. As a client advocate, the nurse is evaluating the client's understanding of the informed consent before witnessing the client's signature on the operative consent form. Which of the following indicates that the nurse needs to contact the surgeon for further communication with the client?

○ 1. "We talked about the effect of my diabetes on healing."

○ 2. "The surgeon explained how the craniotomy was done."

○ 3. "There are no major risks from this surgery."

○ 4. "I will die if the tumor is not removed from my brain."

98. The nurse should ask all clients 65 years or older who are having surgery which of the following questions?

○ 1. "Do you have Medicare Part A to help pay for the hospital reimbursement?"

○ 2. "Do you have an advance directive such as a health care proxy or living will?"

○ 3. "Do you have extra coverage to help pay for medications?"

○ 4. "Do you have Medicare Part B to help pay for your expenses?"

99. The client's identification armband was removed to start an intravenous line as a part of the preoperative preparation. The operating room transport team has arrived to transport the client. What is the nurse's best response?

○ 1. Send the removed armband with the chart and the client to the operating room.

○ 2. Place a new identification armband on the client's wrist before transport.

○ 3. Tape the cut armband back onto the client's wrist.

○ 4. Send the client without an armband because she can verbally identify herself.

100. When a client cannot read or write but is of sound mind, the nurse should read the consent to the client in the presence of two witnesses and

○ 1. have the client's next-of-kin sign the consent.

○ 2. have the client put an "X" on the signature line.

○ 3. have a court appoint a guardian for the client.

○ 4. have a hospital quality management coordinator sign for the client.

Correct Answers and Rationale

The letters in parentheses following the rationale identify the step of the nursing process (A, D, P, I, E) and client needs (1, 2, 3, 4, 5, 6, 7, 8, 9, 10). See the inside front cover for the key.

The Client Who Is Preparing for Surgery

1. 1. A pimple close to the incision site may be reason for the surgeon to cancel the surgical procedure because it increases the risk of infection. If the client had an abnormal ECG, the nurse would notify the anesthesiologist who will be administering the anesthesia. The anesthesiologist is the decision-maker regarding the implications of the anesthesia on the cardiac system. The surgical team should be notified of the client's hearing disability, but the surgeon, who has already met the client, does not need to be notified. The surgical team should be notified of the client's allergy to iodine and it should be documented in all the appropriate places, but the surgeon would not need to be notified in advance of the surgical procedure. (A, 2)

2. 4. When a client has a concern, it is important to decrease her stress as much as possible. The nurse should call the operating room and inform the intraoperative nurse. A special container with correct identification can be prepared so that when the client is anesthetized and her hearing aid is removed, it will not be lost or broken. It is usual policy not to send personal belongings to surgery because they are easily broken or lost in the transfer of an anesthetized client with higher priority needs, but special needs do exist. In some instances the nurse does bring a client's personal belongings to the postanesthesia care unit, but in this case the item involves the client's ability to communicate. Because the trend is to use little premedication, clients are more alert and may want to talk with their surgical team before going to sleep. Decreasing the client's anxieties preoperatively affects the amount of medication used to induce the client and her overall psychological and physiologic status. Telling the client that she won't need to hear is insensitive. (P, 5)

3. 4. The client has deficient knowledge if he smoked a cigarette after 4 AM because, even though he did not have anything to eat or drink, smoking has increased the production of gastric hydrochloric acid, which can increase the risk for aspiration in an anesthetized client. Jello is a clear liquid and is acceptable. Comfort measures such as brushing the teeth without swallowing or holding a cold washcloth against the lips are acceptable for a client who is to have nothing by mouth. (D, 7)

4. 2. Clients who are allergic to shellfish are allergic to iodine skin preparations (Iodophor and Betadine) or any other products with iodine, such as dyes. Clients who are allergic to shellfish do not necessarily have an allergy to any other substances or seafood. (D, 9)

5. 2. The antibiotic is most effective in preventing infection, according to research, if it is given 30 to 60 minutes before the operative incision is made. When the surgeon orders the antibiotic to be given at a specific time related to the scheduled time of the surgical procedure, it is imperative that the antibiotic is given on time. Legally, the nurse considers 30 minutes on either side of the scheduled time to be acceptable for administering medications; but in this situation, giving the antibiotic 30 minutes too soon can make the prophylactic antibiotic ineffective. The postoperative dose of antibiotic is not timed according to the preoperative dose. Peak and titer levels are measured for some antibiotics, but in this case the primary reason is to have the antibiotic infused before the time of the incision. (D, 9)

6. 3. Nurses should provide the preoperative client individual and sincere attention by meeting the client at eye level and introducing themselves by name and role. The nurse should ask the client to tell her full name rather than asking if she is Mrs. Smith, because there might be another client by that name on the schedule. Nurses should not start the physical assessment or ask the client's name without first identifying themselves and their role out of courtesy and to relieve the client's anxiety in the new environment of the surgical experience. (I, 5)

7. 4. The nurse should notify the anesthesiologist, because a serum potassium level of 5.8 mEq/L places the client at risk for dysrhythmias when under general anesthesia. The surgeon may be notified; however, the anesthesiologist will make the decision about whether to proceed with surgery. The nurse should not automatically send a client with abnormal laboratory findings to surgery, because the procedure may be canceled. Once the client is inside the operating room and sterile supplies have opened up for the procedure, the client is usually charged. The nurse should call ahead of time to communicate the abnormal laboratory result instead of placing a note on the front of the chart. A note would not be seen until after the client has been transported to the operating room and the supplies have been opened. (I, 9)

8. 4. Clients should be aware that some questions are asked for verification and safety with each new phase of treatment. (A, 5)

9. 3. The nurse should notify the physician directly for specific orders based on the client's glucose level. The nurse cannot ignore the elevated glucose level. The surgical experience is stressful and the client needs specific insulin coverage during the perioperative period. The nurse should not administer the insulin without checking with the surgeon because there are specific orders to withhold all medications. (I, 7)

10. 3. Psychosocial integrity issues including coping mechanisms, situational role changes, and body image changes are more common in a client who undergoes elective cosmetic surgical procedures. Reduction of risk potential, physiologic adaptation, and health promotion and maintenance are greater needs for clients who are undergoing surgical correction of functional, anatomic, or physiologic defects in nonelective surgical procedures. (P, 5)

11. 1. A client should not elect surgery to meet someone else's needs. The nurse should encourage the client to share his feelings and his perception of the deformity and to clarify his reasons for electing to have the surgery. It is normal to be somewhat afraid, and it is good if a client says he feels "OK" about the surgery. The fact that a client believes that his wife will help him after surgery and that he will also be relatively independent reflects appropriate adaptation. It is a common feeling among preoperative clients that they are ready to "get this over with," indicating that the waiting period is stressful. (D, 5)

12. 2. Brittle nails indicate poor nutrition. Poor posture indicates that the client does not stand up straight and use her muscles to support herself. A dull expression reflects the client's affect and emotional status. The client's weight of 128 pounds is within normal range. (D, 7)

13. 4. The Joint Commission on Accreditation for Hospital Organizations (JCAHO) requires that discharge instructions be written for the postoperative client. The nurse will review all instructions orally and will demonstrate any skill. Clients need to be given discharge instructions both orally and in written form because of stress, medications, and the volume of material to be learned. Explaining all the instructions to a family member is important but does not replace the need for written instructions. (P, 1)

14. 1. The preadmission nurse, the first person in contact with the client, starts the discharge planning for the client undergoing surgery. (P, 1)

15. 3. The nurse should have the client empty his bladder before the premedication is administered. This will be more comfortable and safe for the client. The purpose of the premedication is to decrease anxiety and promote a relaxed state. The client must have an empty bladder before being transferred to the operating room, where he will be immobilized and receive intravenous fluids. The family does not have to be present, but it is usually desired. Shaving the operative area is not generally recommended because it can cause small nicks that harbor bacteria. If the client must be shaved, it is usually done in the operating room holding area. The client should be comfortable at all times and offered a warm blanket whenever he is cool, before or after the premedication. (I, 7)

16. 4. The nurse should immediately think of the congenital metabolic tendency for malignant hyperthermia, which occurs in the presence of certain kinds of anesthetics. Whenever a preoperative client states that a family member has had problems with anesthesia or surgery, the nurse should inquire about the nature of the problems and whether other family members have had similar problems. Reassuring the client that technology has changed will do little to affect her fears and misses the opportunity to evaluate the risk for malignant hyperthermia. Encouraging the client to further express her concerns and reassuring her that her feelings are normal are important, but missing a familial tendency for malignant hyperthermia could be fatal. (A, 4)

17. 2. Clients who are allergic to apples are not known to be at risk for latex allergies. Clients who are allergic to avocados, kiwi, peaches, guava, bananas, water chestnuts, hazelnuts, tomatoes, potatoes, grapes, and apricots are at risk for latex allergies. (A, 4)

18. 1. Clients who have had long-term multiple exposures to latex products, such as would occur with six previous surgeries and recoveries, are at increased risk for latex allergies. The nurse should explore what types of surgeries these were, how involved the client's recoveries were, and whether any signs of latex allergies have occurred in the past. Working as a sales clerk, having type 2 diabetes, or undergoing laser surgery does not expose a client to latex or increase the risk of latex allergy. (D, 4)

19. 3. The nurse should assess the vital signs of the client who exhibits urticaria, rhinitis, and conjunctivitis a few seconds after coming in contact with rubber gloves, a plastic catheter, plastic intravenous tubing, and a plastic intravenous solution bag. The nurse should recognize that these symptoms indicate that a type I allergic reaction is occurring, that the client is responding to the latex, and that the reaction can proceed into anaphylactic shock. The client does not need to be distracted or assessed for pain. Increasing the rate of administration of intravenous fluids is not the correct next action. (A, 10)

20. 4. The nurse would ask the client whether he wears glasses to evaluate his preoperative cognitive–perceptual pattern. Asking about the client's swallowing pattern would evaluate his nutritional–metabolic pattern. Asking about his need for special equipment to walk would evaluate his activity–exercise pattern. Asking the client about his history of smoking would evaluate his health perception–health management pattern. (E, 7)

21. 3. The client is at risk for a difficult intubation, because the neck must be hyperextended to pass the endotracheal tube. Assessment of the pupils should not be limited. (D, 9)

22. 2. The nurse should call the surgeon for a serum creatinine level of 2.6 mg/dL, which is higher than the normal range of 0.5 to 1.0 mg/dL. An elevated serum creatinine value indicates that the kidneys are not filtering effectively and has important implications for the surgical client because many of the anesthesia and analgesia medications need to be filtered out through the renal system. The red blood cell count, hemoglobin level, and blood urea nitrogen level are within normal limits and do not need to be reported to the surgeon. (A, 7)

23. 1. Midazolam hydrochloride (Versed) causes amnesia or decreased ability to remember events that occurred around the time of sedation. Nausea, mild agitation, and blurred vision are side effects of Versed. (P, 8)

24. 3. The client should be encouraged to take slow, deep breaths because midazolam hydrochloride (Versed) is a respiratory depressant. The nurse should assess the client's blood pressure, monitor the pulse oximeter, and keep the client calm and relaxed, but the client will slip into very shallow, ineffective breathing if not encouraged to deep-breathe. (I, 8)

25. 1. The nurse should have an Ambu bag in the client's room, because midazolam hydrochloride (Versed) can lead to respiratory arrest if it is administered too quickly. The client does not need to be shocked back into a normal rhythm or to receive epinephrine unless cardiac compromise developed after the respiratory arrest. The client would receive titrated dosing of flumazenil (Romazicon) to reverse the Versed, but first the nurse would ventilate the client. (P, 8)

26. 2. Metoclopramide (Reglan) is an antiemetic given because of its gastric emptying ability, which is necessary in gastrointestinal procedures. It does not increase gastric pH, reduce anxiety, or inhibit respiratory secretions. (I, 8)

27. 3. Glycopyrrolate (Robinul) is an anticholinergic given for its ability to reduce oral and respiratory secretions before general anesthesia. Increased heart rate and respiratory rate would be adverse effects of the drug. Amnesia should not be an effect of the drug. (P, 8)

28. 1. The nurse can administer atropine sulfate (Atropine), an anticholinergic, to a client with diabetes. Atropine is contraindicated in clients with glaucoma because it increases intraocular pressure. It is contraindicated in clients with urinary retention because it relaxes smooth muscle in the urinary tract and can exacerbate the problem. It is contraindicated in clients with gastrointestinal obstructions because it relaxes smooth muscle in the gut and may worsen the obstruction. (I, 8)

29. 3. Because droperidol (Inapsine) causes tachycardia and orthostatic hypotension, the client should be moved slowly after receiving this medication. Inapsine produces a tranquilizing effect and does affect the central nervous, respiratory, or psychoneurologic system, but the primary reason for moving the client slowly is the potential cardiovascular effects of hypotension. (I, 8)

30. 2. Research findings have shown that enoxaparin (Lovenox) and low-dose heparin given 6 to 12 hours preoperatively reduce the incidence of deep vein thrombosis and pulmonary emboli by 60% in clients who are at risk for deep vein thrombosis, such as those who are placed in the lithotomy position. Lovenox has no effect on red blood cell production, postoperative bleeding, or tissue healing. (D, 8)

31. 4. The nurse does not need to ask about all drugs used in the last 18 months unless the client is still taking them. The nurse does need to know all drugs the client is currently taking, including herbs and vitamins, over-the-counter medications such as aspirin taken in the past 6 weeks, the amount of alcohol consumed, and illegal use of drugs, because these can interfere with the anesthetic and analgesic agents. Steroid use is of concern because it can suppress the adrenal cortex for up to 1 year, and supplemental steroids may need to be administered in times of stress such as surgery. (A, 8)

32. 2. The nurse should notify the surgery department and document the past surgery in the chart in the preoperative notes so that the client's hip is not externally rotated and the hip dislocated while she is in the lithotomy position. The prosthesis should not be a problem as long as the perioperative nurse places the grounding pad away from the prosthesis site. The perioperative nurse will inform the rest of the team, but the primary reason to inform the perioperative nurse is related to safe positioning of the client. The surgeon can handwrite an addendum to the history and initial and date the entry. The history and physical information can then be retyped at a later date. (P, 7)

33. 3. The nurse should notify the anesthesiologist, because supplemental prednisone suppresses the adrenal cortex's natural ability to produce increased corticosteroids in times of stress such as surgery. The anesthesiologist may need to order supplemental steroid coverage dur-

ing the perioperative period. The nurse should document the prednisone with current medications, but it is a priority to inform the anesthesiologist. Because the poison ivy is not in the surgical field, the surgeon does not need to be called regarding the skin disruption. (P, 9)

34. 2. The client who has a significant cigarette smoking history and an operative manipulation close to the diaphragm (the gallbladder is against the liver) is at increased risk for atelectasis and pneumonia. Postoperatively this client will be reluctant to deep-breathe because of pain, in addition to having residual lung damage from smoking. Therefore, the client is at greater-than-average risk for pulmonary complications. The client does not have an increased risk for prolonged immobility unless slowed by a respiratory problem. (D, 9)

35. 3. The circulating nurse is a registered nurse who uses the nursing process (assessment, planning, implementation, and evaluation of client care) during the surgical procedure. The scrub role (passing instruments to the surgeon) can be assumed by a registered nurse or a surgical technologist. Personnel who are not scrubbed can answer the phone. The entire surgical team ensures the sterility of supplies. (I, 1)

36. 4. The purpose of separating the public from the restricted attire area of the operating room is to provide an aseptic environment and prevent contamination of the environment by organisms. The client's privacy is protected, but the main purpose is infection control. (I, 1)

37. 1. The 68-year-old client is at greater risk because an older adult client is more likely to have comorbid conditions, a less-effective immune system, and less collagen in the integumentary system. (A, 9)

38. 1. The child having her 15th laser procedure for a hemangioma should not have a balloon unless it is latex free, because this child has had numerous exposures to latex thus far. If she has not already developed some sensitivity, the nurse should help the family help recognize an awareness of latex products to avoid when possible. A client who is having a tonsillectomy, inguinal hernia repair, or orchiopexy is probably having surgery for the first time and has not been exposed to latex, although it is a good practice is to use latex-free products whenever possible and to inquire about past exposure. (D, 10)

39. 2. An autotransfusion is acceptable for the client who is in danger of cardiac arrest. An autotransfusion can not be collected from a client who has cancer, a contaminated wound, or contamination from *Escherichia coli* because of a ruptured bowel. (D, 9)

40. 2. After a scope or catheter has been inserted into the urethra, the mucosal membrane is irritated and the client feels the need to void even though the bladder may not be full. The nurse should encourage the client to force fluids to make the urine dilute. The client should not ignore the urge to void. The client should be encouraged to use the bathroom; there is no need to use the bedpan. The client does not need assistance to the bathroom, because this procedure does not require any anesthesia except a topical anesthetic for the male client. (P, 9)

41. 4. Early ambulation is the most significant general nursing measure to prevent postoperative complications and has been advocated for more than 40 years. Walking the client increases vital capacity and maintains normal respiratory functioning, stimulates circulation, prevents venous stasis, improves gastrointestinal and genitourinary function, increases muscle tone, and increases wound healing. (I, 9)

The Client Who Is Receiving or Recovering From Anesthesia

42. 4. Airway flow is always the first assessment. Once the nurse establishes that the client has a patent airway, the pulse oximeter is applied to measure the oxygen saturation, the respiratory rate is counted, and the breath sounds are auscultated bilaterally. (A, 10)

43. 1. The last area to regain sensation is the perineal area, and the nurse should check the client for a distended bladder. The client has received a large volume of intravenous fluids since the epidural was inserted, and the client may not feel the urge to void or may be unable to void. In that case, the nurse should obtain an order to catheterize the client before the bladder becomes so distended as to cause bladder spasms. The nurse should assess for a spinal headache, postoperative pain, and the client's ability to move after determining whether the bladder is distended. (D, 7)

44. 3. The nurse should check the client's baseline data to ascertain whether the client's pupil has always been enlarged or this is a new finding. The preoperative assessment is valuable as the baseline for comparison of all subsequent assessments made throughout the perioperative period. The nurse may determine that a more involved neurologic examination is indicated or may choose to administer oxygen or to call the surgeon, but the nurse still needs to know the baseline data before proceeding. (E, 9)

45. 1. The nurse should check the dressing for signs of bleeding to establish a baseline for future assessments of the dressing and to verify that there is no obvious sign of hemorrhage. The nurse does not need to empty peri-incisional drains at this time. All drains should have been emptied and reconstituted by the postanesthesia care nurse before the client was transferred to the surgical floor. Assessing the client's pain level and assessing the bladder are important; however, it is more important to assess the surgical site for bleeding, because hemorrhage is a life-threatening complication of any surgical procedure. (D, 1)

46. 2. Adult clients are induced for general anesthesia by breathing in an inhalant anesthetic mixed with oxygen through a facial mask and receiving intravenous medication to make them sleepy. Clients are not induced with the premedication. Clients usually are not induced with the intravenous infusion or the mask alone. (P, 9)

47. 4. Children are induced for general anesthesia by giving them medication through a facial mask to make them sleepy. Children are not induced with a injection. Children usually are not induced by use of a facial mask with intravenous administration started while they are still awake. (P, 9)

48. 3. Sodium pentothal, a short-acting barbiturate, can cause hypotension, which may be especially problematic for the client with impaired cardiac functioning. Sodium pentothal does not cause bradycardia, complete muscle relaxation, hypertension, or tachypnea. (I, 8)

49. 1. Propofol (Diprivan), a nonbarbiturate anesthetic, causes less nausea and vomiting because of a direct antiemetic action. It does not cause hypotension or skeletal muscle movement, and it does not act slowly. (I, 8)

50. 4. Desflurane (Suprane) and sevoflurane (Ultane) are volatile liquid anesthesia agents that are used for outpatient surgeries primarily because they are rapidly eliminated. They have the added benefits of being better tolerated and nonirritating to the respiratory tract, and they have predictable cardiovascular effects. However, rapid elimination is an important consideration for outpatient procedures. (D, 8)

51. 3. A heart rate of 150 bpm or greater, hypotension, and muscle rigidity are early signs of malignant hyperthermia. The nurse should quickly assemble emergency supplies and personnel, because malignant hyperthermia is potentially and rapidly fatal in more than 50% of cases. Rapid, extreme rise in temperature is a late sign. Another factor influencing the analysis is that the client has a large body frame, and having large, bulky muscles is a risk factor for malignant hyperthermia. The client's vital signs are well out of the range of normal; analysis of the data and swift intervention are indicated. Excessive blood loss secondary to an arthroscopy is unlikely. Although clients do have changes in vital signs when in acute pain, the nurse would expect the client to be hypertensive, not hypotensive. (D, 9)

52. 2. One of the earliest signs of hypoxia is restlessness and agitation. Decreased level of consciousness and somnolence are later signs of hypoxia. Chills can be related to the anesthetic agent used but are not indicative of hypoxia. Urgency is not related to hypoxia. (A, 10)

53. 2. It is important for the nurse to cover this client with warm blankets because he is at high risk for hypothermia secondary to age, spinal anesthesia, placement in a lithotomy position in the cool operating room for 1.5 hours, instillation of 4000 mL of room temperature bladder irrigation, and ongoing bladder irrigation. Spinal anesthesia causes vasodilatation, which results in heat loss from the core to the periphery. The nurse will empty the catheter drainage bag and hang new bags of irrigation as needed, but the client's potential for hypothermia should be addressed first. The client will not be turned at this time. (P, 9)

54. 3. The client who is 5 feet 1 inch tall and weighs 200 pounds would be expected to retain the anesthetic agents longer because adipose tissue absorbs the drug before the desired systemic effect is reached for anesthesia maintenance. Nursing interventions are aimed at encouraging the obese client to turn, cough, and deep-breathe despite feeling sleepy and tired. The sooner this client ambulates, the sooner the retained anesthesia will be worked out of the adipose tissue. (D, 9)

55. 1. The nurse should encourage the client to avoid holding his operated arm, the arm with the intravenous regional nerve block (Bier block), close to her face because she has no motor control over it. With the cast in place she could hit herself in the eye, nose, or mouth and cause soft tissue damage. It is acceptable for the client to hold the operated arm with the unoperated arm or to use the unoperated arm. The nurse should administer the analgesic before the intravenous regional anesthetic completely wears off so that the pain does not peak before pain medication is administered. (I, 9)

56. 3. The nurse should monitor the client's respirations closely for 4 to 6 hours, because naloxone has a shorter duration of action than opioids. The client may need repeated doses of naloxone to prevent or treat a recurrence of the respiratory depression. Naloxone is usually effective in a few minutes; however, it lasts only 1 to 2 hours and ongoing monitoring of the client's respiratory rate will be necessary. The client's dosage of morphine will be decreased or a new drug will be ordered to prevent another instance of respiratory depression. (A, 8)

57. 3. Abnormal coagulation test results have been associated with naloxone (Narcan), and the nurse should monitor surgical clients closely for bleeding. Dizziness, biliary colic, and urinary retention are not associated with naloxone. (A, 8)

58. 3. The client who receives epidural anesthesia is at decreased risk for a headache because a noncutting needle is used instead of a side angle-cutting needle. The epidural needle is a 25- to 27-gauge needle, which is much smaller than a 17-gauge needle. The injection

made for an epidural is an extradural, not a subarachnoid injection as for spinal anesthesia. The onset of spinal anesthesia is faster because a larger dose of medication is usually administered. (D, 9)

59. 3. Spinal anesthesia does not cause parasympathetic blockage. The spinal anesthetic agent usually is injected into the L2 subarachnoid space, where it produces sympathetic, sensory, and motor blockade. (E, 8)

60. 1. Multiply 2.5 mg/5 mg by the unknown x mg/1 mL. Cross-multiply to get $5x = 2.5$ mL. Divide both sides of the equation by 5 to get $x = 0.5$ mL. (I, 8)

61. 3. The nurse should assess the client's temperature every 15 minutes when the client's skin is assessed to prevent burns. (A, 2)

The Client Who Has Had Surgery

62. 4. The nurse should plan for two people, one at each side using a draw sheet, one person at the head, and one person at the feet to transfer an elderly, drowsy client with fragile skin to avoid shearing of the integumentary system. Using only two or three people allows for dragging of some part of the client, which leads to shearing of the dependent part. (P, 7)

63. 3. The client who has not had the gag reflex anesthetized is the client who had a repair of the carpal tunnel syndrome under local anesthesia because the area being anesthetized was the tissue in the wrist. The client who had a bronchoscopy received a local anesthetic on the vocal cords, and the nurse should check the gag reflex or ability to swallow before administering fluids. Clients who had general anesthesia or intravenous conscious sedation received medication for central nervous system sedation, and the nurse should assess the level of consciousness and ability to swallow before administering fluids. (D, 9)

64. 3. When the urine output is less than 30 mL/hour, the nurse should assess for potential causes such as hypovolemia or hemorrhage. The nurse should assess and evaluate the client's vital signs, intake and output, dressing, and available laboratory values and notify the physician. Bowel obstruction, although possible after surgery, is characterized most notably by abdominal distention and absent bowel sounds, not decreased urinary output. The nurse would not expect the client to have hypertension, but rather hypotension. (A, 10)

65. 3. A client who had a left thoracoscopy is placed in the lateral position, in which the most common injury is an injury to the brachial plexus. Numbness and tingling in the arm suggests a brachial plexus injury. (E, 7)

66. 3. Although any client may experience nausea and vomiting secondary to anesthetics or postoperative analgesics, the client who has had manipulation of the abdominal organs is more prone to postoperative nausea and vomiting than the client who has had a procedure such as a total joint replacement, open heart surgery, or a mastectomy. (D, 9)

67. 3. The nurse should inform the client that as the incision heals uneven lumps might appear under the incision line because the collagen is growing new tissue at different rates. Eventually, the lumps will even out and the tissue will be smooth. The client can touch the incision with clean hands as needed to perform incisional care. The client should not clean the incision with hydrogen peroxide, because it may dry out the natural skin oils. The surgeon will remove the staples for the client. (P, 9)

68. 2. When a wound eviscerates (abdominal organs protruding through the opened incision), the nurse should cover the open area with a sterile dressing moistened with sterile normal saline and then cover it with a dry dressing. The surgeon should then be notified to take the client back to the operating room to close the incision under general anesthesia. The nurse should not press the emergency alarm, because this is not a cardiac or respiratory arrest. The nurse should have the visitors and family leave the room to decrease the chance of airborne contamination, but the primary focus should be on covering the wound with a moist sterile covering. (I, 9)

69. 3. After emptying a Jackson-Pratt drainage bulb, the nurse should compress the bulb, plug it to establish suction, and then document the amount and type of drainage emptied. Irrigating a Jackson-Pratt drain is inappropriate because it could contaminate the wound. The Jackson-Pratt drain is not usually connected to wall suction. The purpose of the Jackson-Pratt drain is to remove bloody drainage from the deep tissues of the incision; clamping the drain would be counterproductive. (I, 9)

70. 1. Performing leg exercises, including ankle pumping, ankle rotation, and quadriceps setting exercises, will help prevent stasis of blood in the lower extremities, which can lead to blood clot formation. Encouraging the client to cough and deep-breathe is an important postoperative intervention; however, it is directed at preventing pneumonia, not pulmonary emboli. The nurse should not massage the calves, because a deep vein thrombus could dislodge and travel to the pulmonary vasculature. Antiembolic stockings should be worn continuously during the postoperative period. (I, 10)

71. 2. Naloxone hydrochloride (Narcan) is the antidote for morphine sulfate. The signs of overdose on morphine sulfate are respirations of 2 to 4 breaths/minute, bradycardia, and hypotension. Flumazenil (Romazicon) is the antidote for midazolam (Versed). Doxacurium

(Nuromax) is a nondepolarizing muscle relaxant. Remifentanil (Ultiva) is a narcotic used as an anesthetic adjunct. (D, 8)

72. 2. The client admitted for same-day surgery should not drive home after the surgical procedure because it is unsafe. Even without an anesthetic, the surgical event can be more stressful than anticipated. It is acceptable to have someone arrive after the surgery has started to take the client home. A taxi is permissible but not desirable. (E, 2)

73. 3. The client has deficient knowledge when stating that pain from a laparoscopic cholecystectomy is related to a large incision and manipulation of tissue. The nurse should explain that there are four puncture sites for the incision and that gas is used to distend the abdominal cavity to keep the abdominal organs away from the operative site. There is no real manipulation of tissue to produce pain. The pain that clients do experience from this procedure is related to the gas, which irritates the diaphragm. The client should start on clear liquids and advance to bland foods until the gas is gone. Walking helps to eliminate the gas from the abdominal cavity with 12 to 24 hours after surgery. (I, 7)

74. 3. The urinary output does not have to be checked every 15 minutes for a client who has had an arthroscopy because this client probably does not have a catheter in place. If the client voids, the output would be recorded. Assessments every 15 minutes during the first hour would include vital signs, pulse oximeter values, and pain to monitor the client's comfort level and check for compartment syndrome. Neurovascular checks distal to the operative site are especially vital because a tourniquet was used proximal to the operative site during the surgical procedure and because edema may develop during the postoperative period. (A, 7)

75. 2. Hypotension and tachycardia are common side effects of droperidol (Inapsine) and should be monitored closely by the nurse. Hypotension and tachycardia are not common side effects of ondansetron hydrochloride (Zofran), prochlorperazine (Compazine), or promethazine (Phenergan). (A, 8)

76. 1. The nurse should assess but not disturb the epidural dressing, because the catheter can be easily dislodged and organisms can easily be transmitted into the central nervous system. The nurse should not have to change the dressing at all if a waterproof dressing is applied over the epidural site. Even with strict aseptic technique, a drain into a sterile cavity is a direct route for transmission of organisms and places a client at increased risk of infection. (I, 9)

77. 2. The client who has epidural pain management postoperatively can ambulate because a low concentration of local anesthesia with analgesia causes sensory block-

age only. The epidural catheter is not in place for occasional use only. An analgesic can be used alone, but the real purpose is for the combined dosage of local anesthesia and systemic analgesia. The pain threshold is not affected. (I, 9)

78. 1. The client who develops pruritus and urticaria while receiving an intravenous antibiotic has clinical manifestations of a type I (anaphylactic) reaction. The greatest number of anaphylactic reactions in surgical clients are related to use of intravenous antibiotics. An example of a type II (cytotoxic and cytolytic) reaction would be clumping of incompatible blood in a hemolytic blood transfusion reaction. Clinical manifestation of a type III (immune-complex) reaction depends on the number of complexes and location in the body; common sites are the kidneys, skin, joints, blood vessels, and lungs. Clinical manifestations of type IV (delayed hypersensitivity) reactions include papules, vesicles, and bullae. (D, 10)

79. 2. Hypotension, tachycardia, bronchospasm, and pulmonary edema are clinical manifestations of anaphylaxis. These symptoms are not seen in malignant hyperthermia, contact dermatitis, or cell-mediated responses. (D, 10)

80. 1. The nurse should ask the location of the client's pain because Lortab is a narcotic, which can be constipating. By the third day, many clients become constipated and are feeling distended with sharp, cramping pain that is a gas pain, which is treated with ambulation, not more narcotics. The client's emptying his bladder should not affect his pain level. The nurse should look at the client's chart to determine when the client's last dose of pain medication was administered, rather than asking the client. The client's statement regarding his pain level before the surgery is not relevant to whether the nurse should administer the Lortab. (D, 10)

81. 1. Blood and serous fluid is drained from the operative site to prevent hematoma formation or a collection of fluid that could become a site for infection. This also minimizes postoperative swelling, which can be painful. A simple explanation such as this is appropriate because the client is just waking up from surgery. Blood from the operative site can be collected through an autotransfusion system so that it can be transfused to the client during or immediately after surgery. However, strict guidelines about volume of blood lost, how quickly the device fills, and how long the blood has been out of the client's body govern whether the blood can be transfused. Therefore, although it is possible that the drainage system to which the client refers is an autotransfusion system, it is more likely that the client has a simple Hemovac drain. It is incorrect to tell a client not to worry about something even if she is in the drowsy state of awakening from anesthesia. It is inap-

propriate to ignore the client and give her something to make her drowsy instead of addressing his concerns. (D, 9)

82. 1. The purpose of the Jackson-Pratt drainage tube is to drain off the purulent drainage from the sterile peritoneal cavity and prevent peritonitis. A Jackson-Pratt drain cannot prevent bleeding. The Jackson-Pratt drain has no effect on pressure on the bladder. There is no reason to be concerned about pressure on the gallbladder. (D, 9)

83. 2. Biliary drainage tubes (T-tubes) are placed in the common bile duct and drain bile, which is dark yellow-orange. Serous sanguineous drainage is thin and pinkish red. Bile is not green colored unless it comes in contact with gastric fluid. (I, 9)

84. 1. Urinary elimination in the first 8 hours postoperatively is a requirement before the client who has had an inguinal hernia repair can be discharged from same-day surgery. Ingestion of fluids without nausea and vomiting is important, but eating solid foods is not a requirement for discharge from same-day surgery. Being completely pain free is an unrealistic expectation for the time frame and is not a requirement for leaving same-day surgery. However, the client should be comfortable and his pain should be controlled. It is not a requirement for the client to ambulate in the hallway, but the client should be able to sit up and go to the bathroom without assistance. (E, 7)

85. 3. The ability to self-dose is a requirement for the client to use PCA. Having a family member or court-appointed advocate present is not a requirement for initiating PCA. The nurse teaches the client about how to use the PCA and monitors effectiveness of the pain medication; however, it is not necessary for the nurse to assist with the dosing. (I, 1)

86. 2. The client's body temperature should be assessed every 4 hours during the first 24 hours because the client is still at risk for hypothermia or malignant hyperthermia. The client does not need to be checked every 2 hours unless indicated by an abnormal finding. (A, 2)

87. 2. The postoperative client's temperature should be assessed every 8 hours after the first 24 hours because the client is at risk for an infection. The client does not need to be checked every 6 hours unless indicated by an abnormal finding.(A, 2)

88. 1. The client who has been positioned in the lithotomy position under general anesthesia may experience discomfort in the shoulders postoperatively because the client is placed in the Trendelenberg position to expose the perineal area. The client's weight is then shifted toward the shoulders and the client experiences muscle soreness postoperatively. (A, 9)

89. 2. The client should drink a minimum of 2500 mL of fluid per day (not 1500 mL) to keep secretions liquefied and easier to cough up and eliminate from the upper respiratory tract. The client should use pain medication before coughing. The nurse should monitor the client's breath sounds and temperature to detect early signs of infection. The nurse should assist with early ambulation. (P, 9)

90. 3. The client with thromboembolism does not have coolness. The client with thromboembolism has redness, swelling, increased warmth along the vein, edema, and pain and may have hemoptysis, chest pain, tachycardia, dyspnea, and restlessness. (A, 9)

91. 3. The client should sit in an upright position when doing breathing exercises to allow for full chest expansion of both lungs and all fields and bases. Using an incentive spirometer every hour while awake is appropriate and allows the client visual feedback. Placing his hands lightly over the lower ribs and upper abdomen allows the client to see muscles of inspiration and expiration and is appropriate. Coughing deeply from the lungs after four deep breaths allows the client to effectively cough up secretions. (I, 9)

92. 2. Muscle cramping is a sign of hypokalemia. Potassium is an electrolyte lost with nasogastric suctioning. Confusion is seen with hypercalcemia. Edema is seen with protein deficit or fluid volume overload. Tremors are seen with hypomagnesemia. (A, 9)

93. 3. An indwelling catheter increases the risk of urinary tract infection because microbes ascend the catheter and travel to the bladder. The nurse should try to facilitate the client's ability to void by using the sitting position for a woman or the standing position for a man and by running warm water over the perineum. If such conservative methods fail, the nurse should obtain an order to catheterize the client every 4 hours using a small-French straight catheter until she can void on her own. (I, 9)

Legal and Ethical Issues Associated With Surgery

94. 3. The most critical piece of information is the client identification bracelet. Misidentification of clients can result in serious harm to the client. The nurse also needs the admitting records and Addressograph labels as part of verifying the client's identification. The location of the family is not included in verifying identification. (I, 1)

95. 4. The nurse is not is not required to have the anesthesia note on the chart before the client is transported to the operating room suite. The anesthesia record is on the chart after the surgical procedure is completed and is a good source of client information. The operative

consent, history and physical, and laboratory test results should be on the chart before the client is transported to the operating suite. (I, 1)

96. 2. When the client cannot sign the operative consent and it is a true life-saving emergency, consent may be obtained over the telephone from the client's next-of-kin or guardian. The surgeon must obtain the telephone consent, but if it is a true life-saving emergency the surgeon often is already in surgery, so the nurse makes the telephone call and another nurse witnesses the call. Some institutions have a special consent form for emergency surgery. Consent can be waived in situations where no family is available; however, if the family can be reached by telephone before surgery, verbal consent is legally required. (I, 1)

97. 3. There are risks with both the surgical procedure and the general anesthesia required for a craniotomy. The risks involved in the procedure are a part of the informed consent. Other information that is part of an informed consent includes potential complications, expected benefits, inability of the surgeon to predict results, irreversibility of the procedure (if applicable), and other available treatments. Talking about the effects of the diabetes on healing, explaining how the craniotomy is performed, and explaining the consequences of declining treatment (eg, death if the tumor is not removed) represent appropriate actions to provide information to the client. (E, 1)

98. 2. All health care facilities reimbursed under Medicare and Medicaid are required under the 1991 Patient Self-Determination Act to recognize clients' advance directives such as health care proxies or living wills. Advance directives are an important part of the perioperative care and should be respected by all health care professionals caring for the client. The nurse should not be involved in specific questions regarding how the client is going to pay for health care services except as an advocate addressing the client's psychosocial needs. (I, 1)

99. 2. The client must have an identification bracelet properly secured on her person before being transported to the operating room to ensure correct identification. It is incorrect to send the client without a properly secured identification bracelet. The perioperative nurse must verify the client's identification by checking for the same name on the chart, armband, and schedule and by the client's statement. The preoperative nurse may be asked to physically identify the client and obtain a new armband. (I, 1)

100. 2. When the client cannot read or write, the consent can be read to the client and the client can sign in the present of two witnesses. The client should always sign for himself (not the next-of-kin) unless he is a minor or not of sound mind. The court does not appoint a guardian for a person of sound mind just because he cannot read or write. Hospital personnel would not and could not sign a consent for a client. (I, 1)

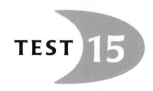
The Client with Health Problems of the Eyes, Ears, Nose, Throat, and Skin

Select the one best answer, and indicate your choice by filling in the circle in front of the option.

The Client With Cataracts

1. A client is admitted to outpatient surgery for a cataract extraction on the right eye. The client asks the nurse, "What causes cataracts in old people?" Which of the following statements should form the basis for the nurse's response? Cataracts most commonly
   ○ 1. are a result of chronic systemic disease.
   ○ 2. are a result of aging.
   ○ 3. are a result of eye injuries sustained early in life.
   ○ 4. are a result of the prolonged use of toxic substances.

2. A client asks, "What does the lens of my eye do?" The nurse should explain that the lens of the eye
   ○ 1. produces aqueous humor.
   ○ 2. holds the rods and cones.
   ○ 3. focuses light rays onto the retina.
   ○ 4. regulates the amount of light entering the eye.

3. The client with a cataract tells the nurse that she is afraid of being awake during eye surgery. Which of the following responses by the nurse would be the most appropriate?
   ○ 1. "Have you ever had any reactions to local anesthetics in the past?"
   ○ 2. "What is it that disturbs you about the idea of being awake?"

   ○ 3. "By using a local anesthetic, you won't have nausea and vomiting after the surgery."
   ○ 4. "There's really nothing to fear about being awake. You'll be given a medication that will help you relax."

4. A client with a cataract would most likely complain of which symptoms?
   ○ 1. Halos and rainbows around lights.
   ○ 2. Eye pain and irritation that worsens at night.
   ○ 3. Blurred and hazy vision.
   ○ 4. Eye strain and headache when doing close work.

5. The nurse is to instill drops of phenylephrine hydrochloride (Neo-Synephrine) into a client's right eye before cataract removal surgery. This preparation acts in the eye to produce
   ○ 1. dilation of the pupil and blood vessels.
   ○ 2. dilation of the pupil and constriction of blood vessels.
   ○ 3. constriction of the pupil and constriction of blood vessels.
   ○ 4. constriction of the pupil and dilation of blood vessels.

6. A short time after cataract surgery, the client complains of nausea. Which of the following represents the nurse's best course of action?

495

○ 1. Instruct the client to take a few deep breaths until the nausea subsides.

○ 2. Explain that this is a common feeling that will pass quickly.

○ 3. Tell the client to call the nurse promptly if vomiting occurs.

○ 4. Medicate the client with an antiemetic, as ordered.

7. The client is discharged on the day of the cataract surgery. Which of the following nursing diagnoses would be most appropriate for the client at this time?

○ 1. Deficient Diversional Activity related to activity limitations after surgery.

○ 2. Chronic Pain related to postoperative incisional discomfort.

○ 3. Risk for Injury related to limited vision after surgery.

○ 4. Feeding Self-Care Deficit related to inability to see food.

8. After returning home, the client will need to continue to instill eye drops in the affected eye. The client is instructed to apply slight pressure against the nose at the inner canthus of the eye after instilling the eye drops. The rationale that supports applying pressure is that it

○ 1. prevents the medication from entering the tear duct.

○ 2. prevents the drug from running down the client's face.

○ 3. allows the sensitive cornea to adjust to the medication.

○ 4. facilitates distribution of the medication over the eye surface.

9. Which of the following activities should be avoided to achieve the goal of decreasing intraocular pressure after eye surgery?

○ 1. Lying supine.

○ 2. Coughing.

○ 3. Deep breathing.

○ 4. Ambulation.

10. After cataract removal surgery, the client is instructed to report any complaints of a sharp pain in the operative eye because this could indicate which of the following postoperative complications?

○ 1. Detached retina.

○ 2. Prolapse of the iris.

○ 3. Extracapsular erosion.

○ 4. Intraocular hemorrhage.

The Client With a Retinal Detachment

11. A client is admitted through the emergency department with a diagnosis of detached retina in the right eye. As the nurse completes the admission history, the client reports that before the physician patched his eye, he saw many spots, or "floaters." The nurse should explain to the client that these spots were caused by

○ 1. pieces of the retina floating in the eye.

○ 2. blood cells released into the eye by the detachment.

○ 3. contamination of the aqueous humor.

○ 4. spasms of the retinal blood vessels traumatized by the detachment.

12. A client with detachment of the retina asks the nurse why it is necessary to patch both of her eyes. The nurse's reply should be based on the knowledge that eye patches serve to

○ 1. reduce rapid eye movements.

○ 2. decrease the irritation caused by light entering the damaged eye.

○ 3. protect the injured eye from infection.

○ 4. rest the eyes to promote healing.

13. The client with retinal detachment in the right eye is extremely apprehensive. He states, "I'm afraid of going blind. It would be so hard to live that way." What factor should the nurse consider before responding to his statement?

○ 1. Repeat surgery is impossible, so if this procedure fails, vision loss is inevitable.

○ 2. The surgery will only delay blindness in the right eye, but vision is preserved in the left eye.

○ 3. More and more services are available to help newly blind people adapt to daily living.

○ 4. Optimism is justified because surgical treatment has a 90% to 95% success rate.

14. Which of the following statements would provide the best guide for activity for a client who has been treated for retinal detachment during her rehabilitation period?

○ 1. Activity is resumed gradually, and the client can resume her usual activities in 5 to 6 weeks.

○ 2. Activity level is determined by the client's tolerance; she can be as active as she wishes.

○ 3. Activity levels will be restricted for several months, so she should plan on being sedentary.

○ 4. Activity can be returned to normal and may include regular aerobic exercises.

15. Which of the following goals would be a priority for a client who has undergone surgery for retinal detachment?

○ 1. Control pain.

○ 2. Prevent an increase in intraocular pressure.

○ 3. Promote a low-sodium diet.

○ 4. Maintain a darkened environment.

16. Scleral buckling, a procedure used to treat retinal detachment, involves

○ 1. removing the torn segment of the retina and stitching down the remaining segment.

○ 2. replacing the torn segment of the retina with a strip of retina from a donor.
○ 3. stitching the retina firmly to the optic nerve to give it support.
○ 4. creating a splint to hold the retina together until a scar can form and seal off the tear.

The Client With Glaucoma

17. The client who has been treated for chronic open-angle glaucoma (COAG) for 5 years asks the clinic nurse, "How does glaucoma damage my eyesight?" The nurse's reply should be based on the knowledge that COAG
○ 1. results from chronic eye inflammation.
○ 2. causes increased intraocular pressure.
○ 3. leads to detachment of the retina.
○ 4. is caused by decreased blood flow to the retina.
18. Which of the following signs or symptoms is most commonly experienced by clients with COAG?
○ 1. Eye pain.
○ 2. Excessive lacrimation.
○ 3. Colored light flashes.
○ 4. Decreasing peripheral vision.
19. Miotics are frequently used in the treatment of glaucoma. The nurse should understand that miotics work by
○ 1. paralyzing ciliary muscles.
○ 2. constricting intraocular vessels.
○ 3. constricting the pupil.
○ 4. relaxing ciliary muscles.
20. Which of the following should the nurse provide as part of the information to prepare the client for tonometry?
○ 1. Oral pain medication will be given before the procedure.
○ 2. It is a painless procedure with no side effects.
○ 3. Blurred or double vision may occur after the procedure.
○ 4. Medication will be given to dilate the pupils before the procedure.
21. The nurse learns that the client uses timolol maleate (Timoptic) eye drops. The nurse would understand that this β-adrenergic blocker helps control glaucoma by
○ 1. constricting the pupils.
○ 2. dilating the canals of Schlemm.
○ 3. reducing aqueous humor formation.
○ 4. improving the ability of the ciliary muscle to contract.
22. The nurse observes the client while he instills his eye drops. The client says, "I just try to hit the middle of my eyeball so the drops don't run out of my eye." The nurse explains to the client that the method he is now using may cause

○ 1. scleral staining.
○ 2. corneal injury.
○ 3. excessive lacrimation.
○ 4. systemic drug absorption.
23. The client with glaucoma is scheduled for a minor surgical procedure. Which of the following orders would require clarification or correction before the nurse carries it out?
○ 1. Administer morphine sulfate.
○ 2. Administer atropine sulfate.
○ 3. Teach deep breathing exercises.
○ 4. Teach leg exercises.
24. Which of the following clinical manifestations would the nurse associate with acute angle-closure glaucoma?
○ 1. Gradual loss of central vision.
○ 2. Acute light sensitivity.
○ 3. Loss of color vision.
○ 4. Sudden eye pain.
25. A client has been diagnosed with an acute episode of angle-closure glaucoma. The nurse plans the client's nursing care with the understanding that acute angle-closure glaucoma
○ 1. frequently resolves without treatment.
○ 2. is typically treated with sustained bed rest.
○ 3. is a medical emergency that can rapidly lead to blindness.
○ 4. is most commonly treated with steroid therapy.

The Client Undergoing Nasal Surgery

26. A 27-year-old woman is admitted for elective nasal surgery for a deviated septum. Which of the following would be an important initial clue that bleeding was occurring even if the nasal drip pad remained dry and intact?
○ 1. Complaints of nausea.
○ 2. Repeated swallowing.
○ 3. Rapid respiratory rate.
○ 4. Feelings of anxiety.
27. The client is ready for discharge after surgery for a deviated septum. Which of the following discharge instructions would be appropriate?
○ 1. Avoid activities that elicit the Valsalva maneuver.
○ 2. Take aspirin to control nasal discomfort.
○ 3. Avoid brushing the teeth until the nasal packing is removed.
○ 4. Apply heat to the nasal area to control swelling.
28. Which one of the following statements would indicate to the nurse that the client who has undergone repair of her nasal septum has understood the discharge instructions?

○ 1. "I should not shower until my packing is removed."
○ 2. "I will take stool softeners and modify my diet to prevent constipation."
○ 3. "Coughing every 2 hours is important to prevent respiratory complications."
○ 4. "It is important to blow my nose each day to remove the dried secretions."

The Client With a Hearing Disorder

29. A 75-year-old client who has been taking furosemide (Lasix) regularly for 4 months tells the nurse that he is having trouble hearing. What would be the nurse's best response to this statement?
○ 1. Tell the client that because he is 75 years old, it is inevitable that his hearing should begin to deteriorate.
○ 2. Have the client immediately report the hearing loss to his physician.
○ 3. Schedule the client for audiometric testing and a hearing aid.
○ 4. Tell the client that the hearing loss is only temporary; when his system adjusts to the furosemide, his hearing will improve.

30. Which of the following best describes the effect of a hearing aid for a client with sensorineural hearing loss?
○ 1. It makes sounds louder and clearer.
○ 2. It has no effect on hearing.
○ 3. It makes sounds louder but not clearer.
○ 4. It improves the client's ability to separate words from background noises.

31. A client states that she was told she has sensorineural hearing loss and asks the nurse what this means. The nurse's response is based on the knowledge that sensorineural hearing loss results from which of the following conditions?
○ 1. Presence of fluid and cerumen in the external canal.
○ 2. Sclerosis of the bones of the middle ear.
○ 3. Damage to the cochlear or vestibulocochlear nerve.
○ 4. Emotional disturbance resulting in a functional hearing loss.

32. A 65-year-old man complains of hearing loss and a sensation of fullness in both ears. The nurse examines his ears with the understanding that a common cause of hearing loss in older adults is related to
○ 1. accumulation of cerumen in the external canal.
○ 2. accumulation of cerumen in the internal canal.
○ 3. external otitis.
○ 4. exostosis.

33. The best method to remove cerumen from a client's ear involves

○ 1. inserting a cotton-tipped applicator into the external canal.
○ 2. irrigating the ear gently.
○ 3. using aural suction.
○ 4. using a cerumen curette.

34. To prepare the irrigation solution used for removal of cerumen, the nurse uses
○ 1. normal saline.
○ 2. sterile water.
○ 3. antiseptic solution.
○ 4. lactated Ringer's solution.

35. A 26-year-old client has a history of chronic otitis media. Which of the following procedures is the most common surgical intervention for chronic otitis media?
○ 1. Ossiculoplasty.
○ 2. Tympanoplasty.
○ 3. Mastoidectomy.
○ 4. Myringotomy.

36. A client is about to have a tympanoplasty. She is asking the nurse what the surgical procedure involves. The nurse begins the conversation by
○ 1. assessing what the client's doctor has told her.
○ 2. describing the surgical procedure.
○ 3. educating the client that the procedure will close the perforation and prevent recurrent infection.
○ 4. informing the client that the procedure will improve her hearing.

37. A 50-year-old man has been taking aspirin regularly for 6 months to prevent a heart attack. He informs the nurse that he has noticed a constant "ringing" in both ears. How should the nurse respond to the client's comment?
○ 1. Tell the client that tinnitus is associated with the aging process.
○ 2. Inform the client he needs a Weber test done.
○ 3. Schedule the client for audiometric testing.
○ 4. Inform the client that the "ringing" may be related to the aspirin he has been taking for his heart.

The Client With Ménière's Disease

38. The classic triad of symptoms associated with Ménière's disease is vertigo, tinnitus, and
○ 1. headache.
○ 2. otitis media.
○ 3. fluctuating hearing loss.
○ 4. vomiting.

39. The client with Ménière's disease is instructed to modify his diet. The nurse would explain that the most frequently recommended diet modification for Ménière's disease is

1. low sodium.
2. high protein.
3. low carbohydrate.
4. low fat.

40. Which of the following statements by the client would indicate that she understands the expected course of Ménière's disease?
    1. "The disease process will gradually extend to the eyes."
    2. "Control of the episodes is usually possible, but a cure is not yet available."
    3. "Continued medication therapy will cure the disease."
    4. "Bilateral deafness is an inevitable outcome of the disease."

41. The potential for injury during an attack of Ménière's disease is great. The nurse should instruct the client to take which immediate action when experiencing vertigo?
    1. "Place your head between your knees."
    2. "Concentrate on rhythmic deep breathing."
    3. "Close your eyes tightly."
    4. "Assume a reclining or flat position."

42. The wife of a client with Ménière's disease expresses concern because her husband has curtailed family activities and evenings out. Based on this information, which of the following would be the most appropriate nursing diagnosis?
    1. Social Isolation related to attacks of vertigo and hearing loss.
    2. Anxiety related to concern about progressive hearing loss.
    3. Self-Care Deficit related to labyrinth dysfunction.
    4. Disturbed Sensory Perception related to labyrinth dysfunction.

43. The nurse would anticipate that all of the following drugs may be used in the attempt to control the symptoms of Ménière's disease *except*
    1. antihistamines.
    2. antiemetics.
    3. diuretics.
    4. glucocorticoids.

44. A client with Ménière's disease continues to have disabling attacks of vertigo and elects to have a labyrinthectomy. A priority nursing diagnosis for the client before surgery is
    1. Deficient Diversional Activity related to inability to participate secondary to vertigo.
    2. Risk for Injury related to vertigo.
    3. Powerlessness related to inability to influence effects of disease process .
    4. Risk for Social Isolation related to hearing loss.

The Client With Adult Macular Degeneration

45. When assessing an older adult with macular degeneration the nurse would expect to find
    1. loss of central vision.
    2. loss of peripheral vision.
    3. total blindness.
    4. blurring of vision.

46. A 75-year-old male client has a history of macular degeneration. While he is in the hospital, the priority nursing goal will be
    1. to provide education regarding community services for clients with adult macular degeneration (AMD).
    2. to provide health care related to monitoring his eye condition.
    3. to promote a safe, effective care environment.
    4. to improve vision.

47. When admitting a female client who is blind to the hospital, the nurse should
    1. ask the client to have someone with her at all times.
    2. encourage her to stay in bed until the nurse can assist.
    3. orient the client to the room environment by providing opportunity to touch the objects.
    4. allow time for the client to orient to the environment.

48. Although all of the following measures might be useful in reducing the visual disability of a client with AMD, which measure should the nurse teach the client primarily as a safety precaution?
    1. Wear a patch over one eye.
    2. Place personal items on the sighted side.
    3. Lie in bed with the unaffected side toward the door.
    4. Turn the head from side to side when walking.

The Client With Cancer of the Larynx

49. After total laryngectomy surgery the client has a feeding tube. The primary rationale for tube feedings is to
    1. meet the fluid and nutritional needs of the client.
    2. prevent aspiration.
    3. prevent fistula formation.
    4. maintain an open airway.

50. Complications associated with a tracheostomy tube include
    1. decreased cardiac output.
    2. damage to the laryngeal nerve.
    3. pneumothorax.
    4. acute respiratory distress syndrome (ARDS).

51. A priority goal for the hospitalized client who 2 days earlier had a total laryngectomy with creation of a new tracheostomy would be to
   ○ 1. decrease secretions.
   ○ 2. instruct the client in caring for the tracheostomy.
   ○ 3. relieve anxiety related to the tracheostomy.
   ○ 4. maintain a patent airway.

The Client With Burns

52. A client is admitted to the hospital after sustaining burns to the chest, abdomen, right arm, and right leg. The shaded areas in Figure 1 indicate the burned areas on the client's body. Using the "rule of nines," the nurse would determine that about what percentage of the client's body surface has been burned?
   ○ 1. 18%.
   ○ 2. 27%.
   ○ 3. 45%.
   ○ 4. 64%.

53. The nurse assesses the client for fluid shifting. Fluid shifts that occur during the emergent phase of a burn injury are caused by fluid moving
   ○ 1. from the vascular to the interstitial space.
   ○ 2. from the extracellular to the intracellular space.
   ○ 3. from the intracellular to the extracellular space.
   ○ 4. from the interstitial to the vascular space.

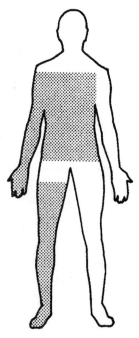

Figure 1.

54. The nurse should recognize that fluid shift in a client with a burn injury results from an increase in the
   ○ 1. permeability of capillary walls.
   ○ 2. total volume of intravascular plasma.
   ○ 3. total volume of circulating whole blood.
   ○ 4. permeability of the kidney tubules.

55. A priority nursing diagnosis category for a client with burns during the emergent period would be
   ○ 1. Excess Fluid Volume.
   ○ 2. Imbalanced Nutrition: Less Than Body Requirements.
   ○ 3. Risk for Injury (falling).
   ○ 4. Risk for Infection.

56. Which of the following activities should the nurse include in the care plan of a client with burn injuries to be carried out about one-half hour before the daily whirlpool bath and dressing change?
   ○ 1. Soak the dressing.
   ○ 2. Remove the dressing.
   ○ 3. Administer an analgesic.
   ○ 4. Slit the dressing with blunt scissors.

57. The client with a major burn injury receives total parenteral nutrition (TPN). The primary reason for this therapy is to help
   ○ 1. correct water and electrolyte imbalances.
   ○ 2. allow the gastrointestinal tract to rest.
   ○ 3. provide supplemental vitamins and minerals.
   ○ 4. ensure adequate caloric and protein intake.

58. The client asks the nurse what the word *eschar* means. Which of the following descriptions by the nurse best defines eschar?
   ○ 1. "Eschar is scar tissue in a developmental stage."
   ○ 2. "Eschar is crust formation without a blood supply."
   ○ 3. "Eschar is burned tissue that has become infected."
   ○ 4. "Eschar is visible living tissue with a rich blood supply."

59. An advantage of using biologic burn grafts, such as porcine (pigskin) grafts, is that they appear to help
   ○ 1. encourage formation of tough skin.
   ○ 2. promote the growth of epithelial tissue.
   ○ 3. provide for permanent wound closure.
   ○ 4. facilitate development of subcutaneous tissue.

60. Which of the following factors would have the *least* influence on the survival and effectiveness of a burn victim's porcine grafts?
   ○ 1. Absence of infection in the wounds.
   ○ 2. Adequate vascularization in the grafted area.
   ○ 3. Immobilization of the area being grafted.
   ○ 4. Use of analgesics as necessary for pain relief.

61. The nurse would plan to begin rehabilitation efforts for the burn client

○ 1. immediately after the burn has occurred.

○ 2. after the client's circulatory status has been stabilized.

○ 3. after grafting of the burn wounds has occurred.

○ 4. after the client's pain has been eliminated.

62. When an individual is burned there is massive cell destruction resulting in a disruption of the normal homeostasis of the body. The nurse anticipates that the client will be susceptible to which of the following in the early phase of burn care?

○ 1. Hypernatremia.

○ 2. Hyponatremia.

○ 3. Metabolic alkalosis.

○ 4. Hyperkalemia.

63. Endotracheal or tracheostomy tubes are placed in clients who have experienced

○ 1. electrical burns of the hands and arms causing dysrhythmias.

○ 2. thermal burns to the head, face, and airway resulting in hypoxia.

○ 3. chemical burns on the chest and abdomen.

○ 4. second-hand smoke inhalation.

64. A newly burned client is admitted to the unit. The nurse measures the client's urine output on an hourly basis, anticipating fluid balance problems related to fluid shifts. Which of the following hourly urinary output rates will alert the nurse to potential problems?

○ 1. 20 mL/hour.

○ 2. 30 mL/hour.

○ 3. 50 mL/hour.

○ 4. 100 mL/hour.

65. After the initial phase of the burn injury, the client's plan of care will focus primarily on

○ 1. helping the client maintain a positive self-concept.

○ 2. promoting hygiene.

○ 3. preventing infection.

○ 4. educating the client regarding care of the skin grafts.

66. The burned client needs fluid replacement because massive amounts of fluid are lost. The rate at which intravenous fluids are infused is based on the burn client's

○ 1. lean muscle mass and body surface area burned.

○ 2. total body weight and body surface area burned.

○ 3. total body surface area and body surface area burned.

○ 4. height and weight and body surface area burned.

67. The nurse is caring for a client with a burn injury and understands that stress reactions can result in hypersecretion of gastric acids. Therefore, the nurse must assess the client for signs and symptoms of

which of the following potential complications?

○ 1. Paralytic ileus.

○ 2. Gastric distention.

○ 3. Hiatal hernia.

○ 4. Curling's ulcer.

68. In the acute phase of burn injury, which pain medication would most likely be given to the client to decrease the perception of the pain?

○ 1. Oral analgesics such as ibuprofen or acetaminophen.

○ 2. Intravenous opioids.

○ 3. Intramuscular opioids.

○ 4. Oral antianxiety agents such as lorazepam (Ativan).

The Client With General Neurosensory Problems

69. The nurse observes that the client's right eye does not close completely. Based on this finding, which of the following nursing interventions would be *most* appropriate?

○ 1. Making sure the client wears her eyeglasses at all times.

○ 2. Placing an eye patch over her right eye.

○ 3. Instilling artificial tears once every shift.

○ 4. Cleansing the eye with a clean washcloth every shift.

70. A potential concern when caring for an older adult who has diminished hearing and vision would be the client's

○ 1. feelings of disorientation.

○ 2. cognitive impairment.

○ 3. sensory overload.

○ 4. social isolation.

71. The nurse is caring for a client with an injury to the thalamus. The nurse should plan to

○ 1. give higher doses of pain medication.

○ 2. keep patches on the client's eyes to prevent corneal abrasion.

○ 3. monitor the temperature of the bathwater.

○ 4. avoid turning the client.

72. The nurse is assigned a patient who has sustained a spinal cord injury. When assessing the client the nurse will expect the client to experience

○ 1. complete anesthesia below the level of the injury.

○ 2. tingling in the fingers.

○ 3. pain below the site of the injury.

○ 4. loss of position and vibratory sense.

73. A client who is paraplegic cannot feel her lower extremities and has been positioned on her side. The nurse would anticipate that which of the following areas would be a pressure point in this position?

○ 1. Sacrum.
○ 2. Occiput.
○ 3. Ankles.
○ 4. Heel.

74. A client is shown a coin and asked to identify it. When the client is not able to recognize the object through his special senses, he is demonstrating which of the following neurologic impairments?
○ 1. Aphasia.
○ 2. Agnosia.
○ 3. Analgesia.
○ 4. Ataxia.

75. The skin can detect superficial sensations including which of the following?
○ 1. Movement, temperature, and vibration.
○ 2. Pressure, touch, vibration, temperature, and pain.
○ 3. Pressure, touch, temperature, and pain.
○ 4. Movement, pressure, touch, and temperature.

The Client With Problems of the Integumentary System

76. The nurse is assessing an older adult's skin. The assessment will involve inspecting the skin for color, pigmentation, and vascularity. The critical component in the nurse's assessment is noting the
○ 1. similarities from one side to the other.
○ 2. changes from the normal expected findings.
○ 3. appearance of age-related wrinkles.
○ 4. skin turgor.

77. Which of the following changes are associated with normal aging?
○ 1. The outer layer of skin is replaced with new cells every 3 days.
○ 2. Subcutaneous fat and extracellular water decrease.
○ 3. The dermis becomes highly vascular and assists in the regulation of body temperature.
○ 4. Collagen becomes elastic and strong.

78. The nurse will anticipate which of the following problems that can result for the older adult undergoing abdominal surgery?
○ 1. Increased scarring.
○ 2. Decreased melanin and melanocytes.
○ 3. Decreased healing.
○ 4. Increased immunocompetence.

79. Health maintenance and promotion activities are especially important for the older adult. Which of the following activities reflects a health maintenance activity for an otherwise healthy older adult?
○ 1. Drinks 1500 mL of fluids per day.
○ 2. Consumes a balanced diet of 1200 calories per day.

○ 3. Walks briskly for 10 minutes three times per week.
○ 4. Sleeps at least 8 hours each night.

80. Which of the following characteristics would put a client at the *greatest* risk for impaired wound healing after abdominal surgery?
○ 1. Age 75 years.
○ 2. Age 30 years, poorly controlled diabetes.
○ 3. Age 55 years, heart attack.
○ 4. Age 60 years, peripheral vascular disease.

81. An 82-year-old woman has several ecchymotic areas on her left arm. The bruises are probably caused by
○ 1. elder abuse.
○ 2. self-inflicted injury.
○ 3. increased capillary fragility and permeability.
○ 4. increased blood supply to the skin.

82. A 90-year-old man complains of feeling cold in his room even though the thermostat is set at 75°F (24°C). The client probably feels cold because older adults have
○ 1. increased cellular cohesion.
○ 2. increased moisture content of the stratum corneum.
○ 3. slower cellular renewal time.
○ 4. decreased ability to thermoregulate.

83. Palpation of the skin provides the nurse useful information regarding
○ 1. bruising of the skin.
○ 2. color of the skin.
○ 3. hair distribution.
○ 4. turgor of the skin.

84. A priority nursing diagnosis for an adult woman who has pruritus and is continuously scratching the affected areas and demonstrates agitation and anxiety regarding the itching sensation would be
○ 1. Altered Comfort related to pruritus.
○ 2. Ineffective Health Maintenance related to lack of knowledge of the disease process.
○ 3. Impaired Skin Integrity related to dehydration from the treatment medications.
○ 4. Social Isolation related to poor self-image.

85. Which of the following factors places a client at greatest risk for skin cancer?
○ 1. Fair skin and history of chronic sun exposure.
○ 2. Caucasian race and history of hypertension.
○ 3. Dark skin and family history of skin cancer.
○ 4. Dark skin and history of hypertension.

86. Malignant melanoma is a result of
○ 1. a lesion arising from a mole.
○ 2. a lesion arising from epidermal basal cells.
○ 3. a tumor arising from squamous cells.
○ 4. a tumor arising in cells producing melanin.

87. In planning an educational presentation for a client with malignant melanoma, the nurse understands that the prognosis of the client depends on

1. the amount of ulceration of the lesion.
2. the color of the lesion.
3. the location of the lesion on the body.
4. the thickness of the lesion.

88. The nurse finds an aide massaging the bony prominences of a client on bed rest. The correct action by the nurse is to
    1. reinforce the aide's use of this intervention over the bony prominences.
    2. explain that massage is effective because it improves blood flow to the area.
    3. inform the aide that massage is even more effective when combined with lotion during the massage.
    4. instruct the aide that massage is contraindicated because it decreases blood flow to the area.

89. A stage 2 pressure ulcer is characterized by
    1. redness in the involved area.
    2. muscle spasms in the involved area.
    3. pain in the involved area.
    4. tissue necrosis in the involved area.

90. Regular oral hygiene is an essential component of nursing care for the client who cannot perform self-care. Which of the following nursing measures would be inappropriate when providing oral hygiene?
    1. Place the client in a supine position with a small pillow under the head.
    2. Keep portable suctioning equipment at the bedside.
    3. Open the client's mouth with a padded tongue blade.
    4. Cleanse the client's mouth and teeth with a toothbrush.

91. An older adult does not want to eat supper and complains that the food does not taste good. Consistent with knowledge about age-related changes to taste, the nurse may find that the client is more willing to eat
    1. sour foods.
    2. salty foods.
    3. sweet foods.
    4. greasy foods.

92. An older adult who had abdominal surgery is being discharged to home. The goal is to maintain and promote adequate nutritional status in the home environment. The nurse anticipates that the client will need additional instruction when she makes which of the following statements?
    1. "I should get approximately 80% of my calories from carbohydrates."
    2. "I should get 25% to 30% of my calories from fat."
    3. "I should use herbs to improve the flavor of foods."
    4. "I should eat a moderate amount of fiber every day."

93. An alert and oriented elderly client is admitted to the hospital for treatment of cellulitis of the left shoulder after an arthroscopy. Which fall prevention strategy is most appropriate for this client?
    1. Keep all the lights on in the room at all times.
    2. Use a nightlight in the bathroom.
    3. Keep all four side rails up at all times.
    4. Place the client in a room with a camera monitor.

94. Prevention of skin breakdown and maintenance of skin integrity among older clients is important because they are at greater risk secondary to
    1. altered balance.
    2. altered protective pressure sensation.
    3. impaired hearing ability.
    4. impaired visual acuity.

95. When assessing an older adult's pain after surgery, the nurse must remember that
    1. pain perception is altered in the older adult.
    2. pain perception varies with the individual.
    3. older clients may be unable to describe their pain.
    4. tolerance to pain is lowered in older adults.

Correct Answers and Rationale

The letters in parentheses following the rationale identify the step of the nursing process (A, D, P, I, E) and client needs (1, 2, 3, 4, 5, 6, 7, 8, 9, 10). See the inside front cover for the key.

The Client With Cataracts

1. 2. Senile cataracts are related to the aging process. The second most common cause of cataracts is a history of eye injury. Systemic diseases (eg, diabetes) and systemic syndromes (eg, Down syndrome) as well as ingestion of injurious or toxic substances (eg, alcohol, smoking, naphthalene, corticosteroids) are associated with cataract development; however, cataracts in older adults are related to the aging process. (D, 3)

2. 3. The lens of the eye is suspended on the suspensory ligaments. The ligaments influence the tension on the lens and thereby focus light rays onto the retina. Accommodation is the ability of the lens to adjust to near and far objects. The ciliary bodies secrete aqueous humor. The retina contains the rods and cones. The iris regulates the amount of light entering the eye. (D, 10)

3. 2. The nurse should give a client who seems fearful of surgery an opportunity to express her feelings. Only after identifying the client's concerns can the nurse intervene appropriately. Asking the client about previous reactions to local anesthetics may be warranted, but it does not address the client's concerns in this instance. Telling the client that she will not have nausea or vomiting ignores the client's feelings of fear and does not provide any data about the client's feelings. More data would help the nurse plan care. Telling the client that there is nothing to be afraid of minimizes her feelings and does not address her concerns. Premature explanations and clichés do not provide needed assessment data and ignore the client's feelings. (A, 5)

4. 3. A client with a cataract usually complains of dimness, blurring, and/or hazy vision. Typically, light scattering occurs and is related to the degree of opacity of the lens. Opacity of the lens blocks light rays from reaching the retina. Eye pain and irritation are not associated with cataracts. Halos and rainbows are usually associated with glaucoma. Eye strain and headache when doing close work is associated with refractive errors. (A, 4)

5. 2. Instilled in the eye, phenylephrine hydrochloride acts as a mydriatic, causing the pupil to dilate. It also constricts small blood vessels in the eye. (P, 8)

6. 4. A prescribed antiemetic should be administered as soon as the client who has undergone cataract extraction complains of nausea. Vomiting can increase intraocular pressure, which should be avoided after eye surgery because it can cause complications. Deep breathing is unlikely to relieve nausea. Postoperative nausea may be common; however, it doesn't necessarily pass quickly and can lead to vomiting. Telling the client to call only if vomiting occurs ignores the client's need for comfort and intervention to prevent complications. (I, 8)

7. 3. Safety of the client is the major concern on the return home. The home environment should be assessed for safety hazards, and steps to decrease potential hazards should be implemented. Arrangements for home care, if necessary, should be made before surgery. The client is usually able to return to the activities of daily living rapidly, so a deficiency of diversional activities or a feeding self-care deficit would not typically be anticipated. Oral pain medication should control the client's discomfort. (D, 2)

8. 1. Applying pressure against the nose at the inner canthus of the closed eye after administering eye drops prevents the medication from entering the lacrimal (tear) duct. If the medication enters the tear duct, it can enter the nose and pharynx, where it may be absorbed and cause toxic symptoms. Eye drops should be placed in the eye's lower conjunctival sac. (P, 8)

9. 2. Coughing is contraindicated after cataract extraction because it increases intraocular pressure. Other activities that are contraindicated because they increase intraocular pressure include turning to the operative side, sneezing, crying, and straining. Lying supine, ambulating, and deep breathing do not affect intraocular pressure. (P, 10)

10. 4. Sudden, sharp pain after eye surgery should suggest to the nurse that the client may be experiencing intraocular hemorrhage. The physician should be notified promptly. Detached retina and prolapse of the iris are usually painless. Extracapsular erosion is not characterized by sharp pain. (A, 10)

The Client With a Retinal Detachment

11. 2. The spots, or floaters, commonly reported by clients with retinal detachment are blood cells released into the vitreous humor by the detachment. (A, 10)

12. 1. Patching the eyes helps decrease random eye movements that could enlarge and worsen retinal detach-

ment. Although clients with eye injuries frequently are light sensitive, and preventing infection is important, the specific goal is to reduce rapid eye movements. Resting the eye is an indirect way of stating the objective. (I, 10)

13. 4. Untreated retinal detachment results in increasing detachment and eventual blindness, but 90% to 95% of clients can be successfully treated with surgery. If necessary, the surgical procedure can be repeated about 10 to 14 days after the first procedure. Many more services are available for newly blind people, but ideally this client will not need them. (A, 10)

14. 1. The scarring of the retinal tear needs time to heal completely. Therefore, resumption of activity should be gradual; the client may resume her usual activities in 5 to 6 weeks. Successful healing should allow the client to return to her previous level of functioning. (P, 7)

15. 2. After surgery to correct a detached retina, prevention of increased intraocular pressure is the priority goal. Control of pain with analgesics is the second goal. Following a low-sodium diet or maintaining a darkened environment is not a goal for this client. (P, 10)

16. 4. A choroidal scar will form a permanent seal to close the hole or tear in the retina. A scleral buckle serves as a splint to bring the two retinal layers in contact with each other until a scar can form. Loss of a portion of the retina or loss of the whole retina would interfere with sight. Retinal transplants are not performed. The retina is never stitched to the optic nerve. (P, 10)

The Client With Glaucoma

17. 2. In COAG, there is an obstruction to the outflow of aqueous humor, leading to increased intraocular pressure. The increased intraocular pressure eventually causes destruction of the retina's nerve fibers. This nerve destruction causes painless vision loss. The exact cause of glaucoma is unknown. Glaucoma does not lead to retinal detachment. (D, 10)

18. 4. Although COAG is usually asymptomatic in the early stages, peripheral vision gradually decreases as the disorder progresses. Eye pain is not a feature of COAG but is common in clients with angle-closure glaucoma. Excessive lacrimation is not a symptom of COAG; it may indicate a blocked tear duct. Flashes of light is a common symptom of retinal detachment. (A, 10)

19. 3. A miotic agent constricts the pupil and contracts ciliary musculature. These effects widen the filtration angle and permit increased outflow of aqueous humor. Miotics also cause vasodilation of the intraocular vessels, where intraocular fluids leave the eye, also increas-

ing aqueous humor outflow. Mydriatics cause cycloplegia, or paralysis of the ciliary muscle. (I, 8)

20. 2. Tonometry, which measures intraocular pressure, is a simple, noninvasive, and painless procedure that requires no particular preparation or postprocedure care and carries no side effects. It is not necessary to dilate the pupils for tonometry. (I, 9)

21. 3. Timolol maleate is commonly administered to control glaucoma. The drug's action is not completely understood, but it is believed to reduce aqueous humor formation, thereby reducing intraocular pressure. (P, 8)

22. 2. The cornea is sensitive and can be injured by eye drops falling onto it. Therefore, eye drops should be instilled into the lower conjunctival sac of the eye to avoid the risk of corneal damage. Systemic absorption occurs when eye drops enter the tear ducts. (A, 8)

23. 2. Atropine sulfate causes pupil dilation. This action is contraindicated for the client with glaucoma because it increases intraocular pressure. The drug does not have this effect on intraocular pressure in people who do not have glaucoma. (P, 8)

24. 4. Acute angle-closure glaucoma produces abrupt changes in the angle of the iris. Clinical manifestations include severe eye pain, colored halos around lights, and rapid vision loss. Gradual loss of central vision is associated with macular degeneration. The loss of color vision, or achromotopsia, is a rare symptom that occurs when a stroke damages the fusiform gyrus. It most often affects only half of the visual field. (A, 10)

25. 3. Acute angle-closure glaucoma is a medical emergency that rapidly leads to blindness if left untreated. Treatment typically involves miotic drugs and surgery, usually iridectomy or laser therapy. Both procedures create a hole in the periphery of the iris, which allows the aqueous humor to flow into the anterior chamber. Bed rest does not affect the progression of acute angle-closure glaucoma. Steroids are not a treatment for acute angle-closure glaucoma; in fact, the are associated with the development of glaucoma. (P, 10)

The Client Undergoing Nasal Surgery

26. 2. Because of the dense packing, it is relatively unusual for bleeding to be apparent through the nasal drip pad. Instead, the blood runs down the throat, causing the client to swallow frequently. The back of the throat can be assessed with a flashlight. An accumulation of blood in the stomach may cause nausea and vomiting, but is not an initial sign of bleeding. Increased respiratory rate occurs in shock and is not an early sign of bleeding in the client after nasal surgery. Feelings of anxiety are not indicative of nasal bleeding. (A, 10)

27. 1. The client should be instructed to avoid any activities that cause Valsalva's maneuver (eg, straining at stool, vigorous coughing, exercise) to reduce stress on suture lines and bleeding. The client should not take aspirin because of its antiplatelet properties, which may cause bleeding. Oral hygiene is important to rid the mouth of old dried blood and to enhance the client's appetite. Cool compresses, not heat, should be applied to decrease swelling and control discoloration of the area. (I, 10)

28. 2. Constipation can cause straining during defecation, which can induce bleeding. Showering is not contraindicated. The client should take measures to prevent coughing. The client should avoid blowing her nose for 48 hours after the packing is removed. Thereafter, she should blow her nose gently using the open-mouth technique to minimize bleeding in the surgical area. (E, 10)

The Client With a Hearing Disorder

29. 2. Furosemide may cause ototoxicity. The nurse should tell the client to promptly report the hearing loss, dizziness, or tinnitus, to help prevent permanent ear damage. Hearing loss is not inevitable, and it is inappropriate to make assumptions about the cause of symptoms without a thorough evaluation. The client's system will not "adjust," and hearing loss will not resolve. (P, 8)

30. 3. Hearing aids have limited use for clients with sensorineural hearing loss because these clients experience problems with sound discrimination as well as volume. A hearing aid can make sound louder but not necessarily clearer. The hearing aid cannot help the client distinguish spoken words from background noises. (A, 7)

31. 3. A sensorineural hearing loss results from damage to the cochlear or vestibulocochlear nerve. Presence of fluid and cerumen in the external canal or sclerosis of the bones of the middle ear results in a conductive hearing loss. Hearing loss resulting from an emotional disturbance is called a psychogenic hearing loss. (A, 3)

32. 1. Cerumen (ear wax) commonly gets impacted in older adults in the external canal. Otalgia is the "fullness" sensation or pain that an older adult may experience when the cerumen becomes impacted. External otitis is an inflammation of the outer ear and would not explain the symptoms the client is experiencing. Exostosis is a bony growth that arises from the surface of a bone and would not explain the symptoms the client is experiencing. (A, 3)

33. 2. Irrigation is the first strategy to loosen cerumen. Successful removal of the cerumen involves gentle irrigation behind the impacted cerumen. The flow of the water must be behind to remove the cerumen out of the canal. A cotton-tipped applicator or other device is not appropriate because it can cause damage to the eardrum. Use of aural suction or a cerumen curette is appropriate only if the impacted cerumen cannot be removed by irrigation. (I, 9)

34. 1. Normal saline is the solution that is generally used to irrigate the ear. Sterile water will cause tissue damage. An antiseptic solution is not typically used unless an infection is present. Lactated Ringer's is a hypertonic solution. (I, 8)

35. 2. Tympanoplasty involves surgical reconstruction of the tympanic membrane and is done to reestablish middle ear function, close perforations, and prevent recurrent infection. Ossiculoplasty is reconstruction of the bones of the middle ear. It is sometimes performed concurrently with tympanoplasty, but it is not as common as tympanoplasty. Mastoidectomy is done to remove a cholesteatoma, a cyst-like mass that can occur in the middle ear secondary to infection. It also is not as common as tympanoplasty. Myringotomy involves making an incision in the tympanic membrane to relieve pressure and drain fluid from the ear. Myringotomy is more common with acute otitis media than chronic otitis media. (P, 9)

36. 1. The nurse should first assess the client's knowledge base. Working within the framework of the client's knowledge and educational level, the nurse then can describe the procedure and its benefits. (D, 9)

37. 4. Tinnitus is a side effect of aspirin. Aspirin contains salicylate, which is an ototoxic drug that can induce reversible hearing loss and tinnitus. The nurse should encourage the client to inform the physician of the symptom. Tinnitus is not a function of aging. The Weber test and audiometric testing are useful for determining hearing loss but are not necessarily helpful in the management or diagnosis of drug-induced tinnitus. (A, 7)

The Client With Ménière's Disease

38. 3. Ménière's disease involves the inner ear and is characterized by episodes of acute vertigo, tinnitus, and fluctuating, progressive hearing loss. The severe vertigo can lead to nausea and vomiting, but vomiting is not considered one of the classic triad of symptoms. Headache is not associated with Ménière's disease. Otitis media is an inflammation of the middle ear. (A, 10)

39. 1. A low-sodium diet is frequently an effective mechanism for reducing the frequency and severity of the disease episodes. About three quarters of clients with Ménière's disease respond to treatment with a low-salt diet. A diuretic may also be ordered. (P, 7)

40. 2. There is no cure for Ménière's disease, but the wide range of medical and surgical treatments allows for adequate control in many clients. The disease often worsens, but it does not spread to the eyes. The hearing loss is usually unilateral. (E, 10)

41. 4. The client needs to assume a safe and comfortable position during an attack, which may last several hours. The client's location when the attack occurs may dictate the most reasonable position. Ideally, the client should lie down immediately in a reclining or flat position to control the vertigo. The danger of a serious fall is real. Placing the head between the knees will not help prevent a fall and is not practical because the attack may last several hours. Concentrating on breathing may be a useful distraction, but it will not help prevent a fall. Closing the eyes does not help prevent a fall. (I, 2)

42. 1. A client with Ménière's disease may curtail social activities out of fear of embarrassment from having a dizzy spell in public. This seems likely in this situation, based on the wife's information, but would need to be validated by the client. However, the wife may be a more reliable source of information about social isolation than the client. (D, 5)

43. 4. A wide variety of medications may be used in an attempt to control Ménière's disease, including antihistamines, antiemetics, tranquilizers, and diuretics. Glucocorticoids play no significant role in disease treatment. (P, 8)

44. 2. The client's risk for injury related to vertigo is the highest priority preoperatively. The client should be instructed how to manage attacks of vertigo safely. Deficient Diversional Activity related to inability to participate secondary to vertigo is an appropriate nursing diagnosis, but it is not a priority. Powerlessness related to inability to influence effects of the disease process is a possible diagnosis, but more data are required before making such a diagnosis. Risk for Social Isolation related to hearing loss is a possible diagnosis for the client after surgery. The client retains the ability to hear with Ménière's disease; however, total hearing loss is a possible complication of labyrinthectomy. (E, 10)

The Client With Adult Macular Degeneration

45. 1. Macular degeneration generally involves loss of central vision. Gradual blurring of vision can occur as the disease progresses and may result in blindness; however, loss of central vision is the most common finding. Tiny yellowish spots, known as *drusen*, develop beneath the retina. Loss of peripheral vision is characteristic of glaucoma. (A, 10)

46. 3. AMD generally affects central vision. Confusion may result related to the changes in the environment and the inability to see the environment clearly. Therefore, providing safety is the priority goal in the care of this patient. Educating him regarding community resources or monitoring his AMD may have been done at an earlier date or can be done after assessing his knowledge base and experience with the disease process. Improving his vision may not be possible. (P, 7)

47. 3. The priority nursing diagnosis for a client with limited eyesight is safety and preventing injury. The initial goal is to orient the client to a new environment. Taking time to identify the objects and where they are located in the room can achieve this goal. It is unrealistic to have someone stay with the client at all times or for the client to stay in bed until the nurse can assist her. (I, 1)

48. 4. To expand the visual field, the partially sighted client should be taught to turn the head from side to side when walking. Neglecting to do so may result in accidents. This technique helps maximize the use of remaining sight. A patch does not address the problem of hemianopia. Appropriate client positioning and placement of personal items will increase the client's ability to cope with the problem but will not affect safety. (I, 2)

The Client With Cancer of the Larynx

49. 1. The goal of postoperative care is to maintain physiologic integrity. Therefore, inserting a feeding tube is a strategy to ensure the fluid and nutritional needs of the client as the surgical site is healing. The feeding tube does help prevent aspiration by preventing ingested fluid from leaking through the wound into the trachea before healing occurs; however, the primary rationale is to meet the client's nutritional and fluid needs. A tracheoesophageal fistula is a rare complication of total laryngectomy and may occur if radiation therapy has compromised wound healing. A feeding tube does not help maintain an open airway. (P, 9)

50. 2. Tracheostomy tubes carry several potential complications, including laryngeal nerve damage, bleeding, and infection. (A, 10)

51. 4. The main goal for a client with a new tracheostomy is to maintain a patent airway. A fresh tracheostomy frequently causes bleeding and excess secretions, and clients may require frequent suctioning to maintain patency. Decreasing secretions may be a component of a client's care after laryngectomy and tracheostomy, and relieving anxiety is always an important goal; however, the primary goal is to maintain a patent airway. Instruction in care of a tracheostomy is a priority later in the client's recovery. (P, 10)

The Client With Burns

52. 3. According to the rule of nines, this client has sustained burns on about 45% of the body surface. The right arm is calculated as being 9%, the right leg is 18%, and the anterior trunk is 18%, for a total of 45%. (A, 10)

53. 1. In a burn injury, the injured capillaries dilate, and there is increased capillary permeability at the site of the burn. Plasma seeps out into the burned tissue, moving from the vascular space into the interstitial space. (A, 10)

54. 1. When a burn occurs, the capillaries and small vessels dilate, and cell damage causes the release of a histamine-like substance. This substance causes the capillary walls to become more permeable, and significant quantities of fluid are lost. The initial fluid derangement after a burn is a shift from the plasma to the interstitial fluid shift. Renal function may be altered as a result of decreased blood flow secondary to blood loss; however, burns do not cause increased permeability of the kidney tubules. (A, 10)

55. 4. Infection is a priority problem for the burned victim because of the loss of skin integrity and alteration in body defenses. Excess fluid or imbalanced nutrition is not a priority during the emergent period. A risk for falling is not a priority for this client because the client would be on bed rest and most likely in a critical care unit. (D, 10)

56. 3. Removing dressings from severe burns exposes sensitive nerve endings to the air, which is painful. The client should be given a prescribed analgesic about one-half hour before the dressing change to promote comfort. The other activities are done as part of the whirlpool and dressing change process and not one-half hour beforehand. (P, 9)

57. 4. Nutritional support with sufficient calories and protein is extremely important for a client with severe burns because of the loss of plasma protein through injured capillaries and an increased metabolic rate. Gastric dilation and paralytic ileus commonly occur in clients with severe burns, making oral fluids and foods contraindicated. Water and electrolyte imbalances can be corrected by administration of intravenous fluids with electrolyte additives, although TPN typically includes all necessary electrolytes. Resting the gastrointestinal tract may help prevent paralytic ileus, and TPN provides vitamins and minerals; however, the primary reason for starting TPN is to provide the protein necessary for tissue healing. (I, 8)

58. 2. Eschar is a crust of dead tissue, heavily contaminated with bacteria and without a blood supply. Eschar has also been defined as devitalized skin. (I, 10)

59. 2. Biologic dressings, such as porcine grafts, serve many purposes for a client with severe burns. They enhance the growth of epithelial tissues, minimize the overgrowth of granulation tissue, prevent loss of water and protein, decrease pain, increase mobility, and help prevent infection. (P, 10)

60. 4. Analgesic administration to keep a burn victim comfortable is important but is unlikely to influence graft survival and effectiveness. Absence of infection, adequate vascularization, and immobilization of the grafted area promote an effective graft. (E, 10)

61. 2. Rehabilitation efforts are implemented as soon as the client's condition is stabilized. Early emphasis on rehabilitation is important to decrease complications and to help ensure that the client will be able to make the adjustments necessary to return to an optimal state of health and independence. It is not possible to completely eliminate the client's pain; pain control is a major challenge in burn care. (P, 7)

62. 4. Immediately after a burn, excessive potassium from cell destruction is released into the extracellular fluid. Hyponatremia is a common electrolyte imbalance in the burned client that occurs within the first week after being burned. Metabolic acidosis usually occurs as a result of the loss of sodium bicarbonate. (P, 9)

63. 2. Airway management is the priority in caring for a burn client. Nasotracheal or endotracheal intubation is anticipated when significant thermal and smoke inhalation burns occur. Clients who have experienced burns to the face and neck usually will be compromised within 1 to 2 hours. Electrical burns of the hands and arms, even with cardiac dysrhythmias, or a chemical burn of the chest and abdomen is not likely to result in the need for intubation. Second-hand smoke inhalation does influence an individual's respiratory status but does not require intubation unless the individual has an allergic reaction to the smoke. (P, 7)

64. 2. The acceptable range for urine output is greater than 30 mL/hour. Less than 30 mL/hour may indicate poor renal perfusion resulting from a hypovolemic state or myoglobin blocking the renal tubules, or both. Increased urine output of 100 mL/hour or more usually occurs after the first 48 hours of a burn. (P, 9)

65. 3. The inflammatory response begins when a burn is sustained. As a result of the burn, the immune system becomes impaired. There is a decrease in immunoglobins, changes in white blood cells, alterations of lymphocytes, and decreased levels of interleukin. The human body's protective barrier, the skin, has been damaged. As a result, the burn patient becomes vul-

nerable to infections. Education and interventions to maintain a positive self-concept would be appropriate during the rehabilitation phase. Promoting hygiene helps the client feel comfortable; however, the primary focus is on reducing the risk for infection. (P, 2)

66. 2. During the first 24 hours, fluid replacement for an adult burned patient is be based on total body weight and body surface area burned. Lean muscle mass considers only muscle mass; replacement is based on total body weight. Total surface area is estimated by taking into account the individual's height and weight. Height is not a common variable used in formulas for fluid replacement. (A, 10)

67. 4. Curling's ulcer or gastrointestinal ulceration occurs in about half of the clients with a burn injury. The incidence of ulceration appears proportional to the extent of the burns and is believed to be caused by hypersecretion of gastric acid and compromised gastrointestinal perfusion. Paralytic ileus and gastric distention do not result from hypersecretion of gastric acid and stress. Hiatal hernia is not necessarily a potential complication of a burn injury. (A, 10)

68. 2. The severe pain experienced by burn clients requires opioid analgesics. In addition, opioids such as morphine sedate and alleviate apprehension. Oral analgesics such as ibuprofen or acetaminophen are unlikely to be strong enough to effectively manage the intense pain experienced by the client who is severely burned. Because of the altered tissue perfusion from the burn injury, intravenous medications are preferred. Antianxiety agents are not effective against pain. (I, 10)

The Client With General Neurosensory Problems

69. 2. When the blink reflex is absent or the eyes do not close completely, the cornea may become dry and irritated. Placing a patch over the eye is the most appropriate intervention to prevent eye injury. Making sure the client wears her eyeglasses at all times will not help protect the eye from injury. A once-per-shift intervention will not adequately relieve the potential for injury from a dry and irritating ocular environment. A normal saline solution should be used to moisten the eye, not tapwater. (I, 10)

70. 4. Social isolation is a concern for an older adult who has diminished hearing and vision. Feeling disoriented may be related to cognitive problems rather than diminished hearing and vision. Diminished hearing and vision is related to the aging process and does not result in impairment of the older adult's thought processes. The client with impaired hearing and vision is unlikely to experience sensory overload. (P, 5)

71. 3. The spinal cord connects the brain to the periphery. The thalamus is located in the midbrain and integrates all sensory impulses except olfaction. The afferent impulses are received and then transmitted from the thalamus. Destruction or interruption of the neurosensory pathway results in loss of communication between the two systems. Monitoring the temperature of the bathwater is important because the client cannot feel whether the water is too hot or too cold. Damage to the thalamus does not result in loss of the corneal reflex. Loss of position and vibratory sense usually occurs with degeneration of the posterior column of the spinal cord; therefore, turning every 2 hours is critical to prevent skin breakdown related to increased capillary pressure. The nurse can give only the prescribed dosage of pain medication. (A, 7)

72. 1. The spinal cord connects the brain to the periphery. Destruction or interruption of the neurosensory pathway results in loss of communication between the two systems. Transsection of the spinal cord renders the individual in a complete state of anesthesia below the level of injury. Tingling in the fingers may be related to spinal cord disease or to improper positioning of the extremity. Loss of position and vibratory sense usually occurs when the individual has degeneration of the posterior column of the spinal cord. (A, 7)

73. 3. Common pressure points in the side-lying position include the ears, shoulders, ribs, greater trochanter, medial and lateral condyles, and ankles. The sacrum, occiput, and heel are pressure points in the supine position. (P, 10)

74. 2. *Agnosia* is the inability to recognize familiar objects. *Aphasia* is the loss of language comprehension or language expression, or both. *Analgesia* is the loss of pain sensation. *Ataxia* is the lack of coordination of movement. (A, 4)

75. 2. The skin registers pressure, touch, vibration, temperature, and pain. The body is composed of the somatovisceral senses. These senses include superficial sensibility (skin), proprioceptive sensation (muscle and joints), and pain sensibility within the body. (A, 3)

The Client With Problems of the Integumentary System

76. 2. Noting changes from the normal expected findings is the most important component when assessing an older adult's integumentary system. Comparing one extremity with the contralateral extremity (ie, comparing one side with the other) is an important assessment step; however, the most important component is noting changes from an expected normal baseline. Noting wrinkles related to age is not of much consequence

unless the client is admitted for cosmetic surgery to reduce the appearance of age-related wrinkling. Noting skin turgor is an assessment of fluid status, not an assessment of the integumentary system. (A, 3)

77. 2. There is a decreased amount of subcutaneous fat, muscle laxity, degeneration of elastic fibers, and collagen stiffening. The outer layer of skin is almost completely replaced every 3 to 4 weeks. The vascular supply diminishes with age. Collagen thins and diminishes with age. (A, 3)

78. 3. Normal aging consists of decreased proliferative capacity of the skin. Decreased collagen synthesis slows capillary growth, impairs phagocytosis among older adults, and results in slow healing. Increased scarring is not a result of age-related skin changes. Both melanin and melanocytes give color to the skin and hair but are increased with aging. There is a decrease in the immunocompetence of the aging adult. (P, 9)

79. 1. Drinking at least six 8-ounce glasses of fluid per day helps the client stay well hydrated. Maintaining optimal fluid balance is important for all body systems. Caloric intake varies according to an individual's size and activity level. An intake of 1200 calories per day may be insufficient for some older adults. Walking 10 minutes per day is useful, but an otherwise healthy older adult should try to walk 20 minutes per day. It is important to get adequate rest; however, the amount of sleep needed varies with the individual. (E, 3)

80. 2. Poorly controlled diabetes is a serious risk factor for postoperative wound infection. Other factors that delay wound healing include advanced age, nutritional deficiencies (vitamin C, protein, zinc), inadequate blood supply, use of corticosteroid drugs, infection, mechanical friction on the wound, obesity, anemia, and poor general health. (D, 9)

81. 3. The aging process involves increased capillary fragility and permeability. Older adults have a decreased amount of subcutaneous fat. Therefore, there is an increased incidence of bruiselike lesions caused by collection of extravascular blood in the loosely structured dermis. In addition, older adults do not always realize that injury has occurred because of a diminished awareness of pain, touch, and peripheral vibration. There are no data to support elder abuse or self-inflicted bruises. Blood supply to the skin declines with aging. (D, 9)

82. 4. Older adults have a decreased thermoregulation that is related to decreased blood supply and reabsorption of body fat. As a result, older adults are at risk for hypothermia. Cellular cohesion and moisture content diminish with age. Cellular renewal time is slowed; however, this does not result in impaired thermoregulation. (D, 3)

83. 4. Assessment of the integumentary system includes both inspection and palpation. Palpation involves assessing temperature, turgor, moisture, and texture. Observing bruises and color and detecting hair distribution are inspection. (A, 3)

84. 1. Risk for Infection related to pruritus is the priority nursing diagnosis because it has been documented that the client continues to scratch the affected areas. Satisfactory control of the itching sensation and discomfort associated with scratching may relieve the agitation and anxiety. More information is required regarding the knowledge level of the client and her disease process, but learning cannot take place when an individual's attention is distracted with pruritus. Impaired Skin Integrity is a potential problem if the client continues to scratch the affected areas and destroys the skin, but the risk for infection deserves priority attention because of the client's anxiety. There are no data to support that the client has a poor self-image. (I, 7)

85. 1. Caucasians who have fair skin and a high exposure to ultraviolet (UV) light are at increased risk for malignant neoplasms of the skin. The other risk factors include exposure to tar and arsenicals and family history. History of hypertension is a coronary artery disease risk factor. (I, 3)

86. 4. Malignant melanoma is a lesion or tumor that arises from melanin-producing cells. Although malignant melanoma may begin in a mole, not all lesions arising in moles are melanomas and melanomas can develop from flat areas of melanin. Lesions arising from the basal cells are called basal cell carcinomas. Lesions arising from squamous cells are called squamous cell carcinomas. (D, 9)

87. 4. Tumor or lesion thickness is the predictive factor for survival. Cutaneous melanoma that is confined to the epidermis layer of the skin has a high cure rate. Asymmetry, border, color, and diameter are known as the "ABCDs" of melanoma. (I, 3)

88. 4. Massaging areas that are reddened due to pressure is contraindicated because it further reduces blood flow to the area. (I, 1)

89. 3. A stage 2 skin breakdown involves epidermal sloughing and pain. Redness without blanching is noted in stage 1. Stage 3 involves tissue necrosis with subcutaneous involvement. Stage 4 involves muscle and/or bone destruction. Muscle spasms are not a criterion used in the staging process. (A, 1)

90. 1. A helpless client should be positioned on the side, not on the back, with the head on a small pillow. This positioning helps secretions escape from the throat and mouth and minimizes the risk of aspiration. (I, 10)

91. 3. Older adults' taste buds retain their sensitivity to carbohydrates. In addition, carbohydrates tend to be food items that are easy to chew. Older adults lose their sensitivity to sour and salty foods. Older adults may find greasy foods harder to digest and therefore may avoid them; however, preference for greasy foods is not related to changes in taste associated with age. (D, 7)

92. 1. In order to maintain or promote nutritional status that promotes healing, the older adult needs a complete balanced diet that includes all of the food groups. Most diets recommend that 50% to 60% of calories come from carbohydrates. Carbohydrates may be easy to chew and taste good, but they cause hyperglycemia, resulting in slow healing. Unless contraindicated by a disorder of gastric hypermotility, moderates amount of fiber should be consumed daily to maintain optimal bowel function. (I, 7)

93. 2. Many falls occur when older adults attempt to get to the bathroom at night. The risk is even greater in an unfamiliar environment. Use of a nightlight in the bathroom enables the older adult client to see the way to the bathroom. Keeping the lights on in the room at all times may contribute to sensory overload and prevent adequate rest. Raised side rails paradoxically contribute to falls when the older adult tries to climb over them to get to the bathroom. The upper side rails may be raised, but it is not recommended that all four side rails be elevated. Camera monitoring can be used but does nothing to prevent a fall. (I, 1)

94. 2. Pressure ulcers usually occur over bony prominences. An alteration in the protective pressure sensation results from a decline in the number of Meissner's and pacinian corpuscles. (D, 8)

95. 2. Pain perception varies with the individual, regardless of age. Although older adults have more physical problems that cause pain, the presence of pain should not be minimized, and both nonpharmacologic and pharmacologic efforts should be used to obtain pain relief. Pain perception is essentially unaltered in the neurologically intact older adult. Older clients can describe their pain as long as they are alert and oriented. (I, 10)

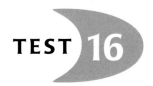

TEST 16
General Client Needs

▶ Pharmacologic and Parenteral Therapies
▶ Growth and Development
▶ Management of Care
▶ Correct Answers and Rationale

Select the one best answer, and indicate your choice by filling in the circle in front of the option.

Pharmacologic and Parenteral Therapies

1. When administering atropine sulfate preoperatively to a client scheduled for lung surgery, the nurse should tell the client which of the following?
   ○ 1. "This medicine will make you drowsy."
   ○ 2. "This medicine will help you relax."
   ○ 3. "This medicine will make your mouth feel dry."
   ○ 4. "This medicine will reduce the risk of postoperative infection."

2. The nurse is preparing to administer digoxin (Lanoxin) 0.125 mg. Scored 0.25-mg tablets are available. How many tablets should the nurse administer?
   ○ 1. 0.5 tablets.
   ○ 2. 1.0 tablets.
   ○ 3. 1.5 tablets.
   ○ 4. 2.0 tablets.

3. Which of the following medications would the nurse anticipate administering in the event of a heparin overdose?
   ○ 1. Warfarin sodium.
   ○ 2. Protamine sulfate.
   ○ 3. Acetylsalicylic acid.
   ○ 4. Atropine sulfate.

4. Chloral hydrate 1000 mg has been ordered. It is available in a syrup containing 0.5 g/5 mL. How many milliliters should the nurse give?
   ○ 1. 1.5 mL.
   ○ 2. 3.0 mL.
   ○ 3. 5.0 mL.
   ○ 4. 10.0 mL.

5. The client is supposed to receive 500 mL of 5% dextrose on 0.45% normal saline (D5/0.45 NS) with 20 mEq of potassium chloride (KCl) over the next 6 hours. The infusion set administers 10 gtt/mL. To what flow rate should the nurse adjust the intravenous flow?
   ○ 1. 14 gtt/minute.
   ○ 2. 18 gtt/minute.
   ○ 3. 21 gtt/minute.
   ○ 4. 25 gtt/minute.

6. What is the primary purpose of administering aminophylline to a client with emphysema?
   ○ 1. To relieve spasms of the diaphragm.
   ○ 2. To relax smooth muscles in the bronchioles.
   ○ 3. To promote efficient pulmonary circulation.
   ○ 4. To stimulate the medullary respiratory center.

7. Diuretic therapy with torsemide (Demadex) is started for a client with heart failure. When calling the client 2 days after the drug therapy is started, the nurse evaluates the torsemide as effective when the client says she has experienced which of the following outcomes?
   ○ 1. She has an improved appetite and is eating better.
   ○ 2. She weighs 6 pounds less than she did 2 days ago.
   ○ 3. She is less thirsty than she was before the drug therapy.
   ○ 4. She has clearer urine since starting the torsemide.

8. Which of the following techniques is correct for the nurse to use when inserting a rectal suppository for an adult client?
   ○ 1. Insert the suppository while the client bears down.
   ○ 2. Place the client in a supine position.
   ○ 3. Position the suppository along the rectal wall.
   ○ 4. Insert the suppository 2 inches into the rectum.

9. A client receiving digoxin (Lanoxin) for congestive heart failure undergoes cardiac catheterization to evaluate his condition further. The procedure reveals a cardiac output of 2.2 L/minute. How would the nurse evaluate this cardiac output?
   ○ 1. High, because of the effects of digoxin.
   ○ 2. Within normal limits, because of the effects of digoxin.
   ○ 3. Within normal limits, but not adequate to support strenuous activity.
   ○ 4. Low, requiring further medical intervention.

10. Clients who are receiving total parenteral nutrition

(TPN) are at risk for development of which of the following complications?
- ○ 1. Hypostatic pneumonia.
- ○ 2. Pulmonary hypertension.
- ○ 3. Orthostatic hypotension.
- ○ 4. Fluid imbalances.

11. The client is receiving propantheline bromide (Pro-Banthine) to treat cholecystitis. The nurse would evaluate the client's response to the medication by observing for which of the following side effects?
- ○ 1. Urinary retention.
- ○ 2. Diarrhea.
- ○ 3. Hypertension.
- ○ 4. Diaphoresis.

12. The nurse is preparing to start an intravenous infusion. Before inserting the needle into a vein, the nurse would apply a tourniquet to the client's arm to accomplish which of the following?
- ○ 1. Distend the veins.
- ○ 2. Stabilize the veins.
- ○ 3. Immobilize the arm.
- ○ 4. Occlude arterial circulation.

13. Prochlorperazine (Compazine) is prescribed postoperatively. The nurse would evaluate the drug's therapeutic effect when the client expresses relief from which of the following?
- ○ 1. Nausea.
- ○ 2. Dizziness.
- ○ 3. Abdominal spasms.
- ○ 4. Abdominal distention.

14. The physician orders Ringer's lactate solution to replace the fluid losses of a client. While the solution is infusing, the nurse should assess for which of the following symptoms that might indicate fluid overload is developing?
- ○ 1. Increased abdominal girth.
- ○ 2. Rapid, thready pulse.
- ○ 3. Moist crackles on auscultation.
- ○ 4. Increased urinary output.

15. The nurse is administering albumin solution to a client. During administration of this solution, the nurse should evaluate the client closely for which of the following complications?
- ○ 1. Excessive diuresis.
- ○ 2. Fluid overload.
- ○ 3. Abnormal weight loss.
- ○ 4. Dehydration.

16. As part of the management of constipation, the client is instructed to take 30 mL of mineral oil orally. Mineral oil facilitates bowel evacuation by
- ○ 1. lubricating and softening the stool.
- ○ 2. increasing the volume of intestinal contents.
- ○ 3. irritating nerve endings in the intestinal mucosa.
- ○ 4. decreasing water retention of stool.

17. A client with a urinary tract infection has been prescribed phenazopyridine (Pyridium) to relieve the dysuria. The nurse tells the client to expect which of the following effects as a result of taking this drug?
- ○ 1. A slight fever.
- ○ 2. Thrush.
- ○ 3. Urinary frequency.
- ○ 4. Reddish-orange urine.

18. The client is to receive an intravenous infusion at 100 mL/hour. The infusion set delivers 15 gtt/mL. What is the flow rate of the infusion?
- ○ 1. 10 gtt/minute.
- ○ 2. 15 gtt/minute.
- ○ 3. 21 gtt/minute.
- ○ 4. 25 gtt/minute.

19. Procaine Penicillin G 600,000 units IM has been ordered. The nurse has available a 1-mL prefilled syringe labeled 600,000 units/mL. How many mL should the nurse administer?
- ○ 1. 0.25 mL.
- ○ 2. 0.50 mL.
- ○ 3. 1.0 mL.
- ○ 4. 2.5 mL.

20. The nurse is administering eye drops to a client with glaucoma. Which of the following is a correct technique for instilling the eye drops? The eye drops are placed
- ○ 1. in the lower conjunctival sac.
- ○ 2. near the opening of the lacrimal ducts.
- ○ 3. on the cornea.
- ○ 4. on the scleral surface.

21. A client has an anaphylactic reaction to penicillin that results in respiratory distress. Which of the following medications would the nurse anticipate administering *first*?
- ○ 1. Dopamine (Intropin).
- ○ 2. Diphenhydramine (Benadryl).
- ○ 3. Cimetidine (Tagamet).
- ○ 4. Epinephrine.

22. A client is using an over-the-counter nasal spray containing pseudoephedrine to treat allergic rhinitis. Which instructions about this medication would be most appropriate for the nurse to provide for the client?
- ○ 1. Prolonged use of nasal spray can lead to nasal infections.
- ○ 2. Pseudoephedrine is an addictive drug and must be used cautiously.
- ○ 3. Overuse of pseudoephedrine can lead to increased nasal congestion.
- ○ 4. A common side effect of pseudoephedrine nasal spray is thrush.

23. The nurse is preparing to give an intramuscular injection. Which one of the following sites has the least amount of blood vessels and major nerves located in the area?

    ○ 1. Deltoid.
    ○ 2. Dorsogluteal.
    ○ 3. Vastus lateralis.
    ○ 4. Triceps.

24. The nurse is planning to teach the client how to properly use a metered dose inhaler to treat asthma. Which of the following instructions should the nurse include in the teaching plan?
    ○ 1. Rinse the mouth after each use of a steroid inhaler.
    ○ 2. Inhale quickly when administering the medication.
    ○ 3. Inhale the medication and then exhale through the nose.
    ○ 4. Cough and deep breath before inhaling the medication.

25. A client is receiving a transfusion of packed red blood cells. Which of the following actions should the nurse implement to safely administer the blood?
    ○ 1. Keep the blood refrigerated on the nursing unit until ready to administer.
    ○ 2. Stay with the client during the first 15 minutes to detect signs of a reaction.
    ○ 3. Do not infuse any blood that has been hanging for more than 6 hours.
    ○ 4. Administer the blood quickly if the client develops a fever to prevent wasting it.

26. A client is receiving a blood transfusion when he begins to complain of difficulty breathing. The nurse notes an elevated blood pressure and a cough. Based on these signs, the nurse suspects which of the following complications?
    ○ 1. Anaphylactic reaction.
    ○ 2. Circulatory overload.
    ○ 3. Sepsis.
    ○ 4. Acute hemolytic reaction.

27. A client has had sucralfate (Carafate) ordered as treatment for peptic ulcer disease. Which of the following statements indicate that the client understands how to take the medication?
    ○ 1. "I should take the Carafate every evening at bedtime."
    ○ 2. "It is important that I take this drug on an empty stomach."
    ○ 3. "I should avoid milk products while taking this drug."
    ○ 4. "I should have my hemoglobin checked monthly while taking Carafate."

28. The nurse administers an intradermal injection to a client. Proper technique has been used if the injection site demonstrates which of the following?
    ○ 1. Minimal leaking.
    ○ 2. No swelling.
    ○ 3. Tissue pallor.
    ○ 4. Evidence of a bleb.

29. The client is prescribed ketorolac (Toradol) 15 mg IM for pain. The nurse has a 1-mL preloaded syringe of Toradol labeled 30 mg/mL. How much of the medication would the nurse administer?
    ○ 1. 0.05 mL.
    ○ 2. 0.5 mL.
    ○ 3. 1.5 mL.
    ○ 4. 2.0 mL.

30. The sudden onset of which of the following signs or symptoms indicates a potentially serious complication for the client receiving an intravenous infusion?
    ○ 1. Noisy respirations.
    ○ 2. Pupillary constriction.
    ○ 3. Halitosis.
    ○ 4. Moist skin.

31. The nurse is planning to initiate a blood transfusion. Which of the following solutions should the nurse select to prime the tubing when preparing to administer the blood?
    ○ 1. Ringer's lactate solution.
    ○ 2. 0.9% normal saline.
    ○ 3. 5% dextrose in 0.45% normal saline.
    ○ 4. 5% dextrose in water.

32. Which of the following actions by the nurse will most likely ensure that the correct client receives a medication?
    ○ 1. Have the client state his or her name.
    ○ 2. Call the client by name.
    ○ 3. Learn to recognize the client.
    ○ 4. Check the client's identification armband.

33. When instructing clients with allergic rhinitis about the use of nasal decongestants, it is important to emphasize that
    ○ 1. the condition will not benefit from environmental changes.
    ○ 2. continuous use for more than 3 days can result in worsening of symptoms.
    ○ 3. the condition requires treatment only during the Spring.
    ○ 4. the condition is self-limited and should not return.

34. The nurse is teaching a client with osteoporosis about taking alendronate (Fosamax). The nurse emphasizes that the client is to take the medication
    ○ 1. at bedtime.
    ○ 2. with food.
    ○ 3. with a full glass of water and remain upright for 30 minutes.
    ○ 4. with a full glass of juice and then rest for 30 minutes.

35. The nurse is inserting an intravenous needle to administer fluids to a client who is going to surgery. The nurse selects the median cubital vein. Using Figure 1, the nurse should insert the needle at
    ○ 1. Point 1.

○ 2. Point 2.
○ 3. Point 3.
○ 4. Point 4.

36. An elderly male client has been taking doxazosin (Cardura) 2 mg daily for 4 weeks for treatment of benign prostatic hypertrophy (BPH). The client complains of feeling dizzy. The nurse should *first*
    ○ 1. take his blood pressure lying, standing, and sitting.
    ○ 2. test his urine for ketones.
    ○ 3. review his other medications.
    ○ 4. report the symptoms to the physician.

37. A client on the burn unit is receiving sulfonamide cream (Silvadene) as topical treatment for her burns. When reviewing the daily laboratory tests, the nurse notices that the client's white blood cell count (WBC) has decreased. The nurse recognizes that
    ○ 1. it is normal to have this response from immunosuppression.
    ○ 2. this is normal; an increased WBC would be a concern.
    ○ 3. this is abnormal; the physician needs to be alerted.
    ○ 4. the WBC should be observed over several days to look for a trend.

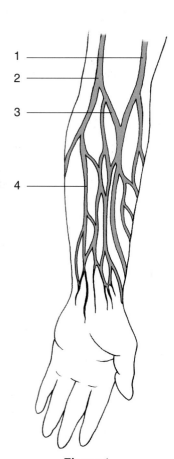

Figure 1.

38. A client with migraine headaches and a history of angina asks the nurse why the physician does not prescribe one of the newer medications for migraine, such as the sumitriptan drugs Imitrex and Zomig. The nurse responds that
    ○ 1. these drugs are very expensive.
    ○ 2. sumitriptan is contraindicated in clients with angina.
    ○ 3. sumitriptan is used only for prophylactic treatment of migraines.
    ○ 4. sumitriptan is used only for migraines with aura.

39. Which medication could predispose a woman to candidiasis?
    ○ 1. Insulin.
    ○ 2. Lisinopril (Zestril).
    ○ 3. Oral contraceptive pills.
    ○ 4. Phenytoin (Dilantin).

40. The nurse is preparing to administer an intramuscular injection to a client and chooses the vastus lateralis muscle for the injection site. Into which part of the thigh would the nurse choose to correctly administer the injection?
    ○ 1. Middle third of the thigh.
    ○ 2. Lower third of the thigh.
    ○ 3. Upper third of the thigh.
    ○ 4. Wherever the thigh is the largest.

41. Which one of the following factors would be most important for the nurse to consider when determining the angle at which to insert the needle for a subcutaneous injection?
    ○ 1. Size of the syringe.
    ○ 2. Tissue turgor.
    ○ 3. Length of the needle.
    ○ 4. Amount of subcutaneous tissue.

42. Trimethoprim (Proloprim) has been ordered for a client with a urinary tract infection. Which of the following instructions should the nurse give the client about taking the medication?
    ○ 1. Take the medication until symptoms subside.
    ○ 2. Return to the office in 3 days so that a urine culture can be obtained.
    ○ 3. Take the medication with meals.
    ○ 4. Report any unusual bleeding or bruising.

43. A 36-year-old woman is admitted to the oncology unit with an infection. It is suspected that the infection may be related to her vascular access device (VAD). The nurse would expect blood cultures to be drawn from which of the following sites?
    ○ 1. A peripheral site and all lumens of the VAD.
    ○ 2. A peripheral site only.
    ○ 3. All lumens of the VAD.
    ○ 4. The proximal lumen of the VAD only.

44. The nurse has been able to draw the daily blood specimen from a client's Hickman catheter only

after requesting that the client raise his arms and cough. The client asks the nurse why he has to do this when his roommate has the same type of catheter and sleeps through the procedure. Which of the following statements represents the nurse's best response?

○ 1. "A fibrin sheath has grown over the tip of the catheter."

○ 2. "The catheter may be lodged against a blood vessel wall."

○ 3. "Your catheter probably is pinched between the clavicle and a rib."

○ 4. "The catheter tends to collapse every time we exert pressure."

45. An emergency department nurse has verbally assessed by telephone triage a client complaining of intense pain and swelling at her Port-A-Cath site. She tells the nurse that she is into her third day of a 5-day regimen of continuous fluorouracil (5-FU) for colon cancer. The nurse immediately suspects that

○ 1. there is infection at the port site.

○ 2. the catheter has migrated and is pinched between the clavicle bone and a rib bone.

○ 3. the port access needle has become dislodged.

○ 4. the port septum has eroded.

46. A nurse requests a 10- or 20-mL syringe to irrigate a Groshong catheter. What is most likely to occur if a 5-mL syringe is used to irrigate the Groshong catheter?

○ 1. Catheter migration.

○ 2. Constriction of the catheter.

○ 3. Leakage around the catheter site.

○ 4. Rupture of the catheter.

47. A client with a history of congestive heart failure is prescribed ketorolac (Toradol) for arthritis. The nurse should include which of the following instructions when teaching the client about the drug?

○ 1. Weigh yourself every morning.

○ 2. Take the medication on an empty stomach.

○ 3. Have your blood pressure checked weekly.

○ 4. Increase your fluid intake to 2000 mL/day.

48. A client with osteoarthritis is learning about his drug therapy. The nurse should instruct the client that which of the following drugs is considered first-line therapy for osteoarthritis?

○ 1. Corticosteroids.

○ 2. Nonsteroidal anti-inflammatory drugs.

○ 3. Acetaminophen.

○ 4. Narcotic analgesics.

49. A client is receiving chrysotherapy (Myochrysine) as treatment for her rheumatoid arthritis. Which of the following is a side effect of the drug that the client should report?

○ 1. Constipation.

○ 2. Jaundice.

○ 3. Urinary retention.

○ 4. Skin rash.

50. The nurse notes that a placebo has been ordered for use when a client requests pain medication. Which of the following statements is most accurate about the use of placebos in the client's plan of care?

○ 1. It is appropriate to substitute placebos when the client requests frequent doses of pain medication.

○ 2. Placebos should be used when it is suspected that the client is addicted to the pain medication.

○ 3. The use of placebos violates the client's right to ethical care.

○ 4. Placebos may be used whenever the nurse believes the client is not really experiencing pain.

51. A client has been diagnosed with a chlamydial infection. Which of the following antibiotics does the nurse anticipate will most likely be prescribed?

○ 1. Pobenecid (Benemid).

○ 2. Ampicillin (Principen).

○ 3. Doxycycline (Vibramycin).

○ 4. Acyclovir (Zovirax).

52. A client is receiving intravenous heparin for treatment of deep vein thrombosis. Which of the following precautions should the nurse incorporate into the client's plan of care as a result of receiving heparin intravenously?

○ 1. Establish a separate intravenous infusion line for administration of other prescribed drugs.

○ 2. Check the client's activated partial thromboplastin time (aPTT) values daily to monitor for therapeutic anticoagulation.

○ 3. Have vitamin K injection available as an antidote to potential heparin overdose.

○ 4. Protect the heparin infusion from light to prevent discoloration of the drug.

53. The nurse wants to prepare a teaching plan for a client who is taking metoclopramide (Reglan). Which of the following is considered a side effect of the drug?

○ 1. Constipation.

○ 2. Urinary retention.

○ 3. Hypotension.

○ 4. Extrapyramidal reactions.

54. A client has been diagnosed with chronic gastritis caused by *Helicobacter pylori*. The nurse anticipates that which of the following drug categories will be most effective in treating the gastritis?

○ 1. Antacids.

○ 2. Antiemetics.

○ 3. Antibiotic combinations.

○ 4. Histamine$_2$-receptor antagonists.

55. A client who has been diagnosed with cirrhosis asks the nurse if there are any specific medications that he should avoid. Which one of the following medications should the nurse specifically tell the client not to take?
○ 1. Acetaminophen (Tylenol).
○ 2. Cimetidine (Tagamet).
○ 3. Neomycin sulfate.
○ 4. Spironolactone (Aldactone).

56. The nurse instructs a client when to take his glipizide (Glucotrol) in order to maximize the effectiveness of the drug. Which of the following instructions by the nurse is accurate?
○ 1. Glipizide should be taken four times a day, at evenly spaced intervals.
○ 2. Glipizide should be taken immediately after meals.
○ 3. Glipizide should be taken 30 minutes before breakfast.
○ 4. Glipizide should be taken as indicated by blood glucose values.

57. A client is taking verapamil hydrochloride (Calan) as an antihypertensive. Which of the following should the nurse tell the client regarding the side effects of verapamil?
○ 1. "A low-residue diet will help prevent the occurrence of diarrhea."
○ 2. "You should obtain a complete blood count routinely to monitor for potential bone marrow depression."
○ 3. "Take your pulse and report any irregular heartbeats."
○ 4. "Restrict your fluid intake to decrease the chance of developing fluid retention."

Growth and Development

58. A home health nurse is giving instructions to a 66-year-old client with a new colostomy. The client states, "I am so tired today; I just cannot think." The nurse's best action for the teaching session is to
○ 1. reschedule the appointment at a time when the client is rested.
○ 2. give the client a written instruction sheet instead of verbal teaching.
○ 3. ask the client to concentrate because the instructions are important.
○ 4. give the teaching session to the spouse instead of the client.

59. An elderly client reports to the nurse that he occasionally takes cimetidine (Tagamet) that he purchases over the counter. The nurse emphasizes that the client should report the occurrence of any
○ 1. nausea.

○ 2. heartburn.
○ 3. ataxia.
○ 4. diarrhea.

60. A physician orders gentamycin (Garamycin) for an elderly client with peritonitis. The client has preexisting impaired vision and hearing. The nurse should
○ 1. give the drug as ordered.
○ 2. question whether the drug is appropriate for treatment of peritonitis.
○ 3. question the order because gentamycin could cause further hearing impairment.
○ 4. question the order because gentamycin could cause further visual impairment.

61. Which of the following is a serious side effect of ibuprofen (Advil, Motrin) in the elderly?
○ 1. Rebound headaches.
○ 2. Neuropathy.
○ 3. Hypoglycemia.
○ 4. Impairment of renal function.

62. Which of the following is a strategy that can be taught to older adults to improve medication compliance?
○ 1. Encourage the use of over-the-counter medications.
○ 2. Avoid confusing dosing schedules.
○ 3. Use a pillbox and system for taking medications.
○ 4. Encourage drug holidays.

63. An elderly client reports that she has asthma. She asks the nurse about the pneumonia vaccine (Pneumovax). The nurse's best response is
○ 1. "You do not need the vaccine."
○ 2. "You will need the vaccine only if you have frequent asthma attacks."
○ 3. "You should receive the vaccine."
○ 4. "You should not have the vaccine because it is contraindicated in asthma."

64. Which of the following clients would the nurse most likely encourage to receive the pneumococcal and influenza vaccination?
○ 1. A 30-year-old pregnant woman.
○ 2. A 75-year-old client with diabetes.
○ 3. A 5-year-old entering school.
○ 4. A 60-year-old man with benign prostatic hypertrophy.

65. A 22-year-old client is admitted to room 13. He states that he does not want to remain in the room because the number will bring him bad luck. Which of the following statements offers the best guide for the nurse in this situation?
○ 1. Move the client; his fears, even when unfounded, can impede recovery.
○ 2. Move the client; superstitions have a good chance of coming true for those who believe them.
○ 3. Do not move the client; having the client use the room will help him overcome an unwarranted fear.

4. Do not move the client; the client may become unmanageable and demanding when he knows he can have his way.

66. A client who was involved in a motor vehicle accident is admitted to the hospital. His wife arrives on the unit 6 hours after her husband's accident, explaining that she has been out of town. She is distraught because she was not with her husband when he needed her. Which of the following is the most appropriate nursing intervention at this time?
    1. Allow her to verbalize her feelings and concerns.
    2. Describe her husband's medical treatment since admission.
    3. Explain to her that her husband's condition is stable.
    4. Reassure her that the important fact is that she is here now.

67. Which of the following clients is most likely to exhibit deficient fluid volume?
    1. A 21-year-old man with profuse diaphoresis after a game of football.
    2. A 75-year-old woman who has been placed on NPO 8 hours before surgery.
    3. An 8-month-old infant with persistent diarrhea for 24 hours.
    4. A 60-year-old man with pneumonia and a temperature of 101°F (38.3°C).

68. When admitting an elderly client for nausea and vomiting that has lasted for 3 days, the nurse assesses for which of the following clinical findings?
    1. Bradycardia.
    2. Polyuria.
    3. Hypertension.
    4. Poor skin turgor.

69. The nurse is evaluating the lifestyle modifications a client has made to prevent gastroesophageal reflux. Which of the following client statements would indicate to the nurse that the client understands how to prevent reflux?
    1. "I lie down and rest for 45 minutes after each meal."
    2. "I sleep on my left side at night to help my stomach empty more quickly."
    3. "I try to eat smaller amounts of food more often throughout the day."
    4. "I have increased my fluid intake at meals to help improve my digestion."

70. Two days after an ileostomy, the client refuses care and requests to be left alone. What should be the nurse's first action?
    1. Encourage the client to verbalize his feelings.
    2. Allow the client the privacy he requests.
    3. Invite a member of the ostomy association for a visit.

4. Tell the client that he must begin to deal with the situation.

71. Which of the following statements *best* explains why the nurse should take the client's cultural background into consideration when developing a plan of care?
    1. Ignoring cultural differences can cause an increase in the cost of the client's care.
    2. Acknowledging cultural differences can help the nurse explain to the client how their health beliefs differ from each other.
    3. Understanding the client's cultural background will prevent the nurse from making embarrassing mistakes when providing care.
    4. Acknowledging the client's cultural background demonstrates the nurse's appreciation of the fact that cultural values are very difficult to change.

72. Which of the following statements *best* explains why the nurse should acknowledge any differences between his or her culture and the client's culture?
    1. The nurse can determine which cultural groups will be noncompliant with their health care.
    2. The nurse can anticipate the client's response to nursing care.
    3. The nurse may hold values that could influence the care of the client.
    4. The nurse can alter his or her beliefs to match the client's.

73. Which one of the following interventions would be *most* appropriate for preventing urinary infections in an elderly female client?
    1. Have the client urinate at least every 6 hours.
    2. Insert an indwelling urethral catheter.
    3. Administer prophylactic antibiotics.
    4. Instruct the client to avoid tight-fitting pants.

74. A 35-year-old woman has been diagnosed with rheumatoid arthritis. During the nursing history and assessment, the nurse notes that the client has bilateral inflamed finger joints with pain, warmth, and limited motion. Although she complains of pain, the client says she is most concerned about her ability to care for her children and home because of her fatigue. Based on these data, which would be the *priority* nursing diagnosis for this client?
    1. Pain related to joint inflammation.
    2. Disturbed Body Image related to joint immobility.
    3. Impaired Home Maintenance related to pain and fatigue.
    4. Activity Intolerance related to fatigue.

75. The nurse assesses an elderly client for signs of dehydration. Which of the following findings would be consistent with a diagnosis of dehydration?
    1. Postural hypotension.

○ 2. Moist crackles.

○ 3. Shortness of breath.

○ 4. Bounding pulse.

76. Which of the following clients is *most* susceptible to infection?

○ 1. A 6-year-old girl with a fractured femur.

○ 2. A 42-year-old man with a recent, uncomplicated appendectomy.

○ 3. An 86-year-old man with burns from using a heating pad.

○ 4. An 18-year-old man with diabetes mellitus.

Management of Care

77. The nurse is assigning care to the unlicensed nursing personnel (UNP) for a client with a nasogastric tube with intermittent suction after gastric surgery. Which of the following interventions cannot be delegated to the UNP?

○ 1. Recording output.

○ 2. Securing the nasal tape.

○ 3. Documenting the color of the drainage.

○ 4. Repositioning the tube.

78. A 42-year-old client was admitted from a homeless shelter with a diagnosis of tuberculosis and alcoholism. It is essential that which of the following health care team members attend the care conference to discuss discharge planning and community resources?

○ 1. Dietitian.

○ 2. Pastoral care.

○ 3. Social worker.

○ 4. Quality management.

79. The charge nurse is making client care assignments for the evening shift. One of the licensed practical/vocational nurses (LP/VNs) is a new graduate in orientation. Which of the following clients would be an appropriate care assignment for this nurse?

○ 1. A 41-year-old client with unstable angina.

○ 2. A 72-year-old client with diverticulitis.

○ 3. A 32-year-old client hospitalized for chemotherapy treatment.

○ 4. A 5-year-old client with Kawasaki's disease.

80. The nursing supervisor of a small community hospital has been called to the emergency department to assist with a 9-month old infant with injuries consistent with suspected child abuse. The nursing supervisor confers with the emergency department physician and must report the incident to

○ 1. A social worker.

○ 2. The medical director of the emergency department.

○ 3. A Children's Protective Services (CPS) representative.

○ 4. A public health nurse.

81. A nurse fails to give the evening dose of an intravenous antibiotic that is to be administered every 12 hours. The nurse's first action is to

○ 1. Report the incident to the physician.

○ 2. Assess the client for increasing signs of infection.

○ 3. Administer the dosage 6 hours late.

○ 4. Call the pharmacist for instructions.

82. An order has just been received for a 72-year-old client with gastrointestinal hemorrhage to have two blood transfusions. The registered nurse caring for the client is a pediatric nurse temporarily assigned to the unit who has never administered blood before. The *best* action of the charge nurse is to

○ 1. ask the nurse to read the policy book before he or she administers the blood.

○ 2. give a thorough explanation of the procedure for blood administration to the nurse.

○ 3. ask the nurse whether he or she feels confident to administer the blood safely.

○ 4. reassign the client to another nurse who is experienced in blood administration.

83. A client with terminal cancer tells the nurse that she is not afraid to die and she is thinking about how to plan her funeral. The most appropriate referral the nurse could suggest would be to the

○ 1. home health care service.

○ 2. social worker.

○ 3. psychologist.

○ 4. pastoral care department.

84. A client with a modified radical mastectomy is being discharged. The client has been very reluctant to discuss the surgery or her situation. The nurse making assignments should delegate the client's care to the

○ 1. UNP, because the client is stable and being discharged.

○ 2. same nurse who has cared for her the past 3 days, for continuity of care.

○ 3. a nurse in orientation who needs experience in discharge instructions.

○ 4. the nurse with the most bed baths, because this client will not need a bath.

85. While giving report to the oncoming night shift, the charge nurse smells alcohol on the breath of one of the nurses. The charge nurse should

○ 1. report this to the nursing supervisor immediately.

○ 2. report this to the head nurse when she arrives in the morning.

○ 3. ask the nurse if she has been drinking.

○ 4. assess the nurse's behavior for signs of intoxication.

86. The Uniform Anatomical Gift Act provides that, before death, a client may give informed consent to

donate body organs. The nurse understands that, under this Act,
- ○ 1. the family must give the final consent before the procedure is performed.
- ○ 2. only those potential donors who have signed a donor card can donate.
- ○ 3. only those potential donors who are younger than 50 years of age can donate.
- ○ 4. persons with clinical evidence of human immunodeficiency virus infection cannot be considered donors.

87. A nurse in a long-term care facility observes bruises in the shape of finger marks around the elbows of an elderly, immobile resident. The course of action the nurse must immediately pursue is
- ○ 1. to report this finding to the nurse who is taking care of the client.
- ○ 2. to report this finding to the physician.
- ○ 3. to document the bruising and continue to assess the area over the next 72 hours.
- ○ 4. to report this finding to the Adult Protective Services (APS).

88. The nurse manager has noticed a sharp increase in the medication errors with intravenous antibiotics over the past 2 months. A good strategy to respond to this situation is to discuss the situation with each nurse involved and
- ○ 1. document it on their evaluation.
- ○ 2. ask them to attend inservice training for administration of intravenous medications.
- ○ 3. report them to the supervisor.
- ○ 4. report the incidents to the hospital attorney.

89. The nurse manager has noticed a sharp increase in the medication errors with intravenous antibiotics over the last 2 months. The group that could offer resources for tracking medication errors and improving care outcomes is the
- ○ 1. Ethics Committee.
- ○ 2. Pharmacy and Products Office.
- ○ 3. Quality Improvement and Risk Management Department.
- ○ 4. Infection Control Committee.

90. The nurse is inserting a nasogastric tube in an adult client. The nurse is estimating the length of tubing to insert. Using the diagram in Figure 2, the correct measurement for inserting the tube in this client is from
- ○ 1. Point 1 to point 2.
- ○ 2. Point 1 to point 3.
- ○ 3. Point 1 to point 4.
- ○ 4. Point 1 to point 5.

91. Because of an outbreak of influenza among nursing staff, the hospital is very short staffed. The nurse manager prioritizes client needs on the surgical unit by which of the following strategies?

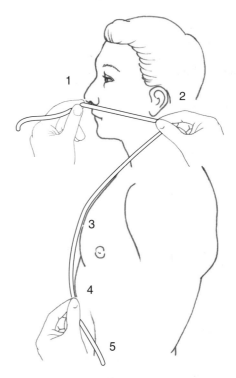

Figure 2.

- ○ 1. Rescheduling surgeries.
- ○ 2. Ensuring that clients receive medications, but omitting full bathing when possible.
- ○ 3. Allowing all medications to be given 2 hours late.
- ○ 4. Allowing UNP to assist in administering analgesics.

92. When reporting to the surgeon that a chest tube is malfunctioning, the nurse is ordered to reposition the tube and obtain a chest radiograph. The nurse should
- ○ 1. inform the surgeon this is not within safe scope of practice.
- ○ 2. report the surgeon to the Ethics Committee.
- ○ 3. report the surgeon to the nursing supervisor.
- ○ 4. follow the order as requested by the surgeon.

93. An Iranian mother and father admitted their 13-month-old son to the pediatric unit for treatment of a Wilms' tumor. When the female pediatric oncologist, who is not Muslim, introduced herself, they became uncooperative and refused treatment. The nurse should be aware that this change of behavior is probably related to
- ○ 1. the gender of the physician.
- ○ 2. fear of being accused of child abuse and neglect by an authority figure.
- ○ 3. religious barriers that prevent the family from accepting care from someone who is not of their religion.

○ 4. aggressiveness of Middle Easterners.

94. The guidelines for evaluating registered nurse professional conduct are contained in the
    ○ 1. Standards of Care.
    ○ 2. Patient's Bill of Rights.
    ○ 3. Code of Ethics.
    ○ 4. Professional certification.

95. The nurse should have the unlicensed assistant obtain the body temperature at what site for the client with a productive cough and difficulty breathing?
    ○ 1. Mouth.
    ○ 2. Ear.
    ○ 3. Rectum.
    ○ 4. Axilla.

96. Before assisting a client to ambulate after surgery, the nurse helps the client to dangle her feet over the side of the bed. Which of the following measures should the nurse carry out before helping the client to dangle her feet?
    ○ 1. Administer a prescribed analgesic.
    ○ 2. Encourage the client to take a short nap.
    ○ 3. Have the client do leg exercises for a few minutes.
    ○ 4. Place the client in a high Fowler's position.

97. As the nurse administers a tapwater enema, the client begins to complain of abdominal cramping. Which of the following actions should the nurse implement *first*?
    ○ 1. Stop infusing the enema, and allow the client to evacuate the fluid.
    ○ 2. Temporarily stop the infusion until the cramping subsides.
    ○ 3. Tell the client to hold his breath, and continue infusing the enema.
    ○ 4. Turn the client onto his back, and continue infusing the enema.

98. A client is to have a nasogastric tube inserted. Which of the following actions by the nurse demonstrates appropriate technique for insertion of the tube?
    ○ 1. Lubricate the tube with petroleum-based lubricant.
    ○ 2. Ask the client to not breathe while the tube is inserted into the nares.
    ○ 3. Place the client in a supine position.
    ○ 4. Have the client flex the head while the tube is advanced past the nasopharynx.

99. Intravenous replacement therapy for a client with a nasogastric tube attached to low suction will be needed primarily to meet which of the following objectives?
    ○ 1. Maintain bladder function.
    ○ 2. Facilitate osmotic diuresis.
    ○ 3. Equalize intake and output.
    ○ 4. Maintain fluid and electrolyte balance.

100. The nurse has asked the unlicensed assistant to help with admitting an elderly client who has been diagnosed with bacterial pneumonia. Which of the following activities is appropriate for the nurse to ask the assistant to perform?
    ○ 1. Assess the client's lung sounds.
    ○ 2. Collect nursing history and assessment data.
    ○ 3. Obtain the client's height and weight.
    ○ 4. Evaluate the client's respiratory status.

101. The nurse has responsibility for the following clients. Based on the information provided, which of these clients would be a priority for the nurse to evaluate when assuming responsibility for their care at the beginning of the evening shift?
    ○ 1. The client who had a total laryngectomy the previous day.
    ○ 2. The client with diabetes who had a fasting blood sugar of 150 mg/dL.
    ○ 3. An elderly client who has Alzheimer's disease and periods of confusion.
    ○ 4. A client with a pneumothorax who had a chest tube inserted earlier in the day.

102. The nurse instructs the unlicensed assistant how to care for a client with chest tubes that are connected to water-seal drainage. Which of the following instructions would be appropriate for the nurse to give the unlicensed assistant?
    ○ 1. Milk the chest tubes every 4 hours.
    ○ 2. Raise the collection apparatus to the height of the bed to measure the fluid level.
    ○ 3. Attach the chest tubes to bed linen to avoid tension on the tubing.
    ○ 4. Mark the time and amount of drainage on the collection container.

103. A client is being prepared for a bronchoscopy. Which of the following preoperative activities would be appropriate for the nurse to delegate to the unlicensed assistant?
    ○ 1. Obtaining the signed consent form.
    ○ 2. Placing the client on NPO (nothing by mouth) status.
    ○ 3. Instructing the client about the procedure.
    ○ 4. Evaluating the client's level of anxiety.

104. A client has a suspected slow gastrointestinal (GI) bleed. Because of this, the nurse specifically instructs the unlicensed assistant to look for and report which of the following symptoms?
    ○ 1. Hypotension.
    ○ 2. Bright red blood in the stools.
    ○ 3. Tarry stools.
    ○ 4. Jaundice.

105. The nurse assigns an unlicensed assistant to provide care for a client with peptic ulcer disease. Concerned about possible ulcer perforation, the nurse instructs the assistant to report which of the following signs immediately?

○ 1. An elevated pulse.
○ 2. Confusion.
○ 3. Severe abdominal pain.
○ 4. Constipation.

106. Of the following interventions, which one should the nurse instruct the unlicensed assistant to perform when providing care for a client with a nasogastric tube?
○ 1. Use a soft toothbrush to clean the teeth and tongue.
○ 2. Provide ice chips to relieve mouth dryness.
○ 3. Rinse the client's mouth every 2 to 4 hours with mouthwash.
○ 4. Provide lemon-glycerin swabs for the client to use to freshen the mouth.

107. The nurse assigns an unlicensed assistant to care for a client who has a newly applied long-leg plaster cast. What should the nurse tell the assistant about proper care of the cast while it is drying?
○ 1. "Keep the cast covered by a sheet to protect it while drying."
○ 2. "Turn the client every 2 hours to promote even drying of the cast."
○ 3. "Use a blow dryer on the cast for 15 minutes every 2 hours until the cast is dry."
○ 4. "Carefully use your fingers to lift the cast and reposition the legs."

108. The nurse is instructing an unlicensed assistant how to correctly position a client who has had a recent total hip replacement. In which position should the nurse tell the assistant to place the operated leg when the client is lying on the nonoperative side?
○ 1. Abduction and flexion.
○ 2. Abduction and extension.
○ 3. Adduction and flexion.
○ 4. Adduction and extension.

109. The nurse is instructing the unlicensed assistant in how to prevent plantar flexion (foot drop) in an immobilized client. Which of the following techniques should the nurse tell the assistant to incorporate into the plan of care?
○ 1. Place a bed cradle at the foot of the bed.
○ 2. Massage lotion onto the feet daily.
○ 3. Encourage active range of motion to unaffected extremities.
○ 4. Place a trochanter roll along the side of the ankle.

110. The nurse assigns an unlicensed assistant to the care of a client who has just returned from surgery for repair of a fractured wrist and application of an arm cast. The nurse should stress to the assistant the importance of reporting which of the following assessments immediately?
○ 1. The client reports he can't move his fingers.

○ 2. Results of hourly neurovascular assessments.
○ 3. Intake and output record for the shift.
○ 4. The client complains of feeling heat from the plaster cast.

111. Which of the following aspects of client care would be most appropriate for the nurse to delegate to an unlicensed assistant?
○ 1. Catheterize a 75-year-old male client who has an enlarged prostate.
○ 2. Change the intravenous fluid bottle for a client whose intravenous fluid level is running low.
○ 3. Obtain a urine specimen for a culture and sensitivity analysis from a client who has a Foley catheter inserted.
○ 4. Administer an antacid to a client after further assessing his complaint of heartburn.

112. The nurse receives report on the assigned clients at the beginning of the second shift. Which of the following clients should the nurse plan to assess first after receiving report?
○ 1. An elderly client with pneumonia who is exhibiting periods of confusion.
○ 2. A client who is scheduled for an abdominal perineal resection in the morning and is visiting with his family.
○ 3. A client receiving total parenteral nutrition via a central line with 400 mL remaining in the intravenous fluid bottle.
○ 4. A young male client with chest tubes placed for treatment of a pneumothorax who is resting comfortably.

113. The nurse is instructing the unlicensed assistant on how to transfer a male client with left-sided weakness from the bed to a wheelchair. Which statement by the assistant tells the nurse that the assistant has understood the instructions?
○ 1. "The wheelchair should be placed at the head of the bed."
○ 2. "I will place the wheelchair behind the client."
○ 3. "The wheelchair should be placed on the right side of the bed."
○ 4. "As long as I assist the client, it does not matter where the wheelchair goes."

114. The nurse is instructing the unlicensed assistant in how to care for a client who is receiving chemotherapy. What self-care precautions should the nurse tell the assistant to take when caring for the client?
○ 1. The assistant must have the nurse handle the disposal of any client excreta.
○ 2. Universal body precautions are sufficient for protecting the assistant.
○ 3. Gowns, mask, and gloves are required for any contact with the client.
○ 4. Wear surgical gloves when handling client's excreta.

115. Which of the following client care activities would be most appropriate for the nurse to delegate to the unlicensed assistant?
- ○ 1. Taking a client's apical pulse before the nurse administers digoxin (Lanoxin).
- ○ 2. Performing a dressing change for a client whose incision is infected and requires irrigation.
- ○ 3. Teaching a client how to change an ileostomy pouch.
- ○ 4. Obtaining a client's routine glucose reading using a glucometer.

116. Which of the following clients would be most appropriate for the nurse to assign to the unlicensed assistant for morning care?
- ○ 1. An elderly client with chronic obstructive pulmonary disease (COPD) who is receiving oxygen therapy for mild dyspnea.
- ○ 2. A middle-aged client who had a laryngectomy 2 days earlier.
- ○ 3. A young client receiving chemotherapy for Hodgkin's disease.
- ○ 4. An elderly client experiencing chest pain due to suspected pulmonary embolus.

Correct Answers and Rationale

The letters in parentheses following the rationale identify the step of the nursing process (A, D, P, I, E) and client needs (1, 2, 3, 4, 5, 6, 7, 8, 9, 10). See the inside front cover for the key.

Pharmacologic and Parenteral Therapies

1. 3. Atropine sulfate is an anticholinergic drug that decreases mucous secretions in the respiratory tract and dries the mucous membranes of the mouth, nose, pharynx, and bronchi. Atropine does not cause drowsiness or relaxation. Moderate to large doses cause tachycardia and palpitations. Large doses cause excitement and manic behavior. Atropine does not reduce the risk of postoperative infection. (I, 8)

2. 1. 0.125 mg / x tablets = 0.25 mg / 1 tablet; x = 0.5 tablets. (I, 8)

3. 2. Protamine sulfate is a heparin antagonist. It is administered intravenously very slowly (over at least 10 minutes). Warfarin sodium (Coumadin) and acetylsalicylic acid (ASA) have anticoagulant properties and would be contraindicated. Atropine sulfate is an anticholinergic drug and would not be effective in treating a heparin overdose. (P, 8)

4. 4. First, convert grams to milligrams: 0.5 g = 500 mg. Then, 1000 mg / x mL = 500 mg / 5 mL; x = 10.0 mL. (I, 8)

5. 1. The intravenous flow rate is determined by the rate of infusion and the number of drops per milliliter of the fluid being administered: gtt/mL × mL/minute = gtt/minute (the intravenous flow rate). 10 gtt/mL × 500 mL/360 minutes = 13.8 gtt/minute. Therefore, the flow rate should be 14 gtt/minute. (I, 8)

6. 2. Aminophylline, a bronchodilator that relaxes smooth muscles in the bronchioles, is used in treatment of emphysema to improve ventilation by dilating the bronchioles. Aminophylline does not have an effect on the diaphragm or the medullary respiratory center and does not promote pulmonary circulation. (I, 8)

7. 2. The primary reason to give a diuretic to a client with heart failure is to promote sodium and water excretion through the kidneys. As a result, the excessive body water that tends to accumulate in a client with heart failure is eliminated, which causes the client to lose weight. Monitoring the client's weight daily helps evaluate the effectiveness of diuretic therapy. The client should be advised to weigh herself daily. An increased appetite or decreased thirst does not establish the effectiveness of the diuretic therapy, nor does having clearer urine after starting the torsemide. (E, 8)

8. 3. The client should be placed in a side-lying position and encouraged to take a deep breath during the insertion of the suppository. Placing the suppository along the rectal wall promotes absorption of the medication and helps avoid placing it into a stool mass. The nurse should insert the suppository 3 to 4 inches into the rectum of an adult client. (I, 9)

9. 4. Normal cardiac output is 4 to 8 L/minute. The value does vary with body size, but 2.2 L/minute is very low and can be life-threatening. For the client with a cardiac output of 2.2 L/minute, the nurse would anticipate that the physician would adjust the medication regimen. The client may experience symptoms of dyspnea and fatigue, requiring nursing intervention. (E, 9)

10. 4. Clients receiving TPN are at risk for a number of complications, including fluid imbalances such as fluid overload and hyperosmolar diuresis. Other common complications include hyperglycemia, sepsis, pneumothorax, and air embolism. Hypostatic pneumonia and pulmonary or orthostatic hypertension are not complications of TPN. (A, 8)

11. 1. Propantheline bromide is an anticholinergic drug. Common side effects include urinary retention and constipation; flushed, dry skin; and dry mouth, nose, and throat. Orthostatic hypotension may also occur. Diarrhea and diaphoresis are side effects of cholinergic drugs. (E, 8)

12. 1. Applying a tourniquet obstructs venous blood flow and, as a result, distends the veins. A tourniquet does not stabilize veins or immobilize the arm, nor is it applied to occlude arterial circulation. (I, 8)

13. 1. Prochlorperazine is administered postoperatively to control nausea and vomiting. Prochlorperazine is also used in psychotherapy because of its effects on mood and behavior. Prochlorperazine is not used to treat dizziness, abdominal spasms, or abdominal distention. (E, 8)

14. 3. Fluid overload or a positive fluid balance can result in increased blood pressure, pulse, and respirations. With fluid volume overload, there can be moist crackles, which may be heard on auscultation. The pulse rate is bounding because of the extra fluid. Increased abdominal girth is usually the result of ascites, which does not develop as a result of intravascular fluid excess from administration of too much intravenous

fluid. An increased urinary output is not an indicator of fluid volume excess. It would be expected that the administration of intravenous fluids in a client with a negative fluid balance would eventually increase the urinary output. (A, 8)

15. 2. The client is at risk for development of fluid overload. Albumin is a hyperosmolar solution and acts to move fluid from the extravascular space into the intravascular space. The solution should be given slowly enough to prevent rapid plasma volume expansion. The client should be monitored closely for signs of fluid overload, such as shortness of breath and moist crackles on auscultation. Administration of albumin would not cause excessive diuresis, abnormal weight loss, or dehydration. (E, 10)

16. 1. Mineral oil is used to soften impacted stool in the management of constipation. It coats the surface of stool and intestine with a lubricant film to allow passage of stool through the intestine. Mineral oil also improves water retention of stool, thereby softening stool and facilitating bowel evacuation. Mineral oil does not work by irritating nerve endings in the intestinal mucosa. Saline cathartics, such as magnesium sulfate and citrate, increase the volume of intestinal content, thus stimulating evacuation. (I, 9)

17. 4. Phenazopyridine is used as a urinary tract analgesic and can cause the urine to turn reddish-orange. A fever is not expected with phenazopyridine administration. If one develops, the client should report it, because it could be an indication of drug toxicity. Thrush occurs with antibiotic therapy. Phenazopyridine should relieve urinary frequency, not cause it. (I, 8)

18. 4. The intravenous flow rate is determined by the rate of infusion and the number of drops per milliliter of the fluid being administered: gtt/mL × mL/minute = gtt/minute (the intravenous flow rate). 15 gtt/mL × 100 mL/60 minute = 25 gtt/minute. (I, 8)

19. 3. 600,000 units / 1 mL = 600,000 units / x mL; x = 1.0 mL. (I, 8)

20. 1. Eye drops are correctly instilled by placing them in the lower conjunctival sac. Eye drops should not be placed near the lacrimal ducts, to decrease the chance of the medication's being systemically absorbed. Placing the drops on the cornea or sclera is uncomfortable for the client and may cause the medication to run out of the eye socket instead of being absorbed. (I, 8)

21. 4. To treat anaphylactic reactions, epinephrine is administered to counteract the effects of histamine. Epinephrine is a rapid-acting sympathomimetic drug that has a bronchodilator effect. Dopamine may be used if hypotension develops. Benadryl may also be given, but not as the initial drug of choice. Cimetidine would not

be administered to treat an anaphylactic reaction resulting in shortness of breath. (P, 8)

22. 3. Overuse of nasal spray containing pseudoephedrine can lead to rhinitis medicamentosa, which is a rebound effect causing increased swelling and congestion after use. Use of pseudoephedrine nasal spray does not cause infections or thrush. Pseudoephedrine is not addictive. (I, 8)

23. 3. The vastus lateralis site is the preferred intramuscular site for all ages because it does not have any major nerves or blood vessels located near it. The deltoid and dorsogluteal muscles have major nerves and blood vessels located nearby. The triceps is not an acceptable muscle for intramuscular injections. (P, 8)

24. 1. Clients should be instructed to rinse their mouths after using a steroid inhaler to avoid developing thrush. Clients should also be instructed to inhale slowly through the mouth and then hold the breath as they count to 10 slowly. It is not necessary for the client to cough and deep breathe before using the inhaler. (P, 8)

25. 2. The nurse should stay with the client during the first 15 minutes of a blood transfusion, because this is when reactions are most likely to occur. Blood products should never be refrigerated on the nursing unit. Blood that has not been infused after 4 hours should not be infused. The blood should be infused over the specific time ordered by the physician. If a fever develops, the blood should be stopped immediately and the blood reaction policy of the institution should be followed. (I, 8)

26. 2. The symptoms of difficulty breathing, elevated blood pressure, and cough are indicative of circulatory overload. Circulatory overload occurs when blood is infused more rapidly than the circulatory system can accommodate. Anaphylactic reactions are manifested by urticaria, wheezing, and shock. Sepsis begins with a rapid onset of chills and fever. Acute hemolytic reaction is typically manifested by chills, fever, low back pain, and flushing. (D, 8)

27. 2. Sucralfate should be taken on an empty stomach 1 hour before or 2 hours after meals, and at bedtime. It is usually taken four times a day. There is no need to avoid milk products while taking the drug. Sucralfate does not affect hemoglobin levels. (E, 8)

28. 4. A properly administered intradermal injection shows evidence of a bleb at the injection site. There should be no leaking of medication from the bleb; it needs to be absorbed into the tissue. Lack of swelling at the injection site means that the injection was given too deeply. The presence of tissue pallor does not indicate that the injection was given correctly. (E, 1)

29. 2. 30 mg / 1 mL = 15 mg / x mL; x = 0.5 mL. Therefore, the nurse should give 0.5 mL of the Toradol preloaded syringe. (I, 8)

30. 1. A serious complication of intravenous therapy is fluid overload. Noisy respirations can develop as a result of pulmonary congestion. Additional symptoms of fluid overload include dyspnea, crackles, hypertension, bounding pulse, and distended neck veins. (D, 8)

31. 2. Only isotonic (0.9%) saline should be used when administering a blood transfusion. The use of dextrose or Ringer's lactate will cause the hemolysis of red blood cells. (P, 8)

32. 4. Checking the client's identification armband is absolutely essential to prevent the administration of medication to the wrong client. Clients can be confused or hard of hearing and may give a wrong name or answer to a wrong name. Learning to recognize a client is not a reliable or safe form of identification. (I, 8)

33. 2. The continual use of nasal decongestants can result in a rebound effect when the agents are discontinued. This leads to a worsening of symptoms due to reflex vasodilation. Environmental changes can affect allergic rhinitis. The client should be instructed on identifying and avoiding exposure to allergens. Allergic rhinitis can occur during any season. It is not self-limited and may require prolonged management. (I, 8)

34. 3. Clients are instructed to take Fosamax on arising, 30 minutes before eating, with a full glass of water. Because it can cause severe esophageal irritation, the client must remain upright for 30 minutes after administration. Taking Fosamax with food or juice significantly reduces absorption. (I, 8)

35. 3. The median cubital vein is a common site for venous access. Point 1 is the cephalic vein; point 2 is the basilic vein; point 4 is the median antebrachial vein. (I, 8)

36. 1. Doxazosin (Cardura) is also used as an antihypertensive agent; the client may be experiencing orthostatic hypotension. The blood pressure readings should be reported to the physician with the client's report of symptoms. (I, 8)

37. 3. Leukopenia, or a decreased WBC, is an adverse reaction of Silvadene cream. A decrease in the WBC should be reported to the physician immediately. The Silvadene cream is discontinued until the WBC returns to normal. (D, 8)

38. 2. Sumitriptan is contraindicated in clients with ischemic heart disease, such as angina, myocardial infarction, or coronary artery disease, because it is a vasoconstrictor. Sumitriptan is used for the abortive treatment of migraines, not prophylactic treatment, and it is effective in treating acute migraines with or without aura. (I, 8)

39. 3. The estrogen content of oral contraceptives may predispose a woman to yeast infections. Poorly managed diabetes, not insulin itself, can increase the risk of candidiasis. (I, 8)

40. 1. The middle third of the thigh is where the body of the vastus lateralis muscle lies, which is approximately one hand's breadth below the greater trochanter and one hand's breadth above the knee. The largest diameter of the thigh is not necessarily where the muscle is located and would be an unsafe criterion to use for selecting the injection site. (P, 8)

41. 4. The amount of subcutaneous tissue is the most important factor to consider when deciding on the angle at which to insert the needle. Thin or emaciated clients with little subcutaneous tissue need to have the needle inserted at less of an angle. Clients who have a large amount of subcutaneous tissue can tolerate up to a 90-degree angle of insertion. Size of syringe has no bearing on the angle used. Tissue turgor can affect the ease with which the needle is inserted, but not the angle. The length of the needle used for subcutaneous injections is between $^3/_8$ and $^5/_8$ inches, which does not provide much variability unless the angle of the injection is also altered by the nurse. (P, 8)

42. 4. Trimethoprim can cause thrombocytopenia, so clients should be instructed to report any unusual bleeding or bruising. Periodic blood counts should be conducted while the client is using this medication. The medication should be taken until the full course of therapy has been completed. A urine culture should be obtained before therapy is implemented. Trimethoprim does not need to be taken with meals. (I, 8)

43. 1. When an infection is suspected from a VAD, blood cultures should be drawn peripherally and from all lumens of the VAD to determine the source of the infection. If the number of organisms is greater from the VAD than in the peripheral culture, the source is determined to be the VAD. (P, 8)

44. 2. The ability to obtain a blood specimen only after the client raises his arms and coughs usually indicates that the catheter is lodged against a vessel wall. The nurse would suspect a fibrin sheath or a pinched or kinked catheter if blood could not be aspirated. (A, 8)

45. 3. Dislodgement of the port access needle allows the intravenous solution to infuse into the port area, which causes pain and swelling. Symptoms of infection could include redness, warmth, discomfort, and exudates. If the catheter were pinched between the clavicle and a rib bone, infusion would cease because the catheter tubing would be obstructed. Port erosion would be very rare and would have been evident 3 days earlier or on the day chemotherapy was initiated. (D, 8)

46. 4. A Groshong catheter can rupture if the maximal pressure is exceeded. To reduce pressure on the catheter, the recommended syringe size to use is 10 to 20 mL. (D, 8)

47. 1. Ketorolac can cause renal impairment and should be used cautiously in clients who have cardiovascular conditions such as congestive heart failure. Clients should be told to weigh every morning and to report any weight gain or peripheral edema. The client does not need to increase fluid intake; instead, the client should maintain a normal intake and be instructed to report any fluid retention. (I, 8)

48. 3. First-line drug therapy for osteoarthritis begins with acetaminophen. Second-line therapy consists of nonsteroidal anti-inflammatory drugs. Corticosteroids are used for intra-articular injections of selected joints but are not recommended for systemic use. Narcotic analgesics are not used to treat osteoarthritis. (P, 8)

49. 4. A common side effect of chrysotherapy is dermatitis and pruritus, and the client should be told to report the development of a skin rash. Diarrhea is another common side effect. Clients do not develop jaundice, but they can develop a gray-blue skin color caused by gold deposits. Urinary retention is not a side effect of chrysotherapy. (A, 8)

50. 3. The client has a right to accurate information and participation in decision making about treatment options. The use of placebos is misleading to the client and unethical because it does not represent full disclosure about the treatment the client is receiving. The nurse cannot determine whether a client is in pain; pain is what the client says it is. (P, 1)

51. 3. Tetracycline antibiotics such as doxycycline are frequently prescribed to treat chlamydia. Probenecid is used to treat gout. Penicillin is frequently prescribed to treat gonorrhea. Acyclovir is used to treat genital herpes. (P, 8)

52. 1. Heparin should never be administered through the infusion lines of other drugs, and other drugs should not be piggybacked onto the heparin line. If other drugs need to be administered intravenously, they require a separate infusion line. The client's blood clotting tests need to be monitored more frequently than daily to maintain blood levels within the therapeutic range. It is recommended that they be monitored every 4 hours for continuous heparin infusions. Vitamin K is the antidote for warfarin (Coumadin); protamine sulfate is the antidote for heparin. It is not necessary to protect the heparin infusion from light. (P, 8)

53. 4. Clients taking metoclopramide should be instructed to report any involuntary movements of the face, eyes, or extremities, because side effects of the drug include extrapyramidal reactions and Parkinsonism-like reac-

tions. Other common side effects include diarrhea and nausea. Occasionally the client may experience transient hypertension. The drug does not typically affect urinary patterns. (P, 8)

54. 3. Currently the treatment of choice to treat chronic gastritis caused by *Helicobacter pylori* is double- or triple-antibiotic combinations. Commonly used antibiotics include amoxicillin, clarithromycin (Biaxin), and omeprazole (Prilosec). Antacids, antiemetics, and histamine$_2$-receptor antagonists can be prescribed in addition to the antibiotics. (P, 8)

55. 1. The client with cirrhosis should be cautioned against taking any over-the-counter medications that may be hepatotoxic, because the liver will not be able to metabolize these drugs. Acetaminophen is an example of such a drug. (I, 9)

56. 3. Glipizide (Glucatrol) is most effective when taken 30 minutes before breakfast. The duration of action is 10 to 24 hours. If the drug needs to be taken more than once a day, the dosage may be divided and taken twice a day before meals. It is not as effective to take the drug after meals. Although blood glucose levels will be monitored, the values do not dictate when the drug should be taken. (I, 8)

57. 3. Verapamil can cause irregular cardiac rhythms. Clients should be taught to take their pulse and report any irregular heartbeats to their health care provider. Diarrhea is not a problem; constipation is the most common side effect of verapamil. Verapamil does not cause bone marrow depression. The client does not need to restrict fluids. Instead, a normal fluid intake is encouraged to prevent constipation. (I, 8)

Growth and Development

58. 1. The client's readiness to learn is compromised by fatigue and lack of concentration. The teaching session should be rescheduled to a better time for improved learning readiness. Written instructions or involving the spouse can supplement verbal instructions but cannot replace teaching the client directly. (P, 1)

59. 3. The use of histamine$_2$ (H$_2$) blockers such as Tagamet can cause paradoxic central nervous system (CNS) stimulation resulting in ataxia in the elderly. Impaired vision, gait, and thinking may also occur. Nausea, heartburn, and diarrhea are not related to CNS effects of H$_2$ blockers. (D, 8)

60. 3. Aminoglycoside antibiotics can cause damage to the eighth cranial nerve and result in ototoxicity. If the client is already hearing impaired, the nurse should question the order with the physician. Another antibiotic may be able to be substituted that would be safer. Giving the drug as ordered would create an unsafe sit-

uation for the client. Gentamycin is an appropriate antibiotic for gram-negative infections such as peritonitis. Gentamycin does not cause visual impairment. (D, 8)

61. 4. Renal function may already be compromised in the elderly, and ibuprofen can further impair renal or liver function. Nonsteroidal anti-inflammatory drugs can also cause nephrosis, cirrhosis, and heart failure in elderly persons. (I, 8)

62. 3. The use of a weekly pillbox and system for taking medications assists older adults in knowing when to take medications and when they have already been taken. It provides an organizing method for taking medications. (I, 3)

63. 3. Elderly clients, especially those with existing respiratory compromise, are good candidates for Pneumovax. This vaccine provides immunity and prophylaxis against pneumococcal pneumonia or bacteremia in adults or children at risk. (I, 8)

64. 2. Clients who have a chronic illness, have experienced a serious illness, reside in long-term care facilities, or are 65 years of age or older are encouraged to obtain pneumococcal and influenza vaccinations. Benign prostatic hypertrophy would not predispose a client to pneumonia or influenza. (I, 4)

65. 1. Fear in adults, even when unfounded, can stand in the way of recovery. When this client expresses a fear of being in room 13 because he thinks the number will bring him bad luck, it would be best for the nurse to try to eliminate the reason for the client's fear. Moving the client because superstitions have a good chance of coming true relies on an unproved phenomenon. A superstition becomes truth only on the basis of chance. Refusing to move the client to another room fails to consider the client's fears. (I, 5)

66. 1. Verbalizing feelings and concerns helps decrease anxiety and allows the wife to move on to understanding the current situation. Describing events or explaining equipment is appropriate when the person is not distraught and is ready to learn. Explaining the client's medical status is appropriate when the person is not distraught. Reassuring the family member does not allow verbalization of feelings and discounts her feelings. (I, 5)

67. 3. Infants and elderly persons have the greatest risk for fluid-related health problems. An infant's body weight is 70% to 80% water content. An infant who is ill and has had persistent diarrhea for 24 hours will quickly lose a significant amount of fluid and electrolytes if the diarrhea is not stopped and replacement fluids given. Healthy young adults have a higher tolerance for fluid loss and can quickly regain their fluid balance when fluids are lost through normal activity. The 75-year-old woman who was placed NPO before surgery is not likely to develop a fluid volume deficit within 8 hours, unless there are other fluid conditions present that would precipitate fluid loss. The 60-year-old client with pneumonia and a fever should be monitored for a fluid volume deficit, but is not as likely to develop one as a client who is actively losing fluids through diarrhea. (D, 10)

68. 4. In a client with persistent nausea and vomiting, the nurse should anticipate that the client may be dehydrated and exhibit signs of a fluid volume deficit. Typical assessment findings would include lethargy, poor skin turgor, dry mucous membranes, tachycardia, weight loss, and decreased urinary output. The blood pressure is usually maintained within normal limits in the case of a mild to moderate fluid volume deficit because of the compensatory mechanisms of sympathetic nervous system stimulation of the heart (causing tachycardia) and peripheral vasoconstriction. (A, 9)

69. 3. To prevent gastric distention and gastroesophageal reflux, the client is encouraged to eat smaller, more frequent meals. The client should not lie down until 2 to 3 hours after a meal. The client should sleep with the head of the bed elevated 4 to 6 inches. These activities facilitate esophageal emptying and decrease episodes of reflux. Fluid intake should be restricted during meals to decrease gastric distention. (E, 9)

70. 1. The nurse's priority action is to encourage the client to verbalize his concerns. It may be appropriate to provide the client some privacy, but not without an understanding of what is motivating his current behavior. Until the client has had a chance to verbalize his concerns, it would be premature to invite a member of the ostomy association to speak with him. Telling the client it is time to deal with his situation is a nontherapeutic response. (I, 5)

71. 4. Cultural beliefs and values are very difficult to change, and developing a plan of care that does not take the client's cultural background into consideration demonstrates a lack of respect for the client's beliefs. A successful plan of care incorporates the client's values. Ignoring cultural differences does not necessarily lead to an increase in the cost of the client's care. The nurse should strive to acknowledge the client's cultural beliefs; however, it is not appropriate for the nurse to explain how his or her belief system differs from the client's. Understanding a client's cultural background may help prevent the nurse from making an embarrassing mistake and offending the client, but that is not the primary purpose for assessing and understanding the client's cultural background. (A, 5)

72. 3. In order to avoid ethnocentric behavior toward the client, it is important that nurses acknowledge what their cultural beliefs are and be careful not to impose

them on the clients they care for, because this could influence the quality of care. It is stereotypic for nurses to assume that they can determine which cultural groups will be noncompliant or that they can anticipate the client's response to care. Nurses need to be aware of their beliefs, not alter them to match the client's culture. (I, 5)

73. 4. To prevent urinary tract infections, clients should be encouraged to wear loose-fitting, cotton underwear to decrease the formation of a warm, moist environment. Clients should void whenever they feel the urge or at least every 4 to 6 hours during the daytime. An indwelling catheter increases the risk for a urinary tract infection. Prophylactic antibiotics are typically not used for urinary tract infections unless the client has experienced repeated episodes within 1 year. (I, 9)

74. 3. The client's primary stated concern is her ability to care for her home and family, which is hampered by her fatigue and pain. It is important for the nurse to develop a plan of care that addresses the client's priorities. There are no data to support a diagnosis of body image disturbance. (D, 10)

75. 1. Postural hypotension or persistent hypotension is present in dehydration, as are poor skin turgor, dry oral mucous membranes, and tachycardia. If the dehydration is severe, the client may also be restless, confused, and complaining of thirst. Most instances of crackles, shortness of breath, and bounding pulse are indicative of excess fluid volume. (A, 9)

76. 3. The very young and the elderly are more susceptible to infection. An elderly client with a break in skin integrity, such as the 86-year-old man with a burn, is at an increased risk for infection. (P, 10)

Management of Care

77. 4. Repositioning the tube in a client who has undergone gastric surgery should be performed (per order of the surgeon) by the registered nurse. Recording output, securing the nasal tape, and documenting the color of the drainage could safely be delegated to the UNP. (P, 1)

78. 3. The social worker is the most essential team member to be involved in discharge planning to meet the client's needs and offer suggestions for the best community resources. (P, 1)

79. 2. A client with diverticulitis will need care that the LP/VN should be able to provide safely. The client with angina is unstable and requires an registered nurse for continuous assessment. The client receiving chemotherapy treatment requires a registered nurse who is certified in chemotherapy administration. A child with Kawasaki's disease must be watched closely

for cardiac complications, and it would be best to assign the child to an experienced pediatric nurse, not a new graduate. (P, 1)

80. 3. Suspected child abuse must be reported to a representative of CPS. Reporting a potential abuse does not indicate guilt, only suspicion or risk. The CPS and the judicial system will follow the correct legal process to establish the need for prosecution and/or counseling. (I, 1)

81. 1. The error must be reported to the physician to obtain a new scheduling order. An incident report should be completed, and the agency policy for medication errors should be followed. Assessing for signs of infection is not the nurse's first action and should be completed routinely for clients receiving antibiotics. The dose should not be administered 6 hours late unless ordered by the physician. The pharmacist is not responsible to give directions for medication omissions. (I, 1)

82. 4. The best option in this situation is to reassign the client to a nurse with experience in blood administration. The policy book and explanation are resources, but the nurse is a pediatric nurse who has never administered blood before, and therefore an unsafe situation is created. An explanation is insufficient teaching for safe and proper blood administration. (P, 1)

83. 4. Spiritual support and planning for a funeral are offered by ministers, priests, and rabbis in pastoral care departments. Home health care or a social worker may be an appropriate referral for discharge planning, but not for funeral plans. The psychologist may be an appropriate referral for meeting the needs of the dying client, but not for planning the funeral. (P, 1)

84. 2. Continuity of care is crucial for this client to feel more comfortable about asking questions and discussing her care at home. (I, 1)

85. 1. This situation should be reported immediately to the nursing supervisor or immediate manager at the time. The nurse is liable to report a suspicious situation that could create an unsafe situation for the clients. Reporting a suspicious situation does not imply actual guilt; it implies identification of a high-risk situation. The supervisor will then follow the correct procedure for management and follow-up of the situation. This situation requires immediate attention and cannot be delayed a shift. The charge nurse, or another staff nurse, should not confront the nurse; this is the responsibility of the nursing supervisor. Assessment of the nurse's behavior is not the nurse's responsibility; reporting the potentially unsafe situation is. (I, 1)

86. 1. The family has the final consent to organ donation before the procedure is performed. The donor's gift will be excluded if the donation causes severe emo-

tional distress to the family. The Act does not limit potential donors. (I, 1)

87. 4. Elderly clients are vulnerable to abuse. Bruising that is not located in areas typical for falls or bumps should be reported to the APS. The location and shape of this bruise is suggestive for abuse. The nurse taking care of this resident and the physician should be alerted to the bruises after the APS is notified. The nurse should continue to assess the areas involved after notifying the APS. (I, 1)

88. 2. Identification of causes of medication errors requires inservice education to inform the staff of strategies to decrease these errors. Errors are frequently the result of systemic problems that can be identified and rectified through problem-solving techniques and changes in procedures. Documenting or reporting the situation would not directly assist the nurses in eliminating errors. Reporting the incidents to the hospital attorney is unnecessary. (I, 1)

89. 3. The Quality Improvement and Risk Management Department is the correct resource to provide tracking and outcome data on any type of error or unsafe incidents. The Ethics Committee reviews ethical issues within an institution. The Pharmacy and Products Office reviews new drug procedures and protocols. The Infection Control Committee tracks nosocomial infections and communicable diseases in the institution. (P, 1)

90. 3. The nurse should measure the nasogastric tube from the tip of the nose to the tip of the ear, and then from the tip of the ear to the xiphoid process. The other measurements will cause the tubing to be misplaced. (I, 9)

91. 2. Daily bathing is not required to meet standards of care. Rescheduling surgeries is not a strategy for meeting nursing care needs of clients. Medications are required to be given as ordered to maintain standards of care and efficacy of the medication. UNP are not licensed to administer analgesics. (P, 1)

92. 1. Initially, the nurse needs to inform the surgeon that the task is outside the scope of nursing practice. If the surgeon still requests the activity, the nurse should refuse to perform the task and should follow the chain of communication for reporting unsafe practice according to the hospital's policy. The nurse must not comply with any order that goes beyond the scope of nursing practice. (I, 1)

93. 1. The Iranian tradition of male authority is still strong. Accepting a woman making life-and-death decisions for their son may be very difficult for these parents. Discussing with the parents other options, such as the idea of turning the case over to a male Muslim oncologist, would be appropriate. The gender issue is a stronger cultural factor than the religious difference.

There is no basis to relate the parents' behavior to fear of being charged with abuse or neglect. Attributing the behavior to Middle Eastern aggressiveness reflects a stereotype, not a cultural value. (I, 1)

94. 1. The Standards of Care identify criteria on which nursing care can be evaluated. The Patient's Bill of Rights outlines rights to protect the client's autonomy and access to care. The Code of Ethics outlines ethical criteria to be followed by professional nurses. Professional certification signifies that the nurse has passed an examination given by a national professional organization. (A, 1)

95. 2. The recommended site for assessing temperature in a client who is coughing and having difficulty breathing is the tympanic site (ear). The mouth is contraindicated because of the client's cough and difficulty breathing. The rectum is not the site of choice because of the invasiveness of the procedure and the client's breathing difficulty. The axillae are used when the oral, tympanic, and rectal sites are contraindicated. (A, 10)

96. 4. Many clients feel faint and weak when helped to ambulate for the first time after surgery. The client's circulatory system needs time to adjust to an upright position before the client is helped to a standing position. This is best done by placing the client into high Fowler's position in bed for a few minutes. After becoming accustomed to a sitting position, the client can then be helped to dangle her legs at the edge of the bed before ambulating. Although analgesics can promote comfort for the postoperative client, they can sedate the client and should not be given at the time the client is assisted out of bed. Having the client nap or do leg exercises will not prepare her to dangle her legs. (I, 10)

97. 2. When the client initially begins to complain of abdominal cramping during an enema, it is usually most appropriate to temporarily stop the infusion until the cramping subsides. If on resuming the flow of enema fluid the client continues to complain of cramping or inability to retain further fluid, the nurse should discontinue the enema. Having the client take slow, deep breaths can help decrease the amount of cramping; telling the client to hold his breath will not relieve cramping and is inappropriate. The client should be placed in a left Sims' position to facilitate flow of the fluid into the colon, not a supine position. (I, 9)

98. 4. The nurse should have the client tilt the head toward the ceiling as the nasogastric tube is inserted. When the tube reaches the nasopharynx, the client should be instructed to bring the head forward a bit by flexing the neck. This technique closes the trachea and opens the esophagus to receive the tube. Correct technique includes lubricating the tube with a water-soluble lubricant and having the client swallow as the tube is

passed into the stomach. The client should not be instructed to hold the breath. The client should be placed in a sitting position. (I, 9)

99. 4. The primary purpose of fluid replacement therapy for a client receiving gastric suction is to maintain fluid and electrolyte balance. Gastric suctioning interrupts the normal intake and absorption of fluids. Fluids and electrolytes are lost through the nasogastric drainage. Intravenous fluids are required to replace the fluid and electrolyte loss. Since the client with a nasogastric tube is also NPO, intravenous fluids will help prevent a fluid volume deficit from developing and will help maintain an adequate urinary output. Intravenous fluids do not maintain bladder function. Postoperatively, intravenous fluids are not typically used to facilitate osmotic diuresis. The administration of intravenous fluids may help balance the client's fluid intake and output, but the primary reason for administering fluids is to maintain fluid and electrolyte balance. (I, 9)

100. 3. It would be appropriate for the assistant to obtain the client's weight and height. It is responsibility of the registered nurse to assess the client's lung sounds, conduct nursing histories and perform assessments, and evaluate client status. (A, 1)

101. 1. Based on the information provided, the client who is on day 1 after a total laryngectomy would be the priority client for the nurse to evaluate. This client is at risk for impaired respiratory status and should be monitored closely. Clients with acute conditions that can affect their respiratory status are a high priority for nursing care. (E, 1)

102. 4. It is appropriate for an unlicensed assistant to mark the time of measurement and fluid level on the collection container. Milking of chest tubes is not routinely recommended, but, if performed, would be the responsibility of the nurse. The collection container should not be raised to bed height, because this can cause fluid to flow back toward the lungs. Chest tubes should not be secured to bed linens, because they could be pulled on when the client moves and turns in bed. (I, 1)

103. 2. It would be appropriate for the nurse to instruct the assistant to place the client on NPO status. It is the responsibility of the physician performing the procedure to obtain the client's informed consent and have the form signed. It is the responsibility of the registered nurse to teach clients and evaluate their health status. These responsibilities cannot be delegated to unlicensed assistants. (I, 1)

104. 3. A client with a suspected slow GI bleed should be observed for tarry (black) stools, which indicate slow bleeding from an upper GI site. The longer the blood remains in the system, the darker it becomes from the degradation of hemoglobin and release of iron.

Hypotension does not occur with a slow GI bleed. Bright red blood indicates bleeding from the lower GI tract or profuse, massive GI bleeding. Jaundice is not a indicator of GI bleeding, but it is an indicator of liver or biliary tract dysfunction. (A, 9)

105. 3. A sign of ulcer perforation is the onset of sudden, severe abdominal pain. The nurse should instruct all assistive personnel to report this symptom immediately, because a perforated ulcer is a medical emergency. (I, 1)

106. 1. A soft toothbrush should be used to regularly clean the client's teeth and tongue. Ice chips should not be given to clients with a nasogastric tube, because their frequent use can promote an electrolyte imbalance. Mouthwash is too astringent and should not be used regularly. Lemon-glycerin swabs can be drying to oral mucosa and can promote bacterial growth. (I, 1)

107. 2. The client should be repositioned every 2 hours to promote even drying of the cast. The cast should be kept uncovered while drying to allow air to circulate around the cast and prevent heat from building up within it. It takes 24 to 72 hours for a plaster cast to dry; a blow dryer is not effective. The palms of the hands, not the fingers, should be used to move a drying cast, to prevent indentations that can cause pressure points to develop. (I, 1)

108. 2. After total hip replacement surgery the leg should be maintained in a position of abduction and extension. A foam abduction pillow is usually placed between the legs to maintain this position. Placing the leg in an adducted and/or flexed position can lead to a dislocation of the prosthesis. (I, 2)

109. 3. Active range of motion should be encouraged to help prevent the development of contractures, including plantar flexion. An unlicensed assistant can help a client perform active range-of-motion exercises to unaffected extremities. A bed cradle relieves the pressure of bedclothes off of the feet but cannot prevent plantar flexion. Massaging lotion helps maintain skin integrity. A trochanter roll is placed at the hips to prevent external rotation. (P, 7)

110. 1. The assistant should be told to report immediately to the nurse any client complaints about inability to move fingers, numbness or tingling, or feelings of tightness, because these may be indicators of impaired neurovascular status. The nurse, not the assistant, is responsible for neurovascular assessments. Intake and output would usually not be particularly significant in a client with a fractured arm. It is normal for the client to feel heat immediately after application of a plaster cast. (I, 1)

111. 3. The most appropriate action to delegate to an unlicensed assistant is collection of a urine specimen for a

culture and sensitivity analysis. The nurse can anticipate that the elderly client with an enlarged prostate
may be difficult to catheterize. It is not within the unlicensed assistant's scope of responsibility to change
intravenous fluids. It is the registered nurses's responsibility to assess a client's complaint of pain; assessment responsibilities cannot be delegated. (P, 1)

112. 1. Because of the elderly client's diagnosis of pneumonia and periods of confusion, there is the potential for
client injury and decreased levels of oxygenation. The
nurse should assess this client first. (A, 1)

113. 3. When assisting a client with a weakness out of bed,
it is important that the client always move toward the
stronger side. This allows the client to assist in the
move as much as he physically can. In this case, the
client will need to move toward his right side to maximize the use of his strong arm and leg. Placing the
wheelchair at the head of the bed or behind the client
does not allow for a safe transfer of the client. The presence of the assistant does not necessarily ensure safety
regardless of the position of the wheelchair. (E, 7)

114. 4. When handling any of the client's excreta during the
administration of chemotherapy, health care personnel
should wear surgical gloves to prevent exposure to any
chemotherapeutic toxin contained in the excreta. It is
not necessary for the nurse to handle the disposal of
any body fluids; assistive personnel must know how to
protect themselves from potential exposure. Universal
body precautions are always used, but it is important
that surgical gloves be used for adequate protection. It
is not necessary to wear gown, gloves, and mask for
every client contact. (I, 2)

115. 4. It is most appropriate for the nurse to delegate the
activity of obtaining a client's routine glucose reading.
The nurse is responsible for performing assessments
and analyzing the data on which treatment decisions
are based; the nurse should assess and evaluate the
client's apical pulse before administering the digoxin.
The dressing of an incision that is infected and requires
irrigation should be changed by the nurse, so that the
nurse can perform the irrigation and evaluate tissue
healing. It is the responsibility of the nurse, not the
unlicensed assistant, to teach the client. (P, 1)

116. 1. The most appropriate client to assign to an unlicensed assistant is the elderly client with COPD and
mild dyspnea because of the relative stability of the
client's chronic condition. The client with a new
laryngectomy requires close observation to maintain
a patent airway, promote comfort, and decrease anxiety. The client who is receiving chemotherapy will
need to be monitored for adverse effects related to the
chemotherapy. The client with a suspected pulmonary embolus is acutely ill and requires close
observation. (I, 1)

Bibliography

Abrams, A. (1998). *Clinical drug therapy: Rationales for nursing practice* (5th ed.). Philadelphia: Lippincott Williams & Wilkins.

Ades, T. B., Pierce, M., Varricchio, C., & Walker, C. (1997). *A cancer source book for nurses* (7th ed.). Boston: Jones & Bartlett.

Altman, G. B., Buchsel, P., & Coxon, V. (2000). *Delmar's fundamental and advanced nursing skills*. Albany, NY: Delmar Thompson Learning.

Andrews, M. M., & Boyle, J. S. (1995). *Transcultural concepts in nursing care* (2nd ed.). Philadelphia: J. B. Lippincott.

Buchsel, P., Miaskowski, C., Nielsen, B., Paice, J., Rostad, M., & Strohl, R. (Eds.) (1993). *The best of oncology nursing*. St. Louis: Mosby–Year Book.

Carignan, J. R., Rosenthal, S., & Smith, B. D. (1993). *Medical care of the cancer patient* (2nd ed.). Philadelphia: W. B. Saunders.

Carpenito, L. (2000). *Nursing diagnosis: Application to clinical practice* (8th ed.). Philadelphia: Lippincott Williams & Wilkins.

Cleveland, L., Aschenbrenner, D. S., Venable, S. J., & Yensen, J. (1999). *Nursing management in drug therapy*. Philadelphia: Lippincott Williams & Wilkins.

Frogge, M. H., Goodman, M., Groenwald, S., & Yarbro, C. H. (2000). (Eds.) *Cancer nursing principles and practice* (5th ed.). Boston: Jones & Bartlett.

Ellis, J. R., & Hartley, C. L. (2000). *Managing and coordinating nursing care* (3rd ed.). Philadelphia: Lippincott Williams & Wilkins.

Ellis, J. R., & Hartley, C. L. (1998). *Nursing in today's world: Challenges, issues, and trends* (6th ed.). Philadelphia: Lippincott Williams & Wilkins.

Grant, M., & McCorkle, R. (1994). *Cancer nursing*. Philadelphia: W. B. Saunders.

Karch, A. (2000). *2000 Lippincott's nursing drug guide*. Philadelphia: Lippincott Williams & Wilkins.

Lewis, S. M., Heitkemper, M., & Dirksen, S. R. (2000). *Medical surgical nursing: Assessment and management of clinical problems* (5th ed.). St. Louis: Mosby–Year Book.

Marquis, B., & Huston, C. (2000). *Leadership roles and management functions in nursing: Theory and application* (3rd ed.). Philadelphia: Lippincott Williams & Wilkins.

Nevidjon, B. M., & Sowers, K. W. (Eds.) (2000). *A nurse's guide to cancer care*. Philadelphia: Lippincott Williams & Wilkins.

Otto, S. (1997). *Oncology nursing* (3rd ed.). St. Louis: Mosby–Year Book.

Purnell, L., & Paulanka, B. J. (1998). *Transcultural health care: A culturally competent approach*. Philadelphia: F. A. Davis.

Reeves, C., Roux, G., & Lockhart, R. (1999). *Medical surgical nursing: A core series*. New York: McGraw-Hill.

Reno, R. (Ed.) (2000). *2000 Standards: Recommended practices and guidelines with AORN official statements*. Denver: American Organization of Operating Room Nurses.

Smeltzer, S., & Bare, B. (2000). *Brunner & Suddarth's textbook of medical-surgical nursing* (9th ed.). Philadelphia: Lippincott Williams & Wilkins.

Wehmer, M. A.. Pulmonary embolism. In Melander, S. (2000). *Case studies in critical care nursing a guide for application and review*. Philadelphia: Lippincott Williams & Wilkins.

The Nursing Care of Clients With Psychiatric Disorders and Mental Health Problems

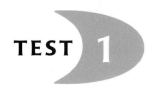
▶ **The Client With Major Depression**

▶ **The Client With Bipolar Disorder, Manic Phase**

▶ **The Client With Suicidal Ideation and Suicide Attempt**

▶ **Correct Answers and Rationale**

Select the one best answer, and indicate your choice by filling in the circle in front of the option.

The Client With Major Depression

1. A client has an Axis I diagnosis of major depression. Which of the following features would be *most* crucial for the nurse to assess?
   ○ 1. Sleep disturbance.
   ○ 2. Feelings of worthlessness.
   ○ 3. Difficulty with concentration.
   ○ 4. Suicidal ideation.

2. A client who has had three episodes of recurrent endogenous depression within the past 2 years states to the nurse, "I want to know why I'm so depressed." Which of the following statements by the nurse would be *most* helpful?
   ○ 1. "I know you'll get better with the right medication."
   ○ 2. "Let's discuss possible reasons underlying your depression."
   ○ 3. "Your depression is most likely caused by a chemical brain imbalance."
   ○ 4. "Members of your family seem very supportive of you."

3. A client diagnosed with major depression spends the majority of the day lying in bed with the sheet pulled over his head. Which of the following approaches by the nurse would be *most* therapeutic?
   ○ 1. Wait for the client to begin the conversation.
   ○ 2. Initiate contact with the client frequently.
   ○ 3. Sit outside the client's room.
   ○ 4. Question the client until he responds.

4. The client exhibits a flat affect, psychomotor retardation, and depressed mood. The nurse attempts to engage the client in an interaction but the client does not respond to the nurse. Which of the following responses by the nurse would be *most* appropriate?
   ○ 1. "I'll sit here with you for 15 minutes."
   ○ 2. "I'll come back a little bit later to talk."
   ○ 3. "I'll find someone else for you to talk with."
   ○ 4. "I'll get you something to read."

5. After a few minutes of conversation, a female client who is depressed wearily asks the nurse, "Why pick me to talk to? Go talk to someone else." Which of the following replies by the nurse would be *best*?
   ○ 1. "I'm assigned to care for you today, if you'll let me."
   ○ 2. "You have a lot of potential, and I'd like to help you."
   ○ 3. "I'll talk to someone else later."
   ○ 4. "I'm interested in you and want to help you."

6. A client is receiving paroxetine (Paxil) 20 mg every morning. After taking the first three doses, the client tells the nurse that the medication upsets his stomach. Which of the following instructions would the nurse give to the client?
   ○ 1. "Take the medication an hour before breakfast."
   ○ 2. "Take the medication with some food."
   ○ 3. "Take the medication at bedtime."
   ○ 4. "Take the medication with 4 ounces of orange juice."

7. The physician orders fluoxetine (Prozac) orally every morning for a 72-year-old client with depression. The nurse would expect the physician to order which of the following dosages for this client?
   ○ 1. 0.5 mg.
   ○ 2. 10 mg.
   ○ 3. 25 mg.
   ○ 4. 30 mg.

8. Which of the following statements by a client taking trazodone (Desyrel) as prescribed by the physician indicates to the nurse that further teaching about the medication is needed?
   ○ 1. "I will continue to take my medication after a light snack."
   ○ 2. "Taking Desyrel at night will help me to sleep."
   ○ 3. "My depression will be gone in about 5 to 7 days."
   ○ 4. "I'll call my doctor if I start to have flu symptoms."

9. A 62-year-old female client with severe depression and psychotic symptoms is scheduled for electroconvulsant therapy (ECT) tomorrow morning. The

client's daughter asks the nurse, "How painful will the treatment be for Mom?" The nurse would correctly respond by saying which of the following?

○ 1. "Your mother will be given something for pain before the treatment."

○ 2. "The physician will make sure your mother doesn't suffer needlessly."

○ 3. "Your mother will be asleep during the treatment and will not be in pain."

○ 4. "Your mother will be able talk to us and tell us if she's in pain."

10. A client with sleep disturbances, feelings of worthlessness, fatigue, and inability to concentrate was let go from her place of employment a month ago. While interacting with the nurse, the client states, "My boss was wonderful! He was understanding and a really nice man." The nurse interprets this statement as indicating which of the following defense mechanisms?

○ 1. Repression.

○ 2. Suppression.

○ 3. Intellectualization.

○ 4. Reaction formation.

11. During a group session, a client who is depressed tells the group that he lost his job. Which of the following responses by the nurse would be *best*?

○ 1. "It must have been very upsetting for you."

○ 2. "Would you tell us about your job."

○ 3. "You'll find another job when you're better."

○ 4. "You were probably too depressed to work."

12. During an interaction with the nurse, a client states, "My husband has supported me every time I've been hospitalized for depression. He'll leave me this time. I'm an awful wife and mother. I'm no good. Nothing I do is right." Based on this information, which of the following nursing diagnoses would the nurse identify when developing the client's plan of care?

○ 1. Impaired Social Interaction related to unsatisfactory relationships as evidenced by withdrawal.

○ 2. Low Self-Esteem related to lack of self-worth as evidenced by negative self-statements.

○ 3. Risk for Self-Directed Violence related to feelings of guilt as evidenced by statements of suicidal ideation.

○ 4. Ineffective Coping related to hospitalizations as evidenced by impaired judgment.

13. A male client who is very depressed exhibits psychomotor retardation, a flat affect, and apathy. The nurse observes the client to be in need of grooming and hygiene. Which of the following nursing actions would be *most* appropriate?

○ 1. Explaining the importance of hygiene to the client.

○ 2. Asking the client if he is ready to shower.

○ 3. Waiting until the client's family can participate in the client's care.

○ 4. Stating to the client that it's time for him to take a shower.

14. A client who is depressed states, "I'm an awful person. Everything about me is bad. I can't do anything right." Which of the following responses by the nurse would be *most* therapeutic?

○ 1. "Everybody around here likes you."

○ 2. "I can see many good qualities in you."

○ 3. "Let's discuss what you've done correctly."

○ 4. "You were able to bathe today."

15. When developing the teaching plan for the family of client with severe depression who is to receive ECT, which of the following would the nurse include?

○ 1. Some temporary confusion and disorientation immediately after a treatment is common.

○ 2. During an ECT treatment session, the client is at risk for aspiration.

○ 3. Clients with severe depression usually do not respond to ECT.

○ 4. The client will not be able to breathe independently during a treatment.

16. Which of the following comments indicates that a client understands the nurse's teaching about sertraline (Zoloft)?

○ 1. "Zoloft will probably cause me to gain weight."

○ 2. "This medicine can cause delayed ejaculations."

○ 3. "Dry mouth is a permanent side effect of Zoloft."

○ 4. "I can take my medicine with St. John's wort."

17. The client with recurring depression has been hospitalized for 3 days on the psychiatric unit. The client obtains a 6-hour pass to go home. Which of the following suggestions to the family would be *best* to help them prepare for the client's visit?

○ 1. Discourage visitors while the client is at home.

○ 2. Provide for a schedule of activities outside the home.

○ 3. Involve the client in usual at-home activities.

○ 4. Encourage the client to sleep as much as possible.

18. A client with major depression is to be discharged home tomorrow. When preparing the client's discharge plan, which of the following areas would be *most* important for the nurse to review with the client?

○ 1. Future plans for going back to work.

○ 2. A conflict encountered with another client.

○ 3. Results of psychological testing.

○ 4. Medication management with outpatient follow-up.

19. A client with major depression and psychotic features is admitted involuntarily to the hospital. He will not eat because his "bowels have turned to jelly," which the client states is just punishment for his wickedness. The client requests to leave the hospital. The nurse denies the request because commitment papers have been initiated by the physician. Which of the following would the nurse identify as a criterion for the client to be legally committable?
    ○ 1. Evidence of psychosis.
    ○ 2. Being gravely disabled.
    ○ 3. Risk of harm to self or others.
    ○ 4. Diagnosis of mental illness.

20. A client who has been taking venlafaxine (Effexor) 25 mg PO, three times a day for the past 2 days states, "This medicine isn't doing me any good. I'm still so depressed." Which of the following responses by the nurse would be *most* appropriate?
    ○ 1. "Perhaps we'll need to increase your dose."
    ○ 2. "Let's wait a few days and see how you feel."
    ○ 3. "It takes about 2 to 4 weeks to receive the full effects."
    ○ 4. "It's too soon to tell if your medication will help you."

21. When teaching the client with atypical depression about foods to avoid while taking phenelzine (Nardil), which of the following would the nurse include?
    ○ 1. Roasted chicken.
    ○ 2. Salami.
    ○ 3. Fresh fish.
    ○ 4. Hamburger.

22. A client is taking phenelzine (Nardil) 15 mg PO, three times a day. The nurse is about to administer the 1 PM dose when the client complains of a throbbing headache. Which of the following would the nurse do *next*?
    ○ 1. Give the client an analgesic ordered PRN.
    ○ 2. Call the physician to report the symptom.
    ○ 3. Administer the client's next dose of phenelzine.
    ○ 4. Obtain the client's vital signs.

23. A female client with severe depression and weight loss has not eaten since admission to the hospital 2 days ago. Which of the following approaches would the nurse include when developing this client's plan of care to ensure that she eats?
    ○ 1. Serving the client her meal trays in her room.
    ○ 2. Sitting with the client and spoon-feeding if required.
    ○ 3. Calling the family to bring the client food from home.
    ○ 4. Explaining the importance of nutrition in recovery.

24. After administering a prescribed medication to a client who becomes restless at night and has diffi-culty falling asleep, which of the following nursing actions would be *most* appropriate?
    ○ 1. Sitting quietly with the client at the bedside until the medication takes effect.
    ○ 2. Engaging the client in interaction until the client falls asleep.
    ○ 3. Reading to the client with the lights turned down low.
    ○ 4. Encouraging the client to watch television until the client feels sleepy.

25. Which of the following behaviors exhibited by a client with depression would lead the nurse to determine that the client is ready for discharge?
    ○ 1. Interactions with staff and peers.
    ○ 2. Sleeping for 4 hours in the afternoon and 4 hours at night.
    ○ 3. Verbalization of feeling in control of self and situations.
    ○ 4. Statements of dissatisfaction over not being able to perform at work.

26. The client with major depression and suicidal ideation has been taking bupropion (Wellbutrin) 100 mg PO four times daily for 5 days. Assessment reveals the client to be somewhat less withdrawn, able to perform activities of daily living with minimal assistance, and eating 50% of each meal. At this time, the nurse would monitor the client specifically for which of the following behaviors?
    ○ 1. Seizure activity.
    ○ 2. Suicide attempt.
    ○ 3. Visual disturbances.
    ○ 4. Increased libido.

27. Which of the following outcomes would the nurse include as an outcome in the initial plan of care for a client who is exhibiting psychomotor retardation, withdrawal, minimal eye contact, and unresponsiveness to the nurse's questions?
    ○ 1. The client will initiate interactions with peers.
    ○ 2. The client will participate in milieu activities.
    ○ 3. The client will discuss adaptive coping techniques.
    ○ 4. The client will interact with the nurse.

28. When preparing a teaching plan for a client about imipramine (Tofranil), which of the following substances will the nurse tell the client to avoid while taking the medication?
    ○ 1. Caffeinated coffee.
    ○ 2. Sunscreen.
    ○ 3. Alcohol.
    ○ 4. Artificial tears.

29. The client with depression who is taking imipramine (Tofranil) states to the nurse, "My doctor wants me to have an ECG in 2 weeks, but my heart is fine." Which of the following responses by the nurse would be most appropriate?

○ 1. "It's routine practice to have ECGs periodically because the drug may cause heart irregularities."

○ 2. "It's probably a precautionary measure because I'm not aware that you have a cardiac condition."

○ 3. "Try not to worry too much about this. Your doctor is just being very thorough in monitoring your condition."

○ 4. "You had an ECG before you were prescribed imipramine and the procedure will be the same."

30. The laboratory calls the nurse stating that a client's imipramine level is within the therapeutic range. The nurse interprets this as indicating that the client's serum concentration is within which of the following ranges?

○ 1. 50 to 150 mg/mL.

○ 2. 151 to 250 mg/mL.

○ 3. 251 to 350 mg/mL.

○ 4. 351 to 450 mg/mL.

31. When assessing a client who is receiving tricyclic antidepressant therapy, which of the following would alert the nurse to the possibility that the client is experiencing anticholinergic effects?

○ 1. Tremors and cardiac arrhythmias.

○ 2. Sedation and delirium.

○ 3. Respiratory depression and convulsions.

○ 4. Urine retention and blurred vision.

32. A client with depression who is taking doxepin (Sinequan) 100 mg PO at bedtime complains of dizziness on arising. Which of the following suggestions would be the *most* appropriate?

○ 1. "Try taking a hot shower."

○ 2. "Get up slowly and dangle your feet before standing."

○ 3. "Stay in bed until you are feeling better."

○ 4. "You need to limit the fluids you drink."

33. The physician orders mirtazapine (Remeron) 30 mg PO at bedtime for a client diagnosed with depression. The nurse is responsible for which of the following?

○ 1. Giving the medication as ordered.

○ 2. Questioning the physician's order.

○ 3. Requesting to give the medication in the morning.

○ 4. Giving the medication in three divided doses.

34. A client taking mirtazapine (Remeron) is very disheartened about a 20-pound weight gain over the past 6 months. The client states, "I stopped taking my antidepressant 5 days ago. I don't want to get depressed again, but I feel awful about my weight." Which of the following responses by the nurse would be *most* therapeutic?

○ 1. "Let's talk about your diet, exercise plan, and daily activities."

○ 2. "Your depression is much better now, so your medication is helping you."

○ 3. "Look at all the positive things that have happened since you've gotten better."

○ 4. "I hear how difficult this is for you and will help you talk with your doctor about it."

35. When developing a teaching plan for a client about the medications prescribed for depression, which of the following components would be *most* important for the nurse to include?

○ 1. Pharmacokinetics of the medication.

○ 2. Current research related to the medication.

○ 3. Management of common side effects.

○ 4. Dosage regulation and adjustment.

36. The client with severe major depression has been taking imipramine (Tofranil) 100 mg PO at bedtime for the past 5 days. To evaluate the therapeutic efficacy of the antidepressant, which of the following would the nurse expect to improve *first*?

○ 1. Suicidal ideation.

○ 2. Agitation.

○ 3. Concentration.

○ 4. Mood.

37. A client who is taking paroxetine (Paxil) 40 mg PO every morning tells the nurse that her mouth "feels like cotton." Which of the following statements by the client would necessitate *further* assessment by the nurse?

○ 1. "I'm sucking on ice chips."

○ 2. "I'm using sugarless gum."

○ 3. "I'm sucking on sugarless candy."

○ 4. "I'm drinking lots of water."

38. A female client whose Axis I diagnosis is major depression with psychotic feature has sleep and appetite disturbances, a flat affect, and psychomotor retardation and is withdrawn. The client has been taking amoxapine (Asendin) 50 mg three times daily for the past 5 days. Which of the following would be *most* important to report to the next shift?

○ 1. The client's speaking about her sins.

○ 2. The client's having a visitor.

○ 3. The client's sleeping from 11 PM to 6 AM.

○ 4. The client's spending the evening in her room.

39. Which of the following would the nurse expect to identify as a good predictor of a client's favorable response to the choice of an antidepressant?

○ 1. The drug's side effect profile.

○ 2. The client's age at diagnosis.

○ 3. The cost of the medication.

○ 4. A favorable response by a family member.

40. For a client with dysthymic disorder, which of the following approaches would the nurse expect to implement?

○ 1. Antidepressant therapy.

○ 2. ECT.

○ 3. Psychotherapeutic approach.
○ 4. Psychoanalysis.

The Client With Bipolar Disorder, Manic Phase

41. The client with an Axis I diagnosis of bipolar disorder, manic phase states to the nurse, "I'm the Queen of England. Bow before me." The nurse interprets this statement as important to document as which of the following areas of the mental status examination?
○ 1. Psychomotor behavior.
○ 2. Mood and affect.
○ 3. Attitude toward the nurse.
○ 4. Thought content.

42. The client is laughing and telling a number of jokes to a group of clients. Suddenly, the client is in tears and talks about a death in the family. A moment later, the client is laughing and joking again. The nurse interprets this behavior as indicative of which of the following?
○ 1. Flat affect.
○ 2. Blunted affect.
○ 3. Labile affect.
○ 4. Normal affect.

43. A client with acute mania exhibits euphoria, pressured speech, and flight of ideas. The client has been talking to the nurse nonstop for 5 minutes and lunch has arrived on the unit. Which of the following would the nurse do *next*?
○ 1. Excuse self while telling the client to come to the dining room for lunch.
○ 2. Tell the client he needs to stop talking because it's time to eat lunch.
○ 3. Do not interrupt the client but wait for him to finish talking.
○ 4. Walk away and approach the client in a few minutes before the food gets cold.

44. A female client with acute mania brings six suitcases and three shopping bags of personal belongings on admission to the unit. On being informed that some of the suitcases and bags will need to be returned home with her husband because of lack of storage space, the client begins to swear and use profanity against the nurse. Which of the following responses by the nurse would be *most* therapeutic?
○ 1. "You are acting very inappropriately."
○ 2. "I will not tolerate your talking to me like that."
○ 3. "Swearing and profanity is unacceptable here."
○ 4. "We don't want to put you in seclusion yet."

45. The husband of a client who is experiencing acute mania and is swearing and using profanity apologizes to the nurse for his wife's behavior. Which of the following replies by the nurse would be most therapeutic?
○ 1. "This must be difficult for you."
○ 2. "It's okay. We've heard worse."
○ 3. "How long has she been like this?"
○ 4. "She needs some medication."

46. The nurse overhears a client with acute mania who is euphoric, flirtatious, and attempts to be sexually inappropriate with other clients talking about a sexual exploit to a group of clients seated at a table. Which of the following would the nurse do *next*?
○ 1. Continue walking down the hall, ignoring the conversation.
○ 2. Speak to the client later in private while saying nothing at this time.
○ 3. Tell the client others may not want to hear about sex, and invite him to play a game of ping-pong.
○ 4. Inform the client that if he continues to talk about sex no one will want to be around him.

47. The client with acute mania states to the nurse, "I'm the prince of peace and can save the world. Those against me will find me and take me to another world. They will come. I know it." The client is beginning to scan the room and starts to repeat his delusion. Which of the following responses by the nurse would be *most* therapeutic?
○ 1. "Describe the people who will come."
○ 2. "The staff and I will protect you."
○ 3. "You are not the prince of peace. Your name is Joe."
○ 4. "Let's walk around the unit for a while."

48. A client with bipolar disorder, manic phase is scheduled for a chest radiograph. Before taking the client to the radiology department, which of the following would be most appropriate for the nurse to do?
○ 1. Give a thorough explanation of the procedure.
○ 2. Explain the procedure in simple terms.
○ 3. Call security to be on standby for possible problems.
○ 4. Cancel the appointment until the client is able to go unescorted.

49. A client exhibiting euphoria, hyperactivity, and distractibility is unable to remain seated at mealtimes long enough to eat an adequate amount of food. When developing the client's plan of care, the nurse anticipates providing the client with "finger food" to eat while moving about the unit. Which of the following foods would the nurse expect to include in the client's plan of care?
○ 1. Bacon, lettuce, and tomato sandwich.
○ 2. Cheeseburger.
○ 3. Ice cream cone.
○ 4. Cut-up vegetables.

50. The client with bipolar disorder, manic phase appears at the nurse's station wearing a transparent shirt, miniskirt, high heels, 10 bracelets, and 8 neck-laces. Her makeup is overdone and she is not wear-ing underwear. A pair of inverted underpants is plopped on her head. Which of the following would be the nurse's *best* response?
    ○ 1. Tell the client to dress appropriately while out of her room.
    ○ 2. Ask the client to put on hospital pajamas until she can dress appropriately.
    ○ 3. Instruct the client to go to her room and change clothes.
    ○ 4. Escort the client to her room and assist with choosing appropriate attire.

51. A client who is diagnosed with bipolar disorder, acute mania, states to the nurse, "Where is my son? I love Lucy. Rain, rain go away. Dogs eat dirt." The nurse interprets these statements as indicating which of the following?
    ○ 1. Echolalia.
    ○ 2. Flight of ideas.
    ○ 3. Neologism.
    ○ 4. Clang associations.

52. The client with mania is skipping up and down the hallway practically running into other clients. Which of the following activities would the nurse expect to include in the client's plan of care?
    ○ 1. Leading a group activity.
    ○ 2. Watching television.
    ○ 3. Reading the newspaper.
    ○ 4. Cleaning the dayroom tables.

53. A client admitted to the unit with bipolar disorder, manic phase is accompanied by his wife. The wife states her husband has been overly energetic and happy, talking constantly, purchasing many unneeded items, and sleeping about 4 hours a night for the past 5 days. When completing the client's daily assessment, the nurse would be especially alert for which of the following findings?
    ○ 1. Exhaustion.
    ○ 2. Vertigo.
    ○ 3. Gastritis.
    ○ 4. Bradycardia.

54. The wife of a client with bipolar disorder, manic phase states to the nurse, "He is acting so crazy. What did he do to get this way?" The nurse bases the response to the client's wife on the understand-ing of which of the following about this disorder?
    ○ 1. It is caused by underlying psychological diffi-culties.
    ○ 2. It is caused by disturbed family dynamics in the client's early life.
    ○ 3. It is the result of an imbalance of chemicals in the brain.

○ 4. It is the result of a genetic inheritance from someone in the family.

55. A client with acute mania has been taking lithium (Lithium Carbonate) 600 mg PO three times daily for 14 days. The nurse analyzes the client's serum lithium level, noting that it is therapeutic when the level is within which of the following ranges?
    ○ 1. 0.5 to 1.5 mEq/L.
    ○ 2. 1.6 to 2.5 mEq/L.
    ○ 3. 2.6 to 3.2 mEq/L.
    ○ 4. 3.3 to 4.0 mEq/L.

56. The client with bipolar disorder, manic phase who is receiving lithium (Lithium Carbonate) 600 mg PO three times daily complains about being thirsty, feel-ing nauseous, and having slight shakiness of the hands. The nurse interprets these findings as indi-cating which of the following?
    ○ 1. An allergic reaction.
    ○ 2. Lithium toxicity.
    ○ 3. Common side effects.
    ○ 4. A drug interaction.

57. The physician orders determination of the serum lithium level tomorrow for a client with bipolar dis-order, manic phase who has been receiving lithium 300 mg PO three times daily for the past 5 days. At which of the following times would the nurse plan to have the blood specimen obtained?
    ○ 1. Before bedtime.
    ○ 2. After lunch.
    ○ 3. Before breakfast.
    ○ 4. During the afternoon.

58. After the nurse teaches a client with bipolar disor-der about lithium therapy, which of the following client statements indicates the need for additional teaching?
    ○ 1. "It's important to keep using a regular amount of salt in my diet."
    ○ 2. "It's okay to double my next dose of lithium if I forget a dose."
    ○ 3. "I should drink about 8 to 10 eight-ounce glasses of water each day."
    ○ 4. "I need to take my medicine at the same time each day."

59. A client with acute mania is to receive lithium (Lithium Carbonate) 600 mg PO three times daily and haloperidol (Haldol) 2 mg PO twice daily. Which of the following would the nurse do?
    ○ 1. Refuse to give the medications as ordered.
    ○ 2. Give the lithium only.
    ○ 3. Request a decreased dosage of lithium.
    ○ 4. Give the medications as ordered.

60. After the nurse teaches a client about bipolar dis-order, which of the following statements indicates that the client has developed insight about her condition?

○ 1. "I enjoy feeling high. I don't need much sleep then and get really creative."

○ 2. "My medicine really helped me. I know I won't need it in about another week."

○ 3. "I'm cured now. I was really wild for a while even though I got into trouble."

○ 4. "I know I'm getting sick when I don't need much sleep and start buying things."

61. During morning community meeting, a client with bipolar disease, manic phase, interrupts others to the point where no one can finish their statements. Which of the following responses by the nurse would be *most* appropriate?

○ 1. "Please stop interrupting others. You can speak when it's your turn."

○ 2. "Stop talking. It's time for you to leave the meeting."

○ 3. "If you can't control yourself, we'll have to take action."

○ 4. "Please behave like an adult. Your behavior is childish."

62. The physician orders valproic acid (Depakene) for a client with bipolar disorder who has achieved limited success with lithium. Which of the following would the nurse anticipate including in the client's medication teaching plan?

○ 1. Follow-up blood tests are unnecessary.

○ 2. The tablet can be crushed if necessary.

○ 3. Drowsiness and upset stomach are common side effects.

○ 4. Consumption of a moderate amount of alcohol is safe.

63. The client with rapid-cycling bipolar disorder who is about to receive the 5 PM dose of carbamazepine (Tegretol) complains of a sore throat and chills. Which of the following would the nurse do *next*?

○ 1. Administer the dose of carbamazepine (Tegretol).

○ 2. Give the client acetaminophen (Tylenol) ordered as PRN.

○ 3. Report the symptoms to the physician in the morning.

○ 4. Call the physician to report the symptoms.

64. A client's wife states, "I don't know what to do sometimes. It's so hard having a husband with a mental illness like bipolar disorder." After talking with the client's wife about her feelings and difficulties, which of the following actions would be *most* appropriate?

○ 1. Suggest that the wife see her physician.

○ 2. Give the wife information about a support group.

○ 3. Recommend that the wife talk with her close friend.

○ 4. Have the wife share her feelings with her husband.

65. The client with bipolar disorder is approaching discharge after being hospitalized with her first episode of acute mania. The client's husband asks the nurse what he can do to help her. Which of the following recommendations for the husband would the nurse anticipate including in the teaching plan?

○ 1. Help the client to be free of worry and anxiety.

○ 2. Communicate openly and offer support.

○ 3. Relieve the client of all responsibilities.

○ 4. Remind the client to control her symptoms.

66. The client with bipolar disorder states to the nurse, "I guess the medication does help me after all. When I stopped taking it, I started to have trouble sleeping and my thoughts were racing." Which of the following replies by the nurse is therapeutic?

○ 1. "I'm happy you realize that you started to get symptoms when you stopped your medication."

○ 2. "Although it took a long time, you finally do understand you need your medication."

○ 3. "Why didn't you go to the community mental health center for help?"

○ 4. "Didn't your family tell you that you were getting sick again?"

67. A client who is acutely manic and very anxious begins to pace, bump into furniture, and preach loudly. Which of the following would be *most* appropriate for the nurse to do?

○ 1. Walk with the client until he calms down.

○ 2. Tell the client to go to his room.

○ 3. Ask the client to sit in on a group therapy session.

○ 4. Administer haloperidol (Haldol) ordered PRN.

68. The client with bipolar disorder, manic phase states, "You're looking good. I'm taking you out to dinner." Which of the following replies by the nurse would be *most* therapeutic?

○ 1. "I don't want to go out to dinner."

○ 2. "I can't go out to dinner with you."

○ 3. "It doesn't matter how I look, the answer is no."

○ 4. "I'm Chris Smith, a nurse working on this unit."

69. After the nurse administers haloperidol (Haldol) 5 mg PO to a client with acute mania, the client refuses to lie down on her bed, runs out on the unit, pushes clients in her vicinity out of the way, and screams threatening remarks to the staff. Which of the following would the nurse do *next*?

○ 1. Follow the client and ask her to calm down.

○ 2. Tell the client to lie down on the sofa in the community room.

○ 3. Seclude and restrain the client.

○ 4. Tell the staff to ignore the client's remarks.

70. As the nurse is turning off the television, a client with bipolar disorder, manic phase says, "I want the TV on so I can watch the late show. I'm not tired and you can't tell me what to do. I want it on!" Which of the following responses by the nurse is *most* therapeutic?
    ○ 1. "I'll let you watch television just this once. Don't tell anyone about this."
    ○ 2. "I'll turn the television off when you get sleepy. Don't ask me to do this again."
    ○ 3. "Television hours are from 7 to 10 PM. It's 10 PM, and the TV goes off so everyone can sleep."
    ○ 4. "The television goes off at 10 PM. I've been telling you this for the past three evenings."

The Client With Suicidal Ideation and Suicide Attempt

71. When developing appropriate assignments for the staff, which of the following clients would the nurse manager judge to be at highest risk for suicide completion?
    ○ 1. An 82-year-old Caucasian man who lives alone after his wife's death.
    ○ 2. A 34-year-old single Hispanic woman who has recently been diagnosed with cancer.
    ○ 3. A 15-year-old African American woman whose boyfriend broke up with her.
    ○ 4. A 52-year-old Asian man who was terminated from his job because of downsizing.

72. When assessing a client for suicidal risk, which of the following methods of suicide would the nurse identify as *most* lethal?
    ○ 1. Aspirin overdose.
    ○ 2. Use of a gun.
    ○ 3. Head-banging.
    ○ 4. Wrist-cutting.

73. The nurse manager overhears two staff members talking in the snack room. One of the staff members states, "Her superficial cuts are just a means of getting our attention. She never should have been admitted. I hope she's out of here soon." Which of the following responses by the nurse manager would be *most* appropriate?
    ○ 1. "It's our job to help her no matter how we feel about her or what she did. She'll be discharged soon."
    ○ 2. "I won't tolerate that kind of discussion from my staff. Now, it is time for you to go back to work."
    ○ 3. "I know it's hard to understand, but we need to do the best we can even though she'll be back."
    ○ 4. "No matter what the intent, all suicidal behavior is serious and deserves our serious consideration."

74. The history of a female client who has just been admitted to the unit and is very depressed reveals a weight loss of 10 pounds in 2 weeks, sleeping 3 hours a night, and poor hygiene. The client states, "I'm no good to anyone. Everyone would be better off without me." Which of the following questions would the nurse ask *first*?
    ○ 1. "What do you mean?"
    ○ 2. "Are you thinking about hurting yourself?"
    ○ 3. "Doesn't your family care about you?"
    ○ 4. "What happened to make you think that?"

75. When developing the plan of care for a client with suicidal ideation, which of the following would the nurse anticipate as the *priority*?
    ○ 1. Self-esteem.
    ○ 2. Sleep.
    ○ 3. Hygiene.
    ○ 4. Safety.

76. Which of the following questions would the nurse use to *best* determine the seriousness of a client's suicidal ideation?
    ○ 1. "Are you planning on harming yourself?"
    ○ 2. "Have you made out a will?"
    ○ 3. "Does your family know you're here?"
    ○ 4. "How long have you been thinking about harming yourself?"

77. The nursing assistant states to the nurse, "My client talks about how awful and useless she is. Sometimes she sounds angry for no reason. I'm tired of listening to her." Which of the following responses by the nurse would be *most* appropriate?
    ○ 1. "I'll switch your assignment to someone who is less depressed and less tiring."
    ○ 2. "It's important for you to listen to her because she needs to verbalize how she is feeling."
    ○ 3. "Don't worry about it. I know you haven't done anything to make her angry."
    ○ 4. "Clients with depression are hard to deal with, but don't take what they say seriously."

78. A client states, "I'm so tired of living and just want to end it all." Which of the following responses would be *most* therapeutic?
    ○ 1. "I'll walk with you to your room so that you can get some rest."
    ○ 2. "Perhaps after your son visits you'll feel better about things."
    ○ 3. "You're in a lot of pain now but you will feel better. I'm here to help you."
    ○ 4. "You are very depressed right now and want to die but you need to focus on life."

79. When developing staff assignments for the unit, the nurse manager would determine that which of the following clients needs one-to-one staff supervision?
    ○ 1. The client who is sometimes preoccupied with death.

○ 2. The client who tries to elope from the unit but is ambivalent about suicide.

○ 3. The client who is impulsive and holds her breath until she faints.

○ 4. The client who is unable to sign a no-harm contract because of hallucinations.

80. A client who was recently discharged from the psychiatric unit, telephones the unit to speak to the nurse. The client states she took her children to the neighbors' house and has turned on the gas to kill herself. She is home alone and gives the nurse her address. Which of the following actions would the nurse do *next*?

○ 1. Refer the caller to a 24-hour suicide hotline.

○ 2. Tell the caller that another nurse will telephone the police.

○ 3. Ask the caller whether she telephoned her physician.

○ 4. Instruct the caller to telephone her family for help.

81. An adolescent walks into the clinic and tells the nurse she wants to die because her boyfriend broke up with her. The client states "I'll show him, he'll be sorry." The nurse interprets the client's statements as an expression of which of the following underlying themes?

○ 1. Loss of self-esteem.

○ 2. Abandonment.

○ 3. Relief of pain.

○ 4. Control.

82. The client has been hospitalized for major depression and suicidal ideation. Which of the following statements indicates to the nurse that the client is improving?

○ 1. "I couldn't kill myself because I don't want to go to hell."

○ 2. "I don't think about killing myself as much as I used to."

○ 3. "I'm of no use to anyone anymore."

○ 4. "I know my kids don't need me anymore since they're grown."

83. The client states to the nurse at the outpatient clinic, "I don't feel ready to go back to work. It's only been a week since I left the hospital." Assessment reveals a flat affect, disheveled appearance, poor posture, and minimal eye contact during interaction. The nurse asks the client whether he is thinking about harming himself. The client tells the nurse he has a loaded revolver at home and will probably use it. Which of the following would the nurse do *next*?

○ 1. Tell the client to go and remove the gun from his home.

○ 2. Ask the client to call the nurse every hour when he gets home.

○ 3. Ask the client to promise not to harm himself.

○ 4. Initiate plans for hospitalization immediately.

84. The widow of a client who successfully completed suicide tearfully says, "I feel guilty because I'm so angry at him for killing himself. It must have been what he wanted." After assisting the widow with dealing with her feelings, which of the following would be *most* helpful?

○ 1. Referring her to group for survivors of suicide.

○ 2. Encouraging her to receiving counseling by a chaplain.

○ 3. Providing her with the local suicide hotline number.

○ 4. Suggesting she receive individual therapy by the nurse.

85. The husband of a client to be discharged from the hospital after an episode of major depression and a suicide attempt asks, "What can I do if she tries to kill herself again?" Which of the following responses would be *most* appropriate?

○ 1. "Don't worry, she'll be okay as long as she takes her medication."

○ 2. "She told me she wants to live so I don't think she'll try again."

○ 3. "Let's talk about some behavioral clues and resources that can help."

○ 4. "Tell her about your concern and just take care of her."

86. A client with depression is exhibiting a brighter affect, ability to attend to hygiene and grooming tasks, and beginning participation in group activities. The nurse asks the client to identify three of her strengths. After much hesitation and thinking, the client is able to state she is usually a nice person, a good cook, and a hard worker. Which of the following would the nurse do *next*?

○ 1. Ask the client to identify an additional three strengths.

○ 2. Volunteer the client to lead the cooking group later in the day.

○ 3. Educate the client about the importance of medication.

○ 4. Praise the client for identifying and sharing her strengths.

87. The friend of a client with depression and suicidal ideation asks the nurse, "How should I act around her?" Which of the following responses by the nurse would be *best*?

○ 1. "Try to cheer her up."

○ 2. "Be caring and genuine."

○ 3. "Control your expressions."

○ 4. "Avoid asking how she's feeling."

88. A client with depression and suicidal ideation voices feelings of self-doubt and powerlessness and is very dependent on the nurse for most aspects of her care.

According to Erickson's stages of growth and development, the nurse determines the client to be manifesting problems in which of the following stages?

○ 1. Trust versus mistrust.
○ 2. Autonomy versus shame/doubt.
○ 3. Initiative versus guilt.
○ 4. Industry versus inferiority.

89. A 68-year-old client has improved with medication and treatment and no longer experiences suicidal ideation. She is able to manage her diabetic care and understands her diet requirements. She will be discharged to live alone in her apartment. Visits by which of the following individuals would be most important for the nurse to arrange before the client's discharge?

○ 1. Psychiatric home care nurse.
○ 2. Medical social worker.
○ 3. Clergy.
○ 4. Unit volunteer.

90. A client who overdosed on barbiturates is being transferred to the inpatient psychiatric unit from the intensive care unit. The nurse receiving the client would anticipate which of the following as a priority?

○ 1. Nutrition.
○ 2. Sleep.
○ 3. Safety.
○ 4. Hygiene.

91. A client is brought to the psychiatric unit from the emergency room escorted by emergency room staff and a security officer. The client's shoulder is bandaged and his arm is in a sling owing to a self-inflicted gunshot wound to his shoulder. Some minutes later, the client's wife follows with a bag of her husband's belongings. Which of the following nursing actions would be *most* appropriate at this time?

○ 1. Tell the wife to take her husband's things home because he is suicidal.
○ 2. Instruct the wife to unpack the bag and put her husband's things in the dresser.
○ 3. Ask the wife whether the bag contains anything dangerous.
○ 4. Inspect the bag and its contents in the presence of the client and his wife.

92. A suicidal client is placed in the seclusion room and given lorazepam (Ativan) because she tried to harm herself by banging her head against the wall. After 10 minutes, the client starts to bang her head against the wall in the seclusion room. Which of the following would the nurse do *next*?

○ 1. Tell the client to stop doing that and act like a responsible adult.
○ 2. Place the client in leather restraints.
○ 3. Call the physician for additional medication orders.

○ 4. Instruct a staff member to sit in the room with the client.

93. A client lives in a group home and visits the community mental health center regularly. During one visit with the nurse, the client states "The voices are telling me to hurt myself again." Which of the following questions by the nurse would be *most* important to ask?

○ 1. "When do you hear the voices?"
○ 2. "Are you going to hurt yourself?"
○ 3. "How long have you heard the voices?"
○ 4. "Why are the voices starting again?"

94. A 20-year-old client diagnosed with paranoid schizophrenia is recovering from his first psychotic break. Before discharge from the hospital, the client becomes depressed and states, "I don't want this illness. I'm about to begin my junior year in college." The nurse determines that the client is planning for the future and is not a risk for self-harm. Which of the following areas would the nurse plan to help the client with in relation to his illness and continuation in college?

○ 1. Disturbed thought processes.
○ 2. Disturbed sensory perception.
○ 3. Communication strategies.
○ 4. Coping abilities.

95. The nurse is teaching unlicensed staff members who are new to the inpatient unit about caring for a client who is suicidal. The nurse determines that additional teaching is needed when which of the following statements is made?

○ 1. "I need to check the client precisely at 15-minute intervals."
○ 2. "Documenting suicide checks is absolutely necessary."
○ 3. "Clients on one-to-one suicide precautions can never be left alone."
○ 4. "All clients using razors must be supervised by staff."

96. Which of the following activities would the nurse recommend to the client who becomes very anxious when thoughts of suicide occur?

○ 1. Watching television.
○ 2. Reading a magazine.
○ 3. Using the exercise bicycle.
○ 4. Meditating.

97. Which of the following amounts would the nurse expect to give a client being treated with imipramine (Tofranil) on an outpatient basis for recurring depression and suicidal ideation?

○ 1. A 30-day supply.
○ 2. A 21-day supply.
○ 3. A 14-day supply.

○ 4. A 2-day supply.

98. The client with recurrent depression and suicidal ideation states to the nurse, "I can't afford this medicine anymore. I know I'll be okay without it." Which of the following would be *most* appropriate for the nurse to do at this time?

○ 1. Inform the physician of the client's statement.

○ 2. Ask the social worker to find assistance for the client.

○ 3. Schedule a follow-up appointment in 3 months.

○ 4. Ask the client whether a family member would help.

Correct Answers and Rationale

The letters in parentheses following the rationale identify the step of the nursing process (A, D, P, I, E) and client needs (1, 2, 3, 4, 5, 6, 7, 8, 9, 10). See the inside front cover for the key.

The Client With Major Depression

1. 4. The nurse must continually assess the client for suicidal ideation because clients with mental health disorders, especially schizophrenia, depression, and alcoholism, are at a higher risk for suicide than the general adult population. Death of psychiatric clients by suicide is of particular importance to the nurse because of the nurse's responsibility for assessment and intervention. Although sleep disturbances, feelings of worthlessness, and difficulty with concentration are associated with major depression, assessment of suicidal ideation is essential. Feelings of worthlessness may contribute to the client's potential for suicidal ideation. (A, 6)

2. 3. Endogenous depression (depression coming from within the person) is biochemical in nature. The biologic theory of depression indicates a neurotransmitter imbalance involving serotonin, norepinephrine, and possibly dopamine. Reactive depression is caused by the occurrence of something happening outside the body, such as the death of a loved one or another significant loss. Stating that the client will improve with the right medication or that family members seem supportive does not address the client's immediate concerns of not knowing the cause of the depression. Discussing possible reasons for the client's depression is nontherapeutic because the depression is endogenous and biochemically based. (I, 6)

3. 2. The nurse should initiate brief, frequent contacts throughout the day to let the client know that he is important to the nurse. This will positively affect the client's self-esteem. The nurse's action conveys acceptance of the client as a worthwhile person and provides some structure to the seemingly monotonous day. Waiting for the client to begin the conversation with the nurse is not helpful because clients who are depressed resist interaction and involvement with others. Sitting outside of the client's room is not productive and not necessary in this situation. If the client were actively suicidal, then a one-on-one client-to-staff assignment would be necessary. Questioning the client until he responds would overwhelm him because he would not be able to meet the nurse's expectations to interact. (I, 6)

4. 1. The most appropriate action is for the nurse to remain with the client even if the client does not engage in conversation with the nurse. A client with severe depression may be unable to engage in an interaction with the nurse because the client feels worthless and lacks the necessary energy to do so. However, the nurse's presence conveys acceptance and caring, thus helping to increase the client's self-worth. Telling the client that the nurse will come back later, stating that the nurse will find someone else for the client to talk with, or telling the client that the nurse will get her something to read conveys to the client that she is not important, reinforcing the client's negative view of herself. Additionally, such statements interfere with the client's development of a sense of security and trust in the nurse. (I, 6)

5. 4. The nurse tells the client that the nurse is interested in her to increase the client's sense of importance, worth, and self-esteem. Also, stating that the nurse wants to help conveys to the client that she is worthwhile and important. Telling the client that the nurse is assigned to care for her is impersonal and implies that the client is being uncooperative. Telling the client that the nurse is there because the client has potential for improvement will not help the client with low self-esteem because most people develop a sense of self-worth through accomplishment. Simply saying that the client has a lot of potential will not convince her that she is worth-while. Telling the client that the nurse will talk to someone else later is not client-focused and does not address the client's question or concern. (A, 6)

6. 2. Nausea and gastrointestinal upset is a common, but usually temporary, side effect of paroxetine (Paxil). Therefore, the nurse would instruct the client to take the medication with food to minimize nausea and stomach upset. Other more common side effects are dry mouth, constipation, headache, dizziness, sweating, loss of appetite, ejaculatory problems in men, and decreased orgasms in women. Taking the medication an hour before breakfast would most likely lead to further gastrointestinal upset. Taking the medication at bedtime is not recommended because Paxil can cause nervousness and interfere with sleep. Because orange juice is acidic, taking the medication with it, especially on an empty stomach, may lead to nausea or increase the client's gastrointestinal upset. (I, 8)

7. 2. Usually, the initial dosage of fluoxetine (Prozac) is 20 mg PO every day. However, lower or less-frequent doses are administered to elderly clients and those hepatic or renal impairment. Typically, elderly clients are prescribed one half of the initial dosage. Therefore, the physician would most likely order 10 mg. (P, 8)

8. 3. Symptom relief can occur during the first week of therapy, with optimal effects possible within 2 weeks. For some clients, 2 to 4 weeks is needed for optimal effects. The client's statement that the depression will be gone in 5 to 7 days indicates to the nurse that clarification and further teaching is needed. Trazodone should be taken after a meal or light snack to enhance its absorption. Trazodone can cause drowsiness, and therefore the major portion of the drug should be taken at bedtime. Trazodone may cause neutropenia and leukopenia. The client should notify the physician of any signs and symptoms of possible infection, such as the flu. (E, 8)

9. 3. The nurse would explain that ECT is a safe treatment and that clients are given an ultra–short-acting anesthetic to induce sleep before the treatment and a muscle relaxant to prevent musculoskeletal complications during the convulsion, which typically lasts 30 to 60 seconds to be therapeutic. Atropine is given before ECT to inhibit salivation and respiratory tract secretions and thereby minimize the risk of aspiration. Medication for pain is not necessary and is not given before or during the treatment. Some clients experience a headache after the treatment and may request and be given an analgesic, such as acetaminophen (Tylenol). Telling the daughter that the physician will ensure that the client does not suffer needlessly would not provide accurate information about ECT. This statement also implies that the client will have pain during the treatment, which is untrue. (I, 8)

10. 4. Reaction formation is a conscious behavior that is the opposite of an unconscious feeling. The client compliments her boss when, unconsciously, she most likely does not like him because he fired her. Repression refers to the unconscious forgetting of painful ideas, events, or conflicts. For example, a car accident victim is currently unable to remember details about the accident but at the time was aware of what had happened. Suppression refers to the voluntary exclusion of anxiety-producing feelings, ideas, and situations from awareness. For example, a client states that he doesn't want to talk about his impending divorce. Intellectualization occurs when the client uses only logical explanations without feelings or an affective component. For example, a client talks about her son's recent bout with leukemia and subsequent death as being mercifully short while at the same time not displaying any signs of sadness. (D, 6)

11. 1. By stating, "It must have been very upsetting for you," the nurse conveys empathy to the client by recognizing the underlying meaning of a painful occurrence. The nurse's statement invites the client to verbalize feelings and thoughts and lets the client know that the nurse is listening to and respects the client. Telling the client to talk about the job disregards the client's feelings and is nontherapeutic for the depressed client because of underlying feelings of worthlessness and guilt that are often present. Telling the client that he will find another job when he is better or that he was probably too depressed to work is inappropriate because it disregards the client's feelings and may promote additional feelings of failure and inadequacy in the client. (I, 6)

12. 2. The client's negative thinking and self-statements are directly related to the psychopathology of depression. The client's views and feelings about herself reflect low self-esteem. Although Impaired Social Interaction, Risk for Self-Directed Violence, and Ineffective Coping are possible nursing diagnoses, there are insufficient data to support these diagnoses. Further assessment is needed to identify supportive data. (D, 6)

13. 4. The client with depression is preoccupied, has decreased energy, and is unable to make decisions, often even simple decisions. Therefore, the nurse presents the situation, "It's time for a shower," and assists the client with personal hygiene to preserve his dignity and self-esteem. Explaining the importance of good hygiene to the client is inappropriate because the client may know the benefits of hygiene but is too fatigued and preoccupied to pay attention to self-care. Asking the client if he is ready for a shower is not helpful because the client with depression often is unable to make even simple decisions. This action also reinforces the client's feeling about not caring about showering. Waiting for the family to visit to help with the client's hygiene is inappropriate and irresponsible on the part of the nurse. The nurse is responsible for making basic decisions for the client until the client is able to make decisions for himself. (I, 6)

14. 4. By saying, "You were able to bathe today," the nurse is pointing out a visible accomplishment or strength, thereby increasing the client's feelings of self-worth and self-esteem. Stating that "everybody around here likes you" or discussing what the client has done correctly is inappropriate because although the client may agree with the nurse, the client still may be depressed. Stating that the nurse sees many good qualities in the client is not helpful because a person's feeling of self-worth is generally determined by accomplishments. Intellectual understanding does not help clients with severe depression. Additionally, the nurse cannot talk a client out of depression because major depression is endogenous and biochemical in nature. Medication should restore the neurotransmitter balance and relieve the depression. (I, 6)

15. 1. The family needs to be informed that some confusion and disorientation will occur as the client emerges from anesthesia immediately after ECT, to lessen their fear and anxiety about the procedure. The nurse will assist the client with reorientation (time, person, and place) and will give clear, simple instructions. Some clients will need to lie down after a treatment because of the effects of the anesthesia. Informing the family that there is a danger of aspiration during ECT is inappropriate and unnecessary information for them. The chances of aspiration occurring during ECT are minimal because food and fluids are withheld for 6 to 8 hours before the treatment. In addition, clients are given atropine to inhibit salivation and respiratory tract secretions. Telling the family that the client will not be able to breathe independently during a treatment may frighten the family unnecessarily. If asked, the nurse should inform the family that the anesthesiologist mechanically ventilates the client with 100% oxygen immediately before the treatment. Clients with severe depression do respond to ECT. Often, ECT is used for those who are severely depressed and not responding to pharmacotherapy and for those who are highly suicidal. (P, 6)

16. 2. Sertraline (Zoloft), like the other selective serotonin reuptake inhibitors (SSRIs), can cause decreased libido and sexual dysfunction such as delay in men and inability to achieve orgasm in women. The SSRIs do not cause weight gain but may cause loss of appetite and weight loss. Dry mouth is a possible side effect, but it is temporary. The client should be told to take sips of water, suck on ice chips, or use sugarless gum or candy. St. John's wort should not be taken with SSRIs because a severe reaction could occur. (E, 8)

17. 3. Involving the client in usual at-home activities provides an opportunity for the client to see how he or she is able to tolerate the home environment with usual activities and interactions with family members. It also gives the client, family, and staff the opportunity to evaluate how the client is able to function at home. This may help determine how soon or whether the client can be discharged to home or to another resource along the continuum of care, such as partial hospitalization or day treatment. Discouraging visitors may not be in the client's best interest because visits with supportive significant others will help reinforce supportive relationships, which are important to the client's self-worth and self-esteem. Providing for a schedule of activities outside the home defeats the purpose of a home visit. Encouraging the client to sleep as much as possible is

nontherapeutic and promotes withdrawal from others. It also defeats the purpose of the home visit. (P, 6)

18. 4. Medication management with outpatient follow-up is of vital importance to discuss with the client before discharge. The nurse teaches and clarifies any questions related to medication and outpatient treatment. The client also has the opportunity to voice feelings related to medication and treatment. The goal is to assist the client in making a successful transition from hospital to home with optimal functioning outside the hospital for as long as possible. The nurse may also need to assist with decreasing any anxiety the client may have related to discharge. Discussing future plans for returning to work or employment is not as immediate a concern as assisting with medication and treatment compliance. Noncompliance with medication is a primary cause of relapse in clients with psychiatric disorders. Reviewing a conflict the client had encountered with another client is not appropriate or therapeutic at this time unless the client brings it to the nurse's attention. The conflict should have been dealt with and resolved at the time it occurred. Reviewing the results of psychological testing is the responsibility of the physician if the physician chooses to do so. (P, 6)

19. 2. Criteria for commitment include being gravely disabled and posing a harm to self or others. This client is not threatening to harm himself in the form of suicide or to harm others. The client is gravely disabled because of his inability to care for himself—namely, not eating because of his delusion. Evidence of psychosis or psychotic symptoms or diagnosis of a mental illness alone does not make the client legally eligible for commitment. (E, 6)

20. 3. The client needs to be informed of the time lag involved with antidepressant therapy. Although improvement in the client's symptoms will occur gradually over the course of 1 to 2 weeks, typically it takes 2 to 4 weeks to get the full effects of the medication. This information will help the client be compliant with medication and will also help in decreasing any anxiety the client has about not feeling better. The client's dose may not need to be increased; it is too early to determine the full effectiveness of the drug. Additionally, such a statement may increase the client's anxiety and diminish self-worth. Telling the client to wait a few days discounts the client's feelings and is inappropriate. Although it is indeed too soon to tell whether the medication will be effective, telling this to the client may cause the client undue distress. This type of statement is somewhat negative because it leaves the door open for the possibility that the medication will not be effective, possibly further compounding the client's anxiety about not feeling better. (I, 8)

21. 2. Phenelzine (Nardil) is a monoamine oxidase inhibitor (MAOI). MAOIs block the enzyme monoamine oxidase, which is involved in the decomposition and inactivation of norepinephrine, serotonin, dopamine, and tyramine (a precursor to the previously stated neurotransmitters). Foods high in tyramine—those that are fermented, pickled, aged, or smoked—must be avoided because, when they are ingested in combination with MAOIs, a hypertensive crisis will occur. Some examples include salami, bologna, dried fish, sour cream, yogurt, aged cheeses, bananas, pickled herring, yogurt, sour cream, caffeinated beverages, chocolate, licorice, beer, Chianti, and alcohol-free beer. The client also needs to avoid caffeinated beverages, chocolate, and licorice. (I, 8)

22. 4. The nurse would first take the client's vital signs, because the client could be experiencing a hypertensive crisis, which requires prompt intervention. Signs and symptoms of a hypertensive crisis include occipital headache, stiff or sore neck, nausea, vomiting, sweating, dilated pupils and photophobia, nosebleed, tachycardia, bradycardia, and constricting chest pain. Giving this client an analgesic without taking the vital signs first would be inappropriate. Once the client's vital signs have been obtained, then the nurse would call the physician to report the client's complaints and vital signs. Administering the client's next dose of phenelzine before taking the vital signs could result in a dangerous situation if the client is experiencing a hypertensive crisis. (I, 8)

23. 2. Clients who are depressed often are not interested in eating because of the psychopathology of the disorder. Therefore, the nurse must take responsibility to ensure that the client eats, including spoon-feeding the client (placing the food on the spoon, putting the food near the client's mouth, and asking the client to eat) if necessary. Serving the client her tray in the room does not ensure that the client will eat. Calling the family to bring the client food from home usually is allowed, but it is still the nurse's responsibility to ensure that the client eats. Explaining the importance of nutrition in recovery is not helpful. The client may intellectually know that eating is important but may not be interested in eating or want to eat. (P, 6)

24. 1. To promote adequate rest (6 to 8 hours per night) and to eliminate hypersomnia and hyposomnia, the nurse should sit with the client at the bedside until the medication takes effect. The presence of a caring nurse provides the client with comfort and security and helps to decrease the client's anxiety. Engaging the client in interaction until the client falls asleep, reading to the client, or encouraging the client to watch television may be too stimulating for the client, consequently increasing rather than decreasing the client's restlessness. (I, 7)

25. 3. The client who verbalizes feeling in control of self and situations no longer feels powerless to affect an outcome but realizes that one's actions can have an impact on self and situations. It is common for clients with depression to feel powerless to affect an outcome and to feel a lack of control over a situation. Although interacting with staff and peers is a positive action, the client could be conversing in a negative or nontherapeutic manner. Sleeping 4 hours in the afternoon and 4 hours at night is evidence of symptomatology and not indicative of improvement or recovery. Verbalizing dissatisfaction over not being able to perform at work indicates that the client is most likely focusing on shortcomings and powerlessness. (E, 6)

26. 2. The nurse must monitor the client for a suicide attempt at this time when the client is starting to feel better, because the depressed client may now have enough energy to carry out an attempt. Bupropion (Wellbutrin) inhibits dopamine reuptake; it is an activating antidepressant and could cause agitation. Although bupropion lowers the seizure threshold for all clients, especially at doses greater than 450 mg/day, and visual disturbances and increased libido are possible side effects, the nurse must closely monitor the client for suicide attempt. As the client with major depression begins to feel better, the client may have enough energy to carry out an attempt. (A, 8)

27. 4. In the initial plan of care, the most appropriate outcome would be that the client will interact with the nurse. First, the client would begin interacting with one individual, the nurse. The nurse would gradually assist the client to engage in interactions with other clients in one-on-one contacts, progressing toward informal group gatherings and eventually taking part in structured group activities. The client needs to experience success according to the client's level of tolerance. Initiating interactions with peers occurs when the client is able to gain a measure of confidence and self-esteem instead of feeling intimidated or unduly anxious. Discussing adaptive coping techniques is an outcome the client may be able to reach when symptoms are not as severe and the client is able to concentrate on improving coping skills. (P, 6)

28. 3. Imipramine, a tricyclic antidepressant, in combination with alcohol will produce additive central nervous system depression. Although caffeinated coffee is safe to use when the client is taking imipramine, it is not recommended for a client with depression who may be experiencing sleep disturbances. Imipramine may cause photosensitivity so the client would be instructed to use sunscreen and protective clothing when exposed to the sun. Reduced lacrimation may occur as a side effect of imipramine (Tofranil). Therefore, the use of artificial tears may be recommended. (P, 8)

29. 1. Telling the client that ECGs are done routinely for all clients taking imipramine, a tricyclic antidepressant, is an honest and direct response. Additionally, it provides some reassurance for the client. Often a client with depression will ruminate, leading needlessly to increased anxiety. Tricyclic antidepressants may cause tachycardia, ECG changes, and cardiotoxicity. Telling the client that it's probably a precautionary measure because the nurse is not aware of a cardiac condition instills doubt and may cause undue anxiety for the client. Telling the client not to worry because the doctor is very thorough dismisses the client's concern and does not give the client adequate information. Explaining that the client had an ECG before initiating therapy with imipramine and that the procedure will be the same does not answer the client's question and is not focused on the client's inquiry. (I, 8)

30. 2. The therapeutic serum concentration level for imipramine is 151 to 250 mg/mL. At the upper limit of the therapeutic range, serious cardiac and central nervous system effects may begin to develop. (D, 8)

31. 4. Anticholinergic effects, which result from blockage of the parasympathetic (craniosacral) nervous system, include urine retention, blurred vision, dry mouth, and constipation. Tremors, cardiac arrhythmias, and sexual dysfunction are possible side effects, but they are caused by increased norepinephrine availability. Sedation and delirium are not anticholinergic effects. Sedation may be a therapeutic effect, because many clients with depression experience agitation and insomnia. Delirium, typically not a side effect, would indicate toxicity, especially in an elderly client. Respiratory depression, convulsions, ataxia, agitation, stupor, and coma are indicative of tricyclic antidepressant toxicity. (A, 8)

32. 2. Doxepin (Sinequan) and other tricyclic antidepressants may cause orthostatic hypotension, especially in the morning. Orthostatic hypotension occurs because the tricyclic antidepressant inhibits the body's natural vasoconstrictive reaction when a person stands. The nurse regularly monitors the client's vital signs, both lying and standing. The nurse should instruct the client to rise slowly and dangle the feet before standing. Advising the client to take a hot shower is detrimental to the client's safety. Heat causes vasodilation, which could further exacerbate the dizziness, placing the client at risk for falls and subsequent injury. Telling the client to stay in bed until feeling better is not helpful and is impractical. The client with depression would rather stay in bed and withdraw from others. Placing the client on fluid restriction is detrimental to the client

with depression whose fluid and food intake may be inadequate. (P, 8)

33. 1. The nurse would give the medication as ordered. Mirtazapine (Remeron) is given once daily, preferably at bedtime to minimize the risk for injury resulting from orthostatic hypotension and sedative effects. Usual dosage ranges from 15 to 45 mg. There is no reason to question the physician's order. The nurse should administer the medication as ordered. Requesting to give the medication in three divided doses is inappropriate and demonstrates the nurse's lack of knowledge about the drug. (I, 8)

34. 4. Stating, "I hear how difficult this is for you and will help you talk with your doctor about it," conveys empathy and is focused on the client's request. Offering to talk to the physician with the client lends support and forms a therapeutic alliance with the client. The client who has stopped taking medication must be taken seriously, because medication noncompliance is an issue here and could result in a recurrence of symptoms of depression, leading to a variety of adverse effects. Discussing the client's diet, exercise, and daily activities may not be helpful at this point, because the client has stopped taking the medication. Pointing out that the medication has helped the client or telling the client that positive things have happened since the depression improved may be true, but these responses do not focus on the client's feelings and needs at the present time. (I, 6)

35. 3. Compliance with medication therapy is crucial for the client with depression. Medication noncompliance is the primary cause of relapse among psychiatric clients in the community. Therefore, the nurse needs to teach the client about managing common side effects to promote compliance with medication. Teaching the client about the medication's pharmacokinetics may help the client to understand the reason for the drug. However, teaching about how to manage common side effects to promote compliance is crucial. Current research about the medication is of more importance to the nurse than to the client. Teaching about dosage regulation and adjustment of medication may be helpful, but typically the physician, not the client, is the person in charge of this aspect. (P, 8)

36. 2. Client manifestations such as sleep, appetite, or psychomotor disturbances (eg, agitation and anxiety) would improve first with pharmacologic therapy. Cognitive symptoms of depression, such as low self-esteem, guilt, pessimism, suicidal thought, lack of concentration, and indecision tend to improve more slowly. Disturbances in the client's ability to concentrate take longer to improve. The client's depressed mood may be the last symptom to demonstrate improvement. (E, 8)

37. 4. Dry mouth is a common, temporary side effect of paroxetine. The nurse needs to further assess the client's water intake when the client states she is drinking lots of water. Excessive intake of water could be harmful to the client and could lead to electrolyte imbalance. Dry mouth is caused by the medication, and drinking a lot of water will not eliminate it. Sucking on ice chips or using sugarless gum is appropriate to ease the discomfort of dry mouth associated with paroxetine. (E, 8)

38. 3. The most important behavior to report to the next shift is that the client was able to sleep from 11 PM to 6 AM. This indicates that improvement in the symptoms of depression is occurring as a result of the pharmacologic therapy. The nurse would expect to observe improvement in sleep, appetite, and psychomotor behavior first, before improvement in cognitive symptoms such as speaking about her sins. The fact that the client had a visitor is not as important as changes in the client's behavior. Spending the evening in the room is a continuation of the client's withdrawn behavior and is important to report but not as important as the improvement in sleep. (E, 6)

39. 4. A favorable response by a family member to a medication and a history of prior response to medication are good predictors of a favorable client response to a medication because the illness is genetic and hereditary. Although the side effects of the drug, the client's age at diagnosis, and the cost of the medication are important factors to consider when choosing antidepressant therapy, this information does not necessarily predict how a client will respond to a specific drug. (A, 8)

40. 3. Dysthymia is a less severe, chronic depression diagnosed when a client has had a depressed mood for more days than not over a period of at least 2 years. Clients with dysthymic disorders benefit from psychotherapeutic approaches that assist the client in reversing the negative self-image, negative feelings about the future, and poor self-esteem that are typically part of the clinical presentation. Antidepressant therapy usually is not prescribed for the client with dysthymic disorder unless the client experiences an episode of major depression. ECT is appropriate treatment for severe depression, not dysthymic disorder. Psychoanalysis is an inappropriate treatment for dysthymic disorders. (P, 6)

The Client With Bipolar Disorder, Manic Phase

41. 4. The client's statement, "I'm the Queen of England. Bow before me," is an example of a grandiose delusion and refers to thought content of the mental status examination. Examples of psychomotor behavior to be documented would include excited, often exaggerated and repetitive physical movements and excessive talking and gesturing. Mood is a subjective feeling state, and affect is an observable expression of emotion. Mood is what a client tells you he or she is feeling, and affect is what you see the client feeling. For example, the client may state that she feels sad or happy in reference to mood. Affect refers to the display of physical emotion, often described as "appropriate" or "flat." Attitude toward the nurse refers to the client's behavior in the presence of the nurse during the mental status examination (eg, pleasant and cooperative, irritable and guarded). (D, 6)

42. 3. The client is exhibiting a labile affect or an affect that quickly changes (eg, from happy to sad). A flat affect refers to an absence of facial expression or an expression that does not change even though the topic of what the client is verbalizing changes. An example would be a client maintaining a flat affect or absence of expression while talking about a party, a television show, and a sad event. A blunted affect is an incomplete expression. For example, the corner of the mouth can indicate a hint of a smile. Normal affect is one that changes appropriately with the topic of conversation. (D, 6)

43. 1. The nurse would excuse himself or herself, showing respect and regard for the client, while telling the client to come to the dining room for lunch. Acutely manic clients need clear, concise comments and directions. Telling the client that he needs to stop talking because it's lunchtime is disrespectful and does not give the client directions for what he needs to do. Using the familiar skill of waiting without interrupting until the person pauses would not be effective with the very talkative, manic client. Walking away and approaching the client after a few minutes before the food gets cold is not helpful because the client would probably continue talking. (I, 6)

44. 3. By stating to the client, "Swearing and profanity is unacceptable here," the nurse is setting limits in a nonpunitive manner for behavior that is inappropriate or threatening to clients and staff. Setting limits helps the client regain self-control, prevents alienation from others, and preserves self-esteem. It is common for the irritable manic client to misperceive the nurse's and other's statements and intentions, feel threatened, and respond in a manner that is out of character for the client when not in a manic phase. Stating that the client is acting very inappropriately or that the nurse will not tolerate the client's swearing and profanity, or threatening to put the client in seclusion, is threatening and punitive and thus nontherapeutic. (I, 6)

45. 1. Stating that this must be difficult for the husband conveys empathy and understanding and offers him the opportunity to voice his feelings to the nurse. Telling the husband that it is okay and that the nurse has heard worse is inappropriate and minimizes the impact of the wife's illness on the husband. Asking about the length of the client's illness or telling the husband that his wife needs some medication ignores the husband's feelings, thereby minimizing his self-respect. (I, 6)

46. 3. Telling the client that others may not want to hear about sex and inviting him to play a game of ping-pong with the nurse informs the client that even though his behavior is unacceptable, the nurse considers him worthy of help. The client's thoughts and action are out of control, and directing him to an activity with the nurse is an appropriate way of regaining control. The nurse is responsible for providing safety and security to this client and others on the unit. Continuing to walk down the hall while ignoring the conversation does nothing to meet the needs of this or other clients. Doing so also diminishes trust in the nurse. Speaking to the client later in private while saying nothing at the time allows the client to continue his provocative behavior instead of focusing his energy toward productive activity. Informing the client that if he continues to talk about sex, no one will want to be around him is not helpful because his behavior is a symptom of his illness and the statement diminishes his self-worth. (I, 6)

47. 4. The nurse suggests an activity such as walking around the unit to distract the client from the paranoid grandiose delusion that could result in loss of control. This action interrupts the client's anxious state and helps to redirect energy and focus on an activity based in reality. The focus must be on the underlying need or feeling of the delusion and not on the content. Asking the client to describe the people who will come challenges the client and forces the client to cling to the delusion. Stating that the nurse and staff will protect the client conveys agreement with the client's belief system, reinforcing the client's delusion. Telling the client that he is not the prince of peace and repeating his name challenges the client and his present belief system. Doing so may lead to decreased trust in the nurse and an aggressive client response, or it may force the client to defend his beliefs. (I, 6)

48. 2. The nurse needs to explain the procedure in simple terms, because the client in a manic phase has difficulty concentrating, is easily distracted, and can misinterpret what the nurse states. Giving a thorough explanation of the procedure is not helpful and can confuse the client. Calling security to be on standby is inappropriate. If the nurse judges that the client might elope or become agitated, the nurse would schedule the appointment for another time. Canceling the appoint-

ment until the client can go unescorted is impractical and may not be in keeping with unit or hospital policy and the client's treatment plan. (I, 6)

49. 2. The nurse needs to provide the client who is unable to sit long enough to eat adequate amounts of "finger foods," or food that can be held and eaten while moving. High-protein and high-carbohydrate foods such as a cheeseburger or a peanut butter sandwich are best for the hyperactive client to help maintain body weight. A bacon, lettuce, and tomato sandwich would not provide the client with adequate protein and carbohydrates. Additionally, this type of sandwich is difficult to carry around and can be dropped easily. An ice cream cone, although high in calories, would not provide the client with adequate protein. Cut-up vegetables are a poor selection because, although they are high in vitamins, they are low in protein, which is necessary for building and repairing body cells and tissues, and low in carbohydrates, which are needed for energy. (P, 7)

50. 4. The nurse escorts the client to her room and assists with choosing appropriate attire to preserve the client's dignity and self-esteem and prevent ridicule from others on the unit. It is common for a client with bipolar disorder, manic phase to exhibit poor judgment, provocative behavior, and hyperactivity. The client in the manic phase often dresses inappropriately and changes clothes many times throughout the day. The nurse needs to assist the client with hygiene, grooming, and proper attire until her judgment improves. Telling the client to dress appropriately while out of her room may be perceived by the client as an attack. Additionally, the client may be incapable of making that decision. Asking the client to put on hospital pajamas until she can dress appropriately is punitive and demeaning. Because of the client's cognitive difficulties, the client may not understand the instructions to go to her room to change clothes. Additionally, the client may become distracted by stimuli on the unit and may not reach her room. (I, 6)

51. 2. Flight of ideas is a speech pattern of rapid transition from topic to topic, often without finishing one idea. It is common in mania. Echolalia refers to the repetition of words heard. For example, when the nurse states, "It is time for bed," the client responds, "Bed, bed, bed, bed." Neologism is a word invented by the client. For example, the client states, "The beefocles are brewing." Clang associations is the use of rhyming words. For example, the client states, "Let's eat lunch, bunch, munch, crunch." (D, 6)

52. 4. The client with mania is very active and needs to have this energy channeled in a constructive task such as cleaning or tidying the dayroom. Because the client is distracted easily and can concentrate only for short

periods, the successful completion of a helpful task would give the nurse the opportunity to thank the client for the help, thereby enhancing the client's self-esteem. Leading a group activity is too stimulating for the client. Participating in this type of activity also would probably cause the client to be disruptive. Watching television or reading the newspaper would be inappropriate for the client who is unable to sit for a period of time. (P, 6)

53. 1. Clients in the manic phase experience insomnia, as evidenced by the client's sleeping only for about 4 hours for the past 5 days. Clients experiencing an acute mania episode are not capable of judging the need for sleep. Therefore, the nurse would need to assess the amount of rest the client is receiving daily to prevent exhaustion. The development of vertigo, gastritis, or bradycardia typically does not result from acute mania. (A, 6)

54. 3. Bipolar disorder is a biochemical disorder caused by an imbalance of neurotransmitters in the brain. Manic episodes seem to be related to excessive levels of nor-epinephrine, serotonin, and dopamine. Psychopharmacologic therapy aims to restore the balance of neurotransmitters. In the past, it was thought that bipolar disorder may have been caused by early psychodynamics or disturbed families, but the current view emphasizes the role of biology. Bipolar disorder could be genetic or inherited from someone in the family, but it is best for the client and family to understand the disease concept related to neurotransmitter imbalance. This understanding also helps them to refrain from placing blame on anyone. Siblings and close relatives have a higher incidence of bipolar disorder and mood disorders in general when compared with the general population. (D, 6)

55. 1. It takes 10 to 21 days to achieve a lithium level within the therapeutic range. During an acute manic episode, the normal therapeutic range is 0.5 to 1.5 mEq/L and the maintenance margin is 0.6 to 1.2 mEq/L. With a level of 1.6 to 3.2 mEq/L, the client would be exhibiting signs and symptoms of toxicity. A level of 3.3 to 4.0 mEq/L is extremely high and toxic. (D, 8)

56. 3. Lithium is associated with some common side effects including thirst, nausea, mild hand tremors, dry mouth, headache, and taste distortion. These side effects usually are transient, subsiding in approximately 6 weeks. An allergic reaction may be manifested by headache, fever, or rash. If the reaction is severe, signs and symptoms of anaphylaxis occur. Lithium toxicity is manifested by coarse hand tremors, vomiting, diarrhea, sedation, muscle weakness, vertigo, blurred

vision, and dilute urine. The symptoms described do not indicate a drug interaction. The client is taking only lithium. Drug interactions (eg, thiazide diuretics) could increase the risk of toxicity by decreasing renal clearance of lithium. (D, 8)

57. 3. Because lithium reaches peak blood levels in 1 to 3 hours, blood specimens for serum lithium concentration determinations are usually drawn before the first dose of lithium in the morning (which is usually 8 to 12 hours after the previous dose) or before breakfast. Stat lithium levels can be drawn at any time, usually when toxicity is suspected. (P, 8)

58. 2. The therapeutic and toxic range of lithium is very narrow. If the client forgets to take a scheduled dose of lithium, the client needs to wait until the next scheduled time to take it, because taking twice the amount of lithium can cause lithium toxicity. The client needs to maintain a regular diet and regular salt intake. Lithium and sodium are eliminated from the body through the kidneys. An increase in salt intake leads to decreased plasma lithium levels as lithium is excreted more rapidly. A decrease in salt intake leads to increased plasma lithium levels. The client needs to drink 8 to 10 eight-ounce glasses of water daily to maintain fluid balance and decrease thirst. Decreased water intake can lead to an increase in the lithium level, and consequently a risk for toxicity. Lithium must be taken on a regular basis at the same time each day to ensure maximum therapeutic effect. (E, 8)

59. 4. Lithium commonly is combined with an antipsychotic agent such as haloperidol (Haldol) or a benzodiazepine such as lorazepam (Ativan). Antipsychotic agents such as haloperidol (Haldol) are prescribed to produce a neuroleptic effect until the lithium, which has a clinical response lag time of 1 to 2 weeks, produces a clinical response. Once a clinical response is achieved, the antipsychotic agent usually is discontinued. Additionally, the dosages of each drug listed are appropriate. Therefore, the nurse would administer the drugs as ordered. (E, 8)

60. 4. The client's statement, "I know I'm getting sick when I don't need much sleep and start buying things," indicates insight into her illness because the client recognizes symptoms that can lead to relapse. The statement, "I enjoy feeling high; I don't need much sleep then and get really creative," gives no indication that the client recognizes the detrimental effects of bipolar disorder. The statements about not needing medicine in another week or being cured indicate the client's lack of understanding about the chronicity of the disorder. Clients are not cured from bipolar disorder, but symptoms of the disorder are usually managed when the clients are stabilized on medication. Medication may be needed by clients for many years or throughout their lives. (E, 6)

61. 1. For this client, the nurse needs to set limits on the client's intrusive, interruptive behavior by saying, "Please stop interrupting others; you can speak when it's your turn." This statement also clearly points out to the client the specific behavior that is unacceptable. The nurse helps the client to attain control and helps the other clients become more tolerant of the situation. Saying "Stop talking; it's time for you to leave the meeting," is not helpful because it leaves the client unaware of what has happened or the behavior that is unacceptable. Also, such a statement may seem punitive. The statement, "If you can't control yourself, we'll have to take action," is threatening to the client and diminishes the client's self-worth. Using the statement, "Please behave like an adult, your behavior is childish," is demeaning and scolding to the client, thereby diminishing the client's self-esteem. (I, 6)

62. 3. Valproic acid (Depakene), an anticonvulsant agent, is used as a mood stabilizer in clients with bipolar disorder. Common side effects include drowsiness and gastrointestinal upset. The client needs to be cautioned not to drive or perform tasks requiring alertness and to take the medication with food or milk or eat small frequent meals. Blood tests are required to evaluate the serum level (usually 50 to 100 μg/mL) and to check for possible hematologic effects. Depakene can cause changes in liver function and blood dyscrasias. The tablet must be swallowed whole and not chewed or crushed, to prevent irritation of the mouth and throat. Alcohol as well as over-the-counter drugs and sleep-inducing agents must be avoided to prevent oversedation. (P, 8)

63. 4. The nurse would call the physician to report symptoms of a sore throat, fever, and chills, because these symptoms may be signs of serious adverse effects of the medication, including potentially fatal hematologic, cardiovascular, and hepatic complications. Giving the dose of carbamazepine (Tegretol) would be contraindicated in this situation. Giving the acetaminophen (Tylenol) ordered PRN would be inappropriate and potentially detrimental to the client's health. Waiting until morning to report the client's symptoms would be a serious error in judgment. (I, 8)

64. 2. The nurse's most appropriate action would be to give the wife information about a support group in her area. The National Alliance for the Mentally Ill (NAMI) has affiliates in every state and many locales. NAMI has separate groups for consumers and family members and offers a 12-week program for family members or caregivers called "Family to Family." The program is psychoeducational in nature, and participants learn, share, and support each other. Family members need

and want education and support. Suggesting that the wife see a physician is not necessary in this situation. She needs support and education. Recommending that she talk with her close friend may be helpful if she so chooses. However, this is not as helpful as attending a support group. Here the wife can learn, share, obtain support from, and provide support to others with similar situations. Having the wife share her feelings with her husband may or may not be appropriate or helpful to her or her husband. The husband may be unable to help his wife with adaptive coping, and therefore the client's self-esteem could be diminished. (I, 6)

65. 2. The nurse would encourage the husband to support and communicate openly with his wife to maintain effective family-client interactions. During any illness, open communication and support helps the relationship between husband and wife. It is unrealistic for any individual to be free of anxiety or worry and impossible for the husband to be able to control what his wife may think or feel. Relieving the client of all responsibilities is unrealistic and not helpful. The client needs to resume activities as soon as she can manage them. Reminding his wife to control her symptoms is not appropriate and indicates that the husband needs further teaching about this condition. (P, 6)

66. 1. The statement, "I'm happy you realize that you started to get symptoms when you stopped your medication" praises the client for realistic self-appraisal and development of insight. Positive reinforcement by the nurse strengthens insight and promotes good judgment in the client. The statements, "Although it took a long time, you finally do understand you need your medication" and "Why didn't you go to the community mental health center for help?" blame the client and diminish the client's self-worth. When clients begin to experience symptoms of relapse, they may not realize what is happening to them and may not have the judgment to seek help at that time. The statement, "Didn't your family tell you that you were getting sick again?" blames the family and makes an unfair assumption. (I, 6)

67. 4. The nurse should administer the haloperidol ordered as PRN to the acutely manic and anxious client to help calm him and reduce the risk of violent or destructive behavior. The manic client is beginning to exhibit behaviors that may escalate and lead to loss of control, thereby causing the client to be a danger to self or others. Walking with the client is not helpful, because his current anxiety is too high and his pacing is not helping him. Telling the client to go to his room is not helpful, because the client is exhibiting a high level of anxiety and hyperactivity and will be unable to stay in his room. Asking the client to sit in on a group therapy session is not helpful because the client is unable to sit for a period of time. The client would be disruptive to the members of the group and his behavior could lead to increased anxiety in the other clients. (I, 6)

68. 4. The nurse should state his or her name and purpose on the unit to clarify his or her identity and to counteract other beliefs the client may have. Stating that the nurse doesn't want to or can't go out to dinner is not therapeutic because it fails to clarify the client's misperceptions or erroneous beliefs, as is the statement, "It doesn't matter how I look, the answer is no." (I, 6)

69. 3. The client is visibly out of control, and other measures have not helped. Therefore, the nurse needs to seclude and restrain the client to protect the client and others from harm. Following the client and asking her to calm down or telling the client to lie down on the sofa is not helpful, because the client's level of anxiety is too high for her to attempt to calm down on her own and she cannot control her behavior. Telling the staff to ignore the client's remarks is not helpful because the client needs external means of control to protect the client, other clients on the unit, and the staff. Safety is the priority. (I, 6)

70. 3. When the client in a manic state attempts to manipulate the nurse or demands privileges, the nurse must restate the unit rules in a calm and matter-of-fact manner. "The television hours are from 7 to 10 PM. It is 10 PM, and the TV goes off so everyone can sleep" is the *most* therapeutic response because it restates the rules and is nonthreatening. During a manic phase, the client is impulsive and has difficulty concentrating. The client needs consistency and structure from the staff. The statement, "I'll let you watch television just this once; don't tell anyone about this," allows the client to manipulate the nurse, as does "I'll turn the television off when you get sleepy; don't ask me to do this again." In addition, the last portion of the statement is a threat. The statement, "The television goes off at 10 PM; I've been telling you this for the past three evenings," is inappropriate because it is authoritative and demeaning to the client. (I, 6)

The Client With Suicidal Ideation and Suicide Attempt

71. 1. High-risk factors that have been related to suicide include hopelessness, Caucasian race, male gender, advanced age, living alone, prior suicide attempts, family history of suicide attempts, family history of substance abuse, general medical illnesses, psychosis, and substance abuse. Psychiatric diagnosis is considered to be the most reliable factor for suicide, especially for those with depression, schizophrenia, and substance disorders. Therefore, an 82-year-old Caucasian male who lives alone after his wife's death is at high risk for suicide completion. (D, 1)

72. 2. A crucial factor in determining the lethality of a method is the amount of time that occurs between initiating the method and the delivery of the lethal impact of the method. Lethal methods of suicide include using a gun, jumping from a high place, hanging, drowning, carbon monoxide poisoning, and overdose with certain drugs such as central nervous system depressants, alcohol and barbiturates. The more detailed the suicide plan, the more lethal and accessible the method, and the more effort that is exerted to block rescue, the greater the chance is for the suicide to be completed. Impulsive attempts at suicide even with rescuers in sight may be lethal depending on the method. Methods that are less likely to be lethal include wrist cutting and overdosing on aspirin. Head-banging is a self-injurious behavior that requires intervention and is not to be taken lightly; however, it is not considered a lethal method of suicide. (A, 6)

73. 4. The statement, "No matter what the intent, all suicide behavior is serious and deserves our serious consideration," is most appropriate because it provides some information for the staff. Certain suicide attempts may be termed suicide gestures to receive attention, not to accomplish self-destruction. Nevertheless, they still are a cry for help and may indicate ambivalence about dying. Clients have accidentally and unintentionally killed themselves because prior attempts were not taken seriously, they acted on impulse, or rescue attempts were foiled. Stating, "It's our job to help her no matter how we feel about her or what she did; she'll be discharged soon" is inappropriate because it does not provide the staff members with information to gain insight about the client's problem. Stating, "I won't tolerate that kind of discussion from my staff; now it is time for you to go back to work" is authoritarian and punitive. Additionally it does not help the staff members gain insight. Stating, "I know it's hard to understand, but we need to do the best we can even though she'll be back" voices agreement with the staff's misperception and lack of knowledge. As such, this statement would be inappropriate. (I, 1)

74. 2. On hearing the client's statement, the nurse must ask the client directly if she plans to kill herself. It is erroneous to think that talking to clients about suicide will drive them to it. Asking directly about suicidal intent is absolutely necessary. Often doing so provides clients with a sense of relief. In addition, the nurse conveys concern for and a sense of worth to the client, thus enabling appropriate planning for care. Asking "What do you mean?" is an indirect method of inquiry that provides the client with the opportunity to evade the nurse's intent. Asking, "Doesn't your family care about

you?" shows poor judgment on the nurse's part and is demeaning to the client. Asking, "What happened to make you think that?" conveys a lack of knowledge of psychopathology. (I, 6)

75. 4. For the client with suicidal ideation, client safety is the priority. The nurse protects the client from self-harm or self-destruction. Although self-esteem, sleep, and hygiene are common areas that require intervention for a client with suicidal ideation, ensuring the client's safety is the most immediate and serious concern. (P, 2)

76. 1. To determine the seriousness of the suicidal ideation, the nurse must ask directly about the intent and the plan. The nurse needs to determine whether the client has a concrete plan and will act on his thoughts. Then the nurse assesses the lethality of the method, immediacy, means to complete suicide, and possibility of rescue. Asking the client, "Have you made out a will?" is not as important and does not necessarily imply that he is planning self-harm. Many individuals have made out wills without planning self-harm. Asking the client, "Does your family know you're here?" provides no information about the client's intent and plan. Asking the client, "How long have you been thinking about harming yourself?" does provide information that the client is thinking about self-harm. However, it does not provide information about the client's intent and plan. (A, 6)

77. 2. The nurse's best response is to teach the nursing assistant about the appropriate intervention and why it is important for the client. Staff members need to be client-focused and to understand why a specific intervention is important and appropriate. Telling the assistant that the assignment will be switched or not to worry about it is not appropriate because it does not teach the nursing assistant about the client's illness and appropriate client care. Although the statement, "Clients who are depressed are hard to deal with but don't take what they say seriously" may be somewhat true, it does not help the staff member understand why listening is important. (I, 1)

78. 3. The most therapeutic response is for the nurse to state, "You're in a lot of pain now but you will feel better and I'm here to help you." The client with active suicidal ideation believes that the solution to his problems is suicide. This statement by the nurse conveys empathy and hope to the client that he will get better and offers the nurse's help in doing so. The statement, "I'll walk with you to your room so that you can get some rest," is inappropriate because it focuses only on the client's use of the word *tired*, not the underlying feeling or intent of the statement. The statement about feeling better after the son visits is inappropriate

because the nurse does not recognize the client's suicidal behavior. The statement, "You are very depressed right now and want to die but you need to think about life" is inappropriate because it will not change the way the client is thinking or feeling. It also minimizes the client's feelings. (I, 6)

79. 4. One-to-one staff supervision is needed for the client who is unwilling or unable to sign a no-harm contract because of an impairment in reality testing due to hallucinations, delusions, dementia, or delirium. Other high-risk clients include those with constant suicidal thoughts, past attempts with high lethality, high risk for elopement, available access to a planned method, and severe depression. The client who is sometimes preoccupied with death or who tries to elope but is ambivalent about suicide is not at high risk for suicide and therefore does not need one-to-one supervision, nor does or the client who is impulsive and holds her breath until she faints This client may be seeking attention and not intending self-harm in the form of suicide. Furthermore, fainting is not a lethal method of suicide. (P, 1)

80. 2. The immediate priority is to save the caller's life. Therefore, the nurse should tell the caller that another nurse will telephone the police. The immediate goal is to rescue the caller because the suicide attempt has begun. Referring the caller to a 24-hour suicide hotline or instructing the caller to telephone her family for help would be appropriate later on, once the client is safe. Asking the caller whether she has telephoned her physician is not appropriate. The nurse is responsible for notifying the physician. (I, 6)

81. 4. The client's statement refers to the suicidal client's wish to use her own death to control others. Loss of self-esteem, abandonment, and relief of pain as well as helplessness, hopelessness, and loneliness are other themes commonly expressed by individuals who are suicidal. For example, a person fails out of college and wants to kill herself; a child loses both parents in a car accident and attempts suicide; or a person with cancer who is terminally ill desires to kill herself because of unbearable physical and psychic pain. (D, 6)

82. 2. The statement, "I don't think about killing myself as much as I used to," indicates a lessening of suicidal ideation and improvement in the client's condition. The statement, "I couldn't kill myself because I don't want to go to hell," indicates that the client will not attempt suicide but could still be thinking about death. The statements, "I'm of no use to anyone anymore," and "I know my kids don't need me anymore since they're on their own," indicate that the client feels worthless and may be experiencing suicidal ideation. (E, 6)

83. 4. Based on the client's statement, the nurse must initiate plans for hospitalization immediately, because the client has suicidal ideation with a definite plan, lethal method, and immediate access to the method. (I, 6)

84. 1. The survivor of suicide, in this situation, would be referred to a group for survivors of suicide to help her with her feelings and to work through the grief reaction. This group provides support and understanding of what the individual is experiencing by members who are experiencing similar reactions including anger and guilt. Depression and unresolved grief can occur when the survivor does not receive appropriate help. Counseling by a chaplain or individual therapy by the nurse may be appropriate in addition to the referral to the group. Giving the survivor the suicide hotline number would be appropriate if the survivor herself were thinking about suicide. (I, 6)

85. 3. The most appropriate response is to discuss the behavior clues and resources, because it provides the husband with important information that he needs to be better able to cope with his wife's condition. Family members are often afraid of future suicidal activity and need helpful information and resources to turn to in a crisis. Telling the husband not to worry minimizes the husband's concern and is not necessarily true. Additionally, past suicide attempts need to be considered when evaluating the client's future risk for suicide. The statement, "She told me she wants to live so I don't think she'll try again" ignores the husband's request and concerns. Additionally, there is no way for the nurse to know whether the client will attempt suicide again. The statement, "Tell her about your concern and just take care of her" is not helpful because the husband needs information and resources to turn to should a crisis develop. (I, 6)

86. 4. After the client identifies and shares her strengths, the nurse praises the client for her ability to evaluate herself in a positive manner. Doing so promotes self-esteem and offers hope for improvement. Asking the client to identify an additional three strengths or volunteering the client to lead the cooking group could be too overwhelming for the client at this time and may increase her anxiety and feelings of worthlessness. Although educating the client about the importance of medication is important, doing so at this time would be inappropriate. (I, 6)

87. 2. The best response would be for the nurse to advise the visitor to be caring and genuine to the client as a friend normally would. Family and friends are often afraid or at a loss about how to act or what to say to someone with a mental illness or to someone who may voice thoughts of self-harm. The statement, "Try to cheer her up" is inappropriate because the client may feel overwhelmed and thus become more despondent when she cannot meet or match the cheerful demeanor. The statement, "Control your expressions" is inappropriate because the client is not helped when interactions are not natural and genuine. The statement, "Avoid asking how she's feeling" is inappropriate because it conveys a lack of interest in and concern for the client. (I, 6)

88. 2. The client with feelings of self-doubt, inability to control her life, and dependency is manifesting problems evident in autonomy versus shame/doubt. Because of illness, regression has occurred and the client's behaviors affect on how the nurse will intervene with the client. With trust versus mistrust, some behaviors reflecting problems include suspiciousness, projection of blame, and withdrawal from others. With initiative versus guilt, some behaviors reflecting problems include excessive guilt, reluctance to show emotions, and passivity. With industry versus inferiority, some behaviors reflecting problems include feelings of being unworthy, poor work history, and inadequate problem-solving skills. (D, 6)

89. 1. The nurse would arrange for a psychiatric home care nurse to visit the client and follow her care. The psychiatric home care nurse will help the client manage her psychiatric disorder, medications for her mental illness and diabetes, diabetic care, and nutrition. A medical social worker may be involved with the client's care after discharge to help with interactions among agencies, and visits by clergy may be helpful, but a psychiatric home care nurse would be most important to help the client manage the many needs associated with her illness. A unit volunteer would be unable to manage the many needs of the client. (P, 6)

90. 3. Client safety is the priority to prevent further self-harm. Nutrition, sleep, and hygiene are important concerns, but they are secondary to safety. (P, 2)

91. 4. The nurse inspects the bag and its contents in the presence of the client and his wife so that they know what is allowed on the unit and what would need to be returned home and why. The nurse is responsible for the client's safety and that of the other clients and staff. Telling the wife to take her husband's things home because he is suicidal diminishes the client's self-worth and is inaccurate. Instructing the wife to unpack the bag and put her husband's things away is inappropriate because it is the nurse's responsibility to manage safety issues pertaining to the client and the unit. Asking the wife whether the bag contains anything dangerous would be poor judgment on the part of the nurse because the wife would not be knowledgeable about the safety factors. (I, 1)

92. 2. The nurse and staff place the client in leather restraints to protect the client from further self-harm. The client's behavior is out of control and necessitates external controls for her safety. Telling the client to stop and act like a responsible adult is ineffective and not therapeutic. Calling the physician for additional medication orders is not appropriate at this time because the lorazepam given by the nurse may take effect if the client remains still. The nurse would be responsible for judging whether additional medication is needed later. Instructing a staff member to sit in the room with the client is unsafe for the client and the staff member. (I, 2)

93. 2. The nurse needs to ask the client whether he is going to hurt himself to determine the client's ability to cope with the voices and to assess the client's impulse control. The nurse's assessment will then determine the course of action to take regarding the client's safety. Asking when the client hears the voices and how long the client has heard them is important but not as important as determining whether the client will act on what the voices are saying. Asking "Why are the voices starting again" would be inappropriate because the client may not know why and may not be able to answer the nurse. (I, 6)

94. 4. The nurse needs to focus on the client's strengths and successful coping strategies to reinforce strengths and teach adaptive coping behaviors to manage his illness and life in college. It is not uncommon for a young man diagnosed with schizophrenia to become depressed when he realizes the impact the illness could have on his life, his hopes, and his ability to succeed and reach his goals. There are no data to support a problem involving disturbed thought processes, disturbed sensory perceptions, or communication strategies at this time. (P, 6)

95. 1. Clients on 15-minute suicide checks must be observed by a staff member every 15 minutes. However, the staff member must stagger the timing of the check so that the client cannot predict the precise time. The staff member could check the client at 10 minutes and then at 8 minutes and so on in order to protect the patient from self-harm. The nurse would further explain the necessity of this procedure to help the staff understand its importance. Documenting that suicide checks have been done is absolutely necessary. Clients on one-to-one suicide precautions can never be left alone. All clients using razors must be supervised by staff. (E, 1)

96. 3. Using an exercise bicycle is appropriate for the client who becomes very anxious when thoughts of suicide occur. This activity helps the client decrease her anxiety through a physical action and provides the client with a means of coping with her emotions. Watching television, reading a magazine, and meditating typically are ineffective in decreasing anxiety for the client with thoughts of suicide. (I, 6)

97. 4. Because the client has a history of recurring depression and suicidal ideation, the nurse would give the client a 2- to 3-day supply of imipramine (Tofranil) to prevent possible overdose. Giving the client a 14-, 21-, or 30-day supply of medication would provide the client with enough medication to complete a suicidal attempt. Tricyclic antidepressants are associated with a higher rate of death than are the selective serotonin-reuptake inhibitors (SSRIs). (I, 8)

98. 2. Because the client is in danger of noncompliance with the medication due to financial concerns, the nurse should contact the social worker to assist with locating available resources for the client to ensure continuation of the medication needed for the recurrent illness. The client needs to continue the medications with no interruptions to minimize the chance of decompensation. Although the physician is the person responsible for ordering the client's medication, routinely the physician is not involved in finding financial assistance for the client's medication needs. The client needs the medication at the present time. Three months is too long to wait for a follow-up appointment. The client could be severely depressed and could even attempt suicide. A family member's assistance may not be a sufficient or a permanent means of financial help for the client in terms of medication needs. (I, 6)

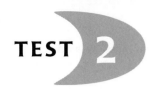

Schizophrenia, Other Psychoses, and Cognitive Disorders

Select the one best answer, and indicate your choice by filling in the circle in front of the option.

The Client With Paranoid Schizophrenia

1. A client who is neatly dressed and clutching a leather briefcase tightly in his arms scans the adult inpatient unit on his arrival at the hospital and backs away from the window. The client requests that the nurse move away from the window. The nurse recognizes that doing as the client requested is contraindicated for which of the following reasons?
   - ○ 1. The action will make the client feel that the nurse is humoring him.
   - ○ 2. The action indicates nonverbal agreement with the client's false ideas.
   - ○ 3. The client will then think that he will have his way when he wishes.
   - ○ 4. The nurse will be demonstrating a lack of composure over the situation.

2. Which of the following nursing diagnoses would the nurse identify for the client reporting thoughts of being followed by foreign agents who are after his secret papers?
   - ○ 1. Disturbed Sensory Perception: Visual related to increased anxiety, as evidenced by inappropriate responses.
   - ○ 2. Disturbed Thought Processes related to increased anxiety as evidenced by delusional thinking.
   - ○ 3. Impaired Verbal Communication related to disordered thinking, as evidenced by loose associations.
   - ○ 4. Social Isolation related to mistrust, as evidenced by withdrawal behaviors.

3. During a conversation with the nurse, a client suddenly jumps up, begins pacing, and wrings her hands. Which of the following would the nurse do *next*?
   - ○ 1. Take the client for a walk to help reduce her restlessness.
   - ○ 2. Change the subject of conversation to the weather.
   - ○ 3. Share the nurse's observations about the client's appearing anxious.
   - ○ 4. Leave after pointing out that the client doesn't appear to want to talk.

4. When assessing an aggressive client, which of the following client behaviors would warrant the nurse's *most* prompt reporting and use of safety precautions?
   - ○ 1. Crying when talking about his divorce.
   - ○ 2. Starting a petition to delay bedtime.
   - ○ 3. Declining attendance at a daily group therapy session.
   - ○ 4. Naming another client as his adversary.

5. When developing the plan of care for a client receiving haloperidol, which of the following medications would the nurse anticipate administering if the client developed extrapyramidal side effects?
   - ○ 1. Lorazepam (Ativan).
   - ○ 2. Benztropine mesylate (Cogentin).
   - ○ 3. Paroxetine (Paxil).
   - ○ 4. Olanzapine (Zyprexa).

6. The parents of a 20-year-old female client with paranoid schizophrenia admitted 4 days ago are attending a family psychoeducation group in the hospital. Which of the following statements by the mother

indicates that she understands her daughter's illness and management?

- 1. "I know that I'll have to do everything for my daughter when she comes home."
- 2. "Tasks as simple as getting out of bed and showering in the morning may be difficult for her."
- 3. "I know that visits from her friends at home should be discouraged for a while."
- 4. "She won't experience a relapse as long as she takes her prescribed medication."

7. While conducting a home visit for a client with paranoid schizophrenia discharged 1 week ago, the client's mother tearfully states, "I can hardly sleep because I'm so worried about my daughter. I'm afraid to leave her alone in the house. What if something should happen while I'm gone?" Which of the following problems related to the caregiver would be *most* appropriate for the nurse to incorporate into the client's plan of care?

- 1. Role strain.
- 2. Anxiety.
- 3. Fear.
- 4. Sleep pattern disturbance.

8. When conducting a mental status examination with a newly admitted client who has an Axis I diagnosis of paranoid schizophrenia, the client states, "I'm being followed; it's not safe. They're monitoring my every move." In which of the following areas of the mental status examination would the nurse document this information?

- 1. Thought content.
- 2. Quality of speech.
- 3. Insight.
- 4. Judgment.

9. The wife of a client diagnosed with paranoid schizophrenia visits 2 days after her husband's admission and states to the nurse, "Why isn't he eating? He's still talking about his food being poisoned." Which of the following appraisals by the nurse would be *most* accurate?

- 1. The wife's inquiry is reasonable.
- 2. Education about her husband's illness is needed.
- 3. Her expectations of her husband are realistic.
- 4. An increase in the client's medication is indicated.

10. A client states that she hears God's voice telling her that she has sinned and needs to be punished. Which of the following nursing diagnoses would be *most* appropriate?

- 1. Disturbed Sensory Perception related to guilt as evidenced by auditory hallucinations.
- 2. Social Isolation related to mistrust, as evidenced by withdrawal behaviors.

- 3. Disturbed Thought Processes related to increased anxiety as evidenced by delusional thinking.
- 4. Impaired Verbal Communication related to disordered thinking as evidenced by loose associations.

11. A client is complaining about blurred vision after 4 days of taking haloperidol (Haldol), benztropine (Cogentin), quetiapine (Seroquel), and buspirone (BuSpar). Which of the following medications would the nurse suspect as the *most* likely cause of this side effect?

- 1. Buspirone (BuSpar).
- 2. Quetiapine (Seroquel).
- 3. Haloperidol (Haldol).
- 4. Benztropine (Cogentin).

12. When developing the plan of care for a client who is isolating himself in his room because he perceives that staff want to harm him, which of the following outcomes would be *most* appropriate?

- 1. Within 2 days the client will complete his activities of daily living.
- 2. Within 3 days the client will participate in recreation with other clients.
- 3. Within 4 days the client will demonstrate an absence of verbal aggression.
- 4. Within 5 days the client will seek out staff to talk about feelings.

13. In addition to experiencing paranoid delusions, a client is withdrawn, unkempt, and unmotivated to get out of bed. Which of the following medications would the nurse expect to be *most* beneficial for the client's symptoms?

- 1. Haloperidol (Haldol).
- 2. Clorpromazine (Thorazine).
- 3. Olanzapine (Zyprexa).
- 4. Trihexyphenidyl (Artane).

14. A pregnant client in her third trimester is started on clorpromazine (Thorazine) 25 mg four times daily. Which of the following instructions would be *most* important for the nurse to include in the client's teaching plan?

- 1. "Do not drive, because there is a possibility of seizures occurring."
- 2. "Avoid going out in the sun without a sunscreen with an SPF of 25."
- 3. "Stop the medication immediately if constipation occurs."
- 4. "Tell your doctor if you experience an increase in blood pressure."

15. A client reports that men in blue clothes keep looking in her window and talking about her. Which of the following responses by the nurse would be *most* appropriate?

- 1. "Those men in blue uniforms are our groundskeepers. They probably are talking about their work, not you."

○ 2. "Don't take things so personally. Not everyone who is talking is talking about you."

○ 3. "Let's not pay attention to the men. Let's play cards instead."

○ 4. "I'll close the drapes so you can't see the men."

16. When preparing the teaching plan for a client who is to be started on clozapine (Clozaril), which of the following would be crucial to include?

○ 1. Description of akathisia and drug-induced parkinsonism.

○ 2. Measures to relieve episodes of diarrhea.

○ 3. The importance of reporting insomnia.

○ 4. An emphasis on the need for weekly blood tests.

17. A client is sitting in the corner of the dayroom cocking his head to one side as if he is hearing something, but no one is nearby. The nurse suspects he is having auditory hallucinations. Which of the following questions would the nurse ask *first*?

○ 1. "Are you seeing someone near you besides me?"

○ 2. "What are you hearing right now?"

○ 3. "What is going on with you right now?"

○ 4. "Do you want to go to the recreation room?"

18. A client who is newly diagnosed with paranoid schizophrenia tells the nurse, "The aliens are telling me that I'm defective and need to be eliminated." Which of the following responses by the nurse would be most appropriate initially?

○ 1. "I know those voices are real to you, but I don't hear them."

○ 2. "You are having hallucinations as a result of your illness."

○ 3. "I want you to agree to tell staff when you hear these voices."

○ 4. "Your medications will help control these voices you are hearing."

19. When administering antipsychotics to a client with paranoid schizophrenia, the nurse understands that the newer atypical antipsychotics such as olanzapine (Zyprexa) and risperidone (Risperdal) are more effective than the older medications in treating the negative symptoms of schizophrenia because of which of the following?

○ 1. Serotonin and γ-aminobutyric acid (GABA) levels are not affected.

○ 2. Dopamine and serotonin receptors are blocked.

○ 3. GABA and norepinephrine levels are increased.

○ 4. Norepinephrine and dopamine receptors are blocked.

20. A client has a history of paranoid schizophrenia and chronic alcohol dependency has been taking risperi-

done (Risperdal) for several months. She stopped drinking 4 days ago. The client is very frightened by the tactile hallucinations of bugs crawling under her skin. Which of the following factors would the nurse incorporate into the plan of care when explaining the tactile hallucinations?

○ 1. Alcohol intoxication.

○ 2. Ineffectiveness of risperidone (Risperdal).

○ 3. Alcohol withdrawal.

○ 4. Interaction of alcohol and risperidone (Risperdal).

21. A newly admitted client with paranoid schizophrenia is pacing and wringing his hands. He states that another client is out to get him. Then he says, "Protect me. Select me. Reject me." Which of the following nursing diagnoses would be *most* appropriate?

○ 1. Disturbed Sensory Perception related to paranoia as evidenced by thinking a client is out to get him.

○ 2. Impaired Verbal Communication related to severe anxiety as evidenced by clang associations.

○ 3. Delayed Growth and Development related to mild anxiety as evidenced by incomplete sentences.

○ 4. Defensive Coping related to noncompliance as evidenced by pacing and wringing of hands.

22. When a client who exhibits feelings of inferiority is asked to attend group activities, she gets more anxious. Within 10 minutes, she begins ridiculing others in the group and receives negative attention. Which of the following statements best reflects the nurse's interpretation of the client's behavior?

○ 1. Increased anxiety levels can cause defensive coping.

○ 2. Negative attention reinforces acting-out behaviors.

○ 3. Negative attention is better than no attention at all.

○ 4. Increased anxiety is a reason to exclude the client from groups.

23. In a family education group for those who have relatives with paranoid schizophrenia, which of the following comments indicates the need for *further* teaching about symptom management?

○ 1. "When the clients get overwhelmed, it is best if they spend some time in their room."

○ 2. "The more we push the clients to spend time with friends, the more their voices decrease."

○ 3. "Until we get the clients up and going, they seem to have no motivation to do anything."

○ 4. "We still have to remind the clients that we don't hear the voices that they do."

24. A client is being successfully treated with clozapine (Clozaril). Which of the following statements by the

client reflects a need for *further* teaching about managing the drug's side effects?

- ○ 1. "If I eat too many fruits, I'll get constipated."
- ○ 2. "I know I still need the weekly blood tests."
- ○ 3. "I have to get up slowly so I don't get dizzy."
- ○ 4. "Sometimes I have to push myself because I'm so sleepy."

25. Which of the following statements indicates increased insight by the client about her newly diagnosed paranoid schizophrenia being stabilized on medications?

- ○ 1. "Now that the voices are gone, I can decrease my medicines."
- ○ 2. "I would feel better if there wasn't still poison in my food."
- ○ 3. "Since I feel so much better, I know I can restart school next week."
- ○ 4. "The voices go away when I tell them to, except if I'm really nervous."

26. A client is aware that he is experiencing auditory hallucinations as a result of his paranoid schizophrenia. At this point, which of the following would be *most* appropriate for the nurse to do?

- ○ 1. "I know you hear voices, but I don't hear them."
- ○ 2. "Time and medicines will make the voices go away."
- ○ 3. "What seems to help make the voices less bothersome?"
- ○ 4 "The only voices I hear right now are yours and mine."

27. A client has been perceiving her roommate's stuffed animal as her own dog at home. The nurse determines that this misperception of reality (illusion) is improving when the client makes which of the following statements?

- ○ 1. "Jan's stuffed dog looks somewhat like my dog, Trixie."
- ○ 2. "Jan's dog and my dog could be twins."
- ○ 3. "I wish Jan hadn't had my dog stuffed."
- ○ 4. "I guess Jan needs a dog as much as I do."

28. A suspicious client states, "I know you nurses are spraying my food with poison as you take it out of the cart." Which of the following actions would most likely be successful?

- ○ 1. Serving foods that come in sealed packages.
- ○ 2. Asking what kind of poison the client suspects is being used.
- ○ 3. Giving the client canned supplements until the delusion subsides.
- ○ 4. Allowing the client to be the first to open the cart and get a tray.

29. The parent of a client with paranoid schizophrenia is asking questions about his son's antipsychotic medication, clozapine (Clozaril). Which of the following statements by the father reflects a need for

further teaching?

- ○ 1. "If he experiences any restlessness or muscle stiffness, he should tell the doctor."
- ○ 2. "I should give him benztropine (Cogentin) to help prevent constipation from the clozapine (Clozaril)."
- ○ 3. "If he doesn't get his weekly blood test, he won't be able to get his prescription refilled."
- ○ 4. "The clozapine (Clozaril) should help him be more motivated and less withdrawn."

The Client With Other Types of Schizophrenia and Psychotic Disorders

30. A client who is very suspicious of others including staff is brought to the hospital wearing a wrinkled dress with stains on the front and appearing confused. Assessment reveals disheveled, uncombed hair; flat affect; and slow movements. Which of the following would the nurse identify as the *initial* priority when planning this client's care?

- ○ 1. Helping the client feel safe and accepted.
- ○ 2. Introducing the client to other clients.
- ○ 3. Giving the client information about the program.
- ○ 4. Providing the client with clean, comfortable clothes.

31. When asked about her stresses before admission, an anxious client stares blankly at the nurse and mutters unintelligibly. Which of the following descriptions of the client's behaviors would the nurse document in the client's chart?

- ○ 1. "Client is not able to answer any questions asked at this time."
- ○ 2. "Client is uncooperative during admission procedure, refusing to answer any questions."
- ○ 3. "Client responded to questions with a blank look and incomprehensible mumble."
- ○ 4. "Client stared at wall when asked questions and was disoriented and incoherent."

32. The nurse identifies a nursing diagnosis of Self-Care Deficit related to apathy, as evidenced by inability to shower and dress self for a female client with schizophrenia. Which of the following outcomes would the nurse expect as *most* therapeutic for the client to achieve by the end of 4 days?

- ○ 1. Verbalize the need to shower and dress herself.
- ○ 2. Recognize the need to shower and dress herself.
- ○ 3. Explain reasons for showering and dressing herself.
- ○ 4. Perform showering and dressing for herself.

33. A client with schizophrenia is brought to the hospital from a group home where he became agitated,

threw a chair at another client, and has been refusing medication for 8 weeks and not caring for his hygiene. The client exhibits a flat affect and has become increasingly withdrawn and asocial. The physician orders treatment with risperidone (Risperdal) to improve the client's negative and positive symptoms of schizophrenia. When evaluating the drug's effectiveness on the client's negative symptoms, the nurse would expect improvement in which of the following?

○ 1. Apathy, affect, social isolation.
○ 2. Agitation, delusions, hallucinations.
○ 3. Hostility, ideas of reference, tangential speech.
○ 4. Aggression, bizarre behavior, illusions.

34. A client with schizophrenia comes to the outpatient mental health clinic 2 days after being discharged from the hospital. The client was given a 1-week supply of clozapine (Clozaril). The client tells the nurse that she has too much saliva and frequently needs to spit. The nurse interprets the client's statement as indicating which of the following?

○ 1. Delusion, requiring further assessment.
○ 2. Unusual reaction to clozapine.
○ 3. Expected side effect of clozapine.
○ 4. Unresolved symptom of schizophrenia.

35. The client with an Axis I diagnosis of schizophrenia, undifferentiated type is acutely psychotic and exhibits religious delusions, hallucinations, loose associations, and concrete thinking. When the nurse offers the client her medication, the client states, "I don't need that. God will heal me." Which of the following responses by the nurse would be *most* appropriate at this time?

○ 1. "God helps those who help themselves."
○ 2. "God wants you to take your medicine."
○ 3. "God is important in your life, but the medicine will help you too."
○ 4. "This medicine will help clear your thinking and decrease the voices."

36. The nurse hands a client who is psychotic and exhibiting concrete thinking the medication cup and tells the client to take his medicine. The client takes the cup, holds it in his hand, and stares at it. Which of the following would the nurse do *next*?

○ 1. Tell the client to put the medicine in his mouth and swallow it with some water.
○ 2. Instruct the client to sit in the dayroom and wait for the nurse to assist him.
○ 3. Ask another staff member to stay with the client until he takes the medication.
○ 4. Say nothing and wait for the client to put the medication in his mouth and swallow it.

37. The client is admitted to the unit with a diagnosis of Axis I delusional disorder, persecutory type. The nurse includes the nursing diagnosis Defensive Coping secondary to suspiciousness as evidenced by the paranoid statement, "Everyone in here is talking about me," in the client's plan of care. Which of the following statements about the client would be an expected outcome specific to the nursing diagnosis?

○ 1. Demonstrate an absence of hostile behavior.
○ 2. Express own needs using assertive communication.
○ 3. Use adaptive coping strategies appropriately.
○ 4. Accurately interpret the behaviors of staff and clients.

38. Which of the following actions would the nurse avoid to prevent increasing the anxiety and suspiciousness in an client who is delusional?

○ 1. Informing the client of schedule changes.
○ 2. Whispering with others where the client can observe.
○ 3. Telling the client gently that the nurse does not share the client's view.
○ 4. Inviting the client to join in leisure activities.

39. A client with undifferentiated schizophrenia tells the nurse that he doesn't go out much because he doesn't have anywhere to go and he doesn't know anyone in the apartment where he's staying. Which of the following actions would be *most* beneficial for the client at this time?

○ 1. Encouraging him to call his family to visit more often.
○ 2. Making an appointment for the client to see the nurse daily for 2 weeks.
○ 3. Thinking about the need for rehospitalization for the client.
○ 4. Arranging for the client to attend day treatment at the clinic.

40. A client with chronic undifferentiated schizophrenia has both positive and negative symptoms of schizophrenia but does not meet the criteria for paranoid, disorganized, or catatonic schizophrenia. Based on the interpretation of this information, the nurse would expect the client to exhibit which of the following as the most likely symptoms?

○ 1. Auditory hallucinations and asocial behaviors.
○ 2. Preoccupation with persecutory delusions and hallucinations.
○ 3. Grossly disorganized behaviors and speech.
○ 4. Immobility and waxy flexibility.

41. The plan of care for an outpatient client with chronic undifferentiated schizophrenia (CUS) includes risperidone (Risperdal) therapy. The nurse prepares to administer this drug based on the understanding of which of the following?

○ 1. The positive symptoms of CUS are usually as prominent as the negative symptoms.

2. Agranulocytosis is less of a risk with risperidone (Risperdal) therapy.
3. Negative symptoms are more prominent than positive symptoms in CUS.
4. Risperidone (Risperdal) is less expensive than traditional antipsychotics.

42. A newly admitted client with an acute exacerbation of psychotic symptoms of CUS is having trouble deciding whether to live in a group home or a supervised apartment. When caring for this client, which of the following activities would be *most* appropriate for the nurse to ask the client to do initially?
    1. List the pros and cons of each housing option.
    2. Choose between apple and orange juice for breakfast.
    3. Identify why the client cannot live in an unsupervised apartment.
    4. Decide which staff member the client would like to have today.

43. A client who has been receiving haloperidol (Haldol) for 2 days develops muscular rigidity, altered consciousness, a temperature of 103°F (39.4°C), and trouble breathing on day 3. The nurse interprets these findings as indicating which of the following?
    1. Neuroleptic malignant syndrome.
    2. Tardive dyskinesia.
    3. Extrapyramidal side effects.
    4. Drug induced parkinsonism.

44. A client with CUS reports to the nurse that he does very little all day except sleep and eat. Which of the following interventions would be *most* appropriate for this client?
    1. Having three meals per day brought in to increase the amount of time client spends out of bed.
    2. Asking a relative to call the client at least 10 times a day to decrease the sleeping.
    3. Helping the client set up a daily activity schedule to include setting a wake-up alarm.
    4. Arranging for the client to move to a group home with structured activities.

45. The nurse notes that a client sitting in a chair has not gotten up in 1 hour. The client does not respond to verbal directions, and her arm has been extended over the armrest for 30 minutes. Which of the following would the nurse do *next*?
    1. Assist the client out of the chair to lead her back to bed.
    2. Give PRN-ordered doses of haloperidol (Haldol) and lorazepam (Ativan).
    3. Ask the client to describe what is being experienced right now.
    4. Sit quietly with the client until she begins to respond.

46. Which of the following would be *most* appropriate as an initial goal for a client with CUS who has been withdrawn from friends and family for 3 weeks?
    1. Calling his mother once a day.
    2. Attending day therapy three times a week.
    3. Allowing two friends to visit every day.
    4. Remaining out of bed for 10 hours a day.

47. For the client with catatonic behaviors, which of the following would the nurse use to determine that the medication administered PRN has been most effective?
    1. The client is able to move all extremities occasionally.
    2. The client walks with the nurse to her room.
    3. The client responds to verbal directions to eat.
    4. The client initiates simple activities without directions.

48. The mother of a client with CUS calls the nurse in the outpatient clinic to report that her daughter has not answered the phone in 10 days. "She was doing so well for months. I don't know what's wrong. I'm worried." Which of the following responses by the nurse would be *most* appropriate?
    1. "Maybe she is just mad at you. Did you two have an argument?"
    2. "She may have stopped taking her medications. I'll check on her."
    3. "Don't worry about this. It happens sometimes."
    4. "Go over to her apartment and see what's going on."

49. During a home visit, the nurse discovers that the client is less verbal, less active, less responsive to directions, severely anxious, and more stuporous. The nurse interprets these findings as indicating that the client is having an exacerbation of which of the following types of schizophrenia?
    1. Disorganized.
    2. Paranoid.
    3. Undifferentiated.
    4. Catatonic.

50. A client diagnosed with disorganized schizophrenia has been well maintained on olanzapine (Zyprexa) for 1 year. Two days ago, the client was found in the back yard without any clothes on, unable to communicate well because of loose associations. His mother died 2 weeks ago. Which of the following would the nurse anticipate as being included in the client's plan of care?
    1. Addition of a short course of haloperidol (Haldol).
    2. A significant increase in the dose of olanzapine (Zyprexa).
    3. Grief counseling.
    4. A switch to risperidone instead of olanzapine (Zyprexa).

51. A client admitted with a diagnosis of schizoaffective disorder, manic phase who is currently taking fluoxetine (Prozac), valproic acid (Depakote), and olanzapine (Zyprexa) as ordered has had an increase in manic symptoms in the last week. The psychiatrist orders a valproic acid blood level to be drawn stat. The nurse understands the rationale for this order as which of the following?
    - ○ 1. All clients taking valproic acid need periodic valproic acid levels drawn.
    - ○ 2. Fluoxetine can decrease the effectiveness of the valproic acid.
    - ○ 3. A decrease in the level of valproic acid could explain the increase in manic symptoms.
    - ○ 4. The valproic acid level is needed before a short course of lorazepam (Ativan) for agitation is ordered.

52. A 22-year-old client is being admitted with a diagnosis of brief psychotic disorder. Two weeks ago, his girlfriend broke off their engagement and cancelled the wedding. Given the *Diagnostic and Statistical Manual of Mental Disorders*, 4th edition, text revised (DSM-IV-TR) criteria for this disorder, the nurse expects to find which of the following data during the interview with the client?
    - ○ 1. Current treatment for pneumonia.
    - ○ 2. Regular use of alcohol and marijuana.
    - ○ 3. Evidence of delusions and hallucinations.
    - ○ 4. A history of chronic depression.

53. A successful real estate agent brought to the clinic after being arrested for harassing and stalking his ex-wife denies any other symptoms or problems except anger about being arrested. The ex-wife reports to the police, "He is fine except for this irrational belief that we will remarry." Which of the following would the nurse expect to include in this client's plan of care?
    - ○ 1. An order for olanzapine (Zyprexa) 10 mg twice daily.
    - ○ 2. A joint session with the client and his ex-wife.
    - ○ 3. An order for fluoxetine (Prozac) 20 mg every morning.
    - ○ 4. Referral to an outpatient therapist.

Clients and Families Affected by Chronic Mental Illnesses

54. When working with clients who are experiencing chronic mental illnesses, which of the following would the nurse expect to be generally unnecessary for this client population?
    - ○ 1. Community-based treatment programs.
    - ○ 2. Psychosocial rehabilitation.

    - ○ 3. Employment opportunities.
    - ○ 4. Custodial care in long-term hospitals.

55. The nurse is offered a position as a psychiatric nurse in a psychosocial rehabilitation program for chronically mentally ill clients. Which of the following strategies would the nurse expect to be *least* beneficial for the client population?
    - ○ 1. Teaching independent living skills.
    - ○ 2. Assisting clients with living arrangements.
    - ○ 3. Helping clients in insight-oriented therapy.
    - ○ 4. Linking clients with community resources.

56. A nurse working at an outpatient mental health center primarily with chronically mentally ill clients receives a telephone call from the mother of a client who lives at home. She reports that the client has not been taking her medication and now is refusing to go to the sheltered workshop, where she has worked for the last year. Which of the following would the nurse do *first*?
    - ○ 1. Call the director of the workshop for information about the client.
    - ○ 2. Reserve an inpatient bed in preparation for the client's admission.
    - ○ 3. Ask to speak to the client now on the phone.
    - ○ 4. Make an appointment for the client to see the doctor.

57. The nurse invites a new client's parents to attend the psychoeducational program for families of the chronically mentally ill. The program would be most likely to help the family with which of the following issues?
    - ○ 1. Feeling more guilty about the client's illness.
    - ○ 2. Developing a support network with other families.
    - ○ 3. Managing their financial concerns and problems.
    - ○ 4. Recognizing the client's weaknesses.

58. When teaching the families of clients with chronic mental illnesses about the primary cause of relapse and rehospitalization, the nurse would include which of the following as a factor?
    - ○ 1. Loss of family support.
    - ○ 2. Noncompliance with medications.
    - ○ 3. Sudden changes in medications.
    - ○ 4. Nonattendance at treatment programs.

59. The director of a workshop program tells the nurse that the client with schizophrenia had done well for 6 months until last week, when a new person started at the workshop. This new person worked faster than the client did and took his place as leader of the group. Based on this information, which of the following interventions would be *most* appropriate?
    - ○ 1. Making a home visit and telling the client that if he does not return to the workshop, he will lose his place there.

○ 2. Asking the director to assign the client to another work group when he returns to the workshop.

○ 3. Making an appointment to meet the client at the mental health center and ask him about the situation.

○ 4. Arranging for the placement of the client in a skill-training program.

60. A 25-year-old client with chronic schizophrenia states, "I stopped my medications a week ago. I was just tired of not being able to drink with my friends. Besides, I feel fine without them." Which of the following responses by the nurse would be *most* appropriate?

○ 1. "It is vitally important for you to go back on your medicines."

○ 2. "I know how difficult it must be to live with the changes caused by your illness."

○ 3. "You will have to talk to your doctor about stopping your medications."

○ 4. "Your buddies will understand that you can't drink anymore."

61. A 23-year-old client with schizophrenia cheerfully announces, "My mom and I are so excited that I'm pregnant. She's willing to help us take care of the baby too." Which of the following reasons would cause the nurse to be concerned about this situation?

○ 1. The client did not say that the father of the baby was excited about this.

○ 2. The mother is not likely to provide enough help for what the client needs.

○ 3. Symptom management will be difficult in early pregnancy without medications.

○ 4. The client will have difficulty financially supporting the baby.

62. Mental health professionals are concerned about chronically ill clients who have aging parents. The primary reason for this concern is associated with which of the following?

○ 1. Clients will have to face grieving issues when one or both parents die.

○ 2. Parents experience much guilt about abandoning their child.

○ 3. Clients will lose a source of emotional support.

○ 4. Parents are frequently providing financial support and/or housing.

63. A set of monozygotic twins who are 23 years old have begun attending groups at a mental health center. One twin is diagnosed with schizophrenia. Her twin has no diagnosis but has been experiencing significant anxiety since becoming engaged. In counseling the engaged twin, it would be crucial to include which of the following facts?

○ 1. Her future children will be at risk for developing schizophrenia.

○ 2. She may have a predisposition for schizophrenia.

○ 3. One of her parents may develop schizophrenia later in life.

○ 4. It is unlikely that she will develop schizophrenia at her age.

64. The discovery of the biochemical hypothesis for the cause of schizophrenia has helped families of ill clients in many ways. Which of the following would the nurse identify as being *most* significant when planning the care of a client and family with schizophrenia?

○ 1. Family dysfunction, if it exists, is viewed as an effect rather than a cause of the disorder.

○ 2. Professionals are more likely to view families as allies than as villains.

○ 3. Families are less likely to participate in "families of schizophrenics" studies.

○ 4. Families are less likely to be involved in providing care to their ill relatives.

65. As a result of the effects of managed care, hospitalization is often reserved for emergency care. Which of the following situations would the nurse recognize as having the *least* priority for admission?

○ 1. Potential for self-harm.

○ 2. Potential for harm to others.

○ 3. Grave disability (unable to care for self).

○ 4. Decline in functioning at work.

66. Given the decrease in length of hospital stay for the chronically mentally ill, the nurse recognizes the increased need for emphasizing discharge planning. For the client who is being discharged before complete stabilization of symptoms, the nurse would anticipate that a client would likely require which of the following?

○ 1. More medical consultations after discharge.

○ 2. Monthly outpatient visits.

○ 3. A wide variety of coordinated services.

○ 4. Caring and supportive follow-up.

67. Clients with chronic mental illness need to develop trust in their care providers, gain education about their illness and its treatment, and have services readily available. Which of the following is the *most* critical need for these clients?

○ 1. Family support.

○ 2. Advocacy for improved mental health statutes.

○ 3. Diligent monitoring for medication compliance.

○ 4. Support groups.

68. When developing a teaching plan for the community about managed care models and their effect on clients with chronic mental illnesses, which of the following factors would the nurse include as *most* critical for this population?

○ 1. Restriction in the range and quantity of services.

○ 2. Hospitalization reserved for emergency services.

○ 3. Nonshifting of allocated funding to outpatient services.

○ 4. Loss of the principle of "least restrictive alternative for care."

69. When developing a community-based service program for clients with chronic mental illnesses, which of the following would be of *least* importance?
   ○ 1. Partial programs.
   ○ 2. Psychiatric home care.
   ○ 3. Residential services.
   ○ 4. Long-term hospitals.

70. With the increasing emphasis on case management for clients with chronic mental illnesses, in addition to the nursing process, which of the following would the nurse also identify as important?
   ○ 1. Master's degree preparation as a clinical specialist.
   ○ 2. Educators to provide for general equivalency diploma (GED) education.
   ○ 3. Families who can pay for clients' medications.
   ○ 4. Advocacy for the needs of the chronically mentally ill.

71. Crisis intervention plays a major role in the management of care for clients with chronic mental illnesses. Although the safety of the client and others is always a priority, these clients typically need crisis intervention in which of the following situations?
   ○ 1. Inability to make outpatient appointments.
   ○ 2. Signs of relapse and decompensation.
   ○ 3. Threat of eviction from housing.
   ○ 4. Unpaid bills and lack of food.

72. The most common reason given by mentally ill clients for noncompliance with medications is their uncomfortable side effects, although benztropine (Cogentin) can relieve some of the side effects of the antipsychotics. When teaching the families, which of the following would the nurse identify as an even greater need?
   ○ 1. Alternative ways to manage the side effects.
   ○ 2. Home visits to set up a week's supply of medications.
   ○ 3. Family monitoring of the administration of medication.
   ○ 4. Outpatient monitoring of medication compliance.

73. The stigma related to having a mental illness, especially a chronic illness, persists despite improvements in the management of illnesses and an increase in public education. The nurse understands that a major reason for the continuation of the stigma relates to which of the following views?

○ 1. Mental illness is hereditary.
○ 2. Mental illnesses have biochemical bases.
○ 3. Clients cannot prevent mental illness if they want to do so.
○ 4. Clients can recover from mental illness if they only use their willpower.

The Client With Cognitive Disorders

74. Transfer data for a client brought by ambulance to the hospital's psychiatric unit from a nursing home indicate that the client has become increasingly confused and disoriented. The client's behavior is found to be the result of cerebral arteriosclerosis. There is no known cure for this disorder, but behaviors may improve with the use of psychotropic medications. Which of the following attitudes would the nursing staff expect to employ to influence the client's behavior?
   ○ 1. Hope.
   ○ 2. Acceptance.
   ○ 3. Concern.
   ○ 4. Nonchalance.

75. A client with early dementia exhibits disturbances in her mental awareness and orientation to reality. The nurse would expect to assess a loss of ability in which of the following other areas?
   ○ 1. Speech.
   ○ 2. Judgment.
   ○ 3. Endurance.
   ○ 4. Balance.

76. The client with dementia states to the nurse, "I know you. You're Margaret, the girl who lives down the street from me." Which of the following responses by the nurse would be *most* therapeutic?
   ○ 1. "Mrs. Jones, I'm Rachel, a nurse here at the hospital."
   ○ 2. "Now Mrs. Jones, you know who I am."
   ○ 3. "Mrs. Jones, I told you already, I'm Rachel and I don't live down the street."
   ○ 4. "I think you forgot that I'm Rachel, Mrs. Jones."

77. Which of the following courses of action would be a priority to be included in the plan of care for an elderly client with cognitive impairment?
   ○ 1. Having two people accompany the client whenever the client is up and about.
   ○ 2. Ensuring the removal of objects in the client's path that may cause him to trip.
   ○ 3. Putting the client's favorite belongings in a safe place so that he will not lose them.
   ○ 4. Giving the client his medications in liquid form to make certain that he swallows them.

78. The nurse manager of a psychiatric unit notices that one of the nurses often avoids a 75-year-old client's

company, preferring to associate with clients of her own age group or younger. Which of the following factors would the nurse manager identify as being *most* likely responsible for this nurse's extreme discomfort with older clients and unconscious avoidance of them?
- ○ 1. Fears and conflicts about aging.
- ○ 2. Dislike of physical contact with older people.
- ○ 3. A desire to be surrounded by beauty and youth.
- ○ 4. Recent experiences with her mother's elderly friends.

79. The nurse observes a client who is reminiscing about his past life. Which of the following effects would the nurse expect reminiscing to have on the client's functioning in the hospital?
- ○ 1. Increase the client's confusion and disorientation.
- ○ 2. Subject the client to the others' impatient responses.
- ○ 3. Decrease the client's feelings of isolation and loneliness.
- ○ 4. Keep the client from participating in therapeutic activities.

The Client With Delirium

80. A client with uremia, admitted to a medical unit, is suddenly experiencing sleep disturbances, inability to focus, memory deficits, altered perceptions, and disorientation to time and place. The psychiatric liaison nurse conducts an evaluation of the client. Based on an analysis of the findings, the psychiatric liaison nurse suspects which of the following?
- ○ 1. Bipolar disorder.
- ○ 2. Dementia.
- ○ 3. General anxiety disorder.
- ○ 4. Delirium.

81. When caring for elderly clients, the nurse would be especially alert for which of the following as the most common cause of delirium?
- ○ 1. Cancer of any kind.
- ○ 2. Impaired hearing.
- ○ 3. Prescription drug intoxication.
- ○ 4. Congestive heart failure.

82. In addition to development over a period of hours or days, the nurse would assess delirium as distinguishable by which of the following characteristics?
- ○ 1. Disturbances in cognition and consciousness that fluctuate during the day.
- ○ 2. The failure to identify objects despite intact sensory functions.
- ○ 3. Significant impairment in social or occupational functioning over time.

- ○ 4. Memory impairment to the degree of being called amnesia.

83. Which of the following would be *most* critical when caring for a client who is experiencing delirium?
- ○ 1. Controlling behavioral symptoms with low-dose psychotropics.
- ○ 2. Correcting the underlying causative condition or illness.
- ○ 3. Manipulating the environment to increase orientation.
- ○ 4. Decreasing or discontinuing any nonessential medications.

84. Which of the following would the nurse identify as a realistic short-term goal to be accomplished in 2 to 3 days for a client with delirium?
- ○ 1. Explain the experience of having a delirium.
- ○ 2. Regain a normal sleep–wake cycle.
- ○ 3. Become oriented to time, place, and person.
- ○ 4. Establish normal bowel and bladder function.

85. Which of the following would the nurse expect to include as a *priority* in the plan of care for a client with delirium based on the nurse's understanding about the disturbances in consciousness associated with this disorder?
- ○ 1. Identifying self and making sure that the nurse has the client's attention.
- ○ 2. Eliminating the client's napping in the daytime as much as possible.
- ○ 3. Engaging the client in reminiscing with relatives or visitors.
- ○ 4. Avoiding arguing with a suspicious client about perceptions of reality.

The Client With Dementia

86. When assessing a client with dementia, which of the following behaviors would the nurse interpret as a manifestation of disinhibition?
- ○ 1. Wandering and getting lost.
- ○ 2. Auditory and/or visual hallucinations.
- ○ 3. Decreased interest in bathing and hygiene.
- ○ 4. Inappropriate language and sexual behaviors.

87. The term *motor apraxia* relates to a decline in motor patterns essential for complex motor tasks. Despite the inability to change a flat tire, the client with severe dementia may be able to perform which of the following actions?
- ○ 1. Balance a checkbook accurately.
- ○ 2. Brush the teeth when handed a toothbrush.
- ○ 3. Use confabulation when telling a story.
- ○ 4. Find misplaced car keys.

88. When communicating with clients who are experiencing dementia and exhibiting decreased attention and increased confusion, which of the following

interventions would the nurse employ as the *first* step?

○ 1. Using gentle touch to convey empathy.

○ 2. Rephrasing questions the client doesn't understand.

○ 3. Eliminating distracting stimuli, such as turning off the television.

○ 4. Asking the client to go for a walk while talking.

89. The daughter of a client with dementia complains that her mother is always distorting things. The nurse understands that the daughter needs *further* teaching about dementia when she makes which of the following statements?

○ 1. "I tell her reality, such as, "That noise is the wind in the trees.""

○ 2. "I understand the misperceptions are part of the disease."

○ 3. "I'll turn off the radio when we're in another room."

○ 4. "I tell her she is wrong and then I tell her what's right."

The Client With Alzheimer's Disease

90. The client in the early stage of Alzheimer's disease (AD) and his adult son attend an appointment at the community mental health center. While conversing with the nurse, the son states, "I'm tired of hearing about how things were 30 years ago. Why does Dad always talk about the past?" The nurse interprets the son's statement to indicate which of the following problems?

○ 1. A lack of knowledge regarding the disease process.

○ 2. Inability to accept the unusual behavior of his father.

○ 3. Misunderstanding of his father's level of anxiety.

○ 4. Misperception of his father's antagonism toward him.

91. The nurse discusses the possibility of a client's attending day treatment for clients with AD. Which of the following would be the *best* rationale for encouraging day treatment?

○ 1. The client would have more structure to the day.

○ 2. Staff are excellent in the treatment they offer clients.

○ 3. The client would benefit from increased social interaction.

○ 4. The family would have more time to engage in their daily activities.

92. When describing AD to a group of nursing students, which of the following would the nurse identify as the characteristic found in AD that distinguishes it from other dementias?

○ 1. Hypoxic destruction of brain cells.

○ 2. Hyperkinesis causing choreiform movements.

○ 3. Neurofibrillary tangles and plaques.

○ 4. An infectious particle called a prion.

93. When developing the plan of care for a client with AD who is experiencing moderate impairment, which of the following types of care would the nurse expect to include?

○ 1. Considerable assistance with activities of daily living.

○ 2. Managing a complex medication schedule.

○ 3. Constant supervision and total care.

○ 4. Supervision of risky activities, such as shaving.

94. Families of clients with AD report that they have the most difficulty in managing their relatives' aggression and wandering. Which of the following suggestions would be *least* important for the nurse to suggest to help manage wandering?

○ 1. A MedicAlert bracelet.

○ 2. Motion and sound detectors.

○ 3. Door alarms.

○ 4. Antidepressant medications.

95. Which of the following would be a priority to include in the plan of care for a client with AD who is experiencing difficulty processing and completing complex tasks?

○ 1. Repeating the directions until the client follows them.

○ 2. Asking the client to do one step of the task at a time.

○ 3. Demonstrating for the client how to do the task.

○ 4. Maintaining routine and structure for the client.

96. Clients with AD may have delusions about being harmed by staff and others. When the client expresses fear of being killed by staff, which of the following responses would be *most* appropriate?

○ 1. "What makes you think we want to kill you?"

○ 2. "We like you too much to want to kill you."

○ 3. "You are in the hospital. We are nurses trying to help you."

○ 4. "Oh, don't be so silly. No one wants to kill you here."

97. When helping the families of clients with AD to cope with vulgar or sexual behaviors, which of the following suggestions would be most helpful?

○ 1. Ignore the behaviors, but try to identify the purposes.

○ 2. Give feedback on the inappropriateness of the behaviors.

○ 3. Employ anger management strategies.

○ 4. Administer the prescribed risperidone (Risperdal).

98. The nurse determines that the son of a client with AD needs further education about the disease when he makes which of the following statements?
- ○ 1. "I didn't realize the deterioration would be so incapacitating."
- ○ 2. "The Alzheimer's support group has so much good information."
- ○ 3. "I get tired of the same old stories, but I know it's important for Dad."
- ○ 4. "I woke up this morning hoping that my old Dad would be back."

99. The husband of a client with AD that was diagnosed 6 years ago approaches the nurse and says, "I'm so excited about the use of donepezil (Aricept) for her illness." The nurse needs to inform the husband of which of the following facts about this drug?
- ○ 1. Improvements seen are usually limited to the early stages.
- ○ 2. The side effects of the drug are numerous.
- ○ 3. The client will attain a functional level of that of 6 years ago.
- ○ 4. Effectiveness in the terminal phase of the illness is scientifically proven.

100. The physician orders risperidone (Risperdal) for a client with AD. The nurse anticipates administering this medication to help decrease which of the following behaviors?
- ○ 1. Sleep disturbances.
- ○ 2. Concomitant depression.
- ○ 3. Agitation and assaultiveness.
- ○ 4. Confusion and withdrawal.

101. Which of the following agents would the nurse expect to administer, if ordered, for an anxious elderly client with AD?
- ○ 1. Oxazepam (Serax).
- ○ 2. Diazepam (Valium).
- ○ 3. Chlordiazepoxide (Librium).
- ○ 4. Nefazodone (Serzone).

102. When providing family education with those who have a relative with AD about minimizing stress, which of the following suggestions would be *most* relevant?
- ○ 1. Allow the client to go to bed four to five times during the day.
- ○ 2. Test the cognitive functioning of the client several times a day.
- ○ 3. Provide reality orientation even if the memory loss is severe.
- ○ 4. Maintain consistency in environment, routine, and caregivers.

Correct Answers and Rationale

The letters in parentheses following the rationale identify the step of the nursing process (A, D, P, I, E) and client needs (1, 2, 3, 4, 5, 6, 7, 8, 9, 10). See the inside front cover for the key.

The Client With Paranoid Schizophrenia

1. 2. The nurse's nonverbal behavior, moving away from the window as the client requests, would indicate agreement with the client's false ideas. The client's behavior is likely to be reinforced if the nurse takes steps to agree with the false ideas he holds. (D, 6)

2. 2. The nursing diagnosis Disturbed Thought Processes related to increased anxiety, as evidenced by delusional thinking, most accurately reflects this client's problem with paranoid delusions. Disturbed Sensory Perception: Visual would be appropriate if the client were experiencing hallucinations. Impaired Verbal Communication would be appropriate if the client were demonstrating less coherent speech. Social Isolation would be appropriate if the client were refusing to come out of his room. (D, 6)

3. 3. When a client becomes restless during a conversation with the nurse, the first course of action is typically to help the client recognize and acknowledge her feelings by sharing observations with her. Walking with the client may be appropriate to help reduce her anxiety once the nurse has shared the observations. Changing the subject of the conversation or leaving the client after pointing out that she doesn't appear to want to talk is inappropriate because this does not help the client to recognize and acknowledge her feelings. Additionally, it does not encourage the client to express her anxiety. (I, 6)

4. 4. The client exhibits aggression against his perceived adversary when he names another client as his adversary. The staff will need to watch him carefully for signs of impending violent behavior that may injure others. Crying about a divorce would be appropriate, not pathologic, behavior demonstrating grief over a loss. A petition to delay bedtime would be a positive, direct action aimed at a bothersome situation. Although declining to attend group therapy needs follow-up, there may be any number of unknown reasons for this action. (A, 2)

5. 2. The drug of choice for a client experiencing extrapyramidal side effects from haloperidol (Haldol) is benztropine mesylate (Cogentin) because of its anti-cholinergic properties. Lorazepam (Ativan) is an antianxiety agent. Paroxetine (Paxil) is an antidepressant. Olanzapine (Zyprexa) antipsychotic agent. (P, 8)

6. 2. Clients with paranoid schizophrenia experience alterations in thought resulting in introspection, confusion, and distraction from external reality. Simple tasks that require concentration and effort, including activities involving self-care, may be difficult for the client, especially during the acute phase of illness. However, the mother should not need to do everything for her daughter. Rather, the mother should be encouraging the daughter to do things for herself with guidance. Visits from friends should be discussed with the client, and the client should be encouraged to visit with friends to minimize the risk for social isolation. Although relapse typically occurs with medication noncompliance, vulnerability to stress, a low threshold for stress, the number of stresses, and the client's lack of adaptive coping behaviors contribute to relapse. (E, 6)

7. 1. The nurse recognizes the mother's feelings of being overwhelmed with the issues concerning the management of her daughter at home. Anxiety, fear, and sleep disturbances all contribute to caregiver role strain. The nurse would help the mother elicit the support of other family members or friends, continue with psychoeducation, and help the family connect with the Alliance for the Mentally Ill for support, reassurance, and education. (D, 5)

8. 1. The client is voicing paranoid delusions of being followed and monitored. Presence of delusions is described in the area of thought content in the mental status examination. The speech section would typically include documentation of disturbances in speech or pressured speech. In the insight section, the nurse would document information reflecting a lack of insight—for example, statements such as "I don't have a problem." In the judgment section, the nurse would document information reflecting a lack of judgment—for example, poor choices, such as buying a gun for self protection. (D, 6)

9. 2. For the client with paranoid schizophrenia, 2 days is too short a time for improvement to be seen. Therefore, the nurse evaluates the client's wife as needing education or knowledge about paranoid schizophrenia, the course of the illness, and medications. Expecting an absence of delusions by the end of the client's second day of hospitalization is unrealistic. Rather, the nurse would reasonably expect delusions to decrease, disap-

pearing by 5 to 9 days of hospitalization. The wife's inquiry is not reasonable because not enough time has elapsed to evaluate the effectiveness of treatment. An increase in the client's medication would be unreasonable because not enough time has elapsed to evaluate the effectiveness of the medication. Generally, a time frame of 5 to 7 days is needed before the effectiveness of medications can be determined. (E, 10)

10. 1. The client is describing an auditory hallucination that is most likely related to unresolved guilt about a perceived "sin." Social Isolation would be supported by evidence indicating that the client refuses to come out of her room. Disturbed Thought Processes would be evidenced, for example, by the client's saying that someone in her life is trying to punish her. Loose associations are reflections of racing thoughts, not problems with verbal communication. (D, 6)

11. 4. Benztropine (Cogentin) frequently causes the side effect of blurred vision. Quetiapine (Seroquel), an atypical antipsychotic, and buspirone (BuSpar), an antianxiety agent, are not likely to produce blurred vision. Although haloperidol (Haldol), a high-potency antipsychotic, may cause blurred vision, this side effect is more common with benztropine. (A, 8)

12. 4. The client is exhibiting suspiciousness of and a lack of trust in the staff, not aggression. Seeking out staff indicates the development of trust and decreased suspiciousness. Although completing activities of daily living and participating in recreation with other clients are important, the major problem presented is related to the client's isolation and perception of being harmed—not, for example, showering, hygiene, or other clients. (P, 6)

13. 3. The client is exhibiting negative symptoms of schizophrenia. Olanzapine (Zyprexa), an atypical antipsychotic, is likely to be effective with negative symptoms. Haloperidol (Haldol), a high-potency antipsychotic agent, and chlorpromazine (Thorazine), a low-potency antipsychotic agent, are effective with the positive symptoms of schizophrenia, such as delusions and hallucinations, but have very little effect on negative symptoms. Trihexyphenidyl (Artane) is an antiparkinson agent, not an antipsychotic agent. (P, 8)

14. 2. Chlorpromazine (Thorazine) is a low-potency antipsychotic that is likely to cause sun-sensitive skin. Therefore the client needs instructions about using sunscreen with an SPF of 25 or higher. Typically, chlorpromazine is not associated with an increased risk for seizures. Although constipation is a common side effect of this drug, it can be managed with diet, fluids, and exercise. The drug does not need to be discontinued. Chlorpromazine is associated with orthostatic hypotension, not

hypertension. Additionally, if orthostatic hypotension occurs, safety measures such as changing positions slowly and dangling before arising, not stoppage of the drug, are instituted. (P, 8)

15. 1. The nurse needs to present the reality of the situation. By explaining that the men are groundskeepers and probably talking about work, the nurse is reinforcing reality to counter the client's illusion (misinterpretation of reality). Additionally, this response voices doubt in the client's paranoid interpretation. Telling the client not to take things personally is flippant and judgmental. Telling the client to not pay attention to the men fails to address the client's misinterpretations and misperceptions. Closing the drapes so that the client doesn't see the men ignores the client's misperceptions and misinterpretation. (I, 6)

16. 4. Clozapine (Clozaril) is associated with agranulocytosis. Therefore, the nurse must instruct the client about the need for weekly blood counts to monitor for this side effect. Akathisia and drug-induced parkinsonism are associated with high-potency antipsychotics. These effects are not common with this atypical antipsychotic agent. Constipation and sedation may occur with this drug. (P, 8)

17. 2. Before intervening with the client experiencing hallucinations, the nurse must validate what the client is experiencing. Asking the client what he is hearing right now accomplishes this. Asking about seeing someone near the client would be appropriate to validate visual hallucinations. Asking the client about what is going on may be helpful. However, the question is too general to validate that the client is experiencing auditory hallucinations. Asking the client if he wants to go to the recreation room might be appropriate once the nurse has validated what the client is experiencing. (I, 6)

18. 3. Clients may act on command hallucinations and harm themselves or others. Therefore, the staff need to know when the client is hearing such commands, to ensure safety first. Telling the client that the voices are real but that the nurse doesn't hear them would be an appropriate response later in the client's hospitalization when the client's safety is not longer an issue because antipsychotics are beginning to take effect. Telling the client that the hallucinations are part of the illness or that medications will help control the voices would be appropriate once the client has developed some insight into the symptoms of the illness. (I, 6)

19. 2. The newer antipsychotics block both dopamine and serotonin receptors. They also block GABA and dopamine receptors. Antidepressants more commonly affect norepinephrine receptors and levels. (D, 8)

20. 3. Tactile hallucinations are more common in alcohol withdrawal than in schizophrenia. Therefore, the nurse would explain that these hallucinations are the result of withdrawal from alcohol. Because the client stopped drinking 4 days ago, the client is not intoxicated. Risperdal has little effect on symptoms of alcohol withdrawal. It is prescribed for symptoms of schizophrenia. Alcohol and risperdal have an additive effect, not one of causing hallucinations. (D, 6)

21. 2. The client is visibly upset and anxious, as demonstrated by his behaviors. In addition, the client's statement reflects clang associations, phrases that rhyme. Panic level anxiety can disturb thought processes, resulting in severely impaired communication such clang associations. Thinking that a client is out to get him is a delusion but reflects less anxiety and impairment. Incomplete sentences are unrelated to growth and development issues. Data such as pacing and wringing of the hands and the client's statements do not indicate noncompliance. (D, 6)

22. 1. Ridiculing others is a defensive coping strategy in response to the client's feelings of increased anxiety. The client's increased level of anxiety is something that can be dealt with in the group. It is not a means or a reason for excluding the client. (D, 6)

23. 2. Pushing a suspicious client into social situations is likely to increase anxiety that increases, not decreases, the hallucinations. The statement about spending some time alone if the client is overwhelmed indicates awareness and understanding of how to intervene when the client is exposed to stress. The statement about lack of motivation indicates awareness and understanding of avolition. The statement about reminding the client that the family doesn't hear the voices indicates awareness and understanding of the client's hallucinations. (E, 6)

24. 1. Clozapine (Clozaril) is the one atypical antipsychotic that is associated with severe anticholinergic side effects, such as constipation. Consuming fruits would not be the cause of the client's constipation. Acknowledging the need for weekly blood tests indicates that the client understands the risk for agranulocytosis, a side effect of clozapine (Clozaril). Getting up slowly indicates that the client understands that orthostatic hypotension may occur with clozapine (Clozaril). The statement about sleepiness indicates that the client understands that sedation may occur with this drug. (E, 8)

25. 4. The statement about the voices occurring if the client is nervous reflects awareness that stress and anxiety can increase the positive symptoms of schizophrenia. Decreasing the medications because the voices are gone reveals a lack of awareness about the need for the medications to control the client's symptoms. Stating that there is still poison in her food demonstrates a lack of insight into the client's delusions. Restarting school in a week reflects an unrealistic expectation for a client who is newly diagnosed and being stabilized on medications. (E, 6)

26. 3. Because the client is aware that he is experiencing auditory hallucinations, he has some insight into his current problem. Therefore, the nurse should help the client take an active role in trying to control the hallucinations. Telling the client that the nurse doesn't hear voices even though the client does is appropriate to help the client gain insight and awareness of the problem. Although time and medications will make the voices go away for most clients, the focus is on helping the client to develop coping strategies to control the hallucinations. Telling the client that the nurse hears only the client's and the nurse's voices is appropriate when the client lacks insight and awareness of the problem. (I, 6)

27. 1. Recognition by the client that there is a difference between the stuffed animal and her live dog indicates that the client is perceiving the reality of the situation. Stating that the stuffed animal and the client's dog could be twins reflects the client's continued misperception of reality, thinking that the stuffed animal and her dog are one and the same. Stating that she wishes her dog hadn't been stuffed reflects her continued misperception of reality. Stating that the roommate needs a dog as much as she does is unrelated to the client's perception or misperception of reality. (E, 6)

28. 4. Allowing the client to be the first to open the cart and take a tray presents the client with the reality that the nurses are not touching the food and tray, thereby dispelling the delusion. Serving foods in sealed packages is unrealistic because most hospital food does not arrive this way. Additionally, if this were possible, the sealing of the packages would further reinforce the client's delusion. Asking the client about the type of poison or giving the client canned supplements confirms the reality of the client's suspiciousness, thereby reinforcing the delusion. (I, 6)

29. 2. Constipation secondary to clozapine is best managed by diet, fluids, and exercise. Benztropine (Cogentin) can increase constipation. However, it may be prescribed for restlessness and stiffness. Restlessness and stiffness should be reported to the physician. Because clozapine is associated with agranulocytosis, it is imperative for the client to comply with weekly blood tests to check the white blood cell count. Clozapine (Clozaril) does help to improve the negative symptoms of schizophrenia, such as avolition. (E, 8)

The Client With Other Types of Schizophrenia and Psychotic Disorders

30. 1. The initial priority for this client is to help her overcome suspiciousness of others including staff, and thereby feel safe and accepted. Introducing the client to others, giving the client information about the program, and providing clean clothes are important, but these are of lower priority than helping the client feel safe and accepted. (P, 6)

31. 3. The nurse must be objective in documenting the client's behavior, recording exactly what the client did or did not say or do in a particular situation. Recording that the client was not able to answer any questions, was uncooperative and refused to answer questions, or was disoriented and incoherent is not true and is a subjective interpretation on the nurse's part. (I, 1)

32. 4. By the end of 4 days, the client should be able to perform showering and dressing for herself. The client with schizophrenia often appears to be apathetic and lack initiative. Therefore, demonstrating the ability to complete the tasks indicates improvement. Although the client may be able to recognize, verbalize, or explain the need to shower and dress herself, she may be unable to do so because of the ambivalence associated with schizophrenia that impedes the client's ability to initiate and complete self-care. Therefore, evidence of improvement would be lacking. (P, 6)

33. 1. When determining the effectiveness of risperidone, the nurse would expect improvement in the client's negative symptoms of apathy, flat affect, and social withdrawal. Delusions, hallucinations, illusions, and ideas of reference are positive symptoms of schizophrenia. Agitation, hostility, and aggression are the result of the positive symptoms. (E, 8)

34. 3. Sialorrhea, excessive salivation, is commonly associated with clozapine therapy. Clients can use a washcloth to wipe the saliva instead of spitting. It is an expected side effect of the drug, not a delusion, an unusual reaction, or an unresolved symptom of schizophrenia. (D, 8)

35. 3. Stating that God is important in the client's life recognizes the client's cognitive and perceptual disturbances and level of anxiety and acknowledges the client's message in a respectful and neutral manner, and stating that the also will medicine clearly and directly states the need for medication. Stating, "God helps those who help themselves" challenges the patient. Stating, "God wants you to take your medicine" is deceitful. Stating, "Medicine will help clear your thinking and decrease the voices" would be helpful to the client later when the client is less acutely psychotic and anxious. (I, 6)

36. 1. The nurse instructs the client clearly and directly to put the medication in his mouth and then to swallow it with some water. Clear, step-by-step directions assist the client to process what the nurse is saying. Telling the client to sit in the dayroom and wait, asking another staff member to stay with the client, or saying nothing is not helpful. (I, 8)

37. 4. Based on the nursing diagnosis of Defensive Coping secondary to suspiciousness, the client's ability to accurately interpret the behaviors of staff and clients would be the expected outcome. The underlying problem is the client's suspiciousness and paranoid statement. Therefore, improvement in this behavior would be the focus of the outcome. Although demonstrating an absence of hostile behavior, developing the ability to express one's own needs assertively, and using adaptive coping strategies are desirable, the focus of the outcome needs to address the client's underlying problem, which is interpretation of the behaviors of others. (P, 6)

38. 2. Whispering and laughing with another person where the client can see or observe the nurse but not hear the conversation increases the client's anxiety and suspiciousness. Therefore, this action should be avoided. Informing the client of schedule changes, telling the client gently that the nurse does not share the client's interpretation of an event, and inviting the client to participate in leisure activities help the client to decrease anxiety and suspiciousness and to focus on actual or realistic events. (I, 6)

39. 4. Because the client is able to live in an apartment setting, further development of independent functioning and the skills to gain as much independence as he is capable of need to be fostered, including getting out and developing new friendships. Family visits and daily nursing visits do not encourage the client to do this. Arranging for participation in day treatment is most beneficial at this time. Day treatment sessions provide activities to promote social skill development, recreation, and psychoeducation in a structured environment. Lack of social relationships is not a sufficient reason for rehospitalization. (I, 6)

40. 1. Hallucinations and asocial behaviors are typical symptoms of undifferentiated schizophrenia. Preoccupation with persecutory delusions and hallucinations are associated with paranoid schizophrenia. Grossly disorganized behaviors and speech are associated with disorganized type of schizophrenia. Immobility and waxy flexibility are associated with catatonic type of schizophrenia. (A, 6)

41. 3. With CUS, negative symptoms are more prominent. Therefore, risperidone therapy is given to help control the negative symptoms. Positive symptoms of CUS initially would be treated with a high-potency antipsychotic agent, such as haloperidol (Haldol). Agranulocytosis is commonly associated with clozapine (Clozaril). Because it is a newer drug, risperidone usually is more expensive than traditional antipsychotics. (P, 8)

42. 2. The client is in an acute psychotic state, unable to process complex decisions or explain complex situations. Therefore, the nurse would focus on decision making involving simple choices. Listing the pros and cons of each housing option and identifying why the client cannot live in an unsupervised apartment are complex decision-making skills. Deciding which staff member to have today is a difficult and threatening decision for a client who is psychotic. (I, 6)

43. 1. The client is exhibiting hallmark signs and symptoms of life-threatening neuroleptic malignant syndrome induced by the haloperidol (Haldol). Tardive dyskinesia usually occurs later in treatment, typically months to years later. Extrapyramidal side effects (eg, dystonia, akathisia) and drug-induced parkinsonism, although common, are not life-threatening. (D, 9)

44. 3. Clients with CUS need more structure every day to improve their functioning. Therefore, helping the client to set up a daily activity schedule would be most appropriate. However, a group home is not necessary. The client is already eating. In fact, it is the one activity that he does do. Having meals brought in would increase the client's dependence, not his activity level. Asking a relative to call the client 10 times per day is unrealistic given the typical daily responsibilities of a healthy relative. (I, 6)

45. 2. The client is exhibiting catatonic behavior, an acutely serious result of severe anxiety and psychosis. In this situation the nurse needs to administer the PRN-ordered doses of haloperidol (Haldol) and lorazepam (Ativan); they can be given together safely. Assisting the client out of the chair to go back to bed or sitting quietly until the client responds ignores the seriousness of the client's condition. It would be unlikely for the client to be able to describe what is being experienced. (I, 6)

46. 1. The client's calling his mother is a first step in getting out of a severe withdrawal. Attending day therapy three times a week or allowing two friends to visit every day would be appropriate if the client is successful with calling his mother once a day. Insufficient information is presented in the scenario to indicate that excessive sleep is a problem. (P, 6)

47. 4. Although all the actions indicate improvement, the ability to initiate simple activities without directions indicates the most improvement in the catatonic behaviors. Moving all extremities occasionally, walking with the nurse to her room, and responding to verbal direc-

tions to eat represent single steps toward the client's initiating her own actions. (E, 8)

48. 2. Noncompliance with medications is common in clients with CUS. The nurse has the responsibility to assess this situation. Asking the mother if they've argued or if the client is mad at the mother or telling the mother to go over to the apartment and see what's going on places the blame and responsibility on the mother and therefore is inappropriate. Telling the mother not to worry ignores the seriousness of the client's symptoms. (I, 6)

49. 4. The client is exhibiting symptoms of becoming immobilized that are classic precursors to catatonic behaviors. Disorganized schizophrenia is characterized by disorganized speech and behaviors. Paranoid schizophrenia is characterized by increased suspiciousness. Undifferentiated schizophrenia is characterized by increased hallucinations and delusions. (D, 6)

50. 1. The client recently lost his mother, causing the client to experience increased stress. This increase in stress can decrease the effectiveness of medications. Therefore, a short course of a fast-acting medication, such as haloperidol (Haldol), would be added to the client's drug therapy regimen. An increase in Zyprexa is not likely to relieve the immediate symptoms quickly. Grief counseling would not be effective until the client's other symptoms are controlled. Changing to a new medication is premature. This would be done only if the client failed to respond to the addition of haloperidol to his drug therapy regimen. (P, 9)

51. 3. Valproic acid is commonly used to treat manic symptoms. Therefore, a decrease in valproic acid level could explain the increase in manic symptoms. Periodic determinations of the valproic level are necessary to determine the effectiveness of the drug. However, the stat nature of the specimen to be drawn indicates an immediate problem. Fluoxetine is not known to decrease the effectiveness of valproic acid. The valproic acid level is not needed before beginning a short course of therapy with lorazepam. (D, 8)

52. 3. According to the DSM-IV-TR criteria, a diagnosis of brief psychotic disorder is made when the client exhibits delusions, hallucinations, and disorganized speech or behaviors in the absence of a mood disorder, substance-induced disorder, or general medical condition. (A, 6)

53. 4. Follow-up counseling is appropriate because of the client's anger and inappropriate behaviors. The goal is to help the client deal with the end of his marriage. A joint session might have been useful before the divorce and arrest, but not after. The client is exhibiting no signs or symptoms of schizophrenia, so olanzapine is

not indicated. The client is not exhibiting any signs of depression, so fluoxetine is not indicated. (P, 6)

Clients and Families Affected by Chronic Mental Illnesses

54. 4. Among the needs of the chronically mentally ill are community-based treatment programs, psychosocial rehabilitation programs, and employment opportunities. During necessary periods of hospitalization, active treatment, rather than custodial care, is needed. (I, 1)

55. 3. The nurse's role in a psychosocial rehabilitation program involves teaching the client to live independently by using interpersonal skills and community resources. Insight-oriented psychotherapy is less beneficial for this client population. (P, 6)

56. 3. The first thing that the nurse should do is to speak with the client on the phone and question her about perceptions or reasons that are interfering with her going to the sheltered workshop. This conveys that the nurse is interested and willing to help the client. The nurse should call the director of the workshop for information only if the nurse receives the client's permission. Making preparations for the client's admission is inappropriate and would not done until the client's needs have been assessed and it is determined that the client requires hospitalization. Making an appointment with the doctor is inappropriate until the nurse has assessed the client's needs. (I, 6)

57. 2. Psychoeducational groups for families help families develop a support network. They provide education about the biochemical etiology of psychiatric disease to reduce, not increase family guilt. These groups also provide information about symptoms and symptom management, medication, and ways of coping with a mentally ill family member. (I, 6)

58. 2. Noncompliance with medications is documented as the primary cause of relapse. Although loss of family support, sudden changes in medications, and nonattendance at treatment programs may contribute to relapse, these factors are not as significant as medication noncompliance as causes of relapse. (I, 6)

59. 3. The most therapeutic action at this time is for the nurse to make an appointment with the client at the mental health center to explore his feelings and behavior. Doing so acknowledges the client's importance and makes him a partner in resolving the problem. The nurse needs to determine what is going on in the situation first, and then plan accordingly. Threatening the client with loss of the position, asking for a new assignment for the client, or arranging for the placement of the client in a skill-training program is inappropriate and premature. (I, 6)

60. 2. By acknowledging the difficulties of living with the illness, the nurse conveys empathy for the client's feelings and opens up the lines of communication. Although it is important for the client to maintain compliance with medication therapy, telling the client that it is vitally important to start taking them again or to talk with the doctor about stopping the medications ignores the underlying feelings of the client's initial statements. Stating that the client's buddies will understand may or may not be true. Additionally, this statement ignores the underlying feelings. (I, 6)

61. 3. Because antipsychotic agents cross the placental barrier and can be teratogenic, they are to be avoided during pregnancy, especially during the first trimester. Later in the pregnancy, low doses of medications may be given if necessary. Although the degree of excitement by the father, the mother's ability to provide help, and the client's financial situation may or may not be of concern, the priority problem in this situation is the safety of the fetus and risks associated with the need for antipsychotic therapy. (A, 6)

62. 4. Although all of the options listed are commonly true, the primary reason for the concern is that parents most frequently provide the financial support and housing for their chronically mentally ill children. The most critical needs after loss of the parents are the lack of financial support and housing, which are hard to replace. (A, 6)

63. 2. A monozygotic twin has a higher risk of developing schizophrenia if the other twin has the disorder. This predisposition may be triggered by the stress associated with marriage or pregnancy. Research reveals that the children of a monozygotic twin whose twin has the disorder have a lower risk for the disorder than their mother does. The parents of monozygotic twins, one of whom has schizophrenia, are at low risk. Women can develop schizophrenia later in life. (I, 6)

64. 2. Families are more likely to be seen as allies in the care of clients because they are no longer viewed as "causing" the illness. Although family dysfunction is viewed as an effect of rather than a cause of the disorder, the most significant aspect is that families are now viewed as allies by health care professionals. Families may or may not be less likely to participate in studies or to be involved in caring for the ill relatives. (P, 6)

65. 4. Although a decline in functioning is important, this situation would have the least priority when compared with other situations that put the client or others in danger of direct or indirect harm. (D, 2)

66. 3. A variety of coordinated services is needed, including medication management, more frequent outpatient visits, day treatment, or some combination of these, to decrease the risk of relapse, which is common among chronically ill clients. Medical consultations (if needed) would be included in the coordinated services provided. Chronically mentally ill clients who are discharged early, before becoming truly stable, typically require more than the usual allotment of monthly outpatient visits because of the high risk for relapse. Caring and supportive follow-up is needed by all clients regardless of their other needs. (P, 6)

67. 3. Noncompliance with medications is the most common cause of relapse and rehospitalization for chronically mentally ill persons. Family support is desirable but is less likely to be available for these clients. Advocacy is a long-term goal. Preventing relapse is a daily goal. Support groups are not always appropriate for chronically ill clients. (A, 6)

68. 1. Without a sufficient range and quantity of services, care is inadequate. Funds were not transferred, but this is a major cause of lack of services that leads to increased hospitalizations. The principle of "least restrictive alternative" is still as relevant as it was before managed care. Hospitalization was reserved for emergency services even before managed care. Nonshifting of allocated funding to outpatient services has increased the problem with the range and quantity of services. (P, 1)

69. 4. For a community-based program, the need for long-term hospitalization is least likely if the other services, such as partial programs, psychiatric home care, and residential services, are available and accessible. (P, 1)

70. 4. Advocacy is a crucial role for all nurses who are working with clients diagnosed with chronic mental illness, to ensure access to a full range of medical and psychiatric services. Although a master's degree–prepared nurse may coordinate care, a variety of professionals are involved in providing services to the chronically mentally ill. Until the client's illness is stabilized, a GED is not realistic. Families, indeed, are important and helpful. However, many resources are needed. (I, 1)

71. 2. Although all of the situations require attention, relapse and decompensation are more likely to be causes of the other situations and warrant immediate attention. (I, 6)

72. 1. Ways to decrease or manage side effects without additional medications is crucial. Although home visits, family monitoring, and outpatient monitoring may help, if the side effects are not controlled the client is less likely to take the drug, which would interfere with its effectiveness. (I, 8)

73. 4. Many Americans still believe that recovery from mental illness is a matter of willpower—for example, "pull yourself up by your bootstraps" or "just get over it." This belief persists despite awareness that mental illness is hereditary and has a biochemical basis. Mental illness can be prevented only if there is early intervention. Clients cannot prevent it just by the desire to do so. (A, 1)

The Client With Cognitive Disorders

74. 1. People of all ages need to have a sense of future well-being. They must have hope for things to come and believe in growth and change to live life to its fullest. Health personnel need to foster this feeling of hopefulness and subscribe to it to help clients attain a sense of well-being, even when the prognosis appears poor. Acceptance and concern would ultimately convey hope. Nonchalance conveys a lack of caring and concern. (P, 6)

75. 2. Clients with chronic cognitive disorders experience defects in memory orientation and intellectual functions, such as judgment and discrimination. Loss of other abilities, such as speech, endurance, or balance, is less typical. (A, 6)

76. 1. Because of the client's short-term memory impairment, the nurse gently corrects the client by stating her name and who she is. This approach decreases anxiety, embarrassment, and shame and maintains the client's self-esteem. Telling the client that she knows who the nurse is or that she forgot can elicit feelings of embarrassment and shame. Saying, "I told you already" sounds condescending, as if the blaming the client for not remembering. (I, 6)

77. 2. When caring for a client with cognitive impairment, the priority is to ensure that all objects in the client's path of ambulation are removed to prevent the client from falling. Additional measures include having two people accompany the client when he ambulates, placing his favorite things in safekeeping, and giving medications in a liquid form to be sure he swallows them. (P, 2)

78. 1. The most likely reason for nurse's discomfort with elderly clients is that she has not examined her own fears and conflicts about aging. Until nurses resolve their fears, it is unlikely that they will feel comfortable with elderly clients. (A, 1)

79. 3. Reminiscing can help reduce depression in an elderly client and lessens feelings of isolation and loneliness. Reminiscing encourages a focus on positive memories and accomplishments as well as shared memories with other clients. An increase in confusion and disorientation is most likely the result of other cognitive and situational factors, such as loss of short-term memory, not reminiscing. Subjecting the client to the others' responses is most likely the result of other cognitive and situational factors, such as hopelessness, fear, or

despair, not reminiscing. Keeping the client from participating in therapeutic activities is most likely the result of other cognitive and situational factors, such as severe depression and dementia, not reminiscing. (P, 6)

The Client With Delirium

80. 4. Based on the assessment findings, delirium is the most likely cause of the sudden onset of symptoms. Uremia is a common cause of delirium resulting from the buildup of toxins in the body. Disorientation and memory deficits are not commonly seen in bipolar or general anxiety disorder. Grandiosity and hyperactivity are more common in bipolar disorder. Dementia has a slow but progressive onset, not a sudden onset as described. (D, 6)

81. 3. Polypharmacy is much more common in the elderly. Drug interactions increase the incidence of intoxication from prescribed medications, especially with combinations of analgesics, digoxin, diuretics, and anticholinergics. With drug intoxication, the onset of the delirium typically is quick. Although cancer, impaired hearing, and congestive heart failure could lead to delirium in the elderly, the onset of the delirium would be more gradual. (A, 9)

82. 1. Fluctuating symptoms are characteristic of delirium. The failure to identify objects despite intact sensory functions, significant impairment in social or occupational functioning over time, and memory impairment to the degree of being called amnesia indicate dementia. (A, 6)

83. 2. The most critical aspect when caring for the client with delirium is to institute measures to correct the underlying causative condition or illness. Controlling behavioral symptoms with low-dose psychotropics, manipulating the environment, and decreasing or discontinuing any nonessential medications also may be helpful while waiting for the delirium to clear. (I, 6)

84. 3. In approximately 2 to 3 days, the client should be able to regain orientation and thus become oriented to time, place, and person. Being able to explain the experience of having delirium is something that the client would be expected to achieve later in the course of the illness, but ultimately before discharge. Regaining a normal sleep–wake cycle and establishing normal bowel and bladder function probably will take longer, depending on how long it takes to resolve the underlying condition. (P, 6)

85. 1. Identifying one's self and making sure that the nurse has the client's attention addresses the difficulties with focusing and maintaining attention. Eliminating daytime napping is unrealistic until the cause of the delir-

ium is determined and the client's ability to focus and maintain attention improves. Engaging the client in reminiscing and avoiding arguing are also unrealistic at this time. (P, 6)

The Client With Dementia

86. 4. Loss of judgment decreases the ability to control impulses and behaviors in social situations. Therefore, the client typically exhibits inappropriate language and sexual behaviors. Wandering and getting lost involve cognitive changes, not disinhibition. (D, 6)

87. 2. Highly conditioned motor skills, such as brushing the teeth, may be retained by the client who has dementia and motor apraxia. Balancing a checkbook involves calculations, a complex skill that is lost with severe dementia. Confabulation is fabrication of details to fill a memory gap. This is more common when the client is aware of a memory problem, not when dementia is severe. Finding keys is a memory factor, not a motor function. (A, 6)

88. 3. Competing and excessive stimuli lead to sensory overload and confusion. Therefore, the nurse should first eliminate any distracting stimuli. Once this is accomplished, then using touch and rephrasing questions are appropriate. Going for a walk while talking has little beneficial effect on attention and confusion. (I, 6)

89. 4. Telling the client that she is wrong and then telling her what is right is argumentative and challenging. Arguing with or challenging distortions is least effective because it increases defensiveness. Telling the client about reality indicates awareness of the issues and is appropriate. Acknowledging that misperceptions are part of the disease indicates an understanding of the disease and an awareness of the issues. Turning off the radio helps to limit environmental stimuli and indicates an awareness of the issues. (E, 6)

The Client With Alzheimer's Disease

90. 1. The son's statements regarding his father's recalling past events is typical for family members of clients in the early stage of AD, when recent memory is impaired. It suggests a lack of knowledge about the disease process. Reminiscing is a positive experience for the client that brings forth familiar feelings and allows the client to engage in social interaction. Memory loss is the problem associated with AD, not anxiety or antagonism. (D, 6)

91. 3. The best rationale for day treatment for clients with AD is the enhancement of social interactions. More daily structure, excellent staff, and allowing caregivers

more time for themselves are all positive aspects, but they are less focused on the client's needs. (I, 6)

92. 3. Neurofibrillary tangles and plaques are found in postmortem examinations of AD clients, distinguishing it from other dementias. Hypoxic destruction of brain cells is associated with multi-infarct dementia. Hyperkinesis causing choreiform movements is associated with Huntington's disease. Evidence of an infectious particle called a prion is associated with Creutzfeldt-Jakob disease. (I, 6)

93. 1. Considerable assistance is associated with moderate impairment when the client is unable to make decisions but can follow directions. Supervision of shaving is appropriate with mild impairment—that is, when the client still has motor function but lacks judgment about safety issues. Managing medications is needed even in mild impairment. Constant care is needed in the terminal phase, when the client is unable to follow directions. (P, 6)

94. 4. Antidepressant medications have little impact on wandering. A Medical Alert bracelet helps in identifying the client should the client wander. Motion and sound detectors and door alarms can alert family members to the possibility of the client's leaving the area. (I, 2)

95. 2. Because the client is experiencing difficulty processing and completing complex tasks, the priority is to provide the client with only one step at a time, thereby breaking the task up into simple steps, ones that the client is able to process. Repeating the directions until the client follows them or demonstrating how to do the task is still too overwhelming to the client because of the multiple steps involved. However, demonstrating one step at a time and then having the client do the step would be helpful. Although maintaining structure and routine is important, it is unrelated to task completion. (P, 6)

96. 3. The nurse needs to present reality without arguing with the delusions. Therefore, stating that the client is in the hospital and the nurses are trying to help is most appropriate. The client doesn't recognize the delusion or why it exists. Telling the client that the staff likes him too much to want to kill him is inappropriate because the client believes the delusions and doesn't know that they are false beliefs. It also restates the word, "kill," which may reinforce the client's delusions. Telling the client not to be silly is condescending and disparaging and therefore inappropriate. (I, 6)

97. 1. The vulgar or sexual behaviors are often expressions of anger or more sensual needs that can be addressed

directly. Therefore, the families should be encouraged to ignore the behaviors but attempt to identify their purpose. Then the purpose can be addressed, possibly leading to decrease in the behaviors. Because of impaired cognitive function, the client is not likely to be able to process the inappropriateness of the behaviors if given feedback. Likewise, anger management strategies would be ineffective because the client would probably be unable to process the inappropriateness of the behaviors. Risperidone (Risperdal) may decrease agitation, but it does not improve social behaviors. (I, 6)

98. 4. The statement about hoping that the old Dad would be back conveys a lack of acceptance of the irreversible nature of the disease. The statement about not realizing that the deterioration would be so incapacitating is based in reality. The statement about the Alzheimer's group is based in reality and demonstrates the son's involvement with managing the disease. Stating that reminiscing is important reflects a realistic interpretation on the son's part. (E, 6)

99. 1. Donepezil (Aricept) is effective primarily in the early stages of the disease. The drug helps to slow the progression of the disease if started in the early stages. After the client has been diagnosed for 6 years, improvement to the level seen 6 years ago is highly unlikely. Data are not available to support the drug's effectiveness for clients in the terminal phase of the disease. When compared with other similar medications, donepezil (Aricept) has fewer side effects. (I, 8)

100. 3. Antipsychotics are most effective with agitation and assaultiveness. Antipsychotics have little effect on sleep disturbances, concomitant depression, or confusion and withdrawal. (I, 8)

101. 1. Oxazepam is the antianxiety drug of choice for the elderly client, because it is one of the safest agents. Diazepam and chlordiazepoxide have an extended half-life and active metabolites. The elderly are less able to break down and excrete these medicines. Nefazodone (Serzone) is an antidepressant and is not used to treat anxiety. (P, 8)

102. 4. Change increases stress. Therefore, the most important and relevant suggestion is to maintain consistency in the client's environment, routine, and caregivers. Although rest periods are important, going to bed interferes with the sleep–wake cycle. Rest in a recliner chair is more useful. Testing of cognitive functioning and reality orientation are not likely to be successful and may increase the stress if memory loss is severe. (I, 6)

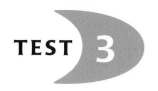
Personality Disorders, Substance-Related Disorders, and Anxiety-Related Disorders

▶ The Client With a Personality Disorder

▶ The Client With an Alcohol-Related Disorder

▶ The Client With Disorders Related to Other Addictive Substances

▶ The Client With an Anxiety-Related Disorder

▶ The Client With a Somatoform Disorder

▶ Correct Answers and Rationale

Select the one best answer, and indicate your choice by filling in the circle in front of the option.

The Client With a Personality Disorder

1. When developing the plan of care for a client with a personality disorder, the nurse expects to assist the client primarily with which of the following?
   ○ 1. Specific dysfunctional behaviors.
   ○ 2. Psychopharmacologic compliance.
   ○ 3. Examination of developmental conflicts.
   ○ 4. Manipulation of the environment.

2. A client with paranoid personality disorder is hospitalized for physically threatening his wife because he suspects her of having an affair with a coworker. Which of the following approaches would the nurse employ with this client?
   ○ 1. Authoritarian.
   ○ 2. Parental.
   ○ 3. Matter-of-fact.
   ○ 4. Controlling.

3. When planning care for a client with schizotypal personality disorder, which of the following would help the client become involved with others?
   ○ 1. Participating solely in group activities.
   ○ 2. Being involved with primarily one-to-one activities.
   ○ 3. Leading a sing-a-long in the afternoon.
   ○ 4. Attending an activity with the nurse.

4. A client is complaining to other clients about not being allowed by staff to keep food in her room. Which of the following interventions would be *most* appropriate?
   ○ 1. Ignoring the client's behavior.
   ○ 2. Setting limits on the behavior.
   ○ 3. Reprimanding the client.
   ○ 4. Allowing the snack to be kept in her room.

5. A client with an Axis II diagnosis of antisocial personality disorder has a potential for violence and aggressive behavior. Which of the following client outcomes to be accomplished in the short term would be *most* appropriate for the nurse to include in the plan of care?
   ○ 1. Use humor when expressing anger.
   ○ 2. Discuss feelings of anger with staff.
   ○ 3. Ask the nurse for medication when upset.
   ○ 4. Use indirect behaviors to express anger.

6. A client with an Axis II diagnosis of antisocial personality disorder has been stealing equipment from his place of employment. He states, "It's not a big deal. My boss can afford a few missing pieces. He doesn't like me." The nurse interprets the client's behavior as indicative of problems in which of the following stages of growth and development defined by Erikson?
   ○ 1. Trust versus mistrust.
   ○ 2. Autonomy versus shame and doubt.
   ○ 3. Initiative versus guilt.
   ○ 4. Industry versus inferiority.

7. Which of the following approaches would the nurse expect to include in the plan of care for a client with antisocial personality disorder who has a history of stealing and jail time?
   ○ 1. Helping the client develop a conscience.
   ○ 2. Teaching the client consequences of her actions.
   ○ 3. Assisting the client with understanding right from wrong.
   ○ 4. Using strategies to help the client become passive.

8. A 28-year-old client with an Axis I diagnosis of major depression and an Axis II diagnosis of dependent personality disorder has been living at home with very supportive parents. The client is

585

thinking about independent living on the recommendation of the treatment team. The client states to the nurse, "I don't know if I can make it in an apartment without my parents." Which of the following responses by the nurse would be *most* therapeutic?
- ○ 1. "You're a 28-year-old adult now, not a child who needs to be cared for."
- ○ 2. "Your parents won't be around forever. After all, they are getting older."
- ○ 3. "Your parents need a break, and you need a break from them."
- ○ 4. "Your parents have been supportive and will continue to be even if you live apart."

9. The client with major depression and dependent personality disorder has made the decision to live independently in an apartment. The nurse and the client meet with his parents to discuss his decision. Which statement by the nurse would be *most* helpful to foster the client's independence?
- ○ 1. "You'll still be able to see your son and help him as much as you want."
- ○ 2. "All of you will gain from his independent living; he needs our support."
- ○ 3. "You'll need to help monitor his medication and clinic appointments."
- ○ 4. "You will live near by and be able to help with meals and laundry."

10. A client who had been living with her family after her boyfriend of 4 weeks told her to leave is admitted to the subacute unit complaining of feeling empty and lonely, being unable to sleep, and hardly eating for the past week. Her arms are scarred from frequent self-mutilation. The nurse interprets these findings as indicating which of the following personality disorders?
- ○ 1. Antisocial personality disorder.
- ○ 2. Avoidant personality disorder.
- ○ 3. Borderline personality disorder.
- ○ 4. Compulsive personality disorder.

11. The client approaches various staff with numerous requests and needs to the point of disrupting the staff's work with other clients. The nurse meets with the staff to decide on a consistent, therapeutic approach for this client. Which of the following approaches would the nurse expect to institute?
- ○ 1. Telling the client to stay in his room until staff approach him.
- ○ 2. Limiting the client to the dayroom and dining area.
- ○ 3. Giving the client a list of permissible requests.
- ○ 4. Having the client address needs to the staff person assigned.

12. The client with borderline personality disorder tells the nurse, "You're the best nurse here. I can talk to you and you listen. You're the only one here that can help me." Which of the following responses by the nurse is *most* therapeutic?
- ○ 1. "Thank you, you're a good person."
- ○ 2. "All of the nurses here provide good care."
- ○ 3. "Other clients have told me that too."
- ○ 4. "Mary and Sam are good nurses too."

13. The client with borderline personality disorder is admitted to the unit after having attempted to cut her wrists with a pair of scissors. The client has several scars on both arms from self-mutilation and suicide gestures. A staff member states to the nurse, "It's just attention that she wants, she's not going to kill herself." Which of the following responses by the nurse would be *most* appropriate?
- ○ 1. "She's here now and we have to do our best."
- ○ 2. "She needs to be here until she can control her behavior."
- ○ 3. "I'm ashamed of you; you know better than to say that."
- ○ 4. "Any attempt at self-harm is serious and safety is a priority."

14. The nurse assesses a client to be at risk for self-mutilation and implements a safety contract with the client. Which of the following client behaviors would indicate that the contract is working?
- ○ 1. The client withdraws to his room when feeling overwhelmed.
- ○ 2. The client notifies staff when anxiety is increasing.
- ○ 3. The client suppresses his feelings when angry.
- ○ 4. The client displaces his feelings onto the physician.

15. The client with borderline personality disorder who is to be discharged soon threatens to "do something" to herself if discharged. Which of the following actions by the nurse would be *most* important?
- ○ 1. Request an immediate extension for the client.
- ○ 2. Ignore the client's statement because it's a sign of manipulation.
- ○ 3. Ask a family member to stay with the client at home temporarily.
- ○ 4. Discuss the meaning of the client's statement with her.

16. A 19-year-old client is admitted to a psychiatric unit with an Axis I diagnosis of alcohol abuse and an Axis II diagnosis of personality disorder NOS (not otherwise specified). The client's mother states, "He's always in trouble, just like when he was a boy. Now he's just a bigger prankster and out of control." In view of the client's history, which of the following would be *most* important initially?
- ○ 1. Letting the client know the staff has the authority to subdue him if he gets unruly.

2. Keeping the client isolated from the other clients until he is better known by the staff.
3. Emphasizing to the client that he will have to pay for any damage he causes.
4. Closely observing the client's behavior to establish a baseline pattern of functioning.

17. The client tells the nurse at the outpatient clinic that she doesn't need to attend groups because she's "not a regular like these other people here." Which of the following responses by the nurse would be *best*?
    1. "Because you're not a regular client, sit in the hall when the others are in group."
    2. "Your family wants you to attend, and they will be very disappointed if you don't."
    3. "I'll have to mark you absent from the clinic today and speak to the doctor about it."
    4. "You say you're not a regular here, but you're experiencing what others are experiencing."

18. After a client with an antisocial personality disorder belches loudly, a staff member asks the client, "Do you wonder why people find you repulsive?" This comment most likely would elicit which of the following client reactions?
    1. Defensiveness.
    2. Remorsefulness.
    3. Shame.
    4. Embarrassment.

19. The client who has a history of using angry outbursts when frustrated begins to curse at the nurse during an appointment after being informed that she will have to wait to have her medication refilled. Which of the following responses by the nurse would be *most* appropriate?
    1. "You are being very childish."
    2. "I'm sorry if you can't wait."
    3. "I will not continue to talk with you if you curse."
    4. "Come back tomorrow and your medication will be ready."

20. Which of the following behaviors would indicate to the nurse that the client with avoidant personality disorder is improving?
    1. Interacting with two other clients.
    2. Listening to music with headphones.
    3. Sitting at a table and painting.
    4. Talking on the telephone.

21. One evening the client takes the nurse aside and whispers, "Don't tell anybody, but I'm going to call in a bomb threat to this hospital tonight." Which of the following actions would be the priority?
    1. Warning the client that his telephone privileges will be taken away if he abuses them.
    2. Offering to disregard the client's plan if he does not go through with it.

3. Notifying the proper authorities after saying nothing until the client has actually completed the call.
4. Explaining to the client that this information will have to be shared immediately with the staff and the physician.

22. When teaching a nursing assistant new to the unit about the principles for the care of a client with a personality disorder, which of the following would the nurse include as the most important basic principle?
    1. The clients are accepted although their behavior may not be.
    2. Clients will need limits on their behavior.
    3. The staff members are the primary ones left to care about these clients.
    4. The staff should use minimal humor when working with these clients.

23. The nurse is talking with a client who has been diagnosed with antisocial personality disorder about how to socialize during activities without being seductive. The nurse would focus the discussion on which of the following areas?
    1. Explaining the negative reactions of others toward his behavior.
    2. Suggesting he apologize to others for his behavior.
    3. Asking him to explain reasons for his seductive behavior.
    4. Discussing his relationship with his mother.

24. The client with an Axis II diagnosis of narcissistic personality disorder tells the nurse he can get an executive position with the best company around anytime he wants. The history reveals that the client, whose highest level of education completed is high school, has held only a series of short-term part-time jobs for the past 2 years. The nurse interprets the client's statement to be an example of which of the following?
    1. Grandiose delusion.
    2. Blatant lie.
    3. Grandiose self-importance.
    4. Sense of entitlement.

25. Which of the following approaches would be *most* appropriate to use with the client who has a narcissistic personality disorder when discrepancies exist between what the client states and what actually exists?
    1. Limit setting.
    2. Supportive confrontation.
    3. Consistency.
    4. Rationalization.

26. The client with a histrionic personality disorder is melodramatic and responds to others and situations in an exaggerated manner. The nurse would recommend which of the following activities for this client?

○ 1. Party planning.
○ 2. Music group.
○ 3. Cooking class.
○ 4. Role playing.

27. When developing the plan of care for a client with an Axis I diagnosis of major depression and an Axis II diagnosis of borderline personality disorder, the nurse would most likely anticipate an order for which of the following medications?
○ 1. A selective serotonin reuptake inhibitor (SSRI).
○ 2. Benzodiazepine.
○ 3. A mood stabilizer.
○ 4. An antipsychotic.

The Client With an Alcohol-Related Disorder

28. An intoxicated client is admitted to the hospital for alcohol withdrawal. Which of the following would the nurse do to help the client become sober?
○ 1. Give the client black coffee to drink.
○ 2. Walk the client around the unit.
○ 3. Have the client take a cold shower.
○ 4. Provide the client with a quiet room to sleep in.

29. A client is entering the chemical dependency unit for treatment of alcohol dependency. Which of the client's possessions will the nurse most likely place in a locked area?
○ 1. Toothpaste.
○ 2. Dental floss.
○ 3. Shaving cream.
○ 4. Antiseptic mouthwash.

30. When obtaining the history from a client entering rehabilitation for alcohol dependency, the nurse questions the client about the amount of alcohol he consumes daily. The client responds, "I just have a few drinks with the guys after work." The nurse interprets this statement as the client's using which of the following as a defense?
○ 1. Projection.
○ 2. Minimization.
○ 3. Denial.
○ 4. Rationalization.

31. While admitting a client to the alcohol treatment program, the nurse asks the client how long she's been drinking this time, how much she's been drinking, and when she had her last drink. The client replies that she has been drinking about a liter of vodka a day for the past week and her last drink was about an hour ago. This information helps the nurse to determine which of the following?
○ 1. The severity of the disease.
○ 2. The severity of withdrawal symptoms.
○ 3. The possibility of alcohol hallucinosis.
○ 4. The occurrence of delirium tremens.

32. The client is feeling better as the symptoms of alcohol withdrawal abate. She refuses information about alcohol rehabilitation and states, "I don't have a problem. I'll never drink like that again. I learned my lesson this time. I guess I'll just have to switch to beer or wine." Which of the following would be *most* effective in decreasing the client's denial?
○ 1. Discussing how alcohol has gotten her into trouble.
○ 2. Explaining the effects of drinking on family.
○ 3. Urging her to attend Alcoholics Anonymous (AA) meetings.
○ 4. Telling her about the physiologic damage that can result.

33. A client who is experiencing alcohol withdrawal exhibits tremors, diaphoresis, and hyperactivity. Blood pressure is 190/87 mm Hg and pulse is 92 bpm. Which of the following medications would the nurse expect to administer?
○ 1. Haloperidol (Haldol).
○ 2. Lorazepam (Ativan).
○ 3. Benztropine (Cogentin).
○ 4. Naloxone (Narcan).

34. Which of the following assessments would provide the *best* information about the client's physiologic response and the effectiveness of the medication prescribed specifically for alcohol withdrawal?
○ 1. Nutritional status.
○ 2. Evidence of tremors.
○ 3. Vital signs.
○ 4. Sleep pattern.

35. A client who had been drinking heavily over the weekend could not remember specific events of where he had been or what he had done. The nurse interprets this information as indicating that the client experienced which of the following conditions?
○ 1. Blackout.
○ 2. Hangover.
○ 3. Tolerance.
○ 4. Delirium tremens.

36. A client is entering the alcohol treatment program for the fourth time in 5 years. Which of the following would be *most* helpful to the client?
○ 1. "I hope you are serious about maintaining your sobriety this time."
○ 2. "I'm Maria, a nurse here. I don't know you from past attempts but you'll get it right this time."
○ 3. "I know someone who was successful after the fifth program."
○ 4. "I'm Maria, a nurse in the program. The staff and I will help you through the program."

37. The wife of a client with alcohol dependency tells the nurse, "I'm tired of making excuses for him to

his boss and coworkers when he can't make it into work. I believe him every time he says he's going to quit." The nurse recognizes the wife's statement as indicating which of the following behaviors?
○ 1. Helpfulness.
○ 2. Self-defeat.
○ 3. Enabling.
○ 4. Masochism.

38. Which of the following statements by the nurse participating in a group confrontation of a coworker would be *most* helpful in reducing the coworker's denial about alcohol being a problem?
○ 1. "Your behavior is unprofessional."
○ 2. "As a nurse you should have sought help earlier."
○ 3. "Nurses are the worst when it comes to asking for help."
○ 4. "You have alcohol on your breath."

39. The husband of a nurse who is being confronted by a group about her problem with alcohol asks the nurse acting as the group leader what he should say during the meeting to his wife. The nurse leader directs the husband to use which of the following statements to facilitate his wife's entrance into treatment?
○ 1. "The children and I want you to get help."
○ 2. "If your parents were alive, they would be extremely disappointed in you."
○ 3. "Either you get help or the kids and I will move out of the house."
○ 4. "You need to enter treatment now or be a drunk if that's what you want."

40. A nurse working in an alcohol rehabilitation program is teaching staff how to give clients constructive feedback. Which of the following statements given as an example illustrates that the staff member has understood the nurse's teaching regarding the use of constructive feedback?
○ 1. "I think you're a real con artist."
○ 2. "You're dominating the conversation."
○ 3. "You interrupted Terry twice in 4 minutes."
○ 4. "You don't give anyone a chance to finish talking."

41. A client ashamedly tells the nurse that he hit his wife while intoxicated and asks the nurse if his wife will ever forgive him. Which of the following replies by the nurse would be *best* in this situation?
○ 1. "Perhaps you could ask her and find out."
○ 2. "That's something you can explore in family therapy."
○ 3. "It would depend on how much she really cares for you."
○ 4. "You seem to have some feelings about hitting your wife."

42. While meeting with the nurse, a client's wife states, "I don't know what else to do to make him stop drinking." The nurse would anticipate initiating a referral for the wife to which of the following organizations?
○ 1. Alateen.
○ 2. Al-Anon.
○ 3. Employee Assistance Program.
○ 4. Alcoholics Anonymous.

43. Which of the following nursing actions is contraindicated for the client who is experiencing severe symptoms of alcohol withdrawal?
○ 1. Ambulating the client.
○ 2. Monitoring intake and output.
○ 3. Assessing vital signs.
○ 4. Using short, concrete statements.

44. Which of the following client statements would indicate to the nurse that the client needs *further* teaching about disulfiram (Antabuse)?
○ 1. "I can drink one or two beers and not get sick while on Antabuse."
○ 2. "I can take Antabuse at bedtime if it makes me sleepy."
○ 3. "A metallic or garlic taste in my mouth is normal when starting on Antabuse."
○ 4. "I'll read the labels on cough syrup and mouthwash for possible alcohol content."

45. While receiving disulfiram (Antabuse) therapy, the client becomes nauseated and vomits severely. Which of the following questions would the nurse ask *first*?
○ 1. "How long have you been taking Antabuse?"
○ 2. "Do you feel like you have the flu?"
○ 3. "How much alcohol did you drink today?"
○ 4. "Have you eaten any foods cooked in wine?"

46. A coworker, new to the chemical dependency unit, questions the use of thiamine for all clients being treated for an alcohol problem. The nurse responds based on the understanding that thiamine is used for which of the following reasons?
○ 1. It prevents the development of Wernicke's encephalopathy.
○ 2. It decreases clients' withdrawal symptoms.
○ 3. It aids clients in regaining their strength sooner.
○ 4. It promotes elimination of alcohol from the body faster.

47. Which of the following client statements indicates an understanding of the signs of alcohol relapse?
○ 1. "I know I can stay dry if my wife keeps alcohol out of the house."
○ 2. "Stopping AA and not expressing feelings can lead to relapse."
○ 3. "I'll have my sponsor at AA keep the list of symptoms for me."
○ 4. "If someone tells me I'm about to relapse, I'll be sure to do something about it."

48. The client sees no connection between her liver disorder and her alcohol intake. She believes that she

drinks very little and that her family is making something out of nothing. The nurse interprets these behaviors as indicative of the client's use of which of the following defense mechanisms?

○ 1. Denial.
○ 2. Displacement.
○ 3. Rationalization.
○ 4. Reaction formation.

49. A client with alcohol dependency is prescribed a B-complex vitamin. The client states, "Why do I need a vitamin? My appetite is just fine." Which of the following responses by the nurse would be *most* appropriate?

○ 1. "Your doctor wants you to take it for at least 4 months."
○ 2. "You've been drinking alcohol and eating very little."
○ 3. "The vitamin is a nutritional supplement important to your health."
○ 4. "The amount of vitamins in the alcohol you drink is very low."

50. The client with alcohol dependency suffers from numbness, itching, and pain in her extremities. Which of the following would the nurse suspect?

○ 1. Neuralgia.
○ 2. Bell's palsy.
○ 3. Neurasthenia.
○ 4. Peripheral neuritis.

51. Which of the following foods would the nurse eliminate from the diet of a client in alcohol withdrawal?

○ 1. Milk.
○ 2. Regular coffee.
○ 3. Orange juice.
○ 4. Eggs.

52. A client with alcohol dependency has peripheral neuropathy. Which of the following areas would be *most* important to include in the client's teaching plan?

○ 1. Washing and drying the feet daily.
○ 2. Massaging the feet with lotion.
○ 3. Trimming the toenails carefully.
○ 4. Avoiding use of an electric blanket.

53. A client who is brought to the emergency room by ambulance begins to thrash about on the stretcher, slapping the sheets and yelling, "Go away, bugs, go away!" Assessment reveals disorientation, a blood pressure of 189/75 mm Hg, and a pulse of 86 bpm. The friend who accompanied the client to the hospital states, "He was drinking a lot when I saw him 4 days ago and asked me for money to get more liquor, but I didn't have any cash to give him." Based on an analysis of these findings, the nurse suspects that the client is experiencing which of the following?

○ 1. Stupor.
○ 2. Mild alcohol withdrawal.
○ 3. Impaired consciousness.
○ 4. Delirium.

54. When a client experiencing alcohol withdrawal thrashes in bed and yells, "Go away, bugs, go away," the nurse would expect to classify this behavior as reflective of which of the following nursing diagnoses?

○ 1. Disturbed Sensory Perception.
○ 2. Disturbed Thought Processes.
○ 3. Risk for Injury.
○ 4. Ineffective Coping.

55. The nurse is teaching unlicensed staff about caring for the client with alcohol dependency. Which of the following statements by the staff indicates the need for additional teaching?

○ 1. "Alcohol dependency affects the entire family."
○ 2. "The client is a weak individual and could stop if he desires."
○ 3. "Alcohol is a problem when it interferes with the client's daily life."
○ 4. "The client who can't stop drinking even though he wants to is alcohol dependent."

56. Which of the following measures would the nurse include in the plan of care for a client with alcohol withdrawal delirium?

○ 1. Using restraints continuously.
○ 2. Touching the client before saying anything.
○ 3. Remaining with the client when she is confused or disoriented.
○ 4. Informing the client about alcohol treatment programs.

57. Which of the following would be an accurate response when a client's asking the nurse about requirements to become a member of AA?

○ 1. "You must be sober for at least a month before joining."
○ 2. "AA is open to anyone who wants sobriety."
○ 3. "The members will interview you and decide if you can join the group."
○ 4. "AA requires daily attendance at meetings."

58. A client is to be discharged from an alcohol rehabilitation program. Which of the following would the nurse emphasize in the discharge plan as a priority?

○ 1. Supportive friends.
○ 2. A list of goals.
○ 3. Family forgiveness.
○ 4. Follow-up care.

59. A client is being admitted to the unit with a dual diagnosis. The nurse would expect that the client's diagnoses would include which of the following?

○ 1. Schizophrenia and dependent personality disorder.
○ 2. Bipolar disorder and suicide attempt.
○ 3. Major depression and alcohol abuse.
○ 4. Chronic paranoid schizophrenia and borderline personality disorder.

60. While caring for a client who has a dual diagnosis of

bipolar disorder and alcohol dependency, which of the following areas would be the priority for daily assessment?
- ○ 1. Sleep pattern.
- ○ 2. Mental status.
- ○ 3. Eating habits.
- ○ 4. Self-care ability.

61. A client diagnosed with schizophrenia and alcohol abuse decides to drink alcohol with his buddies. The nurse interprets this behavior, recognizing which of the following as an underlying dynamic of the client's alcohol use?
- ○ 1. The decision to use alcohol results in a feeling of autonomy and power.
- ○ 2. The decision to drink increases the client's guilt and shame.
- ○ 3. The client abused alcohol before developing a mental illness.
- ○ 4. The client is compelled to drink because of cognitive difficulties.

The Client With Disorders Related to Other Addictive Substances

62. The friend of a client brought to the hospital's emergency room states, "I guess she had some bad junk (heroin) today." The client is drowsy and verbally nonresponsive. Which of the following assessment findings would be of immediate concern to the nurse?
- ○ 1. Respiratory rate of 9 breaths/minute.
- ○ 2. Urinary retention.
- ○ 3. Hypotension.
- ○ 4. Reduced pupil size.

63. The nurse prepares to administer which of the following medications to a client with heroin overdose?
- ○ 1. Haloperidol (Haldol).
- ○ 2. Naloxone (Narcan).
- ○ 3. Lorazepam (Ativan).
- ○ 4. Oxazepam (Serax).

64. Which of the following would the nurse expect to assess for a client who is exhibiting late signs of heroin withdrawal?
- ○ 1. Vomiting and diarrhea.
- ○ 2. Yawning and diaphoresis.
- ○ 3. Lacrimation and rhinorrhea.
- ○ 4. Restlessness and irritability.

65. After administering naloxone (Narcan), a narcotic antagonist, the nurse should monitor the client carefully for which of the following?
- ○ 1. Cerebral edema.
- ○ 2. Kidney failure.
- ○ 3. Seizure activity.
- ○ 4. Respiratory depression.

66. When teaching a client who is to receive methadone therapy for opioid addiction, the nurse would instruct the client that methadone is useful primarily for which of the following reasons?
- ○ 1. It is not an addictive substance.
- ○ 2. A maintenance dose is taken twice a day.
- ○ 3. The client will no longer be addicted to narcotics.
- ○ 4. The client may work and live normally.

67. A client states to the nurse, "I'm not going to any more Narcotics Anonymous meetings. I felt out of place there." Which of the following responses by the nurse would be *best*?
- ○ 1. "Try attending a meeting at a different location; you may feel more comfortable there."
- ○ 2. "Maybe it just wasn't a good day for you. Everybody has bad days now and then."
- ○ 3. "Perhaps you weren't paying close enough attention to what they were saying."
- ○ 4. "Sometimes the meetings can seem like a waste of time, but you need to attend to stay clean."

68. Which of the following would the nurse use as the *best* measure to determine a client's progress in rehabilitation?
- ○ 1. The kinds of friends he makes.
- ○ 2. The number of drug-free days he has.
- ○ 3. The way he gets along with his parents.
- ○ 4. The amount of responsibility his job entails.

69. Which of the following would lead the nurse to suspect that a client is addicted to heroin?
- ○ 1. Hilarity.
- ○ 2. Aggression.
- ○ 3. Labile mood.
- ○ 4. Hypoactivity.

70. A client brought by ambulance to the hospital emergency room after taking an overdose of barbiturates is comatose. The nurse would be especially alert for which of the following?
- ○ 1. Kidney failure.
- ○ 2. Cerebral vascular accident.
- ○ 3. Status epilepticus.
- ○ 4. Respiratory failure.

71. The client's friend reports that the client has been taking about eight "reds" (800 mg of secobarbital [Seconal]) daily, besides drinking more alcohol than usual. The client's friend asks anxiously, "Do you think she will live?" Which of the following responses by the nurse would be *most* appropriate?
- ○ 1. "We can only wait and see. It's too soon to tell."
- ○ 2. "Do you know her well? She's so young."
- ○ 3. "She is very ill and may not live. Some don't pull through."
- ○ 4. "Her condition is serious. You sound very worried about her."

72. Before his hospitalization, a client needed increasingly larger doses of barbiturates to achieve the same euphoric effect he initially realized from their use. From this information, the nurse develops a plan of care that takes into account that the client is most likely suffering from which of the following?
    ○ 1. Tolerance.
    ○ 2. Addiction.
    ○ 3. Abuse.
    ○ 4. Dependence.

73. Which of the following statements by the nurse would be *most* appropriate when addressing a client with a barbiturate overdose who awakens in a confused state and exhibits stable vital signs?
    ○ 1. "I'm here to help you beat your drug habit. But its you who will need to work hard."
    ○ 2. "It's time to get straight and stay clean and put an end to your torture."
    ○ 3. "I'm glad you pulled through; it was touch and go with you for a while."
    ○ 4. "You're in the hospital because of a drug problem; I'm one of the nurses who will help you."

74. During an interaction with the nurse, the client states that her "life has gone down the tubes" since her divorce 6 months ago. Afterwards, she lost her job and apartment and then she "took those pills to sleep and not wake up." From these data, the nurse would identify which of the following nursing diagnoses as the *priority*?
    ○ 1. Low Self-Esteem related to losses.
    ○ 2. Risk for Self-Directed Violence related to suicide attempt.
    ○ 3. Ineffective Coping related to hopelessness.
    ○ 4. Powerlessness related to helplessness.

75. The nurse identifies a nursing diagnosis of Low Self-Esteem for a client who has experienced the loss of her husband through divorce, the loss of her job and apartment, and the development of drug dependency. Which of the following outcomes would be *most* appropriate initially?
    ○ 1. The client will discuss feelings related to her losses.
    ○ 2. The client will identify two positive qualities.
    ○ 3. The client will explore her strengths.
    ○ 4. The client will prioritize problems.

76. The nurse notices that a client recovering from a barbiturate overdose spends most of his time with other young adults who have substance-related problems. This group of clients is a dominant force on the unit, keeping the non–drug users entertained with stories of their "highs." Which of the following methods would be *best* to use when dealing with this problem?
    ○ 1. Providing additional recreation.
    ○ 2. Breaking up drug-oriented discussions.

○ 3. Speaking with the clients individually about their behavior.
○ 4. Discussing the behavior at the daily community meeting.

77. A client recovering from a drug overdose is interacting with the nurse and recounting her exploits at numerous rave parties she's attended. Which of the following actions would be *most* therapeutic?
    ○ 1. Allowing the client to continue with her stories.
    ○ 2. Telling the client you've heard the stories before.
    ○ 3. Questioning the client further about her exploits.
    ○ 4. Directing the conversation to realistic concerns.

78. The nurse is speaking to a sixth grade class about drugs. A student states, "I know someone who smokes marijuana and he says it's safe." Which of the following responses by the nurse would be *most* appropriate?
    ○ 1. "Marijuana isn't safe and it is illegal."
    ○ 2. "Do you really believe him?"
    ○ 3. "That drug causes more damage to your body than regular cigarettes."
    ○ 4. "Marijuana usage can lead to using other chemicals."

79. A client tells the nurse that he "sees sounds and hears colors" when he uses lysergic acid diethylamide (LSD). The nurse interprets this information as indicating that the client has experienced which of the following?
    ○ 1. Impaired judgment.
    ○ 2. Synesthesia.
    ○ 3. Flashback.
    ○ 4. Panic.

80. Which of the following actions would be *most* appropriate for the nurse to do for a client who is experiencing a "bad trip" from LSD use and is frightened and paranoid?
    ○ 1. Staying with the client to talk her down.
    ○ 2. Placing the client in seclusion.
    ○ 3. Leaving the client alone until the "bad trip" subsides.
    ○ 4. Telling another caregiver to check on the client periodically.

81. A client who is a chronic user of cocaine reports that he feels like he has bugs crawling under his skin. His arms are red from scratching. The nurse interprets these findings as possibly indicating which of the following?
    ○ 1. Illusion.
    ○ 2. Formication.
    ○ 3. Confusion.
    ○ 4. Flashback.

82. A client walks into the clinic and tells the nurse she has run out of money for crack, has crashed, and

wants something to help her feel better. Which of the following would be *most* important for the nurse to assess?

○ 1. Suspiciousness.
○ 2. Loss of appetite.
○ 3. Drug craving.
○ 4. Suicidal ideation.

83. A client in the emergency room is diagnosed with amphetamine psychosis. The nurse would most likely prepare to administer which of the following medications?

○ 1. Haloperidol (Haldol).
○ 2. Lorazepam (Ativan).
○ 3. Diazepam (Valium).
○ 4. Chlordiazepoxide (Librium).

84. A client has been taking increased amounts of alprazolam (Xanax) for about 6 months for anxiety. To safely withdraw the client from this drug, the nurse anticipates which of the following to be ordered?

○ 1. Immediate discontinuation of the alprazolam.
○ 2. A slow decrease in dose and frequency of the drug.
○ 3. Administration of alprazolam on an as-needed basis.
○ 4. Tapering off of the drug over a 24-hour period.

85. When caring for a client who has overdosed on phencyclidine (PCP), the nurse would be especially cautious about which of the following client behaviors?

○ 1. Visual hallucinations.
○ 2. Violent behavior.
○ 3. Bizarre behavior.
○ 4. Loud screaming.

86. Which of the following liquids would the nurse administer to a client who is intoxicated on PCP to hasten excretion of the chemical?

○ 1. Water.
○ 2. Milk.
○ 3. Cranberry juice.
○ 4. Grape juice.

87. When assessing a client with possible alcohol poisoning, the nurse would investigate the client's use of which of the following substances while drinking alcohol?

○ 1. Marijuana.
○ 2. LSD.
○ 3. Peyote.
○ 4. Psilocybin.

88. A client with a cocaine dependency is irritable, anxious, highly sensitive to stimuli, and over-reactive to clients and staff on the unit. Which of the following actions would be *most* therapeutic for this client?

○ 1. Secluding and restraining the client as needed.
○ 2. Telling the client to stay in his room until he can control himself.

○ 3. Providing the client with frequent "time-outs."
○ 4. Confronting the client about his behaviors.

89. A client with symptoms of amphetamine psychosis that are improving is anxious and still experiencing some delusions. When developing the client's plan of care, which of the following measures would the nurse include?

○ 1. Assign the client to a group about the physiologic effects of drugs.
○ 2. Advise the client to watch television.
○ 3. Wait for the client to approach the nurse.
○ 4. Invite the client to play a game of ping-pong with the nurse.

90. For the client who has difficulty falling asleep at night because of withdrawal symptoms from alcohol, which are abating, which of the following nursing interventions would be *best*?

○ 1. Inviting the client to play a board game with the nurse.
○ 2. Allowing the client to sit in the community room until she feels sleepy.
○ 3. Advising the client to sleep on the sofa in the dayroom.
○ 4. Teaching the client relaxation exercises to use before bedtime.

The Client With an Anxiety-Related Disorder

91. A client who is pacing and wringing his hands states, "I just need to walk" when questioned by the nurse about what he is feeling. Which of the following responses by the nurse would be *most* therapeutic?

○ 1. "You need to sit down and relax."
○ 2. "Are you feeling anxious?"
○ 3. "Is something bothering you?"
○ 4. "You must be experiencing a problem now."

92. A client is brought to the hospital emergency room by his brother. The client is perspiring profusely, breathing rapidly, and complaining of dizziness and palpitations. Problems of a cardiovascular nature are ruled out, and the client's diagnosis is tentatively listed as panic attack. After the symptoms pass, the client states, "I thought I was going to die." Which of the following responses by the nurse would be *best*?

○ 1. "It was very frightening for you."
○ 2. "We would not have let you die."
○ 3. "I would have felt the same way."
○ 4. "But you're okay now."

93. A client often jumps when spoken to and complains of feeling uneasy. She says, "It's as though something bad is going to happen." Which of the following actions would be *most* beneficial to the client?

○ 1. Leaving her alone.
○ 2. Demonstrating technical competency.
○ 3. Conveying optimistic verbalizations.
○ 4. Reducing environmental stimulation.

94. Which of the following points would the nurse include when teaching a client about panic disorder?
○ 1. Staying in the house will eliminate panic attacks.
○ 2. Medication should be taken when symptoms start.
○ 3. Symptoms of a panic attack are time limited and will abate.
○ 4. Maintaining self-control will decrease symptoms of panic.

95. A client with panic disorder is taking alprazolam (Xanax) 1 mg PO three times daily. The nurse understands that this medication is effective in blocking the symptoms of panic because of its specific action on which of the following neurotransmitters?
○ 1. γ-Aminobutyrate (GABA).
○ 2. Serotonin.
○ 3. Dopamine.
○ 4. Norepinephrine.

96. While a client is taking alprazolam (Xanax), which of the following would the nurse instruct the client to avoid?
○ 1. Chocolate.
○ 2. Cheese.
○ 3. Alcohol.
○ 4. Shellfish.

97. Which of the following statements by a client who has been taking buspirone (BuSpar) as prescribed for 2 days indicates the need for *further* teaching?
○ 1. "This medication will help my tight, aching muscles."
○ 2. "I may not feel better for 7 to 10 days."
○ 3. "The drug does not cause physical dependence."
○ 4. "I can take the medication with food."

98. A week ago, a tornado destroyed the client's home and seriously injured her husband. The client has been walking around the hospital in a daze without any outward display of emotions. She tells the nurse she feels like she's going crazy. Which of the following actions would the nurse use *initially*?
○ 1. Explain the effects of stress on the mind and body.
○ 2. Reassure the client that her feelings are typical reactions to serious trauma.
○ 3. Reassure the client that her symptoms are temporary.
○ 4. Acknowledge the unfairness of the client's situation.

99. After being discharged from the hospital with acute stress disorder, a client is referred to the outpatient clinic for follow-up. Which of the following probably would be *most* important for the client to use for continued alleviation of anxiety?

○ 1. Recognizing when she is feeling anxious.
○ 2. Understanding reasons for her anxiety.
○ 3. Using adaptive and palliative methods to reduce anxiety.
○ 4. Describing the situations preceding her feelings of anxiety.

100. A client with acute stress disorder states to the nurse, "I keep having horrible nightmares about the car accident that killed my daughter. I shouldn't have taken her with me to the store." Which of the following responses by the nurse would be *most* therapeutic?
○ 1. "Don't keep torturing yourself with such horrible thoughts."
○ 2. "Stop blaming yourself. Its only hurting you."
○ 3. "Let's talk about something that is a bit more pleasant."
○ 4. "The accident just happened and could not have been predicted."

101. The client, a veteran of the Vietnam war who has posttraumatic stress disorder (PTSD), tells the nurse about the horror and mass destruction of war. He states, "I killed all of those people for nothing." Which of the following responses by the nurse would be *most* appropriate?
○ 1. "You did what you had to do at that time."
○ 2. "Maybe you didn't kill as many people as you think."
○ 3. "How many people did you kill?"
○ 4. "War is a terrible thing."

102. A client with acute stress disorder has avoided feelings of anger toward her rapist and is unable to verbally express them. The nurse suggests which of the following activities to assist the client with expressing her feelings?
○ 1. Working on a puzzle.
○ 2. Writing in a journal.
○ 3. Meditating.
○ 4. Listening to music.

103. When developing the plan of care for a client with acute stress disorder who lost her sister in a boating accident, which of the following would the nurse expect to initiate?
○ 1. Helping the client to evaluate her sister's behavior.
○ 2. Telling the client to avoid details of the accident.
○ 3. Facilitating progressive review of the accident and its consequences.
○ 4. Postponing discussion of the accident until the client brings it up.

104. A client with PTSD needs to find new housing and wants to wait for a month before setting another appointment to see the nurse. The nurse interprets this action as which of the following?
○ 1. A method of avoidance.

○ 2. A detriment to progress.
○ 3. The end of treatment.
○ 4. A necessary occurrence.

105. The nurse would teach a client with an anxiety disorder who is taking a benzodiazepine about using which of the following in combination with his medication?
   ○ 1. Antacids.
   ○ 2. Acetaminophen (Tylenol).
   ○ 3. Vitamins.
   ○ 4. Aspirin.

106. Which of the following client statements would indicate the need for additional teaching about benzodiazepines?
   ○ 1. "I can't drink alcohol while taking diazepam (Valium)."
   ○ 2. "I can stop taking the drug anytime I want."
   ○ 3. "Valium can make me drowsy, so I shouldn't drive for a while."
   ○ 4. "Valium will help my tight muscles feel better."

107. A client with agoraphobia without panic disorder asks the nurse to advise her on which type of treatment would be best for her illness. Which of the following would the nurse suggest?
   ○ 1. Insight therapy.
   ○ 2. Group therapy.
   ○ 3. Behavior therapy.
   ○ 4. Psychoanalysis.

108. The client with a fear of eating in public places or in front of other people has finished eating lunch in the dining area in the nurse's presence. Which of the following statements by the nurse would reinforce the client's positive action?
   ○ 1. "It wasn't so hard, now was it?"
   ○ 2. "At supper, I hope to see you eat with a group of people."
   ○ 3. "You must have been hungry today."
   ○ 4. "It's a sign of progress to eat in the dining area."

109. The client with agoraphobia refuses to walk down the hall to the group room. Which of the following responses by the nurse would be *most* appropriate?
   ○ 1. "I know you can do it."
   ○ 2. "Try holding onto the wall as you walk."
   ○ 3. "You can miss group this one time."
   ○ 4. "I'll walk with you."

110. A client with obsessive-compulsive disorder (OCD) arrives late for an appointment with the nurse at the outpatient clinic. During the interview, he fidgets restlessly, has trouble remembering what topic is being discussed, and says he thinks he is going crazy. Which of the following statements by the nurse would best deal with the client's feelings of "going crazy"?
   ○ 1. "What do you mean when you say you think you're going crazy?"

○ 2. "Most people feel that way occasionally."
○ 3. "I don't know enough about you to judge."
○ 4. "You sound perfectly sane to me."

111. A client with OCD reveals that he was late for his appointment "because of my dumb habit. I have to take off my socks and put them back on 41 times! I can't stop until I do it just right." The nurse interprets the client's behavior as most likely representing an effort to obtain which of the following?
   ○ 1. Relief of anxiety.
   ○ 2. Control of his thoughts.
   ○ 3. Attention from others.
   ○ 4. Safe expression of hostility.

112. A client with OCD, who was admitted early yesterday morning, must make his bed 22 times before he can have breakfast. Because of his behavior, the client missed having breakfast yesterday with the other clients. Which of the following actions would the nurse institute to help the client be on time for breakfast?
   ○ 1. Tell the client to make his bed one time only.
   ○ 2. Wake the client an hour earlier to perform his ritual.
   ○ 3. Insist that the client stop his activity when it's time for breakfast.
   ○ 4. Advise the client to have breakfast first before making his bed.

113. The nurse notices that a client with OCD must get up and move to another area when someone sits next to her. Which of the following actions by the nurse would be *most* therapeutic?
   ○ 1. Ignoring the client's behavior.
   ○ 2. Questioning the client about her ritual.
   ○ 3. Conveying awareness of the need for the ritual.
   ○ 4. Telling the other clients to follow the client when she moves.

114. The client with OCD is taking clomipramine (Anafranil) for his disorder. The nurse would expect the client to exhibit side effects similar to those of which of the following medications?
   ○ 1. Fluoxetine (Prozac).
   ○ 2. Sertraline (Zoloft).
   ○ 3. Imipramine (Tofranil).
   ○ 4. Fluvoxamine (Luvox).

The Client With a Somatoform Disorder

115. At 10 AM a client with an Axis I diagnosis of pain disorder demands that the nurse call the physician for more pain medication because she's still in pain after the 9 AM analgesic. Which of the following would the nurse do *next*?
   ○ 1. Call the physician as the client requests.
   ○ 2. Suggest the client lie down because she has to wait for the next dosage.

○ 3. Tell the client that the physician will be in later to talk to her about it.

○ 4. Inform the client that the nurse cannot give her additional medication at this time.

116. The nursing assistant tells the nurse that the client is not in the dining room for lunch. The nurse would direct the nursing assistant to do which of the following?

○ 1. Take the client a lunch tray and let the client eat in his room.

○ 2. Tell the client he'll need to wait until supper to eat if he misses lunch.

○ 3. Invite the client to lunch and accompany him to the dining room.

○ 4. Inform the client that he has 10 minutes to get to the dining room for lunch.

117. The client with conversion disorder has a paralyzed arm. A staff member states, "I would just tell the client her arm is paralyzed because she had an affair and neglected her baby's care to the point where the baby had to be hospitalized for dehydration." Which of the following responses by the nurse would be *best*?

○ 1. "Ignore the client's behaviors and treat her with respect."

○ 2. "Pushing insight will increase the client's anxiety and the need for physical symptoms."

○ 3. "Pushing awareness will be helpful and further the client's recovery."

○ 4. "We'll meet with the client and confront her with her behavior."

118. The physician refers a client with somatization disorder to the outpatient clinic because of problems with nausea. The client's past symptoms involved back pain, chest pain, and problems with urination. The client tells the nurse that the nausea began when his wife asked him for a divorce. Which of the following would be *most* appropriate?

○ 1. Asking the client to describe his problem with nausea.

○ 2. Directing the client to describe his feelings about his impending divorce.

○ 3. Allowing the client to talk about the physicians he has seen and the medications he has taken.

○ 4. Informing the client about a different medication for his nausea.

119. A client with pain disorder is talking with the nurse about fishing when he suddenly reverts to talking about the pain in his arm. Which of the following would the nurse do *next*?

○ 1. Allow the client to talk about his pain.

○ 2. Ask the client if he needs more pain medication.

○ 3. Get up and leave the client.

○ 4. Redirect the interaction back to fishing.

120. Which of the following statements indicates to the nurse that the client is progressing toward recovery from a somatoform disorder?

○ 1. "It's okay if I feel nauseous when I'm worried about my divorce."

○ 2. "My stomach pain will go away once I get properly diagnosed."

○ 3. "My headache feels better when I time my medication dose."

○ 4. "I need to find a doctor who understands what my pain is like."

Correct Answers and Rationale

The letters in parentheses following the rationale identify the step of the nursing process (A, D, P, I, E) and client needs (1, 2, 3, 4, 5, 6, 7, 8, 9, 10). See the inside front cover for the key.

The Client With a Personality Disorder

1. 1. The nurse would plan to assist the client who has a personality disorder primarily with specific dysfunctional behaviors that are distressing to self and/or others. The client with a personality disorder has lifelong, inflexible, and dysfunctional patterns of relating and behaving. The client often does not view his behavior as distressful to self. The client becomes distressed because of others' reactions and behaviors toward him, which cause the client emotional pain and discomfort. Psychopharmacologic compliance is not a primary need because medication does not cure a personality disorder. Medication is prescribed if the client has a severe symptom that interferes with functioning, such as severe anxiety or depression, or if the client has an Axis I disorder. Examination of developmental conflicts usually is not helpful because of the ingrained dysfunctional ways of thinking and behaving. It is more useful to help the client with changing dysfunctional behaviors. Although milieu management is a component of care, the client usually is proficient in manipulation of the environment to meet his needs. (P, 6)

2. 3. For this client, the nurse needs to use a calm, matter-of-fact approach to create a nonthreatening and secure environment, because the client is experiencing problems with suspiciousness and trust. Use of "I" statements and responses would be therapeutic to reduce the client's suspiciousness and increase his trust in the staff and the environment. An authoritarian approach is nontherapeutic and inappropriate because the client may perceive this approach as an attack, subsequently responding with anger and threatening behavior. A parental or controlling approach may be perceived as authoritarian, and the client may become defensive and angry. (I, 6)

3. 4. Attending an activity with the nurse assists the client to become involved with others slowly. The client with a schizotypal personality disorder needs support, kindness, and gentle suggestion to improve social skills and interpersonal relationships. The client often has problems in thinking, perceiving, and communicating and appears similar to clients with schizophrenia except that psychotic episodes are infrequent and less severe. Participation solely in group activities or leading a sing-a-long would be too overwhelming for the client, subsequently increasing the client's anxiety and withdrawal. Engaging primarily in one-to-one activities would not be helpful because of the client's difficulty with social skills and interpersonal relationships. However, activities with the nurse could be used to establish trust. Then the client could proceed to activities with others. (I, 6)

4. 2. The nurse needs to set limits on the client's manipulative behavior to help the client control dysfunctional behavior. The manipulative client bends rules to have her needs met without regard for rules or the needs or rights of others. A consistent approach by the staff is necessary to decrease manipulation. Ignoring the client's behavior reinforces or promotes the continuation of the client's manipulative behavior. Reprimanding the client may be perceived as a threat, resulting in aggressive behavior. Allowing the client to keep a snack in her room reinforces the dysfunctional behavior. (I, 6)

5. 2. The nurse assists the client with identifying and putting feelings into words during one-to-one interactions. This helps the client express her feelings in a nonthreatening setting and avoid directing anger toward other clients. A client with an antisocial personality disorder needs to understand how others feel and react to her behaviors and why they react the way they do. The client also needs to understand the consequences of her behaviors. Using humor or indirect behaviors to express anger is a passive–aggressive method that will not help the client learn how to express her anger appropriately. Asking the nurse for medication when upset is a way to avoid dealing with feelings and is not helpful. However, medication may be necessary if talking and engaging in a physical activity have not been effective in lowering anxiety or if the client is about to lose control of her behavior. (P, 6)

6. 3. The client with an antisocial personality disorder is manifesting behavior indicative of problems in Erikson's stage of initiative versus guilt. Typical behaviors of a client with an antisocial personality disorder are engaging in illegal activities, violating rights of others, lack of guilt or remorse, recklessness, impulsiveness, aggressive behavior, and irresponsibility in work and with finances. A lack of guilt or remorse for offenses such as stealing is typically present, as if the client did not have a conscience. This behavior indicates a problem involving the stage of initiative versus guilt. Behaviors indicating problems in the stage of trust versus mistrust include suspiciousness, projection of

blame and feelings, and withdrawal. Behaviors indicating problems in the stage of autonomy versus shame and doubt include self-doubt and self-consciousness, dependency on others for approval, and denial of problems. Behaviors indicating problems in the stage of industry versus inferiority include poor work history, inadequate problem-solving skills, and manipulation of others. (D, 3)

7. 2. The nurse would teach the client consequences of her actions to help the client understand that if she steals she will get into legal trouble and be put in jail. So, if she wants to avoid jail, she needs to not steal. Helping the client to develop a conscience or to understand right from wrong is impossible. However, the client needs to be taught that her actions do lead to consequences. Using strategies to help the client become passive is not helpful, is nontherapeutic for any individual, and does not help the client to understand the consequences of her actions. (P, 6)

8. 4. Some characteristics of a client with a dependent personality are an inability to make daily decisions without advice and reassurance and the preoccupation with fear of being alone to care for self. The client needs others to be responsible for important areas of life. The nurse would respond to this client with the statement, "Your parents have been supportive of you and will continue to be supportive even if you live apart," to gently challenge the client's fears and suggest that they may be unwarranted. Stating, "You're a 28-year-old adult now, not a child who needs to be cared for," or "Your parents need a break, and you need a break from them," is reprimanding and would diminish the client's self-worth. Stating, "Your parents won't be around forever; after all they are getting older," may be true, but it is an insensitive response that may increase the client's anxiety. (I, 6)

9. 2. Stating, "All of you will gain from his independent living; he needs our support," encourages the client's independent behaviors and fosters autonomous functioning for the entire family. The other statements minimize the son's independence and decrease his self-esteem. (I, 6)

10. 3. This client's signs and symptoms are indicative of borderline personality disorder, characterized by impulsivity, self-mutilating behavior, unstable and intense personal relationships, identity disturbances, chronic feelings of emptiness, frantic avoidance of abandonment, and problems with anger. Antisocial personality disorder is characterized by lack of guilt or remorse, engaging in illegal activities, impulsiveness, recklessness, irresponsibility at work, aggressive behavior, and violation of the rights of others. The client with avoidant personality disorder demonstrates social withdrawal, hypersensitivity to criticism, and

reluctance to engage in new activities. The client with compulsive personality disorder is characterized by a preoccupation with details and rules to the exclusion of other life activities, perfectionism, and rigidity. (D, 6)

11. 4. For the client with attention-seeking behaviors, the nurse would institute a behavioral contract with the client to help decrease dysfunctional behaviors and promote self-sufficiency. Having the client approach only his assigned staff person sets limits on his attention-seeking behavior. Telling the client to stay in his room until staff approach him, limiting the client to a certain area, or giving the client a list of permissible requests is punitive and would do nothing to help the client gain control over the dysfunctional behavior. (P, 1)

12. 2. The most therapeutic response is, "All of the nurses here provide good care." This statement corrects the client's unrealistic and exaggerated perception. "Splitting," defined as the inability to integrate good and bad aspects of an individual and the self, is a hallmark behavior of a client with borderline personality disorder. The client sees self and others as all good or all bad. Components of "splitting" include behaviors that idealize and devalue others. It is a defense that allows the client to avoid pain and feelings associated with past abuse and/or a current situation involving the threat of rejection or abandonment. The other statements promote the client's idealistic view and do nothing to help correct the client's distortion. (I, 6)

13. 4. The client with borderline personality disorder is usually in a crisis situation when hospitalized for self-mutilation and suicidal ideation or behavior. The statement, "Any attempt at self-harm is serious and safety is a priority," is the best response, because the misperception that self-mutilation is used to gain attention can result in death for the client. Clients can accidentally commit suicide. Any form of self-harm is an indication that the client is in need of treatment. The statement, "She's here now and we have to do our best," is not helpful and does not educate the staff member about the client's needs. The statement, "She needs to be here until she can control her behavior," may be true but does not provide information about the client's priority needs. The statement, "I'm ashamed of you; you know better than to say that," is punitive, diminishes self-worth, and may not be a correct assumption of the staff member's knowledge. (I, 1)

14. 2. For the client who is at risk for self-mutilation, the nurse develops a contract to assist the client with assuming responsibility for his own behavior and to help the client develop adaptive methods of coping with feelings. Self-mutilation is usually an expression of intense anxiety, anger, helplessness, or guilt; or a means to block psychological pain by inducing physical pain. A typical contract helpful to the client would have the client notify staff when anxiety is increasing.

Withdrawing to his room when feeling overwhelmed, suppressing feelings when angry, or displacing feelings onto the physician is not an adaptive method to help the client deal with his feelings and could still result in self-mutilation. (E, 2)

15. 4. Any suicidal statement must be assessed by the nurse. The nurse would discuss the client's statement with her to determine its meaning in terms of suicide, overwhelming feelings of anxiety, abandonment, or other need which the client is unable to express appropriately. It is not uncommon for a client with borderline personality disorder to make threatening comments before discharge. Extending the hospital stay is inappropriate because it would encourage dependency and manipulation. Ignoring the client's statement on the assumption that it is a sign of manipulation is an error in judgment. Asking a family member to stay with the client temporarily at home is not appropriate and places the responsibility for the client on the family instead of the client herself. (I, 6)

16. 4. The best initial course of action when admitting a client is to observe him to establish baseline information. This assessment provides valuable information about the client's behavior and forms the basis for the plan of care. Telling the client that the staff has authority to subdue him if he gets unruly or that he will have to pay for any damage he causes is threatening and may incite or provoke trouble. Isolating a client is not recommended unless there is a very good reason for it, such as a very active, combative client who is dangerous to himself and others. (A, 6)

17. 4. The best response is, "You say you're not a regular here, but you're experiencing what others are experiencing." This statement helps the client to identify factors that precipitate denial by helping the client to confront that which inhibits compliance. Denial is used to help a client feel better and more secure when a situation provokes a high level of anxiety and is threatening to the client. The statement, "Because you're not a regular client, sit in the hall when the others are in group," agrees with and promotes denial in the client. A statement such as this also interferes with treatment. The statement, "Your family wants you to attend and they will be disappointed if you don't," causes the client to feel guilty and decreases self-esteem. The statement, "I'll have to mark you absent from the clinic today and speak to the doctor about it," is punitive and threatening to the client, subsequently decreasing her self-esteem. (I, 6)

18. 1. When the staff member asks the client if he wonders why others find him repulsive, the client is likely to feel defensive because the question is belittling. The natural tendency is to counterattack the threat to the self-image. Because the client with an antisocial personality disorder is egocentric and unconcerned about his effect on others, he is unlikely to feel ashamed, remorseful, or embarrassed. (A, 6)

19. 3. Stating, "I will not continue to talk with you if you curse," sets limits on the client's behavior and points out the negative effects of her behavior. Therefore, this response is most appropriate and therapeutic. The statement, "You are being very childish," reprimands the client, possibly causing the anger to escalate. The statement, "I'm sorry if you can't wait," fails to provide feedback to the client about her behavior. The statement, "Come back tomorrow and your medication will be ready," ignores the clients' behavior, failing to provide feedback to the client about the behavior. It also shows poor nursing judgment, because the client may need her medication before tomorrow or may not return to the clinic the following day. (I, 6)

20. 1. The client with avoidant personality disorder is showing signs of improvement when interacting with two other clients. A client with avoidant personality disorder is timid, socially uncomfortable, withdrawn, and hypersensitive to criticism. Social contact with others decreases isolation and withdrawal. Listening to music with headphones, sitting at a table and painting, and talking on the telephone are solitary activities and therefore would not indicate improvement, which would be evidenced by social contact. (E, 6)

21. 4. The priority would be to explain to the client that this information will have to be shared immediately with the staff and the physician because of its serious nature. Safety of all is crucial regardless of whether the client follows through on his plan. It is possible that the client is asking to be stopped and that he is indirectly pleading for help in a manner that is very dysfunctional. Bargaining with the client, such as warning him that his telephone privileges will be taken away if he abuses them or offering to disregard his plan if he does not go through with it, is inappropriate. Saying nothing to anyone until the client has actually completed the call and then notifying the proper authorities represents serious negligence on the part of the nurse. (I, 2)

22. 1. The most basic and important idea to convey to a client is that, as a person, he or she is accepted, although his or her behavior may not be. Empathy is conveyed for emotional pain regardless of the client's behavior. Although some clients need limits placed on their behavior, not all clients require limit setting. That the staff members are the primary ones left to care about these clients is not necessarily true, nor is it true that the staff should use very little humor with these clients. Clients who are rigid and perfectionists and who have a restricted affect may need help with displaying humor. (I, 1)

23. 1. The nurse would explain the negative reactions of others toward the client's behaviors to make the client aware of the impact of his seductive behaviors on others. Suggesting that the client apologize to others for his behavior is futile because the client is unable to feel remorse for wrongdoing. Asking him to explain reasons for his seductive behavior is not helpful because this client is skillful at using projection and rationalization. Discussing his relationship with his mother is not helpful, because the focus should be oriented to the present situation and managing his behavior at the present time. (I, 6)

24. 3. The nurse judges the client's statement to be an example of grandiose self-importance, which is not a lie but an overvaluing of one's self. The grandiosity of a client with a narcissistic personality disorder is not a delusion, because it usually is based somewhat in reality. However, it can be distorted, embellished, or convoluted to meet the client's need of self-importance. Sense of entitlement is a symptom of the narcissistic client but refers to deserving to be favored or given special treatment. (D, 6)

25. 2. The nurse would specifically use supportive confrontation with the client to point out discrepancies between what the client states and what actually exists to increase responsibility for self. Limit setting and consistency also may be used. However, limit setting helps the client control unacceptable behavior and consistency helps reduce the frequency of negative behaviors; they do not point out discrepancies. Rationalization is typically used by the client, not the nurse, to blame others, make excuses, and provide alibis for self-centered behaviors. (I, 6)

26. 4. The nurse would use role playing to teach the client appropriate responses to others and in various situations. This client dramatizes events, draws attention to self, and is unaware of and does not deal with feelings. The nurse works to help the client clarify true feelings and learn to express them appropriately. Party planning, music group, and cooking class are therapeutic activities but will not help the client specifically learn how to respond appropriately to others. (I, 6)

27. 1. The client with major depression and borderline personality disorder would probably be taking an SSRI to improve depression and reduce feelings of anger and impulsivity. A benzodiazepine (antianxiety agent) may be used cautiously for anxiety and restlessness. A mood stabilizer would be used for the client with rapid mood swings. An antipsychotic would be used only temporarily and in low doses for the client with transient psychotic symptoms sometimes experienced by clients with borderline personality disorder. (P, 8)

The Client With an Alcohol-Related Disorder

28. 4. The nurse would provide the client with a quiet room to sleep in. Alcohol is destroyed and oxidized in the body at a slow, steady rate. The rate of alcohol metabolism is not influenced by drinking black coffee, walking around the unit, or taking a cold shower. Therefore, it would be best to have the client sleep off the effects of the alcohol. (I, 6)

29. 4. Antiseptic mouthwash often contains alcohol and should be kept in a locked area, unless labeling clearly indicates that the product does not contain alcohol. A client with an intense craving for alcohol may drink mouthwash that contains alcohol. Personal care items such as toothpaste, dental floss, and shaving cream do not contain alcohol, and the client would be allowed to keep them in the room. (P, 2)

30. 2. The client with alcohol dependency is using *minimization* when he states he just has a few drinks with the guys after work. Minimization, projection, denial, and rationalization are defenses that are part of the "stinkin' thinkin'" that permits the client with an alcohol problem to continue drinking. *Projection* involves blaming someone else for one's difficulties. An example is, "My wife keeps getting on my case about nothing. She drives me crazy." *Denial* involves an unconscious refusal to admit an unacceptable idea or behavior. An example is, "I can stop drinking anytime I want. I don't have a problem." *Rationalization* is an attempt to make or prove that one's feelings or behaviors are justifiable. An example is, "If my boss wasn't so hard on me, I wouldn't be so stressed out. I just need a few drinks to relax." (D, 5)

31. 2. The client's response helps the nurse determine the severity of withdrawal symptoms, because the length and extent of drinking alcohol will have an affect on the severity of symptoms the client will experience during withdrawal. Decreased use of alcohol can also result in withdrawal symptoms in the client who has developed a high tolerance to alcohol and is physically dependent. The severity of the disease, the possibility of hallucinations, and the occurrence of delirium tremens are not determined by the information given. The Axis I diagnosis of alcohol dependency is just that—it is not classified as mild, moderate, or severe. Alcohol hallucinosis is a state of auditory hallucinations that develops about 48 hours after the client has stopped drinking. The client hears voices or noises within the context of a clear sensorium, meaning that the auditory hallucination is the only symptom the client experiences. Severe withdrawal symptoms that are not managed medically can progress to delirium tremens or a severe abstinence syndrome. Delirium tremens occurs about 3 to 5 days after the client's last drink and is characterized by confusion, agitation, severe psychomotor activity, hallucinations, sleeplessness, tachycardia, elevated blood pressure, elevated temperature, and possibly seizures. (A, 9)

32. 1. The most effective way to help decrease the client's denial is to point out how alcohol has gotten the client into trouble, using specific, concrete data based on fact, not opinion. Explaining the effects of drinking on family, urging the client to attend AA meetings, and telling her about the physiologic damage that can result are important components of the treatment process but are not as effective in decreasing denial as discussing how alcohol has affected her life until now. (I, 6)

33. 2. The nurse would most likely administer a benzodiazepine, such as lorazepam (Ativan), to the client who is experiencing symptoms of alcohol withdrawal. The benzodiazepine substitutes for the alcohol to suppress withdrawal symptoms. The client experiences symptoms of withdrawal because of the "rebound phenomenon" when sedation of the central nervous system from alcohol begins to decrease. Haloperidol is an antipsychotic and is not indicated for alcohol withdrawal symptoms. Benztropine is used to treat extrapyramidal symptoms associated with antipsychotic therapy. Naloxone is used in opioid overdose to reverse the central nervous system depression caused by the opioid. (P, 8)

34. 3. Monitoring of vital signs provides the best information about the client's overall physiologic status during alcohol withdrawal and the physiologic response to the medication used. Vital signs reflect the degree of central nervous system irritability and indicate the effectiveness of the medication in easing withdrawal symptoms. Although assessment of nutritional status and sleep pattern and assessment for evidence of tremors are important, they provides only indirect information about single aspects of the client's physiologic status. (A, 6)

35. 1. A client is said to be suffering from a blackout when he cannot recall what he did while under the influence of alcohol. A hangover refers to symptoms experienced the next day after a bout of heavy drinking. Common symptoms include headaches and gastrointestinal distress, typically after heavy alcohol consumption. Tolerance refers to the need to increase the amount of the substance or to ingest the substance more often to achieve the same effects. Delirium tremens refers to severe alcohol withdrawal or abstinence syndrome with confusion, psychomotor agitation, sleeplessness, hallucinations, and elevated vital signs. (D, 6)

36. 4. Stating, "I'm Maria, a nurse in the program; the staff and I will help you," is a nonjudgmental, caring approach that promotes trust and the therapeutic relationship. The statement, "I hope you are serious about maintaining your sobriety this time," blames the client, subsequently decreasing the client's self-worth. Saying, "You'll get it right this time" is threatening to the client, possibly leading to decreased self-worth by reinforcing the client's past failures at maintaining sobriety. The

statement, "I know someone who was successful after the fifth program," is impersonal and irrelevant to the client's situation. (I, 6)

37. 3. The wife of the man with alcohol dependency is exhibiting enabling behavior when she makes excuses for her husband's absenteeism. Enabling behavior is not helpful to the client but rescues him from adverse consequences in relation to his employment. Self-defeating behavior would be evidenced by putting one's self in a position that will lead to failure. Masochistic behavior would be evidenced by the need to experience emotional or physical pain to become sexually aroused. (D, 9)

38. 4. To be most helpful, the nurse would calmly and objectively present facts, by saying, "You have alcohol on your breath," to help the coworker overcome denial and resistance. This statement also helps to reinforce the coworker's awareness of the problem. The other statements blame the coworker and may reinforce denial. Blaming, nagging, and yelling diminish self-esteem in the individual with a substance problem who has low frustration tolerance. (I, 6)

39. 3. The nurse leader should direct the husband to say, "Either you get help or the kids and I will move out of the house." This statement facilitates entrance into treatment because it is a direct statement of what the consequences are if the drinking of alcohol continues. The statement, "The children and I want you to get help," is not effective. Most likely, the husband has already made a similar statement before the confrontation session. Saying, "If your parents were alive, they would be extremely disappointed in you," or "You need to enter treatment now or be a drunk if that's what you want," shames the wife and further decreases self-esteem. (I, 6)

40. 3. The statement, "You interrupted Terry twice in 4 minutes," indicates an understanding of the use of constructive feedback by describing specifically what was seen and heard in an objective rather than a judgmental manner. The other statements are judgmental and blame the client without specifying what the objectionable behavior is. (E, 6)

41. 4. The client is feeling remorse about hitting his wife. It is best to make a comment that will help him focus on his feelings and ventilate them. Reflecting what the client has said is a good technique to accomplish these goals. Suggesting the client ask his wife or explore the issue in family therapy is inappropriate because it gives advice and ignores the client's underlying feelings. Saying, "It would depend on how much she really cares for you," is inappropriate because it ignores the client's feelings and reinforces the negative aspects, such as the shamefulness, of the behavior. (I, 6)

42. 2. Al-Anon is a self-help group for spouses and significant others that provides education and support and helps participants learn to lead their own life without feeling responsible for the individual with an alcohol problem. Alateen provides support for teenaged children of a person with an alcohol problem. Employee assistance programs help employees recover from alcohol or drug dependence while retaining their positions or jobs. AA provides support for the individual with alcohol problems to attain and maintain sobriety. (P, 1)

43. 1. Ambulating the client who is experiencing severe symptoms of alcohol withdrawal is contraindicated because increased activity and stimulation may confuse the client and promote hallucinations. The client may also sustain an injury if he or she has a seizure as part of the alcohol withdrawal process. The nurse would monitor intake and output to ensure fluid and electrolyte balance and hydration. The nurse would assess vital signs to assess the physiologic status of the client and the response to medications. The nurse would use short, concrete statements to decrease confusion and ambiguity. (I, 6)

44. 1. Any amount of alcohol consumed while taking disulfiram can cause an alcohol-disulfiram reaction. The reaction experienced is in proportion to the amount of alcohol ingested. The alcohol-disulfiram reaction can begin 5 to 10 minutes after alcohol is ingested. Symptoms can be mild, as in flushing, throbbing in the head and neck, nausea, and diaphoresis. Other symptoms include vomiting, respiratory difficulty, hypotension, vertigo, syncope, and confusion. Severe reactions involve respiratory depression, convulsions, coma, and even death. Disulfiram (Antabuse) can be taken at bedtime if the client feels sleepy from the medication. Some clients experience a metallic or garlic taste when initiating disulfiram treatment. Anything containing alcohol, such as cough medicine, aftershave lotion, or mouthwash, can cause a reaction. Therefore, the client needs to check the labels of these items for their alcohol content. (E, 8)

45. 1. The first question would be to ask the client how much alcohol she has had today, because nausea with severe vomiting is a sign of an alcohol-disulfiram reaction. Asking the client whether she feels like she has flu symptoms would be important after inquiring about alcohol intake. Foods cooked in an alcoholic beverage, such as wine, could also cause a reaction, but the reaction would be less severe because the alcohol dissipates with cooking. Asking how long the client has been taking Antabuse would be least important at this time. (D, 8)

46. 1. Thiamine specifically prevents the development of Wernicke's encephalopathy, a reversible amnestic disorder caused by a diet deficient in thiamine secondary to poor nutritional intake that often accompanies chronic alcoholism. It is characterized by nystagmus, ataxia, and mental status changes. Because the client would rather drink alcohol than eat, the client is depleted of vitamins and nutrients. Alcohol also is an irritant that causes a "malabsorption syndrome" in which vitamins and nutrients are not absorbed properly in the gastrointestinal tract. Thiamine is not associated with decreasing withdrawal symptoms, helping clients regain their strength, or promoting elimination of alcohol from the body. (D, 8)

47. 2. The statement, "Stopping AA and not expressing feelings can lead to relapse," indicates the client's understanding of signs of relapse. The client himself is responsible for sobriety and must understand the signs of relapse. Other antecedents to relapse include severe craving, being around users, and severe emotional crises. The other statements place the responsibility for the client's sobriety on someone else. (E, 9)

48. 1. The client is using *denial*, an unconscious defense mechanism, when she refuses to acknowledge that she has a problem with alcohol. This is further evidenced by the client's inability to connect the liver disorder with alcohol ingestion. *Displacement* involves transfer of a feeling to someone else or to an object. *Rationalization* involves an attempt to make or prove that one's feeling or behavior is justifiable. *Reaction formation* is a conscious behavior that is the exact opposite of an unconscious feeling. (D, 5)

49. 3. Stating that the vitamin is a nutritional supplement important to the client's health is the best response. The client is nutritionally depleted, and the B-complex vitamins produce a calming effect on the irritated central nervous system and prevent anemia, peripheral neuropathy, and Wernicke's encephalopathy. Although the statements about drinking alcohol and eating very little and that there is a low amount of vitamins in the alcohol consumed may be true, but they fail to address the client's concerns directly and fail to provide the necessary information, as does telling the client that the doctor wants the client to take the vitamin for 4 months. (I, 8)

50. 4. The client is most likely experiencing peripheral neuritis secondary to chronic alcohol consumption. Typical symptoms of peripheral neuritis include numbness, itching, and pain in the extremities and a predisposition to footdrop. Neuralgia refers to severe pain along the course of a nerve. Bell's palsy is a type of facial paralysis involving the seventh cranial nerve. Neurasthenia refers to motor and mental fatigue. (D, 6)

51. 2. Regular coffee contains caffeine, which acts as a psychomotor stimulant and leads to feelings of anxiety and agitation. Serving coffee to the client may add to tremors and wakefulness. Milk, orange juice, and eggs are part of a well-balanced, high-protein diet that is needed by the client in alcohol withdrawal, who is nutritionally depleted. (I, 6)

52. 4. The nurse should teach the client with peripheral neuropathy to avoid using an electric blanket, because the client is likely to have decreased sensitivity in the extremities owing to the damaging effects of alcohol on the nerve endings. It is particularly important to guard against burns, because the client may not be able to discern the appropriate degree of heat on the feet. Daily washing and drying, massaging with lotion, and trimming the toenails are appropriate foot care measures for any client. (P, 6)

53. 4. Based on the assessment findings, the nurse would suspect that the client is experiencing delirium, specifically delirium tremens, severe symptoms of withdrawal from alcohol. Delirium tremens is characterized by disorientation, confusion, hallucinations, agitation, and elevated vital signs. *Stupor* refers to a level of consciousness in which a client responds only to repeated verbal stimuli and painful tactile stimuli. Mild alcohol withdrawal is characterized by mild tremors, nausea, nervousness, diaphoresis, rapid heartbeat, and increased blood pressure. Impaired consciousness is characterized by drowsiness, lethargy, loss of recent memory, and slowed thought processes. (D, 6)

54. 1. The client is demonstrating visual hallucinations, one of the defining characteristics of Disturbed Sensory Perception. Although Disturbed Thought Processes, Risk for Injury, and Ineffective Coping may occur in the client experiencing alcohol withdrawal, they are not reflected in the client's statement about bugs. Disturbed Thought Processes refers to the state when the client experiences a disruption in cognitive operations and activities as evidenced by memory problems, hypovigilance or hypervigilance, distractibility, or egocentricity. Risk for Injury is a result of an environmental condition that interacts with a client's adaptive and defensive resources. Ineffective Coping refers to a client's impairment of adaptive behavior and problem-solving ability in meeting life's demands and roles. (D, 6)

55. 2. The statement, "The client is a weak individual and could stop if he desires," is false and indicates a lack of understanding regarding alcohol dependency. The *Diagnostic and Statistical Manual of Mental Disorders*, 4th ed., text revised (DSM-IV-TR) criteria for substance dependency includes the inability to stop using even when wanting to do so. The client cannot stop or control the amount used when dependent on a substance. Alcohol dependency affects individuals from every culture and socioeconomic background and has nothing to do with being a "weak" individual. The devastating affects of alcohol dependency are felt by every member of the family and not just the individual with the alcohol problem. Family members need education

about the physical, physiologic, and psychological effects of alcohol and referrals to self-help groups for support. They have felt and lived with the devastating effects of the disease. A simple and commonly held view of alcoholism is that alcohol is a problem when it interferes with life or disrupts family, work, or social relationships. (E, 1)

56. 3. The client with alcohol withdrawal delirium should not be left unattended when confused, disoriented, or hallucinating. Injury or unintentional suicide is a possibility when the client attempts to get away from hallucinations. Restraints are used only when the client loses control and is a danger to self or others, to protect the client from injury or harm. Touching the client before saying anything is an additional stimulus that would most likely add to the client's agitation. Informing the client about the alcohol treatment program while the client is delirious is inappropriate and shows poor nursing judgment. The client should be given information about alcohol treatment when the withdrawal symptoms are lessening and the client is able to comprehend the information. (P, 2)

57. 2. AA, a self-help program based on 12 steps, is open to anyone whose goal is sobriety. The first step requires that the individual admit that he or she is powerless over alcohol and needs help. Members are in various stages of recovery, and the individual does not have to be sober for at least a month before joining. Potential members are not interviewed. The individual decides how many meetings to attend each week. AA does not require attendance at meetings daily, but some individuals choose to do so, especially at the beginning of recovery. (I, 6)

58. 4. Follow-up care is essential to prevent relapse. Recovery has just begun when the treatment program ends. The first few months after program completion can be difficult and dangerous for the chemically dependent client. The nurse is responsible for discharge plans that include arrangements for counseling, self-help group meetings, and other forms of aftercare. Supportive friends, a list of goals, and family forgiveness may be important and helpful to the client, but follow-up care is essential. (I, 6)

59. 3. The term *dual diagnosis* refers to the presence of at least one psychiatric disorder in addition to a substance abuse or dependency problem. The psychiatric disorder can be a mental illness or a personality disorder (or both). Therefore, major depression and alcohol abuse is a dual diagnosis. (A, 6)

60. 2. The nurse would assess the client's mental status daily to note changes that could occur from exacerbation of the mental illness or withdrawal from alcohol. Changes in mental status would be important for treatment issues such as medication and participation in groups. Assessment of mental status takes priority because mental status affects the client's ability to sleep, eat, and care for self. Flexibility is necessary on the part of nurses and staff members who are working with a heterogeneous client population. (A, 6)

61. 1. The client's decision to drink alcohol results in a feeling of autonomy and a temporary increase in self-esteem. The client feels better, problems are avoided, and he is in temporary control of himself. Guilt or shame may result later, because the client is aware that he should not use alcohol because of his mental illness. The combination of a mental illness and the use of a substance results in increased recidivism and treatment complications. It may not be true that the client abused of alcohol before developing a mental illness or that the client is compelled to drink because of cognitive difficulties. Some clients may be predisposed to development of a substance problem and a mental illness because of their heredity and biologic factors. The largest group of dual diagnosis clients have separate etiologies for their mental illness and substance problem. The client who is not experiencing acute symptoms of his mental illness is probably not impaired cognitively but is able to decide whether he wants to drink alcohol. (D, 6)

The Client With Disorders Related to Other Addictive Substances

62. 1. A respiratory rate of less than 12 breaths/minute is cause for concern because of central nervous system depression. Respiratory depression and arrest is the primary cause of death among clients who abuse opioids. Peripheral nervous system effects associated with opioid abuse include urinary retention, hypotension, reduced pupil size, constipation, and decreased gastric, biliary, and pancreatic secretions. Pinpoint pupils are a sign of opioid overdose. However, respiratory depression is the immediate concern. (A, 6)

63. 2. Heroin is an opioid. Naloxone (Narcan), a narcotic antagonist, is used to treat suspected opioid overdose. Naloxone blocks the neuroreceptors affected by opioids. Usually, the client responds in a few minutes to an intravenous injection of the drug. Respirations improve, but the nurse must monitor the client carefully to determine whether additional naloxone is needed. Haloperidol is an antipsychotic, and lorazepam and oxazepam are antianxiety agents; they would further depress the central nervous system. (P, 8)

64. 1. Vomiting and diarrhea are usually late signs of heroin withdrawal, along with muscle spasm, fever, nausea, repetitive sneezing, abdominal cramps, and backache. Early signs of heroin withdrawal include yawning, tearing (lacrimation), rhinorrhea, and sweating. Intermediate signs of heroin withdrawal are flushing, piloerection, tachycardia, tremor, restlessness, and irritability. (A, 6)

65. 4. After administering naloxone (Narcan), the nurse should monitor the client's respiratory status carefully, because the drug is short-acting and respiratory depression may reoccur after its effects wear off. Cerebral edema, kidney failure, and seizure activity are not directly related to opioid overdose or naloxone therapy. (I, 8)

66. 4. The client takes methadone primarily to be able to work, live normally, and function productively without the mental and physical deterioration caused by opioid addiction. Methadone lessens physiologic dependence on opioids and is used to prevent withdrawal symptoms. Methadone, a substance similar to morphine, is an addictive substance; the client is still considered to be addicted to narcotics. Because methadone has a long half-life of 15 to 30 hours, it can be taken once a day on an outpatient basis. (I, 6)

67. 1. Suggesting that the client try attending a meeting at a different location is a supportive, positive response and encourages the client to continue participating in treatment. Saying, "Maybe it just wasn't a good day for you," or "Perhaps you weren't paying close enough attention," places blame on the client and is not helpful. The statement, "Sometimes the meetings can seem like a waste of time, but you need to attend to stay clean," diminishes the importance of the self-help group and offers little support to the client. (I, 6)

68. 2. The best measure to determine a client's progress in rehabilitation is the number of drug-free days he has. The longer the client is free of drugs, the better the prognosis is. Although the kinds of friends the client makes, the way he gets along with his parents, and the degree of responsibility his job requires could influence his decision to stay clean, the number of drug-free days is the best indicator of progress. (E, 6)

69. 4. The client who is addicted to heroin is most likely to exhibit hypoactivity. Initially, the client feels euphoric. This is followed by drowsiness, hypoactivity, anorexia, and a decreased sex drive. Hilarity, aggression, and labile mood usually are not associated with heroin addiction. (A, 6)

70. 4. Because barbiturates are central nervous system depressants, the nurse would be especially alert for the possibility of respiratory failure. Respiratory failure is the most likely cause of death from barbiturate overdose. Kidney failure, cerebral vascular accident, and status epilepticus are not associated with barbiturate overdose. (A, 9)

71. 4. When a friend asks whether a seriously ill client will live, it is best for the nurse to respond by explaining the seriousness of the client's condition and acknowledging the friend's concern. This type of comment does not offer false hope. Telling the friend to wait and see and that it is too soon to tell is a stereotypical statement that offers no support to the friend. Asking the friend to describe his or her relationship with the client ignores the friend's concern and does not focus on the problem. Simply saying that the client is very ill and may not live and that some don't pull through is harsh and not supportive. (I, 6)

72. 1. *Tolerance* for a drug occurs when a client requires increasingly larger doses to obtain the desired effect. Therefore the plan of care would address the client's state of tolerance. The term *addiction* refers to psychological and physiologic symptoms indicating that an individual cannot control his or her use of psychoactive substances. This term has been replaced with the term *dependence*. *Abuse* refers to the excessive use of a substance that differs from societal norms. Drug *dependence* occurs when the client must takes a usual or increasing amount of the drug to prevent the onset of abstinence symptoms, is unable to keep drug intake under control, and continues to use even though physical, social, and emotional processes are compromised. (P, 6)

73. 4. For a client who is confused when awakening after taking a large dose of barbiturates, the nurse would speak in concrete terms using simple statements in a calm, nonjudgmental, gentle manner to assist the client with cognitive-perceptual impairment, enhance understanding, and decrease anxiety. The other statements contain abstract information and some slang terms that may further confuse the client and thus increase the client's anxiety. (I, 6)

74. 2. The priority nursing diagnosis would be Risk for Self-Directed Violence related to suicide attempt. Although the client may be experiencing a self-esteem disturbance, ineffective coping, or feelings of powerlessness, the priority here is the client's safety. (D, 6)

75. 1. The most appropriate initial outcome for the client would be to discuss thoughts and feelings related to her losses. The nurse would help the client identify and verbalize her feelings so that she can externalize her thoughts and emotions and begin to deal with them. This prevents the client from internalizing feelings, which leads to depression and self-harm. The ability to identify two positive qualities, explore strengths, and prioritize problems would be appropriate once the client has explored her thoughts and feelings, gained awareness of the issues, and then can participate in the treatment plan. (E, 6)

76. 4. The best method to deal with the problem is to discuss observations with clients at the daily community meeting, because the problem involves all of the clients and this provides them with the opportunity to offer their views. Peer pressure is valuable in confronting self-defeating and destructive behaviors. Providing additional recreation avoids or ignores the problem and is damaging to all clients because it decreases trust in the nurse. Breaking up drug-oriented discussions would not be sufficient to stop the behavior. Speaking with the clients individually about their behavior is not as effective as dealing with the problem openly and directly with all clients. (I, 6)

77. 4. The nurse directs the conversation to realistic concerns or issues to decrease denial and focus on rebuilding a substance-free life. Allowing the client to continue with the stories or questioning the client further about her exploits reinforces the denial. Telling the client you've heard the stories before is nondirective. Additionally, these actions do nothing to help the client focus on rebuilding a substance-free life. (I, 6)

78. 3. The statement that marijuana causes more damage to your body than regular cigarettes is a direct, correct, educative response to the student's statement that does not decrease the student's or the friend's self-worth. Marijuana causes harmful pulmonary effects, weakens heart contractions, causes immunosuppression, and reduces serum testosterone and sperm count. Telling the student that marijuana is unsafe and illegal, or that using marijuana leads to using other chemicals, does not provide the student with factual educative information to answer the student's question. Asking whether the student really believes the friend challenges the student and may lead to defensive behavior. (I, 4)

79. 2. Synesthesia is the blending of senses, a phenomenon caused by LSD. The client can taste colors, see sounds, or smell rainbows. Impaired judgment is exhibited by a client who thinks he can fly like a bird. A flashback—the cognitive, emotional, and physical reexperiencing of a traumatic event—can instill panic in a client because he experiences a sense of "going crazy" or paranoia. Acute panic occurs when the client is on a "bad trip" and becomes extremely frightened. (D, 6)

80. 1. When the client experiences a "bad trip" and is frightened and paranoid, the nurse would stay with the client and talk her down. The nurse supports the client through the experience, ensures her safety, and orients her to where she is. The nurse would tell the client that she is experiencing the effects of LSD, she is safe, and the effects of the drug will end. Placing the client in seclusion or leaving the client alone until the "bad trip" subsides is poor judgment and irresponsible on the part of the nurse, possibly leading to increased anxiety, panic, and injury. Telling another caregiver to check on the client periodically demonstrates poor management of the client's care and also unfairness to the caregiver. (I, 2)

81. 2. The feeling of bugs crawling under the skin, termed *formication*, is associated with cocaine use. An *illusion* is misinterpretation of sensory input, such as walking past a tree and thinking it's a ghost. *Confusion* is a state of being bewildered or unclear. A *flashback* is a cognitive, emotional, and physical reexperiencing of a traumatic event. (D, 9)

82. 4. The nurse assesses the client for feelings of depression and suicidal ideation. After experiencing an instantaneous high from crack, a crash immediately follows and the client has an intense craving for more crack. A crash often leads to a cocaine-induced depression when additional crack is unavailable. At times, the depression is so severe that users attempt suicide. Although suspiciousness, loss of appetite, and drug craving are also associated with cocaine use, they are of less priority than suicidal ideation. (A, 6)

83. 1. The nurse would prepare to administer an antipsychotic medication such as haloperidol (Haldol) to a client experiencing amphetamine psychosis to decrease agitation and psychotic symptoms, including delusions, hallucinations, and cognitive impairment. Lorazepam (Ativan) and diazepam (Valium), which are benzodiazepines, and chlordiazepoxide (Librium) are antianxiety agents that would have no effect on the client's symptoms of psychosis. (P, 8)

84. 2. The client is physically dependent on alprazolam. Therefore, the client will be slowly tapered off of the benzodiazepine by decreasing the dose and frequency of the medication over several days. Doing so helps to minimize withdrawal symptoms (similar to those of alcohol withdrawal) while safely withdrawing the client from the medication. Benzodiazepines should never be stopped abruptly because of withdrawal symptoms, especially convulsions and tachycardia. Administering alprazolam on a PRN basis would not help the client to withdraw from the medication. (P, 6)

85. 2. The nurse must be especially cautious when providing care to a client who has taken PCP because of unpredictable, violent behavior. The client can appear to be in a calm state or even in a coma, then become violent, and then return to a calm or comatose state. Visual hallucinations, bizarre behavior, and loud screaming are associated with PCP-intoxicated clients. However, the unpredictable, violent behavior presents a major issue of safety for clients and staff. (I, 6)

86. 3. An acid environment aids in the excretion of PCP. Therefore, the nurse would give the client with PCP intoxication cranberry juice to acidify the urine to a pH of 5.5 and accelerate excretion. (I, 6)

87. 1. Smoking marijuana while using alcohol can lead to alcohol poisoning because marijuana masks the nausea and vomiting associated with excessive alcohol consumption. Marijuana contains tetrahydrocannabinol (THC), which is responsible for suppressing nausea. With the dangerous levels of alcohol in the body, respiratory depression, coma, and death can occur. LSD, peyote, and psilocybin do not contain THC. (A, 6)

88. 3. Providing frequent "time-outs" when the client is highly anxious, sensitive, irritable, and over-reactive is needed to calm the client and reduce the possibility for escalating behaviors and violence. Secluding and restraining the client is not appropriate and would only be used if the client were using threatening behaviors toward others and other alternative actions had been unsuccessful. Telling the client to stay in his room until he can control himself is unrealistic and futile because the client is unable to eliminate behaviors induced by chemicals. Confronting the client about his behaviors would most likely lead to aggression and possibly violent behavior. (I, 2)

89. 4. The nurse would invite the client who is anxious to participate in an activity that involves gross motor movements. Doing so helps to direct energy toward a therapeutic activity. Appropriate activities could include walking, riding a stationary bicycle, or playing volleyball. Assigning the client to an educational group is not helpful because the anxious client would be unable to sit in a group setting and concentrate on what was occurring in group. Watching television may be too stimulating for the client, possibly increasing anxiety. Additionally, the client may be too anxious to sit and focus. Waiting for the client to approach the nurse is not helpful or appropriate. The nurse is responsible for initiating contact with the client. (P, 6)

90. 4. The best action by the nurse to help a client who has difficulty falling asleep would be to teach the client relaxation exercises to use before bedtime to reduce anxiety and promote relaxation. This activity will also be beneficial for the client to use when out of the hospital. Inviting the client to play a board game is inappropriate because this activity can be competitive and thus stimulate the client. Allowing the client to sit in the community room until she feels sleepy is inappropriate because it does nothing to help the client relax; nor does advising the client to sleep on the sofa in the dayroom, which may be against unit policy. (I, 7)

The Client With an Anxiety-Related Disorder

91. 2. Asking, "Are you feeling anxious?" helps the client to specifically label the feeling as anxiety so that he can begin to understand and manage it. Some clients need assistance with identifying what they are feeling so that they can recognize what is happening to them. Stating, "You need to sit down and relax," is not appropriate because the client needs to continue his pacing to feel

better. Asking if something is bothering the client or saying that he must be experiencing a problem is vague and does not help the client to put a label to his feeling and identify it as anxiety. (I, 6)

92. 1. The nurse responds with the statement, "It was very frightening for you," to express empathy, thus acknowledging the client's discomfort and accepting his feelings. The nurse conveys respect and validates the client's self-worth. The other statements do not focus on the client's underlying feelings, convey active listening, or promote trust. (I, 6)

93. 4. Reducing the client's environmental stimulation helps to reduce anxiety. For the client who is already anxious, noise and activity further increase anxiety. Leaving the client alone is not therapeutic because the nurse's presence provides comfort, safety, and support. Making optimistic statements ignores the client's feelings and offers little help when she feels uneasy. Although demonstrating technical competence is helpful to the anxious client, environmental stimulation must be reduced to reduce the client's anxiety. (I, 6)

94. 3. It is important for the nurse to teach the client that the symptoms of a panic attack are time limited and will abate. This helps decrease the client's fear about what is occurring. Clients benefit from learning about their illness, what symptoms to expect, and the helpful use of medication. A simple biologic explanation of the disorder can convince clients to take their medication. Telling the client to stay in the house to eliminate panic attacks is not correct or helpful. Panic attacks can occur "out of the blue," and clients with panic disorder can become agoraphobic because of fear of having a panic attack where help is not available or escape is impossible. Medication should be taken on a scheduled basis to block the symptoms of panic before they start. Taking medication when symptoms start is not helpful. Telling the client to maintain self-control to decrease symptoms of panic is false information, because the brain and biochemicals may account for its development. Therefore, the client cannot control when a panic attack will occur. (I, 6)

95. 1. Alprazolam (Xanax), a benzodiazepine used on a short-term or temporary basis to treat symptoms of anxiety, increases GABA, a major inhibitory neurotransmitter. Because GABA is increased and the reticular activating system is depressed, incoming stimuli are muted and the effects of anxiety are blocked. Alprazolam does not directly target serotonin, dopamine, or norepinephrine. (D, 8)

96. 3. Using alcohol or any central nervous system depressant while taking a benzodiazepine such as alprazolam (Xanax) is contraindicated because of additive depressant effects. Ingestion of chocolate, cheese, or shellfish is not problematic. (I, 8)

97. 1. Buspirone (BuSpar), a nonbenzodiazepine anxiolytic, is particularly effective in treating the cognitive symptoms of anxiety, such as worry, apprehension, difficulty with concentration, and irritability. BuSpar is not effective for the somatic symptoms of anxiety (eg, muscle tension). Therapeutic effects may be experienced in 7 to 10 days, with full effects not occurring for 3 to 4 weeks. This drug is not known to cause physical or psychological dependence. It can be taken with food or small meals to reduce gastrointestinal upset. (E, 8)

98. 2. The nurse initially reassures the client that her feelings and behaviors are typical reactions to serious trauma to help decrease anxiety and maintain self-esteem. Explaining the effects of stress on the body may be helpful later. Telling the client that her symptoms are temporary is less helpful. Acknowledging the unfairness of the client's situation does nothing to address the client's needs at this time. (I, 6)

99. 3. The client with anxiety may be able to learn to recognize when she is feeling anxious, understand the reasons for her anxiety, and be able to describe situations that preceded her feelings of anxiety. However, she is likely to continue to experience symptoms unless she has also learned to use adaptive and palliative methods to reduce anxiety. (E, 6)

100. 4. Saying, "The accident just happened and could not have been predicted," provides the client with an objective perception of the event instead of the client's perceived role. This type of statement reflects active listening and helps to reduce feelings of blame and guilt. Saying, "Don't keep torturing yourself," or "Stop blaming yourself," is inappropriate because it tells the client what to do, subsequently delaying the therapeutic process. The statement, "Let's talk about something that is a bit more pleasant," ignores the client's feelings and changes the subject. The client needs to verbalize feelings and decrease feelings of isolation. (I, 6)

101. 1. The nurse states, "You did what you had to do at that time," to help the client evaluate past behavior in the context of the trauma. Clients often feel guilty about past behaviors when viewing them in the context of current values. The other statements are inappropriate because they do not help the client to evaluate past behavior in the context of the trauma. (I, 6)

102. 2. Writing in a journal can help the client safely express feelings, particularly anger, when the client is unable to verbalize them. Safely externalizing anger by writing in a journal helps the client to maintain control over her feelings. (I, 5)

103. 3. The nurse would facilitate progressive review of the accident and its consequences to help the client integrate feelings and memories and to begin the grieving process. Helping the client to evaluate her sister's

behavior, telling the client to avoid details of the accident, or postponing the discussion of the accident until the client brings it up is not therapeutic and does not facilitate the development of trust in the nurse. Such actions do not facilitate review of the accident, which is necessary to help the client integrate feelings and memories and begin the grieving process. (P, 6)

104. 4. The nurse judges the client's request for an interruption in treatment as a necessary occurrence. A "time-out" is common and necessary to enable the client to focus on emergent problems and solutions. It is not necessarily a method of avoidance, a detriment to progress, or the end of treatment. A problem like housing can be very stressful and require all of the client's energy and attention, with none left for the emotional stress of treatment. (D, 6)

105. 1. Combining a benzodiazepine with an antacid impairs the absorption rate of the benzodiazepine. Acetaminophen, vitamins, and aspirin are safe to take with a benzodiazepine because no major drug–drug interactions occur. (I, 8)

106. 2. Valium, like any benzodiazepine, cannot be stopped abruptly. The client must be slowly tapered off of the medication to decrease withdrawal symptoms, which would be similar to withdrawal from alcohol. Alcohol in combination with a benzodiazepine produces an increased central nervous system depressant effect and therefore should be avoided. Valium can cause drowsiness, and the client should be warned about driving until tolerance develops. Valium has muscle relaxant properties and will help tight, tense muscles feel better. (E, 8)

107. 3. The nurse would suggest behavior therapy, which is most successful for clients with phobias. Systematic desensitization, flooding, exposure, and self-exposure treatments are most therapeutic for clients with phobias. Self-exposure treatment is being increasingly used to avoid frequent therapy sessions. Insight therapy, exploration of the dynamics of the client's personality, is not helpful because the process of anxiety underlies the disorder. Group therapy or psychoanalysis, which deals with repressed, intrapsychic conflicts, is not helpful for the client with phobias because it does not help to manage the underlying anxiety or disorder. (I, 6)

108. 4. Saying, "It's a sign of progress to eat in the dining area," conveys positive reinforcement and gives the client hope and confidence, thus reinforcing the adaptive behavior. Stating, "It wasn't so hard, now was it," decreases the client's self-worth and minimizes his accomplishment. Stating, "At supper, I hope to see you eat with a group of people," will overwhelm the client and increase anxiety. Stating, "You must have been hungry today," ignores the client's positive behavior and shows the nurse's lack of understanding of the dynamics of the disorder. (I, 6)

109. 4. The nurse would walk with the client to activate adaptive coping for the client experiencing high anxiety and decreased motivation and energy. Stating, "I know you can do it," "Try holding on to the wall," or "You can miss group this one time," maintains the client's avoidance, thus reinforcing the client's behavior, and does not help the client begin to cope with the problem. (I, 6)

110. 1. When the client says he thinks he is "going crazy," it is best for the nurse to ask him what "crazy" means to him. The nurse must have a clear idea of what the client means by his words and actions. Using an open-ended question facilitates client description to help the nurse assess the client's meaning. The other statements minimize and dismiss the client's concern and do not give him the opportunity to openly discuss his feelings, possibly leading to increased anxiety. (I, 6)

111. 1. A client who is exhibiting compulsive behavior is attempting to control his anxiety. The compulsive behavior is performed to relieve discomfort and to bind or neutralize anxiety. The client must perform the ritual to avoid an extreme increase in tension or anxiety even though the client is aware that the actions are absurd. The repetitive behavior is not an attempt to control thoughts; the obsession or thinking component cannot be controlled. It is not an attention-seeking mechanism or an attempt to express hostility. (D, 6)

112. 2. The nurse would wake the client an hour earlier to perform his ritual, so that he can be on time for breakfast with the other clients. The nurse provides the client with time needed to perform rituals because the client needs to keep his anxiety in check. The nurse would never take away a ritual, because panic will ensue. The nurse would work with the client later to slowly set limits on the frequency of the action. (I, 6)

113. 3. The nurse conveys empathy and awareness of the client's need to perform the ritual to show acceptance and understanding to the client, thereby promoting trust. Ignoring the behavior, questioning the client about her ritual, or telling the other clients to follow her when she moves is not therapeutic or appropriate. (I, 6)

114. 3. Clomipramine (Anafranil) is used for the treatment of OCD and is related to the tricyclic antidepressants (TCAs). Side effects of anafranil would be similar to those of the TCA imipramine (Tofranil). Fluoxetine (Prozac), sertraline (Zoloft), and fluvoxamine (Luvox) are selective serotonin reuptake inhibitors and have minimal side effects. (A, 8)

The Client With a Somatoform Disorder

115. 4. The nurse sets limits by informing the client in a matter-of-fact manner that the nurse cannot give her additional pain medication at this time. Then the nurse invites the client to participate in a card game to decrease rumination about pain by directing the client's attention to an activity. By telling the client the nurse will call the physician as requested, the nurse is manipulated to do what the client demands. Suggesting that the client lie down because she has to wait for the next dosage or telling the client that the physician will be in later ignores the client and her needs and is not helpful in decreasing rumination about her pain. (I, 6)

116. 3. The nurse instructs the nursing assistant to invite the client to lunch and accompany him to the dining room to decrease manipulation, secondary gain, dependency, and reinforcement of negative behavior while maintaining the client's self-worth. Taking the client a lunch tray and allowing him to eat in his room reinforces negative behaviors and secondary gain. Telling the client he'll need to wait until supper to eat if he misses lunch or informing the client that he has 10 minutes to get to the dining room challenges the client and may increase feelings of anger and the need for physical complaints. (I, 1)

117. 2. Pushing insight or awareness into conflicts or problems increases anxiety and the need for physical symptoms to handle or take care of the anxiety. Awareness or insight must be developed slowly as the client's need for symptoms diminish. Saying, "Ignore the client's behavior and treat her with respect," is not helpful to the staff member or the client. This statement fails to educate the staff member about the client's disorder and simply dismisses the needs of both. It is not true that pushing awareness will be helpful and further the client's recovery; this is the opposite of what is needed. Meeting with the client to confront her behavior is not therapeutic and will greatly increase the client's anxiety and the need for the conversion symptoms. (I, 1)

118. 2. The nurse helps the client to focus on his feelings about his impending divorce so as to decrease the client's anxiety and decrease his focus on physical ailments. The client with a somatoform disorder typically has problems with identifying, describing, and dealing with feelings. Internalizing feelings leads to increased anxiety and the need for protective mechanisms. Asking the client to describe his problem with nausea, allowing the client to talk about the many physicians he has seen and the medications he has taken, and informing the client about a different medication for nausea are counterproductive toward recovery because they reinforce the focus on the symptoms. (I, 6)

119. 4. The nurse would redirect the interaction back to fishing or another focus whenever the client begins to ruminate about physical symptoms or impairment. Doing so helps the client talk about topics that are more therapeutic and beneficial to recovery. Allowing the client to talk about his pain or asking if he needs additional pain medication is not therapeutic because it reinforces the client's need for the symptom. Getting up and leaving the client is not appropriate unless the nurse has set limits previously by saying, "I will get up and leave if you continue to talk about your pain." (I, 6)

120. 1. The client who states, "It's okay if I feel nauseous when I'm worried about my divorce," recognizes the connection between his nausea and the divorce and is developing insight and awareness into his problem. The nurse would then be able to assist the client with developing adaptive coping strategies. The other statements indicate a lack of insight into his disorder and lack of progress toward recovery. The client is still searching for the "right" diagnosis, medication, and doctor. (E, 6)

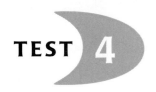

Crisis, Violence, and Disorders in Children and Adolescents

Select the one best answer, and indicate your choice by filling in the circle in front of the option.

The Client in Crisis

1. An anxious teenage girl is brought to the interviewing room of a crisis shelter, sobbing and saying that she thinks she is pregnant but does not know what to do. Which of the following nursing interventions would be *most* appropriate at this time?
   - ○ 1. Ask the client about the type of things that she had thought of doing.
   - ○ 2. Give the client some ideas about what to expect to happen next.
   - ○ 3. Recommend a pregnancy test after acknowledging the client's distress.
   - ○ 4. Question the client about her feelings and possible parental reactions.

2. A potentially pregnant 14-year-old client says that she and her boyfriend have engaged in "mostly heavy petting and necking." Which of the following responses by the nurse would be *best* initially?
   - ○ 1. "You mean you have had sexual intercourse?"
   - ○ 2. "Describe what you mean by heavy petting and necking."
   - ○ 3. "I think we need to talk about what's involved in sexual intercourse."
   - ○ 4. "All you have been doing with your boyfriend is heavy petting and necking?"

3. A 40-year-old client says that she would "rather die than be pregnant." Which of the following responses by the nurse would be *most* helpful?
   - ○ 1. "Try not to worry until after the pregnancy test."
   - ○ 2. "You know, pregnancy is normal event."
   - ○ 3. "You're only 40 years old and not too old to have a baby."

   - ○ 4. "I see you're upset. Take some deep breaths to relax a little."

4. After the results of a pregnancy test for a 15-year-old client are found to be negative, the nurse teaches her about sexual intercourse and contraception. At the end of the teaching session, the client states, "No more fooling around for me!" Which of the following replies by the nurse would be *most* appropriate?
   - ○ 1. "Just in case, why don't you try the pills for a while?"
   - ○ 2. "The last person who said that ended up having a baby."
   - ○ 3. "It's your decision, but if you change your mind, we're here to help you."
   - ○ 4. "Aren't you being a little bit overconfident about it, as attractive as you are?"

5. On a crisis shelter hot line, the nurse talks to two 11-year-old boys who think a friend sniffs glue. They say his breath sometimes smells like glue and he acts drunk. They say they are afraid to tell their parents about the friend. When formulating a reply, the nurse should consider which of the following?
   - ○ 1. The boys probably fear punishment.
   - ○ 2. Sniffing glue is illegal.
   - ○ 3. The boys' observations could be wrong.
   - ○ 4. Glue-sniffing is a minor form of substance abuse.

6. While teaching a group of volunteers for a crisis hot line, a volunteer asks, "What if I'm not sure why someone is calling?" Which of the following statements by the nurse would be *most* helpful?
   - ○ 1. "Ask the caller to tell you why he or she is calling you today."

○ 2. "Tell the caller to make an appointment at the walk-in crisis clinic."

○ 3. "Instruct the caller to go to the nearest emergency room."

○ 4. "Tell the caller to let you speak to anyone else in the house."

7. After teaching a group of students who are volunteering for a local crisis hotline, the nurse judges that *further* education about crisis and intervention is needed when a student states which of the following?

○ 1. "Callers to a crisis line use this service when they're overwhelmed and exhausted."

○ 2. "People use crisis hot lines when they're in the most pain and nothing is working for them."

○ 3. "Most people in crisis will be calling the line once every day for at least a year."

○ 4. "One benefit is that a person will know how to handle stressful situations better in the future."

8. Three months after the death of her husband in an automobile accident, a client is admitted to the hospital after attempting to overdose on her antidepressant. She states, "I can't live without him. It's no use. I just want to die." Which of the following nursing diagnoses would be the priority in the client's plan of care?

○ 1. Dysfunctional Grieving related to husband's death as evidenced by a suicide attempt.

○ 2. Powerlessness related to husband's death as evidenced by statement of "It's no use."

○ 3. Hopelessness related to husband's death as evidenced by the client's statement of inability to live without the husband.

○ 4. Risk for Self-Directed Violence related to husband's death as evidenced by the client's wish to die.

9. A true crisis state, involving a period of severe disorganization, is difficult to endure emotionally and physically. The nurse recognizes that a client will only be able to tolerate being in crisis for which of the following lengths of time?

○ 1. 1 to 2 weeks.

○ 2. 4 to 6 weeks.

○ 3. 12 to 14 weeks.

○ 4. 24 to 26 weeks.

10. The nurse incorporates the underlying premise of crisis intervention, about providing "the right kind of help at the right time," to achieve which of the following goals initially?

○ 1. Regaining of emotional security and equilibrium.

○ 2. Resolution of underlying emotional problems.

○ 3. Development of insight and personal growth.

○ 4. Formulation of more effective support systems.

11. A client is admitted to the emergency department after being found in a daze walking away from her burning car. She was not injured in the fire, but the car is a total loss. She states, "I can't handle it anymore. There's no point to it all." The crisis nurse recommends hospital admission based on the identification of which of the following nursing diagnoses as the priority?

○ 1. Ineffective Coping related to burning of the car as evidenced by walking around in a daze.

○ 2. Decisional Conflict related to burning of the car as evidenced by lack of knowledge of what to do next.

○ 3. Disturbed Thought Processes related to loss of car as evidenced by inability to think clearly.

○ 4. Risk for Suicide related to loss of car as evidenced by statements of helplessness and hopelessness.

12. The nurse understands that with the right help at the right time a client can successfully resolve a crisis and be functioning better than before the crisis, based primarily on which of the following factors?

○ 1. Relinquishment of dysfunctional coping.

○ 2. Reestablishment of lost support systems.

○ 3. Acquisition of new coping skills.

○ 4. Gain of crisis prevention knowledge.

13. A client is being discharged after 3 days of hospitalization for a suicide attempt that followed the receipt of a divorce notice. Which of the following, if verbalized by the client, indicates to the nurse that the client is ready for discharge?

○ 1. A readiness for discharge.

○ 2. Names and phone numbers of two divorce lawyers.

○ 3. A list of support persons and community resources.

○ 4. Emotional stability.

14. Thirty-two children are being brought to the emergency department after a school bus accident. Two children were killed along with the three people in the car that caused the crash. Before the victims arrive, in addition to ensuring that the hospital staff are prepared for the emergency, which of the following would the nurse anticipate doing?

○ 1. Calling the nearest mobile disaster team.

○ 2. Alerting the news media.

○ 3. Notifying the hospital volunteer office.

○ 4. Calling the school for a list of parents' names.

15. A distraught father is waiting for his son to come out of surgery. He accidentally backed the car into his son, causing multiple fractures and a serious head injury. Which of the following statements by the father would alert the nurse to the need for a psychiatric consultation?

○ 1. "My son will be fine, but I may be charged with reckless driving."

○ 2. "His mother is going to kill me when she finds out about this."

○ 3. "I just didn't see him run behind the car."

○ 4. "If he dies, there will be nothing for me to do but join him."

16. A grandson who calls the crisis center expressing concern about his grandmother who lost her husband a month ago states, "She has been in bed for a week and is not eating or showering. She told me that she did not want to kill herself, but it's not like her to do nothing for herself. She won't even talk to me when I visit her." The nurse encourages the grandson to bring his grandmother to the center for evaluation based on which of the following reasons?

○ 1. The behaviors may reflect passive suicidal thoughts.

○ 2. The behaviors reflect altered role performance.

○ 3. Seeing the grandson and grandmother together will be helpful.

○ 4. Refusing to talk to the grandson alone indicates a major problem.

17. A 16-year-old client who is being seen by the crisis nurse after making several superficial cuts on her wrist complains that all her friends are siding with her ex-boyfriend and won't talk to her anymore. She says she knows that the relationship is over, but "If I can't have him, no one will." Which of the following nursing diagnoses would be *most* important?

○ 1. Low Self-Esteem related to rejection of friends as evidenced by friends not talking to her.

○ 2. Risk for Other-Directed Violence related to break-up of the relationship as evidenced by the statement, "If I can't have him, no one else will."

○ 3. Risk for Suicide related to loss of the relationship as evidenced by client's acting-out behaviors.

○ 4. Impaired Adjustment related to rejection by the boyfriend as evidenced by self-mutilation.

18. A client who comes to the crisis center in a very distressed state tells the nurse, "I just can't get over being fired last week. I've asked for help. I've talked to friends. I've tried everything to get through this, but nothing is working. Help me!" Which of the following would the nurse anticipate using as the initial crisis intervention strategy?

○ 1. Referral for counseling.

○ 2. Support system assessment.

○ 3. Emotion management.

○ 4. Unemployment assistance.

19. A major role in crisis intervention is getting a client's significant others involved in helping with the situation as soon as possible. The nurse would determine that the support persons are prepared to help when they verbalize which the following?

○ 1. The names and phone numbers of follow-up counselors.

○ 2. Emergency resources and when to use them.

○ 3. The coping strategies they themselves are using.

○ 4. Long-term solutions they plan to tell the client to use.

20. During the interview, a newly widowed client reveals the wish "to join my husband in Heaven." After the nurse asks the client to sign a "no harm" contract, which of the following statements would be *most* appropriate to say next?

○ 1. "Tell me what feelings you have been experiencing?"

○ 2. "Has your husband's estate been settled yet?"

○ 3. "What was the cause of your husband's death."

○ 4. "Do you have children who are willing to help you out?"

The Client With Problems Expressing Anger

21. A client is admitted to the psychiatric hospital for evaluation after numerous incidents of threatening, angry outbursts, and two episodes of hitting a coworker at the grocery store where he works. The client is very anxious and tells the nurse who admits him, "I didn't mean to hit him. He made me so mad that I just couldn't help it. I hope I don't hit anyone here." Which of the following would be *most* important as the initial action to take to ensure a safe environment?

○ 1. Letting other clients know that he has a history of hitting others so that they will not provoke him.

○ 2. Putting him in a private room and limiting his time out of the room to when staff can be with him.

○ 3. Telling him that hitting others is unacceptable behavior and asking him to tell a staff member when he begins feeling angry.

○ 4. Obtaining an order for a medication to be administered to decrease his anxiety and threatening behavior.

22. Based on a client's history of violence toward others and her inability to cope with anger, which of the following would the nurse use as the *most* important indicator of goal achievement before discharge?

○ 1. Acknowledgment of her angry feelings.

○ 2. Ability to describe situations that provoke angry feelings.

○ 3. Development of a list of how she has handled her anger in the past.

○ 4. Verbalization of her feelings in an appropriate manner.

23. In developing a plan of care for an angry client, the staff decides to take an educational approach. Which of the following steps would be *least* helpful?
    ○ 1. Assisting the client to recognize anger.
    ○ 2. Identifying those with whom the client is angry.
    ○ 3. Identifying alternative ways to express anger.
    ○ 4. Practicing how to express anger.

24. A client is admitted to the hospital because of threatening, aggressive behavior toward his family. In the first group meeting after the client is admitted, another client sits near the nurse and says loudly, "I'm sitting here because I'm afraid of Ted. He's so big, and I heard him talk about hitting people." Which of the following responses by the nurse would be the *most* therapeutic?
    ○ 1. "Everyone is here for different problems. You know you don't have to worry."
    ○ 2. "Ted is new to the group. Let's go around and introduce ourselves to him."
    ○ 3. "You don't know Ted yet. Once you get to know him, I'm sure you won't be afraid."
    ○ 4. "It's frightening to have new people on the unit. We're here to talk about things like being afraid."

25. A female client in an anger management group states, "My doctor tells me I need to get mad more often and not let people tell me what to do. Maybe she thinks I should be more crude." Which of the following would the nurse incorporate in the response to this client as *most* important?
    ○ 1. Denial of anger and lack of assertiveness can be as serious as aggressiveness.
    ○ 2. Assertive behavior in women is not culturally acceptable.
    ○ 3. The client has most likely distorted what the doctor said.
    ○ 4. The client is trying to gain acceptance by the group.

26. The client loses self-control and throws chairs against the wall. Which of the following would the nurse do *next*?
    ○ 1. Ask the client to go to the quiet area and talk about the behavior.
    ○ 2. Administer an oral tranquilizer and prepare for a show of determination.
    ○ 3. Process the incident with the client and discuss alternative behaviors.
    ○ 4. Use restraints and administer an intramuscular tranquilizer.

27. The nurse judges that a client is ready to be released from seclusion and restraints when the client demonstrates which of the following behaviors?
    ○ 1. Is adequately sedated.
    ○ 2. Struggles less against the restraints.
    ○ 3. Stops swearing and yelling.
    ○ 4. Shows signs of self-control.

28. The treatment team recommends that a client take an assertiveness training class offered in the hospital. Which of the following behaviors indicates that the client is becoming more assertive?
    ○ 1. Begins to arrive late for unit activities.
    ○ 2. Asks the nurse to call his employer about his insurance.
    ○ 3. Asks his roommate to put away dirty clothes that are on floor after telling him that this bothers him.
    ○ 4. Follows the nurse's advice of asking his doctor about being passive-aggressive.

29. Which of the following physiologic responses would the nurse expect as *unlikely* to occur when a client is angry?
    ○ 1. Increased respiratory rate.
    ○ 2. Decreased blood pressure.
    ○ 3. Increased muscle tension.
    ○ 4. Decreased peristalsis.

30. Which of the following psychological responses to anger would the nurse expect as *most* common in clients?
    ○ 1. Increased self-esteem.
    ○ 2. Feelings of invulnerability.
    ○ 3. Fear of retaliation.
    ○ 4. Powerlessness.

31. When planning the care of clients experiencing aggression, the nurse incorporates the principle of "least restrictive alternative," meaning that less restrictive interventions must be tried before more restrictive measures are employed. Which of the following measures would the nurse consider to be the *most* restrictive?
    ○ 1. Tension reduction strategies.
    ○ 2. Haloperidol (Haldol) given orally.
    ○ 3. Voluntary seclusion or "time-out."
    ○ 4. Haloperidol (Haldol) given intramuscularly.

32. As an angry client becomes more agitated while talking about his problems, the nurse decides to ask for staff assistance in taking control of the situation when the client demonstrates which of the following behaviors?
    ○ 1. Swearing about his wife's behaviors when discussing marital problems.
    ○ 2. Picking up a pool cue stick and telling the nurse to get out of his way.
    ○ 3. Making a fist and pounding loudly on the table.
    ○ 4. Coming out of his room instead of staying in "time-out."

33. A client who is agitated but not currently psychotic is willing to take a medication ordered as needed (PRN). If all the following medications were ordered

for the client, which would the nurse expect to administer?

- ○ 1. Oral lorazepam (Ativan).
- ○ 2. Oral quetiapine (Seroquel).
- ○ 3. IM haloperidol (Haldol).
- ○ 4. IM fluphenazine (Prolixin).

34. When a client is about to lose control, the extra staff who come to help often stay at a distance from the client unless asked to move closer by the nurse who is talking to the patient. Which of the following *best* explains the primary rationale for staying at a distance initially?

- ○ 1. The client is more likely to act out if there is an audience, even additional staff.
- ○ 2. The nurse talking to the client makes the decisions about other staff actions.
- ○ 3. The client is likely to perceive others as being closer than they are and feel threatened.
- ○ 4. When the extra staff are visible the client is less likely to regain self-control.

35. Psychiatric staff are usually required to participate in an aggression management program annually. Evaluation of such a program would be based *primarily* on which of the following indicators?

- ○ 1. Fewer client injuries during restraint procedures.
- ○ 2. A reduction of complaints by clients' relatives.
- ○ 3. Fewer staff injuries during restraint procedures.
- ○ 4. A reduction in the total number of restraint procedures.

36. When preparing to use seclusion as an alternative to restraint for a client who has not yet lost control, the nurse expects to use a room with limited furniture and no access to dangerous articles. Which of the following would the nurse also consider as *critical*?

- ○ 1. A security window in the door or a room camera.
- ○ 2. Lights that can be dimmed from outside the room.
- ○ 3. A staff member to stay in the room with the client.
- ○ 4. A doctor's order for the seclusion before it is initiated.

37. The nurse is required to restrain all four of a client's extremities initially. For which of the following reasons would the nurse anticipate the need to add a full-length restraint blanket?

- ○ 1. The client complains that restraints are tight and uncomfortable.
- ○ 2. The staff want extra protection for themselves.
- ○ 3. The client is at risk for injury from fighting the restraints.
- ○ 4. Staff assessment reveals that client will feel more secure under the blanket.

38. Which of the following would be the top priority for the client who is placed in restraints?

- ○ 1. Monitoring of the client every 15 minutes.
- ○ 2. Assisting with nutrition and elimination.
- ○ 3. Performing range of motion exercise for each limb, one at a time.
- ○ 4. Changing the client's position every 2 hours.

39. According to hospital protocol, after a client is restrained, the staff meet and discuss the restraint situation. In addition to sharing feelings and offering support, the nurse would identify which of the following at the ultimate goal?

- ○ 1. Providing feedback to each other on how procedures were handled.
- ○ 2. Comparing the perceptions of the various staff members.
- ○ 3. Deciding on when to release the client from restraints.
- ○ 4. Improving the staff's use of restraint procedures.

40. Despite education and role-play practice of restraint procedures, a staff member is injured during an actual restraint. When helping the uninjured staff deal with the incident, the nurse would anticipate addressing which of the following about the injured member?

- ○ 1. The emotional responses may be similar to those of other crime victims.
- ○ 2. The member is likely to resign after experiencing such an injury.
- ○ 3. Legal action against the client will take time and energy.
- ○ 4. The member must debrief with the assaultive client before returning.

The Client With Family Abuse or Violence

41. A married woman has been referred to the mental health center because she is depressed. The nurse notices bruises on her upper arms and asks about them. After denying any problems, the client starts to cry and says, "He didn't really mean to hurt me, but I hate the kids to see this. I'm so worried about them." Which of the following would be the *most* crucial information for the nurse to determine?

- ○ 1. The type and extent of abuse occurring in the family.
- ○ 2. The potential of immediate danger to the client and her children.
- ○ 3. The resources available to the client.
- ○ 4. Whether the client wants to be separated from her husband.

42. A client with suspected abuse describes her husband as a good man who works hard and provides

well for his family. She does not work outside the home and states that she is proud to be a wife and mother just like her own mother. The nurse interprets the family pattern described by the client as *best* illustrating which of the following as characteristic of abusive families?
- ○ 1. Tight, impermeable boundaries.
- ○ 2. Unbalanced power ratio.
- ○ 3. Role stereotyping.
- ○ 4. Dysfunctional feeling tone.

43. When planning the care for a client who is abused, which of the following measures would be *most* important to include?
- ○ 1. Being compassionate and empathetic.
- ○ 2. Teaching the client about abuse and the cycle of violence.
- ○ 3. Explaining to the client his or her personal and legal rights.
- ○ 4. Helping the client develop a safety plan.

44. The nurse is assessing the client's methods of coping. A client who is being abused would be *least* likely to demonstrate which of the following?
- ○ 1. Assertiveness.
- ○ 2. Self-blame.
- ○ 3. Alcohol abuse.
- ○ 4. Suicidal thoughts.

45. During the third session with the nurse, a client who is being abused states, "I don't know what to do anymore. He doesn't want me to go anywhere while he's at work, not even to visit my friends." Which of the following nursing diagnoses would the nurse formulate in respect to this information?
- ○ 1. Risk for Violence related to abusive husband, as evidenced by victim's statement of being battered.
- ○ 2. Low Self-Esteem related to victimization, as evidenced by not being able to leave the house.
- ○ 3. Powerlessness related to abusive husband, as evidenced by inability to make decisions.
- ○ 4. Ineffective Coping related to victimization, as evidenced by crying.

46. After months of counseling, a client abused by her husband tells the nurse that she has decided to stop treatment. There has been no abuse during this time, and she feels better able to cope with the needs of her husband and children. In discussing this decision with the client, it would be *most* important for the nurse to do which of the following?
- ○ 1. Tell the client that this is a bad decision that she will regret in the future.
- ○ 2. Find out more about the client's rationale for her decision to stop treatment.
- ○ 3. Warn the client that abuse often stops when one partner is in treatment, only to begin again later.

- ○ 4. Remind the client of her duty to protect the children by continuing treatment.

47. A third-grade child is referred to the mental health clinic by the school nurse because he is fearful, anxious, and socially isolated. After meeting with the client, the nurse talks with his mother, who says, "It's that school nurse again. She's done nothing but try to make trouble for our family since my son started school. And now you're in on it." Which of the following responses by the nurse would be *most* helpful in developing a relationship with this family?
- ○ 1. "The school nurse is concerned about your son and is only doing her job."
- ○ 2. "We see a number of children who go to your son's school. He isn't the only one."
- ○ 3. "You sound pretty angry with the school nurse. Tell me what has happened."
- ○ 4. "Let me tell you why your son was referred, and then you can tell me about your concerns."

48. The mother of a school-aged child tells the school nurse that for most of the past year her husband was unemployed and she worked a second job to help. Twice during the year, she slapped her son repeatedly when he refused to obey. She says it has not happened again and that the family is "back to normal." After assessing the family, the nurse decides that the child is no longer at risk for abuse. Which of the following observations would *best* support such a decision?
- ○ 1. The parents have a caring and supportive relationship.
- ○ 2. The child has not talked about violence during his visits to the nurse.
- ○ 3. The infrequent episodes were limited to a time of intense family stress.
- ○ 4. The parents have a defensive attitude toward the school nurse.

49. When assessing a client who was the victim of a crime, the nurse understands that crimes, whether they cause physical injury or not, involve a sense of emotional violation and a loss of trust in others. Which of the following would the nurse identify as another developmental stage that is typically affected by crime?
- ○ 1. Autonomy versus shame and doubt.
- ○ 2. Identity versus role diffusion.
- ○ 3. Generativity versus stagnation.
- ○ 4. Integrity versus despair.

50. When caring for a client who was a victim of a crime, the nurse is aware that recovery from any crime can be a long and difficult process depending on the meaning it has for the client. Which of the following would the nurse identify as a victim's ultimate goal in reconstructing his or her life?

○ 1. Getting through the shock and confusion.
○ 2. Carrying out home and work routines.
○ 3. Resolving the grief over any losses.
○ 4. Regaining a sense of security and safety.

51. A client tells the nurse that she has been raped but has not reported it to the police. After determining whether the client was injured, whether it is still possible to collect evidence, and whether to file a report, the nurse's *next* priority is to offer which of the following to the client?
○ 1. Legal assistance.
○ 2. Crisis intervention.
○ 3. A rape support group.
○ 4. Medication for disturbed sleep.

52. In working with any rape victim, which of the following would be *most* important?
○ 1. Continuing to encourage the client to report the rape to the legal authorities.
○ 2. Recommending that the client resume sexual relations with her partner as soon as possible.
○ 3. Periodically reminding the client that she did not deserve and did not cause the rape.
○ 4. Telling the client that the rapist will eventually be caught, put on trial, and jailed.

53. In the process of dealing with the intense feelings about being raped, victims often verbalize that they were afraid they would be killed during the rape and wish that they had been. The nurse would decide that *further* counseling is needed if the client voiced which of the following?
○ 1. "I didn't fight him, but I guess I did the right thing because I'm alive."
○ 2. "Suicide would be an easy escape from all this pain, but I couldn't do it to myself."
○ 3. "I wish they gave the death penalty to all rapists and other sexual predators."
○ 4. "I get so angry at times that I have to have a couple of drinks before I sleep."

54. One of the myths about sexual abuse of young children is that it usually involves physically violent acts. Which of the following behaviors is more likely to be used by the abusers?
○ 1. Tying the child down.
○ 2. Bribery with money.
○ 3. Coercion as a result of the trusting relationship.
○ 4. Asking for the child's consent for sex.

55. A young child is suspected of being sexually abused because he demonstrates self-destructive behaviors of head banging and self-mutilation. Which of the following behaviors would the nurse also commonly expect to assess?
○ 1. Inability to play.
○ 2. Truancy and running away.
○ 3. Substance abuse.
○ 4. Overcontrol of anger.

56. Adolescents and adults who were sexually abused as children commonly mutilate themselves. The nurse interprets this behavior as which of the following?
○ 1. The need to make themselves less sexually attractive.
○ 2. An alternative to bingeing and purging.
○ 3. Use of physical pain to avoid dealing with emotional pain.
○ 4. An alternative to getting "high" on drugs.

57. A young child who has been sexually abused has difficulty putting feelings into words. Which of the following would the nurse employ with the child?
○ 1. Engaging in play therapy.
○ 2. Role-playing.
○ 3. Giving the child's drawings to the abuser.
○ 4. Reporting the abuse to a prosecutor.

58. When working with a group of adult survivors of childhood sexual abuse, dealing with the anger and rage is a major focus. Which of the following strategies would the nurse expect as *least* likely to be successful?
○ 1. Directly confronting the abuser.
○ 2. Using a foam bat while symbolically confronting the abuser.
○ 3. Keeping a journal of memories and feelings.
○ 4. Writing letters about the abuse that are not sent.

59. Once a client reveals a history of childhood sexual abuse, at some point the nurse would need to ask which of the following questions?
○ 1. "What other forms of abuse did you experience?"
○ 2. "How long did the abuse go on?"
○ 3. "Was there a period of time when you did not remember the abuse?"
○ 4. "Does your abuser still have contact with young children?"

60. A client who was sexually abused as a child decides to stop participating in counseling. The nurse will evaluate this as appropriate if the client states which of the following?
○ 1. "It is all out is the open now, and I can be done with it."
○ 2. "It is too hard to deal with all this pain all the time."
○ 3. "I'm functioning OK now, but I know problems will come up again."
○ 4. "Everyone tells me how much better I'm doing and I believe them."

The Client With Anorexia Nervosa

61. When teaching a group of adolescents about anorexia nervosa, the nurse would describe this disor-

der as being characterized by which of the following?
- ○ 1. Excessive fear of becoming obese, near-normal weight, and a self-critical body image.
- ○ 2. Obsession with the weight of others, chronic dieting, and an altered body image.
- ○ 3. Extreme concern about dieting, calorie-counting, and an unrealistic body image.
- ○ 4. Intense fear of becoming obese, emaciation, and a disturbed body image.

62. When developing a teaching plan for a high school health class about anorexia nervosa, which of the following would the nurse include as the primary group affected by this disease?
- ○ 1. Women, age at onset between 12 and 20 years.
- ○ 2. Men, onset during the college years.
- ○ 3. Women, onset typically after 30 years of age.
- ○ 4. Men, onset before 20 years of age.

63. When assessing a client with anorexia nervosa, the nurse would expect to find which of the following?
- ○ 1. Hyperthermia, oliguria, and bradycardia.
- ○ 2. Lanugo, hypothermia, and hypotension.
- ○ 3. Constipation, dysmenorrhea, and hypertension.
- ○ 4. Diarrhea, dry skin, and menorrhagia.

64. The parents of a newly diagnosed 15-year-old with anorexia nervosa are meeting with the nurse during the admission process. Which of the following remarks by the parents would the nurse interpret as typical for a client with anorexia nervosa?
- ○ 1. "We've given her everything and look how she repays us!"
- ○ 2. "She's had behavior problems for the past year both at home and at school."
- ○ 3. "She's been a model child. We've never had any problems with her."
- ○ 4. "We have five children, all normal kids with some problems at times."

65. Which of the following nursing diagnoses would the nurse formulate as the *priority* for a client who is admitted to the mental health unit with a diagnosis of anorexia nervosa and who is 5 feet 4 inches tall and weighs only 82 pounds?
- ○ 1. Low Self-Esteem related to feelings of inadequacy and loss of control.
- ○ 2. Disturbed Body Image related to self-view of being overweight.
- ○ 3. Interrupted Family Processes related to overprotectiveness and avoidance of conflict.
- ○ 4. Imbalanced Nutrition: Less Than Body Requirements related to severe restriction in intake.

The Client With Bulimia

66. A client newly diagnosed with bulimia is attending the nurse-led group at the mental health center. She tells the group that she came only because her husband said he would divorce her if she didn't get help. Which of the following responses by the nurse would be *most* appropriate?
- ○ 1. "You sound angry with your husband. Is that correct?"
- ○ 2. "You will find that you like coming to group. These people are a lot of fun."
- ○ 3. "Tell me more about why you are here and how you feel about that."
- ○ 4. "Tell me something about what has caused you to be bulimic."

67. A client diagnosed with bulimia tells the nurse that she eats excessively when she is upset and then vomits so she won't gain a lot of weight. Which of the following nursing diagnostic categories would be *most* appropriate for this client?
- ○ 1. Disabled Family Coping.
- ○ 2. Ineffective Coping.
- ○ 3. Imbalanced Nutrition: More Than Body Requirements.
- ○ 4. Anxiety.

68. During the initial interview, a client with a compulsive eating disorder remarks, "I can't stand myself and the way I look." Which of the following statements by the nurse would be *most* therapeutic?
- ○ 1. "Everyone who has the same problem feels like you do."
- ○ 2. "I don't think you look bad at all."
- ○ 3. "Don't worry, you'll soon be back in shape."
- ○ 4. "Tell me more about your feelings."

69. When discussing eating disorders with a group of adolescents, the nurse incorporates information that persons living within the culture of the United States often experience difficulty with weight control because they unconsciously equate food with which of the following?
- ○ 1. Love and affection.
- ○ 2. Power and control.
- ○ 3. Status and prestige.
- ○ 4. Survival and growth.

Children and Adolescents With Behavior Problems

70. A 2-year-old child is brought into the physician's office by her parents, who are concerned by her behavior. They state that she resists their affection, twirls around frequently, and refuses to respond to other children and adults. Based on the analysis of these behaviors, which of the following would the nurse suspect?
- ○ 1. Tourette's syndrome.
- ○ 2. Schizophrenia.

   ○ 3. Attention deficit hyperactivity disorder (ADHD).

   ○ 4. Autism.

71. When developing the plan of care for a child diagnosed with ADHD, the nurse would expect to include treatment *most* commonly with a combination of which of the following?

   ○ 1. Antianxiety medications such as buspirone (BuSpar) and home schooling.

   ○ 2. Antidepressant medication such as imipramine (Tofranil) and family therapy.

   ○ 3. Anticonvulsant medications such as carbamazepine (Tegretol) and monthly blood levels.

   ○ 4. Psychostimulant medications such as methylphenidate (Ritalin) and behavior modification.

72. The mental health nurse meets with the mother of a child diagnosed with ADHD. The mother states, "I feel so guilty that he has this disease, like I did something wrong. I feel like I need to be with him constantly in order for him to get better. But still sometimes I feel like I'm going to lose control and hurt him." Which of the following would be *most* appropriate to suggest to the mother?

   ○ 1. Arranging for respite care to watch her child and give herself a regular break.

   ○ 2. Taking a job to allow herself to feel some success because her child won't ever improve.

   ○ 3. Arranging to have coffee with friends daily as a way to begin a support group.

   ○ 4. Considering foster care if she feels that she can't handle her child's problems.

73. The nurse is with the parents of a 16-year-old boy who recently attempted suicide. The nurse cautions the parents to be especially alert for which of the following in their son?

   ○ 1. Expression of a desire to date.

   ○ 2. Decision to try out for an extracurricular activity.

   ○ 3. Giving away valued personal items.

   ○ 4. Desire to spend more time with friends.

74. The parents of a 15-year-old girl bring their daughter for admission to the mental health center. She was recently expelled from school for repeated behavior problems and truancy. She was also arrested for vandalism and prostitution in the past week. Based on an analysis of these findings, the nurse would suspect which of the following as the most likely medical diagnosis?

   ○ 1. ADHD.

   ○ 2. Conduct disorder.

   ○ 3. Oppositional defiant disorder.

   ○ 4. Tourette's syndrome.

75. The nurse at the mental health clinic is meeting a new client who is a 7-year-old boy with Tourette's disorder. Which of the following would the nurse expect to assess?

   ○ 1. Multiple motor and verbal tics.

   ○ 2. Primarily motor tics.

   ○ 3. Isolated verbal tics.

   ○ 4. Alternating simple and complex motor tics.

76. When comparing the signs and symptoms of depression found in children with those found in adults, which of the following would the nurse expect?

   ○ 1. Adults more often display sad behaviors, while children have more somatic complaints and possible acting-out behaviors.

   ○ 2. Adults have more problems performing in the work setting than children have in performing in the school setting.

   ○ 3. Adults typically will not be able to function at work and at home but children continue to succeed in school activities while depressed.

   ○ 4. Adults frequently have few major problems functioning with depression, while children usually are unable to function at school or with tasks at home.

77. Assessment of suicidal risk in children and adolescents requires the nurse to know which of the following?

   ○ 1. Children rarely commit suicide unless one of their parents has already committed suicide, especially in the past year.

   ○ 2. The risk of suicide increases during adolescence, with those who have recently suffered a loss, abuse, or family discord being most at risk.

   ○ 3. Children do have a suicidal risk that coincides with some significant event such as a recent gun purchase in the family.

   ○ 4. Adolescents typically don't choose suicide unless they live in certain geographical regions of the United States including the western states.

78. When counseling a 5-year-old girl who recently suffered the loss of her mother, the nurse understands that which of the following statements reflects the typical understanding about death at this age?

   ○ 1. "My mommy died last week, but I'm going to see her again soon."

   ○ 2. "My daddy said mommy went to heaven and I'm glad Jesus took her there."

   ○ 3. "My dog died and now we got another one."

   ○ 4. "I think Mommy went to heaven and I'll get to see her someday when I die."

79. A child with Asperger's disorder is being referred to the mental health clinic along with his parents. To provide the best care for this family, the nurse remembers that this disorder differs from autism in which of the following areas?

○ 1. Asperger's disorder, often diagnosed earlier than autism, is associated with fewer major problems in interpersonal interactions.

○ 2. In Asperger's disorder, behavior often is similar to that of other children with autism but without the problems with school.

○ 3. Asperger's disorder is recognized later than autism, and interpersonal interaction problems typically become more apparent when the child begins school.

○ 4. There are significant problems with language development, as with autism, but there are no delays or difficulties with motor development.

80. A staff nurse on the mental health unit tells the nurse manager that kids with conduct disorders might as well be jailed because they all end up as adults with antisocial personality disorder anyway. Which of the following would be the *best* reply by the nurse manager?

○ 1. "You really sound burned out. Do you have a vacation coming up soon?"

○ 2. "Actually these children more often have problems with depression and bipolar disorder as adults."

○ 3. "You sound really frustrated. Not all will be diagnosed as antisocial personality disorders as adults."

○ 4. "My experience hasn't been that negative. Let's see what the other staff members think; maybe I'm wrong."

81. The mother of a 14-year-old girl who is diagnosed with oppositional defiant disorder tells the nurse that she has read extensively on this disorder and does not believe the diagnosis is correct for her daughter. Which of the following responses by the nurse would be *most* appropriate?

○ 1. "It sounds like you are very interested in your daughter. Let's focus on what is best for her."

○ 2. "Tell me what you have found in your reading that is leading you to that conclusion."

○ 3. "Your doctor has had many years of education and experience so you can believe he's right."

○ 4. "That doesn't matter now because we just need to help her get better."

82. The father of a 4-year-old boy with the diagnosis of ADHD says to the mental health nurse, "I know that either my wife or I must have caused this disease." Which of the following would be the nurse's *best* response?

○ 1. "ADHD does occur more often within families, suggesting a genetic connection, but no specific causes have been found. There is no evidence that problems with parenting have ever caused this disorder."

○ 2. "What do you think you might have done that could have led to causing this disorder to develop in your son?"

○ 3. "Many parents feel this way, but most of them find that there isn't anything that they did that caused ADHD to develop in their child."

○ 4. "Let's not focus on the cause but rather on what needs to be done to help your son get better. I know that you and your wife are very interested in helping him to improve his behavior."

83. A member of a nurse-led group for depressed adolescents tells the group that she is not coming back because she is now taking medication and no longer needs to talk about her problems. Which of the following responses by the nurse would be *most* appropriate?

○ 1. "I'm glad that you are taking your medication, but how can we know that you will continue to take it? After all, you haven't been on it for very long and you might decide to stop taking it."

○ 2. "I think that it is important to let everyone respond to what you said, so let's go around the group and let everyone give their thoughts about what you have decided."

○ 3. "The purpose of the group is to provide each of you with a place to discuss the problems of being a teenager with depression with others who also are experiencing a similar situation."

○ 4. "You don't have to stay in the group if you don't want to, but if you choose to leave, then you won't be able to change your mind later and return to the group."

84. When assessing a 17-year-old male client with depression for suicide risk, which of the following questions would be *best*?

○ 1. "What movies about death have you watched lately?"

○ 2. "Can you tell me what you think about suicide?"

○ 3. "Has anyone in your family ever committed suicide?"

○ 4. "Are you thinking about killing yourself?"

85. A teacher is talking to the school nurse about a child in her classroom who has a tic disorder. She mentions that the boy often trips other children although no one has ever been hurt. She further states that she ignores him when that happens because it is part of his disorder. Which of the following would be the *best* response by the nurse?

○ 1. "Tripping other children would not be a tic, so you can respond to that as you would in any other child."

○ 2. "I can't believe that you actually allow him get away with that!"

○ 3. "I think that is the best choice unless some parents of the other children start to complain about it."

○ 4. "If no one else is getting hurt then it seems harmless and might prevent the development of a worse behavior."

86. Which of the following medications would the nurse anticipate administering as a treatment for tic disorders, including Tourette's disorder?
    ○ 1. Chlorpromazine (Thorazine).
    ○ 2. Imipramine (Tofranil).
    ○ 3. Lithium.
    ○ 4. Clonidine (Catapres).

87. The nurse leading a group for parents of children diagnosed with oppositional defiant disorder plans on including which of the following recommendations for discipline?
    ○ 1. Avoid limiting the child's use of the television and computer for punishment.
    ○ 2. Be consistent with discipline while assisting with ways for the child to more positively express anger and frustration.
    ○ 3. Use primarily positive reinforcement for good behavior while ignoring any demonstrated bad behavior.
    ○ 4. Use "time-out" as the primary means of punishment for the child regardless of what the child has done.

88. Which of the following children would the nurse identify as being more at risk for an episode of major depression?
    ○ 1. Michael, a 16-year-old, who has been struggling in school, making only C's and D's.
    ○ 2. Lauren, a 13-year-old, who was upset over not being chosen as a cheerleader.
    ○ 3. Cody, a 10-year-old, who has never liked school and basically has a few limited friends.
    ○ 4. Gretchen, a 14-year-old, who recently moved to a new school after her parents' divorce.

89. A 15-year-old sophomore girl is sent to the school nurse with complaints of dizziness and nausea. While assessing the girl, who denies any health problems, the nurse smells alcohol on her breath. Which of the following responses by the nurse would be *most* appropriate?
    ○ 1. "Don't tell me that you have been drinking alcohol before you came to school this morning!"
    ○ 2. "Why don't you tell me the real reason that you are feeling sick this morning?"
    ○ 3. "Tell me everything that you have had to eat and drink yesterday and today."
    ○ 4. "I know that high school is stressful, but drinking alcohol is not the best way to handle it."

90. While coaching a youth soccer team, the nurse has observed one of the teammates bingeing and purging on multiple occasions. The nurse asks the girl's mother to stay after practice and talk privately.

Which of the following ways would be *best* for the nurse to begin the conversation?
    ○ 1. "Thank you for letting your daughter play on the team. She's a very good player and is also pleasant and easy to coach."
    ○ 2. "I have some very bad news for you. Your daughter has a serious problem that is diagnosed as an eating disorder."
    ○ 3. "I am a nurse. I have seen your daughter doing things that are considered to be part of an eating disorder."
    ○ 4. "Let me get right to the point. Your daughter is very sick and needs to see a mental health therapist right away."

91. Parents of a 7-year-old child newly diagnosed with ADHD ask the nurse whether their son will always have to take medication for this condition. Which of the following responses would be *most* appropriate?
    ○ 1. "Yes, almost everyone with this disorder has to continue taking medication forever."
    ○ 2. "Up to 50% of individuals need to continue to take medications as adults."
    ○ 3. "Most people with this disorder do not need to continue taking medications as adults."
    ○ 4. "There is just a small percentage of adults with ADHD who can manage without medications."

92. A 9-year-old client with attention deficit disorder (ADD) tells the nurse, "No one in my class likes me because they think I'm stupid. They're right, I am stupid!" The nurse identifies which of the following nursing diagnoses as relevant for this client?
    ○ 1. Low Self-Esteem related to client's perception of how other's view him.
    ○ 2. Ineffective Coping related to inability to be objective about peers.
    ○ 3. Interrupted Family Processes (disabling) related to the family's difficulty in coping with the child.
    ○ 4. Anxiety related to dislike of client by peers.

93. Which of the following would the nurse expect to include in the teaching plan for the parents of a child who is receiving methylphenidate (Ritalin)?
    ○ 1. Giving the medication at the same time every evening.
    ○ 2. Having the child take two doses at the same time if the last dose was missed.
    ○ 3. Giving the single-dose form of the medication early in the day.
    ○ 4. Allowing concurrent use of any over-the-counter medications with this drug.

94. A 6-year-old female student is brought to the school nurse for refusal to sit in class. She denies feeling sick but insists that her mother be called so she can go home. She is pacing and chewing on a fingernail.

This has occurred daily since school began 4 weeks ago. She tells the nurse that she is afraid something bad is going to happen to her mother. Which of the following would the nurse suspect?

○ 1. Obsessive-compulsive disorder.
○ 2. Major depression.
○ 3. ADD.
○ 4. Separation anxiety disorder.

95. Which of the following children would the nurse assess as demonstrating behaviors that need further evaluation?

○ 1. Joey, age 2, who refuses to be toilet-trained and talks to himself.
○ 2. Adrienne, age 6, who sucks her thumb when tired and has never spent the night with a friend.
○ 3. Curt, age 10, who often tells his mother that he is going to run away whenever they argue.
○ 4. Stephen, age 2, who is indifferent to other children and adults and is mute.

Correct Answers and Rationale

The letters in parentheses following the rationale identify the step of the nursing process (A, D, P, I, E) and client needs (1, 2, 3, 4, 5, 6, 7, 8, 9, 10). See the inside front cover for the key.

The Client in Crisis

1. 3. Before any interventions can occur, knowing whether the client is pregnant is crucial in formulating a care plan. Asking the client about what things she had thought about doing, giving the client some ideas about what to expect next, and questioning the client about her feelings and possible parental reactions would be appropriate once it is determined that the client is indeed pregnant. (I, 6)

2. 2. Because of the client's potential pregnancy, the nurse needs to determine exactly what the client means by the terms "heavy petting and necking" by asking the client describe what she has been doing in sexual encounters with her boyfriend. Asking the client if she means sexual intercourse or telling the client that they need to talk about sexual intercourse makes an assumption that may or may not be appropriate. The nurse needs to determine exactly what the client means by the terms used. Repeating the client's statement does not elicit the necessary information to interpret the client's statement. Additionally, this type of response assumes an understanding of what the client has said. (I, 6)

3. 4. Because people in the midst of emotional crisis find it difficult to focus their thinking, the goal is to return the client to noncrisis functioning. Pointing out and decreasing the client's level of anxiety is the first step in attaining this goal. Telling an obviously distressed person not to worry is ineffective because it ignores the client's distress and concerns. Although pregnancy is normal event, and 40 years of age may not be too old for a pregnancy, these responses also ignore the client's distress and feelings. (I, 6)

4. 3. The client's statement indicates that she needs no more help. Therefore, the nurse needs to inform the client that the door is open for her return. Suggesting that the client try pills for a while imposes the nurse's view on the client without allowing the client to make the decision. The statement that the last person who said that ended up with a baby is condescending, ridiculing, and somewhat threatening. Telling the client that she is overconfident is inappropriate because it is condescending and also somewhat threatening. (I, 5)

5. 1. Telephoning the crisis shelter indicates that the boys are alarmed but are reluctant to talk with their parents. The boys may fear that their parents will assume that they have been sniffing glue and punish them. The nurse should focus on helping the boys talk with their parents. Sniffing glue is included in the *Diagnostic and Statistical Manual of Mental Disorders,* 4th ed., text revised (DSM-IV-TR) as inhalant abuse. Although sniffing glue is dangerous and potentially lethal, it is not illegal. To prove that the observations are incorrect requires an intervention beginning with the boys' parents. (D, 6)

6. 1. The crisis worker needs to use active focusing techniques to determine the crisis-precipitating event or the immediate problem. Asking the caller, "Why are you calling today?" or "What is the immediate problem?" will assist the caller to focus on the specific need or event. Telling the client to make an appointment is inappropriate because the problem might be life-threatening. Telling the caller to go to the nearest emergency room is precipitous and may be unnecessary. Asking to speak to someone else in the home may be futile because the caller might be alone. This action also ignores the caller and his or her feelings. (I, 2)

7. 3. The concern that someone may call the crisis hotline every day for a year indicates that further understanding about crisis and crisis intervention is needed. A crisis situation is time-limited, typically resolving in 4 to 6 weeks if handled effectively. If a person calls the line daily for a year, that person has not been properly dealt with or is probably in a highly disorganized state requiring an alternative intervention. The nurse would need to further review and clarify the material presented. (E, 6)

8. 4. Risk for Self-Directed Violence is the priority nursing diagnosis for a client who has attempted or verbalizes the intent to harm herself. Although the client is depressed and feeling hopeless, powerless, and grieving, these are not the priority concern at this time. (D, 6)

9. 2. Generally, 4 to 6 weeks is viewed as the length of time a client can tolerate the severe level of disturbance of a true crisis. In the first week or two, clients usually are still trying to use their normal coping skills and support systems. After 6 weeks of continuous crisis, a client is probably becoming so physically and emotionally drained that he or she has sought or has been brought by others for medical or psychiatric care. (A, 6)

10. 1. The initial goal in crisis intervention is helping the client regain emotional security and equilibrium. Resolution of the underlying emotional problems, development of insight and personal growth, and formulation of more effective support systems are goals to address as the crisis is subsiding. (D, 6)

11. 4. The client is demonstrating helplessness and hopelessness during a crisis, as evidenced by the her statement, "I can't handle it. There is no point to it." Feelings of helplessness and hopelessness are common factors associated with suicidal ideation. Therefore, the client needs to be hospitalized to ensure safety to herself. Ineffective Coping affects interventions. Not knowing what to do next reflects a request for help in making a decision. However, these diagnoses have less priority when compared with the client's risk for suicide. Disturbed Thought Processes would be evidenced by delusions, such as "The devil set my car on fire," not just the inability to think clearly. (D, 6)

12. 3. Learning new coping skills is the major factor necessary for higher functioning. Better coping is likely to lead to the regaining support systems, giving up dysfunctional coping, and awareness of how to prevent future crises. (A, 6)

13. 3. The risk for suicide can persist for 2 to 3 months even after a crisis has abated. Therefore, it is important for the client to be able to verbalize information about appropriate support persons and community resources and to have this information readily available. Although the client may state that he or she is ready to be discharged, this is not the most reliable indicator. (E, 6)

14. 1. The children and their families are at risk for experiencing a crisis. Disaster teams are available for crisis intervention in such emergencies. Usually the news media monitors emergency radio frequencies and most likely are aware of the accident already. Although volunteers may help in some ways, they are not responsible for crisis intervention. Typically, the school would call the parents to inform them of the accident. The school would have the names of the children on that bus and the emergency contact numbers. (P, 6)

15. 4. The statement about joining the son if he dies indicates potential for self-harm and subsequent suicide, always a risk during crisis. Although the father may be charged with reckless driving, this would not be an indication for a psychiatric consultation. Although the son's mother may be extremely upset and angry about the event, this statement is more likely an overstatement, not a real risk. The statement about not seeing the son run behind the car illustrates the father's attempts at trying to process the situation. (E, 6)

16. 1. Passive suicidal thoughts, such as a wish to die or giving up on self-care, can be as much of a risk as active suicidal ideation (the idea of killing one's self directly), especially for older clients, because they often lack the means, energy, and motivation for an active suicide attempt. Not talking to the grandson and experiencing altered role performance may be real issues, but these are not as critical as the risk for indirect (passive) suicide. (D, 6)

17. 2. The threat toward the ex-boyfriend is the most immediate concern now, as the client turns her anger toward him instead of herself. Although Low Self-Esteem, Risk for Suicide, and Impaired Adjustment are accurate, these nursing diagnoses are less of a concern at this moment. (D, 6)

18. 3. Letting the client express his or her feelings (ie, emotion management) is essential before trying to problem-solve about the situation or deciding what kind of referral is appropriate. A referral for counseling, assessment of the client's support system, and unemployment assistance may be appropriate once the client's anxiety is reduced. (P, 6)

19. 2. During a crisis period, support persons demonstrate preparedness to help the client by verbalizing the emergency resources available and knowing when to use them. Follow-up counseling may be helpful as the crisis subsides. The coping strategies used by the support persons for themselves may or may not be relevant for the client's needs and situation. Long-term solutions and advice may or may not be appropriate. The focus needs to be on the client's immediate needs and situation. (E, 6)

20. 1. The nurse needs to focus on the client and address the client's feelings. Talking about her feelings will help decrease the risk of self-harm. Doing so takes precedence over questions about the husband's estate, the cause of death, and her children's support. (I, 6)

The Client With Problems Expressing Anger

21. 3. The nurse must clearly address behavioral expectations, such as telling the client that hitting is unacceptable and also provide alternatives for the client, such as letting staff members know when he begins to feel angry. Making others responsible for the client's behavior or isolating the client in his room is inappropriate because it does not include the client in managing his behavior. Although medication may be helpful, this action does not involve the client in responsibility for his behavior. (I, 2)

22. 4. Verbalizing feelings, especially feelings of anger, in an appropriate manner is an adaptive method of coping that reduces the chance that the client will act out these feelings toward others. The client's ability to verbalize her feelings indicates a change in behavior, a crucial indicator of goal achievement. Although acknowledging the feelings of anger and describing situations that precipitate angry feelings are important in helping the client reach her goal, they are not appropriate indicators that the client has achieved the goal of actually changing her behaviors. Asking the client to list how she has handled anger in the past is helpful if the nurse discusses coping methods with the client. However, based on this client's history, this would not be helpful because the nurse and client are already aware of the client's aggression toward others. (E, 6)

23. 2. Identifying people with whom the client is angry is less important to the overall plan because this action focuses on the other individuals instead of focusing on the client's responsibility for his or her own behavior. Helping the client to recognize anger, identify alternative ways to express anger, and practice the expression of anger are all steps in the process of teaching the client to recognize and respond appropriately to anger. (P, 6)

24. 4. The nurse needs to acknowledge the client's feelings. In doing so, the nurse helps the group accept a new member. Focusing on "everyone" and telling the client not to worry ignores the client's fears. Having the other group members introduce themselves places the focus on the other clients in the group and does not address the client's fears. Implying that getting to know someone will reduce the fear is false reassurance. (I, 6)

25. 1. Both denial of anger with passive, unassertive behavior and the aggressive expression of anger are dysfunctional behavior patterns. The nurse needs to base the response on this concept. Gender-based stereotypes are not conducive to mental health, and deeming assertive behavior in women culturally unacceptable interferes with the goal of developing assertiveness skills. Thinking that the client has distorted what the doctor has said is an unwarranted assumption. Group acceptance should not be based on whether a client is demonstrating assertive or aggressive behavior. (D, 6)

26. 4. The client is in the crisis phase of the assault cycle. Therefore, the nurse must act immediately, using restraints and an intramuscular tranquilizer to prevent injury to others or further property damage. It is too late to ask the client to go to a quiet area to talk because the client's behavior is past the triggering phase. Giving the client an oral tranquilizer and preparing for a show of determination are nursing interventions used in the escalation phase. Processing the incident with the client and discussing alternative behaviors are interventions used in the postcrisis phase. (I, 6)

27. 4. The client is ready to be released from restraints when he or she shows signs of self-control, decreased anxiety and agitation, reality orientation, mood stabilization, increased attention span, and judgment. Adequate sedation, struggling less against restraints, and not swearing and yelling are not adequate signs of being calm and in control. (E, 6)

28. 3. By requesting that the roommate respect his rights (ie, asking the roommate to put the dirty clothes on the floor away after telling him that this bothers him), the client is asserting himself. Arriving late is often passive resistance and thus not an indicator that the client is becoming assertive. Asking the nurse to call is dependent behavior. Although asking the doctor is more assertive, the client is relying on the nurse's direction to do so. (E, 6)

29. 2. Blood pressure, as well as respiratory rate and muscle tension, increase during anger because of the autonomic nervous system response to epinephrine secretion. Peristalsis also decreases. (A, 6)

30. 3. Fear of retaliation is a common response to anger in clients who lack coping skills and assertiveness. Decreased self-esteem is common because most clients are aware that they have difficulty in responding to anger effectively. Although anger may provide an initial feeling of strength and invulnerability, this is rarely a sustained response. Powerlessness more often leads to anger rather than results from it. (A, 6)

31. 4. Haloperidol (Haldol), when given intramuscularly, is considered most restrictive because it is intrusive and client usually does not receive the drug voluntarily. Haloperidol (Haldol), when given orally, is considered less restrictive because the client usually accepts the pill voluntarily. Tension reduction strategies and voluntary seclusion are considered less restrictive because they are not intrusive and the client usually consents voluntarily to their use. (P, 2)

32. 2. Asking the staff for assistance is appropriate when the client demonstrates behaviors that involve the direct threat of violence. Holding a stick and telling the nurse to move is the most direct threat of violence. Swearing and pounding on a table may be disturbing, but these actions are less of a threat. Coming out of his room may indicate noncompliance with directions. However, further assessment would be needed to determine whether this behavior was a direct threat of violence. (A, 6)

33. 1. An orally administered drug is considered less restrictive than one administered intramuscularly. Lorazepam (Ativan), a benzodiazepine, would be administered for its antianxiety and sedative properties. Quetiapine (Seroquel), haloperidol (Haldol), and fluphenazine (Prolixin) are antipsychotic agents and

would not be administered because the client is not psychotic. (P, 6)

34. 3. The client who is about to lose control is experiencing a high degree of anxiety or agitation, which alters the client's ability to perceive reality. Initially, the client is likely to feel threatened by the presence of others. A client who is out of control is not thinking about having an audience. Although the nurse with the client who is about to lose control is generally the one giving directions, this is not a rationale for staying at a distance. When seeing extra staff, the client may or may not be able to gain self-control. (D, 2)

35. 4. The primary goal of aggression management is the prevention of violence. This goal would be evidenced by a reduction in the total number of restraint procedures used or needed. Although fewer client and staff injuries are important, these goals are secondary to prevention. Reduction in the number of complaints by clients' relatives is affected by more variables than just restraint procedures. (E, 2)

36. 1. When using seclusion, the safety of the client is paramount. Therefore, staff must be able to see the client in seclusion at all times, such as through a security window in the door or with a room camera. Although outside access for dimming the lights to decrease stimuli may be appropriate, it is not critical for the client's safety. Having one staff member stay in a room alone with a potentially violent client is unsafe. A doctor's order for seclusion can be obtained before or after it is initiated. (P, 2)

37. 3. A full-length restraint blanket would be added when the client is at risk for injury from fighting the restraints. The increased degree of restriction is justified only when the risk of client injury increases. Feeling more secure is not a sufficient cause for using a more restrictive measure. Client complaints that restraints are tight and uncomfortable require the nurse to assess the situation and adjust the restraints if necessary to ensure adequate circulation. Four-way restraints already provide adequate protection for the staff. (P, 2)

38. 1. Safety of the client and staff is the utmost priority. Therefore, the client must be monitored closely and frequently, such as every 15 minutes, to ensure that the client is safe and free from injury. Assisting with nutrition and elimination, performing range-of-motion exercises on each limb, and changing the client's position every 2 hours are important once the safety of the client and staff is ensured by close, frequent monitoring. (I, 2)

39. 4. The ultimate goal of the debriefing after restraining a client is to improve aggression management procedures so that prevention of aggression improves and the frequency of restraint use decreases. Providing feedback and comparing perceptions are single aspects that would eventually lead to the ultimate goal of improving aggression management procedures. When a client can be released from restraints is not immediately predictable. (I, 6)

40. 1. Being injured by a client can result in emotional responses similar to those of other crime victims. A resignation after being injured is relatively rare. Legal action against the client is sometimes discussed but rarely initiated. Debriefing with the client may be inappropriate or unnecessary for resolution of the situation. (P, 1)

The Client With Family Abuse or Violence

41. 2. The safety of the client and her children is the most immediate concern. If there is immediate danger, action must be taken to protect them. (A, 2)

42. 3. Although impermeable boundaries, unbalanced power ratio, and dysfunctional feeling tone are all common in abusive families, the traditional and rigid gender roles described by the client are examples of role stereotyping. (D, 3)

43. 4. The client's safety, including the need to stay alive, is crucial. Therefore, helping the client develop a safety plan is most important to include in the plan of care to ensure the client's safety. (P, 2)

44. 1. The nurse would be least likely to find assertiveness in the victim. The victim is usually compliant with the spouse and feels guilt, shame, and some responsibility for the battering. Self-blame, substance abuse, and suicidal thoughts and attempts are possible dysfunctional coping methods used by abuse victims. (A, 6)

45. 3. Based on the client's statements, such as "I don't know what to do anymore," the data here best support the nursing diagnosis of Powerlessness related to abusive husband, as evidenced by inability to make decisions. A nursing diagnosis of Risk for Violence would be appropriate if the client had talked about being beaten up the previous night. A nursing diagnosis of Low Self-Esteem would be appropriate if the client verbalized feelings of embarrassment in leaving the house and worthlessness. A nursing diagnosis of Ineffective Coping would be appropriate if the client was crying or talked about crying herself to sleep at night. (D, 6)

46. 2. The nurse needs more information about the client's decision before deciding what intervention is most appropriate. Judgmental responses could make it difficult for the client to return for treatment should she want to do so. Telling the client that this is a bad decision that she will regret is inappropriate because the nurse is making an assumption. Warning the client that abuse often stops when one partner is involved in treatment may be true for some clients. However, until the nurse determines the basis for the client's decision, this type of response is assumption and therefore inappropriate. Reminding the client about her duty to protect the children would be appropriate if the client had talked about episodes of current abuse by her partner and the fear that her children might be hurt by him. (I, 6)

47. 3. The mother's feelings are the priority here. Addressing the mother's feelings and asking for her view of the situation is most important in building a relationship with the family. Ignoring the mother's feelings will hinder the relationship. Defending the school nurse and the school puts the client's mother on the defensive and stifles communication. (I, 6)

48. 1. A caring, supportive relationship among family members is a characteristic of healthy families. Therefore, evidence of such a relationship would provide data to support the decision that the child is no longer at risk for abuse. Children frequently conceal information about the abuse they are enduring. Therefore, not talking about violence during visits to the nurse would not support the nurse's decision. Episodes of abuse, even if infrequent and occurring only during times of stress, indicate family coping problems if the parents do not have a caring and supportive relationship. A strong defensive reaction by parents to appropriate concern expressed by a teacher or other professional and episodes of abuse, even if infrequent, indicates family coping problems. (D, 3)

49. 1. Autonomy involves the sense of control over oneself and one's life. This area is affected by any crime. The others stages listed are less affected. (A, 6)

50. 4. Ultimately, a victim of a crime needs to move from being a "victim" to being a "survivor." A reasonable sense of safety and security is key to this transition. Getting through the shock and confusion, carrying out home and work routines, and resolving grief over any losses represent steps along the way to becoming a survivor. (P, 6)

51. 2. The experience of rape is a crisis situation. Crisis intervention services, especially with a rape crisis nurse, are essential to help the client begin dealing with the aftermath of a rape. Legal assistance may be recommended if the client decides to report the rape and only after crisis intervention services have been provided. A rape support group can be helpful later in the recovery process. Medications for sleep disturbance, especially the benzodiazepines, should be avoided if at all possible. Benzodiazepines are potentially addictive and can be used in suicide attempts, especially when consumed with alcohol. (I, 6)

52. 3. Guilt and self-blame are common feelings that need to be addressed directly and frequently. The client

needs to be reminded periodically that she did not deserve and did not cause the rape. Continually encouraging the client to report the rape pressures the client and is not helpful. In most cases, resuming sexual relations is a difficult process that is not likely to occur quickly. It is not necessarily true that the rapist will be caught, tried, and jailed. Most rapists are not caught or convicted. (I, 6)

53. 4. Use of alcohol reflects unhealthy coping mechanisms. A client's report of needing alcohol to calm down needs to be addressed. Survival is the most important goal during a rape. The client's acknowledging this indicates that she is aware that she made the right choice. Although suicidal thoughts are common, the statement that suicide is an easy escape but the client would be unable to do it indicates low risk. Fantasies of revenge, such as giving the death penalty to all rapists, are natural reactions and are a problem only if the client intends to carry them out directly. (E, 6)

54. 3. Coercion is the most common strategy used because the child commonly trusts the abuser. Tying the child down usually is not necessary. Typically the abusive person can control the child by his or her size and weight alone. Bribery usually is not necessary because the child wants love and affection from the abusive person, not money. Young children are not capable of giving consent for sex before they develop an adult concept of what sex is. (A, 6)

55. 2. Truancy and running away are common symptoms for both young children and adolescents. The stress of the abuse interferes with school success, leading to the avoidance of school. Running away is an effort to escape the abuse and/or lack of support at home. Rather than an inability to play or a lack of play, play is likely to be aggressive with sexual overtones. Children tend to act out anger rather than controlling it. Substance abuse is a behavior more typically seen with adolescents who are abused. (A, 6)

56. 3. Dealing with the physical pain associated with mutilation is viewed as easier than dealing with the intense anger and emotional pain. The client fears an aggressive outburst when anger and emotional pain increase. Self-mutilation seems easier and safer. Additionally, self-mutilation may occur if the client feels unreal or numb or is dissociating. Here, the mutilation proves to the client that he or she is alive and capable of feeling. The client may want to be less sexually attractive, but this aspect usually is not related to self-mutilation. Bingeing and purging is often done in addition to, not instead of, self-mutilation. Although a few clients report an occasional high with self-mutilation, more often the experience is just relief from the anger and rage. (D, 6)

57. 1. The dolls and toys in a play therapy room are useful props to help the child remember situations and reexperience the feelings, acting out the experience with the toys rather than putting the feelings into words. Role-playing without props often is more difficult for a child. Although drawing itself can be therapeutic, having the abuser see the pictures is usually threatening for the child. Reporting abuse to authorities is a difficult and threatening experience for young children. (I, 6)

58. 1. Directly confronting the abuser is likely to result in further harm because the abusers commonly deny the abuse, rationalize about it, or "blame the victim." Using a foam bat while symbolically confronting the abuser, keeping a journal of memories and feelings, and writing letters about the abuse but not sending them are appropriate strategies because they allow anger to be expressed safely. (P, 6)

59. 4. The safety of other children is a primary concern. It is critical to know whether other children are at risk of being sexually abused by the same perpetrator. (A, 6)

60. 3. The statement about functioning OK now but being aware that problems will come up again indicates insight into problems and the desire for sporadic counseling as new problems arise. Disclosing and feeling done with the work is common in early therapy because of the initial emotional release. It does not reflect the ability to work through problems resulting from the abuse. Stating that it is too hard to deal with all this pain suggests a lack of progress and a wish to escape the pain (perhaps by suicide). Client self-evaluation is more important than relying on the perceptions of others. (E, 6)

The Client With Anorexia Nervosa

61. 4. An intense fear of becoming obese, emaciation, and a disturbed body image all are considered to be characteristic of anorexia nervosa. Near-normal weight is not associated with anorexia. The weight of others is not a primary factor. Concern about dieting is not strong enough language to describe the control of food intake in the individual with anorexia nervosa. (I, 4)

62. 1. Anorexia nervosa occurs most often in girls and women, with the age at onset between 12 and 20 years. It rarely begins after 30 years of age. Although anorexia occurs in men, the prevalence rate is less than 5% to 10%. (P, 6)

63. 2. Lanugo, hypothermia, and hypotension are consistent with anorexia nervosa. Primarily what is found is a decrease or slowing down of bodily functions as starvation occurs. The only function that is increased is urination, and that is to rid the body of the extra waste products. Bradycardia, constipation, and amenorrhea also are associated with anorexia. (A, 10)

64. 3. Parents often describe their child as a model child who is a high achiever and compliant. These adolescents are most often well liked by teachers and peers. It is not typical for behavior problems to be reported. The description about having given the child everything and being repaid is more likely to describe an adolescent who is exhibiting behavior problems. (D, 6)

65. 4. The client is in a state of starvation as evidenced by her body weight compared with height. The priority nursing diagnosis is Imbalanced Nutrition: Less Than Body Requirements because the client is in danger of dying or suffering damage to her body as a result of starvation. Low Self-Esteem, Disturbed Body Image, and Interrupted Family Processes are important and relevant, but the priority is the client's state of starvation and need for refeeding. (D, 6)

The Client With Bulimia

66. 3. Encouraging the client to talk about why she is here and her feelings may reveal more information about what led her to come to the group and what led to her diagnosis. It also provides the nurse with valuable information needed to develop an appropriate plan of care. The comment that the client sounds angry presumes what the client is feeling and focuses her talk on her husband. The focus should be on the client, not the husband. Telling the client that she will like coming to group imposes the nurse's view onto the client. The statement also focuses on having fun in the group instead of stressing the therapeutic value. Having the client tell the nurse something about the cause of her bulimia ignores the client's original statement. In addition, it requires the client to have insight into the cause of her disease, which may not be possible at this point. Also, it may be too early in the relationship to discuss this disorder. (I, 6)

67. 2. Because the client eats excessively whenever she is upset, the best nursing diagnosis is Ineffective Coping. There are no data on the family to support Disabled Family Coping. The client's bingeing and purging behavior occurs in response to her difficulty with coping. If the client were only overeating and not purging, then Imbalanced Nutrition: More than Body Requirements would be an appropriate diagnosis. The client does not report nervousness and tension that would lead to a nursing diagnosis of Anxiety. (D, 6)

68. 4. The nurse needs to explore more about the client's feelings to assess what underlies the eating disorder. The nurse also needs to evaluate the client's suicide risk. The other statements are not therapeutic because they minimize the client's feelings. (I, 5)

69. 1. In the United States, food has been equated with love and affection. Parties and family celebrations usu-

ally include food. When someone is upset, food is often offered as comfort. People rarely share food with enemies. Power and control, status and prestige, and survival and growth may at times be associated with food, but these do not have the universality of association that love and affection both have. (I, 7)

Children and Adolescents with Behavior Problems

70. 4. Problems with interpersonal relationships, such as resisting affection and refusing to respond to others, and repetitive behaviors, such as twirling around frequently, are suggestive of autism. Because the parents did not report any tics, Tourette's syndrome is not suggested. Because the parents did not report any psychotic behaviors, such as hallucinations or delusions, schizophrenia can be ruled out. ADHD is most often portrayed as incessant activity with difficulty completing tasks. (D, 4)

71. 4. ADHD is typically managed by psychostimulant medications such as methylphenidate (Ritalin) and pemoline (Cylert) along with behavior modification. Antianxiety medications, such as busiprone (BuSpar), are not appropriate for treating ADHD. Home schooling often is not a possibility because both parents work outside the home. Antidepressants such as imipramine (Tofranil) are not recommended for use in children. Family therapy may be a part of the treatment. Anticonvulsant medications such as carbamazepine (Tegretol) are not appropriate for ADHD. Also, carbamazepine (Tegretol) levels are obtained weekly early during therapy to avoid toxicity and ascertain therapeutic levels. (P, 6)

72. 1. Suggesting that the mother arrange for respite care so that she can have a regular break would help to alleviate some of the stress that she feels when she is with her child constantly. The mother also could use family and friends to provide some care, thereby helping with giving her a break. The child may improve, so suggesting that the mother take a job to provide a feeling of success would be inappropriate. Having coffee daily with friends may provide some opportunities for socialization. However, friends may not be able to provide the verbal support that the mother needs. Rather, attending a support group of other parents with children with ADHD might be helpful. Placing the child in foster care is an extreme measure that may damage the therapeutic relationship with the nurse and dramatically and negatively affect the relationship between the mother and child. (I, 6)

73. 3. Giving away personal items has consistently been shown to be an indicator of suicide plans in a depressed and suicidal individual. Expression of a desire to date, trying out for an extracurricular activity, or the desire to spend more time with friends would indicate a return of interest in normal adolescent activities. (I, 6)

74. 2. Most likely, the client would be diagnosed with conduct disorder. Conduct disorder is characterized by severe problems with behavior, authority, and the law. The individual with a conduct disorder is not concerned with the rights of others, as demonstrated by vandalism and prostitution. With ADHD, the client would demonstrate constant activity and problems with attention. In oppositional defiant disorder, problems with authority may result in behavior problems, but the core of the disorder is defiance to authority not including legal problems such as vandalism and prostitution. Tourette's syndrome is a tic disorder. However, tics were not described with this individual. (D, 6)

75. 1. Tourette's disorder is characterized by both motor and verbal tics. The disorder begins with simple tics, such as finger twitching, and may progress to a complex tic involving movement of the entire arm. There may also be difficulties with obsessions and compulsions. (A, 6)

76. 1. Children are not as likely as adults to display sad behaviors but instead frequently have somatic complaints and acting-out behaviors. Both adults and children can have problems with performance. (A, 6)

77. 2. Adolescents are more likely than children to attempt or commit suicide. Loss, abuse, and family discord remain significant risk factors. There is no evidence to support that children rarely commit suicide. Additionally, evidence fails to support the belief that children who have lost a parent to suicide will attempt it themselves. Significant events, such as a recent firearm purchase, have not been linked to suicide attempts in children. No geographical region in the United States is free from adolescent suicide. (A, 6)

78. 1. Five-year-old children view death as reversible, so talking about seeing her mother again is a normal statement for a child of this age. A child this age would not usually state that she was glad Jesus took her mom but instead might be afraid that Jesus would also take her or her dad. The idea of replacing her mother with a new one, as hinted in the statement that they got another dog after the dog died, has not been supported by studies of grieving children. Stating that mommy went to heaven and that the child will see her someday when the child dies is reflective of more advanced abstract thinking than a 5-year-old would demonstrate. (D, 3)

79. 3. Asperger's disorder is recognized later than autism, and the interpersonal problems worsen with school attendance. These children usually have restricted and

repetitive patterns of behavior. School problems exist as a result of the interaction difficulties and behavior differences. Motor development may be delayed, but language often progresses normally. (P, 6)

80. 3. The nurse manager needs to focus on the frustration that the nurse is expressing. Additionally, the nurse manager needs to correct any misinformation or misinterpretation that the staff nurse has. Saying that the nurse sounds burned out and asking about a vacation does not focus on the nurse's frustration or address the inaccuracy of the nurse's statement. There is no evidence to suggest that children with conduct disorder have more than the average adult's risk of depression or bipolar disorder. Therefore, this response would be inaccurate and inappropriate. Anecdotal information from personal experience does not supply the nurse with accurate, reliable information. (I, 1)

81. 2. The nurse needs to find out what exactly the mother knows and has read. Reviewing what the mother has found in her reading that is leading her to doubt the diagnosis will help direct the nurse's teaching and clarify any misperceptions or misinformation that the mother may have. The doctor may indeed have many years of education and experience, and the focus should be on the daughter, but the nurse needs to address the mother's concerns at this time. (I, 5)

82. 1. The statement that ADHD occurring more often in families and suggesting of a genetic concern takes the opportunity for teaching while also helping the father realize that he and his wife are not to blame. Parents, who often are blamed by society, need help with education. Questioning the father on what he thinks he may have done implies that the parents played some role in this disorder, possibly contributing to the father's guilt. Telling the father that many parents feel this way or that he should focus on what needs to be done rather than what caused the disorder minimizes the father's concerns and feelings. (I, 6)

83. 3. Focusing on the purpose of the group is the best response. Adolescents are greatly influenced by their peers. Medication alone is not typically the most successful treatment strategy. Questioning whether the client will continue the medication is negative and is not the reason for her to stay in the group. Asking the rest of the group to respond may or may not give the nurse support for the teenager remaining in the group. Groups often have rules regarding movement of members in and out of the group, but this does not address the reasons for the client to remain in the group. (I, 6)

84. 4. Asking whether the client is thinking about killing himself is the most direct and therefore the best way to assess suicidal risk. Knowing whether the client has watched movies on suicide and death, what the client thinks about suicide, and whether other family members have committed suicide will not tell the nurse whether the client is thinking about committing suicide right now. (A, 6)

85. 1. The teacher needs to be informed that this behavior is inappropriate. Therefore, educating the teacher and encouraging her to respond to misbehavior consistently is correct. Telling the teacher that the nurse can't believe the teacher lets the child get away with the behavior is demeaning and condescending. Allowing the child to continue the misbehavior is counterproductive to discipline and could create other problems. (I, 6)

86. 4. Drugs such as clonidine, haloperidol, and pimozide are currently being used for treatment of tic disorders. Risperidone (Risperdal) has also been used in clinical trials, with good results. Chlorpromazine is an antipsychotic, imipramine is an antidepressant, and lithium is used for the management of mania and bipolar disorder. (P, 8)

87. 2. Consistent discipline and alternative methods of anger management are two important tools for parents who have a child with oppositional defiant disorder. Consistent discipline sets limits for the child. Helping the child learn more appropriate ways to manage anger assists the child in living within societal expectations. Avoiding restriction of television and computer time for punishment or using time-out as the primary means of punishment has not been suggested as an appropriate management method. Using a variety of strategies often is more effective. Ignoring bad behavior could be dangerous and does not reinforce to the child that limits on behavior do exist in society. (I, 6)

88. 4. Children who experience serious losses, especially multiple losses, such as old friends or a parent, are more at risk for depression. Girls also are at greater risk than boys during the adolescent years. (D, 4)

89. 3. Asking the client to report everything that she has had to eat and drink yesterday and today is the least judgmental approach and also provides helpful information. Confronting the client about drinking alcohol or asking the client to admit the real reason for feeling sick can put the girl on the defensive and block any further communication. The nurse should avoiding putting the client on the defensive, to facilitate communication that may eventually enable the nurse to get the truth and identify interventions. (I, 6)

90. 3. By telling the mother that the coach is a nurse and relaying the behaviors observed, the nurse gives the mother a chance to recognize the expertise of the coach and introduces the possibility of an eating disorder.

Thanking the mother and complimenting the player doesn't begin to approach the topic. Telling the mother that the nurse has some very bad news is negative and dramatic. Additionally, although the observed behaviors suggest an eating disorder, it would be inappropriate for the nurse to medically diagnose the daughter. Although the daughter may indeed be very sick and need to see a therapist, the nurse should relate the information in a matter-of-fact, nonemotional way. (I, 6)

91. 2. Studies show that usually one third to one half of people diagnosed with ADHD do not need medication as adults. (I, 6)

92. 1. The client is stating that he is stupid like his classmates believe. ADD often causes problems in school, which can lead to problems with self-esteem. Ineffective Coping would be manifested by the client's hitting a peer who laughs at him. Interrupted Family Processes would be evidenced by the parents' not being able to help their son cope or by their own inability to cope with their son and his disorder. Anxiety would be associated with the client's reporting tense or nervous feelings. (D, 6)

93. 3. The single-dose form of methylphenidate (Ritalin) should be taken 10 to 14 hours before bedtime to prevent problems with insomnia, which can occur when the daily or last dose of the medication is taken within 6 hours (for multiple dosing) or 10 to 14 hours (for single dosing) before bedtime. It is recommended that a missed dose be taken as soon as possible; the dose is skipped if it is not remembered until the next dose is due. Any other medication, including over-the-counter medications, should be discussed with the health care provider before use to eliminate the risk of a possible untoward effect. (P, 8)

94. 4. The child's refusal to sit in class, insistence on calling her mother when she isn't ill, fear that something bad is going to happen to her mother, and physical appearance of anxiety best fit separation anxiety disorder. Children with separation anxiety disorder display these types of behaviors for a month or longer. Obsessive-compulsive disorder would be manifested by ritualistic, repetitive behaviors that are excessive and interfere with normal activities. Major depression in children is evidenced by sadness or acting-out behaviors. ADD would be manifested by failure to complete tasks, inability to pay attention during class, and easy distractibility. (A, 6)

95. 4. Indifference to other people and mutism may be indicators of autism and would require further investigation. A 2-year-old who talks to himself and refuses to cooperate with toilet training is displaying behaviors typical for this age. Occasional thumb sucking and not having spent the night with a friend would be normal at age 6. Threats to run away when angry would be considered within the range of normal behaviors for a 10-year-old child. (D, 3)

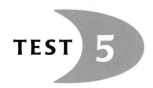
General Client Needs

▶ Pharmacologic and Parenteral Therapies

▶ Management of Care

▶ The Client With Stress, Coping, and Adaptation Issues

▶ The Client Coping With Chronic Illness

▶ The Client Coping With End-of-Life Issues

▶ Correct Answers and Rationale

Select the one best answer, and indicate your choice by filling in the circle in front of the option.

Pharmacologic and Parenteral Therapies

1. Which of the following medications would the nurse expect to administer to a client who is experiencing an oculogyric crisis?
   ○ 1. Chlorpromazine (Thorazine) 50 mg.
   ○ 2. Procyclidine (Kemadrin) 5 mg.
   ○ 3. Thioridazine (Mellaril) 100 mg.
   ○ 4. Benztropine (Cogentin) 1 mg.

2. Which of the following would the nurse include when teaching the family and a client prescribed benztropine (Cogentin), 1 mg PO twice daily, about the drug therapy?
   ○ 1. The drug can be used with over-the-counter cough and cold preparations.
   ○ 2. The client should not discontinue taking the drug abruptly.
   ○ 3. Antacids can be used freely when taking this drug.
   ○ 4. Alcohol consumption with benztropine therapy need not be restricted.

3. Which of the following would the nurse include in a teaching plan that addresses the side effects of antipsychotic medication?
   ○ 1. Information about all potential side effects.
   ○ 2. Research data about rare side effects.
   ○ 3. Side effects that can be seen or felt.
   ○ 4. Percentages associated with each side effect.

4. Clozapine (Clozaril) therapy has been initiated for a client with schizophrenia who has been unresponsive to other antipsychotics. The client states, "Why do I have to have a blood test every week?" Which of the following responses by the nurse would be *most* appropriate?
   ○ 1. "Weekly blood tests are necessary to determine safe dosage and to monitor the effect of the medication on the blood."
   ○ 2. "Weekly blood tests are done so that you can receive another week's supply of the medication."
   ○ 3. "Your physician will want to know how well you are progressing with the medication therapy."
   ○ 4. "Everyone taking clozapine (Clozaril) has to go through the same procedure because it is required by the drug company."

5. The mother of a 28-year-old client who is taking clozapine (Clozaril) states, "Something is wrong. My son is drooling like a baby." Which of the following responses by the nurse would be *most* helpful?
   ○ 1. "I wonder if he's having an adverse reaction to the medicine."
   ○ 2. "Excess saliva is common with this drug; here's a paper cup for him to spit into."
   ○ 3. "Don't worry about it; this is only a minor inconvenience compared to its benefits."
   ○ 4. "I've seen this happen to other clients who are taking clozapine (Clozaril)."

6. A client taking clozapine (Clozaril) states, "I think I'm getting the flu. I have a fever and feel weak." Which of the following would the nurse do *next*?
   ○ 1. Tell the client to wait another day to see if other symptoms of the flu appear.
   ○ 2. Advise the client to take some over-the-counter medication for the flu.
   ○ 3. Discuss the importance of maintaining an adequate fluid intake.
   ○ 4. Report the client's symptoms to the physician after taking the client's temperature.

7. A client taking clozapine (Clozaril) states, "I don't like feeling so sedated during the day. I can hardly keep my eyes open." Which of the following responses by the nurse would be *most* appropriate?

633

○ 1. "Try waking up an hour earlier to see if that helps."

○ 2. "Sleep as long as you need to and nap fairly often."

○ 3. "Let's talk to the doctor about taking most of the drug at bedtime."

○ 4. "Going to bed earlier at night might help."

8. Assessment for which of the following side effects would be the *priority* for a client who is taking risperidone (Risperdal) 1 mg PO twice daily?

○ 1. Insomnia.

○ 2. Headache.

○ 3. Anxiety.

○ 4. Orthostatic hypotension.

9. A client taking risperidone (Risperdal) 2 mg PO twice daily informs the clinic nurse that she will be getting married in 3 months to another client she met at the outpatient clinic. During the client interview, which of the following would be an area of priority concern?

○ 1. Her fiancé's medication compliance.

○ 2. Money management.

○ 3. The possibility of or plan for pregnancy.

○ 4. Living arrangements.

10. A client whose symptoms of schizophrenia are under control with olanzapine (Zyprexa), and who is functioning at home and in her part-time employment, states that she is very concerned about her 20-pound weight gain since she started taking the medication 6 months ago. Which of the following responses by the nurse would be *most* appropriate?

○ 1. Suggest that the client talk with her physician about changing to another antipsychotic.

○ 2. Advise the client to decrease her dosage by one half.

○ 3. Tell the client not to worry because she should stop gaining weight.

○ 4. Discuss nutrition, daily diet, and exercise with the client.

11. The wife of a 67-year-old client who has been taking imipramine (Tofranil) for 3 days asks the nurse why her husband isn't better. Which of the following responses by the nurse would be accurate?

○ 1. "It takes 2 to 4 weeks before the full therapeutic effects are experienced."

○ 2. "Your husband may need an increase in dosage."

○ 3. "A different antidepressant may be necessary."

○ 4. "It can take 6 weeks to see if the medication will help your husband."

12. A 67-year-old client will be discharged to home with imipramine (Tofranil). Which of the following would be *most* important to include when instructing the client and spouse about the medication?

○ 1. Eat a high-fiber diet.

○ 2. Wear sunglasses outdoors.

○ 3. Avoid the ingestion of alcohol.

○ 4. Urinate as soon as the urge is felt.

13. A client has been taking phenelzine (Nardil) for atypical depression. The physician is discontinuing the phenelzine and initiating therapy with fluoxetine (Prozac). When preparing to carry out this order, the nurse would expect to do which of the following?

○ 1. Wait 14 days after stopping the phenelzine before starting the fluoxetine.

○ 2. Stop the phenelzine and then wait 5 weeks before starting fluoxetine.

○ 3. Start the fluoxetine 1 day after stopping therapy with the phenelzine.

○ 4. Taper the client gradually off the phenelzine while beginning therapy with fluoxetine.

14. The nurse is teaching a client and family about phenelzine (Nardil). Which of the following foods would the nurse urge the client to avoid?

○ 1. Eggs.

○ 2. Chicken.

○ 3. American cheese.

○ 4. Sour cream.

15. When preparing the drug teaching plan for a client who is taking phenelzine (Nardil), which of the following signs and symptoms would the nurse stress as *most* important to report to the physician immediately?

○ 1. Urinary hesitancy.

○ 2. Palpitations.

○ 3. Dry mouth.

○ 4. Blurred vision.

16. A client who is taking lithium carbonate complains of nausea, dry mouth, and thirst. Which of the following responses by the nurse would be *most* appropriate?

○ 1. "We need to check the level of lithium in your blood."

○ 2. "These common side effects of lithium will go away after 6 weeks."

○ 3. "Your symptoms really are no cause for concern."

○ 4. "I'll hold off on giving you your lithium until you feel better."

17. After teaching a client and family about lithium therapy, which of the following client statements indicates the need for further teaching?

○ 1. "I need to eliminate salt in my diet."

○ 2. "I should drink 10 to 12 glasses of water daily."

○ 3. "I should avoid driving until I'm stabilized."

○ 4. "I'll report any vomiting, diarrhea, blurred vision, or weakness."

18. A 60-year-old client has a maintenance lithium level of 0.6 mEq/L. Which of the following would the

nurse expect the client to exhibit?
- O 1. Signs and symptoms of lithium toxicity.
- O 2. Manifestations of acute mania.
- O 3. A decrease in manic symptoms.
- O 4. Fairly good control of symptoms of mania.

19. A client's wife states, "I don't think lithium is helping my husband. He's been taking it for 2 days now and he's still so hyper and thinks we're rich." Which of the following responses by the nurse would be *most* accurate?
- O 1. "Because his symptoms are very acute, more time is needed."
- O 2. "I'll be sure to pass on your concern about your husband to the doctor."
- O 3. "It takes 1 to 2 weeks for the drug to build up in the blood to be effective."
- O 4. "Your husband may need to have his dosage increased."

20. A client taking lithium states, "Why can't I double the next dose of lithium if I forget a dose?" Which of the following responses by the nurse would be *most* therapeutic?
- O 1. "Doubling a dose of lithium can lead to lithium toxicity."
- O 2. "It all depends how you are feeling at the time."
- O 3. "You'll need to ask your physician about that."
- O 4. "You weren't listening to what I just explained."

Management of Care

21. Which of the following would the nurse judge to be the *primary* goal of milieu management?
- O 1. Facilitation of clients' growth, rehabilitation, and health restoration.
- O 2. Successful achievement of the needs of staff members.
- O 3. Provision of a sanctuary for helpless clients.
- O 4. Implementation of physicians' orders.

22. A client asks the nurse for medication because she is feeling nervous. With a therapeutic milieu, which of the following would the nurse do *initially*?
- O 1. Talk with the client about her feelings.
- O 2. Suggest that the client play a game with another client.
- O 3. Advise the client to lie down in his room until she feels better.
- O 4. Administer lorazepam (Ativan) 1 mg PO as ordered PRN.

23. A client is playing the stereo loudly in the music room, and other clients are complaining about the volume. Which of the following would the nurse do?

- O 1. Prohibit the use of the stereo for the rest of the day.
- O 2. State to the client what volume is and is not permissible.
- O 3. Turn down the volume and say nothing.
- O 4. Tell the other clients that the time to use the music room is almost over.

24. A 15-year-old male client on the unit shows signs of mild intoxication. When questioned, he states that another client gave him beer, and he refuses to name the client. Which of the following would the nurse do *next*?
- O 1. Telephone the client's parents.
- O 2. Call a community meeting.
- O 3. Urge the client to tell who gave him the beer.
- O 4. Call the physician.

25. When conducting a psychoeducational group session on relapse prevention for clients dually diagnosed with chronic schizophrenia and alcohol abuse or dependency, the nurse would use which of the following approaches?
- O 1. Strong confrontation techniques.
- O 2. A nondirective leadership style.
- O 3. Concrete concepts and simplified material.
- O 4. An unstructured format.

26. One of the clients in group, with a dual diagnosis of chronic schizophrenia and alcohol abuse, states, "I'm not going to take medicine every day." Which of the following responses by the nurse would be *most* appropriate?
- O 1. "Your doctor wants you to take your medication everyday."
- O 2. "Would anyone in group like to discuss this?"
- O 3. "Let's discuss this tomorrow if we have time."
- O 4. "I hear you say that you don't like taking medication daily."

27. The nurse meets with a client in the outpatient clinic who is suicidal and refuses to sign a "no suicide" contract. Which of the following would the nurse do *next*?
- O 1. Arrange for the client to be sent back to the group home.
- O 2. Refer the client to a partial program until the client is no longer suicidal.
- O 3. Arrange for immediate hospitalization on a psychiatric intensive care unit.
- O 4. Arrange for admission to a subacute unit for 2 weeks.

28. The nurse is teaching a group of unlicensed personnel new to psychiatry about balance in a therapeutic milieu. Which of the following statements by a member of the group indicates the need for further teaching?
- O 1. "Balance includes safe and effective treatment for all clients."

○ 2. "Controlling clients helps them feel more comfortable."

○ 3. "We don't fix clients but help them solve their problems."

○ 4. "We need to think of "patients' rights" when working with clients."

29. Two nursing assistants are arguing about which person is responsible for taking the dirty linen bags into the utility room. One nursing assistant approaches the charge nurse and complains about the other. Which of the following actions would the nurse employ?

○ 1. Advise the nursing assistant to be more tolerant of his coworker.

○ 2. Tell the nursing assistant to take care of the linen bags himself.

○ 3. Urge the nursing assistant to discuss the problem with his coworker.

○ 4. Take care of the linen bags to avoid further conflict.

30. The nurse is leading a group about mood disorders. A client in the group is monopolizing the session to the extent that other clients can hardly participate. The nurse would intervene by saying which of the following?

○ 1. "Mrs. Roberts, you've been taking up too much of the group's time. Let's move on."

○ 2. "Mrs. Roberts, you seem to have quite a lot to say today."

○ 3. "Mrs. Roberts, you've done well today, but I'd like to hear from the others."

○ 4. "Mrs. Roberts, it certainly isn't hard for you to talk in group."

31. The nurse is leading an outpatient clinic group composed of clients with chronic schizophrenia. Which of the following statements by the nurse would *most* likely lead to decreased mistrust and anxiety among the members?

○ 1. "It's difficult to talk in group, but I believe everyone here has something to share that can help someone else."

○ 2. "Several of you have been in group before, so you can help out some of the new members."

○ 3. "Let's start by introducing ourselves and sharing one accomplishment since yesterday."

○ 4. "Who can tell me the purpose of our group, what our rules are, and what we do in group?"

32. When working with a client who has a mental illness and her family, which of the following approaches by the nurse would be *best*?

○ 1. Forming an alliance with the client.

○ 2. Helping the client to conform to the family's wishes.

○ 3. Advising each family member on how to deal with the client.

○ 4. Conveying warmth and acceptance to each family member.

33. The nurse would integrate which of the following principles when a client's mental status interferes with his ability to participate in milieu activities?

○ 1. Norms.

○ 2. Structure.

○ 3. Balance.

○ 4. Schedule modification.

34. Which of the following would be an environmental cue that the nurse would use to assist a cognitively impaired client with dementia?

○ 1. Verbal reminders about mealtime.

○ 2. Introduction of self on entering the client's room.

○ 3. Client's name on the bedroom door.

○ 4. Locked doors to the unit.

35. A client is being discharged from the inpatient unit but needs further continuous supervision that is less intense than inpatient hospitalization. The nurse would expect to refer the client to which of the following settings?

○ 1. Partial program.

○ 2. Subacute unit.

○ 3. Daily outpatient visits.

○ 4. Group home.

The Client With Stress, Coping, and Adaptation Issues

36. After teaching a group of nursing students about the neurochemical changes that help facilitate rapid behavioral responses to dangerous situations, which of the following, if stated by the group as important for facilitating rapid responses, indicates effective teaching?

○ 1. Increase in release of endogenous opiates.

○ 2. Increase in noradrenergic and dopaminergic system activity.

○ 3. Decrease in peripheral sympathetic system activity.

○ 4. Decrease in glucocorticoid levels.

37. The experience of anxiety occurs in degrees, from a level that stimulates productive problem solving to a level that is severely debilitating. At a mild, productive level of anxiety, the nurse would expect to see which of the following as a cognitive characteristic of mild anxiety?

○ 1. Slight muscle tension.

○ 2. Occasional irritability.

○ 3. Accurate perceptions.

○ 4. Loss of contact with reality.

38. As a client's level of anxiety increases to a debilitating degree, the nurse would expect which of the fol-

lowing as a psychomotor behavior indicating a panic level of anxiety?
- ○ 1. Suicide attempts or violence.
- ○ 2. Desperation and rage.
- ○ 3. Disorganized reasoning.
- ○ 4. Loss of contact with reality.

39. Nursing interventions with an anxious client change as the anxiety level increases. At a low level of anxiety, the primary focus of interventions is on which of the following?
- ○ 1. Taking control of the situation for the client.
- ○ 2. Learning and problem solving.
- ○ 3. Reducing stimuli and pressure.
- ○ 4. Using tension reduction activities.

40. When coping becomes dysfunctional enough to require the client to be admitted to the hospital, the nurse would expect the client to demonstrate which of the following?
- ○ 1. Objective and rational problem solving.
- ○ 2. Tension reduction activities then some problem solving.
- ○ 3. Anger management strategies with no problem solving.
- ○ 4. Minimal functioning with new problems developing.

41. In addition to teaching assertiveness and problem-solving skills when helping clients to cope effectively with stress and anxiety, which of the following would the nurse also expect to address?
- ○ 1. Suppressing anger.
- ○ 2. Balancing a checkbook.
- ○ 3. Following step-by-step directions.
- ○ 4. Using conflict resolution skills.

42. Which of the following client statements would indicate to the nurse that the client has coped effectively with a relationship problem?
- ○ 1. "My wife will be happy to know that I can spend less time at work now."
- ○ 2. "My wife and I are talking about our likes and dislikes in activities."
- ○ 3. "I can understand how my wife and I see things differently."
- ○ 4. "We are really listening to each other about our different view on issues."

43. In an ongoing assessment, the nurse would identify the client's thoughts and feelings about a situation in addition to which of the following?
- ○ 1. Whether the client's behavior is appropriate in the context of the current situation.
- ○ 2. Whether the client is motivated to decrease dysfunctional behaviors.
- ○ 3. Which of the client's problems have the highest priority.
- ○ 4. Which of the client's behaviors necessitates a "no harm" contract.

44. When developing appropriate short-term goals with clients who are inpatients, which of the following would be the *most* realistic?
- ○ 1. The client will demonstrate a positive self-image.
- ○ 2. The client will describe plans for how to get back into school.
- ○ 3. The client will write a list of strengths and abilities.
- ○ 4. The client will practice assertive skills in a dating situation.

45. When acting in the role of educator and facilitator, the nurse would plan interventions aimed ultimately at which of the following?
- ○ 1. Use of standardized care plans for more efficient client outcome achievement.
- ○ 2. Medication effect and side effect monitoring.
- ○ 3. Medication and treatment compliance by clients.
- ○ 4. Clients learning to solve problems for themselves.

46. When integrating the concepts underlying the cognitive-behavioral model into a client's plan of care, the nurse would expect to focus on which of the following areas?
- ○ 1. Substitution of rational beliefs for self-defeating thinking and behaving.
- ○ 2. Insight into unconscious conflicts and processes.
- ○ 3. Analysis of fears and barriers to growth.
- ○ 4. Reduction of bodily tensions and stress management.

47. Which of the following client statements indicates that a client has gained insight into his use of the defense mechanism of displacement?
- ○ 1. "I can't think about the weekend right now. I've got to study for the exam."
- ○ 2. "I know I'm not very good in sports, but I feel good about my grades."
- ○ 3. "Now when I'm mad at my wife, I talk to her instead of taking it out on the kids."
- ○ 4. "For years I couldn't remember being molested; now I know I have to face it."

48. According to Erikson's developmental model, which of the following interventions would be helpful for a client experiencing a problem with identity versus role confusion?
- ○ 1. Asking for a list of goals related to family and career.
- ○ 2. Discussing productive ways to achieve societal responsibilities.
- ○ 3. Discussing appropriate versus inappropriate social behaviors.
- ○ 4. Asking for a list of benefits and risks for committing in a relationship.

49. When clients are involuntarily committed to a hospital because they are assessed as being dangerous to self or others, which of the following rights is lost?
    ○ 1. The right to refuse medications and treatments.
    ○ 2. The right to send and receive uncensored mail.
    ○ 3. Freedom from seclusion and restraints.
    ○ 4. The right to leave the hospital against medical advice (AMA).

50. In which of the following situations can a client's confidentiality be breached?
    ○ 1. In answer to a request from a client's spouse about the client's medication.
    ○ 2. In a student nurse's clinical paper about a client.
    ○ 3. When a client near discharge is threatening to harm an ex-partner.
    ○ 4. When a client's employer requests the client's diagnosis to initiate medical claims.

51. A client who has not left the bus station for 3 days is brought to the mental health center by a police officer because she had been bothering other people. She denies this, will not give her name, holds tightly to her purse, and refuses to talk to anyone except to say, "You have no right to keep me here. I have money, and I can take care of myself." The police can hold her for disturbing the peace but think she needs psychiatric evaluation. The nurse informs the staff members that the physician is discharging the client because involuntary commitment is not indicated. Another nurse states, "How can her physician be so cruel? She should stay in the hospital instead of the bus station." Which of the following responses would be best for the nurse to make to the peer?
    ○ 1. "I agree with you wholeheartedly. She does have symptoms of mental illness."
    ○ 2. "Although she may have a mental illness, she is not gravely disabled or dangerous to herself or others."
    ○ 3. "The client wants to leave, so the physician is not going to put her through the commitment process."
    ○ 4. "The client has a home to go to and family to support her. She doesn't need to be here."

52. Which of the following is a crucial goal of therapeutic communication when helping clients deal with personal issues and painful feelings?
    ○ 1. Communicating empathy through maintaining gentle touching of the client.
    ○ 2. Conveying client respect and acceptance even if not all of the client's behaviors are tolerated.
    ○ 3. Mutual sharing of information, spontaneity, emotions, and intimacy.
    ○ 4. Guaranteeing total confidentiality and anonymity for the client.

53. Which of the following questions or statements would be appropriate for the nurse to use when planning care?
    ○ 1. "It sounds as if you feeling abandoned by your family."
    ○ 2. "How important is it for you to change this behavior?"
    ○ 3. "Tell me what you want to say to your husband this evening."
    ○ 4. "Which of these two options do you want to try first?"

54. Which of the following questions or statements would the nurse use to encourage client evaluation?
    ○ 1. "I can hear that it is still hard for you to talk about this."
    ○ 2. "So what does this all mean to you now?"
    ○ 3. "What did you do differently with your coworker this time?"
    ○ 4. "What will it take to carry out your new plans?"

55. With shorter lengths of stay in the hospital, a more practical view of the stages of the nurse-client relationship as originally proposed by H. Peplau addresses which of the following?
    ○ 1. The phases involve emphasizing different processes and goals.
    ○ 2. Building of trust is the most that can be accomplished.
    ○ 3. What can be achieved is problem identification and referrals.
    ○ 4. Teaching of new skills becomes most important.

56. Even when the client understands her problems and is motivated to change, she may have fears about failing. Which of the following interventions is most likely to facilitate change?
    ○ 1. Reality testing about the need for change.
    ○ 2. Asking the client about fears that need to be overcome.
    ○ 3. Teaching new communication skills.
    ○ 4. Practicing new behaviors with the nurse.

The Client Coping With Chronic Illness

57. The nurse has been asked to develop a medication education program for clients with chronic mental illness in the rehabilitation program. When developing the course outline, which of the following topics would be *most* important to include?
    ○ 1. A categorization of a wide variety of psychotropic drugs.
    ○ 2. Interventions for common side effects of psychotropic drugs.
    ○ 3. The role of medication in the treatment of acute illness.

○ 4. Effects of combining common street drugs with psychotropic medication.

58. The physician recommends that a client have a partial bowel resection and an ileostomy. Later, the client says to the nurse, "That doctor of mine surely likes to play big. I'll bet the more he can cut, the better he likes it." Which of the following replies by the nurse would be *most* therapeutic?
   ○ 1. "I can tell you more about the surgery if you would like."
   ○ 2. "What do you mean by that statement?"
   ○ 3. "Aren't you being a bit hard on him? He's trying to help you."
   ○ 4. "Does that remark have something to do with the operation he wants you to have?"

59. A client becomes increasingly morose and irritable after being told that she has cancer. She is rude to visitors and pushes nurses away when they attempt to give her medications and treatments. Which of the following would the nurse do when the client has a hostile outburst?
   ○ 1. Offer the client positive reinforcement each time she cooperates.
   ○ 2. Encourage the client to discuss her immediate concerns and feelings.
   ○ 3. Continue with the assigned tasks and duties as though nothing has happened.
   ○ 4. Encourage the client to direct her anger at staff members instead of her visitors.

60. Arrangements are made for a member of the colostomy club to meet with a client before bowel surgery. Which of the following is accomplished by having a representative from the club visit the client preoperatively?
   ○ 1. Letting the client know that he has resources in the community to help him.
   ○ 2. Providing support for the physician's plan of therapy for the client.
   ○ 3. Providing the client with support and realistic information on the colostomy.
   ○ 4. Convincing the client that he will not be disfigured and can lead a full life.

61. A client who was transferred to the medical unit from intensive care after suffering a myocardial infarction 3 days ago states, "My secretary should be here by now. I don't have time to lie around here and do nothing. I've never had time to relax, and I don't plan on starting now." Based on this initial information, which of the following nursing diagnoses would the nurse judge to be of *least* importance?
   ○ 1. Ineffective Coping related to serious illness, as evidenced by the statement about lying around and doing nothing.
   ○ 2. Deficient Knowledge related to cardiac rehabilitation, as evidenced by client's statement

about not planning to relax at present.
   ○ 3. Hopelessness related to serious illness, as evidenced by the client's turning over her work to her secretary.
   ○ 4. Anxiety related to delayed arrival of the client's secretary, as evidenced by the client's statement of expecting that the secretary should already have arrived.

62. The client with atrial fibrillation states to the nurse, "Please hand me the telephone. I need to check on my stocks and bonds." Which of the following responses by the nurse would be *most* therapeutic?
   ○ 1. "You will get more upset if you make that call."
   ○ 2. "You have atrial fibrillations. Let's talk about what that means."
   ○ 3. "You really don't care about the fact that you're sick, do you?"
   ○ 4. "Do you realize you have a life-threatening condition?"

63. The nurse would determine that a client lacks understanding of her acute cardiac illness and the ability to make changes in her lifestyle by which of the following statements?
   ○ 1. "I already have my airline ticket so I won't miss my meeting tomorrow."
   ○ 2. "These relaxation tapes sound okay; I'll see if they help me."
   ○ 3. "No more working 10 hours a day for me unless it's an emergency situation."
   ○ 4. "I talked with my husband yesterday about working on a new budget together."

64. The client with kidney stones refuses to eat lunch and rudely tells the nurse to get out of his room. Which of the following responses by the nurse would be *most* appropriate?
   ○ 1. "I'll leave, but you need to eat."
   ○ 2. "I'll get you something for your pain."
   ○ 3. "Your anger doesn't bother me. I'll be back later."
   ○ 4. "You sound angry. What is upsetting you?"

65. Certain personality traits are often attributed to clients with ulcerative colitis. Based on this theory, which of the following traits would the nurse expect to see in a client with this disorder?
   ○ 1. Self-reliance.
   ○ 2. Decisiveness.
   ○ 3. Perfectionism.
   ○ 4. Ambitiousness.

66. One day, a client receiving dialysis directs a stream of profanities at the nurse, then abruptly hangs his head and pleads, "Please forgive me. Something just came over me. Why do I say those things?" The nurse interprets this as which of the following?
   ○ 1. Punning.
   ○ 2. Confabulation.

○ 3. Flight of ideas.
○ 4. Emotional lability.

The Client Coping With End-of-Life Issues

67. A client who is dying of acquired immunodeficiency syndrome (AIDS) is admitted to the inpatient psychiatric unit because he attempted suicide. His close friend recently died of AIDS. The client begins to talk about his feelings related to his illness and the loss of his friend. He begins to cry. Which of the following responses by the nurse would be *most* appropriate?
    ○ 1. Give the client some tissues and tell him it is okay to cry.
    ○ 2. Tell the client to stop crying and that everything will be okay.
    ○ 3. Sort the client's mail to distract the client.
    ○ 4. Change the subject.

68. A terminally ill client's husband tells the nurse, "I wish we had taken that trip to Europe last year. We just kept putting it off, and now I'm furious that we didn't go." The nurse interprets the husband's statement as indicating which of the following stages of adaptation to dying?
    ○ 1. Anger.
    ○ 2. Denial.
    ○ 3. Bargaining.
    ○ 4. Depression.

69. The nurse who usually is most effective when caring for a dying client and helping the family deal with death is one who has participated in which of the following activities?
    ○ 1. Contemplating his or her own death and mortality.
    ○ 2. Attending continuing education classes on death and dying.
    ○ 3. Providing compassionate and physical care while remaining distant emotionally.
    ○ 4. Viewing dying people as distinct populations of people in need of comfort.

70. Which of the following philosophies would the nurse most likely integrate into the plan of care for a client and family to help them best cope during the final stages of the client's illness?
    ○ 1. Living each day as it comes as fully as possible.
    ○ 2. Reliving the pleasant memories of days gone by.
    ○ 3. Expecting the worst and being grateful when it does not happen.
    ○ 4. Planning ahead for the remaining good times that will be spent together.

71. A 13-year-old boy admitted to the hospital for the third time is diagnosed as having acute lymphatic leukemia. The liaison psychiatric nurse is asked by the team leader to help the nursing staff work more effectively with this terminally ill child and his family. One of the nurses says to the liaison nurse, "Whenever I go to the client's room, I feel that I have to smile and act happy even though I want to cry when I see him." Which of the following responses by the liaison nurse would be *most* appropriate?
    ○ 1. "Call me when you feel that way. We can talk it over at the time."
    ○ 2. "Try not to show emotion, such as crying. You'll upset the client."
    ○ 3. "Keep smiling. The client and his parents need all the support they can get."
    ○ 4. "Tell the client you feel bad because he is ill and cry, too, if it seems appropriate."

72. A client is increasingly prone to outbursts concerning her chemotherapy treatments. Which of the following approaches by the nurse would likely be most helpful in gaining his cooperation?
    ○ 1. Telling the client how the treatment can be expected to help her each time.
    ○ 2. Describing the probable effect on her body that missing a treatment would have.
    ○ 3. Asking her to be "a good patient" and not make the treatment any harder for herself.
    ○ 4. Promising to give her a backrub if she does not make a fuss about the treatment.

73. A 10-year-old client suspects that he will not live. However, others talk about only pleasant matters with him and maintain a persistently cheerful facade around him. The nurse anticipates that the client will most likely feel which of the following as a result of such behavior?
    ○ 1. Relief.
    ○ 2. Isolation.
    ○ 3. Hopefulness.
    ○ 4. Independence.

74. The young sister of a client with leukemia asks, "Can you check my blood? When my sister got the measles, so did I. And I think I have this, too." Which of the following by the nurse would be *inappropriate*?
    ○ 1. Asking the client's physician to take a sample of the sister's blood.
    ○ 2. Explaining to the sister that leukemia is not a communicable disease.
    ○ 3. Discussing the sister's concern with her parents.
    ○ 4. Telling the sister's parents about a group for siblings of clients with terminal illness.

75. When talking with the nurse, the 15-year-old brother of a client with leukemia says, "We used to play pretty rough games together. Maybe some of the bruises he got when I tackled him caused this."

Which of the following would be the nurse's *best* response?

○ 1. "Don't feel guilty. You didn't cause your brother's illness."

○ 2. "I can see you're worried. Let's talk about how people get leukemia."

○ 3. "Here is some information about leukemia for you to read."

○ 4. "Lot's of people worry about things like this. It isn't your fault."

76. During the nursing shift report, the team leader lists tasks and routines completed for a terminally ill client. Which of the following kinds of behavior is the nurse *most* likely demonstrating when emphasizing the technical aspects of caring for a dying client?

○ 1. Tactful behavior.

○ 2. Efficient behavior.

○ 3. Objective behavior.

○ 4. Defensive behavior.

Correct Answers and Rationale

The letters in parentheses following the rationale identify the step of the nursing process (A, D, P, I, E) and client needs (1, 2, 3, 4, 5, 6, 7, 8, 9, 10). See the inside front cover for the key.

Pharmacologic and Parenteral Therapies

1. 4. An oculogyric crisis is a severe dystonic reaction typically caused by the older generation of antipsychotics. The nurse would administer 1 to 2 mg of benztropine (Cogentin) intramuscularly to provide a prompt onset of action and offer the client reassurance. Cogentin is generally used to treat drug-induced extrapyramidal side effects (EPSEs). Chlorpromazine and thioridazine (Mellaril) are traditional antipsychotic agents that would intensify the client's oculogyric crisis. Although procyclidine (Kemadrin) is effective for treating the rigidity and sialorrhea associated with antipsychotics, it is available only in oral form and would not be used in a crisis situation, when a parenteral form is needed for quicker onset of action. (P, 8)

2. 2. The nurse would teach the client and family the importance of not discontinuing benztropine (Cogentin) abruptly. Rather, the drug should be tapered slowly over a 1-week period. Benztropine should not be used with over-the-counter cough and cold preparations because of the risk for an additive anticholinergic effect. Antacids delay the absorption of benztropine, and alcohol in combination with benztropine causes an increase in central nervous system depression; concomitant use should be avoided. (I, 8)

3. 3. The nurse needs to focus on side effects that can be seen or felt, using a simple, brief, written description of the benefits of the medication and a list of common side effects and how to cope with them. The written format helps the client and family feel more in control by participating in treatment. They also can use the written information as a helpful resource for review. Information about all potential side effects, including percentages associated with each, will cause undue anxiety in the client and possibly overwhelm the client and family, negatively affecting compliance. The nurse should use discretion in selecting the content of educational sessions. (P, 8)

4. 1. The client needs specific information about the effects of the drug, specifically its effect on the blood. The statement about weekly blood tests to determine safe dosage and monitoring for effects on the blood gives the client specific information to ensure follow-up with the required protocol for Clozaril therapy. Lack of accurate knowledge can lead to noncompliance with necessary follow-up procedures and noncompliance with medication. (I, 8)

5. 2. Telling the mother that excess saliva is a common side effect of the drug is most helpful because it gives her information about the problem, thereby helping to decrease her anxiety about what is occurring with her son. By offering the paper cup, the nurse also demonstrates concern for the client, thereby leading to increased trust. Saying "I wonder if he's having an adverse reaction to the medicine" shows the nurse's lack of knowledge about the drug, decreases confidence in the nurse, and indicates poor judgment. Saying, "Don't worry about it, it's only a minor inconvenience compared to its benefits," or telling the mother that the nurse has seen this happening to other clients is insensitive and does not assuage the mother's anxiety. (I, 8)

6. 4. The nurse would take the client's temperature and report the symptoms to the physician. Flu-like symptoms of weakness, malaise, fever, sore throat, and lethargy may indicate leukopenia. An elevated temperature could also indicate an infection. Either condition requires medical intervention by the physician. Telling the client to wait another day or to take some over-the-counter flu medication is inappropriate because the client is at risk for leukopenia secondary to clozapine therapy and serious consequences could occur. Although it would be important to encourage the client to consume adequate fluids, the priority is to report the symptoms and check the temperature. (I, 9)

7. 3. Sedation and drowsiness are common side effects of clozapine (Clozaril). Often, taking the majority of the dose at bedtime is helpful. By suggesting that the client and the nurse talk to the physician about taking most of the drug at bedtime, the nurse addresses the client's concern and advocates for the client's needs. The other statements are inappropriate because they minimize the client's concern, possibly leading to noncompliance if the problem continues without appropriate intervention. (I, 8)

8. 4. Significant orthostatic hypotension is associated with risperidone (Risperdal) therapy. The nurse would monitor the client's blood pressure sitting and standing and teach the client interventions to manage this side effect to prevent risk for injury. Although insomnia, headache, and anxiety are possible side effects of

risperidone therapy, they are of less immediate concern than orthostatic hypotension. (A, 8)

9. 3. The nurse would be most concerned about the possibility of or plan for pregnancy for a female client receiving antipsychotic medication. Most antipsychotic medications are contraindicated during pregnancy because of potential injury to the fetus. (I, 8)

10. 4. The nurse would discuss nutrition, daily diet, and exercise with the client concerned about her weight gain while taking olanzapine (Zyprexa). Weight gain is common with this drug therapy. The client would benefit from nutrition and exercise teaching, and the nurse should provide the client with an initial course of action. Suggesting that the client talk with her physician about changing to another antipsychotic may not be in her best interest, because olanzapine (Zyprexa) is keeping the symptoms of her illness under control and she is able to function at home and on the job. Advising her to cut her dose in half may lead to decompensation. Telling her not to worry because she should stop gaining weight minimizes the client's concern. Also, additional weight gain is possible. (I, 8)

11. 1. Imipramine, a tricyclic antidepressant, typically requires 2 to 4 weeks of therapy before the full therapeutic effects are experienced. Because the client has been taking the drug for only 3 days, it would be inappropriate to suggest that the client needs an increase in dosage. (I, 8)

12. 3. Alcohol potentiates the central nervous system depression that can occur with imipramine, leading to increased sedation, confusion, and disorientation, and consequently placing the client at risk for injury. Therefore, instructing the client and spouse about avoiding alcohol is most important. (I, 9)

13. 1. Phenelzine is a monoamine oxidase inhibitor (MAOI), and fluoxetine is a selective serotonin receptor inhibitor (SSRI). A period of 14 days is required between stopping an MAOI and starting an SSRI to decrease the likelihood of the "serotonin syndrome," a potentially lethal consequence. Clients with a serotonin syndrome experience hyperreflexia, myoclonus, and other symptoms suggestive of neuroleptic malignant syndrome (NMS). (P, 8)

14. 4. Because phenelzine is an MAOI, foods high in tyramine need to be avoided to prevent the development of a hypertensive crisis. Some foods high in tyramine include sour cream, aged cheeses, yogurt, chianti, beer, bananas, avocados, salami, sausage, bologna, caffeinated coffee and colas, and chocolate. High-protein foods that have undergone protein breakdown by aging, fermentation, pickling, or smoking should be avoided. A hypertensive crisis, evidenced by occipital headache, stiff neck, nausea and vomiting, sweating, nosebleed, dilated

pupils, tachycardia, and constricting chest pain, can occur with this food-drug combination. (I, 9)

15. 2. Because of the risk for hypertensive crisis with MAOIs such as phenelzine, the client needs to immediately report palpitations to the physician. This symptom could indicate hypertension or a hypertensive crisis caused by ingestion of tyramine-rich food while taking the drug. Although urinary hesitancy, dry mouth, and blurred vision are side effects of phenelzine and should be reported, immediate reporting of possible signs and symptoms of hypertension or hypertensive crisis is crucial. (P, 9)

16. 2. Telling the client that these are common side effects that will go away after 6 weeks is most appropriate. This statement acknowledges the client's concerns, gives the client some information, and provides support. Telling the client that a lithium blood level is needed is inappropriate; the client's complaints reflect common side effects, not indicators of possible lithium toxicity. Telling the client that the symptoms are no cause for concern minimizes the client's feelings and ignores the concerns. Holding the lithium until the client feels better is inappropriate because it ignores the client's concerns. In additional, holding the lithium could lead to a decrease in serum lithium levels and, consequently, the drug's therapeutic effectiveness. (I, 8)

17. 1. Clients receiving lithium need to have a consistent dietary intake of sodium to maintain a therapeutic serum lithium level of 0.6 to 1.2 mEq/L. A decrease in salt intake decreases lithium elimination, causing an increase in the serum lithium level. The client who is taking lithium needs to ingest adequate amounts of fluid, at least 2400 to 3000 mL ($2^{1}/_{2}$ to 3 quarts) per day. Drinking 10 to 12 glasses of water each day would aid in achieving this goal. Because drowsiness and dizziness can occur with this drug, the client should avoiding driving until the effects of the drug are known and the client is stabilized. Calling the doctor if vomiting, diarrhea, blurred vision, and weakness are experienced is important because these symptoms may indicate lithium toxicity. (E, 8)

18. 4. Maintenance serum levels between 0.4 and 0.8 mEq/L are considered appropriate and therapeutic for elderly clients. Therefore, the nurse would expect fairly good control of symptoms of mania with a serum level of 0.6 mEq/L. Signs and symptoms of lithium toxicity would be evidenced with a serum level that is greater than 1.5 mEq/L. Manifestations of acute mania would suggest nontherapeutic serum levels of lithium, as indicated by a serum level of less than 0.4 mEq/L. Manic symptoms abate as the lithium level increases. Typically it takes 7 to 10 days to achieve a clinical response. (A, 8)

19. 3. To be effective, lithium needs to increase in the client's bloodstream gradually to a therapeutic level. This process takes approximately 1 to 2 weeks. Once a therapeutic level is achieved, the symptoms of mania will abate. Telling the wife that the client's symptoms are very acute and more time is needed gives the wife the impression that her husband is more seriously ill than would be expected, possibly causing the wife increased anxiety. Telling the wife that her concerns will be passed on to the physician does not provide the wife with the necessary information about the drug and its action. Telling the wife that an increased dosage may be necessary is inappropriate because the client has been receiving the drug for only 2 days. (I, 8)

20. 1. Lithium must be taken on a regular basis, preferably at the same time each day, to maintain therapeutic blood levels of the drug. If a dose is missed, the client should not take double the dosage the next time, because lithium toxicity can ensue. There is a very fine line between the therapeutic and the toxic level of lithium. Telling the client that it depends on how he or she is feeling provides the client with misinformation that could be detrimental to maintaining a therapeutic lithium level. Telling the client to ask the physician ignores the client's concern, thereby diminishing trust in the nurse. The nurse is responsible for knowing the appropriate information about the drug and therefore is capable of explaining the rationale for not doubling a dose. The statement, "You weren't listening to what I just explained" scolds the client and diminishes the client's self-worth. (I, 9)

Management of Care

21. 1. The primary goal of milieu management is to organize interpersonal and environmental forces to facilitate clients' growth, rehabilitation, and restoration of health. This goal applies to all care settings, including the hospital, community, and home. The nurse is responsible for effectively managing the milieu in all care settings. Meeting the needs of staff is not a goal of milieu management, but all staff in a milieu are responsible for understanding and maintaining a therapeutic environment. Providing a sanctuary for helpless clients is no longer relevant today, as it may have been in the past, when psychiatric hospitals provided a safe haven and custodial care for the mentally ill. A therapeutic milieu reflects social organization, social supports, and community values. Implementation of physicians' orders is not a primary goal of milieu management but a part of treatment to meet the goal of facilitating clients' rehabilitation and restoration to health. (E, 1)

22. 1. In a therapeutic milieu, the nurse would initially talk with the client about her feelings to correctly assess and diagnose before intervening. In a therapeutic milieu, the nurse provides respect, acceptance, and openness to a client, fostering an atmosphere in which thoughts and feelings can be safely shared by the client without fear of ridicule, mockery, or retaliation. Suggesting that the client play a game with another client may be appropriate later on depending on the client's needs and level of anxiety. Advising the client to lie down in her room may be appropriate later if the nurse needs to administer lorazepam. Administering lorazepam (Ativan) orally may be appropriate later on depending on the client's needs and level of anxiety. (I, 6)

23. 2. Setting limits here is essential. The nurse would set limits by stating to the client what volume is and is not permissible. Limit setting is the art of clearly identifying acceptable and unacceptable behaviors that are objective, fair, and reflective of the situation at hand. Limits should be identified clearly and early, especially with clients who may "test the system." Prohibiting the use of the stereo for the rest of the day could be a consequence if the client does not adhere to the limit imposed on the volume. However, it does nothing to establish limits. Turning down the volume and saying nothing does not identify the limits for the client and may lead to repetition of the same behavior. Telling the other clients that the time to use the music room is almost over may cause them to feel that the nurse is unfair and not respectful of their needs. (I, 6)

24. 2. In this situation, the nurse would call a community meeting. The community meeting serves as a forum for clients to voice their opinions about the environment, receive feedback from staff and other clients, and discuss community concerns including exploring the problems of daily living. The community meeting can be used to increase peer support and handle confrontation when necessary. For adolescents, peer pressure is generally more effective in changing behavior than the staff's influence. Telephoning the client's parents or urging the client to tell on his friends is authoritative and may lead to increased mistrust of the staff. Calling a physician is not necessary at this time. Rather, a community meeting would be helpful to discuss the problem. (I, 6)

25. 3. The nurse would use concrete concepts and simplified material when conducting a psychoeducational group for clients with chronic schizophrenia and alcohol abuse or dependency. Clients with dual diagnosis experience difficulties in concentration and memory due to the effects of schizophrenia and the use of alcohol. Groups should be structured with simplified material and concrete concepts. Handouts and simple homework assignments may be helpful for the clients to review and apply concepts learned in the group ses-

sion. Strong confrontation techniques would increase the anxiety level, possibly resulting in clients' being unable to tolerate the group. Appropriate structure is necessary to help clients with cognitive deficits to focus. A nondirective leadership style is inappropriate for this group because a lack of leadership would result in a lack of therapeutic value for the clients. Clients with cognitive deficits would have increased difficulty deriving any benefit from the group. (I, 6)

26. 4. By saying, "I hear you say that you don't like taking medication daily," the nurse accepts the client's statement so that the client feels heard and understood. The nurse demonstrates openness toward hearing unacceptable attitudes to foster further sharing among the clients. The other statements are not helpful or therapeutic. The client is ignored and dismissed, which can lead to increased anxiety, decreased self-esteem, and increase anger toward the nurse and other clients. (I, 6)

27. 3. The nurse would arrange for immediate hospitalization on a psychiatric intensive care unit for the client who is suicidal and refuses to sign a "no suicide" contract. A psychiatric intensive care unit or locked unit is the appropriate setting and least restrictive environment to provide safety for a high-risk client. When clients are treated in an outpatient area, procedures must be in place for swift admission to an inpatient area that has a locked unit. The group home, a partial program, or a subacute unit would not provide the maximum safety that the client needs. (I, 2)

28. 2. The statement, "Controlling clients helps them feel more comfortable," does not reflect an understanding of the concept of balance in a therapeutic milieu. Balance is the careful negotiation of the conflict between dependency and independency in a therapeutic milieu. Clients are dependent when admitted to care but are allowed and encouraged to become independent as they are able to assume responsibility for self. Staff may find it easier to care for the client when they can control the client and may feel needed when the client is dependent on them. In a therapeutic milieu, staff do not solve the clients' problems for them. Rather, they work with the clients to gradually allow independent behaviors and decision making. Understanding clients' rights, legal issues, and ethical concerns are crucial for the skilled used of balance. (E, 1)

29. 3. The nurse would urge the nursing assistant to discuss the problem with his coworker to solve their interpersonal conflict. Many times, the nurse is inappropriately expected to solve interpersonal conflicts when subordinates should be urged to handle their own conflicts. The nurse manager facilitates the resolution of conflicts between others. Advising the nursing assistant to be more tolerant or telling him to take care of the linen bags himself is a method of accommodating.

However, the actual problem is not addressed, so it is a win–lose situation. Taking care of the linen bags is a method of avoiding conflict, but the conflict will reemerge at a later time. Even though it may be easier for the nurse to take care of the linen bags, this does not help staff deal with their interpersonal conflict. Therefore, personal growth does not occur. (I, 1)

30. 3. Saying, "Mrs. Roberts, you've done well in group today, but I'd like to hear from the others," is the appropriate intervention to use with a dominant client. This intervention ends the monopolization without putting the client down, so that others can participate. The other clients may be unable or afraid to handle this client. The nurse is responsible for the integrity of the group. Saying, "Mrs. Roberts, you've been taking up too much of the group's time; let's move on," minimizes the client's contributions and diminishes her self-worth. Saying, "Mrs. Roberts, you seem to have quite a lot to say today," encourages the client to continue talking. Saying, "Mrs. Roberts, it certainly isn't hard for you to talk in group," may be interpreted as a sarcastic remark, thus diminishing to the client's self-worth. (I, 6)

31. 1. The statement, "It's difficult to talk in group, but I believe everyone here has something to share that can help someone else," decreases mistrust and anxiety among members who have difficulty with trust and feel anxious as a group of clients with chronic schizophrenia. The nurse conveys that each client is valuable and able to help someone else, thereby increasing the comfort and self-worth of each client. The other statements challenge clients and increase their anxiety by placing specific expectations on them. (I, 6)

32. 4. When working with a client who has a mental illness and her family, the nurse conveys warmth and acceptance to each family member so that each member feels comfortable in disclosing and sharing problems and feelings. The nurse must resist allying with the client so that the nurse is open to understanding each member's view of living with a mentally ill member and able to develop interventions specific to the family's needs. Helping the client to conform to the family's wishes may not be in the client's best interests. Advising each family member on how to deal with the client demonstrates that the family has not been caring for the client adequately or handling problems appropriately. (I, 6)

33. 4. When a client's mental status interferes with his ability to participate in milieu activities, the nurse uses schedule modification to allow a flexible approach to treatment when the needs of a community member require it. Flexibility on the part of the nurse and the entire milieu is a necessary aspect of a therapeutic milieu. Norms, structure, and balance are necessary for an effective, therapeutic milieu. *Norms* are expectations of behavior that are communicated to clients in direct and indirect ways. *Structure* is the framework for the therapeutic environment. *Balance* refers to the negotiating of dependence versus independence found in psychiatric care. (D, 6)

34. 3. With a cognitively impaired client with dementia, the nurse would use environmental cues to help the client navigate the hospital environment. Examples of environmental cues include names on bedroom doors, clocks, and bulletin boards with the month, day, and year. (I, 6)

35. 2. When inpatient hospitalization is no longer needed, subacute care is the next least restrictive setting when the client requires 24-hour supervision but less extensive and intensive services. Subacute units provide the client with a bed, meals, medication, groups, and activities. The client has autonomy and independence in choosing which groups to attend and can seek employment and housing and apply to school or training. A partial program provides structured activities and ongoing treatment from 4 to 8 hours per day and 1 to 5 days per week. Daily outpatient visits would provide counseling for a small period of time. A group home, temporary or permanent, would provide some supervision, a bed, meals, and laundry facilities. Some group homes provide group therapy and structured activities. However, this would not provide an appropriate level of care for a client who requires 24-hour supervision, structure, and programming. (P, 1)

The Client With Stress, Coping, and Adaptation Issues

36. 2. An increase in the noradrenergic and dopaminergic system activity leads to central nervous system hyperarousal and hypervigilance. An increased release of endogenous opiates allows tolerance of fear and pain rather than increasing activity. A decrease in peripheral sympathetic system activity or glucocorticoid levels would lead to a decrease in behavioral responses. (I, 5)

37. 3. With mild anxiety, perceptions would be accurate. Slight muscle tension would reflect a motor response. Occasional irritability is an emotional response. Loss of contact with reality is a cognitive characteristic of severe anxiety. (A, 5)

38. 1. Suicide attempts and violence are psychomotor responses to a panic level of anxiety. Desperation and rage are emotional responses. Disorganized reasoning and loss of contact with reality are cognitive responses. (A, 5)

39. 2. Mild anxiety motivates the client to focus on issues and resolve them. Therefore, learning and problem

solving can occur at a mild level of anxiety. Taking control for the client is reserved for a near-panic level of anxiety. Severe anxiety interferes with reasoning and functioning. Therefore, reducing stimuli and pressure is crucial at a severe level. Tension reduction is appropriate at a moderate level to help the client think more clearly and engage in problem solving. (I, 5)

40. 4. Minimal functioning, causing new problems to develop, is a reflection of dysfunctional coping. The ability to objectively and rationally problem-solve demonstrates adaptive coping. Tension reduction activities demonstrate palliative coping. However, such activities alone do not solve problems; they must be followed by problem solving. Anger management alone may prevent new problems such as violence toward self or others, but it does not solve problems directly. It is considered maladaptive coping. (A, 5)

41. 4. Because relationships inherently lead to stress and anxiety, conflict resolution skills are essential for solving relationship problems. Dealing with anger is more effective than suppressing it. Suppression is a mechanism that avoids the issue rather than solving it. Balancing a checkbook involves calculations, not coping skills. Following directions is a passive activity that reflects a lack of problem-solving by the client. (P, 5)

42. 4. The client's statement that he and his wife listen to each other reflects improved efforts at communicating about issues. The other statements provides some insight into the need for better communication. However, they are but steps along the way to coping effectively with the problem. (E, 5)

43. 1. Assessment examines the client's thoughts, feelings, and behaviors within a context. Whether the client's behavior is appropriate for the situation is important assessment data. Setting priorities is part of making nursing diagnoses and planning; motivation to change and identifying the need for a "no harm" contract are part of the planning stage. (A, 5)

44. 3. Writing a list of strengths and abilities is short-term, achievable, and measurable. Achieving a positive self-esteem would occur over the long term. Going to school involves complex future steps to a long-term goal. Using skills on a date involves activities after discharge, considered more long-term than short-term. (P, 5)

45. 4. The ultimate outcome is to have clients solve problems by themselves, collaborating in their own care. Standardized plans need to be individualized. The nurse and staff work together to foster individualized care. Medication effect and side effect and compliance monitoring are roles of the staff with some input from the client. (P, 5)

46. 1. Substituting rational beliefs is a major goal when using cognitive-behavioral models, which focus more

on thinking and behaviors than feelings. Unconscious processes are the focus of psychoanalytic models. Analysis of fears and barriers to growth are the focus of developmental models. Tension and stress are targets of the stress models. (D, 5)

47. 3. Displacement refers to a defense mechanism that involves taking feelings out on a less-threatening object or person instead of tackling the issue or problem directly. Talking to his wife directly reflects insight into the client's use of the defense mechanism and his ability to overcome it. Not thinking about the weekend is suppression. Here the client is focusing on the issue with the highest priority. Focusing on academic rather than athletic achievement is compensation, highlighting one's strengths instead of weaknesses. Not remembering the molestation is repression. (E, 5)

48. 1. Lack of goals reflects identity problems. Societal responsibility is related to generativity issues. Social behaviors are learned in the initiative stage. Commitment in relationships is part of intimacy. (I, 5)

49. 4. When a client is committed involuntarily, the right to leave AMA is forfeited. All the other rights are preserved unless there is further court action or a case of imminent danger to self or others (eg, hitting staff, cutting self). (D, 1)

50. 3. Legally there is a duty to warn a potential victim of a client's intent to harm. Staff can be held accountable if the client injures the ex-partner and the staff failed to warn that person. The client's permission is needed to share information with a spouse. Only client initials are used in student papers. Release of information is made directly to the client's insurance company, not to the employer. (I, 1)

51. 2. To be committed involuntarily, a client must not only be suffering from a mental illness but must be gravely disabled (unable to care for self or likely to come to harm if discharged) or dangerous to self or others. Having a mental illness alone is not grounds for commitment. Wanting to leave the hospital is not sufficient cause for discharge, especially if the client is dangerous to self or others or is gravely disabled. Having a supportive family or home but not wanting treatment may still result in involuntary commitment if indicated or necessary to ensure the well-being of the client or another person. (I, 1)

52. 2. The nurse is required to set limits on inappropriate behaviors while conveying respect and acceptance of the person. Doing so conveys to the client that he or she is worthy without posing any harm or embarrassment to the client. Touch is a complex issue that must be used cautiously. Touch may be misinterpreted or misperceived by clients who have been abused or those who have perceptual or thought disturbances. Mutual sharing reflects a social friendship, not a therapeutic one. Total confidentiality is not desirable. For example, treatment team members and insurance companies need selected information to ensure quality services. (P, 5)

53. 4. Encouraging decisions, such as asking the client to pick one of two options, is part of planning. Verbalizing the implied to clarify a message, as in the comment, "It sounds as if you are feeling abandoned by your family," is part of assessment. Asking for meaning and importance, such as, "How important is it for you to change this behavior," is related to nursing diagnosis. Rehearsing new behaviors is part of implementation. (P, 5)

54. 3. Asking for descriptions of changes in behavior (eg, what the client did differently) encourages evaluation. Conveying empathy, such as stating that it is still hard for the client to talk about it, encourages data collection. Asking for meaning helps with nursing diagnosis. Formulating plans is related to planning. (E, 5)

55. 1. With the shorter lengths of stay, the processes and goals of a particular stage are chosen according to the client's current needs and abilities. Building trust (orientation stage) is a priority with psychotic and suspicious clients. It is less crucial for clients who are ready to work on issues. Making referrals (termination stage) is appropriate for all clients regardless of their needs. The other needs will be addressed in counseling after discharge. Teaching skills (working stage) is appropriate for clients with insight and readiness for change. They may not be appropriate for clients with severe psychosis or suspiciousness, especially if denial is present. (I, 5)

56. 4. Practicing new behaviors builds confidence and reinforces appropriate behaviors. Reality testing, asking about fears, and teaching new communication skills are some of the many steps along the way to risking the trying out of new behaviors. (I, 5)

The Client Coping With Chronic Illness

57. 2. The psychotropic drugs used to treat chronic mental illnesses have side effects that often lead to noncompliance. Therefore, teaching the clients measures to deal with the common side effects would be most important. Teaching should be focused on the need for compliance and the specific interests of the target audience. Teaching should concentrate on the medications commonly used to treat chronic mental illness, not on a wide variety of psychotropic drugs or those used in acute illness. Such topics as the role of medication in the treatment of chronic mental illness and the effects of using common street drugs with psychotropic med-

ication should be discussed once the issue of compliance is addressed. (P, 8)

58. 2. When the client seems to be questioning the physician's goals, it is best for the nurse to present an open statement and ask the client what he means. This technique helps the client express his feelings. Telling the client about the surgery is less therapeutic when he is upset. Chastising the client and defending the physician is likely to inhibit communication about the client's needs and feelings. Making assumptions can also interfere with communication, especially if the assumption is incorrect. (I, 5)

59. 2. When this client has hostile outbursts, it is best for the nurse to help her express her feelings. This serves as a release valve for the client. The client needs to express her feelings. Offering positive reinforcement for cooperation does not help the client express herself appropriately. Continuing with assigned tasks ignores the client's feelings and may lead to further escalation. Encouraging the client to direct anger to the staff is inappropriate. The client needs to express her feelings appropriately. (I, 5)

60. 3. Preoperative visits and talks with others who have made successful adjustments to colostomies are helpful and tend to make the client less fearful of the operation and its consequences. Knowing about resources in the community will be helpful as the client approaches discharge. Supporting the physician is less important than supporting the client and giving the client information. The client will have a change in body image, with disfigurement due to the creation of a colostomy. However, the client should be able to lead a full life. (P, 5)

61. 3. Hopelessness would be least appropriate, because the client projects an image of a person who is planning for the future and is usually in charge and productive. Ineffective Coping is an appropriate diagnosis, because the client is rushing to resume her normal activities. Deficient Knowledge is an appropriate diagnosis, because the client indicates a lack of awareness about the need for relaxation. Anxiety is an appropriate diagnosis, because the client is demonstrating impatience and inability to relax. (D, 5)

62. 2. The nurse must present reality to the client about his condition to help decrease his denial about his physical status. By stating the name of the condition and talking about what it means, the nurse provides the client with information and conveys concerns about him and a willingness to help him understand his illness. It may not be true that the client would be made more upset by the call; the news might be good. However, this statement does not provide the client with the reality of his condition. Telling the client that he really doesn't care or asking the client if he realizes that he has a life-threatening condition is belittling and may cause the client to become defensive. (I, 5)

63. 1. Leaving the hospital and immediately flying to a meeting indicates poor judgment by the client and little understanding of what she needs to change regarding her lifestyle. The other statements show that the client understands some of the changes she needs to make to decrease her stress and lead a more healthy lifestyle. (E, 5)

64. 4. The nurse's best response is one that directly expresses the nurse's observations to the client and offers the client the opportunity to talk about his feelings or concerns to decrease somatization (the need to express feelings through physical symptoms). Leaving, offering to provide pain medication, and stating that anger does not bother the nurse ignore the client's needs. (I, 5)

65. 3. Clients with ulcerative colitis commonly have a personality trait described as obsessive-compulsive with behaviors such as perfectionism, conformity, rigidity, and obstinacy. (A, 10)

66. 4. This type of behavior illustrates *emotional lability*, which is a readily changeable or unstable emotional affect. *Punning* is using a word when it can have two or more meanings, or a play on words. *Confabulation* involves replacing memory loss by fantasy to hide confusion; it is unconscious behavior. *Flight of ideas* refers to a rapid succession of verbal expressions that jump from one topic to another and are only superficially related. (D, 5)

The Client Coping with End-of-Life Issues

67. 1. The nurse would give the client a tissue and tell him it's okay to cry to convey acceptance and empathy. He needs to know that it is natural to have tremendous feelings of loss and sadness. Telling the client to stop crying, busying oneself in the client's room, and changing the subject are not helpful to the client because they ignore his needs and inhibit the expression of emotion. (I, 5)

68. 1. The client's husband is experiencing anger, much of which stems from feelings of guilt about not taking the trip. During the stage of denial, the husband is more likely to deny the client's diagnosis and prognosis. During the stage of bargaining, the husband would offer to do certain things in exchange for more time before the client dies. In the stage of depression, the husband is likely to make few or no comments and to act dejected. (D, 5)

69. 1. Nurses who have contemplated or examined their own feelings about death and dying are usually more effective when caring for the dying client and family. Many authorities consider self-examination of one's own finiteness essential before one can successfully meet the needs of a dying client. Continuing education classes on death and dying do not ensure that the nurse truly understands and comprehends death and mortality. Remaining emotionally distant is not helpful for dying clients who need emotional support. Viewing the dying as a separate population is a way of distancing oneself from them. (E, 5)

70. 1. When supporting the friends or family of a terminally ill client, it is best to focus on the present. This can be accomplished by living each day to its fullest. Friends and families also want to know what to expect and want someone to listen to them as they express grief over the approaching death. Focusing on the past can interfere with enjoying the present. Expecting the worst interferes with focusing on day-to-day positive experiences. Planning ahead is inappropriate because of uncertainty when the length of life is unknown. (D, 5)

71. 4. Clients often sense a nurse's feelings. Therefore, when the nurse becomes emotionally upset while caring for a terminally ill child, it is best for her to share her emotions with the child when it seems appropriate. It is also acceptable to cry. It is of little help to the client or the nurse who is upset if the nurse waits until a later time when she can speak to someone about the situation. Trying to smile or not to show emotion is inappropriate. Children are very aware of someone's incongruent mood and behavior. (I, 5)

72. 1. The best course of action when the client has outbursts concerning her treatments is to tell her how the treatment can be expected to help her. Doing so helps motivate the client to get better. Describing the effect on her body if she misses a treatment is a negative approach and may be threatening to the client. The client is likely to feel angry if told to be a "good patient" during treatments. Offering to give the client a backrub if she does not fuss does not give her the information to which she is entitled. It also negatively reinforces the behavior. (I, 5)

73. 2. Children are aware of and show anxieties about death at an earlier age than was once thought, and they recognize false cheerfulness. They tend to experience isolation and loneliness when those around them are trying to hide or mask the truth. They are then left to face the realities of death alone. (D, 5)

74. 1. Taking a blood sample is an unnecessary, invasive procedure that would not directly address the child's fear. Leukemia is not considered a communicable disease. Providing an age-appropriate explanation and alerting the parents to the sibling's concern and the resources available to assist siblings to deal with the terminal illness are all appropriate interventions. (I, 5)

75. 2. A response that acknowledges the brother's concern and provides him with information is most helpful. Therefore, telling the brother that the nurse sees that he is worried and then following this up with a discussion about leukemia is most appropriate. Providing reassurance or information without acknowledging the expressed concern is not as helpful as acknowledging the concern and providing the information. Although acknowledging his worry is appropriate, more importantly, he needs factual information about the disease. (I, 5)

76. 4. The nurse caring for a terminally ill client who reports only tasks and routines completed for the client is probably behaving defensively. This behavior does not convey compassion and caring for the client. It is likely that this nurse has not come to grips with death and dying. (A, 5)

Bibliography

American Psychiatric Association. (2000). *Diagnostic and statistical manual of mental disorders* (4th ed, text revised). Washington, DC: Author.

Andrews, M. M., & Boyle, J. S. (1995). *Transcultural concepts in nursing care* (2nd ed.). Philadelphia: J. B. Lippincott.

Boyd, M. A., & Nihart, M. A. (1998). *Psychiatric nursing: Contemporary practice.* Philadelphia: Lippincott Williams & Wilkins.

Johnson, B. S. (1997). *Psychiatric-mental health nursing: Adaptation and growth* (4th ed.). Philadelphia: Lippincott-Raven.

Karch, A. M. (2001). *2001 Lippincott's nursing drug guide.* Philadelphia: Lippincott Williams & Wilkins.

Schultz, J. M., & Videbeck, S. D. (1998). *Lippincott's manual of psychiatric nursing care plans* (5th ed.). Philadelphia: Lippincott Williams & Wilkins.

Shives, L. R. (1998). *Basic concepts of psychiatric-mental health nursing* (4th ed.). Philadelphia: Lippincott Williams & Wilkins.

Varcarolis, E. M. (1998). *Foundations of psychiatric mental health nursing* (3rd ed.). Philadelphia: W. B. Saunders.

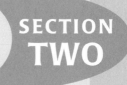

SECTION
TWO

POSTREVIEW TESTS

PART

V

Postreview Comprehensive Tests

COMPREHENSIVE TEST 1

Select the one best answer, and indicate your choice by filling in the circle in front of the option.

1. A client with human immunodeficiency virus infection (HIV) and acquired immunodeficiency syndrome (AIDS) confides that he is homosexual and his employer does not know his HIV status. The nurse's best response to him is
   ○ 1. "Would you like me to help you tell them?"
   ● 2. "The information you confide in me is confidential."
   ○ 3. "I must share this information with your family."
   ○ 4. " I must share this information with your employer."

2. The mother of a child with bronchial asthma tells the nurse that the child wants a pet. Which of the following pets should the nurse tell the mother is most appropriate?
   ○ 1. Cat.
   ● 2. Fish.
   ○ 3. Gerbil.
   ○ 4. Canary.

3. An elderly client is being admitted to same-day surgery for cataract extraction. The client has several diamond rings. The nurse should explain to the client that
   ○ 1. her rings will be taped before the surgery.
   ● 2. she will sign a valuables envelope that will be placed in a safe.
   ○ 3. the rings will be locked in the narcotics box.
   ○ 4. the nursing supervisor will hold onto the rings during the surgery.

4. When an infant resumes taking oral feedings after surgery to correct intussusception, the parents comment that the child seems to suck on the pacifier more since the surgery. The nurse explains that sucking on a pacifier
   ● 1. provides an outlet for emotional tension.
   ○ 2. indicates readiness to take solid foods.
   ● 3. indicates intestinal motility.
   ○ 4. is an attempt to get attention from the parents.

5. A 22-year-old client is brought to the emergency department with his fiancée after being involved in a serious motor vehicle accident. His Glasgow Coma Scale score is 7 and he demonstrates evidence of decorticate posturing. Which of the following would be appropriate for obtaining a permit to place a catheter for intracranial pressure (ICP) monitoring?
   ○ 1. The nurse will obtain a signed consent from the client's fiancée because he is of legal age and they are engaged to be married.
   ○ 2. The physician will get a consultation from one other physician and proceed with placement of the ICP catheter until the family arrives to sign the consent.
   ● 3. Two nurses will receive a verbal consent by telephone from the client's next of kin before inserting the catheter.
   ● 4. The physician will document the emergency nature of the client's condition and that an ICP catheter for monitoring was placed without a consent.

6. A 68-year-old client's daughter is asking about the follow-up evaluation for her father after his pneumonectomy for primary lung cancer. The nurse's best response is which of the following?
   ○ 1. "The usual follow-up is chest x-ray and liver function tests every 3 months."
   ○ 2. "The follow-up for your father will be a chest x-ray and a CT scan of the abdomen every year."
   ○ 3. "No follow-up is needed at this time."
   ● 4. "The follow-up for your father will be a chest x-ray every 6 months."

7. The nurse is preparing to administer blood to an otherwise healthy client who requires postoperative blood replacement. The nurse is aware that the blood administration set must include
   ● 1. a micron mesh filter.
   ○ 2. a nonfiltered administration blood set.
   ○ 3. a special leukocyte-poor filter.
   ○ 4. a microdrip administration set.

8. Under which circumstance may a nurse communicate medical information without the client's consent?
   ○ 1. When certifying the client's absence from work.
   ○ 2. When requested by the client's family.
   ● 3. When treating clients who have a sexually transmitted infection.
   ○ 4. When ordered by another physician.

657

9. During the health history interview, which of the following strategies is the most effective for the nurse to use to help clients feel that they have an active role in their health care?
   - ○ 1. Ask clients to complete a questionnaire.
   - ○ 2. Provide clients with written instructions.
   - ◉ 3. Ask clients for their description of events and for their views concerning past medical care.
   - ○ 4. Ask clients if they have any questions.

10. A client with severe major depression states, "My heart has stopped and my blood is black ash." The nurse interprets this statement to be evidence of which of the following?
    - ○ 1. Hallucination.
    - ○ 2. Illusion.
    - ◉ 3. Delusion.
    - ○ 4. Paranoia.

11. When a client wants to read his chart, the nurse should
    - ○ 1. call the doctor to obtain permission.
    - ◉ 2. give the client the chart and answer questions for him.
    - ○ 3. tell the client that he can read the chart when the doctor makes rounds.
    - ○ 4. ask the client what he wants to know and answer those questions without giving him the chart.

12. A client who has a fractured leg has been instructed to ambulate without weight bearing on the affected leg. The nurse evaluates that the client is ambulating correctly if she uses which of the following crutch-walking gaits?
    - ○ 1. Two-point gait.
    - ○ 2. Four-point gait.
    - ◉ 3. Three-point gait.
    - ○ 4. Swing-to gait.

13. A client with major depression states, "Life isn't worth living anymore. Nothing matters." Which of the following responses by the nurse would be *best?*
    - ◉ 1. "Are you thinking about killing yourself?"
    - ○ 2. "Things will get better, you know."
    - ○ 3. "Why do you think that way?"
    - ○ 4. "You shouldn't feel that way."

14. A client is prescribed atropine, 0.4 mg IM. The atropine vial is labeled gr 1/300 per mL. How much should the nurse plan to administer?
    - ○ 1. 0.5 mL.
    - ○ 2. 0.75 mL.
    - ○ 3. 1.0 mL.
    - ○ 2. 2.0 mL.

15. A multiparous client tells the nurse that she is using medroxyprogesterone (Depo-Provera) for contraception. The nurse instructs the client to increase her intake of which of the following?
    - ○ 1. Folic acid.
    - ○ 2. Vitamin C.
    - ○ 3. Magnesium.
    - ◉ 4. Calcium.

16. The nurse is teaching a client about topical gentamycin sulfate (Garamycin). Which of the following comments by the client indicates the need for additional teaching?
    - ○ 1. "I will avoid being out in the sun for long periods."
    - ○ 2. "I should stop applying it once the infected area heals."
    - ○ 3. "I'll call the physician if the condition worsens."
    - ◉ 4. "I should apply it to over large open areas."

17. A client has been taking imipramine (Tofranil) for his depression for 2 days. His sister asks the nurse, "Why is he still so depressed?" Which of the following responses by the nurse would be *most* appropriate?
    - ○ 1. "Your brother is experiencing a very serious depression."
    - ○ 2. "I'll be sure to convey your concern to his physician."
    - ◉ 3. "It takes 2 to 4 weeks for the drug to reach its full effect."
    - ○ 4. "Perhaps we'll need to change his medication."

18. A multigravid client visiting the prenatal clinic at 16 weeks' gestation exhibits facial swelling, a brownish vaginal discharge, and fundal height of 22 cm. The client's blood pressure is 160/90 mm Hg and her pulse is 80 bpm. The nurse interprets these findings as suggestive of which of the following?
    - ○ 1. Placenta previa.
    - ○ 2. Fetal anemia.
    - ○ 3. Multifetal pregnancy.
    - ◉ 4. Gestational trophoblastic disease.

19. Which of the following responses would be *most* helpful for a client who is euphoric, intrusive, and interrupts other clients engaged in conversations to the point where they get up and leave or walk away?
    - ◉ 1. "When you interrupt others, they leave the area."
    - ○ 2. "You are being rude and uncaring."
    - ○ 3. "You better remember to use your manners."
    - ○ 4. "You know better than to interrupt someone."

20. The nurse coordinates with the laboratory staff to have the gentamycin trough serum level drawn. At what time should the blood be drawn in relation to the administration of the intravenous dose of gentamycin sulfate (Garamycin)?
    - ○ 1. 2 hours before the administration of the next intravenous dose.
    - ○ 2. 3 hours before the administration of the next intravenous dose.

3. 4 hours before the administration of the next intravenous dose.

4. Just before the administration of the next intravenous dose.

21. Older adults with known cardiovascular disease must balance which of the following measures for optimum health?
  1. Diet, exercise, and medication.
  2. Stress, hypertension, and pain.
  3. Mental health, diet, and stress.
  4. Social events, diet, and smoking.

22. A 4-year-old is brought to the emergency department with sudden onset of a temperature of 103°F (39.5°C), sore throat, and refusal to drink. The child will not lie down and prefers to lean forward while sitting up. Which of the following would the nurse do *next*?
  1. Give 600 mg acetaminophen (Tylenol) per rectum as ordered.
  2. Inspect the child's throat for redness and swelling.
  3. Have an appropriate-sized tracheostomy tube readily available.
  4. Obtain a specimen for a throat culture.

23. Assessment of a client taking lithium reveals dry mouth, nausea, thirst, and mild hand tremor. Based on an analysis of these findings, which of the following would the nurse do *next*?
  1. Hold the lithium and obtain a stat lithium level to determine therapeutic effectiveness.
  2. Continue the lithium and immediately notify the physician about the assessment findings.
  3. Continue the lithium and reassure the client that these temporary side effects will subside.
  4. Hold the lithium and monitor the client for signs and symptoms of increasing toxicity.

24. A client asks the nurse how long she will have to take her medicine for hypothyroidism. The nurse's response is based on the knowledge that
  1. lifelong daily medicine is necessary.
  2. the medication is expensive, and the dose can be reduced in a few months.
  3. the medication can be gradually withdrawn in 1 to 2 years.
  4. the medication can be discontinued after the client's thyroid-stimulating hormone (TSH) level is normal.

25. Assessment of which of the following clients would lead the nurse to expect the physician to order an adjustment in lithium dosage?
  1. A client who continues work as a computer programmer.
  2. A client who attends college classes.
  3. A client who is now able to care for his or her children.

4. A client who is beginning training for a tennis team.

26. A client admitted with a gastric ulcer has been vomiting bright red blood. His hemoglobin is 5.11 g/dL, and his blood pressure is 100/50 mm Hg. The client and the family state that their religious beliefs do not support the use of blood products and refuse blood transfusions as a treatment for the bleeding. The nurse would expect that the next step in the treatment plan would be to
  1. discontinue all measures.
  2. notify the hospital attorney.
  3. attempt to stabilize the client through the use of fluid replacement.
  4. give enough blood to keep the client from dying.

27. The parents of a child with cystic fibrosis express concern about how the disease was transmitted to their child. The nurse would explain that
  1. a disease carrier also has the disease.
  2. two parents who are carriers may produce a child who has the disease.
  3. a disease carrier and an affected person will never have children with the disease.
  4. a disease carrier and an affected person will have a child with the disease.

28. A client with angina shows the nurse her nitroglycerin (Nitrostat) that she is carrying in a plastic bag in her pocket. The nurse instructs the client that nitroglycerin should be kept
  1. in the refrigerator.
  2. in a cool, moist place.
  3. in a dark container to shield from light.
  4. in a plastic bag where it is readily available.

29. When teaching a client with bipolar disorder, mania, who has started to take valproic acid (Depakene) about possible side effects of this medication, the nurse would include which of the following in the teaching plan?
  1. Increased urination.
  2. Slowed thinking.
  3. Sedation.
  4. Weight loss.

30. An infant is born with facial abnormalities, growth retardation, mental retardation, and vision abnormalities. These abnormalities are probably caused by maternal
  1. alcohol consumption.
  2. vitamin B_6 deficiency.
  3. vitamin A deficiency.
  4. folic acid deficiency.

31. Nonsteroidal anti-inflammatory drugs (NSAIDs) are frequently used in the treatment of musculoskeletal conditions. It is important for the nurse to remind the client to

○ 1. take NSAIDs at least three times per day.

○ 2. exercise the joints at least one-half hour after taking the medication.

○ 3. take antacids 1 hour after taking NSAID.

○ 4. take NSAIDs with food.

32. The nurse would suspect that the client taking disulfiram (Antabuse) therapy has ingested alcohol when the client exhibits which of the following symptoms?

○ 1. Sore throat and muscle aches.

○ 2. Nausea and flushing of the face and neck.

○ 3. Fever and muscle soreness.

○ 4. Bradycardia and vertigo.

33. The nurse holds the gauze pledget against an intramuscular injection site while removing the needle from the muscle. This technique helps to

○ 1. seal off the track left by the needle in the tissue.

○ 2. speed the spread of the medication in the tissue.

○ 3. avoid the discomfort of the needle pulling on the skin.

○ 4. prevent organisms from entering the body through the skin puncture.

34. A client whose condition remains stable after a myocardial infarction gradually increases his activity. Which the following conditions should the nurse assess to determine whether the activity is appropriate for the client?

○ 1. Edema.

○ 2. Cyanosis.

○ 3. Dyspnea.

○ 4. Weight loss.

35. When a client with alcohol dependency begins to talk about not having a problem with alcohol, the nurse would use which of the following approaches?

○ 1. Questioning the client about how much alcohol she drinks.

○ 2. Confronting the client with the fact that she was intoxicated 2 days ago.

○ 3. Pointing out how alcohol has gotten her into trouble.

○ 4. Listening to what the client states and then asking her how she plans to stay sober.

36. Which of the following correctly describes Medicaid?

○ 1. A program designed to assist ill, low-income older adults.

○ 2. A federal insurance program for pregnant women.

○ 3. A joint federal–state program for low-income persons.

○ 4. A program administered by health maintenance organizations.

37. The nurse is preparing a teaching plan for a 45-year-old client recently diagnosed with type 2 diabetes mellitus. What is the *first* step in this process?

○ 1. Establish goals.

○ 2. Choose video materials and brochures.

○ 3. Assess the client's learning needs.

○ 4. Set priorities of learning needs.

38. A loading dose of digoxin (Lanoxin) is given to a client newly diagnosed with atrial fibrillation. The nurse begins instructing the client about the medication and the importance of monitoring the heart rate. An expected outcome of the education program will be

○ 1. a return demonstration of palpating the radial pulse.

○ 2. a return demonstration of how to take the medication.

○ 3. verbalization of why the client has atrial fibrillation.

○ 4. verbalization of the need for the medication.

39. A multigravid client is scheduled for a percutaneous umbilical blood sampling (PUBS) procedure. The nurse instructs the client that this procedure is useful for diagnosing which of the following?

○ 1. Twin pregnancies.

○ 2. Fetal lung maturation.

○ 3. Rh disease.

○ 4. α-Fetoprotein level.

40. Which of the following is a side effect of vancomycin (Vancocin) and needs to be reported promptly?

○ 1. Vertigo.

○ 2. Tinnitus.

○ 3. Muscle stiffness.

○ 4. Ataxia.

41. Which of the following statements indicates that the client with a peptic ulcer understands the dietary modifications he will need to follow at home?

○ 1. "I should eat a bland, soft diet."

○ 2. "It is important to eat six small meals a day."

○ 3. "I should drink several glasses of milk a day."

○ 4. "I should avoid alcohol and caffeine."

42. The client with a nasogastric tube begins to complain of abdominal distention. Which of the following measures should the nurse implement *first*?

○ 1. Call the physician.

○ 2. Irrigate the nasogastric tube.

○ 3. Check the function of the suction equipment.

○ 4. Reposition the nasogastric tube.

43. A male client has been diagnosed as having a low sperm count during infertility studies. After instructions by the nurse about some causes of low sperm counts, the nurse determines that the client needs further instructions when he says low sperm counts may be caused by which of the following?

○ 1. Varicocele.

○ 2. Frequent use of saunas.

○ 3. Endocrine imbalances.

○ 4. Decreased body temperature.

44. The nurse assesses a client and notes puffy eyelids, swollen ankles, and crackles at both lung bases. The nurse understands that these clinical findings are most specifically associated with fluid excess in which of the following compartments?
    ○ 1. Interstitial compartment.
    ○ 2. Intravascular compartment.
    ○ 3. Extracellular compartment.
    ○ 4. Intracellular compartment.

45. An expected physiologic response to a low potassium level is
    ○ 1. cardiac dysrhythmias.
    ○ 2. hyperglycemia.
    ○ 3. hypertension.
    ○ 4. increased energy.

46. When teaching unlicensed assistive personnel (UAP) about the importance of handwashing in preventing disease, the nurse makes which of the following statements?
    ○ 1. "It is not necessary to wash your hands as long as you use gloves."
    ○ 2. "Handwashing is the best method for preventing cross-contamination."
    ○ 3. "Waterless commercial products are not effective for killing organisms."
    ○ 4. "The hands do not serve as a source of infection."

47. The nurse is performing Leopold maneuvers on a woman who is in her eighth month of pregnancy. The nurse is palpating the uterus as shown in Figure 1. Which of the following maneuvers is the nurse performing?

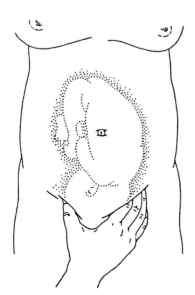

Figure 1.

○ 1. First maneuver.
○ 2. Second maneuver.
○ 3. Third maneuver.
○ 4. Fourth maneuver.

48. A client in a cardiac rehabilitation program states that he would like to make sure he is eating the right foods to ensure adequate endurance on the treadmill. Which of the following nutrients is *most* helpful for promoting endurance during sustained activity?
    ○ 1. Protein.
    ○ 2. Carbohydrate.
    ○ 3. Fat.
    ○ 4. Water.

49. A client's chest tube is connected to a chest tube drainage system with a water seal. The nurse notes that the fluid in the water-seal column is fluctuating with each breath that the client takes. The fluctuation means that
    ○ 1. there is an obstruction in the chest tube.
    ○ 2. the client is developing subcutaneous emphysema.
    ○ 3. the chest tube system is functioning properly.
    ○ 4. there is a leak in the chest tube system.

50. A client with diabetes is explaining to the nurse how she will care for her feet at home. Which statement indicates that the client understands proper foot care?
    ○ 1. "When I injure my toe, I will plan to put iodine on it."
    ○ 2. "I should inspect my feet at least once a week."
    ○ 3. "I do not plan to wear shoes while I am in the house."
    ○ 4. "It is important to dry my feet carefully after my bath."

51. The nurse assesses a client with diverticulitis and suspects peritonitis when which of the following symptoms is noted?
    ○ 1. Hyperactive bowel sounds.
    ○ 2. Rigid abdominal wall.
    ○ 3. Explosive diarrhea.
    ○ 4. Excessive flatulence.

52. When performing chest percussion on a child, which of the following techniques would the nurse use?
    ○ 1. Firmly but gently striking the chest wall to make a popping sound.
    ○ 2. Gently striking the chest wall to make a slapping sound.
    ○ 3. Percussing over an area from the umbilicus to the clavicle.
    ○ 4. Placing a blanket between the nurse's hand and the child's chest.

53. The nurse walks into the room of a client who has a "Do Not Resuscitate" order and finds the client

without a pulse, respirations, or blood pressure. What is the most appropriate action?

○ 1. Stay in the room and notify the nursing team for assistance.

○ 2. Push the emergency alarm to call a code.

○ 3. Dial the hospital phone number for a code.

○ 4. Pull the curtain and leave the room.

54. A client is trying to lose weight at a moderate pace. If the client eliminates 1000 calories per day from his normal intake, how many pounds would he lose in 1 week?

○ 1. 1 pound.

○ 2. 2 pounds.

○ 3. 3 pounds.

○ 4. 4 pounds.

55. A nulliparous client calls the clinic and tells the nurse that she forgot to take her oral contraceptive this morning. Which of the following would the nurse instruct the client to do?

○ 1. Take the medication immediately.

○ 2. Restart the medication in the morning.

○ 3. Use another form of contraception for 2 weeks.

○ 4. Take two pills tonight before bedtime.

56. The nurse recognizes that a client with pain disorder is improving when the client states which of the following?

○ 1. "I need to have a good cry about all the pain I've been in and then not dwell on it."

○ 2. "I need to find another physician who can accurately diagnose my condition."

○ 3. "The pain medicine that you gave me helps me to relax."

○ 4. "I'm angry with all of the doctors I've seen who don't know what they're doing."

57. A client admitted in an acute psychotic states that she hears "terrible voices in the head" and thinks her neighbor is "out to get her." Which of the following would be the nurse's *best* response?

○ 1. "What has your neighbor been doing that bothers you?"

○ 2. "How long have you been hearing these `terrible voices?'"

○ 3. "We won't let your neighbor visit, so you'll be safe."

○ 4. "What exactly are these `terrible voices' saying to you?"

58. The nurse would assess the client with severe diarrhea for which acid–base imbalance?

○ 1. Respiratory acidosis.

○ 2. Respiratory alkalosis.

○ 3. Metabolic acidosis.

○ 4. Metabolic alkalosis.

59. Which of the following outcome criteria would be appropriate for a client with excess fluid volume?

○ 1. A weight resolution of 10% will occur.

○ 2. Pain will be controlled effectively.

○ 3. Arterial blood gas values will be within normal limits.

○ 4. Serum osmolality value will be within normal limits.

60. A 7-year-old child is admitted to the hospital with the medical diagnosis of acute rheumatic fever. Which of the following laboratory blood findings would confirm that the child probably has had a streptococcal infection?

○ 1. High leukocyte count.

○ 2. Low hemoglobin count.

○ 3. Elevated antibody concentration.

○ 4. Low erythrocyte sedimentation rate.

61. A client is scheduled for hip replacement surgery and is interviewed by the nurse in the preadmission testing unit. The client states that he wishes to receive his own blood for the upcoming surgery. What is the nurse's most appropriate response?

○ 1. Document the client's request on the chart.

○ 2. Notify the hematology laboratory.

○ 3. Notify the surgeon's office.

○ 4. Call the blood bank.

62. A client needs surgery to relieve an intestinal obstruction. The day before the surgery, the nurse receives the following set of orders for the client. Which of the following orders should the nurse question before performing?

○ 1. Tapwater enemas until clear.

○ 2. Out of bed as tolerated.

○ 3. Neomycin sulfate 1 g by mouth every 4 hours.

○ 4. Betadine scrub to abdomen twice daily.

63. A client who is NPO is constantly asking for a drink. Which of the following would be the most appropriate nursing intervention?

○ 1. Reexplain to the client why she cannot drink.

○ 2. Offer ice chips every hour to decrease thirst.

○ 3. Offer the client frequent oral hygiene care.

○ 4. Divert the client's attention by turning on the television.

64. A female client is admitted with complaints of fatigue, cold intolerance, weight gain, and muscle weakness. The initial nursing assessment reveals brittle nails, dry hair, constipation, and possible goiter. The client is most likely experiencing signs and symptoms of

○ 1. Cushing's disease.

○ 2. hypothyroidism.

○ 3. hyperthryroidism.

○ 4. a pituitary tumor.

65. A mother visiting the clinic for a routine visit with her 10-year-old daughter reports that her daughter has begun to show symptoms of puberty. The nurse explains to the mother and daughter that after the symptoms of puberty are noticed, menstruation

most typically occurs within which of the following time frames?
- ○ 1. 6 months.
- ○ 2. 12 months.
- ○ 3. 30 months.
- ○ 4. 36 months.

66. While a mother is feeding her full-term neonate 1 hour after birth, she asks the nurse, "What are these white dots in my baby's mouth? I tried to wash them out, but they're still there." After assessing the neonate's mouth, the nurse explains that these spots are which of the following?
- ○ 1. Koplik's spots.
- ○ 2. Epstein's pearls.
- ○ 3. Precocious teeth.
- ○ 4. Thrush curds.

67. Which one of the following factors is most important for healing of an infected decubitus ulcer?
- ○ 1. Adequate circulatory status.
- ○ 2. Scheduled periods of rest.
- ○ 3. Balanced nutritional diet.
- ○ 4. Fluid intake of 1500 mL/day.

68. A client is receiving digoxin (Lanoxin). His pulse range is normally 70 to 76 bpm. After assessing the apical pulse for 1 minute and finding it to be 60 bpm, the nurse should *initially*
- ○ 1. call the physician for orders.
- ○ 2. withhold the digoxin (Lanoxin).
- ○ 3. administer the digoxin (Lanoxin).
- ○ 4. notify the charge nurse.

69. While shopping at a local mall, the nurse hears a pregnant client yell "Oh my! The baby's coming!" After placing the client in a supine position and trying to maintain some privacy, the nurse sees that the neonate's head is crowning. Which of the following would the nurse do *first*?
- ○ 1. Suction the mouth with two fingertips.
- ○ 2. Check for presence of a cord around the neck.
- ○ 3. Tell the client to bear down with force.
- ○ 4. Advise the mother that help is on the way.

70. The nurse is preparing a discharge plan for a 16-year-old who has fractured her femur and ulna. The client asks the nurse how quickly her fractures will heal so she can return to her normal activities. Which of the following responses would be most appropriate for the nurse to make?
- ○ 1. "The healing of your leg will be delayed because you have had a skeletal traction."
- ○ 2. "It will take your arm about 12 weeks to heal completely, but it will take your leg about 24 weeks."
- ○ 3. "Because you are young and healthy, your bones should heal in less than 12 weeks."

- ○ 4. "You will require long-term rehabilitation and should expect it to take at least 8 months for your bones to heal."

71. A client with delirium becomes very anxious and says, "I can't stop what is happening to me. Make it stop, please!" Which of the following would be the nurse's *most* appropriate response?
- ○ 1. "I'll get you some medicines to help you relax. The more you worry, the worse it will get."
- ○ 2. "As soon as we know what's causing this, we can try to stop it. I'll get you some medicine to help you relax."
- ○ 3. "I wish I could do something to make it stop, but unfortunately I can't."
- ○ 4. "I'll sit with you until you calm down a little."

72. After teaching a primigravid client at 10 weeks' gestation about the recommendations for exercise during pregnancy, which of the following client statements indicates successful teaching?
- ○ 1. "While pregnant, I should avoid contact sports."
- ○ 2. "Even though I'm pregnant, I can learn to ski next month."
- ○ 3. "While we are on vacation next month, I can continue to scuba dive."
- ○ 4. "Sitting in a hot tub after exercise will help me to relax."

73. The nurse is caring for a client who has had a myocardial infarction involving a large section of the heart muscle. The nurse anticipates that the client is at risk for
- ○ 1. cardiogenic shock.
- ○ 2. hypovolemic shock.
- ○ 3. neurogenic shock.
- ○ 4. metabolic shock.

74. The nurse is assessing a client who has had a myocardial infarction. The nurse notes the cardiac rhythm shown in Figure 2. The nurse identifies that this rhythm is
- ○ 1. Atrial fibrillation.
- ○ 2. Ventricular tachycardia.
- ○ 3. Premature ventricular contractions.
- ○ 4. Third-degree heart block.

75. The physician has ordered a chemotherapy drug to be administered to a client every day for the next week. The client is on an adult medical–surgical floor but the nurse assigned to the client has not been trained to handle chemotherapy agents. What is the nurse's most appropriate response?
- ○ 1. Send the client to the oncology floor for administration of the medication.
- ○ 2. Ask a nurse from the oncology floor to come to the client and administer the medication.

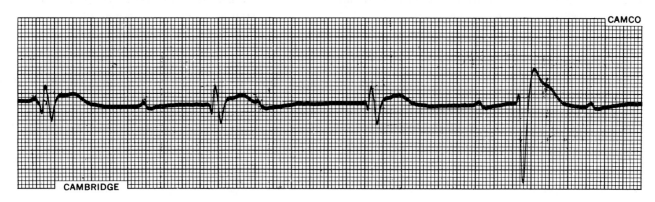

Figure 2.

○ 3. Ask another nurse to help mix the chemotherapy agent.

○ 4. Ask the pharmacy to mix the chemotherapy agent and administer it.

76. Which of the following nursing diagnoses would the nurse identify as a *priority* after surgical repair of a cleft lip?
    ○ 1. Pain.
    ○ 2. Risk for Infection.
    ○ 3. Impaired Physical Mobility.
    ○ 4. Impaired Parenting.

77. Which of the following would be an appropriate expected outcome for a client with rheumatoid arthritis? The client will
    ○ 1. manage joint pain and fatigue to perform activities of daily living.
    ○ 2. maintain full range-of-motion (ROM) in joints.
    ○ 3. prevent the development of further pain and joint deformity.
    ○ 4. take anti-inflammatory medications as indicated by presence of disease symptoms.

78. A client's burn wounds are being cleansed twice a day in a hydrotherapy tub. Which of the following interventions should be included in the plan of care before a hydrotherapy treatment is initiated?
    ○ 1. Limit food and fluids 45 minutes before therapy to prevent nausea and vomiting.
    ○ 2. Increase the intravenous flow rate to offset fluids lost through the therapy.
    ○ 3. Apply a topical antibiotic cream to burns to prevent infection.
    ○ 4. Administer pain medication 30 minutes before therapy to help manage pain.

79. A health care provider has been exposed to hepatitis B through a needlestick. Which of the following drugs would the nurse anticipate administering as postexposure prophylaxis?
    ○ 1. Hepatitis B immune globulin.
    ○ 2. Interferon.

○ 3. Hepatitis B surface antigen.
○ 4. Amphotericin B.

80. When performing an otoscopic examination of the tympanic membrane of a 2-year-old child, the nurse would pull the pinna in which of the following directions?
    ○ 1. Down and back.
    ○ 2. Down and slightly forward.
    ○ 3. Up and back.
    ○ 4. Up and forward.

81. Which of the following findings would the nurse most likely note in the client who is in the compensatory stage of shock?
    ○ 1. Decreased urinary output.
    ○ 2. Significant hypotension.
    ○ 3. Tachycardia.
    ○ 4. Mental confusion.

82. A client has been prescribed hydrochlorothiazide (HydroDIURIL) for treatment of congestive heart failure. For which of the following symptoms should the nurse monitor the client?
    ○ 1. Urinary retention.
    ○ 2. Muscle weakness.
    ○ 3. Confusion.
    ○ 4. Diaphoresis.

83. The son of a client with Alzheimer's disease excitedly tells the nurse, "Mom was singing one of her favorite old songs. I think she's getting her memory back!" Which of the following responses by the nurse is *most* appropriate?
    ○ 1. "She still has long-term memory, but her short-term memory will not return."
    ○ 2. "I'm so happy to hear that. Maybe she is getting better."
    ○ 3. "Don't get your hopes up. This is only a temporary improvement."
    ○ 4. "I'm glad she can sing even if she can't talk to you."

84. The nurse collects a urine specimen from a client for

to see his chart. As a client advocate, the nurse should not make excuses to put the client off in regard to seeing his chart. (I, 1, M)

12. 3. The three-point gait, in which the client advances the crutches and the affected leg at the same time while weight is supported on the unaffected extremity, is the appropriate gait of choice. This allows for non–weight bearing on the affected extremity. The two-point, four-point, and swing-to gaits require some weight bearing on both legs, which is contraindicated for this client. (E, 10, M)

13. 1. When the client verbalizes that life isn't worth living anymore, the nurse needs to ask the client directly about suicide by saying, "Are you thinking about killing yourself?" Asking directly does not provoke suicide but conveys concern, understanding, and the worth of the client. Often, the client experiences a sense of relief that someone finally hears him. It also helps the nurse plan responsible care by identifying the client who is at risk for suicide. The nurse would then evaluate the seriousness of the suicidal ideation by inquiring about the intent and plan. Stating, "Things will get better," offers hope too soon without first evaluating the intent of the suicidal ideation. Asking, "Why do you think that way," implies a lack of understanding and knowledge on the part of the nurse. Major depression usually is endogenous and biochemically based. Therefore, the client may not know why he doesn't want to live. Saying, "You shouldn't feel that way," admonishes the client, decreases self-worth, and conveys a lack of understanding. (I, 6, X)

14. 4. First, convert 0.4 mg to gr 1/150. gr 1/150 / x = gr 1/300 / 1 mL; x = 2.0 mL. (P, 8, M)

15. 4. The nurse should instruct the client to increase her intake of calcium because there is a slight increase in the risk of osteoporosis with this medication. Weight-bearing exercises are also advised. The drug may also impair glucose tolerance in women who are at risk for diabetes. (I, 8, O)

16. 4. The aminoglycoside antibiotic gentamycin sulfate (Garamycin) should not be applied to large denuded areas because toxicity and systemic absorption are possible. The nurse should instruct the client to avoid excessive sun exposure because gentamycin sulfate (Garamycin) can cause photosensitivity. The client should be instructed to apply the antibiotic cream or ointment for only the length of time prescribed, because a superinfection can occur from overuse. The client should contact the physician if the condition worsens after use. (E, 8, M)

17. 3. The nurse needs to inform the sister that there is a lag time of 2 to 4 weeks before a full clinical effect occurs with the drug. The nurse should let her know

that her brother will gradually get better and symptoms of depression will improve. Telling the sister that her brother is experiencing a very serious depression does not give the sister important information about the medication. Additionally, this statement may cause alarm and anxiety. Conveying the sister's concern to the physician does not provide her with the necessary information about the client's medication. Telling the sister that the client's medication may need to be changed is inappropriate because a full clinical effect occurs after 2 to 4 weeks. (I, 8, X)

18. 4. Symptoms of pregnancy-induced hypertension (PIH), such as hypertension and facial swelling, before 24 weeks' gestation and a fundal height larger than expected are suggestive of gestational trophoblastic disease or hydatidiform mole. This condition occurs when the trophoblasts develop abnormally. Ultrasound can confirm the condition. Medical management includes evacuation of the mole and follow-up to detect any malignant changes. Painless vaginal bleeding is suggestive of placenta previa. Fetal anemia is often caused by Rh sensitization. Clients with multifetal pregnancies may exhibit larger fundal heights than expected, but they usually do not have a brownish discharge or symptoms of PIH at this stage of gestation. (D, 9, O)

19. 1. Saying, "When you interrupt others, they leave the area," is most helpful because it serves to increase the client's awareness of how others view him by giving him specific feedback about his behavior. The other statements are punitive and authoritative, possibly threatening to the client, and likely to increase defensiveness, decrease self-worth, and increase feelings of guilt. (I, 6, X)

20. 4. The trough serum level should be drawn just before the administration of the next intravenous dose of gentamycin sulfate (Garamycin). (P, 8, M)

21. 1. Health-promoting strategies for clients with a history of cardiovascular disease requires knowledge in three areas: diet, exercise, and medication. Pain management and management of social activities are not usually features of health promotion activities for these clients. (D, 3, M)

22. 3. The child is exhibiting signs and symptoms of possible epiglottitis. As a result the child is at high risk for laryngospasm and airway occlusion. Therefore, the nurse should have a tracheostomy tube and setup readily available should the child experience an airway occlusion. Although acetaminophen is an antipyretic, the dosage of 600 mg to be administered rectally is too high. A typical 4-year-old weighs approximately 40 pounds. The recommended dose is 125 mg. When any type of respiratory illness, and especially epiglottitis, is suspected, putting any object, including a tongue depressor for inspection or a cotton-tipped applicator to obtain a throat culture, in the back of the mouth or throat or having the child open the mouth is inappropriate because doing so may predispose the child to laryngospasm or occlusion of the airway by a swollen epiglottis. (I, 10, Y)

23. 3. The client is exhibiting the side effects associated with lithium therapy that are temporary. Therefore, the nurse would continue the lithium and explain to the client that he or she is experiencing temporary side effects of lithium that will subside. Common side effects of lithium are nausea, dry mouth, diarrhea, thirst, mild hand tremor, weight gain, bloatedness, insomnia, and lightheadedness. Immediately notifying the physician about these common side effects is not necessary. (D, 8, X)

24. 1. Thyroid replacement is a lifelong maintenance therapy. The medication is usually given as one dose in the morning. It cannot be tapered or discontinued, because the client needs thyroid supplementation to maintain health. The medication cannot be discontinued after the TSH level is normal; the dose will be maintained at the level than normalizes the TSH concentration. (I, 8, M)

25. 4. A client who is beginning training for a tennis team would most likely require an adjustment in lithium dosage because excessive sweating can increase the serum lithium level, possibly leading to toxicity. Adjustments in lithium dosage would also be necessary when other medications have been added, when an illness with high fever occurs, and when a new diet begins. (P, 8, X)

26. 3. The most appropriate response is to continue all treatments and attempt to stabilize the client using fluid replacement without administering blood or blood products. It is imperative that the health care team respect the client's religious belief and wishes, even they are not those of the health care team. Discontinuing all measures is not an option. The health care team should continue to provide the best care possible and does not need to notify the attorney. (D, 1, M)

27. 2. Cystic fibrosis is the most common inherited disease in children. It is inherited as an autosomal recessive trait, meaning that the child inherits the defective gene from both parents. The chances are one in four for each of this couple's pregnancies. (P, 10, Y)

28. 3. Nitroglycerin in all dosage forms (sublingual, transdermal, or intravenous) should be shielded from light to prevent deterioration. Clients should be instructed to keep the nitroglycerin in the dark container that is supplied by the pharmacy, and it should not be removed or placed in any other container. (I, 8, M)

29. 3. Valproic acid (Depakene) causes sedation as well as nausea, vomiting, and indigestion. Sedation is important because the client needs to be cautioned about driving or operating machinery that could be dangerous while feeling sedated from the medication. Depakene does not cause an increase in urination, slowed thinking, or weight loss. However, some clients may experience weight gain. (P, 8, X)

30. 1. These effects and others when seen after birth are known as a cluster of symptoms called *fetal alcohol syndrome*. Vitamin B$_6$ and vitamin A deficiency can affect growth and development but not with these specific effects. Folic acid deficiency contributes to neural tube defects. (A, 7, M)

31. 4. NSAIDs are irritating to the gastric mucosa and should be taken with food. NSAIDs are usually taken once or twice daily. Joint exercise is not related to the drug administration. Antacids may interfere with the absorption of the drug. (I, 8, M)

32. 2. The client who drinks alcohol while taking disulfiram (Antabuse) will experience sweating, flushing of the neck and face, tachycardia, hypotension, a throbbing headache, nausea and vomiting, palpitations, dyspnea, tremor, and/or weakness. (A, 8, X)

33. 3. Holding the gauze pledget against an intramuscular injection site while removing the needle from the muscle avoids the discomfort of the needle pulling on the skin. (I, 8, M)

34. 3. Physical activity is gradually increased after a myocardial infarction while the client is still hospitalized and through a period of rehabilitation. The client is progressing too rapidly if activity significantly changes respirations, causing dyspnea, chest pain, a rapid heartbeat, or fatigue. When any of these symptoms appears, the client should reduce activity and progress more slowly. Edema suggests a circulatory problem that must be addressed but doesn't necessarily indicate overexertion. Cyanosis indicates reduced oxygen-carrying capacity of red blood cells and indicates a severe pathology. It is not appropriate to use cyanosis as an indicator for overexertion. Weight loss is indicative of several factors but not overexertion. (E, 10, M)

35. 3. When a client talks about not having a problem with alcohol, the nurse needs to point out how alcohol has gotten the client into trouble. Concrete, factual information is helpful in decreasing the client's denial that alcohol is a problem. The other approaches allow the client to use defense mechanisms, such as rationalization, projection, and minimization, to explain her actions. Therefore, these approaches are not helpful. (I, 6, X)

36. 3. Medicaid is state funded, with matching federal funds, and provides medical assistance for low-income persons without health insurance. The program for older adults is Medicare. (A, 1, M)

37. 3. Before development and implementation of the teaching plan, it is vital to determine what the client currently knows regarding diabetes and what the client needs to know. (P, 1, M)

38. 1. The goal of the education program is to instruct the client to take his or her pulse; therefore, the expected outcome would be the ability to give a return demonstration of palpation of the heart rate. (E, 9, M)

39. 3. PUBS is a useful procedure for diagnosing Rh disease, obtaining fetal complete blood count, and karyotyping chromosomes to evaluate for genetic disorders. Ultrasound commonly is used to detect twins. A lecithin–sphingomyelin ratio is the procedure of choice to diagnose fetal lung maturation. A maternal blood test is used to determine α-fetoprotein level. (I, 9, O)

40. 2. The client should report tinnitus, because vancomycin (Vancocin) can affect the acoustic branch of the eighth cranial nerve. Vancomycin does not affect the vestibular branch of the acoustic nerve; vertigo and ataxia would occur if the vestibular branch were involved. Muscle stiffness is not associated with vancomycin. (P, 8, M)

41. 4. Caffeinated beverages and alcohol should be avoided because they stimulate gastric acid production and irritate gastric mucosa. The client should avoid foods that cause discomfort; however, there is no need to follow a soft, bland diet. Eating six small meals daily is no longer a common treatment for peptic ulcer disease. Milk in large quantities is not recommended because it actually stimulates further production of gastric acid. (E, 7, M)

42. 3. When a client with a nasogastric tube exhibits abdominal distention, the nurse should first check the suction machine. If the suction equipment is functioning properly, then the nurse should take other steps, such as repositioning the tube or checking tube patency by irrigating it. If these steps are not effective, then the physician should be called. (I, 9, M)

43. 4. Increased, not decreased, body temperature resulting from occupations or infections can contribute to low sperm counts caused by decreased sperm production. Heat can destroy sperm. Varicocele, an abnormal dilation of the veins in the spermatic cord, is an associated cause of a low sperm count. The varicosity increases the temperature within the testes, inhibiting sperm production. Frequent use of saunas or hot tubs may lead to a low sperm count. The temperature of the scrotum becomes elevated, possibly inhibiting sperm production. Endocrine imbalances (eg, thyroid problems) are associated with low sperm counts in men

because of possible interference with spermatogenesis. (E, 7, O)

44. 1. The clinical findings of edema are consistent with fluid excess in the interstitial compartment. The extracellular compartment consists of fluid in two locations, the interstitial (tissue) spaces and plasma (intravascular) spaces. Fluid shifts within the extracellular compartment can occur either from the plasma space to the interstitial space, or from the interstitial space to the plasma space. When fluid shifts from the plasma space into the interstitial space, frequently as a result of abnormal retention of fluids in conditions such as congestive heart failure or renal failure, edema results. The intracellular compartment consists of fluid within the cells. (D, 10, M)

45. 1. Low potassium can cause imbalance at the cellular level that leads to dysrythmias and cardiac arrest. Hyperglycemia is caused by elevated blood sugar. Hypertension is unrelated to potassium levels. Increased energy is unrelated to potassium levels. (A, 9, M)

46. 2. Handwashing with the correct technique is the best method for preventing cross-contamination. The hands do serve as a source of infection. Waterless commercial products containing at least 60% alcohol are as effective for killing organisms as handwashing. (P, 2, M)

47. 3. The third maneuver is used to identify the presenting part. While facing the client, the nurse places the tips of the first three fingers on the side of the woman's abdomen above the symphysis pubis and palpates deeply around the presenting part to identify its contour and size. The first maneuver involves using the tips of the fingers of both hands to palpate the uterine fundus. This maneuver is used to identify the part of the fetus that lies over the inlet to the pelvis. The second maneuver identifies the back of the fetus, and the fourth maneuver identifies the cephalic prominence. (A, 10, O)

48. 2. The stored glucose of muscle glycogen is the major fuel during sustained activity. Glucose production slows as the body begins to depend on fat stores for glucose and fatty acids. Protein is not the body's preferred energy source. Fat is a secondary source of energy. Water is not an energy source, although sufficient water is required to engage in aerobic activity without causing dehydration. (D, 4, M)

49. 3. Fluctuation of fluid with respirations in the water-seal column indicates that the system is functioning properly. If an obstruction were present in the chest tube, fluid fluctuation would be absent. Subcutaneous emphysema occurs when air pockets can be palpated beneath the client's skin around the chest tube insertion site. A leak in the system is indicated when bubbling occurs in the water-seal column. (E, 10, M)

50. 4. It is important to dry the feet carefully after a bath to prevent a fungal infection. Diabetic clients should seek medical attention when they injure their toes or feet to prevent complications. Iodine is highly toxic to the tissues. Diabetic clients should inspect their feet on a daily basis and should wear shoes that support their feet while in the house. (I, 10, M)

51. 2. Diverticular rupture causes peritonitis from the release of intestinal contents (chemicals and bacteria) into the peritoneal cavity. A rigid abdominal wall results from a diverticular cavity. The inflammatory response of the peritoneal tissue produces severe abdominal rigidity and pain, diminished intestinal motility, and retention of intestinal contents (air, fluid, and stool). Hyperactive bowel sounds, explosive diarrhea, and excessive flatulence do not indicate peritonitis. (A, 10, M)

52. 1. The nurse should firmly yet gently strike the chest wall with the hand cupped to make a hollow popping sound. A slapping sound indicates that an incorrect technique is being used. The area over the rib cage is percussed to loosen mucus from the underlying lung passages. The child should wear a thin piece of clothing (eg, T-shirt) over the chest area to protect the skin without diminishing the effect of the percussion. (I, 9, Y)

53. 1. The nurse should call to the desk to ask for assistance. The nurse needs to notify the doctor of the client's death and the family must then be notified. A code should not be called. Nursing personnel should begin postmortem care so that the family does not walk in unannounced to find their loved one deceased and looking disarrayed. (D, 1, M)

54. 2. One pound of weight is approximately equivalent to 3500 calories. Removing 1000 calories per day results in a 2-pound weight loss per week (7000 calories divided by 7 days). If a client wanted to lose 1 pound in a 7-day period, he would need to cut out 500 calories per day (3500 calories divided by 7 days). It is unsafe to try to lose more than 2 pounds per week. (D, 4, M)

55. 1. The nurse should instruct the client to take the medication immediately or as soon as she remembers that she missed the medication. There is only a slight risk that the client will become pregnant when only one pill has been missed, so there is no need to use another form of contraception. However, if the client wishes to increase the chances of not getting pregnant, a condom can be used by the male partner. The client should not omit the missed pill and then restart the medication in the morning because there is a possibility that ovulation can occur, after which intercourse could result in pregnancy. Taking two pills is not necessary and also will result in putting the client off her schedule. (I, 8, O)

56. 1. Pain disorder is a somatoform disorder involving severe pain in one or more anatomic sites causing severe distress or impaired function. The statement, "I need to have a good cry about all the pain I've been in and then not dwell on it," indicates improvement because the client has a realistic view of the physical symptoms and pain and is willing to let them go and move on. The other statements indicate the continued presence of denial, lack of insight, and the need for symptoms to manage anxiety. (I, 6, X)

57. 4. The nurse needs to collect additional information about the client's complaint of hearing voices. Assessing the content of hallucinations is essential to determine whether they are command hallucinations that the client might act on. Asking about what the neighbor has been doing or telling the client that the neighbor won't visit indirectly reinforces the delusion about the neighbor. Although determining the onset and duration of the voices is important, the nurse needs to assess the content of the hallucinations first. (I, 6, X)

58. 3. A client with severe diarrhea loses large amounts of bicarbonate, resulting in metabolic acidosis. Metabolic alkalosis does not result in this situation. Diarrhea does not affect the respiratory system. (A, 10, M)

59. 4. Serum osmolality indicates the water balance of the body. A normal plasma osmolality between 275 and 295 mOsm/kg would indicate that the fluid volume excess has been resolved. A weight reduction of 10% may not necessarily return the client to a state of normal serum osmolality. Clients with excess fluid volume do not necessarily have pain or abnormal arterial blood gas values. (E, 10, M)

60. 3. Exactly why rheumatic fever follows a streptococcal infection is not known, but it is theorized that an antigen–antibody response occurs to an M protein present in certain strains of streptococci. The antibodies developed by the body attack certain tissues, such as in the heart and joints. Antistreptolysin O (ASO) titer findings show elevated or rising antibody levels. This blood finding is the most reliable evidence indicating a streptococcal infection. (A, 9, Y)

61. 3. The nurse should call the surgeon's office so that arrangements can be made for the client to donate a unit of his blood for possible future autotransfusion. This must be done in sufficient time before surgery so that the client is not at risk for being anemic at the time of the scheduled procedure. The client's request must be scheduled through the surgeon's office because the surgeon has ultimate responsibility for the client. The nurse can document that the surgeon's office was notified of the client's request.

Notifying the hematology laboratory would not be an appropriate response. (P, 8, M)

62. 1. High colonic irrigation can increase the risk of perforation in a distended and inflamed colon. Tapwater is hypotonic in the bowel and would draw increased fluid into the area. The other orders are part of standard preparation for intestinal surgery. (I, 9, M)

63. 3. The most appropriate intervention is to offer the client frequent mouth care to moisten the dry oral mucosa. Reexplaining why the client cannot drink may be helpful but will not relieve her thirst. Ice chips cannot be given to a client who is NPO. Diverting the client's attention does not treat her basic complaint. (I, 7, M)

64. 2. This client is demonstrating classic symptoms of hypothyroidism. Primary hypothyroidism results from pathologic changes in the thyroid gland. In this case, the thyroid gland is unable to secrete sufficient amounts of thyroid hormone, leading to a decrease in cellular metabolic activity, decreased oxygen consumption, and decreased heat production. Cushing's disease is manifested by a "buffalo hump," moonface, hypertension, fatigability, and weakness, resulting from the inappropriate release of cortisol. Hyperthyroidism, or Grave's disease, is manifested by increased appetite with weight loss, increased anxiety, hand tremors, palpitations, heat intolerance, and insomnia. A pituitary tumor can manifest in a wide variety of symptoms, depending on the location. (D, 9, M)

65. 3. After the symptoms of puberty, such as increased hair growth and enlargement of the breasts, are noticed, menstruation typically begins within 30 months. (I, 3, O)

66. 2. Epstein's pearls are tiny, hard, white nodules found in the mouth of some neonates. They are considered normal and usually disappearing without treatment. Koplik's spots, associated with measles in children, are patchy and bright red with a bluish-white speck in the middle. Precocious teeth are actual teeth that some neonates have at birth. Usually only one or two teeth are present. *Candida albicans* or thrush is not apparent in the mouth immediately after birth but may appear a day or two later. This infection is manifested by yellowish-white spots or lesions that resemble milk curds and bleed when attempts are made to wipe them away. (I, 3, O)

67. 1. An adequate circulatory status is the most important factor for supporting the healing process of an infected decubitus ulcer. Blood flow to the area must be present to bring nutrients and prescribed antibiotics to the tissues. A fluid intake of 2000 to 3000 mL/day, if not contraindicated, is recommended to provide hydration to the client's tissues. (P, 10, M)

68. 2. The nurse's initial response would be to withhold the digoxin (Lanoxin). The nurse should then notify the physician if the apical pulse is 60 bpm or lower because of the potential for digoxin toxicity. The charge nurse does not need to be notified, but the nurse does need to document the notification and follow-up in the chart. (A, 8, M)

69. 2. In an emergency delivery where the neonate's head is already crowning, the first action by the nurse should be to check for the presence of a cord around the neonate's neck. If the cord present, the nurse should gently remove it from the neck. The client should be told to breathe gently and avoid forceful bearing-down efforts, which could lead to lacerations. Although blood and bodily fluid precautions are always present in client care, this is an emergency. If at all possible, the nurse should don gloves. Suctioning of the mouth can be done once the nurse has checked to ensure that the cord is not around the neonate's neck. Telling the mother that help is on the way is not reassuring, because emergency medical technicians may take some time to arrive. Delivery is imminent because the neonate's head is crowning. (I, 9, O)

70. 2. The ulna will heal in approximately 12 weeks. The femur takes approximately 24 weeks to heal because of the size of the bone and the muscle forces exerted on the femur. Skeletal traction does not delay healing but can actually promote healing by properly aligning the fracture. (P, 10, M)

71. 2. The client needs to know that there is a cause for the delirium, that there is hope for treatment, and that medications can help decrease anxiety. Giving medications can help the anxiety, but the client also needs an explanation about the condition. Saying that the more the client worries, the worse the delirium will get is inappropriate and most likely would add to the client's level of anxiety. (I, 6, X)

72. 1. The client understands the instructions when she says she should avoid contact sports because they may result in injury to the client and/or the fetus. Learning to ski while pregnant is not recommended because injury may occur. Scuba diving should be avoided because depth pressures could cause fetal damage. Hot tubs should be avoided during the first trimester because sitting in them can result in fetal hyperthermia and fetal hypoxia. Mild exercises, such as walking, can help strengthen the muscles and prevent some discomforts, such as backache. (E, 3, O)

73. 1. Cardiogenic shock is a negative outcome of a myocardial infarction that involves a significant amount of cardiac tissue. Lack of blood and oxygen leads to death of the contractile elements of the tissue, resulting in pump failure. Hypovolemic shock results

from blood loss. Neurogenic shock results from loss of sympathetic tone. Metabolic acidosis is commonly caused by uncontrolled diabetes mellitus. (P, 10, M)

74. 4. Third-degree heart block occurs when the atrial stimuli are blocked at the atrioventricular junction. Impulses from the atria and ventricles are conducted independently of each other. The atrial rate is 60 to 100 bpm; the ventricular rate is usually 10 to 60 bpm. (A, 10, M)

75. 1. The nurse should call the oncology unit to institute a transfer. The nurse handling chemotherapy agents should be specifically trained. It is an unwise use of nursing resources to send a nurse from one unit to administer medications to a client on another unit. It is better to centralize and send the clients who need chemotherapy to one unit. Even if the pharmacy mixes the agent, the drug must be administered by a nurse who is trained to do so. (D, 1, M)

76. 2. After surgery, the most important nursing diagnosis should be Risk for Infection. Surgery involves an incision, which is at risk for infection. The infant with this type of procedure does have discomfort, which can be relieved with acetaminophen. Pain would be an important nursing diagnosis but not the priority. The infant may be in arm restraints or have the cuff of the sleeve pinned to the diaper or pants. It is important that the infant not touch the incision line or disrupt the sutures. There is no indication of Impaired Parenting. The parents would be reacting normally with a first reaction of shock. (D, 10, Y)

77. 1. An appropriate expected outcome for clients with rheumatoid arthritis is that they will adopt self-care behaviors to manage their joint pain, stiffness, and fatigue and be able to perform their activities of daily living. ROM exercises can help maintain mobility, but it may not be realistic to expect to be able to maintain full ROM. Depending on the disease progression, there may be further development of pain and joint deformity, even with appropriate therapy. It is important for clients to understand the importance of taking their prescribed drug therapy even if their symptoms have abated. (E, 9, M)

78. 4. Hydrotherapy wound cleansing is very painful for the client. The client should be medicated for pain about 30 minutes before the treatment in anticipation of the increased pain the client will experience. Wounds are debrided but excessive fluids are not lost during the hydrotherapy session. However, electrolyte loss can occur from open wounds during immersion, so the sessions should be limited to 20 to 30 minutes. There is no need to limit food or fluids 45 minutes before hydrotherapy, unless it is an individualized need for a given client. Topical antibiotics are applied after the therapy, not before submersion in the water. (P, 9, M)

79. 1. Hepatitis B immune globulin is given as prophylactic therapy to individuals who have been exposed to hepatitis B. Interferon has been approved to treat hepatitis B. Hepatitis B surface antigen is a diagnostic test used to detect current infection. Amphotericin B is an antifungal antibiotic. (P, 8, M)

80. 1. When examining the tympanic membrane of a child younger than 3 years of age, the nurse should pull the pinna down and back. For an older child, the nurse should pull the pinna up and back to view the tympanic membrane. (A, 9, Y)

81. 3. In the compensatory stage of shock, the client will exhibit moderate tachycardia. If the shock continues to the progressive stage, decreased urinary output, hypotension, and mental confusion will develop as a result of failure to perfuse and ineffective compensatory mechanisms. These findings are indications that the body's compensatory mechanisms are failing. (A, 9, M)

82. 2. Hydrochlorothiazide is a thiazide diuretic. Muscle weakness can be an indication of hypokalemia. Polyuria is associated with this diuretic, not urinary retention. Confusion and diaphoresis are not side effects of hydrochlorothiazide. (E, 8, M)

83. 1. The ability to remember an old song is related to long-term memory, which persists after short-term memory is lost. Therefore, the nurse would respond by providing the son with this information. Stating that the nurse is happy to hear about the change and that the client is getting better is inappropriate and inaccurate. This statement ignores the issue of long-term versus short-term memory. Telling the client not to get his hopes up because the improvement is only temporary is inappropriate. The information provided does not indicate that the client has expressive aphasia, which would be suggested by the statement that the client can't talk to the son. (I, 6, X)

84. 1. A specimen for culture and sensitivity should be sent to the laboratory promptly so that a smear can be taken before organisms start to grow in the specimen. (I, 9, M)

85. 1. The client is in a crisis and has a high anxiety level. Holding the client's hands and encouraging the client to slow down and take a deep breath conveys caring and helps decrease anxiety. Telling the client to calm down or stop worrying offers no concrete directions for accomplishing this task. It is unknown from the data who was at fault in the accident. Therefore, it would be inappropriate for the nurse to state that it wasn't the client's fault. (I, 6, X)

86. 3. Many women who acquire gonorrhea are asymptomatic or experience mild symptoms that are easily ignored. They are not necessarily more reluctant than men to seek medical treatment, but they are more likely

not to realize they have been affected with a disease. Gonorrhea is easily transmitted to all women and can result in serious consequences such as pelvic inflammatory disease and infertility. (I, 2, M)

87. 4. Tingling and numbness of the toes would be the earliest indication of circulatory impairment. Inability to move the toes and cyanosis are later indicators. Complaints of cast tightness should be investigated, because cast tightness can lead to circulatory impairment; it is not, however, an indicator of impairment. (A, 9, M)

88. 3. The nurse notifies the physician because a drooping of one side of the face or a "one-side cry" is associated with facial nerve damage. Additionally, the mother's delivery record and history need to be reviewed for a possible cause. Craniotabes is a softening of the skull bones. The bones are so soft that indentation from the pressure of an examining finger can occur. Meningitis, or inflammation of the meninges, is associated with a rigid neck. Other symptoms may include lethargy, poor sucking reflexes, weak cry, seizures, and apnea. Skull fracture is not associated with a drooping facial appearance. Rather, it would be evidenced by a crack in the skull bone, possibly accompanied by leaking cerebrospinal fluid. (D, 9, O)

89. 3. The client should be encouraged to report any painful urination or urinary retention. Lesions are usually present for 17 to 20 days. The client is capable of transmitting the infection even when asymptomatic, so a barrier contraceptive should be used. Forcing fluids will not stop the lesions from forming. (I, 2, M)

90. 2. Severe hypoperfusion to all vital organs results in failure of the vital functions and then circulatory collapse. Hypotension, anuria, respiratory distress, and acidosis are other symptoms associated with irreversible shock. The client in irreversible shock will not be alert. (P, 10, M)

91. 1. Pulmonary embolism is a potentially life-threatening complication of deep vein thrombosis. The client's change in mental status, tachypnea, and tachycardia are all indicative of a possible pulmonary embolism. The nurse should promptly notify the doctor of the client's condition. Administering a sedative without further evaluation of the client's condition is not appropriate. There is no need to elicit a positive Homan's sign; the client is already diagnosed with a deep vein thrombosis. Increasing the intravenous flow rate may be an appropriate action, but not without first notifying the physician. (I, 9, M)

92. 3. The nurse should always double-check a large dose of insulin before administering it. A nurse should always listen to the client; if a client who has been tak-

ing insulin for a long time suggests that the insulin dose is not right, the nurse should recheck the physician's order. Comparing insulin doses of other clients has no bearing on a particular client's dose. The nurse should not use "U" or "u"; the nurse should specify "unit" to avoid errors. (I, 1, M)

93. 2. Coping with the chronic tinnitus of Ménière's disease can be very frustrating. Providing background sound, such as music, can help camouflage the low-pitched, roaring sound of tinnitus. Maintaining a quiet environment can make the sounds of tinnitus more pronounced. Avoiding caffeine and nicotine is recommended, because this can decrease the occurrence of the tinnitus. However, avoiding these substances does not help the client with coping with tinnitus when it occurs. Taking a sedative does not effect the sounds of the tinnitus. (I, 10, M)

94. 2. The child's signs and symptoms in conjunction with the acute onset suggest possible croup or epiglottitis. The priority diagnosis at this time would be Risk for Injury. The airway may become completely occluded by the epiglottis at any time. Although the child is probably experiencing fear and anxiety, and impaired gas exchange may occur with continued respiratory distress, the immediate priority is a patent airway. No evidence is provided to support aspiration and ineffective airway clearance. (D, 10, Y)

95. 1. In emphysema, the client's lungs lose elasticity and only partially deflate. Air is trapped in the alveoli. As a result of these pathologic changes, the amount of air remaining in the lungs after forced expiration (residual volume) is increased and the amount of air that can be forcibly exhaled (forced expiratory volume) is decreased. Total lung capacity is increased owing to hyperinflation of the lungs. The maximum amount of air that can be exhaled after maximum inhalation (vital capacity) is decreased. (A, 10, M)

96. 4. Diabetic retinopathy involves background and proliferative retinopathy. Both forms are associated with vascular changes in the basement membrane of the arterioles and capillaries of the choroid and retina. Neuropathy is usually associated with the lower extremities. (E, 9, M)

97. 2. The 70-year-old woman with syncopal episodes is at greatest risk for falling. The nurse should assess the client's gait and balance and the syncopal episodes. The 22-year-old man with upper body fractures and the 50-year-old man with angina are not fall risks. The 30-year-old woman could be at risk of falling, but she is at less risk than the 70-year-old client with syncope. (A, 1, M)

98. 3. The baseline laboratory data that are established before a client is started on t-PA or alteplase recombi-

nant (Activase) include hematocrit, hemoglobin, and platelet count. (A, 9, M)

99. 3. The most appropriate long-term goal is for the client with hypertension to commit to lifelong therapy. A significant problem in the long-term management of hypertension is client compliance with the treatment plan. It is essential that the client understand the reasons for modifying lifestyle, taking prescribed medications, and obtaining regular health care. Limiting stress, losing weight, and monitoring blood pressure are important aspects of care for clients with hypertension; however, the treatment plan must be individualized to include aspects of care that are appropriate for each client. (P, 4, M)

100. 1. The nurse should work with the patient to individualize the care plan for managing the client's pain. Cancer pain is best managed with a combination of medications, and each client needs to be worked with individually to find the treatment regimen that works best. Cancer pain is frequently undertreated because of fear of addiction. Clients who are experiencing pain need the appropriate level of analgesic and need to be reassured that they will not become addicted. Cancer pain is best treated with regularly scheduled doses of medication. Administering the medication only when the client asks for it will not lead to adequate pain control. As drug tolerance develops, the dosage of the medication can be increased. (P, 9, M)

101. 4. The client needs further instructions when she says, "I can continue to work at my job at the automobile factory until labor starts." The goal is to avoid preterm labor. Because the client is experiencing severe hydramnios, she will most likely be maintained on bed rest to increase uteroplacental circulation and reduce pressure on the cervix. Hydramnios has been associated with increase weight gain caused by the increased amniotic fluid volume. Hydramnios has been associated with gastrointestinal disorders in the fetus, such as tracheoesophageal fistula with stenosis or intestinal obstruction. The client should continue to eat high-fiber foods and should avoid straining, which could lead to ruptured membranes. Stool softeners may also be ordered. The client should report any symptoms of fluid rupture or labor. (E, 9, O)

102. 1. The stationary bicycle would be the most appropriate training modality because it is a non–weight-bearing exercise. Interval training involves rest and exercise. The time that the individual exercises on the stationary bicycle is increased with improved functional capacity, and the rest time is decreased. (P, 3, M)

103. 1. Nausea and anorexia, and in some situations weight loss, are symptoms experienced by clients with jaundice. Jaundice is associated with high levels of bilirubin in the blood. Causes include hepatitis, yellow fever, and alcoholism. The nursing diagnoses of Pain related to muscle spasms and Ineffective Health Maintenance are not supported by the data. Adult Failure to Thrive is a possible diagnosis; however, more data would be needed to support it. (P, 10, M)

104. 1. The protocol recommended by the Agency for Healthcare Research and Quality is that all clients who are at risk for pressure ulcer development be identified on admission to health care facilities so that preventive actions can be implemented by the nursing staff. These preventive actions need to be individualized to the client, so automatic placement of all at-risk clients on an every-2-hour turning schedule, a specialty bed, or a high-protein, high-carbohydrate diet is not appropriate. (I, 9, M)

105. 3. Visual disturbances are a symptom of digitalis toxicity. These disturbances can include double, blurred, or yellow vision. Cardiovascular manifestations of digitalis toxicity include bradycardia, tachycardia, other dysrhythmias, and pulse deficit. Gastrointestinal symptoms include anorexia, nausea, and vomiting. (I, 8, M)

106. 2. Irradiated skin can become dry and irritated, resulting in itching and client discomfort. The client should be instructed to cleanse the skin gently and apply nonperfumed, nonirritating lotions to help relieve the dryness. Taking an antihistamine does not relieve the skin dryness that is causing the itching. Heat should not be applied to the area, because it can cause further irritation. Medicated ointments, especially corticosteroid ointment, which is controversial, should not be applied to the skin without the order of the radiation therapist. (E, 9, M)

107. 3. Serotonin, a principal neurotransmitter and appetite suppressant, is produced in the brain from tryptophan. Epinephrine and norepinephrine are made from tyrosine. Phenylalanine is an amino acid found in food. (A, 3, M)

108. 3. The mask is too small and is obstructing the nose. Masks that are too large may cover the eyes. Masks should fit snugly against the cheeks and chin. (E, 1, Y)

109. 4. In preparation for a thoracentesis the client should be asked to sit forward and place arms on the bedside table for support. This position provides access to the chest wall and intercostal spaces for insertion of the needle. The supine, Sims', or prone position would not provide adequate access to the chest wall or separate the intercostal spaces sufficiently for needle insertion. (P, 9, M)

110. 4. The anecdote for heparin is 1% protamine sulfate. Vitamin K is the anecdote for warfarin (Coumadin), an oral anticoagulant. Thrombin is a topical anticoagulant. (I, 8, M)

111. 1. At this time, the client's anger is not out of control, so empathy and talking are appropriate to diffuse the anger. Using "time-out" is appropriate when the client's anger is escalating and the client is no longer able to talk about the anger rationally. Restraints are appropriate only when there is imminent risk of harm to self or others. Future strategies are discussed after the initial incident is resolved. (I, 6, X)

112. 2. The client with myasthenia gravis may have impaired ability to swallow. Blood draining down the back of the throat may be aspirated if swallowing is impaired. This client may have an impaired breathing pattern due to weak intercostal muscles; however, the priority is to prevent aspiration. The diagnosis of Risk for Injury is not specific enough in this situation. There are no data to support the diagnosis of Self-Care Deficit. (P, 10, M)

113. 1. The nurse's first action after the removal of a nasogastric tube is to provide the client with oral hygiene. It would then be appropriate to give the client liquids to drink if the client is no longer NPO. There is no association between removal of a nasogastric tube and having the client cough and deep-breathe. Auscultating the client's bowel sounds should be done before removal of the tube, not afterward. (I, 7, M)

114. 3. Heat applications cause vasodilation, which promotes circulation to the area, and increase tissue metabolism and leukocyte mobility. Heat applications do not prevent swelling; applications of cold are used to prevent swelling by causing vasoconstriction. (P, 9, M)

115. 1. Thick, cloudy amniotic fluid is indicative of an intrauterine infection. Typically, the client has a fever, lethargy, and malaise. Greenish-colored amniotic fluid is associated with meconium staining. A strong yellowish color of amniotic fluid is associated with erythroblastosis fetalis, because of the presence of bilirubin and hemolyzed red blood cells. The normal color of amniotic fluid is clear or with a very slight yellow tint later in pregnancy. (D, 9, O)

116. 3. When finishing a 24-hour urine collection, the final voided urine is saved and added to the collection container. The first urine specimen, voided at 7 AM Monday, is discarded. The urine is not sent for a urine culture. It is not necessary to separate each day's collection of urine. (I, 7, M)

117. 2. Hypoalbuminemia occurs in cirrhosis because the liver cannot synthesize albumin. This causes a decrease in colloidal osmotic pressure, resulting in ascites. Hyperkalemia is not an expected electrolyte imbalance of cirrhosis. The AST and ALT values are increased in liver disease. (A, 10, M)

118. 2. At this time, the infant can be given the DTaP and IPV, but not live vaccines. The fact that the child's sibling is immunosuppressed because of chemotherapy

would alert the nurse not to give a live vaccine. The fact that the child has a cold is not grounds for delaying the immunizations. However, if the child had a fever, the immunizations would be delayed. (I, 4, Y)

119. 3. The primary cause of disability and death in children is injury from accidents. Teaching safety measures to children and parents is the best way to decrease injury and accidents. (P, 2, Y)

120. 1. A major goal of postoperative care for the client who has had an incisional cholecystectomy is the prevention of respiratory complications. Because of the location of the incision, the client has a difficult time breathing deeply. Performing leg exercises each shift is not frequent enough; they should be performed hourly. Maintaining a weight reduction diet may be appropriate for the client, but it is not the highest priority in the immediate postoperative phase. Promoting wound healing is important, but respiratory complications are most common after a cholecystectomy. (I, 9, M)

121. 1. In response to hearing a noise, normally hearing infants blink or startle and stop body movements. Shy and withdrawn behaviors are characteristic of older children with hearing impairment. Squealing occurs in 90% of infants by 4 months of age. The majority of infants are able to say "da-da" by 9 months of age. (A, 3, Y)

122. 3. Continuous irrigation, usually consisting of sterile normal saline, is used after a TURP to keep blood clots from obstructing the catheter and impeding the flow of urine. Antibiotics may be instilled in a bladder with the use of an irrigating solution, but this is not the primary reason for using continuous irrigation in TURP. The irrigating solution may secondarily help prevent bladder distention because it keeps the catheter from becoming obstructed. (P, 7, M)

123. 3. A distended bladder produces a dullness when percussed because of the presence of urine. Hyperresonance is a percussion sound that is present in hyperinflated lungs. Tympany, a loud drum-like sound, occurs over gas-filled areas such as the intestines. Flat sounds occur over very dense tissue that has no air present. (A, 10, M)

124. 2. Major accidents can induce feelings similar to those of victims of other kinds of disasters and crime. Therefore, the nurse calls the crisis nurse to assist the passengers with their feelings of victimization. Passengers may mourn the loss of a vacation, but, with no fatalities, major grief reactions are not expected. Other personnel can take calls from relatives while the crisis nurse helps the passengers. Psychiatric hospitalization is a premature assumption. (P, 6, X)

125. 1. When placed on the abdomen, a neonate pulls the legs up under the body, which puts tension on the per-

ineum. Therefore, after surgery, the neonate should be positioned either supine with the legs suspended at a 90-degree angle or on either side with the hips elevated. (P, 10, Y)

126. 1. The child with meningococcal meningitis requires droplet precautions for at least the first 24 hours after effective therapy is initiated to reduce the risk of transmission to others on the unit. Once the child has been placed on droplet precautions, other actions, such as taking the child's vital signs, asking about medication allergies, and inquiring about the health of siblings at home, can be performed. (P, 2, Y)

127. 1. Teenagers usually enjoy activities with peers in preference to socializing with their parents or siblings. Peer relationships help the adolescent develop self-identity. (P, 3, Y)

128. 2. Morphine can cause urinary retention. The nurse should assess the client for urinary hesitancy or retention, and note the urinary output. It is not necessary to take the apical heart rate after each dose of morphine. Mental status should be assessed after each dose, because morphine can cause such effects as sedation, delirium, and disorientation. Assessing for pedal edema is not a necessity. (A, 8, M)

129. 2. Pain is a priority problem for the client with renal calculi. The pain is typically described as excruciating and intermittent, occurring as the stone moves. Analgesics are a major part of therapy. Activity Intolerance is secondary to the excruciating pain. Although the client experiences occasional nausea, there are no data to support a diagnosis of Deficient Fluid Volume or Imbalanced Nutrition. (D, 10, M)

130. 4. Infection would be of the greatest concern to the nurse. Infection occurs more frequently because of the number of procedures performed on patients that require this therapy and people they come in contact with in the hospital. Infection can be reduced if proper infection control techniques are used and human contact is reduced. Deficiencies and toxicities of nutrients are rare because of the use of standard protocols and orders for TPN formulas. Hyperglycemia can occur with TPN administration; however, all clients receiving TPN have their serum glucose concentration monitored frequently, and the hyperglycemia can easily be managed by adding insulin to the TPN solution. An infection is a much more serious complication. (A, 8, M)

131. 2. The nurse should assess for signs of impending shock, such as diaphoresis. The client would have hypotension, dysuria, and cool skin. (A, 9, M)

132. 2. The urinary appliance should be emptied before the pouch is one-third full in order to prevent urinary reflux. The appliance should be attached to a leg bag at night to allow for adequate drainage. It is not appropriate to administer prophylactic antibiotics when incorporating positive self-care activities into the client's routine can prevent most urinary tract infections. The urinary appliance is not changed daily. If no leakage occurs and the client's skin remains free of irritation, the appliance can be left in place for a week or more. (P, 7, M)

133. 1. Preoxygenating the client before suctioning helps prevent the development of hypoxia during the procedure. The suction catheter is inserted about 5 to 6 inches into the cannula. A bolus of 3 to 5 mL of sterile normal saline may be inserted into the cannula before suctioning to stimulate coughing and loosen secretions. The nurse uses sterile technique when suctioning a client. (I, 7, M)

134. 3. Because the toddler has a severe diaper rash, it may be best to change all that the parents are doing. The buttocks need to be washed thoroughly with mild soap and dried well. In fact, it is helpful to leave the diaper off and expose the buttocks to the air. Baby wipes frequently contain additives and perfumes that may be irritating to the baby's sensitive skin. The diaper needs to be changed more often than every 4 to 6 hours. Otherwise, the moist diaper environment will continue to irritate the already irritated area, causing the rash to worsen. Powder has limited absorbing ability and will most likely irritate the already irritated area. In addition, some powders contain perfumes or are scented and can irritate the skin. (I, 7, Y)

135. 2. The toddler is screaming for a reason, so it is most therapeutic to ask the mother why the child is screaming. This type of question is nonaccusatory, just seeking information. Asking the mother what happened between her and the child makes the assumption that something did happen and limits the amount of information to be gained from the question. Asking whether something caused the child to be upset makes an assumption that something happened and limits the answer to a yes or no response, cutting off communication. Asking whether the mother has tried to calm the child is accusatory and also limits the response to yes or no, thus cutting off communication. (I, 3, Y)

136. 4. The client will need to avoid extremes of motion in the hip to avoid dislocation. The hip should not be flexed more than 90 degrees, internally rotated, or legs crossed. It is not possible to safely sit in the bathtub without flexing the hip beyond the recommended 90 degrees. The client can implement the prescribed exercise program at the time of discharge home. The client should take care not to stress the hip for 3 to 6 months after surgery. An elevated toilet seat will be necessary during the recovery from surgery. (E, 9, M)

137. 1. The common presenting symptoms vary greatly but most frequently include fever, malaise, sore throat, and lymphadenopathy. Skin rash, cold symptoms, abdominal pain, and weight loss are less common symptoms. (A, 10, Y)

138. 1. The nurse should place the nondominant hand above the symphysis pubis and the dominant hand at the umbilicus to palpate the fundus. This prevents uterine inversion and trauma, which can be very painful to the client. The nurse should ask the client to assume a supine, not side-lying, position with the knees flexed. The fundus can be palpated in this position and the perineal pads can be evaluated for lochia amounts. The fundus should be massaged gently if the fundus feels "boggy." Vigorous massaging may fatigue the uterus and cause it to become firm and then "boggy" again. The nurse should ask the client to void before fundal evaluation. A full bladder can cause discomfort to the client and can cause the uterus to be deviated to one side. (I, 3, O)

139. 2. A reactive nonstress test is a positive sign indicating that the fetus is doing well at this point in the pregnancy. For a nonstress test to be a reactive test, at least two accelerations (15 beats or more) of the fetal heart rate lasting at least 15 seconds must occur after movement. If the fetus were compromised, the nonstress test would demonstrate no accelerations in fetal heart rate; a contraction stress test would show fetal heart rate decelerations during simulated labor. Late decelerations are associated with a positive or abnormal contraction stress test. No accelerations in a 20-minute period during a nonstress test may mean that the fetus is sleeping; however, this is interpreted as a nonreactive nonstress test. (I, 9, O)

140. 3. Right-sided heart failure causes venous congestion resulting in such symptoms as peripheral (dependent) edema, splenomegaly, hepatomegaly, and neck vein distention. Intermittent claudication is associated with arterial occlusion. Dyspnea and crackles are associated with pulmonary edema, which occurs in left-sided heart failure. (A, 10, M)

141. 1. To help prevent flexion deformities, a client with rheumatoid arthritis should lie in a prone position in bed for about one-half hour several times a day. This positioning helps keep the hips and knees in an extended position and prevents joint flexion. Low Fowler's, modified Trendelenburg, and side-lying positions do not prevent hip flexion. (I, 7, M)

142. 2. Administration of an epidural anesthetic can result in a hypotensive effect on the maternal blood pressure. Therefore, the priority assessment is the mother's blood pressure. Ephedrine or wedging the client to a position to keep pressure off the vena cava, such as on the left side, can be used to elevate the maternal blood pressure should it drop too low. Epidural anesthesia has no effect on the level of consciousness or the client's cognitive function. Although the client's contraction pattern may decrease in frequency after administration of the anesthesia, the priority assessment is the client's blood pressure. Once the blood pressure is maintained, contractions can be assessed. (A, 8, O)

143. 1. The client's assessment findings indicate that the client is in the latent phase of the first stage of labor. Therefore, the nurse should plan to assist the client with comfort measures and breathing techniques to relieve the discomfort. The client is able to move around, walk, or ambulate at this phase of labor. If the client chooses to remain in bed, a left side-lying position provides the greatest perfusion. It is too early for the client to have an epidural anesthetic. Epidural anesthesia is usually administered when the cervix is dilated to 5 to 6 cm. The fetal heart rate is normal, so internal fetal monitoring is not warranted at this time. (P, 3, O)

144. 4. Hypokalemia is one of the most common causes of digitalis toxicity. It is essential that the nurse carefully monitor the potassium levels of clients taking digitalis preparations to avoid digitalis toxicity. Low serum potassium levels can cause cardiac dysrhythmias. (A, 8, M)

145. 1. Clients can develop a drug tolerance to meperidine that necessitates an increase in the dosage. Because the order states that the drug can be administered every 3 hours and the client continues to experience pain, it would be appropriate for the nurse to give the medication on this schedule. It would be inappropriate to urge the client to take the acetaminophen and codeine to prevent addiction. Addiction is a psychological condition in which a client is driven to take drugs for reasons that are not therapeutic. The client is in pain and her need for the meperidine is therapeutic. It is premature to request an increase in dosage, because the nurse has not yet administered the meperidine on the 3-hour time schedule. Although the client may obtain some relief from relaxation exercises, this alone is not sufficient to provide pain relief to the client. (I, 8, M)

146. 1. Infants at age 7 months are not capable of drinking from a cup without spilling. At age 6 months, infants can partially lift their weight on the hands, enjoy imitating sounds, and are developing separation anxiety. (A, 3, Y)

147. 3. According to Erikson, a child of 13 years is normally seeking to meet the need to develop personal identity. Personal values are a component of this identity. Developing a conscience is a component of achieving initiative during the preschool years. Developing a sense of competence is a component of achieving industry of the school-aged years. Developing a lifetime vocation

is a component of achieving generativity in adulthood. (D, 3, X)

148. 4. Cardiac myopathy means that the myocardium is weak and irritable. Amiodarone is an antiarrhythmic and acts directly on the cardiac cell membrane. In this situation, amiodarone would be used to increase the ventricular fibrillation threshold. Amiodarone is contraindicated in sinus node dysfunction, heart block, and severe bradycardia. (P, 10, M)

149. 1. A frothy, purulent vaginal discharge in a sexually active female client is typically caused by a sexually transmitted disease such as trichomonas. Other diseases, such as chlamydia, may also be present. Both the client and the boyfriend need treatment once the disease is determined. Normal variations in female vaginal discharge should be clear to white, not frothy or purulent. Clients should be instructed to wear cotton underwear and avoid pantyhose and tight-fitting garments such as jeans so that air can circulate. (D, 9, O)

150. 4. The single most common factor in skin breakdown is immobility. The right-sided paralysis, in which the client cannot perceive the need to change position and lacks control over the movement of the extremities, is the condition most likely to lead to skin breakdown. It is essential that the nurse plan to change the client's position at least every 2 hours. Nutritional status and urinary incontinence can contribute to skin breakdown, but neither is the most critical factor. Confusion does not directly influence skin breakdown. (P, 9, M)

151. 1. Psychomotor retardation refers to a general slowdown of motor activity commonly seen in a client with depression. Movements appear lethargic, energy is absent or lacking, and performance of activity is slow and difficult. A flat affect reflects a lack of emotion. An unkempt appearance reflects lack of self-care. Avoiding eye contact reflects low self-esteem or suspiciousness. (D, 6, X)

152. 3. A hydrocele, defined as fluid in the processus vaginalis, is determined when the scrotal sac can be transilluminated. A swelling in the scrotal area that can be reduced indicates an inguinal hernia. Both hydroceles and hernias can enlarge the scrotal sac, and both can be either unilateral or bilateral. A hernia typically is more obvious during crying. (D, 10, Y)

153. 1. When cleansing the skin around an incision and drain, the nurse should clean the incision and drain separately to avoid contaminating either wound. This is applying the principle of working from the least contaminated area to the most contaminated area. In this case, both areas are fresh wounds and should be kept separate. (I, 2, M)

154. 4. Any injury to the mouth results in copious amounts of blood because the mouth is a highly vascular area. Because the nurse does not know the mother and does not speak Spanish, the most appropriate action is to give the mother the ice and demonstrate what she is to do. The child will be less fearful if the ice is applied by the mother. Calling for an interpreter is appropriate after caring for the immediate need of the child. Grabbing the child away will probably upset the mother more, further adding to the stress experienced by the child. (I, 10, Y)

155. 4. Having the client deep-breathe hourly is the most appropriate action for the assistant to take to help prevent pulmonary complications. The client should be turned at least every 2 hours. Keeping the client's head elevated will not prevent pulmonary complications. Suctioning the client is not an assistant's responsibility, nor does it prevent pulmonary complications. (E, 1, M)

156. 3. When dextrose is abruptly discontinued, rebound hypoglycemia can occur. The nurse should assess the client for symptoms of hypoglycemia. Essential fatty acid deficiency is very unlikely to occur because some of these fatty acids are stored. Preventing dehydration or malnutrition is not the reason for tapering the infusion rate; the client's hydration and nutritional status and ability to maintain adequate intake must be established before the TPN is discontinued. (D, 8, M)

157. 1. During the third trimester, particularly in the seventh month of pregnancy, the client typically exhibits feelings of vulnerability and fear that the baby will be lost. Confirmation that the fetus is "real" occurs during the second trimester. Ambivalence is typically seen and resolved during the first trimester. Body image disturbance commonly occurs during the second trimester because of the profound changes that occur to the body during this time. (P, 5, O)

158. 2. As the dye is injected, the client may experience a feeling of warmth, flushing of the face, and a salty taste in the mouth. The client should not experience chest pain or cold chills; these would be adverse reactions warranting close monitoring of the client. (E, 9, M)

159. 4. Isoniazid competes for the available vitamin B_6 in the body and leaves the client risk for development of neuropathies related to vitamin deficiency. Supplemental B_6 is routinely prescribed to address this issue. Avoiding sun exposure is a preventive measure to lower the risk for skin cancer. Following a low-cholesterol diet lowers the individual's risk for atherosclerotic plaque development. Rest is important in maintaining homeostasis but has no real impact on neuropathies. (P, 8, M)

160. 2. The interpreter must have gotten delayed somewhere. Therefore, the nurse's best action would be to reschedule the child's appointment when the interpreter can be scheduled as well. Because the mother does not speak English, there is no point to having the pediatric nurse practitioner see the infant because history information is needed and most likely would be too difficult to obtain. Asking the mother to stay longer is rude to her. Also, doing so would probably be difficult because of the communication gap. Paging one more time is a desperate measure and inappropriate. (I, 1, Y)

161. 3. Oxygen concentrations greater than 40% have been found to cause oxygen toxicity in adults.(D, 8, M)

162. 1. Clients who continue on a progressive exercise program at home after a myocardial infarction should be taught to monitor their pulse rates. The pulse rate can be expected to increase with exercise, but exercise should not be increased if pulse rate increases more than about 25 bpm from baseline or exceeds 100 to 125 bpm. Clients should also be taught to decrease exercise if chest pain or dyspnea occurs. (I, 7, M)

163. 1. The nurse's response fails to identify the meaning in what the client has said. The nurse needs to explore the client's statement about hating God for that flood because the meaning of the client's statement is unclear. Also, clichés such as, "Don't feel that way," are not helpful because they ignore the client's feelings and his interpretation of the situation in which he finds himself. Explaining to the client why he may think as he does (ie, offering a rationale) indirectly argues the delusion and thus is inappropriate. The nurse's response fails to identify the meaning in what the client has said and does not add strength to the support systems. Retaining a delusion does not indicate that a client is solving his problems. (I, 5, X)

164. 3. The client who should be assessed first is the multigravid client who has been in labor for 8 hours and whose cervix is 8 cm dilated at 1+ station with contractions every 3 to 4 minutes. A multigravid client typically has a shorter labor than a primigravida, and this client's station is 1+, which means that delivery of the fetus is imminent. (A, 1, O)

165. 2. The nurse should contact the physician and clarify whether the client's usual insulin dose should be given before surgery. Practices vary, and it should not be assumed by the nurse that the usual insulin dose is to be given. It is not the nurse's responsibility to evaluate the client's need for insulin. It is not appropriate for the nurse to defer decision making on this issue until after surgery. (I, 9, M)

166. 4. Immediately after chest tube removal, a petrolatum gauze is placed over the wound and covered with a dry sterile dressing. This serves as an airtight seal to prevent air leakage or air movement in either direction. Bandages or straps are not applied directly over

wounds. Mesh gauze would allow air movement. (I, 2, M)

167. 4. By asking the client to tell more about how she is feeling, the nurse is not making any assumptions about what is troubling the client. The nurse should acknowledge the client's feelings and encourage her to discuss them. Saying that this situation must be frustrating involves assumptions by the nurse about why the client is crying and is not a therapeutic response. Asking how long the client has been unable to comb her hair takes the focus off her feelings and inhibits therapeutic communication. Inquiring why the client's husband hasn't helped insinuates that the husband is not helping enough, which is inappropriate, takes the focus off the client's feelings, and inhibits therapeutic communication. (I, 5, M)

168. 3. Encouraging the client to talk about why she is here and about her feelings may reveal more information about both what led her to come to the group and what led to her diagnosis. It also provides the nurse with valuable information needed to develop an appropriate plan of care. The comment that the client sounds angry presumes what the client is feeling and asks her to talk about her husband. The focus here should be on the client, not the husband. Telling the client that she will like coming to group imposes the nurse's view onto the client. The statement stresses that the group will be fun to be a part of instead of on its therapeutic value. Having the client tell the nurse something about the cause of her bulimia ignores the client's original statement. Additionally, this statement requires the client to have insight into the cause of her disease, which may not be possible at this time. Also, it may be too early in the relationship to discuss this disorder. (I, 6, X)

169. 1. Introduction of medication is the second step, in addition to continuing the lifestyle modifications. Exercise, smoking cessation, and weight reduction are part of the first steps involved in lifestyle modification. (I, 10, M)

170. 2. There is a direct interaction between the effects of insulin and those of β-blockers. The nurse must be aware that there is a potential for increased hypoglycemic effects of insulin when a β-blocker is added to the client's medication regimen. The client's blood sugar should be monitored. Ketoacidosis occurs in hyperglycemia. Although a decrease in the incidence of ketoacidosis could occur when a β-blocker is added, the direct result is an increase in the hypoglycemic effect of insulin. (A, 8, M)

171. 3. Frequently, when a child appears better, the parents stop the medication. Unfortunately, the infection remains. Therefore, the nurse needs to explain that all of the medication is needed to clear up the infection.

Explaining why the medicine should be continued is more helpful to parents than saying it needs to be given. Asking how the mother knows that her child's ears are better is blaming and would diminish the mother's self-esteem. Telling the mother that stopping the medication is not what is best for the child implies blame and is condescending. (I, 8, Y)

172. 4. The nurse should start the intravenous infusion pump at 67 mL/hour to administer 1 g of cefazolin (Ancef) in normal saline 50 mL over 45 minutes. (I, 8, M)

173. 1. Ambivalence is a common reaction, even when the pregnancy was planned. Manifested by conflicting feelings about the pregnancy, it usually resolves during the first trimester. There is no indication of disappointment. A statement such as, "I really don't want to be pregnant," would indicate disappointment. There is no indication that the client desires an abortion, although this is an option for the client. There is no reason to suspect that bonding will be a problem after delivery, unless the client shows no signs of wanting to care for the infant after delivery. (D, 5, O)

174. 2. Increasing estrogen levels during puberty are responsible for breast development. Prolactin is a hormone necessary for milk production during pregnancy and lactation. Progesterone maintains a pregnancy after conception. Testosterone is responsible for male sexual development during puberty. (I, 3, Y)

175. 1. Gastrointestinal hemorrhage occurs in about 25% of clients receiving prolonged mechanical ventilation. Other possible complications include incorrect ventilation, oxygen toxicity, fluid imbalance, decreased cardiac output, pneumothorax, infection, and atelectasis. Immunosuppression and pulmonary emboli are not direct consequences of mechanical ventilation. (A, 10, M)

176. 3. The nurse should encourage the client to sit down or lie down when he has angina. Nitroglycerin relaxes smooth muscles and dilates vascular beds; therefore, nitroglycerin causes hypotension and the client could fall, causing injury. Nitroglycerin should be stored in a dark container. It should be taken once every 5 minutes for three doses and is placed sublingually, not swallowed. (P, 10, M)

177. 2. Before giving information, it is important for the nurse to assess the learner's current level of knowledge. When dealing with parents of an ill child, the nurse considers their emotional strength and the intensity of the situation and deals with them in an accepting, nonthreatening manner. Parents may feel over-whelmed by the events, and they need time to adjust to the situation. (I, 5, Y)

178. 2. The IUD is suitable for clients who desire long-term contraceptive use and are in a monogamous relationship. Because of the increased risk of spread of infection with an IUD if an STD occurs, the device is not appropriate for women with multiple partners or history of STDs. Previous ectopic pregnancy is also a contraindication for an IUD, because the incidence of ectopic implantation is slightly higher. (I, 9, M)

179. 1. One of the main techniques used in crisis intervention in the hospital is helping parents begin to gain an intellectual understanding of SIDS. Numerous theories have been proposed, but no specific cause of SIDS has been identified. Evidence suggests that infants with SIDS have chronic hypoxia, possibly from prolonged periodic apnea. (E, 10, Y)

180. 2. Clients diagnosed with peripheral arterial occlusive disease should be encouraged to participate in a regular walking program to help develop collateral circulation. They should be advised to rest if pain develops and to resume activity when pain subsides. Extremities should be kept in a dependent position to promote circulation; elevation of the extremities will decrease circulation. Heating pads should not be used by anyone with impaired circulation, to avoid burns. Massaging the calf muscles will not decrease pain. Intermittent claudication subsides with rest. (I, 9, M)

181. 4. Toxoplasmosis is a protozoal infection caused by *Toxoplasma gondii*, which is transmitted through ingestion of raw or undercooked meat, through contact with infected cat feces, or across the placental barrier from the mother to the fetus. The mother should be instructed to cook all meats thoroughly, avoid touching the mucous membranes when handling raw meat, thoroughly clean all kitchen surfaces that have come in contact with raw meat, avoid uncooked eggs, and avoid contact with cat litter boxes and cat feces. The disease is not spread by contact with an infected person. Although prophylactic penicillin may be used for pregnant clients who test positive for group B streptococcus, penicillin is not used to treat toxoplasmosis. Toxoplasmosis may be treated with a combination of pyrimethamine (Daraprim) and sulfadiazine, accompanied by folic acid to reduce the toxicity of the other two drugs. However, controversy exists about whether to treat the mother. There is no vaccine for toxoplasmosis. Although a vaccine exists for rubella, this would be given not during pregnancy but within 72 hours postpartum if the client is not immune. (I, 4, O)

COMPREHENSIVE TEST 2

Select the one best answer, and indicate your choice by filling in the circle in front of the option.

1. The unit secretary who transcribes the physicians' orders asks the nurse to interpret an order because he cannot read the writing. The nurse's best action is to
   - ○ 1. interpret the order according to the client's previous medication record.
   - ○ 2. clarify the order with the pharmacist.
   - ○ 3. clarify the order by calling the physician.
   - ○ 4. clarify the client's medications with the client's family.

2. Propantheline bromide (Pro-Banthine) is ordered for a client who has cholecystitis. What is the primary purpose for administering this drug to clients who have cholecystitis?
   - ○ 1. To increase bile production.
   - ○ 2. To decrease biliary spasm.
   - ○ 3. To treat infection.
   - ○ 4. To relieve nausea.

3. The nurse refers the parents of a child with cystic fibrosis to the local chapter of the National Cystic Fibrosis Foundation. The Foundation has been especially beneficial for parents of children with cystic fibrosis by helping them
   - ○ 1. find tutors to educate their children at home.
   - ○ 2. obtain genetic counseling.
   - ○ 3. meet with other parents of children with cystic fibrosis for mutual support.
   - ○ 4. obtain financial assistance to purchase medications for their children.

4. After a bronchoscopy with biopsy, the nurse assesses the client. Which of the following signs should be reported immediately to the physician?
   - ○ 1. Green sputum.
   - ○ 2. Dry cough.
   - ○ 3. Hemoptysis.
   - ○ 4. Laryngeal stridor.

5. A client complains that "the hospital food is horrible." Which of the following is the most appropriate response by the nurse?
   - ○ 1. "The staff is doing the best they can to cook in such large quantities."
   - ○ 2. "I will report this to the physician."
   - ○ 3. "Would you like to speak with the dietitian about the food and meal selection?"
   - ○ 4. "I don't like the hospital cafeteria food either."

6. The nurse must be aware that adverse drug reactions in the elderly may be underestimated because
   - ○ 1. adverse reactions rarely have an atypical presentation.
   - ○ 2. cognitive impairment is an expected finding in the elderly.
   - ○ 3. physical or psychological symptoms are attributed to the effects of aging.
   - ○ 4. excess sedation is difficult to assess in the elderly.

7. An elderly man experiences a thrombotic cerebrovascular accident (CVA) and subsequent flaccid hemiplegia of his right side. When planning his care, rehabilitation begins
   - ○ 1. as soon as anticoagulant therapy is started.
   - ○ 2. when the client is admitted to the hospital.
   - ○ 3. when the client is first able to work cooperatively with health care personnel.
   - ○ 4. as directed by the physical therapist.

8. When considering quality-of-life issues for a client diagnosed with lung cancer, the nurse should be aware that
   - ○ 1. lung cancer is an aggressive disease.
   - ○ 2. small-cell lung cancer has a good prognosis if treated aggressively.
   - ○ 3. a client diagnosed with squamous cell carcinoma can get a complete response with chemotherapy.
   - ○ 4. the overall 5-year survival rate is 45%.

9. An unmarried pregnant teenager tells the nurse that she is undecided about having an abortion or giving the baby up for adoption. The *best* response for the nurse to offer is which of the following?
   - ○ 1. "You should give the baby up so that it can have a better home and opportunities."
   - ○ 2. "Research studies show that babies do better with their natural mothers."
   - ○ 3. "It must be a difficult decision. What have you thought about so far?"
   - ○ 4. "Why don't you try keeping the baby. You can always give it up for adoption later."

10. When administering blood, the nurse must check

the name on the label of the blood with the name on the client's
○ 1. wristband.
○ 2. wristband in the presence of another nurse.
○ 3. medical chart.
○ 4. medication administration record.

11. A client is admitted to the emergency room with crushing chest injuries sustained in a car accident. Which of the following signs would indicate a possible pneumothorax?
○ 1. Cheyne-Stokes breathing.
○ 2. Increased fremitus.
○ 3. Diminished or absent breath sounds on the affected side.
○ 4. A decreased sensation on the affected side.

12. Which of the following statements by a client taking valproic acid (Depakene) for bipolar disorder indicates that *further* teaching about this medication is necessary?
○ 1. "I need to take the pills at the same time each day."
○ 2. "I can chew the pills if necessary."
○ 3. "I can take the pills with food."
○ 4. "I need to call my doctor if I start bruising easily."

13. When obtaining history information from the parent of an infant with suspected acute otitis media, about which of the following would the nurse ask?
○ 1. The position of the infant when taking a bottle.
○ 2. Covering of the infant's ears when out in the cold.
○ 3. Thorough drying of the infant's ears after a bath.
○ 4. The immunization status of the infant.

14. A client is having elective surgery under general anesthesia. Who is responsible for obtaining the informed consent?
○ 1. The nurse.
○ 2. The surgeon.
○ 3. The anesthesiologist.
○ 4. The nurse anesthetist.

15. The family of an elderly client with terminal cancer inquire about hospice services. The nurse explains that hospice care
○ 1. focuses only on the needs of the client.
○ 2. can be only provided in the inpatient setting.
○ 3. is staffed exclusively by professional health care workers.
○ 4. provides medical supervision to clients at all times.

16. A primigravid client at 8 weeks' gestation tells the nurse that she doesn't like milk. To ensure that the client consumes an adequate intake of milk products, the nurse would instruct the client that an 8-ounce glass of milk is equal to which of the following?

○ 1. 2 tablespoons of Parmesan cheese.
○ 2. $^1/_2$ cup of a milkshake.
○ 3. $1^1/_2$ to 2 slices of presliced American cheese.
○ 4. $^1/_2$ cup of cottage cheese.

17. A primigravid client at 35 weeks' gestation is scheduled for a biophysical profile. After instructing the client about the test, which of the following, if stated by the client as one of the parameters of this test, indicates effective teaching?
○ 1. Amniotic fluid volume.
○ 2. Placement of the placenta.
○ 3. Amniotic fluid color.
○ 4. Fetal gestational age.

18. When caring for a child who has been receiving long-term steroid therapy, which of the following would the nurse expect to assess?
○ 1. Usual behavior and temperament.
○ 2. Loss of weight from baseline.
○ 3. Development of truncal obesity.
○ 4. Demonstration of a growth spurt.

19. The nurse manager has assigned a nurse as the circulating nurse for a surgical abortion. The nurse is Roman Catholic and wishes to refuse participation in an abortion. The nurse manager of the operating room should
○ 1. require the nurse to do this assignment.
○ 2. change the assignment, and record the behavior on the nurse's evaluation.
○ 3. change the assignment without comment.
○ 4. change the assignment to circulate, but have the nurse prepare the equipment.

20. A client is taking phenytoin (Dilantin) as an antiepileptic medication. The nurse emphasizes that the client needs
○ 1. increased iron.
○ 2. increased calcium.
○ 3. frequent dental examinations.
○ 4. frequent eye examinations.

21. The nurse should establish baseline data on a client who is starting on long-term gentamycin sulfate (Garamycin) therapy. Which of the following is *not* related to long-term use of this drug?
○ 1. Decreased visual acuity.
○ 2. Altered vestibular function.
○ 3. Decreased renal function.
○ 4. Decreased auditory function.

22. The nurse prepares to discharge a 5-year-old child from the 1-day surgery unit. The nurse leaves the room to get supplies and then, on returning, finds that the child is not breathing. The client is pulseless, and the nurse begins chest compressions. Because effective chest compressions depend on proper technique, the nurse should apply pressure
○ 1. on the lower sternum with the heel of one hand.

○ 2. midway on the sternum with the tips of two fingers.

○ 3. over the apex of the heart with the heel of one hand.

○ 4. on the upper sternum with the heels of both hands.

23. When developing a nutritional plan for a child who needs to increase protein intake, which of the following foods would the nurse be *least* likely to include?

○ 1. Bacon.

○ 2. Cooked dry beans.

○ 3. Peanut butter.

○ 4. Yogurt.

24. The nurse instructs a client with coronary artery disease in the proper use of nitroglycerin (Nitrostat). At the onset of chest pain, the client should

○ 1. call 911 when three nitroglycerin tablets taken every 5 minutes are ineffective.

○ 2. call 911 when five nitroglycerin tablets taken every 5 minutes are ineffective.

○ 3. take three nitroglycerin tablets, 10 minutes apart, and call 911.

○ 4. go to the emergency department if three nitroglycerin tablets are ineffective.

25. A diet high in which of the following food substances contributes to increases in serum cholesterol?

○ 1. Polyunsaturated fat.

○ 2. Saturated fat.

○ 3. Monounsaturated fat.

○ 4. Phospholipid.

26. During the health history, a client bluntly states, "I think I am better off dead." The *best* response by the nurse is which of the following?

○ 1. "Has a family member ever committed suicide?"

○ 2. "When did these feelings begin?"

○ 3. "Do you have someone at home to help you?"

○ 4. "Have you thought about suicide?"

27. A client is taking methotrexate (Rheumatrex) for severe rheumatoid arthritis. The nurse instructs the client that it will be necessary to monitor her

○ 1. serum glucose.

○ 2. serum electrolytes.

○ 3. complete blood count (CBC) with differential and platelet count.

○ 4. sedimentation rate.

28. An elderly client complains to the nurse about constipation and reports that he has never been constipated before. The best response for the nurse to make is which of the following?

○ 1. "Constipation is an expected problem at your age."

○ 2. "You need to eat more fiber."

○ 3. "You need to drink more water."

○ 4. "The new onset of constipation may be a sign of a more serious problem."

29. A nurse is interviewing a client who will begin rehabilitation for alcohol dependency. Which approach by the nurse would be *most* helpful to the client before starting the program?

○ 1. "You need to be very serious about this program."

○ 2. "You need to want to be alcohol free before we can help you."

○ 3. "This program requires you to do a lot of hard work."

○ 4. "We will help you be successful so that you can stay alcohol free."

30. A newly diagnosed type 1 diabetic client asks the nurse, "Why do I have to take two shots of insulin? Shouldn't one shot be enough?" The *best* response for the nurse to make is which of the following?

○ 1. "A single shot of long-acting insulin would be preferable."

○ 2. "You might be able to change to oral medications soon."

○ 3. "Two shots will give you better control and decrease complications."

○ 4. "I will ask the physician to change your insulin schedule."

31. The nurse understands that peak and trough serum levels from a client who is receiving gentamycin sulfate (Garamycin) for used to

○ 1. adjust the dosage to the therapeutic range.

○ 2. avoid allergic reactions.

○ 3. prevent side effects.

○ 4. reach therapeutic levels more quickly.

32. The nurse is helping a client who has heart disease to assess his vitamin needs. The nurse is aware that recent updates to the Recommended Dietary Allowances expanded the description of nutrient needs to include Adequate Intakes, Tolerable Upper Limits, and Estimated Average Requirements. All these recommendations are called

○ 1. Dietary Guidelines.

○ 2. Recommended Daily Allowances.

○ 3. Recommended Daily Intakes.

○ 4. Dietary Reference Intakes.

33. A client with a history of diabetes mellitus and chronic obstructive pulmonary disease (COPD) should have which of the following immunizations?

○ 1. Influenza.

○ 2. Hepatitis A.

○ 3. Measles–mumps–rubella (MMR).

○ 4. Varicella (Varivax).

34. A parent confides to the nurse that she thinks her 8-month-old infant is anxious or nervous. Which of the following suggestions by the nurse would be

most appropriate to help the mother lessen her anxiety about her infant?
- ○ 1. Limit holding of the infant to during feedings.
- ○ 2. Talk quietly to the infant while he is awake.
- ○ 3. Play music in his room for most of the day and night.
- ○ 4. Have a close friend keep the infant for a few days.

35. The parent of a 2-week-old infant brings the child to the clinic for a checkup. The parent expresses concern about the baby's breathing because the infant breathes quickly for a while then breathes slowly. The nurse interprets this finding as an indication of which of the following?
- ○ 1. A normal pattern in infants of this age.
- ○ 2. The need for an apnea monitor.
- ○ 3. A need for close monitoring for the mother.
- ○ 4. The need for a chest radiograph.

36. Which of the following complications is associated with a tracheostomy?
- ○ 1. Decreased cardiac output.
- ○ 2. Damage to the laryngeal nerve.
- ○ 3. Pneumothorax.
- ○ 4. Acute respiratory distress syndrome (ARDS).

37. The nurse who is caring for a client with insulin-dependent diabetes mellitus would use which of the following assessment tools to determine how well the child's insulin, diet, and exercise are balanced?
- ○ 1. Fasting serum glucose level.
- ○ 2. One-week dietary recall.
- ○ 3. Home log of blood glucose levels.
- ○ 4. Glycosylated hemoglobin level.

38. A client is receiving a unit of packed red blood cells. Before the transfusion started, the client's blood pressure was 90/50 mm Hg, pulse rate 100 bpm, respirations 20 breaths/minute, and temperature 98°F (36.7°). Fifteen minutes after the transfusion starts, the client's blood pressure is 92/54 mm Hg, pulse 100 bpm, respirations 18 breaths/minute, and temperature is 101.4°F (38.6°C). The nurse should *first*
- ○ 1. stop the transfusion.
- ○ 2. raise the head of the bed.
- ○ 3. obtain an order for antibiotics.
- ○ 4. offer the client a cool washcloth.

39. Which of the following dietary strategies would best meet the nutritional needs of a client with acquired immunodeficiency syndrome (AIDS)?
- ○ 1. Tell the client to eat large meals frequently.
- ○ 2. Encourage megadoses of nutrient supplements.
- ○ 3. Instruct the client to cook foods thoroughly and adhere to safe food-handling practices.
- ○ 4. Tell the client to prepare food in advance and leave it out to eat small amounts throughout the day.

40. Before a traditional cholecystectomy is performed, the nurse instructs the client in the correct use of an incentive spirometer. Why is incentive spirometry essential after surgery in the upper abdominal area?
- ○ 1. The client will be maintained on bed rest for several days.
- ○ 2. Ambulation is restricted by the presence of drainage tubes.
- ○ 3. The operative incision is near the diaphragm.
- ○ 4. The presence of a nasogastric tube inhibits deep breathing.

41. The nurse is examining a 6-week-old African American infant. There are large spots of deep blue pigmentation across the infant's buttocks. The nurse should identify this sign as characteristic of
- ○ 1. vascular disease.
- ○ 2. telangiectatic nevi.
- ○ 3. milia.
- ○ 4. Mongolian spots.

42. A nulliparous client has been given a prescription for oral contraceptives. Which of the following would the nurse instruct the client to report to her health care provider immediately?
- ○ 1. Blurred vision.
- ○ 2. Nausea.
- ○ 3. Weight gain.
- ○ 4. Mild headache.

43. A client experienced a pneumothorax after the placement of a central venous pressure (CVP) line. Which of the following assessments would support a medical diagnosis of pneumothorax?
- ○ 1. Sudden, sharp pain on the affected side.
- ○ 2. Tracheal deviation toward the affected side.
- ○ 3. Bradypnea and elevated blood pressure.
- ○ 4. Presence of crackles and wheezes.

44. When developing the plan of care for a client who is experiencing a flashback from use of lysergic acid diethylamide (LSD), which of the following approaches would the nurse anticipate using?
- ○ 1. Confronting the client's misperceptions.
- ○ 2. Reassuring the client while presenting reality.
- ○ 3. Secluding the client until the flashback ends.
- ○ 4. Challenging the client's unrealistic statements.

45. The nurse should dispose of a used needle and syringe by
- ○ 1. cutting the needle at the hilt in a needle cutter before disposing of it in the universal precaution container in the client's room.
- ○ 2. placing uncapped, used needles and syringes immediately in the universal precaution container in the client's room.
- ○ 3. recapping the needle and placing the needle and syringe in the universal precaution container in the client's room.
- ○ 4. separating the needle and syringe and placing

both in the universal precaution container in the client's room.

46. An 80-year-old client is admitted with nausea and vomiting. He has a history of congestive heart failure and is being treated with digoxin (Lanoxin). He tells the nurse he has been nauseated for a week and began vomiting 2 days ago. Laboratory values indicate that he has hypokalemia. Because of these clinical findings, the nurse should assess the client carefully for signs of which of the following conditions?
    ○ 1. Chronic renal failure.
    ○ 2. Exacerbation of congestive heart failure.
    ○ 3. Digitalis toxicity.
    ○ 4. Metabolic acidosis.

47. The nurse instructs the client with osteoporosis that food products high in calcium include
    ○ 1. rice.
    ○ 2. broccoli.
    ○ 3. apples.
    ○ 4. meat.

48. A woman is using progestin injections (Depo-Provera, DMPA) for contraception. The nurse instructs the client to return for an appointment in
    ○ 1. 1 month.
    ○ 2. 3 months.
    ○ 3. 4 months.
    ○ 4. 6 months.

49. A client is admitted through the emergency department with third-degree burns. The nurse assesses the client for edema, which can develop as a result of which of the following mechanisms?
    ○ 1. Increase in tissue colloidal osmotic pressure.
    ○ 2. Increase in plasma colloidal osmotic pressure.
    ○ 3. Decrease in capillary hydrostatic pressure.
    ○ 4. Decrease in interstitial fluid pressure.

50. A client exhibits increased restlessness. The results of the arterial blood gas test are as follows: pH, 7.52; PCO_2, 38 mm Hg; HCO_3^-, 34 mg/L. These findings indicate which of the following acid–base imbalances?
    ○ 1. Respiratory alkalosis.
    ○ 2. Respiratory acidosis.
    ○ 3. Metabolic acidosis.
    ○ 4. Metabolic alkalosis.

51. While the nurse is caring for a multigravid client at 39 weeks' gestation in active labor whose cervix dilated to 7 cm and completely effaced at +1 station, the client says, "I need to push!" Which of the following would the nurse do *next*?
    ○ 1. Turn the client to her left side.
    ○ 2. Tell her to push when she has the urge.
    ○ 3. Have her pant quickly during the contraction.
    ○ 4. Tell her to focus on an object in the room to relax.

52. Many antibiotics are nephrotoxic. When teaching a client who is taking antibiotics about signs and symptoms to report, the nurse should encourage the client to promptly report changes in urine output and appearance. Of the following descriptions of urine, which is an expected, normal description?
    ○ 1. Straw-colored.
    ○ 2. Cloudy.
    ○ 3. Smoky.
    ○ 4. Pink.

53. The school nurse is to monitor a child with suspected juvenile hypothyroidism. Which of the following would the nurse expect this child to manifest?
    ○ 1. Short attention span and weight loss.
    ○ 2. Weight loss and flushed skin.
    ○ 3. Rapid pulse and heat intolerance.
    ○ 4. Dry skin and constipation.

54. The nurse would anticipate which of the following medical orders for reducing a client's fluid volume excess?
    ○ 1. Low-sodium diet.
    ○ 2. Serum electrolytes daily.
    ○ 3. Monitor intake and output.
    ○ 4. Elevation of the client's feet.

55. The nurse observes a darkish blue pigment on the buttocks and back of an African American neonate. Which of the following actions would be *most* appropriate?
    ○ 1. Ask the obstetrician to assess the child.
    ○ 2. Assess the child for other areas of cyanosis.
    ○ 3. Document this observation in the child's record.
    ○ 4. Advise the mother that laser therapy will be needed.

56. During a physical examination, the nurse observes a copper bracelet on a client's wrist. The client states that she is wearing it to treat her arthritis. Because the nurse is aware of different cultural beliefs, the nurse recognizes this as a health practice
    ○ 1. in which a protective object is believed to ward off illness.
    ○ 2. that is harmful to the client and must be discontinued.
    ○ 3. that is quackery and should not be tolerated.
    ○ 4. that is medically supported to treat arthritis and other conditions.

57. The heart rate of a newly delivered term neonate is found to be regular at 142 bpm. Which of the following would the nurse do *next*?
    ○ 1. Notify the neonate's pediatrician.
    ○ 2. Check for the presence of cyanosis.
    ○ 3. Assess the heart rate again in 3 hours.
    ○ 4. Document this as a normal neonatal finding.

58. The fetus of a multigravid client at 38 weeks' gestation is determined to be in a frank breech presenta-

tion. The nurse describes this presentation to the client as which of the following fetal parts as coming in contact with the cervix?
- ○ 1. Buttocks.
- ○ 2. Head.
- ○ 3. Both feet.
- ○ 4. Shoulder.

59. The nurse teaches the client that the therapeutic effects of desmopressin (DDAVP) nasal spray are obtained when the client no longer has
- ○ 1. polydipsia.
- ○ 2. nasal congestion.
- ○ 3. headache.
- ○ 4. blurred vision.

60. The nurse advises a 42-year-old client to have a screening mammogram. The client asks why this is necessary, since she performs breast self-examination (BSE) monthly. The nurse's *best* response is
- ○ 1. "All women over 35 should have an annual mammogram."
- ○ 2. "A mammogram can identify breast cancer before it is detectable by BSE."
- ○ 3. "Most women do not perform BSE thoroughly enough to detect cancer."
- ○ 4. "A mammogram can detect other endocrine abnormalities as well."

61. A client is recovering from an infected abdominal wound. Which of the following foods should the nurse encourage the client to eat to support wound healing and recovery from the infection?
- ○ 1. Chicken and orange slices.
- ○ 2. Cheeseburger and french fries.
- ○ 3. Cheese omelet and bacon.
- ○ 4. Gelatin salad and tea.

62. The nurse teaches the client with iron-deficiency anemia that food sources with high iron content include
- ○ 1. cheese.
- ○ 2. squash.
- ○ 3. eggs.
- ○ 4. beef.

63. The mother of a toddler diagnosed with iron-deficiency anemia asks what foods she should give her child. The nurse would evaluate the teaching as successful when the mother later reports that she feeds the toddler which of the following?
- ○ 1. Milk, carrots, and beef.
- ○ 2. Raisins, chicken, and spinach.
- ○ 3. Beef, lettuce, and juice.
- ○ 4. Eggs, cheese, and milk.

64. Four hours after a cast has been applied for a fractured ulna, the nurse assesses that the client's fingers are pale and cool and capillary refill is delayed for 4 seconds. How should the nurse interpret these findings?

- ○ 1. Nerve impairment is developing in the fingers.
- ○ 2. Arterial blood supply to the fingers is decreased.
- ○ 3. Venous stasis is occurring in the fingers.
- ○ 4. The finding is normal for this recovery time period.

65. The nurse is developing a plan of care for a client who has joint stiffness due to rheumatoid arthritis. Which of the following interventions is most likely to be effective in relieving the stiffness?
- ○ 1. A warm shower before performing activities of daily living.
- ○ 2. Aspirin after activity to decrease inflammation.
- ○ 3. A 10-pound weight loss to limit stress on joints.
- ○ 4. Cold compresses to joints for 30 minutes to relieve stiffness.

66. The nurse walks into the room and finds that a client who has just had surgery is diaphoretic, appears to have no respirations, and has a barely palpable pulse. The client is a "full code." What is the most appropriate immediate response?
- ○ 1. Call a code blue.
- ○ 2. Open the airway.
- ○ 3. Start rescue breathing.
- ○ 4. Start cardiac compressions.

67. A client with obsessive–compulsive disorder washes her hands multiple times daily and is late for meals and milieu activities. Which of the following would be *most* appropriate for the nurse to do?
- ○ 1. Totally eliminate the client's ritual.
- ○ 2. Allow the client to decide whether she wants to attend meals and activities.
- ○ 3. Inform the client that absence from meals and activities is not permitted.
- ○ 4. Remind the client about meal and activity times so that the ritual can be completed on time.

68. After discussing preconception needs with an Asian American nulliparous client, which of the following client statements indicates the need for further instruction?
- ○ 1. "I should take folic acid supplements before I get pregnant."
- ○ 2. "If I become pregnant, I can continue to eat sushi twice a week."
- ○ 3. "I should continue to steam my vegetables rather than cooking them for a long time."
- ○ 4. "Eating soy products can increase my protein levels once I am pregnant."

69. A client with osteoarthritis purchased a copper bracelet to wear. He tells the nurse that he feels better since he started wearing it. Which response by the nurse would be most appropriate?
- ○ 1. Tell the client to remove the bracelet because it does not have any therapeutic value.
- ○ 2. Warn the client not to spend any more money on "quackery" such as bracelets.

3. Instruct the client to remove the bracelet because the copper in it can interfere with salicylate metabolism.

4. Acknowledge that the client feels better, but encourage the client to continue with his prescribed therapy.

70. Stanol esters lower cholesterol by
    1. directly lowering cholesterol in the blood.
    2. blocking digestion of cholesterol.
    3. inhibiting lipoprotein lipase.
    4. blocking absorption of cholesterol from the intestine.

71. A man of Chinese descent is admitted to the hospital with multiple injuries after a motor vehicle accident. His pain is not under control. The client states "If I could be with my people, I could receive acupuncture for this pain." The nurse should understand that acupuncture in the Asian culture is based on the theory that it
    1. purges evil spirits.
    2. promotes tranquility.
    3. restores the balance of energy.
    4. blocks nerve pathways to the brain.

72. A client is taking large doses of aspirin daily to treat her rheumatoid arthritis. Which of the following side effects should the nurse instruct her to report?
    1. Abdominal cramps.
    2. Tinnitus.
    3. Rash.
    4. Hypotension.

73. A client is transferred from the coronary care unit to the stepdown unit. Which of the following is not necessary in the transfer report?
    1. The client needs oxygen at 2 L/minute.
    2. The client has a "Do Not Resuscitate" order.
    3. The client uses the bedpan.
    4. The client has four grandchildren.

74. The nurse is assessing fetal presentation in a multiparous client. Figure 1 indicates which of the following types of presentations?
    1. Frank breech.
    2. Complete breech.
    3. Footling breech.
    4. Vertex.

75. A multigravid client at 26 weeks' gestation and with a history of pregnancy-induced hypertension (PIH) asks the nurse about traveling to a village in India by airplane to visit her father, who wishes to see her before she delivers. Which of the following responses by the nurse would be *most* appropriate?
    1. "Air travel at this point in your pregnancy can lead to preterm labor."
    2. "You can travel by airplane as long as you take frequent walks during the trip."

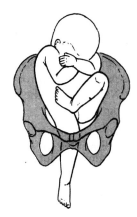

Figure 1.

3. "You need to avoid traveling because of your history of PIH."

4. "You'd be placing yourself and fetus at risk for communicable diseases common in India."

76. To which national food assistance program should the nurse refer a low-income, pregnant client for help in obtaining food for herself and later her infant?
    1. Home-delivered meals.
    2. Congregate meals.
    3. WIC program.
    4. Food bank.

77. The nurse is caring for a client who has received severe burns to the head, neck, trunk, and groin areas. Which client position would be most appropriate for preventing contractures?
    1. High Fowler's.
    2. Semi-Fowler's.
    3. Prone.
    4. Supine.

78. A client sustained an open fracture of the femur from an automobile accident. For which of the following types of shock should the client be assessed?
    1. Cardiogenic.
    2. Hypovolemic.
    3. Neurogenic.
    4. Anaphylactic.

79. A client has various sensory impairments associated with diabetic disease. Which of the following activities is not necessary for the client to follow?
    1. Carefully test the temperature of bathwater.
    2. Avoid kitchen activities that pose a high risk of injury.
    3. Avoid hot water bottles or heating pads.
    4. Inspect the skin daily for injury or pressure points.

80. The father of an adolescent calls to talk to the nurse in the clinic about behaviors he has seen over the

past 6 months in his teenaged son. The father recounts that the adolescent spends lots of time in his room, his grades are falling, and he has given away a few of his most favorite compact disks. Which of the following would be the *most* appropriate action for the nurse?

○ 1. Give the father the telephone number for the local crisis hotline.

○ 2. Have the father take the adolescent to the nearest mental health outpatient facility now.

○ 3. Make a same-day appointment for the adolescent with his usual health care provider.

○ 4. Obtain more history information from the distraught father before making a decision.

81. A 7-year-old child is admitted to the hospital with the medical diagnosis of acute rheumatic fever. If the child develops chorea-like movements, which of the following eating utensils would the nurse suggest the parents *not* allow the child to use?

○ 1. Fork.

○ 2. Spoon.

○ 3. Plastic cup.

○ 4. Drinking straw.

82. A client's catheter is removed 4 days after a transurethral resection of the prostate (TURP). He is experiencing urinary dribbling. Which one of the following nursing interventions is appropriate in this situation?

○ 1. Teach the client Kegel exercises.

○ 2. Obtain a urine culture and sensitivity analysis to screen for a urinary infection.

○ 3. Encourage voiding every hour to prevent dribbling.

○ 4. Inform him that the dribbling will stop after a few days.

83. An adolescent primigravid client at 26 weeks' gestation who has gained 25 pounds since becoming pregnant visits the prenatal clinic for a routine visit. Which of the following is the recommended amount of weight gain during the third trimester?

○ 1. 1 pound a week.

○ 2. 2 pounds per week.

○ 3. 7 pounds per month.

○ 4. 5 to 6 pounds for the trimester.

84. The nurse is preparing to administer 0.1 mg of digoxin (Lanoxin) intravenously. Digoxin comes in a concentration of 0.5 mg/2 mL. How many milliliters should the nurse administer?

○ 1. 0.2 mL.

○ 2. 0.4 mL.

○ 3. 2.2 mL.

○ 4. 2.5 mL.

85. The mother of a 2-month-old infant with colic states, "I don't know what to do anymore. She's up in the middle of the night crying all the time."

Which of the following would be the nurse's *best* suggestion?

○ 1. Walk the floor with the baby at night.

○ 2. Take the infant for a short drive in the car.

○ 3. Allow the infant to cry it out in her crib.

○ 4. Offer cereal to fill the baby's stomach.

86. After the application of an arm cast, the client complains of pain on passive stretching of his fingers, finger swelling and tightness, and loss of function. Based on these data, the nurse anticipates that the client may be developing which of the following?

○ 1. Delayed bone union.

○ 2. Compartment syndrome.

○ 3. Fat embolism.

○ 4. Osteomyelitis.

87. Which of the following cardiac rehabilitation interventions is a priority for a client who has just had a myocardial infarction?

○ 1. Low-back training program.

○ 2. Risk modification education.

○ 3. Strength training program.

○ 4. Jogging exercise program.

88. While assessing a 4-day-old neonate delivered at 28 weeks' gestation, the nurse is unable to elicit the neonate's Moro reflex, which was present 1 hour after birth. The nurse notifies the physician because this may be indicative of which of the following?

○ 1. Postnatal asphyxia.

○ 2. Skull fracture.

○ 3. Intracranial hemorrhage.

○ 4. Facial nerve paralysis.

89. After a TURP, the nurse notices that the client's urine is bright red, has numerous clots, and is viscous. Which nursing action is most appropriate?

○ 1. Irrigate the catheter to remove clots.

○ 2. Milk the catheter tube vigorously.

○ 3. Increase the client's fluid intake.

○ 4. Assess vital signs and notify the surgeon.

90. The nurse is teaching a client about the appropriate use of lorazepam (Ativan) to manage anxiety. Which of the following statements indicates that the client understands the nurse's teaching?

○ 1. "I can take my medicine whenever I feel anxious."

○ 2. "It's okay to double my dose if I need to."

○ 3. "My medicine is not for the everyday stress of life."

○ 4. "It's safe to have a glass of wine while taking this medicine."

91. The physician orders a maternal blood test for α-fetoprotein for a nulligravid client at 16 weeks' gestation. When developing the teaching plan, the nurse bases the explanations on the understanding that this test is used to detect which of the following?

○ 1. Neural tube defects.
○ 2. Chromosomal anomalies.
○ 3. Inborn errors of metabolism.
○ 4. Lecithin–sphingomyelin ratio.

92. A nursing assistant recorded a client's 6 AM blood glucose level as 126 instead of 216. The nursing assistant did not recognize the error until 9 AM but reported it to the nurse right away. The nurse's correct response includes
    ○ 1. reassigning the nursing assistant to another client.
    ○ 2. waiting and observing the client for symptoms of hyperglycemia.
    ○ 3. reprimanding the nursing assistant for the error.
    ○ 4. calling the physician and completing an incident report.

93. A client who is recovering from an abdominal hysterectomy complains of pain in her right calf. Which of the following additional assessments would be appropriate at this time?
    ○ 1. Palpate the calf to note pain.
    ○ 2. Measure the circumference of both calves and note the difference.
    ○ 3. Have the client flex and extend her leg and note presence of pain.
    ○ 4. Raise the right leg and lower it to detect changes in skin color.

94. The nurse is caring for an elderly client who has experienced a sensorineural hearing loss. The nurse anticipates that the client will exhibit which one of the following symptoms?
    ○ 1. Difficulty hearing high-pitched sounds.
    ○ 2. Difficulty with speaking clearly.
    ○ 3. Inability to assign meaning to sound.
    ○ 4. Vertigo when changing positions.

95. A client who was recently diagnosed with lung cancer tells the nurse that she has been having difficulty sleeping and is often preoccupied with thoughts about how her life has changed. She says, "I wish my life could just go on the way it was." Which of the following nursing diagnoses is most appropriate for this client?
    ○ 1. Ineffective Coping related to cancer diagnosis.
    ○ 2. Sleep Pattern Disturbance related to fear of the unknown.
    ○ 3. Anticipatory Grieving related to diagnosis of cancer.
    ○ 4. Anxiety related to need for chemotherapy treatment.

96. The physician orders intravenous nalbuphine (Nubain) for a primigravid client in early active labor. After administering the drug, which of the following would the nurse do *first*?
    ○ 1. Elevate the head of the bed.

○ 2. Cover the client with a blanket.
○ 3. Pull the siderails up.
○ 4. Dim the lights in the room.

97. A client with emphysema has been admitted to the hospital. Which one of the following signs and symptoms would be associated with his emphysema?
    ○ 1. Frequent coughing.
    ○ 2. Bronchospasms.
    ○ 3. Underweight appearance.
    ○ 4. Copious sputum.

98. A 12-year-old boy has a fractured femur and is immobilized in traction as shown in Figure 2. The nurse should
    ○ 1. add additional weight until the foot is only 2 inches from the bed.
    ○ 2. adjust the pulley so that the leg is at a 90-degree angle.
    ○ 3. place a pillow under the fractured leg to provide support.
    ○ 4. provide the boy opportunities for age-appropriate activities.

99. The nurse is participating in a blood pressure screening event. After three separate readings taken at least 2 minutes apart, the nurse determines that a client has a blood pressure of 160/90 mm Hg. Based on the nurse's knowledge of blood pressure screening guidelines, which of the following client recommendations would be appropriate at this time?
    ○ 1. Have blood pressure evaluated within 1 month.
    ○ 2. Begin an exercise program.
    ○ 3. Examine lifestyle to decrease stress.
    ○ 4. Schedule a complete physical immediately.

100. Which of the following activities would be least effective in preventing sensory deprivation during a client's stay in the cardiac care unit?

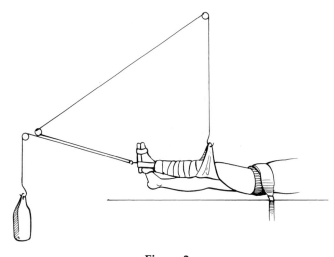

Figure 2

○ 1. Watching television.

○ 2. Visiting with family.

○ 3. Reading the newspaper.

○ 4. Keeping the door closed to provide privacy.

101. The nurse is teaching a client who is taking dexamethasone (Decadron) for cerebral edema about early symptoms of hyperadrenocorticism. Which of the following is a symptom of hyperadrenocorticism?

○ 1. Hypotension.

○ 2. Increased urinary frequency.

○ 3. Increased muscle mass.

○ 4. Easy bruising.

102. A client's wife arrives on the unit 6 hours after her husband's car accident, explaining that she has been out of town. She is distraught because she was not with her husband when he needed her. The most appropriate initial intervention for the nurse to make is to

○ 1. allow her to verbalize her feelings and concerns.

○ 2. describe her husband's medical treatment since admission.

○ 3. explain the nature of the injury and reassure her that her husband's condition is stable.

○ 4. reassure her that the important fact is that she is here now.

103. A client is scheduled to have a graded exercise test. The nurse explains to the client that the test will determine

○ 1. how well he thinks under pressure.

○ 2. how well his body reacts to controlled exercise stress.

○ 3. how far he can walk.

○ 4. how long he can walk.

104. A client tells the nurse that she is afraid to undergo chemotherapy because of what she has heard about the side effects. What would be the nurse's best response to the client's concerns?

○ 1. "Your health has been excellent. It is unlikely that you will experience serious side effects."

○ 2. "We will give you medications to prevent the side effects, so you shouldn't be too concerned."

○ 3. "Each person responds differently to the chemotherapy treatments. We will monitor your responses closely."

○ 4. "It is important for you to accept this treatment. If you refuse your chemotherapy treatments, you will die."

105. The mother of an infant with hemophilia tells the nurse that she is planning to do home teaching when the child reaches school age. She does not want her child in school, because the teacher will not watch the child as well as she would. The mother's comments

represent what common parental reaction to a child's chronic illness?

○ 1. Overprotection.

○ 2. Devotion.

○ 3. Mistrust.

○ 4. Insecurity.

106. A mother tells the nurse that her 17-month-old has been exposed to another child with roseola. After teaching the mother about the illness, which of the following, if stated by the mother as the *most* characteristic sign of roseola, would indicate successful teaching?

○ 1. Fever and sore throat.

○ 2. Normal temperature followed by a low-grade fever.

○ 3. High fever followed by a drop and then a rash.

○ 4. Cold-like signs and symptoms and a rash.

107. A client with acute psychosis, not otherwise specified, has been taking haloperidol (Haldol) for 3 days. When evaluating the client's response to the medication, which of the following comments would reflect the greatest improvement?

○ 1. "I know these voices aren't really real, but I'm still scared of them."

○ 2. "I am feeling so restless, I can't sit still."

○ 3. "Boy, do I need a shower. I think it has been days since I've had one."

○ 4. "I'll be fine if you just let me out of here today."

108. A 78-year-old client who experienced a brief delirium knows that the condition was caused by prescription medication intoxication. Which of the following statements indicates the need for *further* education?

○ 1. "I never realized that taking a little extra medication now and then could cause such a problem."

○ 2. "I get medicines from three different doctors and they don't all know what I'm taking."

○ 3. "I thought that the herbal medicines would help me. I never realized they would make me sick."

○ 4. "I didn't know that cold and flu medicines might not mix with my regular medicines."

109. A physician has asked for intravenous calcium to treat a client with hyperkalemia. What is the nurse's first response?

○ 1. Hand the physician calcium chloride for intravenous use.

○ 2. Check with the physician for his complete order.

○ 3. Hand the physician calcium gluconate for intravenous use.

○ 4. Hand the physician the kind of calcium available on the unit.

110. The nurse is administering an intravenous potas-

sium chloride supplement to a client who has congestive heart failure. When developing a plan of care for this client, which of the following should the nurse incorporate into the care plan?
- ○ 1. Hyperkalemia will intensify the action of the client's digitalis preparation.
- ○ 2. The client's potassium levels will be unaffected by his potassium-sparing diuretic.
- ○ 3. The administration of the intravenous potassium chloride should not exceed 10 mEq/hour or a concentration of 40 mEq/L.
- ○ 4. Metabolic alkalosis will increase the client's serum potassium levels.

111. A client is receiving morphine sulfate by a patient-controlled analgesia (PCA) system after a left lower lobectomy about 4 hours ago. The client complains of moderately severe pain in his left thorax that worsens when he coughs. The nurse's *first* course of action is to
- ○ 1. reassure the client that the PCA is working and will relieve his pain.
- ○ 2. encourage the client to rest; no further assessment is needed.
- ○ 3. assess the pain systematically with the hospital-approved scale.
- ○ 4. encourage the client to ignore the pain and sleep, because pain is expected after this type of surgery.

112. Which of the following factors can alter tissue tolerance and lead to the development of a pressure ulcer?
- ○ 1. Client's age.
- ○ 2. Exposure to moisture.
- ○ 3. Presence of hypertension.
- ○ 4. Smoking.

113. The nurse is screening clients for cancer prevention. Which of the following is the recommended screening protocol for colon cancer in clients who have a low-risk profile?
- ○ 1. Guaiac testing of stools should be performed annually after 50 years of age.
- ○ 2. Digital rectal examinations are recommended annually after 40 years of age.
- ○ 3. Sigmoidoscopy is recommended if symptoms of colon problems are present.
- ○ 4. a low-fat diet should be implemented by 50 years of age.

114. The nurse is evaluating the effectiveness of antipsychotic medications in a client with severe Alzheimer's disease. Which of the following changes would indicate improvement resulting from medications?
- ○ 1. Adjustment to the structured daily routine.
- ○ 2. Improvement in the client's short-term memory.
- ○ 3. Decrease in verbal and physical aggression.
- ○ 4. Diminished resistance with activities of daily living done one step at a time.

115. After vaginal delivery of a term neonate, the nurse determines that the placenta is about to separate when which of the following occurs?
- ○ 1. The uterus becomes oval shaped.
- ○ 2. The uterus enlarges.
- ○ 3. A sudden gush of dark blood occurs.
- ○ 4. The client expends efforts pushing.

116. The nurse should complete which of the following assessments on a client who has received tissue plasminogen activator (t-PA) or alteplase recombinant (Activase) therapy?
- ○ 1. Neurologic signs every 30 minutes from the second through the eighth hours.
- ○ 2. Excessive bleeding every hour for the first 8 hours.
- ○ 3. Blood glucose level.
- ○ 4. Hemoglobin level.

117. During the emergent phase of burn management, the nurse would anticipate which of the following fluid and electrolyte imbalances to occur?
- ○ 1. Hypokalemia, hyponatremia.
- ○ 2. Hyperkalemia, increased hematocrit.
- ○ 3. Decreased hematocrit, hypernatremia.
- ○ 4. Hypocalcemia, increased hematocrit.

118. A 6-year-old child is to have a cardiac catheterization and asks the nurse if it will hurt. Which of the following statements provides the nurse with the *best* guide for responding to the child's question?
- ○ 1. The medication used to numb the insertion site will sting.
- ○ 2. A momentary sharp pain usually occurs when the catheter enters the heart.
- ○ 3. Most 6-year-olds feel some discomfort during the procedure.
- ○ 4. It is a painless procedure, although a tingling sensation may be felt in the extremities.

119. A 10-year-old with a history of recent respiratory infection comes to the clinic and reports swelling around the eyes in the morning and dark urine. Which of the following would the nurse ask *first*?
- ○ 1. Has the child had a rash and fever?
- ○ 2. Has the child had a sore throat?
- ○ 3. Does the child have any allergies?
- ○ 4. Does the child drink lots of liquids?

120. After a nasogastric tube has been inserted, the nurse can most accurately determine that the tube is in the proper place if which of the following can be demonstrated?
- ○ 1. The client is no longer gagging or coughing.
- ○ 2. The pH of the aspirated fluid is measured.
- ○ 3. Thirty milliliters of normal saline can be injected without difficulty.
- ○ 4. A "whooshing" sound is auscultated when 10 mL of air is inserted.

121. A nulligravid client at 40+ weeks' gestation visits

the emergency room of the hospital because she thinks she is in labor. Which of the following would be the *best* indication that the client is in true labor?

○ 1. Fetal descent into the pelvic inlet.

○ 2. Cervical dilation and effacement.

○ 3. Painful contractions every 3 to 5 minutes.

○ 4. Leaking amniotic fluid clear in color.

122. Which of the following should be considered the *highest* priority during the first 24 hours postoperatively for the client who had a total laryngectomy due to cancer of the larynx?

○ 1. Provide adequate nourishment.

○ 2. Prevent skin breakdown.

○ 3. Maintain proper bowel elimination.

○ 4. Maintain a patent airway.

123. It has been 5 months since a client lost his wife and child in a car–train accident. The nurse would determine that the client needs continuing counseling if he makes which of the following statements?

○ 1. "I'm sleeping, eating, and working pretty well, but I still get so sad at times."

○ 2. "I miss them so much, but I can tell I am getting better day by day."

○ 3. "I wish I didn't have to sleep. I hate the nightmares about what the car looked like."

○ 4. "I never thought I'd get over this, but I am working with my congressman for train crossing safety."

124. A client is hearing voices that are telling her to kill herself. She is demanding a knife to use on her wrists. Which of the following would be *most* appropriate at this time?

○ 1. Put the client in restraints after giving an intramuscular dose of PRN medication.

○ 2. Ask the client to talk about her anger and what is causing it.

○ 3. Give oral PRN doses of Haloperidol (Haldol) and lorazepam (Ativan) as ordered.

○ 4. Search the client's room for potential weapons after locking the unit kitchen.

125. The nurse should adjust a client's heparin dose according to a prescribed anticoagulation order based on maintaining which laboratory value at what therapeutic level for anticoagulant therapy?

○ 1. Activated partial thromboplastin time (aPTT), 1.5 to 2.5 times the normal control.

○ 2. Prothrombin time (PT), 1.5 to 2.5 times the normal control.

○ 3. International normalized ratio (INR), 2 to 3 seconds.

○ 4. Thrombin clotting time, 10 to 15 seconds.

126. Which of the following measures would be contraindicated when the nurse assists a child who has leukemia with oral hygiene?

○ 1. Applying petroleum jelly to the lips.

○ 2. Cleaning the teeth with a toothbrush.

○ 3. Swabbing the mouth with moistened cotton swabs.

○ 4. Rinsing the mouth with a nonirritating mouthwash.

127. The nurse realizes that a medication error has been made and a client has received the wrong medication. What should be the nurse's first action when realizing an error has been made?

○ 1. Assess the client's condition.

○ 2. Notify the physician of the error.

○ 3. Complete an incident report.

○ 4. Report the error to the unit manager.

128. The nurse has been assigned to a client who has had diabetes for 10 years. The nurse gives the client's usual dose of Humulin Regular insulin at 7 AM. At 10:30 AM, the client complains of lightheadedness and sweating. The nurse suspects that the client is experiencing

○ 1. metabolic acidosis.

○ 2. hyperglycemia.

○ 3. hypoglycemia.

○ 4. ketoacidosis.

129. A 6-year-old boy is being treated in the emergency department for injuries inflicted by his stepfather. The client's mother says, "This never happened before. Jim got fired today. He got drunk and came home in a tirade. I'm so sorry that Jason got hurt, but I don't think it will ever happen again." Which of the following responses would be *most* appropriate initially?

○ 1. "I'm sorry too, but I agree it probably won't happen again."

○ 2. "I'm not as forgiving are you are. I think you need to file charges on Jim."

○ 3. "This is child abuse and I have to file a report with Child Protective Services."

○ 4. "I want to know more about your situation. Let's sit and talk."

130. The nurse administers a tapwater enema to a client. While the solution is being infused, the client begins to complain of abdominal cramping. What should be the nurse's first response to the client's complaint?

○ 1. Clamp the tubing and carefully withdraw the tube.

○ 2. Temporarily stop the infusion and have the client take deep breaths.

○ 3. Raise the height of the enema container.

○ 4. Rub the client's abdomen gently until the cramps subside.

131. In preparing for insertion of a peripheral intravenous catheter, the nurse must select an appropriate site. Which of the following areas should the nurse try first if an appropriate vein is found?

○ 1. Back of the hand.
○ 2. Inner aspect of the elbow.
○ 3. Inner aspect of the forearm.
○ 4. Outer aspect of the forearm.

132. The nurse administers lactulose to a client with cirrhosis. What is the expected outcome from the administration of the lactulose?
   ○ 1. Stimulation of peristalsis of the bowel.
   ○ 2. Reduced peripheral edema and ascites.
   ○ 3. Reduced serum ammonia levels.
   ○ 4. Prevention of hemorrhage.

133. A 12-month-old child is seen in the neighborhood clinic for a regular checkup. The child's mother states that the child is caught up with immunizations. The nurse interprets this statement as indicating that the toddler has already received which of the following?
   ○ 1. DtaP #1 and 2; Hep B #1 and 2.
   ○ 2. DtaP #1, 2, and 3; Hep B #1, 2, and 3; IPV #1 and 2.
   ○ 3. DtaP #1 and 2; Hep B #1, 2, and 3; OPV #1 and 2.
   ○ 4. DtaP #1, 2, and 3; HIB #1 and 2; OPV #1 and 2.

134. When conducting a health promotion class with a group of women, the nurse should include which of the following strategies to help reduce the risk of developing osteoarthritis?
   ○ 1. Follow a high-protein diet.
   ○ 2. Exercise at least three times per week.
   ○ 3. Prevent obesity.
   ○ 4. Take a multivitamin supplement daily.

135. A deficiency of which of the following vitamins is thought to be the first step in the formation of plaque and oxidative changes?
   ○ 1. Vitamin C.
   ○ 2. Vitamin A.
   ○ 3. Vitamin E.
   ○ 4. Vitamin B_6.

136. A neonate circumcised with a Plastibell 1 hour ago is brought to his mother for feeding. The nurse instructs the mother to do which of the following?
   ○ 1. Read a pamphlet about circumcision care.
   ○ 2. Remove the Vaseline gauze in 24 hours.
   ○ 3. Tell the nurse when the neonate voids.
   ○ 4. Place petroleum jelly over the site every 2 hours.

137. A client has been diagnosed with early alcoholic cirrhosis. The client should be taught that incorporating which of the following behaviors into his lifestyle could potentially reverse the pathologic changes occurring in the liver?
   ○ 1. Avoid overexertion and fatigue.
   ○ 2. Avoid drinking alcohol.
   ○ 3. Eliminate smoking.
   ○ 4. Eat a high-carbohydrate, low-fat diet.

138. A child is to receive dexamethasone (Decadron) intravenously at the ordered dosage of 7.6 mg. The drug concentration in the vial is 4 mg/mL. Which of the following amounts would the nurse administer?
   ○ 1. 0.05 mL.
   ○ 2. 0.72 mL.
   ○ 3. 1.9 mL.
   ○ 4. 3.8 mL.

139. A 40-year-old primigravid client with type AB-positive blood visits the outpatient clinic for an amniocentesis at 16 weeks' gestation. The nurse determines that the most likely reason for the client's amniocentesis is to determine if the fetus has which of the following?
   ○ 1. Cri du chat syndrome.
   ○ 2. ABO incompatibility.
   ○ 3. Erythroblastosis fetalis.
   ○ 4. Down syndrome.

140. The nurse is assessing a client who has benign prostatic hypertrophy (BPH). Which symptom is the client most likely to exhibit?
   ○ 1. Impotence.
   ○ 2. Flank pain.
   ○ 3. Difficulty starting the urinary stream.
   ○ 4. Hematuria.

141. Which of the following would be the *most* helpful strategy to use for anger management when dealing with a verbally aggressive client?
   ○ 1. Role-playing assertive statements with the nurse.
   ○ 2. Watching a videotape about assertiveness.
   ○ 3. Describing feelings that occur after aggressive outbursts.
   ○ 4. Discussing situations that appear to be threatening.

142. Which of the following actions would the nurse anticipate using when caring for a term neonate diagnosed with transient tachypnea at 2 hours after birth?
   ○ 1. Monitoring the neonate's color and cry every 4 hours.
   ○ 2. Feeding the neonate with a bottle every 3 hours.
   ○ 3. Obtaining extracorporeal membrane oxygenation equipment.
   ○ 4. Providing warm, humidified oxygen in a warm environment.

143. A client is to receive Gantrisin 1.5 g every 6 hours orally. The Gantrisin comes in an elixir of 300 mg in 2 mL. How many milliliters should the nurse give?
   ○ 1. 1.0 mL.
   ○ 2. 2.0 mL.
   ○ 3. 5.0 mL.
   ○ 4. 10.0 mL.

144. The skin tone of a client of Vietnamese descent with

dark skin who has early signs of iron-deficiency anemia appears

○ 1. reddish-brown.

○ 2. yellowish-brown.

○ 3. black-brown.

○ 4. whitish-brown.

145. Which of the following laboratory findings would be present in nephrotic syndrome?

○ 1. Decreased total serum protein.

○ 2. Hypercalcemia.

○ 3. Hyperglycemia.

○ 4. Decreased hematocrit.

146. While caring for several preterm infants in the special care nursery, which of the following actions would be *most* important for preventing nosocomial infections in these neonates?

○ 1. Using sterile supplies for all treatments.

○ 2. Performing thorough handwashing before giving infant care.

○ 3. Donning cover gowns for nurses and visitors to the unit.

○ 4. Wearing a mask, and changing it frequently when giving care.

147. Which of the following types of restraints would be best for the nurse to use for a child in the immediate postoperative period after cleft palate repair?

○ 1. Safety jacket.

○ 2. Elbow restraints.

○ 3. Wrist restraints.

○ 4. Body restraints.

148. When preparing to present a community program about women who are victims of physical abuse, which of the following would the nurse stress about the incidence of battering?

○ 1. Death from battering is rare.

○ 2. Battering is a major cause of injury to women.

○ 3. Lower socioeconomic groups are primarily affected.

○ 4. Battering rarely involves pregnant women.

149. A client undergoes a nephrectomy. In the immediate postoperative period, which nursing intervention has the *highest* priority?

○ 1. Monitoring blood pressure.

○ 2. Encouraging the use of the incentive spirometer.

○ 3. Assessing urinary output hourly.

○ 4. Checking the flank dressing for urinary drainage.

150. A nulliparous client tells the nurse that during her last pelvic examination the physician said that her uterus was in a severe retroverted position. The nurse determines that the client may experience which of the following?

○ 1. Frequent vaginal infections.

○ 2. Pain from endometriosis.

○ 3. Severe menstrual cramping.

○ 4. Difficulty conceiving a child.

151. A mother tells the nurse that she wants her 4-year-old to stop sucking her thumb. When developing the teaching plan for this mother, which of the following would the nurse expect to suggest?

○ 1. Apply a special medicine that tastes terrible on the thumb.

○ 2. Get the child to agree to stop the thumb sucking.

○ 3. Remind the child every time the mother sees the thumb in her mouth.

○ 4. Put the child in "time-out" every time the mother observes thumb sucking.

152. A client in severe respiratory distress is admitted to the hospital. When assessing the client, the nurse should

○ 1. conduct a complete health history.

○ 2. complete a comprehensive physical examination.

○ 3. delay assessment until client's respiratory distress is resolved.

○ 4. focus assessment on the respiratory system and distress.

153. A client has had a total hip replacement. Which of the following signs would most likely indicate that the hip has dislocated?

○ 1. Abduction of the affected leg.

○ 2. Loosening of the prosthesis.

○ 3. External rotation of the affected leg.

○ 4. Shortening of the affected leg.

154. A client with paranoid schizophrenia is withdrawn and suspicious of others and projects blame. The client's behavior reflects problems in which of the following stages of development as identified by Erikson?

○ 1. Trust versus mistrust.

○ 2. Autonomy versus shame and doubt.

○ 3. Initiative versus guilt.

○ 4. Intimacy versus isolation.

155. During the initial interview, a client with a compulsive eating disorder remarks, "I can't stand myself and the way I look." Which of the following statements by the nurse would be *most* therapeutic?

○ 1. "Everyone who has the same problem feels like you do."

○ 2. "I don't think you look bad at all."

○ 3. "Don't worry, you'll soon be back in shape."

○ 4. "Tell me more about your feelings."

156. A client with a new ileal conduit asks the nurse when he will need to wear his appliance. Which of the following responses by the nurse is correct?

○ 1. "You will need to wear your appliance all the time."

○ 2. "You will need to wear your appliance after you irrigate."

○ 3. "It is only necessary to wear your appliance at night."

○ 4. "The appliance must be worn after your meals."

157. A child who is admitted after having suffered trauma

has also been exposed to varicella. Which of the following would the nurse institute for infection control?
- ○ 1. Airborne precautions.
- ○ 2. Droplet precautions.
- ○ 3. Contact precautions.
- ○ 4. Indirect contact precautions.

158. Which of the following expected outcomes would be appropriate for a client with multiple myeloma?
- ○ 1. Achieve effective management of bone pain.
- ○ 2. Recover from the disease with minimal disabilities.
- ○ 3. Decrease episodes of nausea and vomiting.
- ○ 4. Monitor for signs of hyperkalemia.

159. A client with major depression is completing his morning care independently. When the nurse approaches the client with his medication, he tells the nurse that he is a failure as a husband and a father and is worthless. His wife told the nurse previously that the client is a good provider and a wonderful father and husband. Which of the following responses by the nurse would be *most* appropriate?
- ○ 1. "You were able to shower and dress without any help this morning."
- ○ 2. "Your wife told me that you are a good husband and father."
- ○ 3. "You don't have any reason why you should feel that way."
- ○ 4. "This medication will help your thinking."

160. The nurse uses Montgomery straps primarily to achieve which of the following client outcomes?
- ○ 1. The client is free from falls.
- ○ 2. The client is free from bruises.
- ○ 3. The client is free from skin breakdown.
- ○ 4. The client is free from wandering.

161. After an episode of severe pain, a client says to the nurse, "The pain really frightened me. I thought I was going to die." Which statement would be the most appropriate response from the nurse?
- ○ 1. "I understand that pain can be a frightening experience."
- ○ 2. "Why were you frightened? You have had pain before."
- ○ 3. "There's no need to be frightened of pain."
- ○ 4. "Pain cannot cause you to die. Try to relax."

162. A child returns to the pediatric unit after a bowel resection. Which of the following actions has the *highest* priority?
- ○ 1. Administer intravenous fluids.
- ○ 2. Keep the child NPO.
- ○ 3. Monitor vital signs frequently.
- ○ 4. Assess the child's pain level.

163. During a health history, a 59-year-old male client is being evaluated for possible type 2 diabetes mellitus. Which of the following client statements supports the diagnosis of type 2 diabetes?

- ○ 1. "I have some shortness of breath when I exercise."
- ○ 2. "No matter how much I drink, I'm still thirsty all the time."
- ○ 3. "I wake up early in the morning and can't return to sleep."
- ○ 4. "In the past couple of weeks, I've been having a lot of trouble urinating."

164. A common nursing diagnosis for a client who has hypothyroidism and is complaining of fatigue, muscular weakness, and muscle cramping would be
- ○ 1. Activity Intolerance.
- ○ 2. Anxiety.
- ○ 3. Hopelessness.
- ○ 4. Ineffective Family Coping.

165. A client is diagnosed with metastatic bone cancer. Because of this diagnosis, which of the following abnormal laboratory values would the nurse expect to see?
- ○ 1. Hypocalcemia.
- ○ 2. Elevated serum alkaline phosphatase.
- ○ 3. Elevated aspartate aminotransferase (AST).
- ○ 4. Hypokalemia.

166. A 25-year-old man has been diagnosed with hypertrophic cardiomyopathy. The nurse plans to assess the client for
- ○ 1. angina.
- ○ 2. fatigue and shortness of breath.
- ○ 3. abdominal pain.
- ○ 4. hypertension.

167. The nurse would advise the mother of a toddler suspected of having pinworms to do the cellophane tape test at which of the following times?
- ○ 1. Before bathing.
- ○ 2. After a bowel movement.
- ○ 3. While the child is asleep.
- ○ 4. After a meal.

168. Which of the following conditions occurring in a mother's pregnancy would provide a clue that the newborn might have a gastrointestinal tract anomaly?
- ○ 1. Meconium in the amniotic fluid.
- ○ 2. Low implantation of the placenta.
- ○ 3. Increased amount of amniotic fluid.
- ○ 4. Toxemia in the last trimester.

169. As part of the treatment plan, a client is prescribed steroids to treat ulcerative colitis. The nurse should assess the client for which of the following common complications related to steroid therapy?
- ○ 1. Peptic ulcer.
- ○ 2. Hypoglycemia.
- ○ 3. Tachycardia.
- ○ 4. Renal failure.

170. A client's abdominal incision eviscerates. The nurse's priority action on detecting the evisceration is to

○ 1. take the client's vital signs and call the physician.
○ 2. lower the client's head and elevate the feet.
○ 3. cover the incision with a dressing moistened with sterile saline.
○ 4. start an emergency infusion of intravenous fluids.

171. What is the priority nursing intervention for a client who is admitted to the emergency department with burns over an estimated 27% of the body surface area?
○ 1. Insert a large-caliber intravenous line.
○ 2. Administer morphine intramuscularly.
○ 3. Establish an airway.
○ 4. Administer tetanus toxoid.

172. Which of the following clients would the nurse expect to place on one-to-one suicide precautions?
○ 1. A client who is withdrawn and anorectic.
○ 2. A client who refuses to sign a "no suicide" contract.
○ 3. A client who is visibly crying.
○ 4. A client who refuses his medication.

173. To prepare a client who has a fractured femur for ambulation, the nurse teaches her how to do quadriceps setting exercises. Which of the following client instructions is most accurate?
○ 1. "Contract and relax your buttocks."
○ 2. "Try to lift your legs up when I press against your feet."
○ 3. "Press the back of your knee against the bed."
○ 4. "Flex and extend your toes."

174. A client with an ileostomy calls the nurse to report that she is experiencing abdominal cramps, vomiting, and watery discharge from her ileostomy. What would be the nurse's best response?
○ 1. Tell the client to take 30 mL of milk of magnesia.
○ 2. Encourage the client to increase her fluid intake.
○ 3. Have the client measure her abdominal girth.
○ 4. Notify the physician immediately.

175. Which of the following signs and symptoms would indicate that a client with HIV infection has developed acquired immunodeficiency syndrome (AIDS)?
○ 1. Severe fatigue at night.
○ 2. Pain on standing and walking.
○ 3. Weight loss of 10 pounds over 3 months.
○ 4. Herpes simplex ulcer persisting for 2 months.

176. The nurse has been teaching a client with genital herpes how to care for the lesions. Which of the following statements by the client indicates that she needs additional instruction?
○ 1. "I will use a sitz bath to decrease the inflammation of the sores."
○ 2. "I will wear occlusive underwear to prevent transmission of the virus."
○ 3. "I can use a hair dryer to dry the lesions as long as I use a cool setting."
○ 4. "It is important that I drink plenty of fluids."

177. The client has been taking propantheline bromide (Pro-Banthine) at home. The nurse prepares a teaching plan for the client indicating that the medication acts primarily to achieve which of the following?
○ 1. Suppress gastric secretions.
○ 2. Neutralize acid in the stomach.
○ 3. Shorten the time required for digestion in the stomach.
○ 4. Improve the mixing of foods and gastric secretions.

178. Which of the following dietary changes should the nurse emphasize to a client with fibrocystic breast disease?
○ 1. Increase sodium consumption.
○ 2. Use only bottled water.
○ 3. Decrease consumption of caffeine.
○ 4. Decrease calcium intake.

179. A very obese client would like to lose weight and attends an introductory class on how to eat properly. The nurse provides him with a brochure that contains information, updated every 5 years, that guides healthy eating. This brochure is called
○ 1. *The Dietary Guidelines for Hearty Eating.*
○ 2. *The Dietary Guidelines for Americans.*
○ 3. *The Guidelines and Goals for Americans.*
○ 4. *Food for Lifestyle.*

180. A client with an Axis I diagnosis of bipolar disorder, mania, states to the nurse, "I'm the Prince of Wales and you will be my Queen Anna. Get ready for our wedding." Which of the following replies by the nurse would be *most* appropriate?
○ 1. "Sorry, but I am already happily married and won't be getting ready for a wedding."
○ 2. "No, you know better, we are not going to be married. There will be no wedding."
○ 3. "You are Sam Smith, a client here in the hospital, and I'm Marjorie, a nurse here on the unit."
○ 4. "You are not a prince and I cannot be your queen. We are not going to be married."

181. A client with a new colostomy tells the nurse she thinks she is ready to learn how to care for it. Which of the following interventions would most likely be effective in preparing the client to look at the colostomy?
○ 1. Tell her how quickly other clients have adjusted to caring for their colostomies.
○ 2. Encourage her to handle the colostomy appliance.
○ 3. Ask a female member of the local ostomy club to visit her.
○ 4. Show the client pictures that illustrate how a colostomy looks and functions.

Correct Answers and Rationale

The letters in parentheses following the rationale identify the step of the nursing process (A, D, P, I, E), client needs (1, 2, 3, 4, 5, 6, 7, 8, 9, 10), and nursing care area (O, Y, M, X). See the inside front cover for the key.

1. 3. Illegible writing is one of the most common reasons for medication errors. The physician should be called to clarify the order. The previous medication record should not be used as a substitute for the exact order written by the physician. The pharmacist or the client's family cannot be asked to interpret an order written by a physician. (I, 1, M)

2. 2. Propantheline bromide is an anticholinergic used to decrease biliary spasm. Decreasing biliary spasm aids in the reduction of pain in cholecystitis. Propantheline does not increase bile production or have an antiemetic effect, and it is not effective in treating infection. (P, 8, M)

3. 3. An important function of the National Cystic Fibrosis Foundation is to put parents of children with cystic fibrosis in touch with each other. Other parents are often able to offer support and help. In some instances, the Foundation gives parents financial assistance for equipment required for home care of their child with cystic fibrosis (but not for medications). The Foundation does not obtain tutors for children or provide genetic counseling for parents. (I, 1, Y)

4. 4. Laryngeal stridor is characteristic of respiratory distress from inflammation and swelling after a bronchoscopy. It must be reported immediately. Green sputum would be indicative of infection and would occur 3 to 5 days after the bronchoscopy. A mild cough or hemoptysis would be usual after a bronchoscopy. If a tissue biopsy specimen was obtained, sputum may be blood-streaked for several days. (A, 9, M)

5. 3. Strategies for meeting client satisfaction include involving hospital department personnel to improve service. Saying, "The staff is doing the best they can," or, "I will report this to the physician," does not offer a practical resolution to the client's complaint. Expressing a personal dislike for the food negates the client's complaint and does not offer a solution. (I, 1, M)

6. 3. Aging clients frequently present with vague or atypical responses to medications and diseases that are erroneously attributed to aging. A new cognitive change needs to be investigated and is not an expected change with aging. Changes in a client's behavior should be investigated to see whether there is a relation to excessive sedation. The nurse can interview the family members to obtain information. (A, 3, M)

7. 2. Rehabilitation for a client who has sustained a CVA begins at the time the client is admitted to the hospital. The first goal of rehabilitation should be to help prevent deformities. This goal is achieved through such techniques as positioning the client properly in bed, changing his position frequently and supporting all parts of his body in proper alignment. Passive range-of-motion (ROM) exercises may also be started, unless contraindicated. (P, 7, M)

8. 1. Lung cancer is a very aggressive disease. Small cell lung cancer is frequently metastatic at the time of diagnosis. The client with non–small-cell lung cancer may have a longer survival time, but lung cancer continues to be an aggressive disease that disseminates rapidly. The overall 5-year survival rate for all types of lung cancer is 10% to 13%. (D, 10, M)

9. 3. The nurse's response should suggest exploration of the difficult decision-making process the client must go through. The client should be encouraged to verbalize the various options in order to make the choice that is right for her. Telling the client that she should give the baby up so it can have a better home or that research shows babies do better with their birth mothers is judgmental and does not place the control of the decision with the client. Suggesting that the client try keeping the baby at first minimizes the situation and also does not put the control of the decision with the client. (I, 5, M)

10. 2. Two nurses must verify the name and label of the blood with the client's wristband. (I, 8, M)

11. 3. Accumulation of air in the pleural cavity after a crushing chest injury may be assessed by unilateral diminished or absent breath sounds. Cheyne-Stokes respirations with periods of apnea often precede death. They are indicative of heart failure or brain death. Fremitus is increased with lung consolidation and decreased with pleural effusion or pneumothorax. Pain occurs at the injury site and increases with inspiration. (A, 9, M)

12. 2. Chewing the pill or capsule form of valproic acid can cause irritation of the mouth and throat and is contraindicated. Taking the pills at the same time each day is important to maintain therapeutic effectiveness of the drug. Taking the pills with food is appropriate if the client is experiencing gastrointestinal upset. Valproic acid may cause clotting problems; therefore, bruising should be reported. (E, 8, X)

13. 1. A significant association between feeding position and otitis media exists. Those children fed in a supine position have a high incidence of otitis media because of the reflux of milk into the eustachian tubes during feedings. Keeping the infant's ears covered when out in the cold or thoroughly drying the ears after a bath has not be associated as a contributing factor to an infant's development of ear infections. Although the infant's immunization status is always important to ascertain, other factors, such as the position of the infant when taking a bottle, have more impact. (A, 9, Y)

14. 2. It is the role of the surgeon or the person performing the procedure to obtain the informed consent. This consists of informing the client about the procedure, the risks of treatment, the side effects, other types of treatments available, and the effects without the procedure. (I, 1, M)

15. 4. Medical care is available at all times in a hospice program. Hospice care includes the dying client and the family. Care for the family may continue throughout the bereavement period. Hospice care involves care of the client at home as well as in an inpatient setting. Although professional care is provided in hospice, family members, volunteers, and unlicensed nursing personnel also participate in the care of the client. (P, 1, M)

16. 3. An 8-ounce glass of milk is the equivalent of $1^1/_2$ to 2 slices of presliced American cheese. Two tablespoons of Parmesan cheese or $^1/_2$ cup of milkshake is equivalent to 4 ounces of milk, and $^1/_2$ cup of cottage cheese is equivalent to 2 ounces of milk. (I, 7, O)

17. 1. The biophysical profile typically measures five parameters to assess the fetus: fetal breathing, movement, and tone; amniotic fluid volume; and fetal heart reactivity. The test uses a scale of 0 to 2 for each parameter with a maximum score of 10. (E, 10, O)

18. 3. One of the side effects of steroid therapy is fat deposition on the trunk and face, producing classic Cushingoid signs. Therefore, the nurse would expect to find truncal obesity. Steroids also can cause altered moods or mood swings. Typically, long-term steroid use results in a weight gain. Steroids may inhibit the action of growth hormone. Therefore, a growth spurt is not likely. (I, 8, Y)

19. 3. The nurse should not be required to participate in an abortion if it is contradictory to the nurse's religious beliefs. The behavior should not be reflected negatively on the nurses' evaluation. Preparing equipment and supplies for the case may be viewed as the same as circulating for the case. The nurse has a right not to participate in an abortion unless it is an absolute emergency and no one else is available to care for the client. (P, 1, M)

20. 3. Phenytoin (Dilantin) causes hyperplasia of the gums, and the client needs frequent dental examinations and meticulous oral hygiene. Dilantin therapy may contribute to a folic acid deficiency, but it is not related to iron or calcium metabolism. A need for frequent eye examinations is not related to the side effects of phenytoin. (I, 8, M)

21. 1. Visual acuity is not affected by long-term gentamycin sulfate (Garamycin) therapy. The nurse should establish baseline data for vestibular, renal, and auditory function because gentamycin sulfate is ototoxic and renotoxic. (A, 8, M)

22. 1. The chest is compressed with the heel of one hand positioned on the lower sternum, two fingerbreadths above the sternal notch. Fingertips are used to compress the sternum in infants, and the heels of both hands are used in adult cardiopulmonary resuscitation. (I, 10, Y)

23. 1. Bacon is high in fat and therefore a poor choice for protein. Yogurt, dry beans, and peanut butter all contain protein in amounts that make them good sources of protein for the child. (P, 7, Y)

24. 1. Nitroglycerin (Nitrostat) tablets should be taken 5 minutes apart for three doses; if this is ineffective, 911 should be called to obtain an ambulance to take the client to the emergency department. The client should not drive or have a family member drive the client to the hospital. (I, 8, M)

25. 2. Saturated fats raise blood cholesterol. Polyunsaturated fats maintain blood cholesterol. Monounsaturated fats may help to maintain or lower blood cholesterol. Phospholipids do not have an effect on cholesterol but act as emulsifiers, keeping fats dispersed in water. (D, 4, M)

26. 4. The depressed client who voices death wishes must be asked directly about thoughts of suicide and specific suicide plans. The other questions are important history questions but are not crucial to address the follow-up needed when the client verbalizes a death wish. (A, 9, M)

27. 3. This client should be monitored for blood dyscrasias, evidenced by decreased platelet count and white blood cell count with changes in the CBC differential. (I, 8, M)

28. 4. The new onset of constipation may be a sign of a tumor from colon cancer. Constipation is not an expected change of aging. Increased fiber and fluid intake is helpful with constipation, but in this case the client needs to be seen by a health care provider to rule out colon cancer. (A, 4, M)

29. 4. Saying, "We will help you be successful so that you can stay alcohol-free," conveys interest in the client as a worthwhile individual who needs help and treatment. This statement also helps to build trust and enhances self-esteem. The other statements confront the client and may result in the client's feeling belittled, judged, and rejected. (I, 6, X)

30. 3. Research has shown that at least two injections daily provide improved blood glucose control and decreased incidence of target end-organ damage. Type 1 diabetes requires insulin replacement and cannot be managed with oral medications alone. It would be inappropriate to ask the physician to change the insulin schedule. (I, 8, M)

31. 1. Peak and trough serum levels are used to adjust the dosage within a therapeutic range. (D, 8, M)

32. 4. Dietary Reference Intakes (DRIs) are sets of nutrient intake values suggested for the dietary intakes of healthy people in the United States and Canada. The DRIs were developed to establish levels of nutrient intake required to prevent chronic disease. The DRIs are meant to replace the Recommended Daily Allowances (RDAs), which represented the minimum amount required to prevent symptoms of deficiency. The Dietary Guidelines describe food choices that promote good health. (A, 4, M)

33. 1. Clients with diabetes and chronic respiratory conditions are most at risk for influenza and should receive the vaccine yearly. Diabetes and chronic respiratory conditions do not increase the risk of hepatitis A. An adult client is not as likely to need MMR or Varivax, but titers can be checked if the client has not had childhood immunizations or the disease. (I, 8, M)

34. 2. Infants are sensitive to stress in their caretakers. The best way to handle an anxious infant is to talk quietly to him, thereby soothing the infant. Limiting holding of the infant to feeding periods interferes with meeting the infant's needs for close contact, possibly compromising his ability to develop trust. Playing music in the room for most of the day and night will make it difficult for the infant to differentiate days from nights. Having a friend take the infant for several days will not necessarily take care of the problem, because when the infant returns to the mother the same behaviors will recur unless the mother makes some changes. (I, 5, Y)

35. 1. The infant is exhibiting periodic breathing, which normal in infants of this age. The infant typically alternates short periods of rapid, louder respirations with periods of slower, quieter respirations. (D, 3, Y)

36. 2. Tracheostomy tubes are associated with several potential complications, including laryngeal nerve damage, bleeding, and infection. Tracheostomy tubes do not cause decreased cardiac output, pneumothorax, or ARDS. (A, 10, M)

37. 4. A glycosylated hemoglobin level gives the nurse data about the average blood glucose concentration over 2 to 3 months, providing a picture of the client's overall glucose control. A fasting serum glucose level gives a picture of the child's recent glucose level, not the overall effectiveness of the child's therapeutic regimen. A 1-week diet recall is not always accurate. Although a home log would provide some information about the child's overall control and compliance, the log may not have all of the glucose levels recorded. (E, 10, Y)

38. 1. The nurse's first action should be to clamp off the transfusion, because the client is having a transfusion reaction. It is most important that the client not receive any more blood. Other measures may be appropriate after the blood has been stopped. The nurse should raise the head of the bed if the client becomes short of breath. A blood sample for culture and sensitivity analysis should be taken before an antibiotic is started so that an antibiotic-specific agent can be administered. The nurse can provide a cool washcloth for a headache or fever; however, this is not a priority. (E, 8, M)

39. 3. People with AIDS are immunocompromised, and food safety is an important concern. Foodborne illnesses and infections can be devastating to the client with AIDS. Large, frequent meals are not necessary. Megadoses of vitamins can result in toxicities that may aggravate the patient's clinical condition. Leaving food out encourages growth of microorganisms. (I, 7, M)

40. 3. The incisions made for upper abdominal surgeries, such as cholecystectomies, are near the diaphragm and make deep breathing painful. Incentive spirometry, which encourages deep breathing, is essential to prevent atelectasis after surgery. The client is not maintained on bed rest for several days. The client is encouraged to ambulate by the first postoperative day, even with drainage tubes in place. Nasogastric tubes do not inhibit deep breathing and coughing. (I, 10, M)

41. 4. This finding describes Mongolian spots, which are common in newborns of African, Asian, or Latin descent. Telangiectatic nevi, or "stork bites," are pink lesions most often found on the back of the neck. Milia are small white papules over the nose and cheek that are indicative of blocked sebaceous glands. (A, 3, M)

42. 1. Blurred vision is a serious adverse effect of oral contraceptives, possibly because of severe hypertension as a result of the medication. If the client experiences blurred vision, she needs to contact her health care provider immediately. Nausea, weight gain, and mild headache are common and possibly bothersome side effects and should be noted. However, they do not need to be reported immediately unless they are severe, prolonged, or accompanied by other symptoms. (I, 8, O)

43. 1. Signs and symptoms of a pneumothorax include sudden, sharp pain with breathing or coughing on the affected side, tachypnea, dyspnea, diminished or absent breath sounds on affected side, tachycardia, anxiety, and restlessness. Tracheal deviation away from the affected side indicates the presence of a tension pneumothorax, which is a medical emergency. (A, 9, M)

44. 2. When a client is experiencing a flashback, the nurse should stay with the client, offer reassurance, and present reality in a nonthreatening manner to minimize the client's anxiety and agitation. The client needs to be told that she is experiencing an effect from LSD and that she is safe and the flashback will end. Confronting the client's misperceptions or challenging her unrealistic statements could increase her anxiety and agitation, possibly leading to aggressive behavior. Secluding the client until the flashback ends usually is not necessary or appropriate unless the client threatens or demonstrates aggression toward self or others. (P, 6, X)

45. 2. The nurse should dispose of any used needle and syringe by immediately placing uncapped, used needles and syringes in the universal precaution container. (I, 8, M)

46. 3. Nausea and vomiting, along with hypokalemia, are likely indicators of digitalis toxicity. Hypokalemia is a common cause of digitalis toxicity; therefore, serum potassium levels should be carefully monitored if the client is taking digoxin. The earliest clinical signs of digitalis toxicity are anorexia, nausea, and vomiting. Bradycardia, other dysrhythmias, and visual disturbances are also common signs. Chronic renal failure usually causes hyperkalemia. With persistent vomiting, the client would be more likely to develop metabolic alkalosis than metabolic acidosis. (A, 8, M)

47. 2. Food sources high in calcium include steamed broccoli, dairy products, and fortified cereals. Rice, apples, and meat are not calcium-rich sources. Menopausal women need 1500 mg of calcium daily. (I, 9, M)

48. 2. At the time a client receives a Depo-Provera injection, a follow-up appointment should be made for 3 months later. The nurse should emphasize the need to adhere to the medication schedule to prevent an unplanned pregnancy. One of the most common reasons for failure of this contraceptive is lack of adherence to the appointment schedule for injections every 3 months. (I, 8, M)

49. 1. In major burns, there is a significant initial shift of fluid out of the plasma space into the interstitial spaces. This is the result of increased capillary permeability. Because of the increased permeability of capillary walls, water, sodium, and plasma protein escape into the tissues, increasing the tissue colloidal osmotic pressure and causing edema. Plasma colloidal pressure is decreased as a result of protein loss. A decrease in capillary hydrostatic pressure does not result in edema; an increase does. As fluid escapes into the tissues, it creates an increase in interstitial fluid pressure, not a decrease. (A, 10, M)

50. 4. The pH of 7.52 indicates that the body is in a state of alkalosis. The PCO_2 value is normal and the HCO_3^- value is elevated. The increased HCO_3^- value indicates that the acid–base imbalance is metabolic alkalosis. Restlessness can be a clinical finding in metabolic alkalosis. (D, 10, M)

51. 3. Panting will alleviate the client's urge to push. The client risks edema or tearing of the cervix if pushing begins before complete cervical dilation (10 cm) is achieved. Although turning the client to her left side improves uteroplacental blood flow, it will have no effect on diminishing the client's urge to push. Although focusing on an object in the room may help the client to relax, it will have no effect on diminishing the client's urge to push due to the pressure of a fetus at +1 station. (I, 3, O)

52. 1. The client who is taking potentially nephrotoxic antibiotics does not need to report straw-colored urine because this is normal. The client needs to report if the urine is cloudy, smoky, or pink; early signs of nephrotoxicity are manifested by changes in the color of urine. (P, 8, M)

53. 4. Clinical manifestations of juvenile hypothyroidism include dry skin, constipation, sparse hair, and sleepiness. Short attention span, weight loss, moist flushed skin, rapid pulse, and heat intolerance would suggest hyperthyroidism. (A, 10, Y)

54. 1. In clients with excess fluid volume, sodium restriction may be necessary to promote fluid loss. Monitoring electrolytes daily may be appropriate but will not reduce the excess of fluid. Maintaining a record of the client's intake and output is also an independent nursing intervention. Elevating the client's feet helps promote venous return and fluid reabsorption but in itself will not reduce the volume of excess fluid. The nurse can elevate the client's feet without a medical order. (P, 10, M)

55. 3. The bluish pigment on the buttocks and back of an African American infant is a common finding and should be documented as Mongolian spots in the child's record. These spots typically fade by the time the child is 5 or 6 years of age. Additional assessment by the physician is not indicated. Laser therapy is not used. Rather, laser therapy is useful for port wine stains, which are dark purple and disfiguring. (I, 3, O)

56. 1. Clients might wear objects as a protection against specific medical disorders. Typically these practices bring no harm to the client and should not be discouraged. The client should continue to be encouraged to follow the medical guidance of her health care provider. If the practice is not harming the client, it is inappropriate to label it quackery and demand that the client discontinue it. There is no medical evidence to support the wearing of a copper bracelet. (I, 5, M)

57. 4. Normally, a neonate's heart rate should be between 120 and 160 bpm shortly after birth. The nurse should document this as a normal neonatal finding. The physician does not need to be notified. Assessing for cyanosis is a routine assessment at birth, but with the neonate's heart rate at 142 bpm, cyanosis should be minimal and typically located in the hands and feet. Heart rate assessments are performed routinely according to the institution's protocol. For example, the heart rate is assessed soon after birth, then every 15 minutes for 1 hour, then every 30 minutes for 1 hour, and then every 4 hours. (I, 3, O)

58. 1. In a frank breech, the buttocks alone present to the cervix, while the knees are extended to rest on the chest. In a cephalic presentation, the head is the fetal body part first coming in contact with the cervix. Both feet presenting to the cervix is termed double footling breech. In a shoulder presentation, one of the shoulders (actually the acromion process) presents to the cervix. Typically, the fetus is lying horizontally (transverse lie). (I, 3, O)

59. 1. The therapeutic effects of desmopressin (DDAVP) nasal spray are relief of polydipsia and control of polyuria and nocturia in clients with diabetes insipidus. Side effects include nasal congestion and headache. Blurred vision is not related to desmopressin. (I, 8, M)

60. 2. A mammogram can detect a lesion the size of a pinhead, and a lump is about 2 cm in size before it can be detected on BSE. The American Cancer Society guidelines recommend a mammogram yearly after 40 years of age. A mammogram will not detect other endocrine abnormalities. (A, 4, M)

61. 1. Protein and vitamin C are particularly important in promoting wound healing and recovery from infection. A diet high in carbohydrates is also essential. Because clients with infections frequently do not feel like eating, it is important that what they are encouraged to eat should be nutritious. Chicken and orange slices would help meet the client's protein and vitamin needs. A meal of cheeseburger and fries or cheese omelet and bacon is high in fat and low in vitamins. Gelatin salad and tea contain minimal nutrients. (I, 7, M)

62. 4. Beef, liver, iron-fortified cereals, and spinach are iron-rich foods. Cheese, squash, and eggs are not significant sources of iron. (I, 9, M)

63. 2. Good sources of dietary iron include red meats, poultry, green leafy vegetables, and dried fruits such as raisins. Milk products are poor sources of iron. Carrots are high in vitamin A. (E, 10, Y)

64. 2. The pallor and cool temperature of the fingers and the decreased return time for capillary refill are indicative of decreased arterial blood supply to the fingers. These findings are not normal for any time in the recovery process. Nerve impairment would include numbness, tingling, and impaired movement of the fingers. Signs of venous stasis would include edema and reddening of the fingers, not pallor and cool temperature. (D, 9, M)

65. 1. Warm showers, baths, or hand soaks can help relieve joint stiffness and allow the client to more comfortably perform activities of daily living. Aspirin or other anti-inflammatory drugs should be taken before activity to help decrease inflammation and reduce joint pain and inflammation. Although weight loss may decrease stress on joints, pain and stiffness will continue to be a problem. Cold compresses are most effective for relieving joint pain, whereas moist heat is useful for decreasing pain and stiffness. When cold compresses are applied, their use should be limited to 10 to 15 minutes at a time to decrease the chance of tissue damage. (P, 10, M)

66. 2. The most appropriate immediate response is to open the airway. The nurse then would look, listen, and feel for respirations. Noting none, the nurse would attempt two quick breaths and call a code blue. (D, 10, M)

67. 4. The nurse would remind the client about meal and activity times so that the ritual could be completed beforehand and not interfere with meals and activities. The client must be allowed to complete her rituals because they are a way to keep anxiety in check. Totally eliminating the client's ritual will increase the client's anxiety and the need for the handwashing. Allowing the client to decide whether she wants to attend meals and activities is not appropriate or in the client's best interests, because the client must perform the ritual to assuage anxiety. Informing the client that absence from meals and activities is not permitted scolds the client, increasing her anxiety and her need for the ritual. (I, 6, X)

68. 2. The client needs further instructions when she says, "If I become pregnant, I can continue to eat sushi twice a week." Raw fish, including tuna, should be avoided while the client is pregnant because of the risk of contamination with mercury and other potential teratogens. Folic acid supplements taken before the client gets pregnant and during pregnancy can help reduce the risk of neural tube defects. Steaming the vegetables reduces the risk that vitamins will be lost in the cooking water. Soy products can increase the client's protein levels. (E, 3, O)

69. 4. The nurse should acknowledge that the client feels better, but should also remind the client to continue his drug therapy and other self-care activities of rest, exercise, joint protection, and adequate nutrition. Wearing the bracelet is not harmful, and the nurse should not instruct the client to remove it or label it "quackery." Copper bracelets do not interfere with salicylate metabolism. (I, 5, M)

70. 4. Stanol esters are not recognized by the intestine and bind up dietary cholesterol from being absorbed. Stanol esters do not enter the blood and cannot, therefore, directly lower cholesterol. Stanol esters do not block digestion of cholesterol, only its absorption. They do not inhibit lipoprotein lipase. (D, 4, M)

71. 3. Acupuncture, like acumassage and acupressure, is performed in certain Asian cultures to restore the energy balance within the body. Pressure, massage, and fine needles are applied to "energy pathways" to help restore the body's balance. Acupuncture is not based on a belief in purging evil spirits. Although pain relief through acupuncture can achieve promote tranquility, acupuncture is performed to restore energy balance. In the Western world, many researchers think that the gate-control theory of pain may explain the success of acupuncture, acumassage, and acupressure. (D, 7, M)

72. 2. Tinnitus or ringing in the ears is a sign of aspirin toxicity and should be reported. Clients should be instructed to take aspirin as prescribed and to avoid overdosage. Gastrointestinal symptoms associated with aspirin include nausea, heartburn, and epigastric discomfort caused by gastric irritation. Abdominal cramps, rash, and hypotension are not related to aspirin therapy. (I, 8, M)

73. 4. The nurse does not need to know that the client has four grandchildren in the transfer report, because this is not information needed to help with the client's continuity of care. (D, 1, M)

74. 3. Although breech presentations are rare, footling breech occurs when there is an extension of the fetal knees and one or both feet protrude through the pelvis. In frank breech there is flexion of the fetal thighs and extension of the knees. The feet rest at the sides of the fetal head. In complete breech there is flexion of the fetal thighs and knees; the fetus appears to be squatting. Vertex position occurs in 95% of deliveries; in such cases, the head is engaged in the pelvis. (D, 10, O)

75. 3. Traveling is not advised because of the client's history of PIH. The client may be in jeopardy if complications occur and medical care is not available. In some cases, insurance companies will not cover costs of medical care in foreign countries. Air travel is not associated with preterm labor, although some airlines advise clients who are at 28 weeks or beyond not to travel by air. Any travel that causes fatigue should be avoided. Additionally, any pregnant client should get frequent exercise while traveling to avoid venous stasis from prolonged sitting. The client is not at any greater risk for communicable diseases. The priority is the client's history of PIH, which, if it occurs, could lead to complications. (I, 9, O)

76. 3. WIC, or Women, Infants, and Children Supplemental Food Program, would be the best option. Home-delivered and congregate meals are for adults older than 60 years of age. The food bank foods would not ensure adequate intake of the appropriate nutrients during pregnancy. (P, 7, M)

77. 4. A supine position in extension is the position most likely to prevent contractures. Clients who have experienced burns will find a flexed position most comfortable. However, flexion promotes the development of contractures. The high Fowler's and semi-Fowler's positions create hip flexion. The prone position would be contraindicated in this client because of head and neck burns. In clients with head and neck burns, pillows should not be used under the head or neck, because this will promote neck flexion contractures. (I, 9, M)

78. 2. A fractured femur, especially an open fracture, can cause much soft tissue damage and lead to significant blood loss. Hypovolemic shock can develop. Cardiogenic shock occurs when cardiac output is decreased as a result of ineffective pumping. Neurogenic shock occurs as a result of an impaired autonomic nervous system function. Anaphylactic shock is the result of an allergic reaction. (A, 10, M)

79. 2. Safety concerns are essential for a client with sensory impairment. Water temperature should be tested carefully, hot water bottles should be avoided, and the skin should be inspected regularly. Independence and self-care are also important; the client should not be instructed to avoid kitchen activities out of fear of injury. (I, 2, M)

80. 3. These behaviors suggest that the adolescent is thinking of suicide. Because the behaviors have been going on with the adolescent for a period of time, it would be imperative for the adolescent to see his health care professional as soon as possible to determine whether he is indeed experiencing suicidal thoughts. Once the nurse makes the appointment, then obtaining more information would be appropriate. Giving the father the telephone number for the local crisis hotline is appropriate once the appointment is made, to ensure that the father has additional support should the adolescent's behavior escalate and an emergency situation arises. Taking the adolescent to the nearest mental health outpatient facility now is not warranted unless the adolescent's behavior escalates. (I, 5, Y)

81. 1. For a child with chorea-like movements, safety is of prime importance. Feeding the child may be difficult. Forks should be avoided because of the danger of injury to the mouth and face with the tines. (P, 2, Y)

82. 1. After a TURP, sphincter tone is poor, resulting in dribbling or incontinence. Kegel exercises can increase sphincter tone and decrease the dribbling. Voiding every hour will not prevent dribbling or improve sphincter tone. It may take up to 12 months for urinary continence to be regained. (I, 9, M)

83. 1. The pattern of weight gain is often more important than the amount. Clients should be advised to gain a total of 25 to 35 pounds if they are of average weight when becoming pregnant. The recommended pattern is 1 pound per month in the first trimester, then 1 pound per week in the second and third trimester. A sudden increase in weight gain is associated with pregnancy-induced hypertension, whereas a sudden weight loss may indicate an illness. (I, 3, O)

84. 2. The nurse should administer 0.4 mL to administer 0.1 mg of digoxin (Lanoxin) intravenously if it comes in a concentration of 0.5 mg/2 mL, or 0.25 mg/mL. (I, 8, M)

85. 2. Numerous things have been tried by mothers with babies crying with colic. However, research has identified that the motion of a car is soothing to a baby with colic, frequently quieting the infant. The more the infant cries, the more air is swallowed, adding to the colic pain. Cereal should not be offered until the infant is 4 to 6 months of age because of the increased risk of food allergies. Additionally, cereal has not been found to help with colic. (I, 10, Y)

86. 2. Compartment syndrome, caused by compression of blood vessels and nerves, can lead to irreversible muscle and nerve damage if not detected early. Common signs of compartment syndrome in the arm include pain unrelieved by analgesics, pain on passive extension of fingers, loss of function, numbness and tingling, pallor, coolness of the extremity, and decreased or absent peripheral pulse. Delayed bone union does not cause symptoms of neurovascular impairment. Fat embolism is characterized primarily by confusion and respiratory symptoms. Osteomyelitis is infection of the bone and is manifested by signs and symptoms of inflammation and infection. (D, 9, M)

87. 2. Inpatient cardiac rehabilitation includes client and family education and individualized activity counseling. Generally, the educational programs focus on presenting all of the coronary artery risk factors associated with coronary artery disease. Low-back training would be associated with a back injury recovery program. A strength training or jogging exercise program would not be appropriate immediately after a cardiac event but could be associated with outpatient cardiac rehabilitation goals. (P, 7, M)

88. 3. When the nurse is unable to elicit the Moro reflex of a 4-day-old preterm infant and the Moro reflex was present at birth, intracranial hemorrhage or cerebral edema should be suspected. Other symptoms include lethargy, bulging fontanels, and seizure activity. Confirmation can be made by ultrasound. Postnatal asphyxia would be suggested by respiratory distress, grunting, nasal flaring, and cyanosis. A skull fracture can be confirmed by radiography. However, it is unlikely to occur in a preterm neonate. Rather, it is more common in neonates who are large for gestational age. Facial nerve paralysis is indicated when there is no movement on one side of the face. This condition is more common in large-for-gestational-age neonates. (D, 9, O)

89. 4. Blood clots are normal after TURP surgery, but bright red urine can indicate a hemorrhage. The nurse should assess the client's vital signs and notify the surgeon. Irrigation of the catheter may help remove clots, but it does not decrease bleeding. Milking a urinary catheter or increasing fluid intake is not effective for controlling bleeding or decreasing clots. (I, 9, M)

90. 3. The statement, "My medicine is not for the everyday stress of life," indicates an accurate understanding of the nurse's teaching about the use of lorazepam (Ativan). Antianxiety agents like the benzodiazepines are used to treat anxiety that is unmanageable by other means and beyond the client's ability to cope. For the drug to be effective, it must be taken as prescribed. Lorazepam can cause physical and psychological dependence. Tolerance can occur, and doubling the dose of Ativan may increase the chance of tolerance. Lorazepam is a central nervous system depressant. When it is taken in combination with alcohol, this depressant effect increases, posing danger to the client. (E, 8, X)

91. 1. A blood test for α-fetoprotein is recommended at 15 to 20 weeks' gestation to screen for neural tube defects such as spina bifida. Chorionic villi sampling is used to detect chromosomal anomalies. Amniotic fluid amino acid determination would be used to detect inborn errors of metabolism, such as phenylketonuria. An amniocentesis is used to determine the lecithin–sphingomyelin ratio. Fetal lung maturity is indicated by a ratio of 2:1. (P, 9, O)

92. 4. The error should be reported to the physician promptly for orders. The nurse should complete an incident report because an unusual occurrence happened during the client's care. The nurse should observe the client for symptoms of hyperglycemia but first must call the physician and complete an incident report. The nursing assistant does not need to be reas-

signed for this error. The nurse does not need to reprimand the nursing assistant for the error, because the nursing assistant already knows an error was made. (D, 1, M)

93. 2. After abdominal pelvic surgery, clients are especially prone to thrombophlebitis. Measuring calf circumference can help detect edema in the affected leg. The calf should not be rubbed or palpated, because a clot could be loosened and travel to the lungs as a pulmonary embolism. Homan's sign, which is calf pain on dorsiflexion of the foot when the leg is raised, is sometimes associated with thrombophlebitis. Having the client flex and extend the leg does not provide useful assessment data; the leg will not change color when raised and lowered. (A, 9, M)

94. 1. Clients who experience a sensorineural hearing loss have difficulty hearing high-pitched sounds. Aging and ototoxicity are two causes of sensorineural hearing loss. The client's ability to speak is not affected. Clients who cannot assign meaning to sound have experienced a central hearing loss. Vertigo is frequently an indication of an inner ear problem, not a hearing loss. (P, 10, M)

95. 3. Anticipatory Grieving best describes the client as she grieves for the changes occurring in her life since her cancer diagnosis. The other diagnoses may be appropriate, but Anticipatory Grieving is the most applicable diagnosis for this client. (P, 5, M)

96. 3. Nalbuphine (Nubain) is an analgesic that is used for clients in labor. It has a sedative effect and can slow the respiratory rate. After administering the drug, the nurse should first put the siderails up to prevent injury to the client and then assess the vital signs. Then the nurse can lower the head of the bed slightly to allow the client to sleep, cover the client with a blanket, and dim the lights. (I, 8, O)

97. 3. The client with emphysema is frequently underweight in appearance. It is theorized that weight loss is caused by the increased energy required to support the work of breathing. Frequent coughing, bronchospasms, and copious sputum are clinical manifestations of chronic bronchitis. (A, 10, M)

98. 4. The traction is set up correctly. Additional weights are not needed, and the angle of leg extension is appropriate. A pillow under the leg would negate the effects of the traction. Because the adolescent will be positioned in this way for an extended period, the nurse can help by finding activities that interest this client. (I, 7, Y)

99. 1. It is recommended by that individuals with a systolic blood pressure of 160 to 179 mm Hg be evaluated by a health care professional within 1 month of the screening. Individuals with a diastolic blood pressure of 90 to 99 mm Hg should be rechecked within 2 months. Exercise and reduction of stress may be desir-

able activities, but it is first necessary to evaluate the cause of elevated blood pressure. In the absence of other symptoms, it is not necessary to have the client evaluated immediately. (I, 4, M)

100. 4. Keeping the client's door closed is likely to contribute to feelings of isolation and sensory deprivation. Such activities as watching television, visiting with a relative, and reading a newspaper help prevent sensory deprivation and yet do not require physical effort. (I, 5, M)

101. 4. The client taking dexamethasone (Decadron) needs to know the early signs of hyperadrenocorticism, which include easy bruising, moonface, buffalo hump, and osteoporosis. The nurse instructs the client to report any of these signs to the physician. Hypertension is a symptom of hyperadrenocorticism, and muscle mass is decreased. Increased urinary frequency is not a symptom of hyperadrenocorticism. (P, 9, M)

102. 1. Verbalizing feelings and concerns helps decrease anxiety and allows the family member to move on to understanding the current situation. Describing events or explaining equipment is appropriate when the person is not distraught and is ready to learn. Reassuring the family member does not allow verbalization of feelings and discounts the person's feelings. (I, 5, M)

103. 2. Graded exercise testing is a diagnostic and prognostic tool used to determine the physiologic responses to controlled exercise stress. Information gained from a graded exercise test can achieve diagnostic, functional, and therapeutic objectives for the clients. Graded exercise tests involve use of a treadmill, stationary bicycle, or arm ergometry. Thinking under pressure, distance walked, and duration of walking are not the purpose of a graded exercise test. (I, 10, M)

104. 3. It is normal for clients who are beginning chemotherapy to be anxious and fearful about possible side effects. It is important that the nurse listen to the client's concerns, correct any misconceptions, and explain the supportive care that will be provided during the chemotherapy treatments. Clients need to understand that individuals do respond differently to the treatments, and their experiences may be very different from those of other people they know. A previously excellent health record does not necessarily ensure that the client will not experience side effects. Medications may lessen but not prevent the side effects, so client concerns should not be dismissed. Telling the client that she will die if she refuses treatment does nothing to allay her fears and concerns. (I, 5, M)

105. 1. Overprotection is a typical parental reaction to chronic illness in a child. Characteristics include sacrifice of self and family for the child, failure to recognize the child's capabilities and sense of responsibility, placement of overly stringent restrictions on play and peer friendship, and a lack of confidence in other peoples' capabilities. (D, 5, Y)

106. 3. Children with roseola have a high fever for 3 days, which drops suddenly. Then a nonpuritic rash appears, typically lasting for 1 to 2 days. High fever followed by a rash is a characteristic sign. Associated symptoms include cold symptoms, cough, and lymphadenopathy. (E, 10, Y)

107. 1. Knowing that the voices are not real is a reflection that the haloperidol (Haldol) is effective in decreasing the psychosis. Restlessness may be a side effect of haloperidol, not an indication of improvement. Awareness of need for activities of daily living is an indicator of improvement. However, recognizing that the voices are not real demonstrates a greater awareness of the client's disorder than the need for hygiene does. Wanting discharge reflects denial of illness. (E, 8, X)

108. 2. Older clients often have multiple physicians. The client needs to inform every doctor about all the medications being prescribed by all of them. (E, 8, X)

109. 2. The nurse should first check with the doctor for the complete order of calcium, because calcium chloride has a concentration of 13.6 mEq calcium per gram and calcium gluconate has 4.65 mEq calcium per gram. The nurse can always offer the doctor the type of calcium available once the conversion in calcium has been made; otherwise the error could be fatal. (D, 8, M)

110. 3. When administering potassium chloride intravenously, the administration should not exceed 10 mEq/hour or a concentration of 40 mEq/liter via a peripheral line. These limits are extremely important to prevent the development of hyperkalemia and the possibility of cardiac dysrhythmias. In some situations, with dangerously low serum potassium levels, the client may need cardiac monitoring and more than 10 mEq of potassium per hour. Potassium-sparing diuretics may lead to hyperkalemia because they affect the kidney's ability to excrete excess potassium. Metabolic alkalosis can cause potassium to shift into the cells, thus decreasing the client's serum potassium levels. Hypokalemia can lead to digoxin toxicity. (P, 8, M)

111. 3. Systematic pain assessment is necessary for adequate pain management in the postoperative client. Guidelines from the Agency for Healthcare Research and Quality recommend that institutions adopt a pain assessment scale to facilitate pain management. Even though the client is receiving morphine sulfate by PCA, assessment is needed if he is experiencing pain. Encouraging the client to rest or to ignore pain without further assessment is not sufficient intervention. (A, 7, M)

112. 2. Exposure to moisture can lead to maceration and the development of pressure ulcers. It is important for the client's skin to be kept clean and dry with prompt attention to cleanliness after incidents of incontinence. Client age and presence of hypertension are not factors leading to pressure ulcers. Smoking affects the oxygen status of the client but does not directly lead to the development of pressure ulcers. (A, 9, M)

113. 2. In clients who are determined to have a low-risk profile for the development of colon cancer, digital rectal examinations are recommended annually after 40 years of age. Guaiac testing of stools is also recommended annually after age 40. A baseline sigmoidoscopy is recommended at age 50. A low-fat diet is not a screening protocol but is good dietary advice for any adult client. (I, 4, M)

114. 3. A low dose of an antipsychotic can decrease aggression. Adjustment to the structured daily routine and diminished resistance with activities of daily living are improvements related to the nursing care given, not the medications. No medications currently given to treat Alzheimer's disease affect short-term memory. (E, 8, X)

115. 3. A sudden gush of dark blood, a lengthening of the umbilical cord, a smaller uterus, and changing of the uterus to a round or spherical shape are impending signs of placental separation. Pushing effort from the client is not a reliable indicator for impending placental separation, nor is it necessary for placental expulsion. (A, 3, O)

116. 1. The nurse needs to assess neurologic signs every 30 minutes from the second through the eighth hours on the client who has received t-PA or alteplase recombinant (Activase) therapy. The nurse must check for bleeding every 30 minutes for the first 8 hours. The nurse needs to check the hematocrit level, not the hemoglobin level. The blood glucose level does not need to be evaluated. (A, 9, M)

117. 2. In the emergent phase of burn management, hyperkalemia develops as a result of the destruction of red blood cells. The hematocrit is increased in response to the plasma loss that has occurred and the resulting hemoconcentration. Initially, hyponatremia may occur as sodium shifts into the interstitial spaces. (P, 10, M)

118. 1. The nurse should explain that the child will feel a stinging when the numbing medicine is inserted into the area around the introduction site of the catheter. There may also be a feeling of pressure when the catheter is introduced. Because the child will be sedated and will feel little during the procedure, telling the child that a momentary sharp pain is felt on entering the heart would be inappropriate. A tingling sensation in the extremities is not felt. (I, 9, Y)

119. 2. In conjunction with the child's history of recent respiratory infection and report of dark urine, swelling around the eyes would lead the nurse to suspect acute glomerulonephritis. Therefore, the nurse would ask about a recent sore throat, because a child with glomerulonephritis typically would have had a sore throat in the past 10 days. Drinking lots of liquids is unrelated to the periorbital edema. (A, 10, Y)

120. 2. Measuring the pH of the aspirated gastric fluid is the most accurate determination of the placement of the nasogastric tube. A pH lower than 4 indicates that the tube is in the stomach. Whether or not the client is gagging or coughing is not an accurate way to determine if the tube is placed correctly. No fluids should be inserted into the tube until the placement has been determined. Inserting air into the tube and listening for the resulting "whoosh" can be used, but this is not as accurate as pH measurement. (E, 9, M)

121. 2. True labor is present when cervical dilation and effacement are occurring. Fetal descent into the pelvic inlet is an indication that labor will begin soon. However, for a nulligravid client, this may take 1 to 2 weeks. Painful contractions every 3 to 5 minutes may be Braxton Hicks contractions. Contractions that disappear when the client lies down are a sign of false labor. Although leaking amniotic fluid should be reported, it is not a sign of true labor. (A, 3, O)

122. 4. During the first 24 hours after a total laryngectomy, maintaining a patent airway is a priority goal. After a total laryngectomy, the client will have a tracheostomy with increased secretions and will require suctioning and tracheostomy care. Providing adequate nutrition, preventing skin breakdown, and maintaining proper bowel elimination will be appropriate as the client recovers, but maintaining a patent airway is the initial priority goal. (P, 10, M)

123. 3. Not sleeping to avoid nightmares reflects inadequate grief resolution. The client is not letting go or resolving the vivid memories of the trauma as expected. Statements that the client gets sad at times but is able to function in daily activities, or that the client still misses his family but acknowledges improvement, indicate that the client is recovering and continued counseling would not be necessary. Working for train crossing safety indicates motivation to help others escape what he has experienced. This action also denotes a goal for the future, indicating recovery. (E, 6, X)

124. 3. Haloperidol (Haldol) and lorazepam (Ativan) together will decrease the hallucinations and the agitation, thus decreasing the risk for self-harm. Putting the client in restraints is premature, because danger is not imminent. Asking the client to talk about her anger is inappropriate because the client is beyond rational conversation. A room search is appropriate only after the crisis with the client is handled. (I, 6, X)

125. 1. The nurse should adjust the heparin dose to maintain the client's activated aPTT between 1.5 and 2.5 times the normal control. The PT and INR are used to maintain therapeutic levels of warfarin (Coumadin), oral anticoagulation therapy. The thrombin clotting time is used for confirmation of disseminated intravascular coagulation. (A, 9, M)

126. 2. The oral mucous membranes are easily damaged and are often ulcerated in clients with leukemia. It is better to provide oral hygiene without using a toothbrush, which can easily damage sensitive oral mucosa. Applying petrolatum jelly to the lips, swabbing the mouth with moistened cotton swabs, and rinsing the mouth with a nonirritating mouthwash are appropriate oral care measures for a child with leukemia. (I, 7, Y)

127. 1. The nurse's first response to the error is to assess the client for any untoward reactions as a result of the error. Notifying the physician and unit manager of the error, as well as completing an incident report, are all appropriate later actions, but the first action is to assess the client. (I, 1, M)

128. 3. The peak action of Regular insulin is approximately 2 to 3 hours after administration. The client is having typical hypoglycemic symptoms. Acidosis results from uncontrolled diabetes mellitus, with hyperpnea (Kussmaul respirations) as the outstanding symptom. The hallmark symptoms of hyperglycemia are increased thirst, fruity breath, and glucosuria. The signs and symptoms of diabetic ketoacidosis include Kussmaul respirations, fruity breath, tachycardia, abdominal pain, nausea, vomiting, headache, thirst, dry skin, and dehydration. (A, 8, M)

129. 4. The nurse needs to obtain more information before plans are developed. Therefore, asking to know more about the situation is most appropriate. The nurse has no way of predicting whether abuse will occur again. Therefore, it would be inappropriate for the nurse to agree with the mother, stating that the abuse probably will not happen again. Filing charges and a Child Protective Services report may be needed, but more information is needed first. These actions would not be done without the mother's understanding why. (I, 6, X)

130. 2. If the client begins to experience abdominal cramping during administration of the enema fluid, the nurse's first action is to temporarily stop the infusion and have the client take a few deep breaths. Once the cramping subsides, the nurse can continue with the enema solution. If the cramping does not subside, the nurse should clamp the tubing and remove it. Raising the height of the container will increase the flow of fluid and cause the cramping to increase. Rubbing the

abdomen while infusing the enema fluid will not cause the cramping to stop. (I, 7, M)

131. 1. When inserting an intravenous catheter needle, the nurse initially uses veins low on the hand or arm if available, unless contraindicated. Should the intravenous fluid infiltrate or the vein become irritated at this insertion site, veins higher on the arm would still be available for use. After a vein higher up on the arm has been damaged, veins below it cannot be used. (I, 8, M)

132. 3. Lactulose is used to treat hepatic encephalopathy by reducing serum ammonia levels. It is not used to stimulate bowel peristalsis, even though diarrhea can be a side effect of the drug. Lactulose does not have any effect on edema, ascites, or hemorrhage. (E, 8, M)

133. 2. A 12-month-old whose immunizations are current would have received three diphtheria, tetanus, and pertussis (DTaP); three hepatitis B (Hep B); and two inactivated poliovirus (IPV) immunizations. Oral polio vaccine (OPV) is not used routinely. HIB is administered at 2, 4, and 6 months, and a booster is given at 12 to 15 months. (D, 3, Y)

134. 3. Obesity is a risk factor for osteoarthritis because it places increased stress on the joints. A high-protein diet, regular exercise, and vitamin supplements will not reduce a client's risk for development of osteoarthritis. (P, 4, M)

135. 3. Vitamin E is a powerful antioxidant that helps to prevent oxidation of the cell membrane. Vitamins C, A, and B_6 are helpful in the prevention of heart disease, but vitamin E plays a more important role. (D, 4, M)

136. 3. The nurse should instruct the mother to report the first voiding after the circumcision, because edema could cause a urinary obstruction. Although reading a pamphlet about circumcision care may be helpful, it may not be appropriate for all mothers. Some mothers could have difficulty reading or understanding the information. Vaseline gauze is used with Gomco clamp circumcisions, not Plastibells. Petroleum jelly should not be used with Plastibell circumcision methods, because the bell prevents any further bleeding. (I, 3, O)

137. 2. Alcoholic cirrhosis is associated with excessive alcohol intake. In the early stages of the disease, the liver develops fatty changes. If alcohol intake is stopped, the fatty changes can be reversed. Avoiding overexertion is important in the client with cirrhosis, but it does not reverse the disease. Stopping smoking is a positive, healthy lifestyle change, but it does not have any impact on the cirrhosis. A diet that is high in carbohydrates and low in fat is also recommended for the client with cirrhosis, but the diet does not reverse the pathologic changes that have occurred in the liver. (P, 9, M)

138. 3. Using the ratio-proportion method, the equations are as follows: 4 mg / 1 mL = 7.6 mg / x mL; $4x = 7.6$; $x = 7.6 / 4 = 1.9$ mL. (I, 8, Y)

139. 4. Because of the client's age, the amniocentesis is most likely being done to evaluate for Down syndrome (trisomy 21). Women older than 35 years are at higher risk for having a child with Down syndrome. Cri du chat syndrome is a genetic disorder involving a short arm on chromosome 5. This disorder is not associated with mothers who are older than 35 years of age. The client is AB-positive, so the amniocentesis is not being done for ABO incompatibility, in which the mother is type O and the fetus is type A, B, or AB. The amniocentesis is not being done to detect erythroblastosis fetalis, because the mother is Rh-positive. (D, 9, O)

140. 3. The symptoms of BPH are related to obstruction as a result of an enlarged prostate. Difficulty in starting the urinary stream is a common symptom, along with dribbling, hesitancy, and urinary retention. Impotence does not result from BPH. Flank pain is most commonly related to pyelonephritis. Hematuria occurs in urinary tract infections, renal calculi, and bladder cancer, to name some of the most common causes. (A, 10, M)

141. 1. Having the client role-play assertive statements assists the client in learning how to use assertiveness and practicing appropriate behaviors in a safe environment. Watching a videotape on assertiveness or discussing situations that appear threatening is a step toward actually using assertive techniques. Describing feelings that occur after an angry outburst motivates the client to make changes in behavior. (I, 6, X)

142. 4. Symptoms of transient tachypnea include respirations as high as 150 breaths/minute, retractions, flaring, and cyanosis. Treatment is supportive and includes provision of warm, humidified oxygen in a warm environment. The nurse should continuously monitor the neonate's respirations, color, and behaviors to allow for early detection and prompt intervention should problems arise. Feedings are given by gavage rather than bottle, to decrease respiratory stress. Obtaining extracorporeal membrane oxygenation equipment is not necessary but may be used for neonates diagnosed with meconium aspiration syndrome. (P, 9, O)

143. 4. Convert 1.5 g to 1500 mg. 1500 mg / x mL = 300 mg / 2 mL; $x = 10$ mL. (E, 8, M)

144. 2. One of the early signs of iron-deficiency anemia in a client of Vietnamese descent with dark skin is yellowish-brown skin tones. The nurse can assess for petechiae or jaundice, which may be observed in the conjunctiva or buccal mucosa. (A, 9, M)

145. 1. A decreased total serum protein occurs as extensive amounts of protein are excreted from the body through the urine. Clients may develop hypocalcemia. Hyper-

glycemia is not a finding related to nephrotic syndrome. A decreased hematocrit is not a finding related to nephrotic syndrome. (A, 10, M)

146. 2. The number one cause of nosocomial infections in hospital units is not washing the hands. Nosocomial infections can be significantly reduced by thorough handwashing before caring for each different infant. Sterile supplies are not necessary for all treatments. Cover gowns and masks, although helpful in reducing the risk of exposure to blood and body fluids, do not decrease the risk of nosocomial infection. (I, 2, O)

147. 2. Recommended restraints for a child who has had palate surgery would be elbow restraints. They minimize the limitation placed on the child but still prevent the child from injuring the repair with fingers and hands. A safety jacket or wrist or body restraints restrict the child unnecessarily. (I, 2, Y)

148. 2. Battering is a major cause of injury to women. Although battering occurs in all socioeconomic groups, it may appear to be more common in members of lower socioeconomic groups because they are more likely to use emergency room services. Pregnant women are frequent victims of battering. Death from battering is not rare. (P, 6, X)

149. 3. After a nephrectomy, a specific aspect of immediate postoperative management includes monitoring the urinary output at least hourly. Monitoring blood pressure and encouraging the use of incentive spirometry are other important considerations, but because of the surgical disruption of the urinary system, urinary output is a priority. Measurement of urinary output should also include an estimation of the amount of urine drainage on the flank dressing. (I, 9, M)

150. 4. Severe retroversion or anteversion may lead to infertility or difficulty conceiving a child because these positions can block the deposition or migration of sperm. The normal position of the uterus is tipped slightly forward. Frequent vaginal infections commonly are associated with diabetes or human immunodeficiency virus (HIV) infection, not abnormal uterine positions. Pain from endometriosis (abnormal myometrial growth outside the uterus) is not associated with abnormal uterine positions. Severe menstrual cramping or dysmenorrhea (primary) is caused by increased prostaglandin production, not abnormal uterine positions. Secondary dysmenorrhea is associated with pelvic inflammatory disease or endometriosis. (D, 3, O)

151. 2. A 4-year-old is old enough to be able to cooperate and stop the behavior. Therefore, the first step is to obtain the child's cooperation. Once this has occurred, then the mother makes sure it is okay to remind the child when the behavior is viewed. The mother also should be encouraged to praise the child when she sees her not engaging in the behavior. (P, 3, Y)

152. 4. During an episode of acute respiratory distress, it is important that the nurse focus the assessment on the client's respiratory system and distress in order to quickly address the client's problem. Conducting a complete health history and a comprehensive physical examination can be deferred until the client's condition is stabilized. It is not appropriate to delay all assessments until the respiratory distress is resolved, because the nurse must have data to guide treatment of the respiratory distress. (A, 10, M)

153. 4. The most likely indication of a dislocated hip is a shortening of the affected leg. Other indications of dislocation include increasing pain, loss of function to the extremity, and deformity. Abduction of the leg after total hip replacement is a desirable position to prevent dislocation. Loosening of the prosthesis does not necessarily indicate that the hip has dislocated. External rotation of the hip can occur without the hip's being dislocated. However, a neutral position of rotation is the desired position. (A, 9, M)

154. 1. The client who is withdrawn, is suspicious, and projects blame is exhibiting problems in trust versus mistrust. Shame and doubt would be reflected as low self-esteem and suspiciousness. Guilt would be reflected in self-blame for all problems. Isolation would be reflected in a lack of long-term relationships. (D, 3, X)

155. 4. The nurse needs to explore more about the client's feelings to assess what underlies the eating disorder. The nurse also needs to evaluate the client's suicide risk. The other statements are not therapeutic because they minimize the client's feelings. (I, 5, X)

156. 1. An ileal conduit is a urinary diversion that requires the client to wear an appliance, or pouch, at all times because the urine will drain continually. Ileal conduits are not irrigated. The urinary drainage is affected by fluid intake, not meals. (I, 7, M)

157. 1. Children with varicella or suspected varicella should be treated under airborne precautions in addition to standard precautions. Varicella is transmitted by airborne nuclei. Droplet precautions are indicated for conditions such as pertussis, meningococcal pneumonia, and rubella. Contact precautions are indicated for conditions such as draining major abscesses, acute viral conjunctivitis, and *Clostridium difficile* gastroenteritis. Indirect contact is not a method of controlling infection. Rather it is a mode of transmission involving contamination via some intermediate object, such as an instrument, needle, or dressing, or by hands that are not washed or gloves that are not changed between clients. (I, 2, Y)

158. 1. In multiple myeloma, neoplastic plasma cells invade the bone marrow and begin to destroy the bone. As a result of this skeletal destruction, the pain can be significant. There is no cure for multiple myeloma. Nausea and vomiting are not characteristics of the disease, although clients may experience anorexia. The client should be monitored for signs of hypercalcemia resulting from bone destruction, not for hyperkalemia. (E, 10, M)

159. 1. Stating, "You were able to shower and dress without any help this morning," points out a visible, realistic accomplishment and strength to the client with self-deprecatory statements, thereby helping to increase the client's self-worth. The statements, "Your wife told me that you are a good husband and father," and, "You don't have any reason why you should feel this way," are not helpful because logical statements are ineffective in changing the thinking of a client who is depressed. The client may agree with what the nurse states but be just as depressed because intellectual understanding does not help severely depressed clients. The statement, "This medication will help your thinking," although true, does not recognize the client's accomplishment and will have no positive effect on self-esteem. (I, 6, X)

160. 3. The nurse uses Montgomery straps primarily to avoid the removal of long-term abdominal dressing tape and ultimate skin breakdown. (I, 7, M)

161. 1. The nurse's most appropriate response is to acknowledge and validate the client's concerns. Questioning the client's fears is not a therapeutic response and can make the client feel defensive. False reassurance that the client should not be afraid disregards the client's fears and does not promote further communication between client and nurse. Dismissing the client's feelings and telling the client to relax does not encourage sharing of feelings. (I, 5, M)

162. 3. In a child with abdominal surgery it would be important to check the vital signs frequently to assess for internal bleeding. Administering intravenous fluids, assessing pain, and keeping the child NPO are all important, but monitoring vital signs frequently is the priority. (I, 9, Y)

163. 2. Polydipsia, or increased thirst, is a classic clinical manifestation of diabetes. The excessive loss of fluids is the result of the osmotic diuresis that occurs with glycosuria. It is unlikely that shortness of breath, early awakening, or trouble urinating is related to diabetes mellitus. (A, 10, M)

164. 1. Activity Intolerance would be a common diagnosis for clients with hypothyroidism. Cellular metabolism and oxygen consumption are decreased. Anxiety is a symptom of hyperthyroidism, and Hopelessness is associated with depression; they are not supported by the data given here. Ineffective Family Coping could be relevant at some point, but not based on the facts given. (D, 9, M)

165. 2. The client's serum alkaline phosphatase, which is produced by the osteoblasts in the bone, will be elevated in bone cancer. Hypercalcemia may occur in bone cancer. An elevated AST is present in liver disease. Potassium levels are not affected in bone cancer. (A, 10, M)

166. 3. Cardiac myopathy is a broad term that includes three major forms: dilated, hypertrophic, and restrictive cardiac myopathies. The underlying etiology of hypertrophic cardiomyopathy is unknown; it is typically observed in young men but is not limited to the male population. Common symptoms are fatigue, low tolerance to activity related to the low ejection fraction, and shortness of breath. Angina may be observed if coronary artery disease is present. Abdominal pain and hypertension are not common. (A, 10, M)

167. 3. Pinworms come out of the rectum during the nighttime and early morning hours. Therefore, the best time to apply the tape to get results is while the child is asleep. (I, 10, Y)

168. 3. Maternal hydramnios occurs when the fetus has a congenital obstruction of the gastrointestinal tract, such as occurs in the presence of a tracheoesophageal fistula. The fetus normally swallows amniotic fluid and absorbs the fluid from the gastrointestinal tract. Excretion then occurs through the kidneys and placenta. Most fluid absorption occurs in the colon. Absorption cannot occur when the fetus has a gastrointestinal obstruction. Meconium in the amniotic fluid, low implantation of the placenta, and toxemia could occur but are more specifically associated with fetal hypoxia. (A, 3, Y)

169. 1. A common complication of steroid therapy is gastric irritation and peptic ulcers. Hyperglycemia is a potential complication. Tachycardia and renal failure are not associated with steroid therapy. (A, 8, M)

170. 3. When an incision eviscerates, it is a medical emergency. The nurse's first response is to apply a sterile dressing that has been moistened with sterile normal saline. The client should also be placed in a semi-Fowler's position to release any tension on the abdominal area. Vital signs should be taken, and an intravenous line may be started for emergency treatment; however, the first action is to protect the wound and abdominal contents. (I, 9, M)

171. 3. Establishing a patent airway is the priority intervention. Prophylactic intubation is initiated if heat has been inhaled or if the neck, head, or face is involved. Swelling of the upper airways can progress to obstruction. Fluid replacement can best be achieved using a large-caliber peripheral intravenous catheter, and morphine sulfate is appropriate for analgesia in a burn client. Although these are priorities, they are secondary

to establishing a patent airway. Administering tetanus toxoid is a secondary priority. (I, 9, M)

172. 2. The client who refuses to sign a "no suicide" contract is an immediate and serious threat for suicide. Therefore, the nurse would place this client on one-to-one suicide precautions to protect the client from self-harm. Although a client who is withdrawn and anorectic or visibly crying may have symptoms of depression, these symptoms alone do not warrant one-to-one suicide precautions. Refusal of medication indicates a lack of insight by the client into his illness and lack of participation in treatment, but it is not an immediate suicide threat. However, the nurse must be alert for the "cheeking" and hoarding of medication as a possible means for self-harm. (A, 6, X)

173. 3. Quadriceps setting exercises help the immobilized client keep the quadriceps muscles strong and ready for resuming ambulation. Pressing the back of the knee against the bed promotes tightening of the quadriceps muscle. (E, 7, M)

174. 4. The physician should be notified immediately, because the client's symptoms indicate that an intestinal obstruction may have developed. Taking milk of magnesia or any laxatives with a suspected obstruction can worsen the client's condition. Increasing oral fluids while the client is vomiting will not be effective. Measuring the abdominal girth is not an essential activity at this time. (D, 9, M)

175. 4. Herpes simplex with skin ulcerations persisting longer than 1 month is categorized as an AIDS-defining illness. The Centers for Disease Control and Prevention lists opportunistic diseases that, when found in people with laboratory evidence of HIV infection, are diagnostic of AIDS. (A, 10, M)

176. 2. The client should wear loose, cotton underwear to promote cleanliness and dryness in the genital area. Sitz baths can promote cleanliness and decrease inflammation in the area. A hair dryer, set on a cool setting, can be used to carefully dry the lesions in the perineal area. Drinking plenty of fluids is advised to decrease the dysuria, which accompanies genital herpes. (E, 9, M)

177. 1. Propantheline bromide is an anticholinergic drug that reduces secretion by the gastric, salivary, bronchial, and sweat glands. Anticholinergic drugs act by blocking ganglionic action in the autonomic nervous system. (P, 8, M)

178. 3. Methylxanthines, a chemical found in coffee, tea, cola, and chocolate, contribute to fibrocystic breast disease in many women. Although the response has not been universal, decreasing caffeine intake has been very beneficial for many women in helping treat fibrocystic breast disease. In the absence of other health conditions, a woman would not be advised to increase sodium or decrease calcium. A woman would not be advised to use bottled water. (I, 4, M)

179. 2. *The Dietary Guidelines for Americans* discusses healthy nutritional guidelines. Dietary Reference Intakes include protein, vitamin and mineral needs but do not address energy and health guidelines. (A, 3, M)

180. 3. The nurse needs to clarify the reality of the situation in response to the client's grandiose delusions. The statement, "You are Sam Smith, a client here in the hospital, and I'm Marjorie, a nurse here on the unit," clarifies the client's identity and status and that of the nurse. The other statements do not help to clarify the identity of the client and nurse and do not address the reality of the situation, thereby correcting the client's grandiose delusions. The statement, "You know better; we are not going to be married," is blaming. (I, 6, X)

181. 4. When the client demonstrates a readiness to look at and learn about the colostomy, providing literature that shows the client how the colostomy looks and functions is a helpful teaching tool. Telling the client how others have adjusted to caring for their colostomy does not focus on the client's feelings as an individual. Handling colostomy appliances will be important before the client learns to care for the colostomy, but it is not essential to preparing the client to look at the stoma. Having a member of the local ostomy club visit can be beneficial, but it will probably be more effective once the client has looked at the colostomy and has some knowledge of how it functions. (I, 5, M)

COMPREHENSIVE TEST 3

Select the one best answer, and indicate your choice by filling in the circle in front of the option.

1. A primigravid client at 10 weeks' gestation tells the nurse that she eats fruits and vegetables but isn't very fond of them. After teaching the client about possible serving sizes, the nurse determines that the teaching has been successful when the client states that one serving of vegetables is equivalent to which of the following?
   - ○ 1. One fourth of a cantaloupe.
   - ○ 2. 3 ounces of vegetable juice cocktail.
   - ○ 3. 3 tomatoes.
   - ○ 4. 1 raw apricot.

2. A nurse performs care on the client's Hickman catheter according to hospital policy. The client develops an infection and is considering litigation. The nurse's practice is
   - ○ 1. malpractice.
   - ○ 2. *respondeat superior.*
   - ○ 3. negligent.
   - ○ 4. tort.

3. A Hispanic client is admitted to the surgical unit from the emergency department for an appendectomy. The nurse conducts the preoperative preparations and determines that the client has difficulty understanding English. The surgeon needs to obtain the client's informed consent. The best course for obtaining the client's informed consent is to
   - ○ 1. have the client call a family member to act as interpreter.
   - ○ 2. have the client sign the Spanish surgical consent form.
   - ○ 3. call the Spanish interpreter to translate the surgeon's explanation of the procedure, risks, and alternatives to obtain the client's consent and to answer the client's questions.
   - ○ 4. notify the surgical charge nurse of the situation.

4. A client who has glaucoma has been prescribed timolol (Timoptic) eye drops. Which of the following instructions should the nurse give the client about the administration of the eye drops?
   - ○ 1. Instill the eye drops whenever the eyes feel irritated.
   - ○ 2. The medication may cause some transient eye discomfort.
   - ○ 3. Keep the medication refrigerated between doses.
   - ○ 4. The need to use the eye drops will be reevaluated after 1 month.

5. A 6-year-old child is admitted to the hospital for heart surgery to repair tetralogy of Fallot. The child asks the nurse if the cardiac catheterization will hurt. Which of the following statements offers the nurse the best guide for responding to the child's question?
   - ○ 1. The medication used to numb the insertion site will sting.
   - ○ 2. Momentary sharp pain will usually occur when the catheter enters the heart.
   - ○ 3. It is usual for a 6-year-old to feel discomfort during the procedure.
   - ○ 4. It is a painless procedure, although a tingling sensation may be felt in the extremities.

6. The nurse is assessing a 55-year-old client with chronic obstructive pulmonary disease. The client weighs 200 pounds and is 6 feet tall. Using the diagram in Figure 1, the nurse should record in the health history that the client's chest is
   - ○ 1. Barrel-shaped.
   - ○ 2. Muscular.
   - ○ 3. Normal for the client's age, height, and weight.
   - ○ 4. Showing the effects of long-term use of bronchodilators.

7. A diabetic primigravid client at 38 weeks' gestation asks the nurse why she had a fetal acoustic stimulation during her last nonstress test. Which of the following would the nurse include as the rationale for this test?
   - ○ 1. To listen to the fetal heart rate.
   - ○ 2. To startle and awaken the fetus.
   - ○ 3. To stimulate mild contractions.
   - ○ 4. To confirm amniotic fluid amount.

8. The mother of an older infant reports stopping the prescribed iron supplements after 2 weeks of treatment. Which of the following responses by the nurse would be *most* appropriate?
   - ○ 1. "Bring the child in so that we can retest him."
   - ○ 2. "You need to continue the iron for several more weeks."

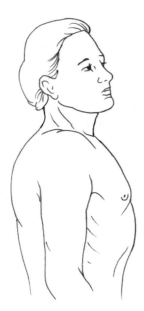

Figure 1.

○ 3. "Let's start a diet that high in iron foods."
○ 4. "No more medication is needed at this time."

9. A Jewish client requests an orthodox diet while she is hospitalized. The nurse should refer this request to the
○ 1. dietary department and dietitian.
○ 2. physician.
○ 3. nursing supervisor.
○ 4. rabbi in pastoral care.

10. A mother reports to the nurse that she cannot afford the antibiotic azithromycin, which was ordered by the physician for her toddler's otitis media. The nurse's best response is to
○ 1. instruct the mother on the importance of the medication.
○ 2. ask the mother if she knows anyone who could loan her the money.
○ 3. confer with the physician as to whether a less expensive drug could be ordered.
○ 4. consult with the social worker.

11. The doctor has prescribed nitroglycerin to a client with angina. The client also has closed-angle glaucoma. The nurse contacts the physician to discuss the potential for
○ 1. decreased intraocular pressure.
○ 2. increased intraocular pressure.
○ 3. hypotension.
○ 4. hypertension.

12. A client states she thinks she is experiencing premenstrual syndrome (PMS). The nurse instructs the client that common symptoms of this syndrome are
○ 1. menstrual cycle irregularity with increased menstrual flow.

○ 2. mood swings immediately after menses.
○ 3. tension and fatigue before menses and through the second day of the menstrual cycle.
○ 4. midcycle spotting and abdominal pain at the time of ovulation.

13. For which of the following should the nurse closely assess in a client who is reversing from a general anesthesia and receiving colistimethate sodium (Coly-Mycin)?
○ 1. Tachycardia.
○ 2. Respiratory depression.
○ 3. Hypotension.
○ 4. Renal failure.

14. The nurse is helping a client who has heart disease to assess his vitamin needs. The nurse is aware that recent updates to the Recommended Dietary Allowances have included expansion of the nutrient needs to include Adequate Intakes, Tolerable Upper Limits, and Estimated Average Requirements. All of these recommendations are called
○ 1. Dietary Guidelines.
○ 2. Recommended Daily Allowances.
○ 3. Recommended Daily Intakes.
○ 4. Dietary Reference Intakes.

15. A nulliparous client visiting the clinic tells the nurse that she stopped taking oral contraceptives 6 months ago but doesn't think she is ovulating. Which of the following would the nurse anticipate that the physician would order if the client is anovulatory?
○ 1. Dienestrol (Ortho Dienestrol).
○ 2. Clomiphene citrate (Clomid).
○ 3. Medroxyprogesterone (Depo-Provera).
○ 4. Norgestrel (Ovrette).

16. A client who has been recently diagnosed with AIDS inquires about hospice services. The nurse explains that hospice care is appropriate
○ 1. for clients with an inevitable death within weeks to months.
○ 2. for all clients with AIDS at any stage.
○ 3. only for clients with cancer.
○ 4. when the client is ready to discuss his or her prognosis.

17. While assessing a neonate at 24 hours of age, the nurse observes several irregularly shaped, red, flat patches on the back of the neonate's neck. The nurse interprets this finding as which of the following?
○ 1. Storkbite.
○ 2. Port wine stain.
○ 3. Newborn rash.
○ 4. Café au lait spot.

18. A Mexican mother brings her 2-month old son to the emergency department with a high fever and possible sepsis. A lumbar puncture is ordered, but the mother will not sign the consent until the father arrives to give permission. The nurse is aware that

○ 1. this needs to be reported to the social worker.

○ 2. this needs to be reported to the Children's Protective Services.

○ 3. the Mexican man is considered the family head and makes the major decisions.

○ 4. this behavior is unusual for Mexican cultural norms.

19. A client with Alzheimer's disease is being started on a low dose of lorazepam (Ativan) because of agitation and a sleep disturbance. While monitoring the client for possible adverse effects, the nurse would expect to find which of the following as *most* common?

○ 1. Confusion and nighttime agitation.

○ 2. Extrapyramidal side effects.

○ 3. Vomiting and profuse sweating.

○ 4. Anticholinergic side effects.

20. A postmenopausal client with an intact uterus asks the nurse why her hormone medicine has two drugs, estrogen and progesterone. Which of the following statements by the nurse provides the client with accurate information?

○ 1. "The progesterone will help prevent cervical cancer."

○ 2. "The progesterone will help prevent breast cancer."

○ 3. "The progesterone will help prevent liver disease."

○ 4. "The progesterone will help prevent endometrial cancer."

21. The nurse will turn the client on bed rest every 2 hours to prevent the development of pressure ulcers. In addition, the nurse will

○ 1. ambulate the client at least twice a day.

○ 2. insert an indwelling urinary catheter.

○ 3. monitor the serum albumin.

○ 4. monitor the white blood cell count.

22. A client has been hospitalized with congestive heart failure. He is receiving digoxin (Lanoxin) and furosemide (Lasix) intravenously. He tells the nurse that he hears a continuous ringing in his ears and that he has never had this problem before. What is the appropriate action for the nurse to take at this time?

○ 1. Obtain a digitalis level to check for digitalis toxicity.

○ 2. Note the observation in the chart and plan to reassess in 2 hours.

○ 3. Ask the client if he has been taking any aspirin in addition to his other medications.

○ 4. Discontinue the furosemide and notify the physician.

23. A client receives an intravenous (IV) dose of gentamycin sulfate (Garamycin). How long after the completion of the IV dose of the antibiotic should the peak serum concentration level be measured?

○ 1. 10 minutes.

○ 2. 20 minutes.

○ 3. 30 minutes.

○ 4. 40 minutes.

24. A client with hydrocephalus complains of a headache in the morning on arising, but it disappears later in the day. The nurse is aware that intracranial pressure is highest in

○ 1. the early morning.

○ 2. the late afternoon.

○ 3. the evening.

○ 4. the middle of the night.

25. A primigravid client visits the clinic for a routine examination at 35 weeks' gestation. The client's blood pressure is near the baseline of 120/74 mm Hg with no proteinuria or evidence of facial edema. The client asks the nurse "What should I take if I get an occasional headache after looking at my computer at work all day?" The nurse instructs the client that she can occasionally take which of the following?

○ 1. Acetaminophen (Tylenol).

○ 2. Aspirin (Bufferin).

○ 3. Ibuprofen (Advil).

○ 4. Naproxen (Aleve).

26. A 19-year-old client has undergone an examination and had evidence collected after being raped. Her father is overheard yelling at his daughter, "You are going to tell me who did this to you. I am going to kill them." Which of the following would be the nurse's *most* immediate action?

○ 1. "Please come with me, sir. I need some important information."

○ 2. "Stop yelling. You're being inappropriate."

○ 3. "Please be quiet. You're not helping your daughter this way."

○ 4. "If you don't stop yelling, I'll have to call Security."

27. Which of the following groups is more likely to develop severe hypertension?

○ 1. Asian.

○ 2. African American.

○ 3. European.

○ 4. American Indian.

28. During a neonate's assessment shortly after birth, the nurse observes a large pad of fat at the back of the neck, widely set eyes, simian hand creases, and epicanthal folds. Which of the following actions would be *most* appropriate?

○ 1. Notify the physician immediately.

○ 2. Ask the mother to consent to genetic studies.

○ 3. Explain these deviations to the newborn's mother.

○ 4. Document these findings as minor deviations.

29. A client with severe arthritis has been receiving maintenance therapy of prednisone 10 mg/day for

the past 6 weeks. The nurse should instruct the client to immediately report symptoms of
○ 1. respiratory infection.
○ 2. joint pain.
○ 3. constipation.
○ 4. joint swelling.

30. A 90-year-old client discloses that he has two guns at home. The nurse asks him whether he has any grandchildren who come to visit, or other school-aged visitors, because the most common risk factor for school-aged children associated with injury or death from firearms is
○ 1. an argument with a stranger.
○ 2. firearm access.
○ 3. substance use.
○ 4. peer pressure.

31. A 7-year-old child is admitted to the hospital with the medical diagnosis of acute rheumatic fever. During the acute phase of the illness, it would be *least* desirable to interest the child in which of the following diversional activities?
○ 1. Reading a book to the father.
○ 2. Playing with a doll with the nurse.
○ 3. Watching the television with a sibling.
○ 4. Playing checkers with a roommate.

32. A woman is taking oral contraceptives. The nurse teaches the client to report which of the following danger signs?
○ 1. Breakthrough bleeding.
○ 2. Severe calf pain.
○ 3. Mild headache.
○ 4. Weight gain of 3 pounds.

33. Which of the following is the most essential goal for the hospitalized client with a new tracheostomy?
○ 1. Decrease secretions.
○ 2. Provide client teaching regarding tracheostomy care.
○ 3. Relieve anxiety related to the tracheostomy.
○ 4. Maintain a patent airway.

34. Immediately after the client received an injection of bupivacaine (Marcaine), he became restless and nervous and reported a feeling of impending doom. Which of the following actions by the nurse would be appropriate at this time?
○ 1. Ask the client to talk more about what he is feeling.
○ 2. Reassure the client that it is normal to feel restless before a procedure.
○ 3. Assess the client's vital signs.
○ 4. Administer epinephrine.

35. A menopausal woman is taking hormone replacement therapy. The nurse teaches the client that a warning sign for endometrial cancer that needs to be reported is
○ 1. hot flashes.

○ 2. irregular vaginal bleeding.
○ 3. urinary urgency.
○ 4. dyspareunia.

36. When teaching a group of students in health class about cystic fibrosis, which of the following would the school nurse use when explaining how this disorder is transmitted?
○ 1. Both parents have the recessive gene.
○ 2. The gene is carried on the X chromosome.
○ 3. The disease is restricted to males, implicating the Y chromosome.
○ 4. It usually happens by chance; neither parent has the gene.

37. A client complains of a severe vulvar pruritus and a yellow-green, malodorous vaginal discharge. The nurse recognizes that the symptoms suggest
○ 1. Gonorrhea.
○ 2. Syphilis.
○ 3. Chlamydia.
○ 4. Trichomoniasis.

38. To evaluate the effectiveness of the client's use of an incentive spirometer, the nurse should understand that this device is used primarily to accomplish which of the following objectives?
○ 1. Stimulate circulation.
○ 2. Prepare the client for ambulation.
○ 3. Strengthen abdominal muscles.
○ 4. Increase respiratory effectiveness.

39. A client was talking with her husband by telephone; then she began swearing at him. The nurse interrupts the call and offers to talk with the client. She says, "I can't talk about that bastard right now. I just need to destroy something." At this point, which of the following would the nurse do *next*?
○ 1. Tell her to write her feelings in her journal.
○ 2. Urge her to talk with the nurse now.
○ 3. Ask her to calm down or she will be restrained.
○ 4. Offer her a phone book to "destroy" while staying with her.

40. The nurse is caring for a multigravid client in active labor when the nurse detects variable fetal heart rate decelerations on the electronic monitor. The nurse interprets this as indicating compression of which of the following structures?
○ 1. Head.
○ 2. Chest.
○ 3. Umbilical cord.
○ 4. Placenta.

41. Two days after placement of a pleural chest tube, the tube is accidentally pulled out of the chest wall. The nurse should *first*
○ 1. immerse the tube in sterile water.
○ 2. apply an occlusive dressing such as petroleum jelly gauze.
○ 3. instruct the client to cough to expand the lung.

○ 4. auscultate the lung to determine whether it is collapsed.

42. A client is admitted to the hospital with a diagnosis of a pulmonary embolism. Which of the following client problems would the nurse address first?
○ 1. Nonproductive cough.
○ 2. Activity intolerance.
○ 3. Ineffective breathing pattern.
○ 4. Impaired gas exchange.

43. Which of the following is characteristic of cardiogenic shock?
○ 1. Hypovolemia.
○ 2. Increased cardiac output.
○ 3. Decreased myocardial contractility.
○ 4. Infarction.

44. The nurse is reviewing the laboratory results of a client with hypothyroidism. An expected finding would be
○ 1. decreased T_4 and increased TSH levels.
○ 2. decreased TSH and increased T_4 levels.
○ 3. decreased CPK levels.
○ 4. absence of antithyroid antibodies.

45. The mother of a 7-month-old child born 6 weeks early asks the nurse which play activities and toys would be appropriate for her child. Which of the following would the nurse suggest?
○ 1. Picture books.
○ 2. Peek-a-boo.
○ 3. Rattle.
○ 4. Colored blocks.

46. Which of the following is the most accurate method of determining the extent of a client's fluid loss?
○ 1. Measuring intake and output.
○ 2. Assessing vital signs.
○ 3. Weighing the client.
○ 4. Assessing skin turgor.

47. The nurse is counseling a client regarding treatment of the client's newly diagnosed depression. The nurse emphasizes that during the acute phase antidepressant therapy will
○ 1. require 6 months before resolution of the acute phase of depression.
○ 2. take 3 to 4 weeks before a significant improvement occurs.
○ 3. usually bring complete remission from depression in the near future.
○ 4. not be effective without counseling.

48. A 70-year-old, previously well client asks the nurse, "I have noticed I have tremors. Is this just normal for my age?" The best response for the nurse to make is which of the following?
○ 1. "I would not be worried, because this is common with aging."
○ 2. "You should report this to the physician, because it may indicate a problem."

○ 3. "You should drink orange juice when this occurs."
○ 4. "You should have your blood pressure checked when this occurs."

49. A school-aged child diagnosed with attention deficit hyperactivity disorder (ADHD) is prescribed methylphenidate hydrochloride (Ritalin). Assessment of which of the following would alert the school nurse to the possibility that the child is experiencing a common side effect of the drug?
○ 1. Growth retardation.
○ 2. Vomiting.
○ 3. Photosensitivity.
○ 4. Weight gain.

50. A client complains of a dull headache and dizziness and has an increased pulse rate. The results of the arterial blood gas test are as follows: pH, 7.26; pCO_2, 50 mm Hg; HCO_3, 24 mEq/L. These findings indicate which of the following acid–base imbalances?
○ 1. Respiratory alkalosis.
○ 2. Respiratory acidosis.
○ 3. Metabolic acidosis.
○ 4. Metabolic alkalosis.

51. Which of the following interventions would be appropriate for a client who is experiencing metabolic alkalosis?
○ 1. Monitor serum potassium levels.
○ 2. Maintain the client on bed rest.
○ 3. Have the client inhale CO_2 using a paper bag.
○ 4. Administer sodium bicarbonate as ordered.

52. Which of the following demonstrates that a client needs further instruction after being taught about ciprofloxacin (Cipro)?
○ 1. "I must drink 1000 to 1500 mL of water a day."
○ 2. "I should not take an antacid before taking the Cipro."
○ 3. "I should let the doctor know if I start vomiting from the Cipro."
○ 4. "I may get lightheaded from the Cipro."

53. When developing the plan of care for a client with Alzheimer's disease, which of the following activities would be of *least* benefit to the client?
○ 1. Reminiscence group.
○ 2. Walking.
○ 3. Pet therapy.
○ 4. Stress management.

54. Which of the following nursing diagnoses would the nurse implement as part of the long-term care for a child with hemophilia?
○ 1. Deficient Knowledge.
○ 2. Risk for Injury.
○ 3. Low Self-Esteem.
○ 4. Pain.

55. When preparing a 3-year-old child to have blood

specimens drawn for laboratory testing, which of the following would the nurse do?

○ 1. Explain the procedure well in advance.

○ 2. Explain why the blood needs to be drawn.

○ 3. Use distraction techniques during the procedure.

○ 4. Provide verbal explanations about what will occur.

56. The client has been prescribed lisinopril (Prinivil) as treatment for hypertension. Which of the following electrolyte imbalances may occur in clients who take this drug?

○ 1. Hyponatremia.

○ 2. Hypocalcemia.

○ 3. Hyperkalemia.

○ 4. Hypermagnesemia.

57. A client with a chronic mental illness who does not always take her medications is separated from her husband and receives Supplemental Security Income. She lives with her mother and older sister and manages her own medication. The client's mother is in poor health and receives Social Security benefits. The client's sister works outside the home, and the client's father is dead. Which of the following issues would the nurse need to address *first*?

○ 1. Family.

○ 2. Marital.

○ 3. Financial.

○ 4. Medication.

58. A client is receiving total parenteral nutrition (TPN). The nurse notices that the bag of TPN solution has been infusing for 24 hours but has 300 mL of solution left. What would be the most appropriate action for the nurse to take?

○ 1. Continue the infusion until the remaining 300 mL is infused.

○ 2. Change the filter on the tubing and continue with the infusion.

○ 3. Notify the physician and obtain orders to alter the flow rate of the solution.

○ 4. Discontinue the current solution, change the tubing, and hang a new bag of TPN solution.

59. A client with a history of cardiac problems complains of severe chest pain. What should be nurse's *first* response?

○ 1. Notify the physician.

○ 2. Administer an analgesic to control the pain.

○ 3. Assess the client's pain.

○ 4. Start oxygen at 2 L/minute via nasal cannula.

60. Which of the following characteristics would the nurse include in the teaching plan for a multiparous client after delivery of a neonate who is diagnosed with trisomy 13?

○ 1. Webbed neck.

○ 2. Small testes.

○ 3. Congenital heart defects.

○ 4. Polydactyly.

61. A client is being treated for acute low back pain. Which of these clinical manifestations must be reported to the physician immediately?

○ 1. Diffuse, aching sensation in the L4–5 area.

○ 2. New onset of foot drop.

○ 3. Pain in the lower back when the leg is lifted.

○ 4. Pain in the lower back that radiates to the hip.

62. An insulin-dependent diabetic client asks the nurse whether he can take ginseng at home. The nurse's best response to the client is which of the following?

○ 1. "No, ginseng is not good for people."

○ 2. "No, taking ginseng will increase the risk for hypoglycemia."

○ 3. "Yes, ginseng is good for you, and will help your memory."

○ 4. "I am not certain."

63. The nurse teaches the client with hepatitis that the expected effect of lactulose (Cephulac) is

○ 1. One regular bowel movement a day.

○ 2. Two to three soft stools per day.

○ 3. Four to five loose stools per day.

○ 4. Five to six loose stools per day.

64. The nurse is evaluating the laboratory results of a client who was recently admitted to the hospital. Which one of the following laboratory results would indicate the presence of inflammation?

○ 1. Decreased sedimentation rate.

○ 2. Thrombocytopenia.

○ 3. Leukocytosis.

○ 4. Erythrocytosis.

65. The nurse is assessing teenaged girls at a well child clinic. The nurse should describe the girl shown in Figure 2 as having

○ 1. Normal posture for a teenaged girl.

○ 2. Kyphosis.

○ 3. Scoliosis.

○ 4. Lordosis.

66. A client complains of pain in his casted left arm that is unrelieved by pain medication. The nurse assesses the arm and notes that the fingers are swollen and difficult to separate. Which action would be most appropriate for the nurse to take at this time?

○ 1. Administer meperidine (Demerol) 100 mg IM.

○ 2. Apply an ice bag to the fingers to relieve pain.

○ 3. Elevate the arm on two pillows and reassess in 30 minutes.

○ 4. Call the physician to report swelling and pain.

67. A primiparous client develops uterine atony and postpartum hemorrhage 1 hour after a vaginal delivery. The physician has ordered prostaglandin-$F_{2\alpha}$ IM. After administration of the medication, the nurse should observe the client for which of the following?

○ 1. Tachycardia.

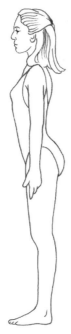

Figure 2.

○ 2. Hypotension.
○ 3. Constipation.
○ 4. Abdominal distention.

68. While caring for a mother and her 1-day-old neonate delivered vaginally at 30 weeks' gestation, the nurse explains about the neonate's need for gavage feeding at this time instead of the mother's plan for bottle feeding. Which of the following would the nurse include as the rationale for this?
    ○ 1. The neonate has difficulty coordinating sucking, swallowing, and breathing.
    ○ 2. A high-calorie formula, presently needed at this time, is more easily delivered via gavage.
    ○ 3. Gavage feedings can minimize the neonate's increased risk for development of hypoglycemia.
    ○ 4. This type of feeding, easily given in the isolette, decreases the neonate's risk for cold stress.

69. The nurse is evaluating the client's ability to manage the fatigue associated with her rheumatoid arthritis. Which statement by the client indicates she understands how to manage her fatigue?
    ○ 1. "I sleep for 8 to 10 hours every night so that I will have the energy to care for my children during the day."
    ○ 2. "I schedule afternoon rest periods for myself in addition to sleeping 10 hours every night."
    ○ 3. "I spend one weekend day a week resting in bed while my husband cares for the children."
    ○ 4. "I get up early in the morning and get all my household chores completed before my children wake up."

70. The school nurse is caring for a child with hemophilia who is actively bleeding from the leg. Which of the following would the nurse apply?
    ○ 1. Direct pressure, checking every few minutes to see if the bleeding has stopped.
    ○ 2. Ice to the injured leg area several times a day.
    ○ 3. Direct pressure to the injured area continuously for 10 minutes.
    ○ 4. Ice bag with elevation of the leg twice a day.

71. Which of the following is *not* a danger associated with pancytopenia?
    ○ 1. Anemia.
    ○ 2. Bleeding.
    ○ 3. Infection.
    ○ 4. Hypothyroidism.

72. A client suspected of being a victim of abuse returns to the emergency department and, sobbing, tells the nurse, "I guess you really know that my husband beats me and that's why I have bruises all over my body. I don't know what to do. I'm afraid he'll kill me one of these times." Which of the following responses would *best* demonstrate that the nurse recognizes the client's needs at this time?
    ○ 1. "The fear that your husband will kill you is unfounded."
    ○ 2. "We can begin by discussing various options open to you."
    ○ 3. "You can legally leave your husband because he has no right to hurt you."
    ○ 4. "We can begin by listing ways to avoid making your husband angry with you."

73. A client has just returned from surgery for a gastrectomy. The nurse should position the client in which position?
    ○ 1. Prone.
    ○ 2. Supine.
    ○ 3. Low Fowler's.
    ○ 4. Right or left Sims'.

74. A child with heart disease is to start on oral digoxin (Lanoxin). When preparing to administer the medication, which of the following would the nurse do *first*?
    ○ 1. Check the last serum electrolyte results for the child.
    ○ 2. Verify the dosage with the LPN/LVN the nurse is working with today.
    ○ 3. Ask the mother if she would be willing to administer the medication.
    ○ 4. Teach the mother how to measure the child's heart rate.

75. The nurse is caring for a client who has suffered deep partial-thickness and full-thickness burns. During the emergent (resuscitative) phase of burn management, the nurse would anticipate a fluid shift

○ 1. from the intracellular to extracellular compartment.

○ 2. from the extracellular to intravascular compartment.

○ 3. from the interstitial to the intracellular compartment.

○ 4. from the intravascular to the interstitial compartment.

76. The nurse is evaluating the effectiveness of fluid resuscitation during the emergent period of burn management. Which of the following indicates that adequate fluid replacement has been achieved in the client?

    ○ 1. An increase in body weight.

    ○ 2. Fluid intake is less than urinary output.

    ○ 3. Urinary output greater than 35 mL/hour.

    ○ 4. Blood pressure of 90/60 mm Hg.

77. A client who comes to the emergency department with multiple bruises on her face and arms, a black eye, and a broken nose says that these injuries occurred when she "fell down the stairs." The nurse suspects that the client may have been physically assaulted. Which of the following would the nurse do *next*?

    ○ 1. Ask the client specifically about the possibility of physical abuse.

    ○ 2. Tell the client that it is difficult to believe that such injuries resulted from a fall.

    ○ 3. Ask the client what she did to make someone beat her so badly.

    ○ 4. Discuss with the client what she can do to deescalate the situation next time.

78. What is the primary goal for the care of a client who is in shock?

    ○ 1. Achieve adequate tissue perfusion.

    ○ 2. Preserve renal function.

    ○ 3. Prevent hypostatic pneumonia.

    ○ 4. Maintain adequate vascular tone.

79. A 2-year-old child is brought into the physician's office by his parents, who are concerned by his behavior. They describe how the child resists their affection, twirls around frequently, and refuses to respond to other children and adults. Based on the analysis of these behaviors, which of the following would the nurse suspect?

    ○ 1. Tourette's syndrome.

    ○ 2. Schizophrenia.

    ○ 3. ADHD.

    ○ 4. Autism.

80. Which of the following is appropriate to include in an incident report?

    ○ 1. An interpretation of the likely cause of the incident.

    ○ 2. What the nurse saw and did.

    ○ 3. The client's statement about the incident that occurred.

○ 4. The extenuating circumstances involved in the situation.

81. To reduce urethral irritation, where should the nurse tape the female client's Foley catheter?

    ○ 1. Inner thigh.

    ○ 2. Groin area.

    ○ 3. Lower abdomen.

    ○ 4. Lower thigh.

82. The physician has determined that a primigravid client in active labor requires a cesarean delivery because of cephalopelvic disproportion. After the delivery of a male neonate, for which of the following would the nurse assess *first*?

    ○ 1. Nasopharyngeal secretions.

    ○ 2. High-pitched cry.

    ○ 3. Skull fracture.

    ○ 4. Decreased muscle tone.

83. The nurse understands that most accidental scaldings of young children occur

    ○ 1. on the back of the body.

    ○ 2. on the front of the body.

    ○ 3. in a circular or glove pattern.

    ○ 4. on the buttocks.

84. A 17-year-old client visits the clinic at 36 weeks' gestation. The client's blood pressure is 130/90 mm Hg. On previous visits, her blood pressure ranged from 100 to 110 mm Hg systolic, 70 to 80 mm Hg diastolic. Further assessment reveals slight edema of her hands and 1+ proteinuria. The nurse anticipates that the physician will most likely order which of the following?

    ○ 1. Intravenous magnesium sulfate.

    ○ 2. Labetalol hydrochloride (Normodyne).

    ○ 3. Bed rest with bathroom privileges.

    ○ 4. Hourly blood pressure checks.

85. The nurse observes that an area in the mouth of a child with leukemia is bleeding. Which of the following items would the nurse use because it is most effective for promoting homeostasis over the lesion?

    ○ 1. Karaya gum.

    ○ 2. A cotton ball imbedded with petroleum jelly.

    ○ 3. A nonsticking gauze sponge.

    ○ 4. A dry tea bag.

86. Which of the following interventions would be appropriate for the nurse to include in a plan for the prevention of pressure ulcers?

    ○ 1. Daily skin cleansing with soap and hot water.

    ○ 2. Gentle massage of bony prominences every shift.

    ○ 3. Encourage clients to sit up as much as possible.

    ○ 4. Systematic skin assessment at least once a shift.

87. Which of the following acid–base imbalances would the nurse anticipate developing in the client with a nasogastric tube inserted?

    ○ 1. Respiratory alkalosis.

○ 2. Respiratory acidosis.

○ 3. Metabolic alkalosis.

○ 4. Metabolic acidosis.

88. A nulligravid client at 36 weeks' gestation tells the nurse, "I've been having a lot of backaches lately." After giving instructions about how to decrease the backaches, the nurse determines that the client needs *further* instruction when she says which of the following?

○ 1. "I should walk with my pelvis tilted backward."

○ 2. "I may need to put a board under my mattress."

○ 3. "I should squat and not bend to pick up objects."

○ 4. "I should wear flat or low-heeled shoes."

89. Which of the following is usually the initial clinical manifestation of gonorrhea in men?

○ 1. Impotence.

○ 2. Scrotal pain.

○ 3. Penile lesion.

○ 4. Urethral discharge.

90. A client's blood pressure was elevated at 160/90 mm Hg when the physician ordered "clonidine (Catapres) 1 mg by mouth now." The nurse sent the order to pharmacy at 7:10 AM, but the medication still had not arrived at 8 AM. The most appropriate responses of the nurse include all but which of the following?

○ 1. Check all appropriate places on the unit to which the drug could have been delivered.

○ 2. Check the client's blood pressure.

○ 3. Call the pharmacy.

○ 4. Go to the pharmacy to obtain the drug.

91. The client with major depression states, "I'm too tired to get out of bed to go to group. I just want to rest." Which of the following would be the nurse's *best* response?

○ 1. "Perhaps you will feel better later on."

○ 2. "I'll let you rest for as long as you need."

○ 3. "Attending group is an important part of your treatment plan."

○ 4. "You've been in bed long enough and need to get up."

92. After teaching the mother of a 7-month-old diagnosed with bronchiolitis, the nurse determines that the teaching has been effective when the mother states which of the following as a sign to report immediately?

○ 1. Seven wet diapers a day.

○ 2. Temperature of 100°F (37.8°C) for 2 days.

○ 3. Clear nasal discharge for longer than 2 days.

○ 4. Longer periods of sleep than usual.

93. Which of the following clients would benefit from the application of warm moist heat?

○ 1. A client with appendicitis.

○ 2. A client with a recently sprained joint.

○ 3. A client with a suspected malignancy.

○ 4. A client with low back pain.

94. A 65-year-old client is newly diagnosed with pernicious anemia. The nurse emphasizes to the client the need to increase vitamin B_{12} intake by

○ 1. increasing dietary intake of B_{12}.

○ 2. taking oral B_{12} replacement.

○ 3. taking B_{12} injections or nasal spray replacement.

○ 4. chelation therapy.

95. A client with major depression and suicidal ideation is suddenly calmer and more energetic. Which of the following conclusions would the nurse reach?

○ 1. The client is improving.

○ 2. The client's medication dosage is too high.

○ 3. The client is overstimulated.

○ 4. The client is imminently suicidal.

96. A multigravid client at 38 weeks' gestation is scheduled to undergo a contraction stress test. Which of the following would the nurse include in the explanation as the purpose of this test?

○ 1. Evaluation of fetal lung maturity.

○ 2. Determination of the fetal biophysical profile.

○ 3. Assessment of fetal ability to tolerate labor.

○ 4. Determination of fetal response during movements.

97. The nurse is caring for a client who has been diagnosed with atypical pneumonia. When conducting a client assessment, which of the following symptoms would the nurse anticipate observing?

○ 1. High fever.

○ 2. Tachypnea.

○ 3. Dry cough.

○ 4. Severe chills.

98. The nurse is teaching a client with emphysema how to do pursed-lip breathing. What is the primary reason for clients with emphysema to use pursed-lip breathing?

○ 1. To increase oxygenation.

○ 2. To prolong exhalation.

○ 3. To prevent respiratory infection.

○ 4. To decrease shortness of breath.

99. The advantages of using automated medication dispensing equipment include which of the following?

○ 1. It facilitates the change-of-shift count of narcotics.

○ 2. It keeps a record of narcotic usage.

○ 3. It allows nurses unmonitored access to narcotics.

○ 4. It cancels the charges for narcotics.

100. A 21-year-old male client is transported by ambulance to the emergency department after a serious automobile accident. He complains of severe pain in

his right chest where he struck the steering wheel. He also has a compound fracture of his right tibia and fibula and multiple lacerations and contusions. The primary client goal at this point should be to

○ 1. reduce the client's anxiety.

○ 2. maintain adequate oxygenation.

○ 3. decrease chest pain.

○ 4. maintain adequate circulating volume.

101. While assessing a primiparous client 8 hours after delivery, the nurse inspects the episiotomy site, finding it edematous and slightly reddened. Which of the following interpretations by the nurse would be *most* appropriate?

○ 1. The client needs application of an ice pack.

○ 2. The episiotomy site is probably infected.

○ 3. A hematoma will likely develop.

○ 4. The client has had a repair of a vaginal laceration.

102. When administering an intramuscular injection, the nurse uses the Z-tract technique when the medication

○ 1. takes a long time to absorb.

○ 2. takes effect very quickly.

○ 3. is irritating to tissues.

○ 4. is viscous in consistency.

103. A client with an Axis I diagnosis of bipolar disorder, mania is monopolizing the use of the telephone by making several calls each day, interfering with the ability of other clients to use the telephone. Which of the following actions would be *most* appropriate?

○ 1. Instructing the other clients to be patient.

○ 2. Limiting the amount of calls the client can make each day.

○ 3. Reminding the client that others need to use the telephone.

○ 4. Taking away the client's telephone privileges.

104. When preparing a 20-month-old with a foreign body in the nasal passage for removal of the foreign body by the health care provider, which of the following would be *most* appropriate for this child?

○ 1. Jacket restraint.

○ 2. Elbow restraint.

○ 3. Use of father to hold.

○ 4. Papoose board.

105. The nurse auscultates the lungs of a client who has been diagnosed with lung cancer and notes auscultatory wheezing over one lung. The nurse understands that the most likely cause of this clinical finding is

○ 1. the presence of exudate in the airways.

○ 2. the result of the client's history of smoking.

○ 3. an indication of pleural effusion.

○ 4. obstruction of the airway by a tumor.

106. The nurse is teaching a client who is taking insulin about the signs of hyperglycemia. The signs of hyperglycemia include

○ 1. Kussmaul breathing.

○ 2. excessive hunger.

○ 3. dry, flaky skin.

○ 4. high blood pressure.

107. A nurse at the outpatient clinic receives a lithium level report of 1.0 mEq/L for a client who has been taking lithium for 2 months. The nurse would interpret this level to indicate which of the following?

○ 1. An error in reporting.

○ 2. Too low to be therapeutic.

○ 3. Too high, indicating toxicity.

○ 4. Within the therapeutic range.

108. A 16-year-old Latina nulligravid client at 10 weeks' gestation has been diagnosed with mild iron-deficiency anemia. The client tells the nurse that she doesn't like to eat much meat. Which of the following foods would the nurse suggest to provide the client with the greatest amount of iron in her diet?

○ 1. 1 cup of lentils.

○ 2. 1 cup of sunflower seeds.

○ 3. $1^1/_2$ ounces of hard cheese.

○ 4. 2 poached eggs.

109. A client has been receiving radiation therapy for 3 weeks for treatment of his cancer. He is complaining of fatigue. Which of the following should be considered as the nurse plans interventions to help the client cope with the fatigue?

○ 1. Fatigue is a temporary problem that requires no active intervention.

○ 2. The client should be closely examined to determine the cause of fatigue.

○ 3. Fatigue indicates that the client's cancer is not under control.

○ 4. The client should be encouraged to maintain activity to combat the fatigue.

110. Which of the following nutrients provides the base for the Food Guide Pyramid?

○ 1. Fat.

○ 2. Protein.

○ 3. Carbohydrate.

○ 4. Table sugar.

111. When educating unlicensed assistants on how to prevent the development of pressure sores, the nurse should emphasize that most tissue injuries related to shearing can be prevented by implementing which of the following activities?

○ 1. Close adherence to a turning schedule.

○ 2. Keeping the skin clean and dry.

○ 3. Proper positioning and moving of the client.

○ 4. Use of skin lubricants.

112. When using crutches, the client should be instructed to bear weight primarily

○ 1. on the axillae.

○ 2. on the elbows.

○ 3. on the upper arms.

○ 4. on the hands.

113. Which of the following nursing diagnoses would be

a priority for the family whose child is dying of leukemia?
- ○ 1. Disabled Family Coping.
- ○ 2. Impaired Parenting.
- ○ 3. Fear.
- ○ 4. Anticipatory Grieving.

114. Which of the following would the nurse do *first* for a toddler just admitted with croup?
- ○ 1. Monitor vital signs.
- ○ 2. Assess respiratory status.
- ○ 3. Ensure adequate fluid intake.
- ○ 4. Place a tracheostomy set at the bedside.

115. Before the nurse administers an IV bag of 5% dextrose in water (D_5W) with potassium chloride, what nursing intervention must first be completed?
- ○ 1. Gently rotate the bag.
- ○ 2. Invert the bag several times.
- ○ 3. Obtain the bag early from pharmacy.
- ○ 4. Add the potassium chloride on the unit.

116. Homocysteine may be cleared from the blood with the help of which of the following vitamins?
- ○ 1. Vitamin C.
- ○ 2. Vitamin E.
- ○ 3. Vitamin K.
- ○ 4. Vitamin B_6.

117. Which of the following signs and symptoms would be an early indication that a client has developed hypocalcemia?
- ○ 1. Tingling in the fingers.
- ○ 2. Depressed reflexes.
- ○ 3. Ventricular dysrhythmias.
- ○ 4. Memory changes.

118. The nurse is auscultating the lung sounds of a client with long-standing emphysema. Which of the following abnormal lung sounds would the nurse anticipate hearing?
- ○ 1. Fine crackles.
- ○ 2. Diminished breath sounds.
- ○ 3. Stridor.
- ○ 4. Pleural friction rub.

119. A client with a paranoid personality disorder sees some clients laughing during a group activity and asks the nurse, "Why are they laughing at me? I bet they're making fun of me." Which of the following responses by the nurse would be *most* appropriate?
- ○ 1. "You shouldn't let yourself get so upset."
- ○ 2. "Don't worry about them; they don't mean any harm."
- ○ 3. "Look. They seem to be having fun."
- ○ 4. "They're laughing at a joke John told; they were not laughing at you."

120. Mebendazole (Vermox) is prescribed for an 8-year-old child with pinworms. The child has an 18-month-old brother and a 4-year-old sister. The nurse

would expect to treat which of the following family members with this drug?
- ○ 1. Both of the child's siblings.
- ○ 2. The child's parents and brother.
- ○ 3. Everyone who lives in the household.
- ○ 4. The parents and sister.

121. When planning a presentation on the topic of osteoporosis to a group of middle-aged women, which of the following would the nurse expect to include?
- ○ 1. An early symptom of osteoporosis is the "dowager's hump."
- ○ 2. African American and Latina women are at greater risk.
- ○ 3. Loss of height is an early symptom of the disease.
- ○ 4. Conventional radiographs are usually used to confirm the disease.

122. Which of the following statements best explains why the nurse should evaluate gastric residual before administering the client's next enteral feeding?
- ○ 1. To determine how well nutrients are being absorbed.
- ○ 2. To determine if the client is receiving enough feeding.
- ○ 3. To prevent over-distention of the stomach.
- ○ 4. To prevent the mixing of undigested formula with partially digested formula.

123. Which of the following serologic tests should the nurse have on the chart before a client is started on tissue plasminogen activator (tPA) or alteplase recombinant (Activase)?
- ○ 1. Activated partial prothrombin time (aPTT).
- ○ 2. Potassium level.
- ○ 3. Lee-White clotting time.
- ○ 4. Fibrin split product (FSP).

124. An older adult man has been referred by his physician to participate in the cardiac rehabilitation program. The client is a diabetic and has complaints of bilateral leg discomfort with walking. The nurse would use a stationary bicycle and intermittent training because of the client's
- ○ 1. diabetic neuropathy.
- ○ 2. muscle atrophy.
- ○ 3. Raynard's disease.
- ○ 4. transient ischemic attacks.

125. The client with borderline personality disorder spends much time around the nurse's station, making numerous minor requests. The nurse interprets these behaviors as indicative of which of the following?
- ○ 1. Fears of abandonment and attention seeking.
- ○ 2. Enjoyment of bothering the staff.
- ○ 3. Boredom suggesting the need for something to do.
- ○ 4. Lack of desire for involvement in milieu activities.

126. A client has soft wrist restraints on to prevent her from pulling out her nasogastric tube. Which of the following nursing interventions should be implemented while the restraints are on the client?
    ○ 1. Instruct the client not to move while the restraints are in place.
    ○ 2. Remove the restraints every 4 hours to provide skin care.
    ○ 3. Secure the restraints to siderails of the bed.
    ○ 4. Check on the client every 30 minutes while the restraints are on.

127. A client with alcohol dependence states, "I feel so bad because of what I've done to my wife and kids. I'm just no good." Which of the following responses by the nurse would be *most* appropriate?
    ○ 1. "You'll need to make up for a lot of things."
    ○ 2. "They will need to forgive your shortcomings."
    ○ 3. "Alcohol dependence is a disease that can be treated."
    ○ 4. "Alcoholism is painful for everyone involved."

128. After teaching the parents of a toddler about appropriate snack foods for their child, the nurse would judge that the instructions about not giving the child raisins for snacks are effective when the father states which of following?
    ○ 1. "Raisins are low in nutritive value."
    ○ 2. "Raisins can increase tooth decay."
    ○ 3. "Raisins are easy to choke on."
    ○ 4. "Raisins are hard to digest entirely."

129. A client has been diagnosed with atrial fibrillation. The physician ordered warfarin sodium (Coumadin) to be taken on a daily basis. The nurse will instruct the client to avoid using which of the following over-the-counter medications while taking warfarin?
    ○ 1. Aspirin.
    ○ 2. Benadryl.
    ○ 3. Lanoxin.
    ○ 4. Sudafed.

130. The nurse should inform a client taking carbamazepine (Tegretol) that it can effect other medications in which of the following ways?
    ○ 1. It decreases the effects of oral anticoagulants.
    ○ 2. It decreases the serum concentration of verapamil (Calan).
    ○ 3. It increases the serum concentration of other anticonvulsants.
    ○ 4. It increases the effects of oral contraceptives.

131. A client has been diagnosed with viral hepatitis. Which of the following expected outcomes would be most appropriate for the client?
    ○ 1. Achieve control of abdominal pains.
    ○ 2. Increase activity levels gradually.
    ○ 3. Be able to breathe without difficulty.
    ○ 4. Experience relief from edema.

132. Which of the following activities by the mother would offer the *most* support to the child during the first few days after surgery to repair cleft lip?
    ○ 1. Holding and cuddling the child.
    ○ 2. Helping the child play with some toys.
    ○ 3. Reading some of the child's favorite stories.
    ○ 4. Staying at the bedside and holding the child's hand.

133. Which of the following would be the public health nurse's *best* strategy to reduce the number of children involved in automobile accidents who were not wearing seat belts?
    ○ 1. Contact the local state representative to discuss new legislation about child seat belts.
    ○ 2. Attend a school board meeting to advocate for classes teaching children seat belt safety.
    ○ 3. Call the town mayor's office with this information so that the mayor can discuss it with the media.
    ○ 4. Start a letter-writing campaign to the school superintendent about seat belt importance.

134. A basic principle of any rehabilitation program, including a cardiac rehabilitation program, is that rehabilitation begins
    ○ 1. on discharge from the hospital.
    ○ 2. on discharge from the cardiac care unit.
    ○ 3. on admission to the hospital.
    ○ 4. 4 weeks after the onset of illness.

135. A child is admitted to the emergency department with dyspnea related to bronchospasms. The nurse should place the client in which of the following positions?
    ○ 1. High Fowler's.
    ○ 2. Side-lying.
    ○ 3. Prone.
    ○ 4. Supine.

136. The nurse is preparing to administer intramuscular (IM) morphine sulfate to a client who is experiencing pain. On checking the physician's order, the nurse notes that the order states "Morphine sulfate 60 mg IM every 4 hours as needed for pain." The nurse understands that a usual IM dose of morphine is 10 to 15 mg. What would be the most appropriate action for the nurse to take?
    ○ 1. Administer the medication as ordered.
    ○ 2. Reduce the ordered dosage to 20 mg and give that.
    ○ 3. Contact the physician to verify the order.
    ○ 4. Ask another nurse to review the order.

137. The nurse is preparing a client for a paracentesis. Which of the following activities should the nurse complete in preparation for this test?
    ○ 1. Have the client void before the procedure.
    ○ 2. Prepare the client's abdomen with Betadine solution.

○ 3. Position the client supine.

○ 4. Make the client NPO 4 hours before the procedure.

138. A nurse working in a community health center suspects that a 20-month-old is being abused. Which of the following behaviors would lead the nurse to suspect this?

○ 1. Absence of crying during the examination.

○ 2. Clinging to parent during the examination.

○ 3. Playing with toys on the examination room floor.

○ 4. Talking easily with the nurse.

139. Which of the following would the nurse plan to include when teaching the client and family about a substance abuse problem?

○ 1. The role of the family in perpetuating the problem.

○ 2. The family's responsibility for the client.

○ 3. The physical, physiologic, and psychological effects of substances.

○ 4. The reasons that could have led the client to use the substance.

140. A client who has had a laparoscopic cholecystectomy receives discharge instructions from the nurse. Which statement indicates that the client has understood the instructions?

○ 1. "I will need to maintain a low-fat diet for the next 6 months."

○ 2. "I can remove the dressing from my incision tomorrow and take a shower."

○ 3. "I can anticipate some nausea for several days after surgery."

○ 4. "I will be able to return to work in 4 to 6 weeks."

141. The nurse should recognize that Mexican-American culture most highly values

○ 1. children.

○ 2. materialism.

○ 3. first-born sons.

○ 4. the elderly.

142. A client comes into the emergency department complaining of extreme fatigue. He is malnourished, and laboratory tests reveal that he is severely anemic. Based on an understanding of how vitamin and mineral deficiencies are associated with anemia, the nurse asks the client about his intake of food high in which of the following nutrients?

○ 1. Vitamins A, E, and C.

○ 2. Vitamins B_6, B_{12}, folate, iron, and copper.

○ 3. Thiamin, riboflavin, and niacin.

○ 4. Vitamins A and B.

143. The nurse is assessing a neonate born to a diabetic mother. Which of the following findings would the nurse expect to see in the infant?

○ 1. Hypertonia

○ 2. Hyperactivity

○ 3. Large size

○ 4. Scaly skin

144. A client who had a transurethral resection of the prostate (TURP) complains of dribbling urine after his Foley catheter is removed on the second postoperative day. The nurse notes that the client had 200 mL of urine output in the last 8 hours with a 1000 mL intake. Which of the following interventions is a priority for the nurse at this time?

○ 1. Apply a condom catheter.

○ 2. Assess for bladder distention.

○ 3. Obtain a urine specimen for culture.

○ 4. Teach the client Kegel exercises.

145. A client has atrial fibrillation. The nurse should monitor the client for

○ 1. cardiac arrest.

○ 2. cerebral vascular accident.

○ 3. heart block.

○ 4. ventricular fibrillation.

146. A child diagnosed with tinea is being treated with griseofulvin (Grifulvin V). Which of the following instructions would the nurse give to the parents?

○ 1. Give the medication before a meal.

○ 2. Have the child avoid intense sunlight.

○ 3. Give the medication for 10 days.

○ 4. Encourage increased fluid intake.

147. The nurse is teaching a client who had a myocardial infarction about her diet. What percentage of calories should come from fat?

○ 1. 10%.

○ 2. 20%.

○ 3. 30%.

○ 4. 40%.

148. After going through the necessary procedures for collecting physical evidence after a rape, a client is crying and talking about what happened to her. Which of the following actions would be *most* appropriate?

○ 1. Advising the client to try to forget about what happened.

○ 2. Recommending that the client be thankful for the fact that she's alive.

○ 3. Questioning the client about what she could have done to deter the attack.

○ 4. Listening to the client's descriptions about what occurred.

149. A client undergoes a cystoscopy with biopsy of the bladder. After the procedure, which assessment is most appropriate for the nurse to make?

○ 1. Assess the patency of the Foley catheter.

○ 2. Assess the urine for excessive bleeding.

○ 3. Percuss the bladder for distention.

○ 4. Obtain a urine specimen for culture.

150. When a client of Mexican American descent tells the

nurse that she treated her infection by drinking milk, the nurse interprets the client's remark as
○ 1. confusion from fever.
○ 2. use of the hot disease concept.
○ 3. use of milk as a laxative.
○ 4. the need for a dietitian to assist her with meal planning.

151. A female client with paranoid schizophrenia has been hearing negative voices and "getting special messages from various sources." Which of the following interventions would be *most* appropriate for the client's symptoms?
○ 1. Asking her to make simple decisions.
○ 2. Being matter-of-fact with her.
○ 3. Monitoring her reactions to television programs.
○ 4. Reinforcing appropriate dress and hygiene.

152. A 20-year-old client who reports vaginal itching and a thick, white, cheese-like vaginal discharge beginning 2 days ago tells the nurse that she has been taking oral contraceptives for 2 months. The nurse determines that the client is most likely exhibiting signs of which of the following?
○ 1. Trichomonas vaginalis.
○ 2. Candidiasis.
○ 3. Herpes genitalis.
○ 4. Gonorrhea.

153. The nurse judges that the parents of a newborn with imperforate anus know what a low defect is when the father says that the rectum
○ 1. is below the abdominal rectus muscle.
○ 2. is above the abdominal rectus muscle.
○ 3. has descended through the puborectalis muscle.
○ 4. has ascended through the puborectalis muscle.

154. A 75-year-old man is receiving meperidine (Demerol) after surgery. For which of the following side effects of meperidine should the nurse carefully evaluate the client?
○ 1. Respiratory depression.
○ 2. Dysrhythmias.
○ 3. Constipation.
○ 4. Seizures.

155. A client with iron-deficiency anemia is taking iron supplements. The nurse emphasizes to the client that the drug will have increased absorption if taken with
○ 1. milk.
○ 2. orange juice.
○ 3. food.
○ 4. β-carotene.

156. When obtaining the nursing history of a client who has diabetes mellitus, the nurse would identify which of the following as a potential early symptom of renal insufficiency?
○ 1. Polyuria.
○ 2. Dysuria.

○ 3. Hematuria.
○ 4. Oliguria.

157. A client is planning to be treated for infertility with the zygote intrafallopian transfer (ZIFT) method. Which of the following would the nurse include when teaching the client about this type of treatment method?
○ 1. Fertilization takes place outside of the body.
○ 2. ZIFT is helpful for clients with bilateral blocked fallopian tubes.
○ 3. Ova and sperm are needed for instillation into the fallopian tube.
○ 4. Fertilized ova are instilled into the vagina to enter the uterus.

158. When assessing for oxygenation in a client with dark skin, the nurse should examine the client's
○ 1. skin.
○ 2. buccal mucosa.
○ 3. nape of the neck.
○ 4. forehead.

159. Which of the following rehabilitative measures should the nurse teach the client to perform after chest surgery to prevent shoulder ankylosis?
○ 1. Turn from side to side.
○ 2. Raise and lower the head.
○ 3. Raise the arm on the affected side over the head.
○ 4. Flex and extend the elbow on the affected side.

160. A client with a tracheostomy tube coughs and dislodges the tracheostomy tube. The nurse' first action should be to
○ 1. call for emergency assistance.
○ 2. attempt reinsertion of tracheostomy tube.
○ 3. position the client in semi-Fowler's position with the neck hyperextended.
○ 4. insert the obturator into the stoma to reestablish the airway.

161. An infant is to return to the clinic for a regular checkup and receive immunizations. In preparation for this next visit, which of the following would the nurse suggest to the parents?
○ 1. "Be prepared for the infant to be very fussy."
○ 2. "Give the infant acetaminophen (Tylenol) before coming."
○ 3. "Plan to keep the infant out of day care for that day."
○ 4. "Bring someone else to the appointment to support you."

162. A first-time mother is concerned that her 6-month-old infant is not gaining enough weight. The *best* response for the nurse to make is which of the following?
○ 1. "Birth weight doubles by 6 months of age."
○ 2. "Birth weight doubles by 3 months of age."
○ 3. "The baby will eat what he needs."
○ 4. "You need to make sure the baby finishes each bottle."

163. In accurately assessing a client who reports a back injury, it is critical for the nurse to question the client concerning which of the following?
    ○ 1. Family history of back problems.
    ○ 2. Previous hospitalizations.
    ○ 3. Personal history of illness.
    ○ 4. Mechanism of injury.

164. The nurse realizes that an antihypertensive medication functions to
    ○ 1. lower the individual's blood pressure.
    ○ 2. alter cardiac output.
    ○ 3. alter cardiac output or peripheral vascular resistance.
    ○ 4. alter peripheral vascular resistance.

165. The nurse is examining a client with possible early rheumatoid arthritis. Which of the following symptoms would the nurse most likely observe?
    ○ 1. Nausea.
    ○ 2. Joint swelling.
    ○ 3. Fatigue.
    ○ 4. Limitation of movement.

166. The nurse instructs the client in mixing and administering Regular and NPH Insulin. Which of the following statements indicates that the client needs additional instruction?
    ○ 1. "I draw up the Regular insulin first."
    ○ 2. "I shake the bottle of NPH insulin before drawing it up."
    ○ 3. "I store the insulin in a cool place."
    ○ 4. "I insert the needle at a 90-degree angle."

167. The mother of a child with newly diagnosed Duchenne's muscular dystrophy asks how her child developed the disease. The nurse formulates a response incorporating which of the following statements about its transmission?
    ○ 1. It is an autosomal recessive genetic disorder.
    ○ 2. It is a genetic disorder carried by males and transmitted to male children.
    ○ 3. It is a disorder primarily transmitted by males in the family.
    ○ 4. It is a disorder usually carried by females and transmitted to male children.

168. Which of the following would the nurse identify as a *priority* nursing diagnosis for an infant with intussusception?
    ○ 1. Deficient Fluid Volume.
    ○ 2. Diarrhea.
    ○ 3. Impaired Skin Integrity.
    ○ 4. Pain.

169. The physician orders Kefzol 1 g IV for a client. In preparing to administer the Kefzol, the nurse notes that the client is allergic to penicillin. Based on this information, what would be an appropriate action for the nurse to take?

1. Continue to prepare to administer the Kefzol as ordered.
    ○ 2. Notify the physician of the client's allergy to penicillin.
    ○ 3. Administer the Kefzol, staying at the client's bedside during the infusion.
    ○ 4. Call the pharmacist to verify that the Kefzol should be administered as ordered.

170. When a client has a tearing of tissue with irregular wound edges, the nurse should document this as a
    ○ 1. contusion.
    ○ 2. abrasion.
    ○ 3. laceration.
    ○ 4. colonization.

171. A client with schizophrenia is responding well to risperidone (Risperdal) and is no longer psychotic. After teaching the client about managing his illness, which of the following statements reflects a need for *further* education?
    ○ 1. "I just don't know if I can afford to keep taking medicines everyday."
    ○ 2. "When my thoughts start racing, I know I need to relax more."
    ○ 3. "I can name the side effects of Risperdal, but I'm not having any."
    ○ 4. "I don't listen to my mom's religious beliefs about not using medicines."

172. When preparing to give medications, the nurse should review the "five rights" of medication administration to ensure client safety. The "five rights" include which of the following?
    ○ 1. Person, route, dose, drug, and time.
    ○ 2. Person, action, route, dose, and time.
    ○ 3. Person, room, route, dose, and time.
    ○ 4. Person, drug, dose, time, and expiration date.

173. Which of the following symptoms would the nurse expect to find as an early symptom of chronic congestive heart failure?
    ○ 1. Fatigue.
    ○ 2. Pedal edema.
    ○ 3. Nocturia.
    ○ 4. Irregular pulse.

174. The nurse instructs the client with gastroesophageal reflux disease (GERD) regarding dietary measures. The recommended dietary changes for clients with GERD include
    ○ 1. eliminating spicy foods.
    ○ 2. avoiding chocolate and coffee.
    ○ 3. eliminating cucumbers and other foods with seeds.
    ○ 4. avoiding steamed foods.

175. Signs and symptoms of which of the following would be a priority when caring for a newly delivered term neonate diagnosed as small for gestational age?
    ○ 1. Iron-deficiency anemia.

○ 2. Birth asphyxia.
○ 3. Persistent pulmonary hypertension.
○ 4. Hyperglycemia.

176. At what rate should the nurse start an IV infusion if the order is for 1 g of vancomycin (Vancocin) to be given in 180 mL of D_5W over 60 minutes? The drip rate factor is 15 drops/mL.
○ 1. 27 drops/minute.
○ 2. 30 drops/minute.
○ 3. 45 drops/minute.
○ 4. 90 drops/minute.

177. A mother of a child with food allergies expresses concern that her child's 2-month-old sibling may also have food allergies. When discussing feeding techniques for the infant, the nurse should suggest that the mother
○ 1. give only rice cereal to the child.
○ 2. use only apple juice as a supplementary fluid.
○ 3. introduce new foods to the infant one at a time.
○ 4. discontinue formula feedings when the infant begins to eat baby food.

178. The nurse enters a client's room and finds the client crying. Which of the following is the nurse's *most* appropriate response?
○ 1. "It's OK to cry."
○ 2. "Is there someone I can call for you?"
○ 3. "Here's a tissue."
○ 4. "Do you want to talk about it?"

179. A 23-year-old client is experiencing PMS symptoms. Which of the following dietary choices is appropriate for relieving symptoms of PMS?
○ 1. Decreasing sodium and increasing calcium.
○ 2. Limiting fat to 9 g/day.
○ 3. Increasing vitamins A and C.
○ 4. Increasing proteins and decreasing carbohydrates.

180. A client with a fractured tibia has a long leg plaster cast. The cast is still damp, and the client complains that it feels hot to him. What should be the nurse's response?
○ 1. Notify the physician, because this is an indication that the cast is applying pressure to soft tissue.
○ 2. Explain to the client that this feeling is a normal part of the drying process for plaster casts.
○ 3. Elevate the casted leg on two pillows.
○ 4. Administer prescribed pain medication to decrease discomfort.

181. A 28-year-old woman is learning about breast self-examination (BSE). The nurse teaches the woman that the best time of each month to examine her breasts is during
○ 1. the week before menstruation occurs.
○ 2. the week that menstruation occurs.
○ 3. the first week after menstruation.
○ 4. the week that ovulation occurs.

Correct Answers and Rationale

The letters in parentheses following the rationale identify the step of the nursing process (A, D, P, I, E), client needs (1, 2, 3, 4, 5, 6, 7, 8, 9, 10), and nursing care area (O, Y, M, X). See the inside front cover for the key.

1. 1. One serving of a vegetable or fruit is equivalent to one fourth of a cantaloupe. The client would need 6 ounces of a vegetable juice cocktail, 2 tomatoes, or 2 raw apricots to meet one vegetable serving. (E, 7, O)

2. 2. *Respondeat superior* is Latin for "The master is responsible for the acts of his servants." The nurse, as an employee of the hospital, was acting according to the established policy of the hospital. Because the nurse followed hospital policy, it is unlikely that this incident involved malpractice, negligence, or tort law. (I, 1, M)

3. 3. The surgeon is required to give the client explanations and have questions answered. The nurse has no way of assessing the client's understanding without the interpreter. The client should sign the Spanish consent form only after receiving an explanation of the procedure, its risks, and alternatives. A family member cannot be relied on to translate the surgeon's instructions. The nurse is often asked to witness the explanation and to obtain the client's signature on the informed consent form. Informed consent is the provision of information concerning the procedure and its risks, not obtaining the client's signature on the form. The surgical charge nurse does not need to be notified. (I, 1, M)

4. 2. Timolol can cause some eye discomfort when administered. It is important for the client to continue to take the drug. Glaucoma eye drops should be administered as prescribed, not whenever the client desires. Clients with glaucoma will need to take eye medication on an ongoing basis in order to control the disorder and prevent vision damage. There is no need to refrigerate the drug. (I, 8, M)

5. 1. The nurse's best response when a child asks if cardiac catheterization is painful is to explain that the child will feel a little stinging when the numbing medicine is inserted into the area around the introduction site of the catheter. There may also be a feeling of pressure when the catheter is introduced. The child's trust in the nurse will be quickly lost if the nurse is untruthful. Most children are sedated and feel little during the procedure. (I, 9, Y)

6. 1. This client has a barrel chest. The anterior-posterior diameter of the chest is larger than the transverse diameter, as is characteristic of clients with chronic obstructive pulmonary disease. Although the client may be muscular, the barrel chest is not associated with the client's age, height, or weight. Use of bronchodilators will not change the shape of this client's chest. (A, 10, M)

7. 2. Fetal acoustic stimulation involves the use of an instrument that emits sound levels of approximately 80 dB at a frequency of 80 Hz. The sharp sound startles and awakens the fetus and is used with nonstress testing as a method to evaluate fetal well-being. A fetoscope or Doppler stethoscope is used to listen to the fetal heart rate. Nipple stimulation or intravenous oxytocin is used to stimulate contractions. Ultrasound testing is used to determine amniotic fluid volume. (I, 9, O)

8. 2. Typically, iron supplements are needed for at least 1 month. By the end of this time, there should be a significant rise in the hemoglobin and hematocrit. Therefore the mother needs to continue the iron supplements for several more weeks. Testing the child after only 2 weeks of treatment may not be beneficial. A significant rise in hemoglobin and hematocrit usually requires approximately 1 month of therapy. An iron-rich diet should have been started when the diagnosis was made and continued for at least the duration of iron supplement therapy. (I, 8, Y)

9. 1. The dietary department should meet with the client to ensure that the foods are available and prepared according to her religious beliefs. On admission, all clients should be asked whether they have special dietary needs. The dietary department should be notified of these special needs, and a dietary representative should meet with the client and/or family when possible. The physician should be consulted if a requested food is contrary to a prescribed diet restriction. The nursing supervisor does not need to be contacted regarding a dietary request. The rabbi is not involved in dietary requests. (I, 1, M)

10. 3. The nurse must act as an advocate for the client when the client cannot afford treatment. It is possible to substitute a less expensive antibiotic. Correct procedure would include contacting the physician to explain the mother's economic situation and request a substitution. For example, amoxicillin is much more economical than azithromycin. (I, 8, M)

11. 2. Nitroglycerin causes vasodilation, which results in increased intraocular pressure. The vasodilatory effects of the medication can trigger an attack, causing pain and loss of vision. Hypotension is a common side effect of nitroglycerin, which dilates the blood vessels, but is not a concern in clients with glaucoma. (E, 8, M)

12. 3. The timing of symptoms is important to the diagnosis of PMS. The client should keep a 3-month log of symptoms and menses. With PMS, the symptoms begin 3 to 7 days before menses and resolve 1 to 2 days after the menstrual cycle has started. Menstrual cycle irregularity and mood swings after menses are not related to PMS, and other causes should be investigated. Midcycle spotting and pain are related to ovulation. (A, 4, M)

13. 2. The client who has received general anesthesia has also received a muscle relaxant. A side effect of the antibiotic colistimethate sodium (Coly-Mycin) is neuromuscular blockade. The combined effect of the medications places the client at increased risk and the nurse should assess the client closely for respiratory depression or paralysis. The nurse will be monitoring the client's heart rate, blood pressure, and urinary output, but not specifically because of potential drug interactions and side effects of colistimethate sodium. (A, 8, M)

14. 4. Dietary Reference Intakes (DRIs) are sets of nutrient intake values suggested for the dietary intakes of healthy people in the United States and Canada. The DRIs were developed to establish levels of nutrient intake required to prevent chronic disease. The DRIs are meant to replace the Recommended Daily Allowances (RDAs), which represented the minimum amount required to prevent symptoms of deficiency. The Dietary Guidelines describe food choices that promote good health. (A, 4, M)

15. 2. When ovulation is suppressed for 6 to 8 months after oral contraceptive use, the physician may prescribe clomiphene citrate (Clomid) to stimulate ovulation. Clomiphene acts to give the hypothalamus the signal to increase secretion of follicle-stimulating hormone and luteinizing hormone, thereby stimulating ovulation. Dienestrol is an estrogen applied topically to treat atrophic vaginitis and kraurosis vulvae in postmenopausal women. Medroxyprogesterone is a progesterone derivative that prevents maturation of the follicle and ovulation. Norgestrel is a progesterone-only contraceptive that is believed to alter the cervical mucus, possibly suppress ovulation in some women, and interfere with implantation in the uterus. (P, 8, O)

16. 1. Hospice programs are appropriate programs for clients with any type of terminal illness when death is imminent within weeks up to 6 months. Clients may discuss their prognosis of a terminal illness long before it progresses to the terminal stage when a referral to hospice care is indicated. (P, 1, M)

17. 1. Several irregularly shaped red patches, common skin variations in neonates, are termed "stork bites." They will eventually fade away as the neonate grows older. Port wine stains are disfiguring darkish red or purplish skin discolorations on the scalp and face that may need laser therapy for removal. Newborn rash is typically generalized over the body, not localized to one body area, and is often raised. Café au lait spots are brown in color, typically found anywhere on the body. More than six spots or spots larger than 1.5 cm are associated with neurofibromatosis, a genetic condition of neural tissue. (D, 3, O)

18. 3. In the traditional Mexican household, the man is the head of the family and makes the major decisions. Efforts should be made to reach the father as soon as possible to acquire his permission. Contacting the social worker does not reflect the nurse's need to understand a client's cultural values and how they affect medical care decisions. This is not a situation of suspected child abuse. (I, 1, M)

19. 1. In cognitively impaired clients, benzodiazepines, such as lorazepam, can increase confusion and nighttime agitation. Extrapyramidal side effects are more common with antipsychotics. Vomiting and sweating are signs of benzodiazepine withdrawal. Anticholinergic side effects are more likely with antipsychotics and tricyclic antidepressants. (A, 8, X)

20. 4. A woman with a uterus who takes unopposed estrogen has an increased risk of endometrial cancer. The addition of progesterone prevents the formation of endometrial hyperplasia. (I, 8, M)

21. 3. The nurse will monitor the client's serum albumin. A decreased serum albumin indicates malnutrition and is considered a risk factor of the development of pressure ulcers. Other risk factors include immobility, incontinence, and decreased sensation. Ambulating the client and inserting an indwelling Foley catheter will require a physician's order. The white blood cell count would be monitored if an infection were present. (P, 10, M)

22. 4. The nurse should recognize the ringing in the ears, or tinnitus, as a sign of ototoxicity probably caused by the furosemide. The appropriate action is for the nurse to stop the furosemide and notify the physician. If the drug is stopped soon enough, permanent hearing loss can be avoided and the tinnitus should subside. The nurse should note the observation in the chart but should not delay action. Tinnitus is not a symptom of digitalis toxicity. Aspirin can cause tinnitus, but the nurse should first investigate the obvious cause of tinnitus, which in this case is the furosemide. (I, 8, M)

23. 3. The peak serum dose of an antibiotic is drawn 30 minutes after the completion of the IV dose of the antibiotic. (P, 8, M)

24. 1. Intracranial pressure is highest in the early morning. If the client has a headache on arising, this should be reported to the physician. The client with hydrocephalus may be experiencing signs of increased intracranial pressure that need to be treated. (A, 4, M)

25. 1. The nurse should instruct the client that symptoms from an occasional headache due to eye strain or continuous work at a computer can be relieved by acetaminophen (Tylenol). Although this drug causes prostaglandin inhibition, this effect is rapidly reversed and cleared with no apparent harmful effects in pregnancy. If the headaches become more frequent or severe, the client should be instructed to contact her health care provider immediately. Aspirin should be avoided during pregnancy because it inhibits prostaglandin synthesis. It also decreases uterine contractility and may delay the onset of labor or prolong pregnancy and labor. Aspirin decreases platelet aggregation, possibly increasing the risk of bleeding. Ibuprofen and naproxen can lead to premature closure of the fetal ductus arteriosus and decreased amniotic fluid with prolonged use. They may also prolong pregnancy or labor because of their antiprostaglandin effects. (I, 8, O)

26. 1. With this level of anger in a crisis, the father needs simple but firm directions to leave the room, calm down, and then to talk. Doing so relieves the daughter of any pressure from her father. Telling the father to stop yelling or be quiet provides no concrete directions to the father and may embarrass him in front of his daughter. Telling the father that if he doesn't stop yelling, the nurse will call Security is a threat, possibly leading to an escalation of the situation. (I, 6, X)

27. 2. Epidemiologic and experimental research studies indicate that African Americans are more likely to develop severe hypertension. (D, 4, M)

28. 1. A large pad of fat at the back of the neck, widely set eyes, a simian crease in the hands, and epicanthal folds are typically associated with Down syndrome. The nurse should notify the physician immediately. The physician should obtain consent for genetic studies and is responsible for explaining these deviations to the parents. However, the nurse may need to provide additional teaching to the mother and to answer any questions that may arise. (A, 3, O)

29. 1. Clients receiving chronic steroid therapy can become immunosuppressed and are prone to infections. Signs of infection can also be masked with prednisone. Signs and symptoms of infections should be reported immediately. Joint pain, constipation, and joint swelling are not related to side effects of steroid therapy. (I, 8, M)

30. 2. Injury and death from firearms is a major public health problem in the United States. One reason that this is such an epidemic is that children, grandchildren, and neighbor children have easy access to firearms. (A, 9, M)

31. 4. School-aged children enjoy board games and are commonly intense about following rules. Their play can often become emotional. Adequate rest is of utmost importance during the acute stage of rheumatic fever. Therefore, playing a game with another child probably would be too strenuous. Such diversional activities as reading a book, playing with a doll, and watching television would be more satisfactory. (P, 3, Y)

32. 2. Women who take oral contraceptives are at increased risk for thromboembolic conditions. Severe calf pain would need to be investigated as a potential sign of deep vein thrombosis. Breakthrough bleeding, mild headache, or weight gain may be a common benign side effect that accompanies oral contraceptive use. The client may be monitored for these side effects without change in treatment. (I, 8, M)

33. 4. The main goal for a client with a new tracheostomy is to maintain a patent airway. A new tracheostomy frequently causes bleeding and excess secretions, and clients may require frequent suctioning to maintain a patent airway. (P, 10, M)

34. 3. The nurse should assess the client's vital signs, because the client is most likely having a reaction to the bupivacaine (Marcaine). If the client's vital signs are abnormal, immediate intervention may be necessary. Although the nurse may ask the client to continue to describe how he is feeling, this is not likely to be a psychosocial reaction. Simple reassurance is inappropriate in most clinical situations and can be dangerous if physiologic causes for restlessness are overlooked. The nurse should not administer epinephrine until the vital signs have been assessed. (D, 8, M)

35. 2. Endometrial cancer has very few warning signals; irregular bleeding may be the only sign. Any irregular bleeding in a menopausal woman should be investigated, and an endometrial biopsy may be ordered. Hot flashes result from the decreased estrogen levels that accompany menopause. Urinary urgency should be monitored and treated as a separate problem. Dyspareunia is the occurrence of pain in the labial, vaginal, or pelvic areas during or after sexual intercourse. It may be caused by inadequate vaginal lubrication in the menopausal woman. (I, 8, M)

36. 1. Cystic fibrosis is an autosomal recessive genetic disorder. This means that both parents have the gene. There is a one in four chance with each pregnancy from such parents that the child will have cystic fibrosis. (I, 10, Y)

37. 4. Trichomoniasis is caused by a protozoan. Although a few clients do not have symptoms, the classic presentation of trichomoniasis is a malodorous, yellow-green discharge. Gonorrhea, syphilis, and chlamydia do not frequently manifest as a vaginal discharge. (A, 4, M)

38. 4. Incentive spirometry promotes lung expansion and increases respiratory function. When used properly, an incentive spirometer causes sustained maximal inspiration and increased cardiac output. (E, 10, M)

39. 4. At this level of aggression, the client needs an appropriate physical outlet for the anger. She is beyond writing in a journal. Urging the client to talk to the nurse now or making threats, such as telling her that she will be restrained, is inappropriate and probably would lead to an escalation of her anger. (I, 6, X)

40. 3. Variable decelerations are associated with compression of the umbilical cord. The nurse should alter the client's position and increase the IV fluid rate. Fetal head compression is associated with early decelerations. Severe compression of the fetal chest, such as during the process of vaginal delivery, may result in transient bradycardia. Compression or damage to the placenta, typically from abruptio placenta, results in severe late decelerations. (D, 9, O)

41. 2. If the chest tube is accidentally pulled out (a rare occurrence), a petroleum jelly gauze and sterile 4- × 4-inch dressing should be applied over the chest wall insertion site immediately. The dressing should be covered with adhesive tape and be occlusive, and the surgeon should be notified. The lungs can be auscultated and vital signs can be taken after the dressing is in place and the surgeon has been called. (I, 9, M)

42. 4. Emboli obstruct blood flow, leading to a decreased perfusion of the lung tissue. Because of the decreased perfusion, a ventilation-perfusion mismatch occurs, causing hypoxemia to develop. Arterial blood gas analysis typically will indicate hypoxemia and hypocapnia. A priority objective in the treatment of pulmonary emboli is maintaining adequate oxygenation. A nonproductive cough and activity intolerance are not indicative of impaired gas exchange. The client does not demonstrate an ineffective breathing pattern; rather, the problem of impaired gas exchange is caused by the inability of blood to flow through the lung tissue. (D, 10, M)

43. 3. Cardiogenic shock occurs when myocardial contractility decreases and cardiac output greatly decreases. The circulating blood volume is within normal limits or increased. Infarction is not always the cause of cardiogenic shock. (A, 10, M)

44. 1. The nurse would expect to find decreased levels of thyroxine (T_4) and triiodothyronine (T_3) and increased thyroid-stimulating hormone (TSH). An elevated creatine phosphokinase (CPK) concentration and the presence of antithyroid antibodies are other indicators of hypothyroidism. (D, 10, M)

45. 3. Although chronologically the infant is 7 months old, because of being born 6 weeks early, the child is only $5^1/_2$ months old developmentally. Appropriate activities for a 5- to $5^1/_2$-month-old infant include placing a rattle or ball in the infant's hand. Picture books are an appropriate choice for an infant older than 9 months of age. Playing peek-a-boo would be appropriate for a 9- to 12-month-old infant. Colored blocks would be appropriate for a toddler approximately 15 to 18 months of age. (I, 3, Y)

46. 3. Accurate daily weights provide the best measure of a client's fluid status: 1 kg (2.2 pounds) is equal to 1000 mL of fluid. To be accurate, weights should be obtained at the same time every day, with the same scale, and with minimal clothing on. (I, 10, M)

47. 2. An adequate trial of an antidepressant medication to induce remission requires about 4 weeks on an adequate dose. Antidepressant medications usually do not bring complete remission from depression quickly. They may be more effective in combination with counseling. (I, 8, M)

48. 2. Fine tremors are the first symptom reported in 70% of clients with Parkinson's disease. A new onset of tremors needs to be investigated by the physician. Tremors are not an expected change with aging. (A, 4, M)

49. 1. One of the more common side effects associated with methylphenidate hydrochloride (Ritalin) is growth retardation and loss of appetite. Children are monitored for these side effects as well as for hypertension. Although nausea is associated with this drug, vomiting is not. Photosensitivity is not associated with this drug. However, it may occur with some antibiotics and drugs used in chemotherapy regimens. Weight loss is associated with Ritalin. (A, 8, Y)

50. 2. The pH of 7.26 indicates that the body is in a state of acidosis. The elevated CO_2 value accompanied by a normal HCO_3 value indicates that the acid–base imbalance is respiratory acidosis. The additional clinical findings of a headache, dizziness, and increased pulse rate, resulting from the elevated CO_2 concentration, further supports this diagnosis. (D, 10, M)

51. 1. With a client in metabolic alkalosis, the nurse should monitor for hypokalemia. Metabolic alkalosis can cause potassium to shift into the cells, resulting in a decrease of serum potassium. In metabolic alkalosis, the body tries to compensate by conserving CO_2, so there is no need to have the client inhale CO_2, as would be the case if hyperventilation were occurring. There is already a base bicarbonate excess with this condition, so the nurse would not expect to administer sodium bicarbonate. Unless client symptoms dictate, the client does not necessarily need to be placed on bed rest. (I, 10, M)

52. 1. To reduce the risk of crystalluria, the client should drink 2000 to 3000 mL of water a day, not 1000 to 1500 mL. The client should not take an antacid before taking ciprofloxacin (Cipro). An antacid will decrease the absorption of ciprofloxacin. The client should let the doctor know if vomiting occurs from the medication. The client may get lightheaded from the ciprofloxacin. If so, the client should not drive a motor vehicle and should contact the physician. (E, 8, M)

53. 4. Stress management would not be beneficial to the client with Alzheimer's disease because of cognitive impairment, confusion, and short-term memory loss. Reminiscence group, walking, and pet therapy would be beneficial. (P, 6, X)

54. 2. The priority long-term nursing diagnosis for this child would be Risk for Injury. This is always a concern for children with hemophilia. As with all children who have chronic illnesses, there is a potential for self-esteem problems, but no data are presented to support this diagnosis. The parents should have a good understanding of the disease process and realize the importance of obtaining regular health care for their child. Pain would be an appropriate diagnosis of the child who has bleeding into a joint, but this would be a transient situation. (D, 9, Y)

55. 3. A 3-year-old child responds best to distraction during a procedure because of the typical level of cognitive development of a 3-year-old and the fear of painful events. Preparation for the procedure should be done immediately beforehand, so that the child will not become too frightened. A 3-year-old is not concerned about the "why" of the procedure but about whether the procedure will hurt. This child is too young for verbal explanations alone because of the limited verbal abilities at this age and the fear of a painful event. (I, 3, Y)

56. 3. Lisinopril is an angiotensin-converting enzyme (ACE) inhibitor. Hyperkalemia can be a side effect of ACE inhibitors. Because of this side effect, ACE inhibitors should not be administered with potassium-sparing diuretics. (A, 8, M)

57. 4. Medication noncompliance is a primary cause of exacerbation in chronic mental illnesses. Of the issues listed, medications should be addressed first. Other issues, such as family, marriage, and finances can be addressed as client stabilization is maintained. (P, 6, X)

58. 4. Intravenous fluids should not be infused for any longer than 24 hours because of the potential for bacterial growth in the solution. The appropriate action for the nurse to take is to discontinue the current TPN solution, change the tubing, and hang a new bag of

solution. Changing the filter does not decrease the chances of contamination. Notifying the physician for a change in flow rate is not an acceptable solution. (I, 8, M)

59. 3. The nurse's first response is to further assess the client's pain. After a thorough assessment, additional appropriate actions may be to notify the physician, administer an analgesic, and administer oxygen. (I, 10, M)

60. 4. Trisomy 13 (Patau's syndrome) is an autosomal disorder. Characteristics include cleft lip and palate, polydactyly, malformed ears, and mental retardation. These neonates typically die during infancy. A webbed neck is associated with Turner's syndrome (45 total chromosomes). Small testes and absence of sperm are associated with Klinefelter's syndrome (47 chromosomes). Congenital heart defects are associated with trisomy 21 (Down syndrome) and trisomy 18 (Edward's syndrome). (I, 9, O)

61. 2. Neurologic symptoms such as foot drop or bowel or bladder changes should be reported to the physician immediately. When musculoskeletal strain causes the back pain, these symptoms may take 4 to 6 weeks to resolve. As an accompanying symptom of acute low back pain, the client may have a diffuse, aching sensation in the L4–5; pain in the lower back when the leg is lifted; or pain that radiates to the hip. (A, 4, M)

62. 2. Taking ginseng when on insulin is not encouraged because ginseng increases the risk for hypoglycemia. Ginseng can be therapeutic in certain situations. If the nurse does not know about the interaction, it would be appropriate to ask the pharmacist. (E, 8, M)

63. 2. The expected effect of lactulose (Cephulac) is for the client to have two to three soft stools a day in order to help reduce the pH and serum ammonia levels, which will prevent portal–systemic encephalopathy. (P, 8, M)

64. 3. Leukocytosis, an increased white blood cell count, indicates the presence of inflammation, infection, or a leukemia process. In inflammation and infection, the client's sedimentation rate is increased. Thrombocytopenia, a platelet deficiency, occurs in clients with leukemia, immunocompromise, aplastic anemia, or other conditions. Erythrocytosis, an elevation of the red blood cell count, occurs in polycythemia vera. (E, 10, M)

65. 4. This girl has an exaggeration of the lumber spine, swayback, or lordosis. Kyphosis is an increased convexity or roundness of the curve of the thoracic spine. Scoliosis is a lateral curvature of the spine. (D, 3, Y)

66. 4. The most appropriate action is to report the swelling, loss of mobility, and unrelieved pain to the physician. These symptoms are indicators of neurovascular impairment. Administering meperidine will not eliminate the cause of the problem, which is unrelieved pressure on nerves and blood supply. If prompt action (eg, cutting

the cast) is not taken to relieve the pressure, permanent muscular and neurologic injury may result. Applying the ice bag would have been appropriate earlier to decrease or prevent swelling, but applying it at this time could actually lead to further decreased circulation. The arm should be elevated, but the nurse cannot wait 30 minutes to reassess the client without risking permanent damage. (I, 9, M)

67. 1. Prostaglandin $F_{2\alpha}$ promotes uterine contractions, thereby minimizing uterine atony and subsequent hemorrhage. Possible side effects include nausea, tachycardia, hypertension, and diarrhea. Abdominal distention is not associated with the use of prostaglandin $F_{2\alpha}$. (A, 8, O)

68. 1. Before 32 weeks' gestation, the majority of neonates have difficulty coordinating sucking and swallowing reflexes along with breathing. Increased respiratory distress may occur with bottle feeding. Bottle feedings can be given once the neonate shows sucking and swallowing behaviors. High-calorie formulas can be given by bottle or by gavage feeding. Although frequent feeding prevents hypoglycemia, the feeding does not have to be given via a gavage tube. Although these neonates can be stressed by cold, they can be kept warm with blankets while being bottle-fed or fed while in the warm isolette environment. (I, 3, O)

69. 2. Regularly scheduled rest periods during the day along with 8 to 10 hours of sleep at night will help relieve the fatigue, pain, and stiffness associated with rheumatoid arthritis. Even with mild rheumatoid arthritis the client may find it difficult to perform activities of daily living without some rest periods. Spending one day a week in bed to relieve fatigue does not adequately manage the disease. Clients must recognize their need for rest before feeling exhausted, because overexertion can cause exacerbations of the arthritis. In addition, prolonged periods of inactivity can increase joint stiffness and pain. Getting up early to do household chores before the children are awake does not allow for adequate rest. (E, 9, M)

70. 3. For the child with hemophilia who is actively bleeding, the nurse should apply direct pressure to the injured area for 10 minutes continuously along with elevating the leg. The continuous application of direct pressure aids in stopping the bleeding. Elevating the leg reduces blood flow to the area, thereby minimizing the extent of blood loss. Although ice will cause local vasoconstriction and slow the bleeding, applying continuous direct pressure is essential. (I, 10, Y)

71. 4. Hypothyroidism is not associated with pancytopenia. Various anemias are associated with pancytopenia owing to the reduction in all cellular elements of the blood. Bleeding and clotting difficulties can be associated with pancytopenia. Infection is a common danger associated with pancytopenia. (I, 2, M)

72. 2. The client's return to the emergency department and her statement about not knowing what to do about being abused by her husband indicate that the client is asking for help. The nurse's best course of action is to explain the various options available to her. This helps the client make decisions based on appropriate knowledge. Research reveals that women are more likely to be killed by partners than by strangers. Although the client can legally leave her husband, this answer provides the client with no safety options. Listing ways to avoid making the husband angry ignores the dynamics of abuse and blames the victim. (I, 6, X)

73. 3. The nurse places a postoperative client who has had abdominal surgery in low Fowler's position. This position relaxes abdominal muscles and promotes maximum respiratory and cardiovascular function. (I, 10, M)

74. 1. It is most important to know the child's serum potassium level when administering digoxin. Digoxin increases contractility of the heart and increases renal perfusion, resulting in a diuretic effect with increased loss of potassium and sodium. Hypokalemia increases the risk of digoxin toxicity. Verifying the dosage is specified by the institution's policy and varies from institution to institution. Although the child may take the medication better from the mother than from the nurse, asking the mother to give the medication is not necessary. In addition, this would be done after the nurse has checked the electrolyte levels. Teaching the parent how to measure the child's heart rate can be done at any time, not necessarily when preparing to give the medication. (P, 8)

75. 4. During the emergent phase of burn management, there is a massive shift of fluid from the blood vessels (intravascular compartment) into the tissues (interstitial compartment). The result of this shift is hypovolemic shock and edema formation. The fluid shift, which occurs between the intravascular and interstitial extracellular compartments, is caused by increased capillary permeability that allows water, sodium, and protein to shift to the tissues. As the emergent period ends and capillary permeability returns to normal, the fluid in the interstitial compartment will return to the intravascular compartment. (P, 10, M)

76. 3. A urinary output of 30 to 50 mL/hour is considered to be an indicator of adequate fluid replacement in burn clients. An increase in body weight may indicate fluid retention. A urinary output that is greater than fluid intake does not represent a fluid balance. Depending on the client, a blood pressure of 90/60 mm Hg could indicate the presence of a hypovolemic state; by

itself, it does not indicate adequate fluid replacement. (E, 10, M)

77. 1. Many clients who experience abuse are hesitant to talk about it and need help to do so. The nurse should ask the client directly about abuse when it is suspected, using a sensitive, empathic, and compassionate approach. In this way, the client can feel comfortable revealing information about the abuse. Telling the client that it's difficult to believe her injuries resulted from a fall is not helpful because it is blameful and puts the client on the defensive. Asking the client what she did to make someone hit her or discussing what she can do the next time blames and alienates the client. (I, 6, X)

78. 1. A primary goal for the care of the client in shock is to achieve adequate tissue perfusion, thus avoiding multiple organ dysfunction. The lungs are susceptible to injury, especially acute respiratory distress syndrome. Vasoconstriction occurs as a compensatory mechanism until the client enters the irreversible stage of shock. (P, 10, M)

79. 4. Problems with interpersonal relationships, such as resisting affection and refusing to respond to others, and repetitive behaviors, such as twirling around frequently, are suggestive of autism. Because the parents did not report any tics, Tourette's syndrome is not suggested. No psychotic behaviors, such as hallucinations or delusions, were reported, so schizophrenia can be ruled out. ADHD is most often portrayed as incessant activity with difficulty completing tasks. (D, 4, X)

80. 2. The incident report includes only what the nurse saw and did—the objective data. The nurse does not try to interpret the likely cause of the incident, include statements from the client about the incident, or comment on extenuating circumstances. (D, 1, M)

81. 1. To reduce urethral irritation and allow drainage, the nurse should tape the Foley catheter to a female client's inner thigh. Taping the catheter also prevents excessive traction against the bladder neck. Taping the catheter to the groin or lower abdomen would not allow for proper drainage and would cause urethral discomfort. Taping the catheter to the lower thigh would pull on the catheter and cause urethral irritation. (I, 9, M)

82. 1. A neonate delivered by cesarean delivery has not had the benefit of the chest-squeezing action of a vaginal delivery, which helps remove some of the nasopharyngeal secretions. The nurse should place the neonate under the radiant warmer and suction the mouth and nares with a bulb syringe to remove nasopharyngeal secretions. A high-pitched cry is associated with neurologic involvement or neonatal drug withdrawal and is unrelated to cesarean delivery. Skull fractures may occur with difficult vaginal deliveries

and are not typically seen with cesarean deliveries. Decreased muscle tone is associated with oversedation or neurologic impairment, not cesarean delivery. (A, 3, O)

83. 2. Accidental scaldings are usually splash-related and occur on the front of the body. Any burns on the back of the body or in a well-defined circular or glove pattern may indicate physical abuse. Immersion burns on the buttocks are also suspicious injuries. (A, 3, M)

84. 3. A client who is exhibiting mild preeclampsia will initially be treated with activity restriction. Bed rest, or lying on the left side, decreases pressure on the vena cava and improves circulatory blood flow. Restriction of visitors and a quiet environment are also necessary. Intravenous magnesium sulfate, a central nervous system depressant, is usually ordered for clients with severe preeclampsia. Labetalol hydrochloride is used for clients with severe preeclampsia. Frequent monitoring of the client's blood pressure is important. However, hourly blood pressure checks are more routinely ordered for clients with severe preeclampsia. Additionally, the client needs to rest, and checking her blood pressure hourly could interfere with her ability to rest. (P, 9, O)

85. 4. A dry tea bag placed on the bleeding area can be effective to control bleeding from lesions on the oral mucosa. The tannic acid in the tea apparently helps control bleeding. (I, 7, Y)

86. 4. The best treatment for a pressure ulcer is prevention. If a client has been determined to be at risk for development of a pressure ulcer, a systematic skin assessment should be conducted at least once a shift. Other preventive measures include daily gentle cleansing of the skin, avoiding harsh soaps and hot water, which are damaging to the skin. Massage of bony prominences is not done, because it can actually increase damage to the underlying tissue. Clients should be encouraged to change position at least every 2 hours to avoid pressure on any one area for a prolonged period. (I, 9, M)

87. 3. Nasogastric suctioning removes gastric acid from the gastrointestinal tract, thus creating a base bicarbonate excess and a state of metabolic alkalosis. The respiratory system is not affected by the presence of a nasogastric tube. Metabolic acidosis is not created when gastric acid is removed. (P, 10, M)

88. 1. The client needs further instructions when she says, "I should walk with my pelvis tilted backward." Walking in this position puts greater strain on the back. The client should walk with her pelvis tilted forward. Pelvic tilt exercises can also help the client with backaches. Putting a board under the mattress will make the mattress firmer and provide more support. Squatting and not bending to pick up objects will help decrease

back strain. Squatting involves the use of the large thigh muscles rather than those of the back. Flat or low-heeled shoes provide better balance and greater support and can help decrease backaches. (E, 7, O)

89. 4. Urethritis is usually the initial clinical manifestation of gonorrhea in men. The symptoms include a profuse, purulent discharge and dysuria. Complications are uncommon, but they include prostatitis and sterility. Impotence, scrotal pain, and penile lesions are not associated with gonorrhea. (A, 2, M)

90. 4. Although the nurse needs to obtain and administer the medication as soon as possible, it is inappropriate for the nurse to go down to the pharmacy and request the drug without first calling the pharmacy and checking to see whether the medication was delivered. The drug may have been delivered to a number of appropriate spots on the unit, such as the client's drug bin, the transport system, or the delivery box. The nurse should assess the client's blood pressure to determine the immediacy of the condition for which the medication was ordered. (D, 2, M)

91. 3. The client with major depression suffers from lack of energy and withdrawal. The nurse would emphasize the importance of group involvement for the client to gain support from others and to see that others have similar problems and concerns. Attendance at group sessions and activities decreases social isolation and destructive rumination. The other statements are not therapeutic and interfere with increasing the client's involvement with others. (I, 6, X)

92. 4. An infant's sleeping longer than usual can indicate that the child is expending too much energy to breathe and is tiring, suggesting that the child's condition is getting worse. This would need to be reported to the physician. Fewer than seven wet diapers a day would indicate the child is not drinking enough. A temperature of 100°F (37.8°C) for longer than 2 days should be reported. Clear nasal drainage would be normal. However, a yellow nasal drainage lasting longer than 24 hours should be reported. (E, 9, Y)

93. 4. Direct application of warm moist heat would benefit a client with low back pain, because the heat relaxes muscle spasms. Heat should not be applied to a client who has appendicitis, because it can lead to rupture of the appendix and peritonitis. Ice is applied to recently sprained joints to help decrease the formation of edema. Applying heat to the area of a suspected malignancy can increase blood flow to the tumor and promote nourishment of the cancer cells. (P, 7, M)

94. 3. The client with pernicious anemia will require life-long supplementation of B_{12}, available through injection or nasal spray administration. It must be given in these forms to ensure absorption. Oral B_{12} would not be absorbed, because the client lacks the intrinsic factor in the stomach necessary for absorption. Chelation therapy is used to extract metals at toxic levels, such as occurs in lead poisoning. (I, 8, M)

95. 4. When a client with major depression and suicidal ideation displays a sudden elevation in mood, seems calmer, has more energy, and is more peaceful, the nurse would judge these behaviors as an indication that a suicide attempt is imminent. These client symptoms may indicate relief from ambivalent thoughts about suicide or that the client has an immediate plan for killing himself. (D, 6, X)

96. 3. The purpose of a contraction stress test is to determine the fetal response during labor. If late decelerations are noted with the contractions, the test is considered positive or abnormal. Fetal lung maturity is evaluated through amniocentesis to obtain the lecithin–sphingomyelin ratio. The nonstress test is part of the biophysical profile. Determining fetal response during movements is evaluated as part of the nonstress test. (I, 9, O)

97. 3. Atyptical pneumonia is characterized by a gradual onset of symptoms such as dry cough, headache, sore throat, fatigue, nausea and vomiting. Typical pneumonia is characterized by tachypnea, fever, chills, and productive cough with purulent sputum. (A, 10, M)

98. 2. The primary reason for instructing clients with emphysema how to pursed-lip breathe is to prolong exhalation. Prolonging exhalation helps to prevent bronchiolar collapse and the trapping of air. It does not directly prevent respiratory infection. Because pursed-lip breathing affects the expiratory phase of the respiratory cycle, it does not affect oxygenation. It may decrease shortness of breath, but this is not the primary reason for the technique. (I, 9, M)

99. 2. The primary purpose of the automated dispensing machine for nurses is to keep an up-to-date record of the narcotic usage and count. The automated dispensing machine has eliminated the need for change-of-shift counts for narcotics. It does not include unmonitored access by nurses to narcotics, which would not be considered an advantage. The pharmacy has direct information about the narcotics being used on the individual clients at what intervals and by whom, and it automatically records the charges of narcotics used. Not recording the charges would not be an advantage. (P, 1, M)

100. 2. Blunt chest trauma can lead to respiratory failure. Maintenance of adequate oxygenation is the priority for the client. Decreasing the client's anxiety is related to maintaining effective respirations and oxygenation. Although pain is distressing to the client and can increase anxiety and decrease respiratory effectiveness,

pain control is secondary to maintaining oxygenation, as is maintaining adequate circulatory volume. (P, 10, M)

101. 1. An episiotomy that is edematous and slightly reddened 8 hours after delivery is normal. Therefore, the nurse should offer the client an ice pack to provide some relief from the perineal pain for the first 24 hours. An infection is present if greenish, purulent drainage is observed from the site. The edema and discoloration of the episiotomy at this time after delivery are normal and do not indicate that a hematoma is likely to develop. Sutures usually are present when a laceration has been repaired. (D, 3, O)

102. 3. The Z-track technique is used with medications that are irritating to tissues. It allows the medication to be trapped in the muscle and prevents it from leaking back through the tissues. (P, 8, M)

103. 2. The nurse would limit the amount of telephone calls the client would be allowed to make. Setting limits for a client with bipolar disorder, mania helps to control the hyperactive client who has excessive goal-directed activity, especially when it interferes with the rights of other clients. Instructing the other clients to be patient is neither fair to them nor helpful to the hyperactive client in managing behavior. Reminding the client that others need to use the telephone will probably be futile because the client with mania is experiencing cognitive impairment and needs to be active. Taking away the client's telephone privileges would not be the best action because the client has a right to use the telephone. The nurse is responsible for helping the client manage behavior by setting constructive limits. (I, 6, X)

104. 4. Because toddlers are strong and move frequently, the child needs to be restrained during the removal procedure by a total body restraint. To protect the child, the papoose board is best because the arms, legs, chest, and head can be fully restrained. A jacket restraint would immobilize only the child's upper body. Elbow restraints would immobilize only the child's arms. The father should be available to provide comfort before and after the procedure, not to hold the child down during the procedure. (P, 2, Y)

105. 4. Auscultatory wheezing over one lung in the presence of lung cancer is most likely caused by obstruction of the airway by a tumor. Exudate would be more likely to cause crackles. The client's history of smoking would not cause unilateral wheezing. Pleural effusion would be most likely to produce diminished or absent breath sounds. (A, 10, M)

106. 1. The client with hyperglycemia exhibits Kussmaul breathing, as well as flushed skin and low blood pressure. The client with hyperglycemia does not have excessive hunger. (A, 9, M)

107. 4. For the client who has been receiving lithium therapy for the past 2 months, a maintenance serum lithium level of 0.6 to 1.2 mEq/L would be considered therapeutic. A maintenance level greater than 1.2 mEq/L would be considered suggestive of toxicity. (D, 8, X)

108. 2. One cup of sunflower seeds contains 15 mg of iron. During pregnancy, 30 mg of iron is recommended daily. One cup of lentils provides the equivalent of 6.9 mg of iron. One and one-half ounces of hard cheese provides the equivalent of the amount of calcium in one cup of milk. Two poached eggs would provide only 2 mg of iron. (I, 7, O)

109. 4. The plan of care to treat fatigue associated with radiation therapy should include encouraging the client to remain active and to plan scheduled rest periods as necessary before activity. Engaging in activities, such as walking, has been shown to decrease the cycle of fatigue, anxiety, and depression that can occur during treatment. Fatigue is a very common side effect of radiation therapy that typically begins during the third or fourth week of treatment and persists until after treatment ends. The presence of fatigue does not mean that the cancer is not responding to treatment or that the client has developed another health problem. (P, 9, M)

110. 3. Carbohydrate is the base of the diet; it is found in grains, fruits, vegetables, and milk. Carbohydrate provides the base because it is the primary fuel for energy in the human body. Protein is near the top of the food pyramid, above carbohydrates and fruits and vegetables, indicating it should be used moderately. Fats and sweets are at the very top of the pyramid, indicating that they should be used sparingly. (A, 4, M)

111. 3. Shearing forces occur because of improper movement and positioning, which causes the underlying tissues and capillary blood supply to be pulled and disrupted. This leads to tissue trauma and the potential beginning of skin breakdown. To prevent shearing, clients should be moved with the use of lift sheets and other devices, thus preventing dragging of the skin across the mattress and linens. Clients should also be positioned and supported to prevent pulling or tension of the skin across bony prominences. Turning a client, if not done properly, can cause shearing injuries. Keeping the skin clean, dry, and lubricated is an important aspect of care, but care must be used to decrease the amount of pulling forces exerted on the tissues. (I, 9, M)

112. 4. The proper use of crutches requires supporting the body weight primarily on the hands. Improper use of crutches can cause nerve damage from excess pressure on the axillary nerve. (I, 9, M)

113. 4. Because this family is waiting for the child to die, the most appropriate nursing diagnosis would be Antici-

patory Grieving. Families grieve at the time of diagnosis, as well as during the illness, as the child is dying, and after death has occurred. This is a normal process and does not indicate Disabled Family Coping, Impaired Parenting, or Fear. (D, 5, Y)

114. 2. For the child with croup, assessing the child's respiratory status is the priority. It is especially important to assess airway patency, because laryngeal spasms can occur suddenly. Once the nurse has assessed the toddler's respiratory status, having a tracheostomy set at the bedside would be the next priority action. Monitoring vital signs is important, as is ensuring adequate fluid intake to keep secretions loose, but assessing the respiratory status is key. (I, 10, Y)

115. 2. It is essential that the nurse invert the IV bag of D_5W with potassium chloride several times to mix the contents well. When concentrated potassium chloride enters the vein, sclerosing of the vein and fatal dysrhythmias can occur. The nurse can add the potassium chloride on the unit, but concentrated potassium chloride for injection should be stored in a designated area that is clearly labeled and should not be dispensed outside the pharmacy. (P, 8, M)

116. 4. Research indicates that vitamin B_6, vitamin B_{12}, and folate may help to clear homocysteine from the blood. Elevated homocysteine correlates with a high incidence of heart and artery disease. (D, 4, M)

117. 1. Neuromuscular irritability is usually the first indication that a client has developed a low serum calcium level. Numbness and tingling around the mouth, as well as in the extremities, is an early sign of neuromuscular irritability. Depressed reflexes, decreased memory, and ventricular dysrhythmias are indications of hypercalcemia. (A, 10, M)

118. 2. In emphysema, the anteroposterior diameter of the chest wall is increased. As a result, the client's breath sounds may be diminished. Fine crackles are present when there is fluid in the lungs. Stridor occurs as a result of a partially obstructed larynx or trachea; stridor can be heard without auscultation. A pleural friction rub is present when pleural surfaces are inflamed and rub together. (A, 10, M)

119. 4. Clients with paranoid personality disorder interpret the actions of others as personal threats and feel very vulnerable. They question and are overly sensitive to others' motives. Saying "They're laughing at a joke John told; they were not laughing at you," is a simple explanation of others' behavior which helps to decrease the client's suspiciousness and promote trust. The other statements do not help the client to realistically interpret situations and the behaviors of others and are not helpful in reducing the client's suspicions or mistrust. (I, 6, X)

120. 4. Mebendazole (Vermox) is prescribed for household members older than 2 years of age. Although the child's 18-month-old brother would not receive the drug, his 4-year-old sister and parents would. (P, 8, Y)

121. 3. Loss of height and back pain are early indications of the disease that are caused by collapse of the vertebrae. Later signs include the dowager's hump and loss of the waistline. The dowager hump is a later signs of osteoporosis that occurs when the vertebrae can no longer support the upper body in an upright position. Fair-skinned, small-boned, white and Asian women are at greater risk for osteoporosis. Conventional radiographs are of little help because more than 30% of the bone mass must be lost before the disease is detected. High-density bone scans can detect the disease earlier. (P, 9, O)

122. 3. The primary reason for evaluating gastric residual is to determine whether gastric emptying has been delayed and the stomach is becoming overdistended from the feeding. With delayed gastric emptying, the possibility of aspiration of the feeding into the lungs is increased. It is not possible to determine how well the client's body is absorbing nutrients or whether the client is receiving enough feeding by simply checking the gastric residual. It is not necessary to keep partially digested formula separate from undigested formula. (E, 7, M)

123. 1. The baseline values of the client's aPTT, bleeding time, and protrombin time (PT) should be obtained. Potassium levels are not indicative of a client's coagulation time. The Lee-White clotting time or baseline FSP does not need to be established before starting tPA or alteplase recombinant. (A, 9, M)

124. 1. A common complication of diabetes is diabetic neuropathy. Diabetic neuropathy results from the metabolic and vascular factors related to hyperglycemia. Damage leads to sensory deficits and peripheral pain. Muscle atrophy can result from disuse, but it is not a direct consequence of diabetes. Raynard's disease is associated with vasospasms in the hands and the feet. Transient ischemic attacks involve the cerebrum. (D, 9, M)

125. 1. Clients with borderline personality disorder have fears of abandonment and seek attention. Clients are dependent and fear being alone; this stems from disapproval, feelings of being abandoned, and not having needs met earlier in their life. The nurse intervenes by reducing attention-seeking behaviors and the clients' abandonment fears to help the client with irrational feelings and emotions. (D, 6, X)

126. 4. The application of restraints places the client in a vulnerable, confined position. The nurse should check on the client every 30 minutes while she is restrained to

make sure that the client's needs are being met and she is safe. The client should be able to move while the restraints are in place. The restraints should be removed every 2 hours to provide skin care and exercise the extremities. Restraints should not be secured to the siderails; they should be secured to the movable bed frame so that when the bed is adjusted the restraints will not be pulled too tightly. (I, 2, M)

127. 3. The most appropriate response is, "Alcohol dependence is a disease that can be treated," because it conveys hope. It also emphasizes that the client has a treatable illness, which is helpful in reducing denial and guilt and encouraging the client to seek and comply with treatment. The other statements are judgmental and guilt-producing, possibly leading to denial and furthering the need for alcohol. (I, 6, X)

128. 2. Raisins are high in nutritive value but are sticky and have a high sugar content. The raisin can stick to the teeth and act like high-sugar foods in promoting tooth decay. Although anything can be aspirated, round, hard, smooth foods are more easily aspirated than raisins, which are soft and chewy. Raisins need to be chewed thoroughly for maximum nutritive value. (E, 7, Y)

129. 1. Aspirin is an antiplatelet medication. The use of aspirin is contraindicated while taking Coumadin because it will potentiate the effects of the warfarin sodium. Benadryl and Sudafed do not affect blood coagulation. Lanoxin is not an over-the-counter medication and needs a physician's order. (P, 10, M)

130. 1. The nurse should inform the client that carbamazepine (Tegretol) can decrease effects of oral anticoagulants. Tegretol can increase the serum concentration of verapamil (Calan) and can decrease the serum concentration of other anticonvulsants and the effects of oral contraceptives. (P, 8, M)

131. 2. Viral hepatitis causes fatigue. It is important for the client to rest to allow the liver to recover. Activity levels are resumed gradually as the client begins to recover. Abdominal pain is not a common manifestation of hepatitis. The client typically does not have difficulty breathing or experience edema. (E, 10, M)

132. 1. The mother should be encouraged to hold and cuddle her child to provide needed emotional support. Such activities as helping the child play with toys, reading stories, and staying with the child would not be contraindicated but do not offer as much emotional support as holding and cuddling. (P, 5, Y)

133. 2. The best strategy to affect child seat belt safety would be to attend the school board meeting and advocate for educational programming. The programming could be simple and done quickly. This action also targets the best audience. (I, 4, Y)

134. 3. A basic principle of rehabilitation, including cardiac rehabilitation, is that rehabilitation begins on hospital admission. Early rehabilitation is essential to promote maximum functional ability as the client recovers from an illness. Delaying rehabilitation activities is associated with poorer client outcomes. (P, 7, M)

135. 1. The goal of the intervention is to decrease the child's work of breathing by decreasing pressure on the diaphragm and increase chest expansion by increasing the pull of gravity on the diaphragm. Placing the client in a high Fowler's position accomplishes this. Side-lying positions make it more difficult to expand the side of the lung closest to the bed. The prone or supine position does not decrease the work of breathing unless the head of the bed is raised. (I, 10, Y)

136. 3. The most appropriate action is to contact the physician to verify that the order is correct. Although 60 mg of morphine is a significant dose, the amount of morphine administered to a client can vary widely, especially if a client has been taking morphine for an extended period and has developed a tolerance to the medication. The safest approach is for the nurse to always verify orders that do not appear to fall within the norm. Administering the medication without verification would be unsafe. The nurse cannot arbitrarily decide to reduce the amount of a prescribed medication without an order. Asking another nurse to review the order is not inappropriate; however, checking with the physician to verify the order should be done. (I, 8, M)

137. 1. Before a paracentesis, the client is asked to void. This is done to collapse the bladder and decrease the risk of accidental perforation of the bladder. The abdomen is not prepared with Betadine. The client is placed in a Fowler's position. The client does not need to be made NPO before the procedure. (P, 9, M)

138. 1. Children who are being abused may demonstrate behaviors such as withdrawal, apparent fear of parents, and lack of an appropriate reaction such as crying and attempting to get away when faced with a frightening event (eg, an examination or procedure). (A, 5, Y)

139. 3. The nurse would include teaching the client and family about the physical, physiologic, and psychological effects of substances to educate them about the potential injury, illness, and disability that can result from substance use. Teaching about the role of the family in perpetuating the problem, the family's responsibility for the client, or the reasons that could have led the client to use the substance is inappropriate and based on an erroneous assumption. Including these topics blames the family for the problem and attempts to rationalize the use of substance. (P, 6, X)

140. 2. Postoperative care after a laparoscopic cholecystectomy includes removal of the dressing from the inci-

sional site the day after surgery and allowing the client to bathe or shower. The client can resume a normal diet but may wish to follow a low-fat diet for a few weeks after surgery. Nausea is not expected to last for several days after surgery. Most clients can return to work within 1 week. (E, 9, M)

141. 1. Children are highly valued and are closely protected by godparents. The tradition of the family is all-encompassing, and the health care provider gains trust and improved compliance rates by including the family in teaching and health care matters. (D, 5, M)

142. 4. Many vitamin and mineral deficiencies can result in anemia. All of these vitamins and minerals would need to be assessed preferably through a nutrition assessment. Deficiencies of vitamins A, B_6, and C all result in a small cell, microcytic anemia. Folate and vitamin B_{12} deficiencies result in large cell, macrocytic anemia. Iron, copper, and vitamin E deficiencies can also result in anemia. (A, 10, M)

143. 3. Women with diabetes mellitus generally have neonates who are large but physically immature. Other common findings in these infants are hypoglycemia, hypocalcemia, hyperbilirubinemia, polycythemia, renal thrombosis, and congestive anomalies. The neonates do not exhibit hypertonia, hyperactivity, or scaly skin. (O, A, 3)

144. 2. The imbalance between the client's intake and output indicates that the client may be retaining urine since the removal of his Foley catheter. The nurse's first action is to validate this assumption by assessing for bladder distention. Applying a condom catheter will not relieve urinary retention; condom catheters are meant to be used for incontinence. A urine specimen for a culture is obtained if a urinary infection is suspected, but this is not a priority at this point. Kegel exercises are helpful in controlling urinary dribbling but do not treat retention. (A, 7, M)

145. 2. Because of the poor emptying of blood from the atrial chambers, there is an increased risk for clot formation around the valves. The clots become dislodged and travel through the circulatory system. As a result, cerebral vascular accident is a common complication of atrial fibrillation. (P, 10, M)

146. 2. Griseofulvin is associated with photosensitivity reactions. Therefore, the nurse should instruct the parents to have the child avoid intense sunlight. Griseofulvin is best absorbed when it is administered after a high-fat meal, not before a meal. Treatment with griseofulvin typically lasts for at least 1 month. There are no indications that increased fluid intake affects absorption. (I, 8, Y)

147. 3. Based on the National Cholesterol Education Program Expert Panel of Detention, Evaluation and Treat-

ment of High Blood Cholesterol in Adults, 30% of the diet should come from fats. (P, 4, M)

148. 4. The nurse would actively listen to the client's descriptions and details about being raped and allow her to talk about the trauma. This allows the client to vent, decreases feelings of isolation, and guides the nurse to potential areas that could be problematic for the client. The nurse is a safe person to confide in, thus helping to decrease the client's apprehension about disclosing intimate details and feelings. Advising the client to try to forget about what happened, recommending that she be thankful for being alive, or questioning her about what she could have done to deter the attack is contraindicated for the victim of violence. These responses blame the victim and tend to increase her guilt, as if somehow she is to blame or would have be capable of preventing the rape. (I, 6, X)

149. 2. After a cystoscopy with biopsy, the nurse would assess for excessive hematuria, which might indicate hemorrhage caused by the biopsy. Catheters are not routinely inserted after a cystoscopy. The nurse would not assess for bladder distention unless the client was having difficulty voiding. Urine cultures are not routinely ordered after cystoscopies. (A, 9, M)

150. 2. The nurse interprets the client's statement as use of the hot disease concept in the Mexican American culture, where the belief of a hot and cold balance of the body exists. A hot disease such as an infection is treated with the opposite, a cold food such as milk. The nurse should focus on the cultural differences and be sensitive to the cultural diversity. (A, 4, M)

151. 3. A client who is "getting special messages" (ideas of reference) often misinterprets content presented on television as containing messages for the client. Therefore, it would be most important for the nurse to monitor the client's reactions to television programs. (I, 6, X)

152. 2. A thick, white, cottage cheese-like vaginal discharge along with vaginal itching is most likely candidiasis. This condition is associated with oral contraceptive use, diabetes, and systemic antibiotic therapy because the normal vaginal flora is altered. Candidiasis is treated with miconazole (Monistat). Trichomonas vaginalis typically is characterized by a greenish discharge. Herpes genitalis is associated with blisters and pain. Although women may not experience symptoms related to gonorrhea, the most common symptom is a purulent vaginal discharge. (D, 3, O)

153. 3. In a low anorectal anomaly, the rectum has descended normally through the puborectalis muscle. In an intermediate anomaly, the rectum is at or below the level of the puborectalis muscle; in a high anomaly, the rectum ends above the puborectalis muscle. (E, N, 10)

154. 1. It is especially important for the nurse to carefully assess the elderly client for respiratory depression after administering a dose of meperidine. It may be necessary to reduce the dosage to prevent respiratory depression. Dysrhythmias, constipation, and seizures are all potential side effects of meperidine, but respiratory depression is most significant in the elderly. (A, 10, M)

155. 2. Ascorbic acid (vitamin C) increases absorption of iron. Taking iron with a food rich in ascorbic acid, such as orange juice, increases absorption. Milk will delay iron absorption. It is best to give iron on an empty stomach to increase absorption. β-Carotene does not affect iron absorption. (I, 8, M)

156. 1. In early renal insufficiency, the kidneys lose the ability to concentrate urine, resulting in polyuria. Oliguria occurs later. Dysuria and hematuria are not associated with renal insufficiency. (A, 10, M)

157. 1. The zygote intrafallopian transfer method (ZIFT) requires that fertilization take place outside the body. Once fertilization has occurred, the fertilized eggs are transferred by laparoscopy to the open end of the fallopian tube. At least one tube must be patent for this procedure to succeed, so it is not beneficial if the client has bilateral blocked fallopian tubes. Ova and sperm are instilled in the fallopian tube for fertilization when the gamete intrafallopian transfer method (GIFT) is used. With in vitro fertilization, a fertilized ovum is instilled into the vagina to enter the uterus for implantation. (I, 3, O)

158. 2. The nurse should examine the buccal mucosa, along with the conjunctiva and sclera, nailbeds, palms, soles, lips, and tongue to assess for oxygenation in a client with dark skin. (A, 7, M)

159. 3. A client who has undergone chest surgery should be taught to raise the arm on the affected side over the head to help prevent shoulder ankylosis. This exercise helps restore normal shoulder movement, prevents stiffening of the shoulder joint, and improves muscle tone and power. (I, 7, M)

160. 2. The nurse's first action should be to attempt to replace the tracheostomy tube immediately so that the client's airway is reestablished. Although the nurse may also call for assistance, there should be no delay before attempting reinsertion of the tube. The client would be placed in a supine position with the neck hyperextended to facilitate reentry of the tube. The obturator is inserted into the replacement tracheostomy tube to guide insertion and is then removed to allow passage of air through the tube. (I, 9, M)

161. 2. Many parents are advised to administer acetaminophen before the child receives immunizations to minimize local and systemic reactions. Typically, infants should not be very fussy after receiving immuniza-

tions. There is no reason to keep the infant out of day care that day; the child is not contagious. Although it may be helpful to the parents to have someone with them at the appointment, advising them to give the infant acetaminophen would be more important. (P, 3, Y)

162. 1. A general growth parameter is that the birth weight doubles in 6 months and triples in a year. Telling the mother that the baby will eat what he needs is not appropriate. The nurse needs to investigate whether the baby's weight is within the normal parameters of infant weight gain. A bottle-fed baby should not be forced to complete the bottle, because this may contribute to obesity. (I, 3, M)

163. 4. The mechanism of injury is always the most critical information to obtain from a client with a musculoskeletal injury. In the event of a back injury, the mechanism of injury will provide the greatest clue as to the extent of injury and the proper treatment plan. The other questions are important but will not give the critical information needed related to this specific complaint and injury. (D, 10, M)

164. 3. Mechanisms for regulating blood pressure involve cardiac output and peripheral vascular resistance. Therefore, the way to modify the client's blood pressure is to prescribe medications that alter one of these two variables. Alteration of the blood pressure is the result of the antihypertensive medication, but this answer does not explain the mechanism of action. (A, 8, M)

165. 3. Typical early signs of rheumatoid arthritis are nonspecific and not necessarily related to specific arthritic joint complaints. Common early symptoms include fatigue, anorexia, weight loss, and generalized feelings of stiffness. Joint swelling and limitation of movement usually occur as joint involvement becomes more specific. Nausea is not typically associated with the disease process but can be related to medications prescribed to treat rheumatoid arthritis. (A, 10, M)

166. 2. NPH Insulin should be rolled between the palms to mix it before drawing it up; shaking it will introduce air bubbles into the solution, which can cause inaccurate dosing. (I, 8, M)

167. 4. The gene for Duchenne's muscular dystrophy is carried by women and transmitted to their male children. It involves an X-linked inheritance pattern. About one third of new cases involve mutations. (D, 10, Y)

168. 4. Because of the colic-like abdominal pain, Pain would be the priority nursing diagnosis. There are no data to indicate a skin problem or dehydration. Diarrhea or constipation may precede the appearance of currant-jelly stools. (A, 10, Y)

169. 2. The nurse should notify the physician that the client is allergic to penicillin before giving the Kefzol. Cephalosporins are contraindicated in clients who are

allergic to penicillin. Clients who are allergic to penicillin may have a cross-allergy to cephalosporins. (I, 8, M)

170. 3. The nurse should document a tearing of tissue with irregular wound edges as a laceration. A contusion or a bruise is a closed wound caused by a blunt object resulting in bleeding in underlying tissue. An abrasion is a superficial wound from a rubbing or a scraping of the surface of the skin, such as from a fall. Colonization is a wound containing microorganisms. (A, 2, M)

171. 1. The major cause of relapse is noncompliance. If the client states that he's not sure he can afford to keep taking his medicines, it is a warning sign to the nurse that the client may be at risk for noncompliance. Therefore, the nurse needs to stress the need for compliance to prevent relapse. If money is a problem, a referral to a social worker may be necessary. (E, 6, X)

172. 1. The "five rights" of medication administration include the right person, right drug, right dose, right route, and right time. By checking these five factors before giving medications, nurses can greatly reduce medication errors. (I, 8, M)

173. 1. Fatigue is often the earliest symptom of chronic congestive heart failure; it is caused by a decreased cardiac output and decreased tissue oxygenation. Pedal edema and nocturia are both symptoms of congestive heart failure, but they occur later in the course of the condition. An irregular pulse can be a complication of congestive heart failure, but it is not necessarily an early indication of the condition. (A, 10, M)

174. 2. Chocolate, tea, cola, and caffeine lower the esophageal sphincter pressure, thereby increasing reflux. Clients do not need to eliminate spicy foods unless such foods bother them. Foods with seeds are restricted in diverticulosis. Steamed foods are encouraged to retain vitamins and decrease fat intake. (I, 10, M)

175. 2. The nurse would assess for signs and symptoms of birth asphyxia as a priority. Birth asphyxia is a common problem for small-for-gestational-age neonates because they have undeveloped chest muscles and a risk of meconium aspiration syndrome due to anoxia during labor. Iron-deficiency anemia is not a typical problem for the small-for-gestational-age neonate. However, the neonate may have polycythemia due to anoxia during intrauterine life. Persistent pulmonary hypertension is a problem for preterm neonates, not small-for-gestational-age neonates. Hypoglycemia, not hyperglycemia, is a problem for small-for-gestational-age neonates. (A, 9, O)

176. 3. The nurse should administer 45 mL/minute, not 27, 30, or 90. The formula is to divide 180 mL by 60 minutes, which yields 3 mL/minute; 3 mL/minute × 15 drops = 45 drops/minute. (I, 8, M)

177. 3. When introducing solid foods to infants, only one new food should be added at a time; if an allergic reaction occurs, the food allergen can be easily identified. In the absence of evidence of allergy, all foods are appropriate except mixed foods, which should be avoided to facilitate allergen identification. Infant formula is a major source of nutrition for the first year and should not be eliminated when solids are introduced. Rice cereal is usually recommended as the starter cereal, but other cereals, such as oatmeal, are also recommended. (I, 2, Y)

178. 4. The most appropriate response for the nurse is to ask the client to verbalize his feelings because venting is therapeutic for the client. The client does not need anyone's permission to cry. Asking if there is someone the nurse can call implies that the nurse is not willing to listen to the client. The nurse should not offer the client a tissue, because it implies that the nurse is not comfortable with the client's crying. (I, 5, M)

179. 1. Studies have shown that decreasing sodium and increasing calcium improve PMS symptoms such as fluid retention, breast tenderness, and mood changes. (I, 10, M)

180. 2. The nurse should explain that the feeling of heat is a normal part of the process for a plaster cast. The sensation is not an indication that the cast is applying pressure to soft tissue. Keeping the cast exposed to room air will help facilitate drying and dissipate the heat. Elevating the casted leg is an appropriate action, but it does nothing to decrease heat. Administering pain medication also does not relieve the feeling of heat. (I, 7, M)

181. 3. It is recommended that a woman examine the breasts during the first week after menstruation. During this period the breasts are least likely to be tender or swollen, because the secretion of estrogen, which prepares the uterus for implantation, is at its lowest level. (I, 3, M)

COMPREHENSIVE TEST 4

Select the one best answer, and indicate your choice by filling in the circle in front of the option.

1. A primigravida at 26 weeks' gestation asks the nurse what causes heartburn during pregnancy. The nurse should explain to the client that heartburn during pregnancy is usually caused by which of the following?
   - ○ 1. Increased peristaltic action during pregnancy.
   - ○ 2. Displacement of the stomach by the diaphragm.
   - ○ 3. Decreased secretion of hydrochloric acid.
   - ○ 4. Backflow of stomach contents into the esophagus.

2. A client at a follow-up appointment after having a miscarriage 2 weeks previously yells at the nurse, "How could God do this to me? I've never done anything wrong." Which of the following responses by the nurse would be *most* appropriate at this time?
   - ○ 1. "God can handle your anger. It's OK."
   - ○ 2. "I know you are angry. It's so hard to lose your baby."
   - ○ 3. "It isn't God's fault. It was an accident."
   - ○ 4. "You're a strong person. You will get through this."

3. A client with cancer has been advised by the physician that he should have chemotherapy. The client is concerned about chemotherapy and wants to take herbal treatments instead. The nurse's best response to the client is which of the following?
   - ○ 1. "You are making a mistake and placing your life in jeopardy."
   - ○ 2. "Herbal treatments are not approved by the FDA."
   - ○ 3. "Herbal treatments have not been researched with cancer."
   - ○ 4. "Tell me about your concerns with chemotherapy."

4. A 4-year-old child is admitted for a cardiac catheterization. Which of the following is *most* important to include as the nurse teaches this child about the cardiac catheterization?
   - ○ 1. A plastic model of the heart.
   - ○ 2. A catheter that will be inserted into the artery.
   - ○ 3. The parents.
   - ○ 4. Other children undergoing a catheterization.

5. A client has a reddened area over a bony prominence. The nurse finds a nursing assistant massaging this area. The nurse should
   - ○ 1. reinforce the nursing assistant's use of this intervention over the bony prominence.
   - ○ 2. explain to the nursing assistant that massage is effective because it improves blood flow to the area.
   - ○ 3. inform the nursing assistant that massage is even more effective when combined with the use of lotion.
   - ○ 4. instruct the nursing assistant that massage is contraindicated because it decreases blood flow to the area.

6. A worried mother confides in the nurse that she wants to change physicians because her infant is not getting better. The best response of the nurse is which of the following?
   - ○ 1. "This doctor has been on our staff for 20 years."
   - ○ 2. "I know you are worried, but the doctor has an excellent reputation."
   - ○ 3. "You always have an option to change. Tell me about your concerns."
   - ○ 4. "I take my own children to this doctor."

7. A recently widowed, elderly male client is receiving chemotherapy. He tells the nurse that he does not like to cook for himself. A community resource for this client is
   - ○ 1. Hospice Association.
   - ○ 2. Visiting Nurses' Association (VNA).
   - ○ 3. Meals on Wheels.
   - ○ 4. American Association of Retired Persons (AARP).

8. The nurse assists the doctor in inserting a temporary pacemaker into the client. The nurse knows that it will be critical to document
   - ○ 1. the client's cardiovascular status.
   - ○ 2. the client's emotional state.
   - ○ 3. the type of sedation used.
   - ○ 4. pacemaker information: rate, type, settings.

9. The nurse judges that the mother of a 9-month-old infant in a hip spica cast understands how to feed her child when she states which of the following?

○ 1. "I can lay my child flat and feed that way."

○ 2. "I'll raise my child's head up and leave the hips and legs on a pillow."

○ 3. "I can borrow a special feeding table to use."

○ 4. "It will take two of us, one to hold and one to feed."

10. The nurse is assessing a client who has had a myocardial infarction. The nurse notes the cardiac rhythm shown in Figure 1. The nurse identifies this rhythm as

○ 1. atrial fibrillation.

○ 2. atrial tachycardia.

○ 3. premature ventricular contractions.

○ 4. ventricular tachycardia.

11. The nursing staff have finished a particularly difficult restraint with an adolescent client. In addition to determining whether anyone was injured, the staff are mandated to evaluate the incident to obtain which of the following ultimate outcomes?

○ 1. Coordinate documentation of the incident.

○ 2. Resolve negative feelings and attitudes.

○ 3. Improve the use of restraint procedures.

○ 4. Calm down before returning to the other clients.

12. The nurse is caring for a client who has experienced severe multiple trauma. The client's arterial blood gases reveal low arterial oxygen levels that are not responsive to high concentrations of oxygen. The nurse is aware that this finding is a major indicator of the development of which of the following conditions?

○ 1. Hypostatic pneumonia.

○ 2. Hypovolemic shock.

○ 3. Acute respiratory distress syndrome (ARDS).

○ 4. Asthma.

13. A client asks the nurse why he was asked to complete an advance directive when he entered the hospital. The nurse's best response is which of the following?

○ 1. "This will provide a substitute for informed discussion with the physician."

○ 2. "It is a legal requirement for all clients entering a hospital to be offered the chance to make an advance directive."

○ 3. "The physician will make the best decisions for you in an emergency."

○ 4. "Are you worried that extraordinary means will be taken if you are dying?"

14. When witnessing the client's signature on a consent for a procedure, the nurse verifies that the consent was obtained in an appropriate manner. Which of the following is an unrealistic expectation for the nurse to verify?

○ 1. That there was adequate disclosure of information.

○ 2. That there was sufficient comprehension of information.

○ 3. That there was voluntary consent on the client's part.

○ 4. That the client has full awareness of the rehabilitation process.

15. An elderly client is diagnosed with temporal arteritis. The medication of choice is

○ 1. Prednisone (Deltasone).

○ 2. Naproxen (Naprosyn).

○ 3. Aspirin.

○ 4. Azathioprine (Imuran).

16. A pregnant woman at 12 weeks' gestation is diagnosed with gonorrhea. The physician orders doxycycline. The *first* action of the nurse should be to

○ 1. instruct the client about the effects of the drug.

○ 2. make sure the record notes that the baby must receive eye drops when born.

○ 3. have the physician add a single dose of ceftriaxone (Rocephin).

○ 4. discuss with the physician the need to change the order.

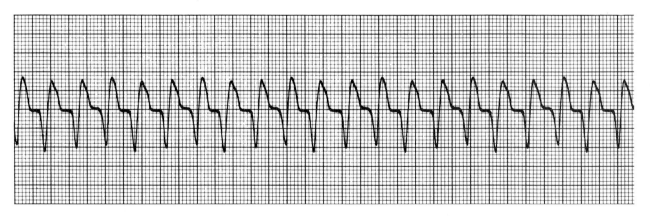

Figure 1.

17. After a client undergoes a contraction stress test that is negative, which of the following would the nurse assess *next*?
    ○ 1. Evidence of ruptured membranes.
    ○ 2. Viability status of the fetus.
    ○ 3. Indications that contractions have ceased.
    ○ 4. Fetal heart rate variability.

18. The infant is at risk for an ileus after surgery to correct intussusception. Which observation would the nurse *not* include in an assessment for this complication?
    ○ 1. Measurement of urine specific gravity.
    ○ 2. Assessment of bowel sounds.
    ○ 3. Characteristics of the first stool.
    ○ 4. Measurement of gastric output.

19. A client with asthma asks the nurse if she should use her salmeterol (Serevent) inhaler when she exercises and experiences wheezing and shortness of breath. The nurse's best response is which of the following?
    ○ 1. "Yes, use the inhaler immediately for these symptoms."
    ○ 2. "No, this drug is a maintenance drug, not a rescue inhaler."
    ○ 3. "Use the inhaler 5 minutes before you exercise to prevent the wheezing."
    ○ 4. "This inhaler is for allergic rhinitis, not asthma."

20. When assessing a client who is receiving clozapine (Clozaril), the nurse finds a pulse rate of 148 bpm. Which of the following would the nurse do *next*?
    ○ 1. Give the clozapine, and tell the client to lie down.
    ○ 2. Withhold the clozapine, and tell the client to go to exercise group.
    ○ 3. Administer the clozapine, and notify the physician.
    ○ 4. Withhold the clozapine, and notify the physician.

21. A client has been diagnosed with absence seizures. The nurse would expect the physician to prescribe which of the following drugs?
    ○ 1. Valproic acid (Depakote).
    ○ 2. Phenytoin (Dilantin).
    ○ 3. Gabapentin (Neurontin).
    ○ 4. Paroxetine (Paxil).

22. The nurse is watching two siblings, ages 7 and 9 years, verbally arguing over a toy. The nurse has counseled the mother before about how to handle this situation. The nurse would judge that the teaching has been effective when the mother does which of the following?
    ○ 1. Tells the siblings to stop arguing and shake hands.
    ○ 2. Ignores the arguing and continues what she is doing.

○ 3. Tells the children they will be punished when they go home.
○ 4. Says they will not go out to lunch now since they have argued.

23. A 64-year-old man is admitted with palpitations, hyperventilation, a choking sensation, and tightness in the chest. The nurse analyzes the results of arterial blood gas studies. Which of the following metabolic factors will be depleted?
    ○ 1. Sodium.
    ○ 2. Oxygen.
    ○ 3. Potassium.
    ○ 4. Carbon dioxide.

24. A client is diagnosed with genital herpes, (herpes simplex virus type 2, or HSV-2). The nurse should instruct the client that
    ○ 1. using occlusive ointments may decrease the pain from the lesions.
    ○ 2. reducing stressful life events may decrease the incidence of herpetic outbreaks.
    ○ 3. there are no effective drug therapies to manage herpes symptoms.
    ○ 4. herpes is transmitted to partners only when lesions are weeping.

25. The client is having ototoxic effects of the vestibular branch of the acoustic nerve. Which clinical manifestation would *not* be associated with this problem?
    ○ 1. Vertigo.
    ○ 2. Tinnitus.
    ○ 3. Nausea and vomiting with motion.
    ○ 4. Ataxia.

26. A young male client presents to the clinic with a bite he received in a fight. He has a bite mark on his forearm and the skin is broken. His last tetanus shot was about 8 years ago. Recommended treatment should include
    ○ 1. administration of 0.5 mL of tetanus toxoid IM.
    ○ 2. administration of 0.5 mL of tetanus toxoid IV.
    ○ 3. closure of the wound with sutures.
    ○ 4. withholding medication to see if signs of infection develop.

27. At 6 weeks postpartum, the nurse instructs a primiparous client scheduled to received prescribed subdermal hormonal implants after delivery of a term neonate about the advantages of this method of contraception. Which of the following, if stated by the client as an advantage, indicates successful teaching?
    ○ 1. Lack of the side effects associated with progesterone therapy.
    ○ 2. A slowed return of fertility after being discontinued.
    ○ 3. Continuation of breast-feeding without adverse effects.
    ○ 4. Protection against sexually transmitted diseases.

28. In the care and treatment of a client with heart failure, the nurse would expect the client to be taking which of the following types of drugs?
    ○ 1. Selective serotonin reuptake inhibitors (SSRIs).
    ○ 2. Nonsteroidal anti-inflammatory drugs (NSAIDs).
    ○ 3. Diuretics.
    ○ 4. Steroids.

29. A mother who is visibly upset tells the nurse she wants to take her child home because the child is dying. Which of the following would be the nurse's *best* response?
    ○ 1. "I know how you feel, but the medication will make your child feel better."
    ○ 2. "I can't let you do this without calling your physician first."
    ○ 3. "Can you tell me why you want to take your child home now?"
    ○ 4. "I can imagine how hard this is for you, but its not what's best for the child."

30. Clients with chronic obstructive pulmonary disease (COPD) may be bedridden at home and get little exercise. Which of the following is a normal physiologic reaction to prolonged periods of bed rest and inactivity?
    ○ 1. Increased sodium retention.
    ○ 2. Increased calcium excretion.
    ○ 3. Increased insulin use.
    ○ 4. Increased red blood cell production.

31. Which of the following parameters would indicate to the nurse that a 5-month-old weighing 15 pounds and being treated for dehydration has a normal urine output?
    ○ 1. 1 to 2 mL/kg per hour.
    ○ 2. 3 to 5 mL/kg per hour.
    ○ 3. 6 to 8 mL/kg per hour.
    ○ 4. 10 to 12 mL/kg per hour.

32. A 24-year-old client has been diagnosed with acute osteomyelitis in the left leg. He complains of acute pain in the leg that intensifies when he moves it. The client has a temperature of 101°F (38.3°C) and a reddened, warm area in the midcalf region over the shaft of the tibia. Based on this information, which of the following nursing diagnoses would be *most* appropriate for this client?
    ○ 1. Anticipatory Grieving related to possible left lower leg amputation.
    ○ 2. Activity Intolerance related to severe left leg pain.
    ○ 3. Disturbed Body Image related to left leg swelling and inflammation.
    ○ 4. Deficient Fluid Volume related to elevated temperature of 101°F (38.3°C).

33. A client has undergone a vasectomy. The nurse instructs the client that he can begin having unprotected intercourse
    ○ 1. when desired, because sterilization is immediate.
    ○ 2. as soon as scrotal edema and tenderness resolves.
    ○ 3. when the sperm count reflects sterilization.
    ○ 4. after 6 to 10 ejaculations.

34. Long-term administration of gentamycin sulfate (Garamycin) to a client has been discontinued. The client should be instructed to have which of the following assessments?
    ○ 1. Hemoglobin level in 2 weeks.
    ○ 2. White blood cell count in 2 weeks.
    ○ 3. Vestibular check in 3 to 4 weeks.
    ○ 4. Serum potassium level in 1 week.

35. Which of the following nursing interventions would best accomplish the goal of preventing atelectasis and pneumonia in a postoperative client?
    ○ 1. Administer oxygen therapy as needed to maintain adequate oxygenation.
    ○ 2. Offer pain medication 30 minutes before having the client cough and deep-breathe.
    ○ 3. Encourage the client to cough, deep-breathe, and turn in bed once every 4 hours.
    ○ 4. Force fluids to 2000 mL every 24 hours.

36. A 7-year-old child is admitted to the hospital with the medical diagnosis of acute rheumatic fever. When discussing long-term care for the child with the parents, the nurse should teach them that a necessary part of this care is
    ○ 1. physical therapy.
    ○ 2. antibiotic therapy.
    ○ 3. psychological therapy.
    ○ 4. anti-inflammatory therapy.

37. The nurse is assessing the perineal changes of a woman in the second stage of labor. Figure 2 represents which of the following perineal changes?
    ○ 1. Anterior-posterior slit.
    ○ 2. Oval opening.
    ○ 3. Circular shape.
    ○ 4. Crowning.

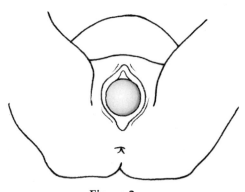

Figure 2.

38. A client is admitted to the hospital with a diagnosis of suspected pulmonary embolism. Physician orders include the following: oxygen 2 to 4 L/minute per nasal cannula, oximetry at all times, and intravenous administration of 5% dextrose in water (D5W) at 100 mL/hour. The client complains of increasing dyspnea and has a respiratory rate of 32 breaths/minute. What is the nurse's first response to this situation?
    - ○ 1. Increase the oxygen flow rate from 2 to 4 L/minute.
    - ○ 2. Call the physician immediately.
    - ○ 3. Provide reassurance to the client.
    - ○ 4. Obtain a sample for arterial blood gas analysis.

39. The mother of a 10-month-old child calls the nurse because her child has cold symptoms. The mother asks how she can clear the infant's nose. Which of the following would be the nurse's *best* recommendation?
    - ○ 1. Use a cool air vaporizer with plain water.
    - ○ 2. Use saline nose drops and then a bulb syringe.
    - ○ 3. Blow into the child's mouth to clear the infant's nose.
    - ○ 4. Administer a nonprescription vasoconstrictive nose spray.

40. Clinical symptoms of metastatic lung cancer may include
    - ○ 1. diarrhea.
    - ○ 2. constipation.
    - ○ 3. voice hoarseness.
    - ○ 4. weight gain.

41. A client is at risk for development of metabolic alkalosis because of persistent vomiting. Which of the following symptoms is indicative of metabolic alkalosis?
    - ○ 1. Confusion.
    - ○ 2. Hyperventilation.
    - ○ 3. Diarrhea.
    - ○ 4. Edema.

42. Which of the following would *first* alert the nurse that a child is hemorrhaging after a tonsillectomy?
    - ○ 1. Mouth breathing.
    - ○ 2. Frequent swallowing.
    - ○ 3. Requests for a drink.
    - ○ 4. Increased pulse rate.

43. Nursing interventions for a client having a transfusion reaction include all but which of the following?
    - ○ 1. Discontinue the current intravenous site and restart the infusion at a different site.
    - ○ 2. Start a normal saline infusion at 30 mL/hour.
    - ○ 3. Assess vital signs every 10 minutes.
    - ○ 4. Send the blood bag and blood slip to the blood bank.

44. The nurse is to administer chloramphenicol 50 mg IV in 100 mL of D5W over 30 minutes. The infusion set administers 10 gtt/mL. What is the flow rate of the infusion?
    - ○ 1. 21 gtt/minute.
    - ○ 2. 27 gtt/minute.
    - ○ 3. 33 gtt/minute.
    - ○ 4. 35 gtt/minute.

45. A client's belief in her "special mission from God" can be referred to as a religious delusion of grandeur. The nurse incorporates this delusion into the client's plan of care based on the understanding that the primary purpose of such a delusion is to provide which of the following?
    - ○ 1. Sexual outlet.
    - ○ 2. Comfort.
    - ○ 3. Safety.
    - ○ 4. Self-esteem.

46. A client who has been vomiting for 2 days has a nasogastric tube inserted. The nurse notes that over the past 10 hours the tube has drained 2 L of fluid. The nurse should plan to implement treatment that will prevent which of the following electrolyte imbalances?
    - ○ 1. Hypermagnesia.
    - ○ 2. Hypernatremia.
    - ○ 3. Hypokalemia.
    - ○ 4. Hypocalcemia.

47. During the clinical breast examination, which of the following is a normal finding?
    - ○ 1. Pronounced unilateral venous pattern.
    - ○ 2. Peau d'orange breast tissue.
    - ○ 3. Long-term, bilateral nipple inversion.
    - ○ 4. Breast tissue that is darker than the areolae.

48. A child with sickle cell crisis is being discharged. As part of discharge teaching to prevent further crisis, the nurse advises the parent to do which of the following?
    - ○ 1. Encourage the child to drink lots of liquids.
    - ○ 2. Take the child's temperature every morning.
    - ○ 3. Weigh the child every day.
    - ○ 4. Offer the child a high-protein diet.

49. While assessing a neonate 30 minutes after birth, the nurse observes that the child has a short neck covered with webbing. The nurse notifies the pediatrician based on the interpretation that this usually indicates which of the following?
    - ○ 1. Genetic deviations.
    - ○ 2. Cleft palate.
    - ○ 3. Potter's syndrome.
    - ○ 4. Neural tube defects.

50. In a client with severe diarrhea, the nurse would conclude that the client was experiencing hypokalemia if which of the following signs were observed?
    - ○ 1. Muscle spasms.
    - ○ 2. Thirst.

○ 3. Arrhythmia.

○ 4. Confusion.

51. The nurse identifies clinical manifestations of a superimposed infection when a client who has been taking an antibiotic returns to the medical clinic. Which of the following is *not* associated with a superinfection?

○ 1. Black, hairy tongue.

○ 2. Pruritus.

○ 3. Glossitis.

○ 4. Anal itching.

52. Which of the following is the most reliable indicator of the existence and intensity of acute pain?

○ 1. The client's vital signs.

○ 2. The client's self-report of pain.

○ 3. The nurse's assessment of the client.

○ 4. The severity of the condition causing the pain.

53. The nurse advises a mother with a 2-year-old child to avoid encouraging excessive milk consumption (more than 3.5 cups per day) by the infant because excess milk consumption can lead to

○ 1. vitamin C deficiency.

○ 2. iron deficiency.

○ 3. biotin deficiency.

○ 4. folate deficiency.

54. The nurse is caring for a client with a fracture of a long bone. Which of the following assessments would be the earliest symptom of a fat embolism?

○ 1. Respiratory distress.

○ 2. Confusion.

○ 3. Petechiae.

○ 4. Fever.

55. A client tells the nurse, "Everybody smiles at me because they know that I was chosen by God for this mission." The nurse interprets this statement as which of the following?

○ 1. Idea of reference.

○ 2. Thought insertion.

○ 3. Visual hallucination.

○ 4. Neologism.

56. To test the hearing ability of a neonate at 12 hours of age, the nurse claps the hands while standing away from the neonate at approximately which of the following distances?

○ 1. 3 inches.

○ 2. 6 inches.

○ 3. 12 inches.

○ 4. 24 inches.

57. The physician decides to change a client's current dose of intramuscular (IM) meperidine hydrochloride (Demerol) to an oral dosage. The current IM dose is 75 mg every 4 hours as needed. What dosage of oral meperidine hydrochloride will be required to provide an equivalent analgesic dose?

○ 1. 25 to 50 mg every 4 hours.

○ 2. 75 to 100 mg every 4 hours.

○ 3. 125 to 140 mg every 4 hours.

○ 4. 150 to 300 mg every 4 hours.

58. Which of the following nursing measures is most useful in preventing the development of osteoporosis in a client who is immobilized?

○ 1. Beginning weight-bearing activities as soon as possible.

○ 2. Increasing the client's calcium intake in the diet.

○ 3. Performing passive range-of-motion exercises four times a day.

○ 4. Teaching the client to perform isometric exercises.

59. The mother of a toddler asks the nurse what she should do with her toddler when he has a temper tantrum. Which of the following suggestions would be *most* appropriate?

○ 1. Move the toddler to a time-out chair.

○ 2. Try to talk the toddler out of the tantrum.

○ 3. Leave the toddler alone during the tantrum as long as he is safe.

○ 4. Punish the toddler for having a temper tantrum.

60. The nurse who is stuck by a used needle but has not completed the hepatitis B immunization should receive

○ 1. both active and passive immunization.

○ 2. active immunization.

○ 3. passive immunization.

○ 4. immunization only after a blood titer has been drawn.

61. Which of the following nursing interventions is appropriate for preventing pressure ulcers?

○ 1. Cleanse the skin daily using mild soap and hot water.

○ 2. Perform a systematic skin assessment at least once a day.

○ 3. Massage bony prominences gently every shift.

○ 4. Encourage the client to sit in a chair as much as possible.

62. The nurse is evaluating the pin insertion site of a client's skeletal traction. Which of the following signs would be indicative of a complication?

○ 1. Presence of crusts around the pin insertion site.

○ 2. Serous drainage on the dressing.

○ 3. Pin moves slightly at insertion site.

○ 4. Client does not feel pain at insertion site.

63. On the night before a 58-year-old wife and mother is to have a lobectomy for lung cancer, she remarks to the nurse, " I am so scared of this cancer. I should have quit smoking years ago. Now I've brought all this fear and sadness on myself and now my family." What would be the nurse's best response to the client?

1. "It's normal to be scared. I would be too. We'll help you through it."
2. "Do you feel guilty because you smoked?"
3. "Don't be so hard on yourself. You don't know if your smoking caused the cancer."
4. "It's okay to be scared. What is it about cancer that you're afraid of?"

64. The nurse is caring for an elderly client who has hip pain related to rheumatoid arthritis. The nurse knows that the client is practicing appropriate self-care activities when the client chooses to sit which of the following chairs?
    1. Recliner chair with arms to support wrists and hands.
    2. Couch with soft cushions to support thighs.
    3. Straight-back chair with elevated seat.
    4. Curved-back rocking chair.

65. The nurse is with the parents of a 16-year-old boy who recently attempted suicide. The nurse cautions the parents to be especially alert for which of the following in their son?
    1. Expression of a desire to date.
    2. Decision to try out for an extracurricular activity.
    3. The giving away of valued personal items.
    4. Desire to spend more time with his friends.

66. Which of the following responses would be *most* appropriate for the nurse when comforting a primiparous client whose critically ill neonate delivered at 25 weeks dies while the mother is present?
    1. "This is probably for the best because his organs were so immature."
    2. "You should try to get pregnant again soon to get over this loss."
    3. "You can stay with your baby as long as you want and say anything you want."
    4. "If you want me to, I can call the chaplain to stay with you."

67. A 32-year-old woman recently diagnosed with Hodgkin's disease is admitted to the hospital outpatient clinic for staging by undergoing a bone marrow aspiration and biopsy. The nurse assesses the client's nutrition status. Which of the following blood examinations would be most helpful in determining whether the client's diet lacks protein?
    1. Red blood cell count.
    2. Direct and indirect bilirubin levels.
    3. Reticulocyte count.
    4. Albumin level.

68. The nurse teaches a client taking desmopressin (DDAVP) nasal spray about how to manage treatment. The nurse determines that the client needs additional instruction when he makes which of the following comments?
    1. "I should check for sores in my nose while taking this medication."
    2. "I should use the same nostril each time I take the medicine."
    3. "I should report nasal congestion."
    4. "I should report any signs of respiratory infection."

69. The nurse has an order to administer ampicillin 250 mg IM. After reconstituting the ampicillin with sterile water for injection, the solution available is 500 mg/mL. How many milliliters should the nurse administer?
    1. 0.05 mL.
    2. 0.4 mL.
    3. 0.5 mL.
    4. 1.0 mL.

70. The nurse assesses a client and notes that he has a weak, irregular pulse, as well as soft, flabby muscles. These findings are indicative of which electrolyte imbalance?
    1. Hypercalcemia.
    2. Hypernatremia.
    3. Hypokalemia.
    4. Hypomagnesemia.

71. A primipara at 48 hours postpartum is to be given medroxyprogesterone acetate (Depo-Provera) before discharge. Which of the following would the nurse include in the teaching plan before administering this medication?
    1. There is an increased risk of ovarian cancer.
    2. Amenorrhea is common during the first 6 months.
    3. Heavy menstrual bleeding may occur.
    4. The client may experience periods of increased energy.

72. The nurse establishes the goal of preventing the development of a stress ulcer in a burn client. Which of the following interventions would most likely contribute to the achievement of this goal?
    1. Implementing relaxation exercises.
    2. Administering a sedative as needed.
    3. Providing a soft, bland diet.
    4. Administering cimetidine (Tagamet) as ordered.

73. A parent of a child with acquired immunodeficiency syndrome (AIDS) asks the nurse how to look for signs and symptoms of infection. The nurse responds that they need to be especially alert for which of the following?
    1. Erythema around the infected area.
    2. Rectal temperature higher than 100.5°F (38°C).
    3. Tenderness of the infected area.
    4. Warmth of the infected area.

74. The nurse is teaching a group of unlicensed personnel new to psychiatry about providing care to clients with depression. To care effectively for these clients, the nurse would emphasize that caregivers demonstrate which of the following behaviors?

○ 1. Cheerful demeanor.
○ 2. Empathetic concern.
○ 3. Serious, business-like affect.
○ 4. Humorous lightheartedness.

75. When fluids by mouth are appropriate for the infant after surgery to correct intussusception, the nurse most likely would initiate feeding with
    ○ 1. cereal-thickened formula.
    ○ 2. full-strength formula.
    ○ 3. half-strength formula.
    ○ 4. oral electrolyte solution.

76. A client is taking paroxetine (Paxil) 20 mg orally every morning. The nurse would monitor the client for which of the following side effects?
    ○ 1. A hypertensive crisis.
    ○ 2. Sexual problems.
    ○ 3. Sleep disturbance.
    ○ 4. Orthostatic hypotension.

77. The Dietary Approaches to Stop Hypertension (DASH) diet, includes ensuring the adequate intake of very specific nutrients. These specific nutrients include
    ○ 1. magnesium, potassium, vitamin C, and calcium.
    ○ 2. vitamins B_6, B_{12}, E, and A.
    ○ 3. iron, zinc, vitamin D, and vitamin K.
    ○ 4. biotin, protein, riboflavin, and pantothenic acid.

78. Which of the following neurologic changes indicates that the client is in the progressive stage of shock?
    ○ 1. Restlessness.
    ○ 2. Confusion.
    ○ 3. Incoherent speech.
    ○ 4. Unconsciousness.

79. The code team and crash cart arrive in the room of a client who has had a cardiac arrest. What is the first piece of monitoring equipment applied to the client by the code team members?
    ○ 1. Electrocardiogram (ECG) electrodes.
    ○ 2. Pulse oximeter.
    ○ 3. Blood pressure cuff.
    ○ 4. Doppler for pulse check.

80. The nurse is talking to a group of parents about drug abuse among adolescents. One parent says he has heard that you can tell which drug a person is using by how the eyes look. The parent asks how you could tell a person was taking heroin. Which of the following would the nurse use to describe the eyes of a person using heroin?
    ○ 1. Whites red and bloodshot.
    ○ 2. Pupils small and constricted.
    ○ 3. Pupils large and dilated.
    ○ 4. Drooping eyelids.

81. When performing routine health evaluations in school-aged children, which of the following would alert the school nurse to pediculosis capitis (head lice)?

○ 1. Spotty baldness.
○ 2. Wheals with scalp blistering.
○ 3. Frequent scalp scratching.
○ 4. Dry, scaly patches on the skin.

82. Which of the following best indicates that a client's peristaltic activity is returning to normal after surgery?
    ○ 1. The client passes flatus.
    ○ 2. The client says that she is hungry.
    ○ 3. Bowel sounds are hypoactive on auscultation.
    ○ 4. Peristalsis can be felt on abdominal palpitation.

83. A client appears flushed and has shallow respirations. The arterial blood gas report shows the following: pH, 7.24; pCO_2, 49 mm Hg; HCO_3^-, 24 mEq/L. These findings are indicative of which of the following acid–base imbalances?
    ○ 1. Metabolic acidosis.
    ○ 2. Metabolic alkalosis.
    ○ 3. Respiratory acidosis.
    ○ 4. Respiratory alkalosis.

84. Which of the following measures is *most* important for pain management for a client after a lobectomy?
    ○ 1. Reposition the client immediately after administering pain medication.
    ○ 2. Reassess the client 30 minutes after administering pain medication.
    ○ 3. Reassure the client after administering pain medication.
    ○ 4. Readjust the pain medication dosage as needed.

85. The nurse is evaluating a female client's understanding of how to prevent sexually transmitted diseases (STDs). Which of the following statements indicates that the client understands how to protect herself?
    ○ 1. "I will be sure my partner uses a condom."
    ○ 2. "I need to be sure to take my birth control pills."
    ○ 3. "I will always douche after sexual intercourse."
    ○ 4. "I will be sure to take antibiotics to prevent an STD."

86. While assessing a multigravid client at 10 weeks' gestation, the nurse notes a purplish color to the vagina and cervix. The nurse documents this finding as which of the following?
    ○ 1. Goodell's sign.
    ○ 2. Chadwick's sign.
    ○ 3. Hegar's sign.
    ○ 4. Melasma's sign.

87. A client with bipolar disorder, mania has flight of ideas and grandiosity and becomes easily agitated. To prevent harmful behaviors, which of the following would the nurse do *initially*?
    ○ 1. Encourage the client to stay in his room.
    ○ 2. Seclude the client at the first sign of agitation.

 3. Tell the client to seek out staff when feeling agitated.
 4. Instruct the client to ask for medication when agitated.

88. The nurse is preparing written information for a client. Which of the following represents a sound approach to providing information?
 1. Use charts to help convey information.
 2. Prepare information at an eighth-grade reading level.
 3. Use short words.
 4. Print the material in a medium-sized type.

89. A nurse is evaluating the proper use of crutches by a client who has fractured her right leg. Which statement by the client indicates that she is using the correct technique?
 1. "I move my left leg forward first as I swing forward on my crutches."
 2. "I need to increase my arm strength, because my arms tingle after I use my crutches."
 3. "I padded the tops of my crutches so that I can lean more comfortably on my crutches."
 4. "I feel pressure on the palms of my hands when I am walking with my crutches."

90. Which of the following factors is a priority when evaluating discharge plans for a 68-year-old man after a lower left lobectomy for lung cancer?
 1. The distance the client lives from the hospital.
 2. Support available for assisting the client at home.
 3. The client's ability to do home blood pressure monitoring.
 4. The client's knowledge of the causes of lung cancer.

91. A primiparous client planning to breast-feed her term neonate delivered vaginally asks, "When will my `real' milk come in?" The nurse explains to the client that after delivery breasts begin to fill with milk within which of the following periods?
 1. 12 hours.
 2. 24 hours.
 3. 2 to 4 days.
 4. 7 days.

92. The nurse is caring for an elderly, debilitated client who has been bedridden for an extended period. Which of the following is the predominant clinical finding indicating that the client has developed pneumonia?
 1. Fever and chills.
 2. Productive cough.
 3. Confusion.
 4. Pleuritic chest pain.

93. A child with rheumatic fever has polyarthritis and chorea. An echocardiogram shows swelling of the cardiac tissue. Which of the following would the nurse include in the child's plan of care?
 1. Explaining that the chorea will disappear over time.
 2. Performing neurologic checks every 4 hours until the chorea subsides.
 3. Promoting ambulation by administering aspirin every 4 hours.
 4. Keeping the child in a slightly cool environment.

94. A 19-year-old unmarried college student who is visiting the clinic and is found to be approximately 8 weeks pregnant asks, "If I have an abortion in the next 2 or 3 weeks, how will it be done?" The nurse instructs the client that at this gestational age an abortion is usually performed by which of the following techniques?
 1. Dilation and curettage.
 2. Menstrual extraction.
 3. Dilation and vacuum extraction.
 4. Saline induction.

95. The nurse is performing a respiratory assessment on a client who has a pleural effusion. Which of the following findings would the nurse anticipate finding to support this diagnosis?
 1. Decreased chest movement on the affected side.
 2. Normal bronchial breath sounds.
 3. Hyperresonance on percussion.
 4. Fever.

96. Which of the following is an expected client outcome related to one of the nursing diagnoses made for the child with intussusception: Acute Pain related to cramping? The client
 1. exhibits no manifestations of discomfort.
 2. is very still.
 3. has a normal bowel movement.
 4. has not vomited in 3 hours.

97. Garamycin 25 mg IM has been ordered every 6 hours. Garamycin 40 mg/mL is available. How many mL should the nurse administer?
 1. 0.55 mL.
 2. 0.6 mL.
 3. 1.0 mL.
 4. 1.6 mL.

98. Assessment of a 36-year-old woman complaining of malaise and dysuria reveals a temperature of 100°F (37.4°C) and painful blisters on the outside of her vagina. The client tells the nurse she had intercourse with a new partner 5 days ago. Which of the following would the nurse suspect as *most* likely?
 1. Human immunodeficiency virus (HIV) infection.
 2. *Chlamydia trachomatis* infection.
 3. Syphilis.
 4. Herpes genitalis.

99. A child with leukemia fails to respond to therapy. Which of the following statements offers the nurse the *best* guide in making plans to assist the parents in dealing with their child's imminent death?
    ○ 1. Knowing that the prognosis is poor helps prepare relatives for the death of children.
    ○ 2. Relatives are especially grieved when a child does well at first but then declines rapidly.
    ○ 3. Trust in health personnel is most often destroyed by a death that is considered untimely.
    ○ 4. It is more difficult for relatives to accept the death of a 10-year-old than the death of a younger child whose family membership has been short.

100. A client who states that he is allergic to penicillin has an order to receive cefazolin (Ancef). The nurse's initial response is to
    ○ 1. ask the client if he has taken cefazolin (Ancef) before.
    ○ 2. consult with the physician or a clinical pharmacist.
    ○ 3. administer cefazolin (Ancef) immediately.
    ○ 4. observe the client closely for urticaria.

101. A client with chronic renal failure tells the nurse that her skin feels dry and is constantly itching. Based on these data, which of the following is an appropriate nursing diagnosis?
    ○ 1. Ineffective Health Maintenance related to poor hygiene.
    ○ 2. Chronic Pain related to skin irritation.
    ○ 3. Risk for Impaired Skin Integrity related to severe pruritus.
    ○ 4. Ineffective Coping related to manifestations of chronic illness.

102. When preparing the teaching plan for a client and his family about lithium therapy, the nurse would expect to include teaching about which of the following?
    ○ 1. Maintaining an adequate sodium intake.
    ○ 2. Discontinuing sodium in the diet.
    ○ 3. Buying foods labeled "low in sodium."
    ○ 4. Increasing sodium in the diet.

103. A client who is undergoing radiation therapy develops mucositis. Which of the following interventions should be included in the client's plan of care?
    ○ 1. Increase mouth care to twice per shift.
    ○ 2. Provide the client with hot tea to drink.
    ○ 3. Promote regular flossing of teeth.
    ○ 4. Use half-strength hydrogen peroxide on mouth ulcers.

104. A parent calls the Poison Control Center because her 3-year-old has eaten 10 to 12 chewable acetaminophen tablets. The nurse instructs the parent to take the child to the emergency department after doing which of the following *first*?

○ 1. Giving the child a large glass of milk.
○ 2. Giving the child water with syrup of ipecac.
○ 3. Giving the child baking soda in 4 ounces of water.
○ 4. Not allowing the child to drink any fluids.

105. While waiting for the physician, the parent of a preschool-aged child tells the nurse that the child is hyperactive and something needs to be done. Which of the following responses would be *most* appropriate initially?
    ○ 1. "What makes you think your child is hyperactive?"
    ○ 2. "What do you think needs to be done ?"
    ○ 3. "How does your child behave normally?"
    ○ 4. "Why not wait and see what the doctor says?"

106. When preparing for the discharge of a newborn after surgery to correct tracheoesophageal fistula (TEF), the nurse teaches the parents about the need for long-term health care because their child has a high probability of developing which of the following?
    ○ 1. Recurrent mild diarrhea with dehydration
    ○ 2. Esophageal stricture
    ○ 3. Speech problems
    ○ 4. Ulcers

107. A young man with Hodgkin's disease has been readmitted to the hospital because of his aggressive disease that is unresponsive to multiple therapies. Death appears imminent. One goal for this client is to
    ○ 1. reduce feelings of isolation.
    ○ 2. reduce fear of pain.
    ○ 3. reduce fear of more aggressive therapies.
    ○ 4. reduce feelings of social inadequacy.

108. A nulligravid client is admitted in early active labor at 39 weeks' gestation with intact membranes. When assessing the fetal heart rate, the nurse locates the heart sounds above the client's umbilicus at midline. The nurse would suspect that the fetus is lying in which of the following positions?
    ○ 1. Cephalic.
    ○ 2. Frank breech.
    ○ 3. Face.
    ○ 4. Transverse.

109. The nurse is caring for a client who has been diagnosed with pernicious anemia. Which of the following statements by the client indicates an understanding of the treatment of pernicious anemia?
    ○ 1. "I will need to increase my dietary intake of foods that are high in vitamin B_{12}."
    ○ 2. "I will receive my first injection of vitamin B_{12} tomorrow, and I will return for a follow-up injection in 1 month."
    ○ 3. "I understand that the oral form of vitamin B_{12} is preferred because it is safer and less expensive than the injection form."

○ 4. "I will need to take vitamin B_{12} replacements for the rest of my life."

110. A client's 12:00 noon blood glucose concentration was inaccurately documented as 301 instead of 130. This error was not noticed until 1:00 PM. The nurse administered the sliding scale insulin for a blood sugar of 310 instead of 130. What should the nurse do *first*?
    ○ 1. Notify the physician.
    ○ 2. Take orange juice to the client.
    ○ 3. Consult with the clinical pharmacist.
    ○ 4. Call the charge nurse.

111. An older infant who has been injured in an automobile accident has to wear a splint on the injured leg. The mother reports that the infant has become mobile even while wearing the splint. The nurse would advise the mother to do which of the following?
    ○ 1. Notify the physician immediately to adjust the treatment plan.
    ○ 2. Confine the infant to one room in the apartment.
    ○ 3. Keep the infant in the splint at night, removing it during the day.
    ○ 4. Remove any unsafe items from the area in which the infant is mobile.

112. While preparing a client for surgery, the nurse assesses for psychosocial problems that may cause preoperative anxiety. Which of the following is believed to be the most distressing fear a preoperative client is likely to experience?
    ○ 1. Fear of the unknown.
    ○ 2. Fear of changes in body image.
    ○ 3. Fear of the effects of anesthesia.
    ○ 4. Fear of being in pain.

113. A 56-year-old woman is admitted for a modified radical mastectomy. The client appears anxious and asks many questions. The nurse's *best* course of action is to
    ○ 1. tell the client as much as she wants to know and is able to understand.
    ○ 2. delay discussing the client's questions with her until the convalescent phase of her care.
    ○ 3. delay discussing the client's questions with her until her apprehension subsides.
    ○ 4. explain to the client that she should discuss her questions with her physician.

114. The nurse asks the client to sign a consent form before undergoing surgery. The client indicates that he was not told about the risks of the surgical procedure. Which of the following statements by the nurse is most appropriate?
    ○ 1. "What are your concerns? I can answer any questions that you have."
    ○ 2. "You can go ahead and sign the form. I will be sure to tell the surgeon you have questions."
    ○ 3. "It is important that your questions are answered before you consent to the procedure. I will contact the surgeon."

○ 4. "Actually, the risks associated with this procedure are minimal. The surgeon has performed this surgery many times."

115. The nurse is assessing fetal position in a 32-year-old woman in her eighth month of pregnancy. From Figure 3, the fetal position can be described as
    ○ 1. left occipital transverse.
    ○ 2. left occipital anterior.
    ○ 3. right occipital transverse.
    ○ 4. right occipital anterior.

116. The father of an infant states that the physician told him that his child has a urinary tract infection. The father calls the clinic to ask about the signs and symptoms that he should watch out for in the future to indicate a recurrence. Which of the following would the nurse tell the father?
    ○ 1. Increased urine output and clear urine.
    ○ 2. Loss of appetite and fussiness.
    ○ 3. Feeding problems and jaundice.
    ○ 4. Fever and dysuria.

117. After teaching a mother about the neonate's positive Babinski's reflex, the nurse determines that the mother understands the instructions when she says that a positive Babinski's reflex indicates
    ○ 1. possible partial paralysis
    ○ 2. possible lower limb defect
    ○ 3. immature central nervous system
    ○ 4. possible injury to nerves that innervate the legs

118. The nurse should instruct a client who is taking dexamethasone (Decadron) and furosemide (Lasix) to observe for signs of hypokalemia, which include
    ○ 1. excitability.
    ○ 2. muscle weakness.

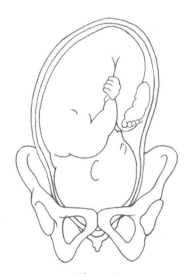

Figure 3.

○ 3. diarrhea.

○ 4. increased thirst.

119. A client with a suspected diagnosis of lung cancer has a bronchoscopy with biopsy. Which of the following interventions would be appropriate after the procedure?
    ○ 1. Encourage the client to gargle with oral lidocaine to decrease throat irritation.
    ○ 2. Monitor the client for signs of pneumothorax.
    ○ 3. Administer pain medication as needed to relieve mediastinal discomfort.
    ○ 4. Advise the client not to talk until the gag reflex returns.

120. A child is to receive 500 mL of an IV solution over 12 hours via tubing that delivers microdrips at 60 drops/mL. The nurse would infuse the solution at which of the following rates?
    ○ 1. 21 drops/minute.
    ○ 2. 42 drops/minute.
    ○ 3. 63 drops/minute.
    ○ 4. 84 drops/minute.

121. Which of the following techniques is correct when administering a subcutaneous injection?
    ○ 1. Use a 1-inch needle for injection.
    ○ 2. Insert the needle at a 45-degree angle to the skin.
    ○ 3. Spread the skin tightly at the injection site.
    ○ 4. Draw 0.2 mL of air into the syringe before administration.

122. Which of the following is a *priority* nursing diagnosis for the client presenting with pelvic inflammatory disease?
    ○ 1. Imbalanced Nutrition: Less than Body Requirements.
    ○ 2. Bathing/Hygiene Self-Care Deficit.
    ○ 3. Acute Pain.
    ○ 4. Impaired Skin Integrity.

123. After talking with the mother of a child, the nurse determines that the child has a difficult temperament. Which of the following would the nurse expect to include when developing this child's plan of care?
    ○ 1. Allow the child to determine when feeding should occur.
    ○ 2. Ensure that the child is fed even though crying does not occur.
    ○ 3. Provide structured feeding times and bedtimes.
    ○ 4. Instruct the mother to take extra safety precautions around the house.

124. Which of the following steps is appropriate for the nurse to include when giving a client a tube feeding?
    ○ 1. Warm the feeding solution before administration.
    ○ 2. Position the client side-lying on the left side.
    ○ 3. Aspirate residual gastric contents before the feeding and discard.
    ○ 4. Verify position of the tube before beginning feeding.

125. A multiparous client 48 hours postpartum who is breast-feeding tells the nurse, "I'm having a lot of cramping. This didn't happen when I nursed my first baby." Which of the following would be the nurse's *best* response?
    ○ 1. "I will notify your doctor. It's possible there are some placental fragments remaining."
    ○ 2. "I need to check your lochial flow. You may have a clot that is being dislodged."
    ○ 3. "You must have gotten a heavy dose of oxytocin (Pitocin). It should wear off soon."
    ○ 4. "The cramping is normal and is caused by your baby's sucking, which stimulates the release of oxytocin."

126. The mother of a child with moderate diarrhea calls the clinic to find out how to manage her child's illness. Which of the following would the nurse suggest?
    ○ 1. Begin clear liquids for 24 hours.
    ○ 2. Feed the child bananas, rice, applesauce, and toast.
    ○ 3. Offer foods that are low in fat.
    ○ 4. Continue the child's regular diet.

127. The nurse is performing routine tracheostomy care. Which of the following steps would be appropriate for the nurse to include in the performance of the procedure?
    ○ 1. Remove the inner cannula every 2 hours for cleaning.
    ○ 2. Secure the tracheostomy ties with a square knot.
    ○ 3. Use cut gauze under the neck plate to protect the skin.
    ○ 4. Suction the inner cannula on completion of the procedure.

128. What is the nurse's most appropriate response when finding a sealed container of IV 50% dextrose in a catch-all bin on the unit?
    ○ 1. Leave it where found and notify risk management.
    ○ 2. Send it to pharmacy.
    ○ 3. File an incident report.
    ○ 4. Discard it in a sharps container.

129. To reduce the risk of pressure ulcer formation, which of the following activities would the nurse teach the client who is wheelchair-bound as a result of a spinal cord injury?
    ○ 1. Bathe daily.
    ○ 2. Eat a high-carbohydrate diet.
    ○ 3. Shift your weight every 15 minutes.
    ○ 4. Move from the bed to the wheelchair every 2 hours.

130. A nulligravid client in the second stage of labor has had no anesthesia or analgesia. Anatomically, which of the following would be the *most* effective position for the client to begin pushing?
    ○ 1. Squatting with body curved in a C shape.

○ 2. Side-lying while keeping the head elevated.

○ 3. In the knee–chest position while keeping the head down.

○ 4. Squatting with the back arched.

131. A client with antisocial personality disorder tells the nurse, "I punched the guy out because he deserved it and then the cops arrested me." Which of the following responses would be *most* helpful to the client?

○ 1. "It's wrong to punch others."

○ 2. "If you punch people out, you'll get into trouble."

○ 3. "I wouldn't do that again if I were you."

○ 4. "Don't ever do that again; you're an adult."

132. The nurse is teaching unlicensed personnel about the care of clients with self-mutilation. Which of the following, if stated by the unlicensed personnel about self-mutilation, demonstrates that the teaching has been effective?

○ 1. "It is a means of getting what the person wants."

○ 2. "It is a nonserious event that can be ignored."

○ 3. "It is a way to express anger and rage."

○ 4. "It is a form of manipulation."

133. The nurse has obtained the nursing history of a client diagnosed with hepatitis C. What would be considered a potential risk factor for acquiring hepatitis C?

○ 1. Drinking contaminated water.

○ 2. Traveling to India.

○ 3. Having a tattoo.

○ 4. Eating shellfish.

134. A client is experiencing symptoms of early alcohol withdrawal. His blood pressure is 150/85 mm Hg and his pulse is 98 bpm. The nurse would expect to administer which of the following medications?

○ 1. Lorazepam (Ativan).

○ 2. Naltrexone (ReVia).

○ 3. Methadone (Dolophine)

○ 4. Imipramine (Tofranil).

135. After a child returns from the postanesthesia care unit after surgery, which of the following would the nurse assess *first*?

○ 1. The intravenous fluid access site.

○ 2. The child's level of pain.

○ 3. The surgical site dressing.

○ 4. The functioning of the nasogastric tube.

136. A critical nursing intervention to protect a client who has received tissue plasminogen activator (t-PA) or alteplase recombinant (Activase) therapy includes

○ 1. using the radial artery to obtain blood gas samples.

○ 2. maintaining arterial pressure for 10 seconds.

○ 3. administering intramuscular injections.

○ 4. encouraging physical activity.

137. Two clients have been following low-sodium diets for several weeks. One of the clients states that his blood pressure has not changed and asks the nurse why not. The nurse should base the response on the fact that the percentage of the population that are able to lower their blood pressure through a sodium-restricted diet is only which of the following?

○ 1. 10%.

○ 2. 25%.

○ 3. 50%.

○ 4. 70%.

138. A client is admitted with acute pancreatitis. Which laboratory value is indicative of pancreatitis?

○ 1. Decreased urinary amylase.

○ 2. Hypercalcemia.

○ 3. Hypoglycemia.

○ 4. Increased serum amylase and lipase.

139. For the client with a substance abuse problem, which of the following would be *most* helpful to aid the client in dealing with feelings and concerns related to alcohol and drugs?

○ 1. Individual therapy.

○ 2. Group sessions.

○ 3. Solitary activities.

○ 4. Recreation.

140. Which of the following assessment findings would the nurse expect to observe in a client with cystitis?

○ 1. Flank pain.

○ 2. Oliguria.

○ 3. Nausea and vomiting.

○ 4. Foul-smelling urine.

141. A client with acute stress disorder is telling the nurse about the tornado that leveled his house and killed his wife and baby while he was out of town on business. He states, "If only I'd been at home, I could have saved them." Which of the following responses would be *most* appropriate?

○ 1. "Don't blame yourself; you'll only feel worse."

○ 2. "It's not your fault; so stop feeling so guilty."

○ 3. "You might not have been at home."

○ 4. "You couldn't have prevented the tornado; it just happened."

142. On the first postpartum day, the nurse is caring for a primiparous client who has recently emigrated from Japan to the United States and speaks only a little English. The nurse observes that the client has been bottle-feeding her neonate on occasion, but most of the neonatal care is being performed by the client's mother-in-law. Which of the following actions would be *most* appropriate?

○ 1. Notify the social worker because bonding may be affected.

○ 2. Document the unusual maternal behavior in the client's chart.

3. Determine whether this is a cultural practice for the client and her family.

4. Obtain an order to make a home visit after the client's discharge.

143. A client is scheduled for a creatinine clearance test. Which one of the following preparations is appropriate for the nurse to make?

1. Instruct the client about the need to collect urine for 24 hours.

2. Prepare to insert an indwelling urethral catheter.

3. Provide the client with a sterile urine collection container.

4. Instruct the client to force fluids to 3000 mL/day.

144. When the nurse is assessing a client's cultural adaptation, which of the following statements is *least* sensitive to the client's needs?

1. "What are some of your favorite foods?"

2. "Describe any health problems in your past."

3. "Please tell me how you would like to be addressed."

4. "Your eyes look dark; is this normal for you?"

145. After several months of taking olanzapine (Zyprexa), the client reports that he is no longer hearing voices of any kind. Which of the following would confirm that the client is developing insight into his illness?

1. "That Zyprexa is the best medicine I have ever had."

2. "I didn't realize how sick I could get from a chemical brain imbalance."

3. "My mom is proud of me for staying on my medicines."

4. "I think I may be able to get a little part-time job soon."

146. A client who is a computer operator has developed carpal tunnel syndrome. The nurse explains to the client that carpal tunnel syndrome is caused by which of the following pathophysiologic conditions?

1. Decreased circulation to the brachial nerve.

2. Muscle atrophy resulting from disuse.

3. Median nerve compression.

4. Progressive flexion contracture of the wrist.

147. In addition to milk and eggs, which of the following foods is most often implicated in allergic reactions?

1. Peanuts.

2. Soy.

3. Fish.

4. Orange juice.

148. A client who is recovering from a transurethral resection of the prostate (TURP) experiences urinary incontinence. He tells the nurse that he has decreased his fluid intake because of the incontinence. What would be the nurse's best response to the client?

1. "Yes, limiting your fluids can decrease your incontinence."

2. "Limiting your fluids will cause kidney stones."

3. "Drink 8 glasses of water a day and urinate every 2 hours."

4. "If your incontinence continues, we will reinsert your catheter."

149. An infant has surgery to correct a tracheoesophageal fistula. The most appropriate nursing diagnosis for the nurse to identify after surgery is

1. Risk for Infection.

2. Acute Pain.

3. Constipation.

4. Impaired Physical Mobility.

150. The nurse teaches girls 10 to 12 years of age about self-care during menses. The nurse emphasizes that a risk factor for toxic shock syndrome (TSS) is

1. changing tampons every 3 hours.

2. avoiding use of deodorized tampons.

3. alternating tampons with sanitary pads.

4. using only tampons at night.

151. A client with a history of cystitis is admitted to the hospital with a diagnosis of pyelonephritis. Which of the following assessment findings specifically supports a diagnosis of pyelonephritis?

1. Suprapubic pain.

2. Dysuria.

3. Urinary retention.

4. Costovertebral tenderness.

152. A woman is taking oral contraceptives. The nurse teaches the client that medications that may interfere with oral contraceptive efficacy include

1. antihypertensives.

2. antibiotics.

3. diuretics.

4. antihistamines.

153. A 28-year-old female client is prescribed danazol (Danocrine) for endometriosis. Which of the following would the nurse include as a side effect when teaching the client about the drug?

1. Headaches.

2. Weight loss.

3. Increased libido.

4. Hair loss.

154. To which of the following unlicensed personnel should the nurse assign a male client of Mexican American descent who needs complete morning care?

1. Mary, who has 2 complete morning care clients.

2. Joe, who has 1 complete morning care client.

3. Jill, who has 4 partial morning care clients.

4. Jim, who has 5 partial morning care clients.

155. A client with chronic renal failure is experiencing central nervous system (CNS) changes caused by uremic toxins. Which nursing intervention would be *most* appropriate for addressing the changes?
    ○ 1. Allow the client to grieve for body image changes.
    ○ 2. Restrict foods that are high in potassium.
    ○ 3. Restrict fluid intake to 1000 mL/day.
    ○ 4. Assess the client's mental status regularly.

156. The nurse is preparing to give a subcutaneous injection to an elderly, emaciated client. Which needle length and angle would the nurse plan to use to administer the injection safely?
    ○ 1. A ³/₈-inch needle at a 90-degree angle.
    ○ 2. A ⁵/₈-inch needle at a 45-degree angle.
    ○ 3. A ¹/₂-inch needle at a 15-degree angle.
    ○ 4. A ⁵/₈-inch needle at a 90-degree angle.

157. A young female client comes into the emergency department with complaints of flank pain, dysuria, frequency, burning on urination, and malaise. The nurse obtains a urine specimen because the nurse anticipates that the client's symptoms are related to
    ○ 1. pelvic inflammatory disease.
    ○ 2. renal calculi.
    ○ 3. urinary tract infection.
    ○ 4. renal failure.

158. A multigravid client at 38 weeks' gestation is admitted to the hospital's birthing center with dark, scant vaginal bleeding and abdominal pain. The nurse observes frequent low-amplitude uterine activity while the client's contraction pattern is externally monitored. Which of the following would the nurse suspect?
    ○ 1. Abruptio placenta.
    ○ 2. Placenta accreta.
    ○ 3. Placenta previa.
    ○ 4. Battledore placenta.

159. A female client is treated for trichomoniasis with metronidazole (Flagyl). The nurse instructs the client that
    ○ 1. the medication should not alter the color of the urine.
    ○ 2. she should discontinue oral contraceptive use during this treatment.
    ○ 3. she should avoid alcohol during treatment and for 24 hours after completion of the drug.
    ○ 4. her partner does not need treatment.

160. A client is in the advanced stages of osteoarthritis. Which of the following best describes the pain that occurs in the advanced stage of the disease?
    ○ 1. Pain occurs with minimal activity.
    ○ 2. Crepitation develops and intensifies pain.
    ○ 3. Joints are symmetrically affected by pain.
    ○ 4. Fatigue accompanies pain.

161. A family may request to have a client of Vietnamese descent transferred to die at home because it is traditionally believed that
    ○ 1. it is disloyal to their loved one to be left in the hospital.
    ○ 2. the hospital cannot be trusted.
    ○ 3. the family can provide more comfort at home.
    ○ 4. reincarnation will not occur in the hospital.

162. A client has just been admitted with acute delirium of unknown etiology. The client's daughter states that she is worried about her mom because she has never been this sick before. Which of the following would be the *most* helpful statement to make to the daughter?
    ○ 1. "Please don't worry. We will take good care of your mother."
    ○ 2. "The doctor will order tests to find out what is causing her condition."
    ○ 3. "We can help you learn how to take care of her after she is discharged."
    ○ 4. "It helps if you avoid arguing when she talks about seeing people who aren't there."

163. A client with dementia is going to live with his daughter who does not work outside of the home. The nurse would evaluate that the daughter needs *further* education when she makes which of the following statements?
    ○ 1. "I've put special locks on all the doors that Dad won't be able to unlock."
    ○ 2. "Dad said that what he missed most while he was here was using his aftershave."
    ○ 3. "Dad will be in a bedroom that has nothing for him to trip over getting to the bathroom."
    ○ 4. "I've taken the knobs off of the stove so he won't be able to turn it on."

164. Allopurinol (Zyloprim) is prescribed for a client who has chronic gout. Which of the following comments indicates that the client understands how to take the allopurinol?
    ○ 1. "I will take the medication whenever my joints hurt."
    ○ 2. "I must take this drug on an empty stomach."
    ○ 3. "I should drink plenty of fluids when taking allopurinol."
    ○ 4. "I should not take aspirin when taking allopurinol."

165. A client complains of severe vulvar itching. The nurse recognizes that a client with moniliasis (*Candida albicans*) has a vaginal discharge that is
    ○ 1. yellow-green in color.
    ○ 2. thick and white.
    ○ 3. fishy smelling.
    ○ 4. purulent.

166. The next-door neighbor of a nurse comes over to say that her toddler just got burned on the arm. The nurse should advise the mother to *first*

○ 1. pack the arm in ice, then take the child to the closest emergency room.

○ 2. rub the burned area with an antibacterial ointment, then call the doctor.

○ 3. run cool water over the burned area, then wrap it in a clean cloth.

○ 4. call the child's health care provider immediately, then wrap the arm in a clean cloth.

167. The nursing assessment of a client with osteomyelitis of the left great toe reveals pain with partial weight bearing, unsteady gait, and complaints of general weakness. Based on these data, the *priority* nursing diagnosis for the client is

○ 1. Impaired Physical Mobility.

○ 2. Impaired Skin Integrity.

○ 3. Ineffective Coping.

○ 4. Risk for Injury.

168. A client receiving a blood transfusion begins to complain of chills and headache within the first 15 minutes of the transfusion. Based on these data, what should be the nurse's first response to the client's complaints?

○ 1. Administer acetaminophen.

○ 2. Take the client's blood pressure.

○ 3. Discontinue the transfusion.

○ 4. Check the infusion rate of the blood.

169. A 72-year-old client is referred for counseling. During the initial nursing assessment, the client denies the need for counseling. The nurse would agree with her if she made which of the following comments?

○ 1. "My doctor just put me on an antidepressant, and I'll be fine in a week or so."

○ 2. "My daughter sent me here. She's mad because I don't have the energy to take care of my grandkids."

○ 3. "Since I've gotten over the death of my husband, I've had more energy and been more active than before he died."

○ 4. "My son got worried because I made this silly comment about wanting to be with my husband in heaven."

170. A client takes isosorbide dinitrate (Isordil) as an antianginal medication. Which of the following statements indicates that the client understands the side effects of the drug?

○ 1. "I should take my pulse before taking the medication."

○ 2. "I should take Isordil with food."

○ 3. "I will need to change positions slowly so I won't get dizzy."

○ 4. "It is important that I report any swelling in my ankles."

171. The nurse is working on discharge plans with a client who is diagnosed with intermittent explosive disorder, characterized by sudden angry outbursts. The nurse determines that the client is ready for discharge when he makes which of the following comments?

○ 1. "I'm just not going to let myself get angry anymore."

○ 2. "Drinking doesn't help, but I like being with my buddies at the bar."

○ 3. "I'll be taking valproic acid (Depakote) and propranolol (Inderal) forever to help stay in control."

○ 4. "It would help if my mom would stop getting on my case all the time."

172. The nurse walks into a client's room to administer the 9 AM medications and notices that the client is in an awkward position in bed. What is the nurse's first action?

○ 1. Ask the client his name.

○ 2. Check the client's name band.

○ 3. Straighten the client's pillow behind his back.

○ 4. Give the client his medications.

173. Which of the following would be an expected outcome for a client 24 hours after an abdominal hysterectomy?

○ 1. Bowel sounds will be heard on auscultation.

○ 2. The perineal pad will have a minimal amount of serous drainage.

○ 3. The client will express feelings of a positive body image.

○ 4. The client will perform leg exercises hourly.

174. A client has been prescribed furosemide (Lasix) 80 mg twice daily. The cardiac monitor technician informs the nurse that the client has started having rare premature ventricular contractions (PVC) followed by runs of bigeminy lasting 2 minutes. During the assessment, the nurse determines that the client is asymptomatic and has stable vital signs. Which of the following actions should the nurse perform next?

○ 1. Call the physician.

○ 2. Check the client's potassium level.

○ 3. Summon the nurse manager.

○ 4. Administer potassium.

175. During a home visit 3 weeks after delivery of a term neonate, a primiparous client tells the nurse that she has had tremendous mood swings, uncontrollable crying, loss of energy, and no appetite. Based on an analysis of the client's assessment findings, which of the following would the nurse suspect?

○ 1. Postpartum blues.

○ 2. Postpartum depression.

○ 3. Postpartum psychosis.

○ 4. Normal postpartum adjustment.

176. After a child with leukemia dies, the mother asks the nurse, "What if we had brought her in when she first complained of an earache?" Which of the following would be the nurse's *best* response to the mother?

○ 1. Explain that nothing could have helped the child.

○ 2. Provide comfort by saying that the child is no longer suffering with an incurable illness.

○ 3. Reassure the mother that all possible care was given.

○ 4. Explain that infections are often the result of leukemia rather than the cause of it.

177. The nurse has received the following information from unlicensed assistant personnel about various clients. Which of the following clients should the nurse assess immediately?

○ 1. A postoperative client who has a temperature of 100°F (37.8°C).

○ 2. A client who had a TURP and complains of bladder spasms with 60 mL of urine output from his catheter.

○ 3. A client with an ileal conduit who has a urinary appliance pouch that is one-third full of urine.

○ 4. A client recovering from a bronchoscopy with a biopsy who expectorates a small amount of bloody sputum.

178. The physician orders 500 mL of D5W to be administered over 10 hours. Using a microdrip administration set, to what flow rate would the nurse adjust the IV?

○ 1. 50 gtt/minute.

○ 2. 60 gtt/minute.

○ 3. 75 gtt/minute.

○ 4. 100 gtt/minute.

179. A client who had been taking phenelzine (Nardil) is being switched to fluoxetine (Prozac) by the physi-

cian. Which of the following facts would the nurse emphasize with the client?

○ 1. The client must wait 14 days before he can start taking fluoxetine (Prozac).

○ 2. The client must have his blood levels drawn every week while taking fluoxetine (Prozac).

○ 3. The client must notify his physician before taking any over-the-counter medication.

○ 4. The client must report symptoms of headache and nausea to the physician immediately.

180. The nurse would evaluate that a client is coughing effectively after surgery if the nurse observes which of the following activities?

○ 1. The client breathes through her nose, holds her breath, and then exhales slowly before coughing.

○ 2. The client takes short, panting breaths and coughs from the throat to expectorate sputum.

○ 3. The client takes a deep abdominal breath and then "huff" coughs three or four times.

○ 4. The client takes three deep breaths and then coughs forcefully.

181. A 14-year-old nulligravid client with no history of prenatal care is admitted to the birthing unit in active labor. On admission, the client's cervix is dilated to 9 cm, completely effaced, at 1+ station. The client is thrashing in the bed, screaming and crying, and tells the nurse, "Do something for the pain!" Which of the following would the nurse do *first*?

○ 1. Tell the client to calm down immediately.

○ 2. Tell the client to breathe deeply with each contraction.

○ 3. Get the client's attention by looking her in the eyes.

○ 4. Call the physician for an order for analgesia.

Correct Answers and Rationale

The letters in parentheses following the rationale identify the step of the nursing process (A, D, P, I, E), client needs (1, 2, 3, 4, 5, 6, 7, 8, 9, 10), and nursing care area (O, Y, M, X). See the inside front cover for the key.

1. 4. Heartburn is caused when stomach contents enter the distal end of the esophagus, producing a burning sensation. To avoid heartburn during pregnancy, the client should avoid spicy foods; eat smaller, more frequent meals; and avoid lying down after eating. Peristalsis usually decreases during the latter half of pregnancy. Displacement of the stomach by the uterus, not the diaphragm, may contribute to heartburn. Increased, not decreased, secretion of hydrochloric acid also contributes to heartburn during pregnancy. (I, 3, O)

2. 2. Acknowledging the anger and its source encourages communication about the client's feelings. Although anger at God is common after a loss, the client is displacing the anger that she needs to deal with more directly. Telling the client that the miscarriage was an accident or that she is a strong person and will get through this ignores the client's feelings of anger and loss, thereby cutting off communication. (I, 5, X)

3. 4. Asking the client to speak about his concerns encourages open discussion. Telling the client that he is making a mistake is judgmental of the client's wishes and eliminates opportunities for the client to explore the situation and discuss various treatment options. Saying that herbal treatments have not been approved by the FDA or that they have not been researched is irrelevant, places a value judgment on the client's wishes, and provides no opportunity for discussion. (I, 1, M)

4. 3. The most important aspect of teaching a preschooler is to have the family members there for support. Preschoolers are able to understand information that is individualized to their level. Including a plastic model of the heart and a catheter as part of the preoperative preparation may be helpful. The other family members will understand the heart model and catheter better than the preschooler will. (P, 9, Y)

5. 4. Massaging a area that is reddened due to pressure is contraindicated because it further reduces blood flow to the area. In the past, massaging reddened areas was thought to improve blood flow to the area, and some nursing personnel may still believe that massaging the area is effective in preventing pressure ulcer formation. (I, 1, M)

6. 3. Asking the mother to talk about her concerns acknowledges the mother's rights and encourages open discussion. The other responses negate the parent's concerns. (I, 1, M)

7. 3. The Meals on Wheels program delivers meals to clients once a day in their home. In addition to the improved nutrition, it is often valued as a means to check on elderly persons who live alone. Hospice care involves daily needs for the terminally ill at home. VNA provides skilled nursing care to clients at home. AARP is a national organization for retired people, not a health care organization. (P, 1, M)

8. 1. The cardiovascular status of the client is the first information documented. This information will validate the effectiveness of the temporary pacemaker. The client's emotional state and the type of sedation are important but not a high priority. The nurse will need to document the pacemaker information (settings of the pacemaker); this will be considered part of the cardiovascular information. (I, 10, M)

9. 3. Using a special feeding table or modified high chair is the best method for an infant who is used to sitting up for feedings. The child should not be flat because of the danger of aspiration. Raising the child's head will not work as well as using a feeding table because the child is not used to lying down to eat. Two people are not necessary. (E, 7, Y)

10. 4. Ventricular tachycardia is recognized by a wide QRS complex; the rhythm may be regular or irregular. The P waves, if observed, are not related to the QRS complex. Ventricular tachycardia is a major dysrhythmia and must be treated immediately. (A, 10, M)

11. 3. Although coordinating documentation, resolving negative feelings, and calming down are goals of debriefing after a restraint, the ultimate outcome is to improve restraint procedures. (E, 1, X)

12. 3. ARDS frequently develops after a major insult to the body. The major diagnostic indicator is low arterial oxygen levels that are not responsive to the administration of high concentrations of oxygen. Early recognition of ARDS is important to increase the client's chances of recovery. The oxygen levels of clients with hypostatic pneumonia, hypovolemic shock, or asthma would be expected to improve with oxygen administration. (D, 10, M)

13. 2. By federal law, all clients entering a hospital or hospice program are offered the chance to make an advance directive, so that their wishes will be known

and followed in an emergency. The directive is not a substitute for informed discussion with the physician. Worry about extraordinary means being taken can be discussed with the client later, but the client needs to be informed that the directive is a federal requirement to protect the client's autonomy. (I, 1, M)

14. 4. The role of the nurse in witnessing the signing of the consent is not to witness that the client is fully aware of the rehabilitation. The nurse's role is to witness that the client is informed of the procedure, understands the information, and is signing of his or her own free will. (I, 1, M)

15. 1. Temporal arteritis, often seen in the elderly, can result in blindness if not treated quickly with steroids. The dose is individualized and depends on the elevation of the sedimentation rate. The client may need to take steroids for several weeks to months. (I, 8, M)

16. 4. Doxycycline is contraindicated in pregnancy because it can stain the teeth and affect the bones of the developing fetus. The nurse should hold the drug and notify the physician to change the order. All neonates are given prophylactic ophthalmic ointment for the prevention of ophthalmic neonatorum, conjunctivitis caused by gonorrhea. (I, 8, M)

17. 3. The contraction stress test simulates labor and determines the fetal response to the labor process and the mother's contractions. Therefore, determining that contractions have ceased after the test is important. Although spontaneous rupture of membranes is a possibility after a contraction stress test, it is not a typical occurrence. The test should not affect the viability of the fetus. Fetal viability is related to gestational age. A fetus of at least 23 weeks' gestation is considered viable, or capable of extrauterine life. A negative contraction stress test should not affect or alter fetal heart rate variability. (A, 9, O)

18. 1. A postoperative ileus is a functional obstruction of the bowel. Assessment of bowel sounds, the first stool, and the amount of gastric output provide information about the return of gastric function. Measurement of urine specific gravity provides information about fluid and electrolyte status. (A, 9, Y)

19. 2. Salmeterol is a β_2-agonist, a maintenance drug that the asthmatic client uses twice daily, every 12 hours. Albuterol (Proventil) is used as the "rescue inhaler" for bronchospasms. Serevent can be used to prevent exercise-induced bronchospasms, but it should be taken 30 to 60 minutes before exercise. If the client is taking Serevent twice daily, it should not be used in additional doses before exercise; twice daily is the maximum dose. Indications for Serevent include only asthma and bronchospasm induced by chronic obstructive pulmonary disease. (I, 8, M)

20. 4. Because clozapine can cause tachycardia, the nurse should hold the medication if the pulse rate is greater than 140 bpm and notify the physician. Giving the drug or telling the client to go exercise could be detrimental to the client. (I, 8, X)

21. 1. Valproic acid is the treatment of choice for absence seizures. Dilantin is used for major motor seizures. Neurontin is indicated for partial seizures. Paxil is indicated for depression and panic disorders. (D, 8, M)

22. 2. The best approach by the mother is not to interfere. The children need to learn how to solve disagreements on their own. If the parent always intervenes, then the children do not learn how to do this. Siblings will disagree and argue as part of normal development. Punishment, including telling the children that they will not go out to lunch, is not warranted. (E, 3, Y)

23. 4. Hyperventilation causes the excessive loss of carbon dioxide. This results in a decreased carbonic acid content of the blood. The kidneys will try to compensate by eliminating bicarbonate to maintain a normal ratio of carbonic acid to bicarbonate, but this takes several days. If compensatory efforts are insufficient, the client will develop respiratory alkalosis. Hyperventilation does deplete oxygen levels. Arterial blood gas studies do not evaluate sodium or potassium levels. (E, 9, M)

24. 2. Managing stressful life events can decrease the incidence of outbreaks of HSV-2. Occlusive ointments should not be applied. Antiviral therapies will not cure herpes, but they can manage symptoms and decrease the incidence of outbreaks. Clients with HSV-2 should use condoms to prevent HSV transmission. Cells can be shed at other times, not only when the vesicles are weeping. (I, 7, M)

25. 2. Tinnitus or a ringing in the ears is a clinical manifestation of altered function of the auditory branch of the eighth cranial nerve, not the vestibular branch. Ototoxic side effects affecting the vestibular branch of the acoustic nerve include vertigo, nausea and vomiting with motion, and ataxia. (A, 8, M)

26. 1. Tetanus toxoid is indicated, since there has been no booster in the last 5 years. Tetanus is not administered intravenously. With a human bite there is a potential of severe infection. The closure of the wound should be delayed until it is determined that there is no infection, in approximately 24 to 48 hours. (I, 8, M)

27. 3. One of the advantages of subdermal hormonal implants for contraception is that this form can be used by a client who is breast-feeding 6 weeks after delivery without adverse effects on the neonate. Subdermal hormonal implants are progesterone based. Therefore, the same side effects as those associated with progesterone

therapy may occur. After subdermal hormonal implants are discontinued (removed), fertility returns rapidly because ovulation resumes quickly. Subdermal hormonal implants do not offer protection against sexually transmitted diseases. Only condoms or abstinence offers such protection. (E, 8, O)

28. 3. Diuretics and digoxin are first-line therapy for symptom control and management of heart failure. SSRI are used to treat depression. (A, 8, M)

29. 3. With a parent who is visibly upset, it is best to try to determine what the cause is. Therefore, asking the mother about why she wants to take the child home can provide insight into what the problem is. The nurse cannot stop the mother from taking her child home. However, the physician should be notified about the mother's decision and efforts are needed to explain the ramifications of taking the child home. It is inappropriate for the nurse to say "I know how you feel" or "I can imagine how hard this is" unless the nurse has had the same experience. (I, 5, Y)

30. 2. Prolonged inactivity causes the body to excrete excessive calcium. This leads to breakdown of bone tissue; as a result, the bones become brittle and fracture easily, a condition known as osteoporosis. The excessive calcium excretion that occurs during bed rest also predisposes the client to formation of renal calculi. Prolonged bed rest does not increase sodium retention, insulin use, or red blood cell production. (A, 10, M)

31. 1. Normal urine output for an infant is 1 to 2 mL/kg/hour. (A, 10, Y)

32. 2. Based on the data given, the most appropriate nursing diagnosis is Activity Intolerance related to severe left leg pain. The other diagnoses are not supported by the data presented. There is no clinical indication that the leg will need to be amputated or that the client is experiencing a disturbance in body image. A temperature of 101°F (38.3°C) would be unlikely to produce a fluid volume deficit in this client. (D, 10, M)

33. 3. After vasectomy, a sperm analysis will be performed every 4 to 6 weeks. A sperm-free analysis is necessary before the man can be considered sterile. Sperm gradually disappear from the ejaculate. Clients must be informed that conception is possible in the immediate postvasectomy period. (I, 9, M)

34. 3. Garamycin is ototoxic; therefore, the client should have a vestibular and auditory check 3 to 4 weeks after discontinuing the drug. This is the most likely time for deafness to occur. It is not necessary to check the client's hemoglobin level, white blood cell count, or serum potassium level solely on the basis of having been taking gentamycin. The blood urea nitrogen level and the creatinine level will be checked to assess renal function, if necessary. (I, 9, M)

35. 2. Coughing and deep-breathing are more effective when pain is minimal. A client in severe pain tends to limit movement and to breathe shallowly to decrease the pain. Enough pain medication should be given to decrease pain without depressing respirations; this allows the client to cough effectively. Administration of oxygen or forcing fluids will not prevent atelectasis or pneumonia. Deep-breathing exercises should be performed at least every 2 hours. (I, 10, M)

36. 2. A child who has had rheumatic fever is likely to develop the illness again after a future streptococcal infection. Therefore, it is advised that such a child receive antibiotic prophylaxis for at least 5 years and sometimes even longer after the acute attack to prevent recurrence. (I, 8, Y)

37. 4. Crowning occurs when the fetal head is visible. Anterior-posterior slit occurs as the perineum flattens and is followed by an oval opening. As labor progresses, the perineum takes on a circular shape, followed by crowning. (A, 10, O)

38. 1. The first action is to increase the oxygen flow rate from 2 to 4 L/minute to help ensure adequate oxygenation for the client. Although it is important to notify the physician for additional orders and to obtain further assessment data such as arterial blood gas measurements, it is a priority to support the client's cardiopulmonary system. It would be appropriate to reassure the client while these other interventions are occurring. (I, 9, M)

39. 2. Although a cool air vaporizer may be recommended to humidify the environment, using saline nose drops and then a bulb syringe before meals and at nap and bed times will allow the child to breathe more easily. Saline helps to loosen secretions and keep the mucous membranes moist. The bulb syringe then gently aids in removing the loosened secretions. Blowing into the child's mouth to clear the nose introduces more organisms to the child. A nonprescription vasoconstrictive nasal spray is not recommended for infants, because if the spray is used for longer than 3 days a rebound effect with increased inflammation occurs. (I, 9, Y)

40. 3. Voice hoarseness may indicate metastatic disease to the recurrent laryngeal nerve and is most often noted with left upper lobe lung tumors. Diarrhea and constipation are not associated with lung cancer. Weight loss can be a symptom of extensive disease. (A, 10, M)

41. 1. A client with metabolic alkalosis may exhibit confusion, nervousness, or irritability, which can be the result of hypoventilation and increased carbon dioxide retention. Hyperventilation is a clinical manifestation of respiratory alkalosis. Diarrhea is a possible clinical finding in metabolic acidosis. Edema is not specifically associated with an acid–base imbalance. (a, 10, M)

42. 2. An initial sign of hemorrhaging after a tonsillectomy is swallowing frequently as mucus and blood combine to increase secretions. Increased pulse rate is a later sign of hemorrhage. Mouth breathing is expected after surgery because the child's mouth is very dry and the throat is sore. Because the child has been without fluids for a period of time, the child usually is thirsty and asks for a drink. (A, 9, Y)

43. 1. The nurse should not restart a new intravenous catheter at a different site. The nurse should keep the catheter patent at the original blood transfusion site so that a normal saline drip can be started immediately in case of hypotension and the need for emergency intravenous medication. (I, 8, M)

44. 3. The flow rate is determined by the rate of infusion and the number of drops per milliliter of the fluid being administered: drops/mL × mL/minute = IV flow rate (drops/minute). Therefore, 10 gtt/mL × 100 mL/30 minutes = 33 gtt/minute. (I, 8, M)

45. 4. Delusions of grandeur provide the client with an exaggerated sense of self-esteem that is unrelated to the client's actual achievements. Other, less grandiose, religious delusions may provide comfort or meaning for the client. Delusions of persecution are frequently related to safety issues. Delusions may also be related to sexual issues. (D, 6, X)

46. 3. Loss of electrolytes from the gastrointestinal tract through vomiting, diarrhea, or nasogastric suction is a common cause of potassium loss, resulting in hypokalemia. Hypermagnesia does not result from excessive loss of gastrointestinal fluids. Common causes of hypernatremia are water loss (as in diabetes insipidus or osmotic diuresis) and excessive sodium intake. Common causes of hypocalcemia include chronic renal failure, elevated phosphorus concentration, and primary hypoparathyroidism. (P, 10, M)

47. 3. It is a normal variation for women to have long-term, bilateral nipple inversion. A woman who has a unilateral nipple inversion that is a new change is at risk for a tumor; the weight of the tumor causes pulling on the nipple. A pronounced unilateral venous pattern, peau d'orange breast tissue, and breast tissue darker than the areolae are definite warning signals for breast cancer that must be reported to the physician immediately. (D, 4, M)

48. 1. It is important for children with sickle cell disease to drink lots of fluids to help prevent a crisis. Dehydration precipitates sickling and a crisis. Although taking the child's temperature may provide information about the child's status, it will do nothing to prevent a crisis, nor would weighing the child daily. Offering the child a high-protein diet will not prevent a crisis, nor is it recommended. (I, 10, Y)

49. 1. The nurse notifies the pediatrician because a short, webbed neck is associated with genetic deviations, such as chromosomal disorders. Cleft palate is associated with embryonic developmental failures and an abnormal opening in the palate. Potter's syndrome (renal agenesis) is characterized by an atypical facial appearance consisting of a flat nose, recessed chin, epicanthal folds, low-set abnormal ears, limb abnormalities, and pulmonary hypoplasia. Neural tube defects are associated with spina bifida or myelomeningocele. (D, 9, O)

50. 3. Clinical manifestation of hypokalemia include an irregular pulse, fatigue, muscle weakness, flabby muscles, decreased reflexes, nausea, vomiting, and ileus. Muscle spasms are not seen in hypokalemia. Thirst is a symptom of hypernatremia. Confusion can be seen in hyponatremia and hypocalcemia. (E, 10, M)

51. 2. Pruritus, or skin itching, is not one of the clinical manifestations of a superinfection, which is a new infection caused by microorganisms different from the ones causing the initial infection. A black, hairy tongue; glossitis; and anal itching are clinical manifestations of a superinfection. (A, 8, M)

52. 2. The client's self-report of pain is the most reliable indicator of the existence and intensity of the pain. Client response to pain is highly individualized and subjective. The nurse must respect the client's self-report. (A, 10, M)

53. 2. Excessive milk consumption can often lead to the displacement of iron-rich foods in the diet. This can result in iron-deficiency anemia. (A, 4, M)

54. 2. Although all the symptoms listed can manifest in cases of fat embolism syndrome, confusion is the earliest symptom noted. The confusion is caused by a low arterial oxygen level. (A, 10, M)

55. 1. An idea of reference is a person's view that other people recognize that she has an important characteristic or power. Thought insertion refers to a person's belief that others, or a specific other, can put thoughts into her mind. Visual hallucinations involve seeing objects or persons not based in reality. A neologism is a word or phrase that has meaning only to the person using it. (D, 6, X)

56. 3. To test the hearing ability of a neonate, the nurse should position himself or herself approximately 12 inches away from the neonate and make a loud noise, such as clapping the hands. (A, 9, O)

57. 4. The equianalgesic dose of oral meperidine hydrochloride is up to four times the IM dosage. Meperidine hydrochloride can be given orally, but it is much more effective when given by the IM route. (D, 8, M)

58. 1. In order to prevent disuse osteoporosis, it is important to implement weight-bearing activities as soon as medically allowed. Increasing the client's calcium will not prevent the development of osteoporosis without the inclusion of weight-bearing activity. Passive range-of-motion exercises and isometric exercises do not provide the bone stress necessary to reduce the risk of osteoporosis. (I, 9, M)

59. 3. Toddlers have temper tantrums in their attempt to develop autonomy. Toddlers should be left alone as long as they are safe during a tantrum. Moving the child to a "time-out" chair or punishing the child reinforces the behavior and is to be avoided. Attempting to talk to the toddler also reinforces the behavior. Additionally, at this cognitive level, toddlers do not understand as well as older children do. (I, 3, Y)

60. 1. When a nurse has been stuck by a used needle and has not completed the hepatitis B vaccination, he or she should receive both active and passive immunization. (I, 4, M)

61. 2. Daily skin inspection is essential in preventing pressure ulcers. Hot water is irritating to skin and should be avoided. Massaging bony prominences is contraindicated and may actually promote skin breakdown. Prolonged, uninterrupted chair sitting should be avoided; the client's position should be adjusted at least every hour. (I, 9, M)

62. 3. Skeletal pins should not be loose and able to move. Any pin loosening should be reported immediately. Slight serous drainage is normal and may crust around the insertion site or be present on the dressing. The pin insertion site should be cleansed with aseptic technique according to institution policy. Pin insertion sites are typically not painful; pain may be indicative of an infection and should be reported. (E, 9, M)

63. 4. Acknowledging the basic feeling that the client expressed and asking an open-ended question allows the client to explain her fears. Saying, "It's normal to be scared. We'll help you through it," does not focus on the client's feelings; rather, it gives reassurance. Asking if the client feels guilty for having smoked assumes guilt, which might be present, but additional information is needed to confirm. Telling the client not to be so hard on herself does not acknowledge the client's feelings at all. (I, 5, M)

64. 3. It is important that clients with rheumatoid arthritis maintain proper posture and body alignment to support joints and decrease pain and stiffness. Clients with hip pain will be most comfortable when sitting in a straight-back chair with an elevated seat. Elevated seats avoid excessive hip flexion and place less stress on the hip joints. (E, 9, M)

65. 3. Giving away personal items has consistently been shown to be an indicator of suicidal plans in the depressed and suicidal individual. The other behaviors indicate a return of interest in normal adolescent activities. (I, 6, X)

66. 3. When a neonate dies, the mother should be allowed to stay with the baby as long as she wants and say anything she wants. She is grieving and needs time with the neonate. A photograph should be taken in case the mother wants a photograph at a later time. Telling the mother that this is for the best is inappropriate because such a statement discounts the mother's feelings. Advising the mother to get pregnant again to get over the loss is not helpful because the mother needs time to grieve and be with the neonate. The nurse should remain near the mother and not delegate this responsibility to the hospital's chaplain. A chaplain or other religious member can be contacted if the mother desires. (I, 5, O)

67. 4. Serum albumin levels help determine whether protein intake is sufficient. Proteins are broken down into amino acids during digestion. Amino acids are absorbed in the small intestine, and albumin is built from amino acids. The red blood cell count, bilirubin levels, and reticulocyte count do not indicate protein intake. (A, 4, M)

68. 2. The client who is taking desmopressin (DDAVP) nasal spray should not use the same nares for administration each time. The client should alternate nares every dose. The client should observe for and report promptly signs of nasal ulceration, congestion, or respiratory infection. (I, 8, M)

69. 3. 500 mg/mL = 250 mg / x mL; x = 0.5 mL. (I, 8, M)

70. 3. Common clinical manifestations of hypokalemia include ventricular dysrhythmias, weak and irregular pulse, soft and flabby muscles, and decreased deep tendon reflexes. Hypercalcemia causes confusion and decreased memory, bone pain, polyuria, and nausea, vomiting, and constipation. Hypernatremia causes signs of fluid volume deficit. Hypomagnesemia is manifested by tremors, confusion, hyperactive deep tendon reflexes, and seizures. (A, 10, M)

71. 3. As with other contraceptives that are progestin based, heavy menstrual bleeding may occur. Other side effects include rash, acne, alopecia, fluid retention, edema, and sudden loss of vision. Depression and weight gain have been reported. For clients taking this drug, the risk of endometrial or ovarian cancer is decreased. Amenorrhea has been reported after receiving four injections 3 months apart for 1 year. Depression and loss of energy have been reported. (P, 8, O)

72. 4. Clients with burns are susceptible to the development of Curling's ulcer, a gastroduodenal ulcer that is caused by a generalized stress response. The stress response results in increased gastric acid secretion and a decreased production of mucus. Prevention is the best treatment, and clients are frequently treated prophylactically with antacids and H_2 histamine blockers such as cimetidine. (P, 9, M)

73. 2. Fever is a cardinal manifestation of infection in people with AIDS. Because the major physiologic alteration in AIDS is generalized immune system dysfunction, typical indicators of the body's response to infection (eg, erythema, warmth, tenderness) may be absent. (I, 10, Y)

74. 2. To care effectively for clients with depression, the nurse would teach the importance of demonstrating empathetic concern. Caregivers must accept clients as they are even though many will be angry and negative, acknowledge their emotional pain, and offer to help them work through their pain. For the client who is depressed, using a cheerful demeanor or a humorous, lighthearted approach may be overwhelming because the client will be unable to meet the caregiver's expectations, subsequently leading to decreased self-worth. A serious, business-like affect may threaten the client and inhibit the development of trust. (I, 1, X)

75. 4. When a child is ready to take fluids by mouth postoperatively, clear liquids are given initially. If clear liquids are tolerated, the concentration and amount of oral feedings are gradually increased. This means advancing to half-strength and then to full-strength formula while increasing the amount given with each feeding. (I, 7, Y)

76. 2. The nurse would monitor the client taking paroxetine (Paxil), an SSRI, for sexual problems such as decreased libido, impotence, and ejaculatory disturbances, because these side effects can occur frequently and lead to medication noncompliance. Sleep disturbances can occur with an SSRI such as paroxetine. However, this client is taking the drug every morning, which would not affect nighttime sleep. A hypertensive crisis is associated with the ingestion of foods rich in tyramine when a client is taking a monoamine oxidase inhibitor (MAOI). Orthostatic hypotension is a potential side effect with tricyclic antidepressants (TCAs). (I, 8, X)

77. 1. This diet is based on experimental research indicating that diets low in potassium are often associated with hypertension. Higher-potassium diets appear to prevent and correct hypertension. Magnesium deficiency causes artery walls and capillaries to constrict and therefore raises blood pressure. Magnesium intake within the normal range lowers blood pressure. Vitamin C helps to normalize blood pressure. Calcium lowers blood pressure in healthy people and in those with hypertension. (D, 4, M)

78. 2. In the progressive stage of shock, the client can display listlessness or agitation, confusion, and slowed speech. Restlessness occurs in the compensatory stage. Incoherent speech and unconsciousness are clinical manifestations of the irreversible stage. (A, 10, M)

79. 1. When the crash cart arrives, ECG electrodes are applied to the client's chest. If the client is found to be in ventricular fibrillation, the immediate priority is to defibrillate the client. Pulse oximetry is not an immediate priority. The client's oxygenation is evaluated in a code situation using arterial blood gas analysis. The client's blood pressure is evaluated after the ECG rhythm has been established. A portable Doppler ultrasound unit may be needed to check for the presence of a pulse or to check the blood pressure in a code situation. (D, 10, M)

80. 2. Heroin causes pupils to be pinpoints. Marijuana causes the eyes to appear red and bloodshot. Cocaine use causes pupils to dilate. Drooping of the eyelids is not typically associated with the use of any substance. (I, 6, Y)

81. 3. A typical sign of pediculosis capitis (head lice) is frequent scratching of the scalp, because the condition causes severe itching. Scratch marks are usually easily visible. Because head lice are easily transmitted to others, the child's family members and peers also should be examined for infestation. Spotty baldness, wheals, and scaly lesions are often allergic in nature. (A, 10, Y)

82. 1. Passing flatus indicates the return of peristalsis, as does active bowel sounds. Hunger is not the best indicator of peristaltic return. Hypoactive bowel sounds indicate that there is some peristaltic activity but it is limited and not yet normal. Palpitation is not an appropriate method of assessing bowel activity. (E, 10, M)

83. 3. The pH of 7.24 indicates that the client is acidotic. The pCO_2 value of 49 mm Hg is elevated. The HCO_3^- value of 24 mEq/L is normal. The client is in uncompensated respiratory acidosis. Hypoventilation and a flushed appearance are additional clinical manifestations of respiratory acidosis. (D, 10, M)

84. 2. It is essential for the nurse to evaluate the effects of pain medication after it has had time to act. Although other interventions may be appropriate, continual reassessment is most important to determine effectiveness and the need for additional intervention, if any. Repositioning could provide some comfort, but assessment of the client's pain level is essential. Reassuring the client is important, but it will be of no value unless the nurse evaluates the client's pain level. To readjust pain dosage is appropriate only if titration is prescribed by the physician. (E, 10, M)

85. 1. Barrier contraceptives must be used to protect against STDs. Birth control pills and douching are not

effective for prevention of STDs. Prophylactic antibiotics are not used to prevent the acquisition of STDs. (E, 2, M)

86. 2. A purplish-blue discoloration of the vagina and cervix is termed Chadwick's sign; it is caused by increased vascularity of the vagina during pregnancy. It is considered a probable sign of pregnancy. Goodell's sign, considered a probable sign of pregnancy, refers to a softening of the cervix during pregnancy. Hegar's sign, also a probable sign of pregnancy, refers to a softening of the lower uterine segment. Melasma, the mask of pregnancy, refers to the pigmentation of the skin on the face during pregnancy. Melasma is considered a presumptive sign of pregnancy. (A, 3, O)

87. 3. Initially, the nurse would tell the client to seek out staff when feeling agitated or upset to prevent violent episodes. Doing so helps the client to redirect negative feelings in an appropriate manner (eg, talking). Encouraging the client to stay in his room is inappropriate because it does not help the client to deal with his feelings. Secluding the client at the first sign of agitation is not indicated and may be perceived by the client as punishment. Instructing the client to ask for medication when agitated would not be the initial course of action. The nurse would interact with the client and direct the client to an activity to decrease his anxiety before intervening with any PRN medication. (I, 6, X)

88. 3. The nurse should use short words, sentences, and paragraphs and avoid medical jargon. Correct terminology should be used when appropriate (eg, type 1 diabetes, not "sugar diabetes"). The format should be as simple as possible; charts are not necessary and may be confusing to some clients. Information should be prepared at a fifth-grade reading level. The information should be presented in large-sized type. (P, 5, M)

89. 4. It is normal for the client to feel pressure on the palms of the hands when walking with crutches. The client should move her affected (right) leg forward first as she swings forward with the crutches. Leaning on the crutches can apply pressure to the axillae, leading to neurovascular impairment. If the client's arms are tingling after she uses her crutches, she is probably applying pressure on her axillae when walking. (E, 7, M)

90. 2. Because clients are discharged as soon as possible from the hospital, it is essential to evaluate the support for assistance and self-care at home. (D, 1, M)

91. 3. If the client begins breast-feeding early and often after delivery, the breasts begin to fill with milk within 48 to 96 hours, or 2 to 4 days. The breasts secrete colostrum for the first 24 to 48 hours, which is beneficial to the neonate because of the immunoglobulins contained in colostrum. (I, 3, O)

92. 3. The predominant clinical finding in elderly or debilitated clients indicating that they have developed pneumonia is confusion, which results from hypoxia. Fever and chills, productive cough, and pleuritic chest pain could be present, but confusion is the predominant development. (A, 1, M)

93. 1. It is important for the child and family to understand that chorea associated with rheumatic fever is not permanent. Therefore, the nurse would explain that the chorea will disappear over time. It is not necessary to assess the child's neurologic status, because the chorea is self-limited and nonprogressive. Because the child has cardiac involvement, ambulation is contraindicated. Aspirin is used primarily as an anti-inflammatory drug and secondarily for pain relief. A slightly cool environment is unnecessary. Environmental temperature does not affect the child's polyarthritis and chorea. (P, 10, Y)

94. 1. When the gestation is less than 13 weeks, a therapeutic abortion is usually performed by the dilation and curettage method. Menstrual extraction, or suction evacuation, is the easiest method, but it is used only when the client is between 5 and 7 weeks' gestation. Dilatation and vacuum extraction is used when clients are between 12 and 16 weeks' gestation. Saline induction, used for clients between 16 and 24 weeks' gestation, involves instillation of a hypertonic saline solution into the amniotic sac to initiate expulsion. Oxytocin infusion may also be used with saline induction. (I, 3, O)

95. 1. A pleural effusion is a collection of fluid between the pleural layers of the lung. The effusion decreases chest wall movement on the affected side. The nurse would expect the breath sounds to be decreased or diminished over the affected area. Because of the presence of fluid, percussion would elicit dullness, not hyperresonance. Fever may be present if emphysema has developed, but not in the case of a nonpurulent pleural effusion. (A, 10, M)

96. 1. An expected client outcome relative to the nursing diagnosis of Pain related to cramping is that the client exhibits no manifestations of discomfort, such as crying or drawing the legs to the abdomen. Being very still may indicate either a pain state or a state of relaxation. (P, 10, Y)

97. 2. 40 mg/mL = 25 mg / x mL; x = 0.6 mL. (I, 8, M)

98. 4. The client is exhibiting symptoms of herpes genitalis, which include painful blisters or vesicles that appear 2 to 20 days after transmission of the disease. The client was most likely exposed from her new partner. Vulvar pain, dyspareunia, dysuria, and flu-like symptoms also may be present. HIV infection is commonly manifested by numerous signs and symptoms such as persistent

candidiasis, anogenital condyloma, and herpes simplex infections. *Chlamydia trachomatis* infection is asymptomatic, often going undetected by affected women. Symptoms, when present, include a grayish-white discharge and vulvar itching. Syphilis typically is manifested by chancre occurring about 10 days after exposure. The chancre is usually deep but painless. (A, 9, O)

99. 2. It has been found that parents are more grieved when optimism is followed by defeat. The nurse should recognize this when planning various ways to help the parents of a dying child. It is not necessarily true that knowing about a poor prognosis for years helps prepare parents for a child's death, that trust in health personnel is destroyed when a death is untimely, or that it is more difficult for parents to accept the death of an older child than that of a younger child. (P, 5, Y)

100. 1. A client who has an allergy to penicillin may have a cross-sensitivity to cefazolin (Ancef), a first-generation cephalosporin, and the drug should be given with caution. The nurse should ask the client whether he has taken cefazolin before. The nurse should inform the pharmacy of the client's allergy after asking the client about prior use of cefazolin. The medication should not be administered until the nurse first inquires about the client's exposure to cefazolin and then consults with the pharmacist or physician. Observing the client for urticaria is appropriate but is not an initial response. (D, 2, M)

101. 3. Clients with chronic renal failure are susceptible to uremia, an accumulation of nitrogenous waste products in the blood. Clinical manifestations include dry, itchy skin that can be severe in nature. Because of the irritation of the skin and the inclination to scratch, clients are prone to impaired skin integrity. The pruritus is not a result of poor hygiene. Chronic pain is not a likely result of the pruritus and is not a priority nursing diagnosis. The data do not support the nursing diagnosis of Ineffective Coping. (D, 7, M)

102. 1. The nurse would teach the client taking lithium and his family about the importance of maintaining adequate sodium intake to prevent lithium toxicity. Because lithium is a salt, a reduced sodium intake could result in lithium retention with subsequent toxicity. Increasing sodium in the diet is not recommended and may be harmful. Increased sodium levels result in lower lithium levels. Therefore, the drug may not reach therapeutic effectiveness. (P, 8, X)

103. 3. Mucositis is a inflammation of the oral mucosa caused by radiation therapy. It is important that the client with mucositis receive meticulous mouth care, including flossing, to prevent the development of an infection. Mouth care should be provided before and after each meal, at bedtime, and more frequently as needed. Extremes of temperature should be avoided in food and drink. Half-strength hydrogen peroxide is too harsh to use on irritated tissues. (I, 9, M)

104. 2. The first treatment for ingestion of nonprescription medication is to empty the stomach. This can be achieved by giving syrup of ipecac and water. If the child does not vomit in 30 minutes, then the dose should be repeated. It is important that the parent attempt to empty the child's stomach before or during transport to the emergency department. (I, 8, Y)

105. 1. The best approach by the nurse is to determine why the parent thinks the child is hyperactive. Some children are very active but do not have the necessary defining characteristics of hyperactivity. Asking what the parent thinks needs to be done or how the child behaves normally would be an appropriate follow-up question once more information is gathered from the parent to determine whether the child indeed is hyperactive. Telling the parent to wait for the physician ignores the parent's concern and does not deal with the parent's issue. (I, 10, Y)

106. 2. Dilation at the anastomosis site is needed during the first years of childhood in about 50% of children who have had corrective surgery for TEF. Recurrent mild diarrhea with dehydration is not likely to develop with this surgery. Speech problems can occur if other abnormalities are present to produce them; the larynx and structures of speech are not affected by TEF. Dysphagia and strictures may decrease food intake, and poor weight gain may be noted, but gastric ulcers should not develop from surgery to repair TEF. (Y, I, 9)

107. 1. Terminally ill clients most often describe feelings of isolation because they feel ignored. The terminally ill client may sense any discomfort that family and friends feel in the client's presence. Nursing interventions include spending time with the client, encouraging discussion about feelings, and answering questions openly and honestly. Reducing fear of pain or fear of more aggressive therapies is secondary to lessening the client's feelings of isolation. Reducing feelings of social inadequacy is not relevant to the terminally ill client. (P, 5, M)

108. 2. When the fetus is in a breech position, the fetal heart rate most often is located above the umbilicus, because the fetal heart is near the top of the mother's uterus. The heart of a fetus in the cephalic position is typically located on either the left or the right side of the client's uterus. Also, because the fetal heart typically is located in the lower portion of the mother's uterus, the sounds would be heard below the umbilicus. With a face presentation, fetal heart sounds are typically located on

either the left or the right side of the client's uterus; in addition, because the fetal heart typically is located in the lower portion of the mother's uterus, the sounds would be heard below the umbilicus. When the fetus is in a transverse position, the fetal heart sounds typically would be located below the umbilicus and in the midline. (D, 3, O)

109. 4. Clients who have been diagnosed with pernicious anemia are lacking adequate amounts of the intrinsic factor (IF) that is secreted by the gastric mucosa. IF is necessary for the absorption of cobalamin (vitamin B_{12}) in the distal ileum. Without the presence of IF, dietary intake of vitamin B_{12} is useless because it cannot be absorbed. Treatment of pernicious anemia includes intramuscular injections of cobalamin, at first daily for 2 weeks, then weekly until the anemia is corrected. A maintenance schedule of monthly injections is then implemented. The injections will need to be continued for the rest of the client's life. (E, 10, M)

110. 2. The nurse should first take orange juice to the client, because a hypoglycemic reaction is likely to occur. The nurse (charge nurse or otherwise) should notify the physician for orders to prevent or treat severe hypoglycemia. The nurse could consult with the clinical pharmacist until able to contact the physician. The nurse should ask for assistance so that the client can be monitored by a nurse while someone prepares a longer-acting carbohydrate or protein. (D, 7, M)

111. 4. Safety is the priority in caring for this infant. Infants adapt easily, increasing mobility even with a splint in place. Therefore, the mother needs to ensure that the area in which the infant is mobile is safe. There is no need to contact the physician to alter the treatment plan. Confining the infant to one room may not allow the child to achieve normal development. The child needs different environments for maximum development. The infant needs to wear the splint as ordered by the physician to ensure optimal healing. (I, 2, Y)

112. 1. Anxiety in a preoperative client may be caused by many different fears, such as fear of the effects of anesthesia, the effects of surgery on body image, separation from family and friends, job loss, disability, pain, or death. However, fear of the unknown is most likely to be the greatest fear, because the client feels helpless. Therefore, an important part of preoperative nursing care is to assess the client for anxieties and explore possible causes. Emotional support can then be offered, so that the client is in the best possible psychological condition for surgery. (A, 5, M)

113. 1. An important nursing responsibility is preoperative teaching. The recommended guide for teaching is to tell the client as much as she wants to know and is able to understand. Delaying discussion of issues or concerns

will most likely increase the client's anxiety. Telling the client to discuss questions with the physician avoids acknowledging the client's concerns. (I, 5, M)

114. 3. The client must have adequate disclosure of the risks associated with the surgery before signing the consent form. It is the physician's responsibility to explain the risks of any procedures and to obtain the client's informed consent. If the nurse suspects that the client has not been truly informed, it is the responsibility of the nurse to act as a client advocate and contact the surgeon to provide additional information to the client. It is not appropriate to have the client sign the consent form if the client has questions. The nurse should not minimize the procedure or dismiss the client's concerns. (I, 1, M)

115. 4. In right occipital anterior lie, the occiput faces the right anterior segment of the woman's pelvis. In left occipital transverse lie, the occiput faces left the woman's left hip. In left occipital anterior lie, the occiput faces the left anterior segment of the woman's pelvis. In right occipital transverse lie, the occiput faces the woman's right hip. (D, 10, O)

116. 2. Urinary tract infections in infants are a bit hard to diagnose because symptoms may be subtle, such as loss of appetite and fussiness. Dysuria and fever may also occur, but dysuria is harder to recognize in an infant. Increased urine output may occur, but it would be very difficult for the parent to actually determine this. Typically, urine is cloudy in appearance in an infant with a urinary tract infection. Feeding problems may occur, but jaundice would be a late sign. (I, 10, Y)

117. 3. A positive Babinski's reflex in a neonate is a normal finding demonstrating the immaturity of the central nervous system in corticospinal pathways. A neonate's muscle coordination is immature, but the Babinski's reflex does not help determine this immaturity. A positive Babinski's reflex does not indicate a defect in the spinal cord or an injury to nerves that innervate the legs. There is no evidence to suggest partial paralysis. A positive Babinski's reflex in an adult indicates disease. (O, E, 3)

118. 2. The nurse should instruct the client who is taking dexamethasone (Decadron) and furosemide (Lasix) to observe for signs of hypokalemia, such as malaise, muscle weakness, vomiting, and a paralytic ileus, because both dexamethasone and furosemide deplete the serum potassium. (P, 8, M)

119. 2. After a bronchoscopy with a biopsy, the nurse should monitor the client for signs of pneumothorax as well as hemorrhage. The client should not gargle with oral lidocaine; this will not allow the gag reflex to return. The client should not have any mediastinal discomfort after a bronchoscopy; if pain does occur it should be re-

ported promptly to the physician. It is not necessary to tell the client not to talk until the gag reflex returns. (I, 9, M)

120. 2. The number of drops the client should receive each minute is determined as follows: 500 mL / 12 hours = between 41 and 42 mL to be infused each hour; 42 mL × 60 (drop factor) = 2520 drops to be infused each hour; 2520 drops / 60 minutes = 42 drops to be infused every minute. (I, 8, Y)

121. 2. Subcutaneous injections are administered at an angle of 45 to 90 degrees, depending on the size of the client. Subcutaneous needles are typically $^3/_8$ to $^5/_8$ inches in length. The skin should be pinched up at the injection site to elevate the subcutaneous tissue. Air is not drawn into the syringe for a subcutaneous injection. (I, 8, M)

122. 3. Acute Pain is a priority nursing diagnosis for the client with pelvic inflammatory disease because the disease is associated with severe pain. Imbalanced Nutrition, Self-Care Deficit, and Impaired Skin Integrity are not priority nursing diagnoses associated with pelvic inflammatory disease. (D, 10, M)

123. 3. Children with difficult temperaments do better in structured environments than in environments with daily changes. This helps to teach them what to expect. Easy children do well with flexible feeding times. Children with easy temperaments do not cry often, and parents need to remember to feed them. Children with high activity levels, another type of temperament, who are always on the go, need to be watched more closely and need extra safety precautions taken around the house. (P, 3, Y)

124. 4. The position of the tube should be verified before the feeding is implemented. Warming the solution is not necessary or desirable because it can encourage bacterial growth. The client should be lying down with the head elevated or sitting upright during administration of the feeding. Gastric residual should be aspirated and then reinstilled to prevent electrolyte losses. (I, 9, M)

125. 4. The cramping is caused by the baby's sucking and subsequent stimulation for the release of oxytocin. This cramping is normal. With each subsequent pregnancy, the uterus becomes "stretched" and the release of oxytocin causes the uterus to contract, resulting in the feeling of cramping. Continued moderate to large amounts of lochia rubra is indicative of retained placental fragments. Cramping indicates that the uterus is contracting and most likely firm. A boggy uterus, continued moderate to heavy lochia, mild vasoconstriction, and restlessness and anxiety suggest delayed postpartum hemorrhage due to subinvolution of the placental site, retained placental tissue, or infection. Most clients

receive a standard dose of oxytocin (Pitocin) after delivery. Oxytocin has a duration of action of 60 minutes. Therefore, the effects of the drug would have worn off by 24 hours postpartum. (I, 3, O)

126. 4. The current recommendations for children experiencing mild to moderate diarrhea are to continue the child's regular diet. With this diet plan, children seem to get well faster. Clear liquids, such as juices, colas, and gelatin, are high in carbohydrates but low in electrolytes, as are foods such as bananas, rice, applesauce, and toast. Foods low in fat also typically lack the electrolytes that the child needs. (I, 9, Y)

127. 2. When performing tracheostomy care, it is important that the tracheostomy ties be securely tied to prevent dislodgment of the tube. It is not necessary to remove the inner cannula every 2 hours for cleaning. Routine cleansing is usually performed every 8 hours. The nurse should use precut tracheostomy dressings under the neck plate to protect the skin surrounding the stoma. Cutting and using a gauze dressing can cause loose gauze fibers to enter the airway. The inner cannula should be suctioned before cleansing, not afterward. (I, 7, M)

128. 2. The nurse should send the sealed container of IV 50% dextrose found in the catch-all bin to the pharmacy. A concentrated medication such as 50% dextrose could be lethal if inadvertently administered and should be not be stored outside the pharmacy. An incident report is not necessary in this situation. The sharps container is not the appropriate method for disposal of this medication. (D, 1, M)

129. 3. The client who is wheelchair-bound with a spinal cord injury should be taught to make small weight shifts, lifting off the sacral area every 15 minutes. This decreases the risk of pressure ulcer formation. Bathing daily promotes skin cleanliness, but by itself it will not prevent pressure ulcer formation. Eating a well-balanced diet that includes proteins and carbohydrates promotes good skin integrity. Moving from the bed to the wheelchair every 2 hours is not desirable because the client should not spend excessive amounts of time in bed. Pressure sores can develop in less than 2 hours. (I, 10, M)

130. 1. Anatomically, the squatting position enlarges the pelvic outlet and uses the force of gravity during pushing. The mother should curve her body into a C shape for the greatest effectiveness. (I, 3, O)

131. 2. Saying, "If you punch people out, you'll get arrested," helps the client by pointing out the negative consequences of his behavior. Clients with antisocial personality disorder are aggressive, impulsive, and reckless; engage in illegal activities; and lack guilt or remorse. The nurse teaches the client that there are con-

sequences to his irresponsible behavior and that the way to stay out of trouble is to change his behavior. Saying, "It's wrong to punch others," is not helpful since the client does not feel guilt or remorse. Saying, "I wouldn't do that again if I were you" or "Don't ever do that again," is authoritative and scolds the client without helping him. (I, 6, X)

132. 3. Self-mutilation is a way to express anger and rage, commonly seen in clients with borderline personality disorder. It typically is a cry for help, an expression of intense anger, helplessness, or guilt. When a client is experiencing numbness or feelings of unreality, self-mutilation induces physical pain which validates the person's being alive because of the ability to feel the physical pain. Self-mutilation is not a means of getting what the person wants. It is not used as a form of manipulation, although it is often misinterpreted as such. Self-mutilation is a serious behavior that is harmful to the self and cannot be ignored. (E, 6, X)

133. 3. Hepatitis C is transferred by percutaneous exposure, such as tattooing. Hepatitis A is acquired through contaminated water, exposure in underdeveloped countries, or shellfish in contaminated waters. (A, 9, M)

134. 1. Lorazepam (Ativan), a benzodiazepine, is commonly used to decrease the symptoms of central nervous system irritability in the client who is experiencing symptoms of alcohol withdrawal. Diazepam (Valium) and chlordiazepoxide (Librium), also benzodiazepines, may be used in some instances. Naltrexone (ReVia) is an opioid-receptor antagonist that interferes with opioid functioning and reduces the craving for alcohol and narcotics. It is used as an adjunct for treating alcohol or narcotic dependence. Methadone (Dolophine) is an opioid similar to morphine. It is used to treat opioid dependence. Imipramine (Tofranil) is a tricyclic antidepressant used to treat major depression. It also may be used as a substitute for heroin and narcotics in clients who want to terminate drug use. (P, 8, X)

135. 3. After surgery, the nurse's initial assessment is the surgical site dressing to determine whether there is any bleeding or drainage. Once this assessment is completed, then the nurse would assess the other areas such as the intravenous access site, pain, and nasogastric tube function. (A, 10, Y)

136. 1. The nurse should use the radial artery to obtain blood gas samples, because it is easier to maintain firm pressure there than on the femoral artery. Nursing interventions to protect the client who has received t-PA or alteplase recombinant (Activase) therapy include maintaining arterial pressure for 30 seconds, because it takes longer for coagulation to occur with the thrombolytic agent onboard. Intramuscular injections are contraindicated during thrombolytic therapy. The

nurse should prevent physical manipulation of the client, which can cause bruising. (I, 10, M)

137. 3. Experimental and epidemiologic research indicates that approximately 50% of all patients with hypertension can lower their blood pressure through dietary sodium reduction. (D, 4, M)

138. 4. Serum amylase and lipase are increased in pancreatitis, as is the urinary amylase. Other abnormal laboratory values include hypocalcemia, hyperglycemia, and hyperlipidemia. (A, 10, M)

139. 2. For the client with an alcohol or drug problem, group sessions are helpful in dealing with emotions and concerns about alcohol and drugs. Clients with substance abuse problems identify with each other's similar experiences and can best help each other deal with these feelings and emotions. Additionally, the members of the group are able to support and confront each other. Individual therapy is not as helpful as group sessions because group members offer peer support and confrontation when needed. Solitary activities and recreation lead to increased avoidance of the issues that must be faced and dealt with by the client. These are often areas that the client must learn to develop and manage while in recovery. (I, 9, X)

140. 4. Foul-smelling urine is indicative of cystitis. Other symptoms include dysuria, frequency, and urgency. Flank pain, nausea, and vomiting indicate pyelonephritis. (A, 10, M)

141. 4. By saying, "You couldn't have prevented the tornado, it just happened," the nurse helps the client to develop an objective perspective and promotes a better understanding of the event. The other statements tell the client how to feel, possibly causing resistance and thus delay therapeutic healing. Guilt and self-blame will not be decreased. (I, 6, X)

142. 3. In many Asian cultures, the 30 days after the birth of the neonate is a time for the mother to heal from the delivery. The appropriate action by the nurse is to determine whether this is a cultural practice for this client and her family. If so, then the client is behaving within her cultural practices. Teaching should be provided to both the mother and her mother-in-law. There is no indication that bonding is not taking place. Lack of bonding might be indicated if the client did not show any interest in the neonate. Documenting the client's maternal behavior in her chart is a routine task. However, the nurse should not assume that this behavior is unusual, because it may be reflective of the client's cultural framework. A home visit is not warranted unless there is evidence of infant neglect or the family needs additional follow-up or teaching. (I, 3, O)

143. 1. A creatinine clearance test is a 24-hour urine test that measures the degree of protein breakdown in the body.

The collection is not maintained in a sterile container. There is no need to insert a Foley catheter as long as the client is able to control urination. It is not necessary to force fluids. (A, 7, M)

144. 4. The statement, "Your eyes look dark," is the least sensitive statement because it points out an obvious difference for no real purpose. The nurse has a reason to ask the client about favorite foods and needs to know about past health problems. Also, it is appropriate for the nurse to ask the client how she wishes to be addressed. (D, 6, M)

145. 2. Insight into the illness is demonstrated when the client recognizes the relationship between the chemical imbalance and his illness and symptoms. Stating that the olanzapine is the best medicine or that the client's mother is proud of him for staying on his medicines reflects awareness about the effect of medications and the need for compliance. Stating that he may be able to get a part-time job indicates an awareness of his increased capacity for work. (E, 6, X)

146. 3. Carpal tunnel syndrome is a condition in which the median nerve becomes compressed in the wrist. The brachial nerve is not affected. Carpal tunnel syndrome may be the result of a systemic disease such as rheumatoid arthritis or diabetes mellitus, or it may be an occupational hazard for people whose jobs require repetitive hand movements. It is not a condition resulting from disuse. The wrists do not develop flexion contractures with carpal tunnel syndrome. (I, 9, M)

147. 1. Seventy-five percent of all food allergies are caused by milk, eggs, or peanuts. (A, 9, M)

148. 3. Clients who have undergone a TURP need to be instructed to maintain an adequate fluid intake despite urinary dribbling or incontinence. The client should be advised to drink at least 8 glasses of water a day to dilute the urine and help prevent urinary tract infections. Maintaining a voiding schedule of every 2 hours can help decrease incidents of incontinence. Teaching the client Kegel exercises is also beneficial for strengthening sphincter tone. The nurse should not encourage the client to decrease fluids. It is not necessarily true that a decreased intake will cause renal calculi. Threatening the client with a catheter is not beneficial, and it is not the treatment of choice for a client who is experiencing incontinence from a TURP. (I, 10, M)

149. 1. Risk for Infection would be a priority nursing diagnosis after surgery. With any type of incision, the immediate concern is preventing infection at the site. Pain is also a diagnosis of concern and would be next in order of priority. The infant would be partially restrained to prevent disturbance of the IV infusion and nasogastric tube. Bowel elimination should begin in a few days. (D, 10, Y)

150. 4. Risk factors for TSS include the use of tampons at night, when the tampon would be in place for 7 to 9 hours. TSS can occur in other situations, but it is most often associated with women during menses, particularly women who use tampons. The longer the tampon is left in place, the greater the risk for TSS. Changing tampons every 3 hours or more frequently, avoiding use of deodorized tampons, and alternating tampons with sanitary pads are actions that decrease the risk for TSS. (I, 4, M)

151. 4. Costovertebral tenderness occurs on the side of the affected kidney in pyelonephritis. Dysuria, suprapubic pain, and urinary retention may occur in pyelonephritis but do not specifically support a diagnosis of pyelonephritis. Dysuria, suprapubic pain, and urinary retention are symptoms of cystitis, which can lead to pyelonephritis if not treated. (A, 10, M)

152. 2. Broad-spectrum antibiotics can cause decreased efficacy of contraceptives, placing the client at risk for an unplanned pregnancy. When a client is prescribed a course of antibiotics, a back-up method of contraceptive should be used. Antihypertensives, diuretics, and antihistamines do not interfere with oral contraceptive efficacy. (I, 8, M)

153. 1. Side effects of danazol (Danocrine) include headaches, dizziness, irritability, and decreased libido. Masculinization effects such as deepened voice, facial hair, and weight gain may occur. (I, 8, O)

154. 2. The nurse should assign the male client of Mexican American descent who needs complete morning care to Joe. Modesty is a high priority for this client. The nurse must also consider case load, and Joe has the lightest assignment. (I, 5, M)

155. 4. CNS changes include such symptoms as apathy, lethargy, and decreased concentration. Seizures and coma can also occur. The nurse should assess the client's level of consciousness at regular intervals and maintain client safety. Allowing the client to express feelings related to body image changes and restricting foods high in potassium and fluid intake are all appropriate activities, but they are not related to the CNS changes. (I, 10, M)

156. 3. Elderly individuals have less subcutaneous tissue. An elderly, emaciated client will require a short needle and a shallow angle to avoid hitting an underlying bone. The nurse should choose the shortest subcutaneous needle available, at the least angle. (P, 8, M)

157. 3. This situation describes the classic symptoms of urinary tract infection. Urinalysis and culture and sensitivity studies would be helpful information for this diagnosis. Pelvic inflammatory disease is manifested by severe suprapubic pain and vaginal discharge. Renal calculi are accompanied by severe, colicky flank pain and hematuria. Renal failure is manifested by hypertension, pruritus, anorexia, nausea, and vomiting. (P, 10, M)

158. 1. Scant dark vaginal bleeding, abdominal pain, and frequent low-amplitude uterine activity are associated with *abruptio placenta*. The client needs a cesarean delivery to prevent hypovolemic shock. *Placenta accreta* is an unusually deep attachment of the placenta to the myometrium and usually is not discovered until delivery. Hysterectomy is usually the treatment. *Placenta previa* refers to an abnormal implantation of the placenta. Typically, painless, bright red vaginal bleeding is seen. *Battledore placenta* occurs when the cord is inserted marginally rather than centrally, and it is of no clinical significance. (D, 9, O)

159. 3. Flagyl can cause an Antabuse-like reaction if it is taken with alcohol. Tachycardia, nausea, vomiting, and other serious interaction effects can occur. Flagyl will make the urine a darker color. Oral contraceptives should never be discontinued with trichomoniasis. The partner also requires treatment to prevent retransmission of infection. (I, 8, M)

160. 1. In the advanced stages of osteoarthritis, pain can occur with minimal activity or even when the client is at rest. Crepitation can be present at any stage of the disease and does not exacerbate pain. Joints are not symmetrically affected by the disease. Symmetric joint involvement and fatigue are characteristics of rheumatoid arthritis. (A, 10, M)

161. 3. The traditional belief of Vietnamese Americans is that the family can provide more comfort for their loved one at home. It is not seen as being disloyal if their loved one dies in the hospital. The request is not based on a feeling that the hospital cannot be trusted. The Vietnamese Americans accept death as a part of life and do not think that reincarnation is prevented in the hospital. (I, 5, M)

162. 2. It is important for the daughter to know that there is an underlying cause for what her mother is experiencing and that it is treatable. Telling her not to worry is a useless cliché and does nothing to inform the daughter. Talking about care after discharge implies that the delirium is irreversible. Delirium is a reversible condition. Although not arguing with hallucinations is valid, this response ignores the daughter's concern. (I, 6, X)

163. 2. The client with dementia should not have access to toiletries that could be swallowed (eg, aftershave) unless closely supervised. Putting special locks on all the doors is appropriate to prevent wandering, thus maintaining the client's safety. Placing the client in a room that has nothing to trip over is appropriate to reduce the client's risk for falling. Taking the knobs off of the stove is appropriate to prevent possible burns. (E, 6, X)

164. 3. It is important that the client force fluids to 3000 mL/day to avoid the development of renal calculi when taking allopurinol. Allopurinol must be taken consistently to be effective in the treatment of gout. The drug should be taken after meals to avoid gastrointestinal distress. Although the client can take aspirin when taking allopurinol, both drugs can cause gastrointestinal irritation and the practice is not recommended if the client is sensitive to the medications. (E, 8, M)

165. 2. A white, cottage cheese–like discharge accompanied by severe itching is characteristic of *Candida* infection. Trichomonas has a yellow-green discharge. Bacterial vaginosis often has a positive, fishy odor. A purulent discharge should be investigated, cultured, and treated immediately. (A, 4, M)

166. 3. The best advice for the nurse to give the child's mother is to run cool water over the burned area to stop the burning process. Then the area should be wrapped in a clean cloth. Once these initial actions are completed, the mother can call the child's doctor. Packing the arm in ice may cause more damage to the burned area, because cold can cause burns just as heat can. For most burns, it is not advised to apply any ointment until the area has been evaluated. (I, 9, Y)

167. 4. The priority nursing diagnosis for this client is Risk for Injury. The goal in this situation is to prevent falling. Impaired Physical Mobility contributes to the risk for injury and is an applicable diagnosis but does not address the client's safety needs, which are the priority. Impaired Skin Integrity and Ineffective Coping are not applicable diagnoses at this time. (D, 9, M)

168. 3. Chills and headache are signs of a febrile, nonhemolytic blood transfusion reaction and the nurse's first action should be to discontinue the transfusion as soon as possible and then notify the physician. Antipyretics and antihistamines may be ordered. The nurse would not administer acetaminophen without an order from the physician. The client's blood pressure should be taken after the transfusion is stopped. Checking the infusion rate of the blood is not a pertinent action; the infusion needs to be stopped regardless of the rate. (D, 8, M)

169. 3. Resolving grief and having increased energy and activity convey good mental health, indicating that counseling is not necessary at this time. Taking an antidepressant or having less energy and involvement with grandchildren reflects possible depression and the need for counseling. Wanting to be with her dead husband suggests possible suicide ideation that warrants serious further assessment and counseling. (A, 5, X)

170. 3. Common side effects of isosorbide are lightheadedness, dizziness, and orthostatic hypotension. Clients should be instructed to change positions slowly to prevent these side effects and to avoid fainting. Ankle swelling is not related to the isosorbide. The client's pulse does not need to be taken before taking the medication. The medication does not need to be taken with food. (E, 8, M)

171. 3. Valproic acid (Depakote) and propranolol (Inderal) are often prescribed to help manage explosive anger. Recognizing the need for medications indicates readiness for discharge. Not ever getting angry is difficult, impractical, and unrealistic without specific anger management strategies. Drinking does not address anger control and suggests a risk for continued drinking. Blaming others, such as the client's mother, does not address anger control and indicates a lack of responsibility for the client's own behavior. (E, 6, X)

172. 3. The nurse should first help the client into a position of comfort even though the primary purpose for entering the room was to administer medication. After attending to the client's basic care needs, the nurse can proceed with the proper identification of the client, such as asking the client his name and checking his armband, so that the medication can be administered. (I, 7, M)

173. 4. During the first 24 hours after an abdominal hysterectomy, the client is at risk for development of thrombophlebitis because of potential interference with pelvic and leg circulation. Leg exercises are essential to promote circulation and prevent a thrombus. Bowel sounds may not be heard immediately after surgery. It may take up to 48 hours for peristalsis to return. Perineal pads are used after a vaginal hysterectomy, not an abdominal hysterectomy. In the early phases of recovery, the client will be more likely to focus on expressing feelings of discomfort rather than a positive body image. (E, 10, M)

174. 2. The client is asymptomatic but has had a change in heart rhythm. More information is needed before calling the physician. Because the client is taking furosemide (Lasix), a potassium-wasting diuretic, the next action would be to check the client's potassium level. The nurse would then call the physician with a more complete database. The physician will need to be notified after the nurse checks the latest potassium level. Calling the nurse manager is not indicated at this time. Administering potassium requires a physician's order. (P, 10, M)

175. 2. Depression is the most common affective disorder during the postpartum period, affecting 10% to 15% of all women. It is characterized by mood swings, uncontrollable crying, anorexia, and feelings of sadness. It is diagnosed when the transient "blues" persists beyond 2 weeks postpartum. Postpartum blues generally lasts only a few days and then resolves. Postpartum psychosis exists when the client loses touch with reality and requires hospitalization. Commonly, postpartum adjustment is resolved within a few days after delivery. (D, 6, O)

176. 4. Just as with the child, it is best to answer relatives honestly when they ask questions about their loved one's condition. The nurse answers the questions honestly when explaining that infections are often a result of leukemia rather than a cause of it. It is less satisfactory to tell the parents that everything possible has been done for their child, that the child is no longer suffering from the illness, or that nothing could have helped their child. (I, 10, Y)

177. 2. After a TURP, a client can be prone to bladder spasms. Because of the spasms and the decreased urinary output, it is important for the nurse to evaluate the client to determine whether the bladder spasms have been caused by blood clots that are obstructing the flow of urine from the catheter. The client will be acutely uncomfortable until the situation is resolved. The febrile client will need to be assessed for the possible source of the fever, but this assessment can be delayed until the client with bladder spasms has received care. The client with the ileal conduit needs to have the pouch emptied of urine; this activity can be delegated to the assistant. A small amount of hemoptysis after a bronchoscopy with biopsy is to be expected and does not require immediate follow-up. (D, 1, M)

178. 1. Microdrip administration sets have a drop factor of 60 gtt/mL. Therefore, 60 gtt/mL × 500 mL / 600 minutes = 50 gtt/minute. (I, 8, M)

179. 1. The client must wait 14 days between stopping phenelzine (Nardil) and starting fluoxetine (Prozac) because of the risk for serotonin syndrome, a potentially lethal condition manifested by hyperreflexia, hyperthermia, myoclonus, and other symptoms suggesting neuroleptic malignant syndrome. The client does not need to have blood levels drawn every week while taking fluoxetine. Weekly blood draws are needed especially when lithium or clozapine therapy is initiated. Notifying the physician before taking any over-the-counter medication is not usually necessary unless other conditions warrant it. Headache and nausea are common side effects of fluoxetine and do not require immediate physician notification. However, severe headaches or nausea should be reported. (I, 8, X)

180. 3. Taking a deep abdominal breath and then "huff" coughing is the most effective manner of coughing. This technique helps facilitate removal of secretions and conserves energy for the client. The client should breathe slowly but not hold her breath. Short panting breaths and then coughing from the throat does not promote expectoration of sputum from the lungs. Coughing forcefully can cause alveoli to collapse; "huff" coughing prevents this. (E, 9, M)

181. 3. The first objective is for the nurse to get the client's attention. This can be done by looking the client in the eyes and speaking in a calm voice. Once the nurse has her attention, the nurse can instruct the client in breathing techniques. Modified pace breathing can be used during the contractions. The nurse may need to assist the client to breathe with each contraction. Telling the client to calm down or to breathe with each contraction is not helpful if the client isn't listening to the nurse. The nurse needs to get the client's attention first. Analgesia is not warranted at this phase of labor because the neonate may experience respiratory depression if delivery occurs within 1 to 2 hours. (I, 5, O)

COMPREHENSIVE TEST 5

Select the one best answer, and indicate your choice by filling in the circle in front of the option.

1. A nurse has been working with a battered woman who is being discharged to her husband. The nurse says, "All this work with her has been useless. She's just going back to him as usual." Which of the following statements by a nursing colleague would be *most* helpful to this nurse?
   - 1. "Her reasons for staying are complex. She can leave only when she is ready and can be safe."
   - 2. "I know it is frustrating to work with clients who don't follow our advice."
   - 3. "You did your best. You will see her again and have another chance."
   - 4. "These women almost never leave for good because of their emotional and financial dependency."

2. Ergonovine maleate (Ergotrate) 200 μg IM has been ordered. The ampule label reads 0.2 mg/mL. How many milliliters should the nurse administer?
   - 1. 0.2 mL.
   - 2. 0.5 mL.
   - 3. 1.0 mL.
   - 4. 2.0 mL.

3. The nurse in a community hospital has been notified that a 6-month-old infant is being admitted from the emergency department with dehydration secondary to viral gastroenteritis. Which of the following room assignments is the most appropriate for this infant?
   - 1. A semiprivate room with an 8-year-old child who has had an appendectomy.
   - 2. A semiprivate room with a 10-year-old child with a closed head injury.
   - 3. A private room.
   - 4. A semiprivate room with a 4-year-old child with leukemia.

4. For which of the following would the nurse be especially alert when caring for a term neonate, who weighed 10 pounds at birth, 1 hour after a vaginal delivery?
   - 1. Hyperglycemia.
   - 2. Hypercalcemia.
   - 3. Hypermagnesemia.
   - 4. Hyperbilirubinemia.

5. A female client with infertility related to anovulatory cycles is prescribed menotropins (Pergonal). Which of the following, if stated by the client as a possible adverse effect of this medication, indicates successful teaching?
   - 1. Pulmonary edema.
   - 2. Ovarian enlargement.
   - 3. Visual disturbances.
   - 4. Breast tenderness.

6. A family has been notified that their son is brain dead, and the physician has discussed the possibility of donating organs. The nurse is aware that the referral sources responsible for organ recovery in the United States are the
   - 1. Organ and Tissue Procurement Organizations.
   - 2. American Transplant Association.
   - 3. American Hospice Foundation.
   - 4. American Association of Critical Care Nurses.

7. The nurse is involved in preoperative teaching with a client who will be undergoing a lung resection. The client is told that two chest tubes will be placed during surgery. The nurse explains that the purpose of the lower chest tube is to
   - 1. prevent clots.
   - 2. remove air.
   - 3. remove fluid.
   - 4. facilitate "milking" of the tubes.

8. Depression in an older adult differs from depression in a younger person because
   - 1. sadness of mood is usually present but it is masked by other symptoms.
   - 2. impairment of cognition usually is not present.
   - 3. psychosomatic tendencies do not tend to dominate.
   - 4. traditional antidepressant therapies are less effective.

9. A primary concern of the hospitalized adolescent would be
   - 1. respect for the need for privacy.
   - 2. allowing friends to visit after hours.
   - 3. wearing a hospital gown.
   - 4. the fear of loss of control when in pain.

10. A 20-year-old single parent brings her 3-year-old

son into the emergency department because he "fell." The child has bruises on his face, arms, and legs; his mother says that she did not witness the fall. The nurse suspects child abuse. While examining the child, the mother says, "Sometimes I guess I'm pretty rough with him. I'm alone, and I just don't know how to manage him." The nurse would anticipate referring the mother to which of the following types of programs?
- ○ 1. A program for single parents.
- ○ 2. A parenting education program.
- ○ 3. A women's support group.
- ○ 4. A support group for abusive parents.

11. A nurse who fails to check a client's armband before administering his medications is
- ○ 1. *res judicata.*
- ○ 2. negligent.
- ○ 3. *stare decisis.*
- ○ 4. vicariously liable.

12. Before administering morphine to a client, the nurse should assess the client's
- ○ 1. blood pressure.
- ○ 2. respiration rate.
- ○ 3. pulse.
- ○ 4. temperature.

13. A mother states that she is very angry with the physician who diagnosed her child with leukemia. The nurse is aware that
- ○ 1. anger is a natural result of a sense of loss and helplessness.
- ○ 2. parents of sick children are usually unable to control their anger.
- ○ 3. anger is rarely demonstrated by parents when coping with a sick child.
- ○ 4. the mother cannot overcome her anger in an acceptable manner.

14. Which of the following nursing strategies would be effective in managing a resident in a long-term care facility who has Alzheimer's disease and wanders?
- ○ 1. Encourage participation in activities such as bingo.
- ○ 2. Discourage wandering by allowing the behavior at selected intervals.
- ○ 3. Involve the client in activities that promote walking.
- ○ 4. Promote safety by restricting the client in a geriatric chair.

15. A child who had a cast applied to his arm earlier this morning is complaining that his fingers are numb. Which of the following actions by the nurse would be *most* appropriate?
- ○ 1. Notify the physician who applied the cast.
- ○ 2. Cut the cast to loosen it.
- ○ 3. Assess the circulation to the fingers.
- ○ 4. Ensure that the arm is positioned correctly.

16. The major advantage of second-generation antihistamines such as loratadine (Claritin) and fexofenadine (Allegra) is
- ○ 1. decreased cost.
- ○ 2. increased effectiveness.
- ○ 3. delayed absorption.
- ○ 4. they are nonsedating.

17. The client with newly diagnosed low back pain (LBP) is very worried. The nurse emphasizes that the most common cause of low back pain is
- ○ 1. osteoporosis.
- ○ 2. herniated disk.
- ○ 3. muscle strain.
- ○ 4. spondylosis.

18. While helping clients brought to a crisis center during a severe flood, the nurse interviews a client whose pregnant wife is missing and whose home has been destroyed. The client keeps talking rapidly about his experience and says, "I can't see how I can ever rebuild my life." Which of the following responses by the nurse would be *most* appropriate?
- ○ 1. "If you start organizing your life now, I'm sure all will be fine."
- ○ 2. "This has been a terrible experience. Tell me more about how you feel."
- ○ 3. "Let me note a few of the things you said before you continue with your story."
- ○ 4. "Tonight, think some more of what happened, so that we can continue with this tomorrow."

19. A client with asthma has been prescribed beclomethasone (Beclovent) via metered dose inhaler. The nurse instructs the client to rinse her mouth after using the beclomethasone inhaler because
- ○ 1. this helps prevent gingival hyperplasia.
- ○ 2. this helps prevent oral candidiasis.
- ○ 3. this helps prevent absorbing too large a dose.
- ○ 4. this is needed to prevent dental caries.

20. The nurse finds a client lying on the floor next to the bed. After returning the client to bed, assessing for injury, and notifying the physician, the nurse fills out an incident report. Which of the following is the nurse's next action?
- ○ 1. Give the incident report to the nurse manager.
- ○ 2. Place the incident report on the chart.
- ○ 3. Call the family to inform them.
- ○ 4. Omit mentioning the fall in the chart documentation.

21. The mother of 2-year-old who has been bitten by the family dog asks the nurse what to do about the bite. Which of the following would be the *most* appropriate recommendation to this mother?
- ○ 1. "You need to take the child to the local urgent care center immediately."
- ○ 2. "Wash the bite area with lots of running water, and then check the injury."

○ 3. "Determine when the child's latest tetanus vaccine was administered."

○ 4. "Make an appointment to see the child's physician now to start rabies shots."

22. A multigravid client at 36 weeks' gestation who has insulin-dependent diabetes is scheduled for a biophysical profile in the morning. The nurse explains to the client that which of the following is one of the fetal parameters to be assessed?
○ 1. Biparietal diameter.
○ 2. Bilirubin levels.
○ 3. Contraction stress test.
○ 4. Breathing movements.

23. A schoolteacher calls the nurse and asks whether all the children at school need treatment after exposure to a 7-year-old child with *Hemophilus influenzae* meningitis. The nurse responds that chemoprophylaxis should be given to
○ 1. all children at the school.
○ 2. all household contacts and close contacts.
○ 3. the entire community.
○ 4. household contacts only.

24. The mother of an 18-month-old boy is concerned about the number of persons with heart disease in her family. She asks the nurse when she should start her infant on a diet to lower the risk for heart disease. The nurse tells her that the American Heart Association provides recommendations for children to prevent heart disease. For what age do they begin providing recommendations?
○ 1. At birth.
○ 2. At age 2 years.
○ 3. At age 5 years.
○ 4. At age 10 years.

25. A client is being treated for severe pediculosis. The nurse teaches the client to treat the problem in the eyebrows and eyelashes by
○ 1. applying petroleum jelly to lashes and brows three to four times a day.
○ 2. applying a pediculicide with a cotton-tipped swab three to four times a day.
○ 3. applying lindane ointment to the lashes and eyebrows three times daily.
○ 4. applying bacitracin ointment to the lashes and brows three times daily.

26. The nurse is discussing safety and accident prevention with the mother of a 9-month-old. The nurse knows that the teaching has been effective when the mother states which of the following?
○ 1. "I make sure that I keep my cleaning supplies locked up."
○ 2. "Sometimes she plays in the bathroom when I'm cleaning in there."
○ 3. "Occasionally she gets under the chair and plays with the telephone cord."

○ 4. "I've found that those child-protective cabinet locks don't work very well."

27. The nurse knows that atypical signs and symptoms of appendicitis could occur in
○ 1. children older than 5 years of age.
○ 2. pregnant women in the first trimester.
○ 3. adolescents.
○ 4. clients who are taking steroids.

28. The nurse instructs the client who is talking gentamycin to monitor factors related to renal function. The nurse determines that the client needs *additional* instruction when he makes which of the following statements?
○ 1. "I should call you if I notice that I'm not urinating as much."
○ 2. "I should call you if my urine looks dark or unusual."
○ 3. "I should call you if my legs swell or I notice my skin looks puffy around my eyes."
○ 4. "I should call you if I have a fever."

29. A 15-month-old child is admitted to the pediatric unit with the diagnosis of pneumonia and is placed in a mist tent. Which of the following toys would be appropriate for this child?
○ 1. A pull toy.
○ 2. Story books.
○ 3. Crayons and paper.
○ 4. Plastic blocks.

30. When teaching a group of parents about the potential for febrile seizures in children, which of the following facts would the nurse include?
○ 1. The exact cause is known.
○ 2. The seizures occur as the fever rises.
○ 3. Children older than 3 years of age are most at risk.
○ 4. These seizures commonly occur after immunization administration.

31. The nurse should instruct a woman taking folic acid supplements for folic acid–deficiency anemia that
○ 1. it will take several months to notice an improvement.
○ 2. folic acid should be taken on an empty stomach.
○ 3. iron supplements are contraindicated with folic acid supplementation.
○ 4. oral contraceptive use, pregnancy, and lactation increase daily requirements.

32. The nurse makes a home visit to a primiparous client and her neonate at 1 week after a vaginal delivery. Which of the following findings should be reported to the physician?
○ 1. A scant amount of maternal lochia serosa.
○ 2. The presence of a neonatal tonic neck reflex.
○ 3. A nonpalpable maternal fundus.
○ 4. Neonatal central cyanosis.

33. Which of the following is the most common systemic antibiotic used in the treatment of severe acne?

○ 1. Isoretinoin.
○ 2. Cephalexin (Keflex).
○ 3. Azithromycin.
○ 4. Tetracycline.

34. Which of the following is *not* a risk factor for osteoporosis?
    ○ 1. Heavy use of alcohol.
    ○ 2. Excessive antacid use.
    ○ 3. A diet very high in fiber.
    ○ 4. Adequate vitamin K intake.

35. The nurse tells a rape victim that even if she was protected against pregnancy by a contraceptive and has no intention of taking any legal action against her assailant, she should still be checked by a physician. The nurse recommends this postrape physical examination *primarily* for early detection of which of the following?
    ○ 1. Venereal disease.
    ○ 2. Anxiety reaction.
    ○ 3. Periurethral tears.
    ○ 4. Menstrual difficulties.

36. A client in a private room fell on the floor and sustained a small laceration on her hand that required stitches. The intern asks for bupivacaine (Marcaine) with epinephrine and a suture kit in order to suture the laceration. The nurse should question which of the following?
    ○ 1. The intern's ability to suture.
    ○ 2. The client's room as an aseptic environment.
    ○ 3. The marcaine with epinephrine as the local anesthetic.
    ○ 4. The cosmetic effect from suturing.

37. Which of the following signs and symptoms experienced by a child with suspected appendicitis would the nurse correctly judge to be unrelated to the transient sympathetic effects caused by the acute abdominal pain?
    ○ 1. Tachycardia.
    ○ 2. Chills.
    ○ 3. Rapid breathing.
    ○ 4. Dilated pupils.

38. When assessing a dark-skinned client for cyanosis, the nurse should examine which of the following?
    ○ 1. The client's retinas.
    ○ 2. The client's nail beds.
    ○ 3. The client's oral mucous membranes.
    ○ 4. The inner aspects of the client's wrists.

39. Betamethasone (Celestone) syrup 0.9 mg has been ordered. It is available in a 0.6 mg/5 mL solution. How many milliliters should the nurse administer?
    ○ 1. 2.5 mL.
    ○ 2. 6.0 mL.
    ○ 3. 7.5 mL.
    ○ 4. 10.0 mL.

40. A nulligravid client at 37 weeks' gestation is scheduled for a biophysical profile. Which of the following would the nurse instruct the client to do before the test?
    ○ 1. Drink 1 to 2 L of fluid.
    ○ 2. Remain NPO (take nothing by mouth) after midnight before the test.
    ○ 3. Plan to remain in the clinic for 4 hours after the test.
    ○ 4. Eat a high-fiber meal after the test.

41. The nurse on the obstetrical unit has been notified by staff in the emergency room that a primigravid client with a history of sickle cell disease is to be admitted at 32 weeks' gestation with a diagnosis of sickle cell crisis. The nurse anticipates that the physician will order an infusion of which of the following?
    ○ 1. Platelets.
    ○ 2. Granulocytes.
    ○ 3. Packed red cells.
    ○ 4. Whole blood.

42. A working mother is concerned about the amount of snacking her teenaged boy is doing. She is concerned that this behavior could lead to obesity. Which of the following is an appropriate percentage of the daily diet to be obtained from snacks?
    ○ 1. 10%.
    ○ 2. 25%.
    ○ 3. 40%.
    ○ 4. 50%.

43. The client complains of sore nares while a nasogastric tube is in place. Which of the following nursing measures would be most appropriate to help alleviate the client's discomfort?
    ○ 1. Reposition the tube in the nares.
    ○ 2. Irrigate the tube with a cool solution.
    ○ 3. Apply a water-soluble lubricant to the nares.
    ○ 4. Have the client change position more frequently.

44. The nurse is instructing a Hindu client to increase protein in the diet. Which of the following meal plans is appropriate for a Hindu client?
    ○ 1. Lentil soup and fish sandwich.
    ○ 2. Hamburger.
    ○ 3. Steak.
    ○ 4. Veal cutlet.

45. A child with partial- and full-thickness burns is admitted to the pediatric unit. Which of the following would be the *priority* at this time?
    ○ 1. Preventing wound infection.
    ○ 2. Evaluating vital signs frequently.
    ○ 3. Maintaining fluid and electrolyte balance.
    ○ 4. Managing the child's pain.

46. A normal, healthy infant is brought to the clinic for the first immunization against polio. The nurse should administer Sabin's vaccine by what route?

○ 1. Oral route.
○ 2. Intramuscular route.
○ 3. Subcutaneous route.
○ 4. Intradermal route.

47. The nurse observes that a client who has received midazolam (Versed) for local anesthesia is having shallow respirations. Which of the following actions is *inappropriate* for the nurse to do?
○ 1. Encourage the client to deep-breathe.
○ 2. Have respiratory resuscitation equipment in the room.
○ 3. Administer oxygen as ordered.
○ 4. Administer naloxone (Narcan).

48. The nurse is planning to assist the physician with a thoracentesis for a client who has a pleural effusion. Which of the following positions would be appropriate for the client to assume?
○ 1. Lying supine with arms extended.
○ 2. Lying prone with head supported by arms.
○ 3. Sitting upright and leaning on an overbed table.
○ 4. Side-lying with knees drawn up to the abdomen.

49. The nurse is preparing a presentation on nutrition to a group of pregnant adolescents. Which of the following would be important for the nurse to include in the teaching plan?
○ 1. Spinach is an excellent source of calcium in the diet.
○ 2. Two to four servings of whole-grain products is recommended.
○ 3. Three or more servings of dairy products meets the calcium requirement.
○ 4. Vitamin A supplements may be necessary for clients who are vegetarian.

50. The nurse anticipates an expected outcome of viral (coxsackie B) or *Trypanosoma* (parasite) infection is
○ 1. myocarditis.
○ 2. myocardial infarction.
○ 3. renal failure.
○ 4. liver failure.

51. Which of the following compensatory actions by the body would occur if a client were in respiratory acidosis?
○ 1. excretion of HCO_3^- by the kidneys.
○ 2. retention of HCO_3^- by the kidneys.
○ 3. increase in respiratory rate by the lungs.
○ 4. decrease in respiratory rate by the lungs.

52. A client has started taking amiodarone (Cordarone). The nurse should inform the client that periodic laboratory tests will be done to monitor the client's
○ 1. hemoglobin.
○ 2. liver enzymes.
○ 3. creatine phosphokinase (CPK) concentration.
○ 4. urinalysis.

53. The father of a 9-month-old child diagnosed with a first ear infection asks whether he should do anything else to help the child. Which of the following would be the nurse's *best* response?
○ 1. "Your child should also take an antihistamine."
○ 2. "The antibiotic is the only medicine necessary."
○ 3. "Cotton in the ears helps the discomfort."
○ 4. "Over-the-counter ear drops often are helpful."

54. A child's plan of care lists increasing protein intake as a goal. Which of the following foods that the child likes would the nurse encourage the child to eat?
○ 1. A bacon, lettuce, and tomato sandwich.
○ 2. Fruit-flavored yogurt.
○ 3. Nacho chips and salsa.
○ 4. Crackers with butter and jelly.

55. The clinical findings of prominent neck veins, hypertension, and bounding pulse are specifically indicative of fluid excess in which body compartment?
○ 1. Interstitial compartment.
○ 2. Intravascular compartment.
○ 3. Intracellular compartment.
○ 4. Extracellular compartment.

56. Which of the following laboratory findings would the nurse anticipate will *not* be affected by ciprofloxacin (Cipro)?
○ 1. Theophylline level.
○ 2. Prothrombin time (PT).
○ 3. Activated partial thromboplastin time (aPTT).
○ 4. Total iron-binding capacity (TIBC).

57. A 10-year-old child is diagnosed with pediculosis. The mother is concerned about the spread of the lice to children who have been in contact with her child. Which of the following activities would cause the *most* concern?
○ 1. Sharing craft supplies.
○ 2. Having contact during a swimming class.
○ 3. Sharing of batting helmets.
○ 4. Showering after football practice.

58. A 24-year-old nulligravid client with a history of irregular menstrual cycles visits the clinic because she suspects that she is "about 6 weeks pregnant." An ultrasound is scheduled for the client 2 weeks from today. When teaching the client about the procedure, which of the following would the nurse include as the *most* likely reason for this client to have the procedure?
○ 1. Assessment of gestational age.
○ 2. Determination of a multifetal pregnancy.
○ 3. Identification of the gender of the fetus.
○ 4. Assessment of maternal pelvic adequacy.

59. A client with a history of peptic ulcer disease is admitted to the hospital. Initial assessment reveals that his blood pressure is 96/60 mm Hg, his pulse rate is 120 bpm, and he has vomited coffee-ground material. Based on this assessment, what is the nurse's priority action?

- ○ 1. Administer an antiemetic.
- ○ 2. Prepare to insert a nasogastric tube.
- ○ 3. Collect data regarding recent client stressors.
- ○ 4. Place the client in a modified Trendelenburg position.

60. A male client has intermittent episodes of third-degree heart block and complains of shortness of breath and chest pain. The nurse anticipates that the client will undergo

- ○ 1. cardiac catheterization.
- ○ 2. coronary artery bypass surgery.
- ○ 3. insertion of a temporary pacemaker.
- ○ 4. insertion of an aortic balloon pump.

61. As of 1999, all refined grain products such as cereal, pasta, flour, rolls, buns, farina, grits, and rice are fortified with which of the following?

- ○ 1. Vitamin C.
- ○ 2. Niacin.
- ○ 3. Vitamin B_{12}.
- ○ 4. Folic acid.

62. In the early postoperative period, the nurse notes a bright red, 3- by 5-inch area of drainage on the client's abdominal laparotomy dressing. What should be the nurse's first action be in response to this observation?

- ○ 1. Ignore it, because drainage is normal.
- ○ 2. Increase the intravenous flow rate.
- ○ 3. Take the client's vital signs.
- ○ 4. Change the dressing.

63. Knowing that the infant with pyloric stenosis is at risk because of decreased circulating fluid volume, the nurse should assess for which of the following disorders?

- ○ 1. Inappropriate antidiuretic hormone release.
- ○ 2. Acute renal failure.
- ○ 3. Paralytic ileus.
- ○ 4. Adrenal insufficiency.

64. The nurse understands that when a client has a massive bleed from esophageal varices, the *immediate* priority is to

- ○ 1. control hemorrhaging.
- ○ 2. replace fluids.
- ○ 3. relieve the client's anxiety.
- ○ 4. maintain a patent airway.

65. Which of the following areas would be *most* important for the nurse to include in the teaching plan for a client who is taking phenelzine (Nardil)?

- ○ 1. Eating a normal amount of salt in the diet.
- ○ 2. Drinking 10 to 12 glasses of water each day.
- ○ 3. Taking 10 days to 4 weeks to achieve therapeu-

tic effects.
- ○ 4. Avoiding foods high in tyramine.

66. The nurse should closely monitor the client with an open fracture for which of the following complications?

- ○ 1. Avascular necrosis.
- ○ 2. Compartment syndrome.
- ○ 3. Osteomyelitis.
- ○ 4. Fat embolism syndrome.

67. Which of the following would be a *priority* nursing diagnosis for a client who has had a total laryngectomy?

- ○ 1. Risk for Impaired Skin Integrity.
- ○ 2. Excess Fluid Volume.
- ○ 3. Ineffective Thermoregulation.
- ○ 4. Impaired Verbal Communication.

68. When conducting a screening session for hypertension at a retirement center, the nurse encounters a client who has a long history of uncontrolled hypertension. The nurse should teach the client that chronic hypertension can damage which area of the eye?

- ○ 1. Iris.
- ○ 2. Cornea.
- ○ 3. Retina.
- ○ 4. Sclera.

69. While preparing to provide neonatal care instructions to a primiparous client who delivered a term neonate 24 hours ago, which of the following would be included in the client's teaching plan?

- ○ 1. Term neonates generally have few creases on the soles of their feet.
- ○ 2. Strawberry hemangiomas—deep, dark red discolorations—require laser therapy for removal.
- ○ 3. Milia are white papules from plugged sebaceous ducts that disappear by 2 to 4 weeks of age.
- ○ 4. If erythema toxicum is present, it will be treated with antibiotic therapy.

70. Two days after the fracture of his femur, a client suddenly complains of chest pain and dyspnea. The nurse also notes some confusion and an elevated temperature. Based on these assessment findings, the nurse suspects which of the following complications?

- ○ 1. Osteomyelitis.
- ○ 2. Compartment syndrome.
- ○ 3. Venous thrombosis.
- ○ 4. Fat embolism syndrome.

71. While assessing a neonate at 4 hours after birth, the nurse observes an indentation with a small tuft of hair at the base of the neonate's spine. The nurse would document this finding as which of the following?

- ○ 1. Spina bifida cystica.
- ○ 2. Spina bifida occulta.

3. Meningocele.

4. Myelomeningocele.

72. The primary purpose of instilling 5 mL of normal saline before suctioning a tracheostomy tube is to
    1. thin the secretions to be suctioned.
    2. stimulate the client to cough.
    3. help the catheter to slide down the tracheostomy tube.
    4. provide humidification to the respiratory tract.

73. A client with emphysema is receiving continuous oxygen therapy. Depressed ventilation is likely to occur unless the nurse ensures that the oxygen is administered in which of the following ways?
    1. Cooled.
    2. Humidified.
    3. At a low flow rate.
    4. Through nasal cannula.

74. A nulligravid client at 12 weeks' gestation tells the nurse that she is a vegetarian and eats "lots of rice." To help meet the client's needs for protein during pregnancy, the nurse suggests that the client combine the rice with which of the following?
    1. Beans.
    2. Soy milk.
    3. Yogurt.
    4. Corn.

75. A client with rheumatoid arthritis tells the nurse that she feels "quite alone" in adjusting to changes in her lifestyle. Which one of the following nursing actions is most appropriate in response to this statement?
    1. Refer the client and her husband for counseling to decrease her sense of isolation.
    2. Suggest that the client develop a hobby to occupy her time.
    3. Tell the client about her community's arthritis support group.
    4. Suggest that the client discuss her feelings with her minister.

76. Which of the following would the nurse expect to include in the plan of care to ensure adequate nutrition for a very active, talkative, and easily distractable client who is unable to sit through meals?
    1. Direct the client to his room to eat.
    2. Offer the client nutritious finger foods.
    3. Ask the client's family to bring his favorite foods from home.
    4. Ask the client about his food preferences.

77. A client is very dependent on the staff but is able to make simple decisions. The client asks, "Would you do my laundry? I don't know how the machine works." Which of the following responses would be *best*?
    1. "Sure, I have time; I can do it for you."
    2. "You'll have to wait; I don't have time now."
    3. "Can your family do it for you?"
    4. "Get your laundry; I'll show you how the machine works."

78. The nurse is caring for a client with chronic renal failure. Knowing that the client is a candidate for development of hypermagnesemia, for which of the following signs and symptoms would the nurse closely monitor the client?
    1. Flushed skin.
    2. Lethargy.
    3. Severe thirst.
    4. Tremors.

79. A newly diagnosed diabetic informs the nurse that she has not been eating to try and better control her blood sugar. The nurse tells her that this is not a solution to blood glucose control because blood glucose is regulated not only by insulin but by glucagon, which is stimulated to raise blood glucose when a person has not eaten. Glucagon causes a rise in glucose by stimulating
    1. glycogen breakdown and release from the muscles.
    2. the intestine to absorb glucose.
    3. the liver to release glucose into the blood.
    4. the brain to release glucose.

80. When giving a change of shift report, which of the following statements by the nurse is *not* considered appropriate?
    1. "Randi Smith is a 38-year-old female client of Dr. Born with cholecystitis and cholelithiasis."
    2. "Mrs. Jones' pain is best relieved in the left lateral Sims' position."
    3. "Mr. Levi is just contrary today and nothing is going to please him."
    4. "Mr. Emmert was able to walk around the unit twice today with no complaint of dizziness."

81. The nurse is teaching unlicensed personnel about caring for a client who is withdrawing from alcohol and street drugs. Which of the following communication techniques would the nurse include in the teaching?
    1. Matter-of-fact manner and short sentences.
    2. Cheerful tone and humor.
    3. Abstract terms and a loud voice tone.
    4. Clear, lengthy explanations in a quiet voice.

82. What is the primary goal of nursing care during the emergent phase after a burn injury?
    1. Replace lost fluids.
    2. Prevent infection.
    3. Control pain.
    4. Promote wound healing.

83. The nurse assesses for euphoria in a client with multiple sclerosis, looking for which of the following characteristic clinical manifestations?
    1. Inappropriate laughter.

○ 2. An exaggerated sense of well-being.

○ 3. Slurring of words when excited.

○ 4. Visual hallucinations.

84. The client with a burn injury is assessed using the "rule of nines" to determine which of the following?

○ 1. Amount of body surface area burned.

○ 2. Rehabilitation needs.

○ 3. Respiratory needs.

○ 4. Type of intravenous fluids required.

85. When assessing a 2-month-old infant, the nurse feels a "click" when abducting the infant's left hip. Which of the following would the nurse do *next*?

○ 1. Document the finding as normal for a 2-month-old.

○ 2. Check the lengths of the femurs to see if they are equal.

○ 3. Instruct the mother to keep the leg in an adducted position.

○ 4. Reschedule the child for a follow-up assessment in 3 weeks.

86. Which of the following laboratory tests would the nurse monitor when the client is receiving warfarin sodium (Coumadin) therapy?

○ 1. PTT.

○ 2. Serum potassium.

○ 3. Arterial blood gases.

○ 4. PT.

87. A client who had a transurethral resection of the prostate (TURP) 2 days earlier is complaining of lower abdominal pain. Which nursing intervention should the nurse perform *first*?

○ 1. Auscultate the abdomen for bowel sounds.

○ 2. Administer an oral analgesic.

○ 3. Have the client use a sitz bath for 15 minutes.

○ 4. Assess the patency of the urethral catheter.

88. The nurse would identify which of the following as a *priority* nursing diagnosis for the family of a neonate with cleft lip?

○ 1. Altered Family Processes.

○ 2. Anticipatory Grieving.

○ 3. Ineffective Coping.

○ 4. Anxiety.

89. The nurse is ready to administer a partial fill of imipenem–cilastatin (Primaxin) in the IV pump when a full partial fill bag of imipenem–cilastatin (Primaxin) is found hanging at the client's bedside. Which of the following is *not* an appropriate response for the nurse when recognizing that the previous dose was not administered 8 hours ago to the client with pneumonia?

○ 1. Discard the full partial fill of imipenem–cilastatin (Primaxin) found hanging at the client's bedside.

○ 2. Check the identifying information of the full partial fill of imipenem–cilastatin (Primaxin) found hanging at the client's bedside.

○ 3. Follow-up on the legal documentation of the client's previous administration of imipenem–cilastatin (Primaxin).

○ 4. Administer the new partial fill of imipenem–cilastatin (Primaxin).

90. A client with a moderate level of anxiety is pacing quickly in the hall. As the nurse approaches, he states, "Help me, I can't take it anymore." Which of the following would be the *best* response initially?

○ 1. "It would be best if you would lie down until you're calmer."

○ 2. "Let's go to a quieter area where we can talk if you want."

○ 3. "Try doing your relaxation exercises to calm down."

○ 4. "I'll get some medicine to help you relax."

91. The nurse should plan to teach a client who is taking warfarin sodium (Coumadin) to do which of the following?

○ 1. Consult the physician before having dental work.

○ 2. Avoid the use of a toothbrush during oral hygiene.

○ 3. Use rectal suppositories to treat constipation.

○ 4. Eat green leafy vegetables.

92. A 30-year-old client is hospitalized with a fractured femur which is being treated with skeletal traction. He states that he has not had a bowel movement for 2 days. Which of the following interventions is most appropriate at this time?

○ 1. Administer a tapwater enema.

○ 2. Place the client on the bedpan every 2 to 3 hours.

○ 3. Increase the client's fluid intake to 3000 mL/day.

○ 4. Perform range-of-motion movements to all extremities.

93. A 62-year-old client with a 29-pack-year history is admitted with a diagnosis of lung cancer. She reports "no appetite" and exhibits symptoms of anorexia. The client is 5 feet 8 inches tall and weighs 112 pounds. The client is now scheduled for a left lung lobectomy. Which of the following would increase the client's risk of developing postoperative pulmonary complications?

○ 1. The client tends to keep her real feelings to herself.

○ 2. The client ambulates and can climb one flight of stairs without dyspnea.

○ 3. The client is 62 years of age.

○ 4. The client is 5 feet, 8 inches tall and weighs 112 pounds.

94. When developing the plan of care for a 12-year-old child who is to receive 48 hours of chemotherapy that is associated with nausea and vomiting, at

which of the following times would the nurse anticipate administering an antiemetic?

○ 1. 30 minutes after the chemotherapy has started, then every 4 to 6 hours.

○ 2. 30 minutes before the chemotherapy starts, then every 4 to 6 hours.

○ 3. When the 12-year-old requests medication for nausea, then every 4 hours as needed.

○ 4. On starting the chemotherapy infusion, and then routinely every 8 hours.

95. The membranes of a multigravid client in active labor rupture spontaneously, revealing greenish-colored amniotic fluid. The nurse interprets this finding as related to which of the following?

○ 1. Passage of meconium by the fetus.

○ 2. Maternal intrauterine infection.

○ 3. Rh incompatibility between mother and fetus.

○ 4. Maternal sexually transmitted disease.

96. A client's arterial blood gas values are as follows: pH, 7.24; pCO$_2$, 35 mm Hg; HCO$_3$$^-$, 15 mEq/L. The client also has Kussmaul respirations. These findings are indicative of which of the following acid–base imbalances?

○ 1. Metabolic acidosis.

○ 2. Metabolic alkalosis.

○ 3. Respiratory acidosis.

○ 4. Respiratory alkalosis.

97. A client is suspected of having a slow gastrointestinal bleed. The nurse should evaluate the client for which sign or symptom?

○ 1. Increased pulse.

○ 2. Nausea.

○ 3. Tarry stools.

○ 4. Abdominal cramps.

98. Which of the following suggestions would the nurse give to an adolescent football player with Osgood-Schlatter disease of the left knee?

○ 1. Apply ice on the knee after playing.

○ 2. Use crutches until healing has occurred.

○ 3. Stop playing until healing has occurred.

○ 4. Make an appointment with a physical therapist.

99. The nurse instructs a client who is taking iron supplements that

○ 1. iron supplements should be taken on an empty stomach.

○ 2. a daily bulk laxative such as psyllium hydrophilic mucilloid (Metamucil) should be avoided.

○ 3. the stools will become darker.

○ 4. liquid iron supplements will not discolor teeth.

100. Which of the following would the nurse teach a client with generalized anxiety disorder to help the client cope with anxiety?

○ 1. Cognitive and behavioral strategies.

○ 2. Issue avoidance and denial of problems.

○ 3. Rest and sleep.

○ 4. Withdrawal from role expectations and role relationships.

101. After a lobectomy, clients are instructed to perform deep-breathing exercises to

○ 1. decrease blood flow to the lungs for rest and increased surface alveoli ventilation.

○ 2. elevate the diaphragm to enlarge the thorax so that the lung surface area available for gas exchange is increased.

○ 3. control the rate of air flow to the remaining lobe to decrease the risk of hyperinflation.

○ 4. expand the alveoli and increase lung surface available for ventilation.

102. Which of the following would demonstrate the correct technique for applying an Ace bandage to a leg?

○ 1. Increase tension with each successive turn of the bandage.

○ 2. Start at the distal end of the extremity and move toward the trunk.

○ 3. Secure the bandage with a clips over the area of the inner thigh.

○ 4. Overlap each layer twice when wrapping.

103. A nulliparous client says that she and her husband plan to use a diaphragm with spermicide to prevent conception. Which of the following would the nurse include as the action of spermicides when teaching the client?

○ 1. Destruction of spermatozoa before they enter the cervix.

○ 2. Prevention of spermatozoa from entering the uterus.

○ 3. A change in vaginal pH from acidic to alkaline.

○ 4. Slowing of the movement of the migrating spermatozoa.

104. A client with acquired immunodeficiency syndrome (AIDS) is admitted because of paranoia and visual hallucinations probably related to progressive dementia. In addition to continuing all of the client's AIDS-related medications, which of the following medications would the nurse expect the physician to add?

○ 1. Methylphenidate (Ritalin).

○ 2. Lorazepam (Ativan).

○ 3. Nefazodone (Serzone).

○ 4. Haloperidol (Haldol).

105. Which of the following assessment findings would a nurse expect to find in a client with bacterial pneumonia?

○ 1. Increased fremitus.

○ 2. Bilateral expiratory wheezing.

○ 3. Resonance on percussion.

○ 4. Vesicular breath sounds.

106. A client is admitted with complaints of severe

abdominal pains and the diagnosis of acute pancreatitis. The plan of care during the acute phase of pancreatitis will involve interventions targeting which of the following problems?

○ 1. Drug and alcohol abuse.
○ 2. Risk for injury.
○ 3. Severe pain.
○ 4. Ineffective airway clearance.

107. An infant with increased intracranial pressure on a regular diet vomits while eating dinner. Which of the following would the nurse do *next*?

○ 1. Make the child NPO for 4 hours.
○ 2. Call to report this event to the physician.
○ 3. Wait a few minutes, then refeed the child.
○ 4. Administer the prescribed antiemetic.

108. When the nurse prepares to draw up 2 units of a short-acting insulin and 3 units of a long-acting insulin in the same syringe, the nurse should

○ 1. inject air in the vial with the long-acting insulin first.
○ 2. draw up the clear insulin first.
○ 3. draw up either insulin first.
○ 4. use a high-dose insulin syringe.

109. The mother of an infant with iron-deficiency anemia asks the nurse what she could have done to prevent the anemia. The nurse should teach the mother that it is helpful to introduce solid foods into the infant's diet at age

○ 1. 1 to 2 months.
○ 2. 5 to 6 months.
○ 3. 8 to 10 months.
○ 4. 10 to 12 months.

110. The nurse is caring for a client who is having an acute asthma attack. Which of the following symptoms should the nurse be most concerned about while caring for the client?

○ 1. Loud wheezing.
○ 2. Tenacious, thick sputum.
○ 3. Decreased breath sounds.
○ 4. Persistent cough.

111. A client who is in the end stage of cardiac myopathy asks the nurse about having a transplant. The nurse explains that the client could be a candidate for a

○ 1. heart transplant.
○ 2. liver transplant.
○ 3. lung transplant.
○ 4. kidney transplant.

112. Which of the following skin care instructions would be appropriate for a client receiving radiation therapy?

○ 1. Avoid shaving with straight-edge razors.
○ 2. Cleanse the skin daily with antibacterial soap.
○ 3. Apply moisturizing lotion before and after each treatment.
○ 4. Keep the radiated area covered with a sterile gauze dressing.

113. A client has returned to the unit after a heart catheterization. Her left femoral dressing has a moderate amount of bloody drainage, and the client is complaining of severe pain in that area. What is the priority nursing intervention?

○ 1. Assess the airway.
○ 2. Administer oxygen.
○ 3. Apply pressure to the site.
○ 4. Assess the pulse in the left extremity.

114. The nurse tells the parent of a child who is taking valproic acid (Depakene) that the child will need to have routine blood analyses consisting of which of the following?

○ 1. Complete blood count and alkaline phosphate level.
○ 2. Cholesterol and platelet levels.
○ 3. Electrolytes and complete blood count.
○ 4. Platelet and fibrinogen levels.

115. Bacterial conjunctivitis has affected several children at a local day care center. A nurse consultant is contacted for help. Which of the following would the nurse consultant most likely advise to minimize the risk for infection?

○ 1. Close the day care center for 1 week to control the outbreak.
○ 2. Restrict the infected children from returning for 48 hours after treatment.
○ 3. Perform thorough handwashing before and after touching any child in the day care center.
○ 4. Set up a conference with the parents of each child to explain the situation carefully.

116. The nurse is evaluating the client's potential for development of a pressure sore. Which of the following individual characteristics would be the best indicator of risk for the client's developing a pressure sore?

○ 1. The client's nutritional status.
○ 2. The client's circulatory status.
○ 3. The client's mobility status.
○ 4. The client's orientation status.

117. A patient with acute pancreatitis is made NPO, with the intent of not stimulating the pancreas. The client is prescribed an intravenous infusion of D5 ½ NS at 120 mL/hour. After 3 days of this regimen, the nurse should observe the client for which of the following metabolic conditions?

○ 1. Ketosis.
○ 2. Hyperglycemia.
○ 3. Metabolic syndrome.
○ 4. Lactic acidosis.

118. The nurse is assisting a client to ambulate as part of his cardiac rehabilitation program. He complains of midsternal burning. From an earlier assessment, the nurse knows that this is a typical complaint of the client and decides to

○ 1. stop and assess the client further.

○ 2. measure the client's blood pressure and heart rate.

○ 3. call for help and place the client in a wheelchair.

○ 4. administer nitroglycerin.

119. The nurse evaluates a client's knowledge as deficient when the client makes which of the following statements about the drug dexamethasone (Decadron)?

○ 1. "I cannot stop the Decadron all at one time."

○ 2. "If I forget a dose, it's no big deal, I'll just take it when I remember it."

○ 3. "When I get a cold, I need to let my doctor know."

○ 4. "I need to watch for an allergic reaction when I first start taking Decadron."

120. A 3-month-old is admitted to the pediatric unit with moderate dehydration. Which of the following would the nurse expect to assess?

○ 1. Oliguria.

○ 2. Rapid, thready pulse.

○ 3. Decreased skin elasticity.

○ 4. Pale skin color.

121. The nurse is assessing a client who is suspected of being in the early symptomatic stages of HIV infection. Which of the following symptoms of infection would the nurse most likely detect during this stage?

○ 1. Whitish-yellow patches in the mouth.

○ 2. Dyspnea.

○ 3. Bloody diarrhea.

○ 4. Raised, hyperpigmented lesions on the legs.

122. A primiparous client who is breast-feeding develops endometritis on the third postpartum day. Which of the following instructions would the nurse give to the mother?

○ 1. The neonate will need to be bottle-fed for the next few days.

○ 2. The condition typically is treated with intravenous antibiotic therapy.

○ 3. The client's uterus may become "boggy," requiring frequent massage and oxytocics.

○ 4. The client needs to remain in bed in a side-lying position as much as possible.

123. After instructing a primipara client who is breast-feeding how to prevent nipple soreness during feedings, the nurse determines that the client needs *further* instruction when she states which of the following?

○ 1. "I should position the baby the same way for each feeding."

○ 2. "I should make sure the baby grasps the entire areola and nipple."

○ 3. "I should air dry my breasts and nipples for 10 to 15 minutes after the feeding."

○ 4. "I shouldn't use a hand breast pump if my nipples get sore."

124. A client who has Ménière's disease is experiencing an acute attack of vertigo. Which of the following interventions should the nurse include in the care plan?

○ 1. Darken the client's room and provide a quiet environment.

○ 2. Provide a low-sodium, bland diet.

○ 3. Administer a narcotic to relieve headache.

○ 4. Encourage fluid intake to prevent dehydration.

125. During a home visit to a primiparous client 1 week postpartum who is bottle-feeding her neonate, the client tells the nurse that her mother has suggested that she feed the neonate cereal so he will sleep through the night. Which of the following would be the nurse's *best* response?

○ 1. "It is permissible to give the baby cereal if it is really thinned with formula."

○ 2. "The time for starting cereal varies, so check with your pediatrician."

○ 3. "Formula is the food best digested by the baby until about 4 to 6 months of age."

○ 4. "If cereal is given too early in life, the undigested food can lead to a need for surgery."

126. When a client states that he is allergic to amoxicillin (Ampicillin), even though his medication administration record and armband to do not indicate medication allergies, the nurse should do which of the following measures?

○ 1. Administer the prescribed medication.

○ 2. Withhold the amoxicillin (Ampicillin).

○ 3. Administer another, similarly acting, antibiotic.

○ 4. Call the family to verify the client's statement.

127. While assessing a term neonate on a home visit to a primiparous client 2 weeks after a vaginal delivery, the nurse observes that the neonate is slightly jaundiced and the stool is a pale, light color. The nurse notifies the physician, because these findings are indicative of which of the following?

○ 1. Biliary atresia.

○ 2. Rh isoimmunization.

○ 3. ABO incompatibility.

○ 4. Esophageal varices.

128. A 6-year-old child is admitted to the hospital for heart surgery to repair tetralogy of Fallot. The nurse should anticipate that when the child goes home the parents will most likely have a concern about

○ 1. allowing the child to lead a normal, active life.

○ 2. persuading the child to get enough rest.

○ 3. having the child develop postoperative complications.

○ 4. having the child out of school for a month.

129. A client is recovering from abdominal surgery and

has a nasogastric tube inserted. The nurse understands that the primary reason that the tube is in place is to achieve which of the following functions in the gastrointestinal tract?
○ 1. Compression.
○ 2. Lavage.
○ 3. Decompression.
○ 4. Gavage.

130. The nurse teaches the mother of a toddler who has had cleft palate repair that her child is at risk for developing which of the following in the future?
○ 1. Hearing problems.
○ 2. Poor self-concept.
○ 3. Speech defect.
○ 4. Chronic sinus infections.

131. The nurse assesses a client who is receiving a tube feeding. Which of the following situations would require prompt intervention from the nurse?
○ 1. The client is sitting upright in bed while the feeding is infusing.
○ 2. The feeding that is infusing has been hanging for 8 hours.
○ 3. The client has a gastric residual of 25 mL.
○ 4. The feeding solution is at room temperature.

132. A client has been taking furosemide (Lasix) for 2 days. The nurse realizes that a possible side effect of this type of diuretic is
○ 1. an elevated blood urea nitrogen (BUN).
○ 2. an elevated potassium level.
○ 3. a decreased potassium level.
○ 4. an elevated sodium level.

133. When suctioning the respiratory tract of a client, it is recommended that the suctioning period not exceed how many seconds?
○ 1. 5 seconds.
○ 2. 10 seconds.
○ 3. 15 seconds.
○ 4. 20 seconds.

134. An 80-year-old client with severe kidney damage is placed on life support and dialysis. Care decisions are being made by his wife, who is showing signs of early Alzheimer's disease. The client's daughter arrives from out of town with a copy of the client's living will, which states that the client did not want to be on life support. Which of the following would be *most* appropriate for the nurse to do?
○ 1. Immediately inform the physician about the living will.
○ 2. Suggest to the daughter that she discuss her father's wishes with her mother.
○ 3. Prepare to remove the client from life support.
○ 4. Make a copy of the living will and give it to the client's wife.

135. Clients must meet certain criteria to be eligible for plasminogen activator (t-PA) or alteplase recombi-

nant (Activase) therapy. Which one of the following conditions makes the client ineligible to receive t-PA or alteplase recombinant therapy?
○ 1. Age greater than 65 years.
○ 2. No symptoms of a stroke.
○ 3. Hypotension.
○ 4. Current, active internal bleeding.

136. When caring for a client with myasthenia gravis who is receiving anticholinesterase drug therapy, the nurse must be able to distinguish cholinergic crisis from myasthenic crisis. Which of the following symptoms is *not* present in a cholinergic crisis?
○ 1. Improved muscle strength after intravenous administration of edrophonium chloride (Tensilon).
○ 2. Increased weakness.
○ 3. Diaphoresis.
○ 4. Increased salivation.

137. The nurse identifies the type of presentation shown in Figure 1 as which of the following?
○ 1. Frank breech.
○ 2. Compound breech.
○ 3. Complete breech.
○ 4. Incomplete breech.

138. Which of the following client statements indicates that the client with hepatitis B understands his discharge teaching?
○ 1. "I will not drink alcohol for at least 1 year."
○ 2. "I must avoid sexual intercourse."
○ 3. "I should be able to resume normal activity in a week or two."
○ 4. "Because hepatitis B is a chronic disease, I know I will always be jaundiced."

139. Which of the following examples would the nurse use to describe bulimia to a group of parents at a local community center?
○ 1. An adolescent male who uses calorie-counting to maintain his weight in the desirable range for his height.
○ 2. A college-age male who uses regular exercise to

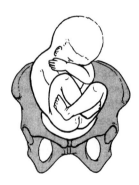

Figure 1.

be able to eat and drink what he wants without gaining weight.

○ 3. A middle-age female who uses diet pills occasionally to help her lose 10 pounds.

○ 4. A college-age female who uses bingeing and purging to keep her weight close to her normal range.

140. An early sign of Hodgkin's disease is
○ 1. difficulty breathing.
○ 2. swollen cervical lymph nodes.
○ 3. difficulty swallowing.
○ 4. feeling of fullness over the liver.

141. An intravenous infusion is to be administered through a scalp vein on an infant's head. The nurse should prepare the parents for the procedure by explaining that
○ 1. it will be necessary to remove a small amount of hair from the infant's scalp.
○ 2. a sedative will be given to the infant to help keep the child quiet.
○ 3. visiting the infant will be delayed until the infusion has been completed.
○ 4. holding the infant will be contraindicated while the infusion is being administered.

142. Which of the following goals would be most expected for a client with acute pancreatitis?
○ 1. The client reports minimal abdominal pain.
○ 2. The client regains a normal pattern for bowel movements.
○ 3. The client limits alcohol intake to two to three drinks per week.
○ 4. The client maintains normal liver function.

143. A nurse is caring for a child with diabetes mellitus at camp. The child presents as being irritable and complaining of a headache. Which of the following would the nurse do *first*?
○ 1. Administer 2 ounces of orange juice.
○ 2. Notify the physician about the child's complaints.
○ 3. Check the child's blood glucose level.
○ 4. Send the child back to the planned activities.

144. A client tells the nurse that her bra fits more snugly at certain times of the month and she is concerned this may be a sign of breast cancer. The *best* response for the nurse is to explain that
○ 1. a change in breast size should be checked by her physician.
○ 2. benign cysts tend to cause the breast to vary in size.
○ 3. it is normal for the breast to increase in size before menstruation begins.
○ 4. a difference in size of her breasts is related to normal growth and development.

145. Which of the following is an example of traditional Chinese medicine found in Asian American culture?

○ 1. Health is described as harmony between family members.
○ 2. Illness is caused by an imbalance of the yin and yang.
○ 3. Exercise to the point of overexertion can improve health.
○ 4. Illness is caused by a change in eating habits.

146. A client is scheduled for an intravenous pyelogram (IVP). Which of the following questions would be most important for the nurse to ask the client in preparation for the procedure?
○ 1. "Have you ever had an IVP before?"
○ 2. "Do you have any allergies to shellfish?"
○ 3. "When was your last bowel movement?"
○ 4. "Have you ever experienced any urinary incontinence?"

147. Which oral contraceptive is considered safe for use while breast-feeding because it will not affect the breast milk or breast-feeding?
○ 1. Estrogen.
○ 2. Estrogen and progestin.
○ 3. Progestin.
○ 4. Testosterone.

148. A multigravid client at 36 weeks' gestation who is visiting the clinic for a routine visit begins to sob and tells the nurse, "My boyfriend has been beating me up once in a while since I became pregnant—but I can't bring myself to leave him because I don't have a job and I don't know how I would take care of my other children." Which of the following actions would be the priority at this time?
○ 1. Contact a social worker for assistance and family counseling.
○ 2. Help the client make concrete plans for the safety of herself and her children.
○ 3. Tell the client that she shouldn't allow anyone to hit her or her children.
○ 4. Provide the client with brochures on the statistics about violence against women.

149. Sulfadiazine has been ordered for a client who has a urinary tract infection (UTI). Which of the following nursing interventions is most appropriate for administering sulfonamides?
○ 1. Encourage the client to take the medication with meals.
○ 2. Instruct the client to drink at least 8 glasses of water a day.
○ 3. Measure the client's urinary output.
○ 4. Instruct the client that the urine may turn reddish-orange.

150. A client with chronic undifferentiated schizophrenia is having an acute exacerbation of symptoms. The client states, "Black cats and black hats. Where does the time go?" Which of the following would be *most* important for the nurse to do?

○ 1. "Halloween is getting close, isn't it."
○ 2. "Do you have a black cat?"
○ 3. "What's the connection between cats, hats, and time?"
○ 4. "Time certainly does go faster these days."

151. A client has been diagnosed with multi-infarct (or vascular) dementia (MID). Although there is no cure, there are ways to slow the progression of the disease. When preparing a teaching plan for the client and family, which of the following would be the *most* critical factor for slowing MID?
○ 1. Administering anticoagulants such as warfarin (Coumadin).
○ 2. Administering benzodiazepines such as lorazepam to decrease choreiform movements.
○ 3. Managing related symptoms such as depression.
○ 4. Managing the symptoms by increasing dopamine availability.

152. While performing cardiopulmonary resuscitation (CPR) on a 5-year-old child, the nurse palpates for a pulse. Which of the following sites is best for checking the pulse during CPR in a 5-year-old child?
○ 1. Femoral.
○ 2. Carotid.
○ 3. Radial.
○ 4. Brachial.

153. The clinical manifestations of nephrotic syndrome include which of the following?
○ 1. Hematuria.
○ 2. Massive proteinuria.
○ 3. Increased serum albumin.
○ 4. Weight loss.

154. A child with tetralogy of Fallot and a history of severe hypoxic episodes is to be admitted to the pediatric unit. Which of the following would be *most* important for the nurse to have at the bedside?
○ 1. Morphine sulfate in a syringe ready to administer.
○ 2. Oxygen tubing and gauge plugged in.
○ 3. Blood pressure cuff and stethoscope.
○ 4. Suction tubing and equipment.

155. Which attitude would most likely be seen in a Mexican American client with pain?
○ 1. "Enduring pain is a part of God's will."
○ 2. "This pain is killing me."
○ 3. "I've got to see a doctor right away."
○ 4. "I can't go on in pain like this any longer."

156. A client tells the nurse that he is voiding small amounts of urine every 30 to 60 minutes. Which of the following actions is the nurse's first priority?
○ 1. Palpate for a distended bladder.
○ 2. Catheterize the client for a residual urine.
○ 3. Request a urine specimen for culture.
○ 4. Encourage an increased fluid intake.

157. Which of the following interventions would be most appropriate for a client with chronic renal failure?
○ 1. Apply corticosteroid creams to relieve itching.
○ 2. Achieve pain control with analgesics.
○ 3. Maintain a low-sodium diet.
○ 4. Measure abdominal girth daily.

158. An 18-month-old, previously well child presents to the physician's office with severe respiratory distress. The father was babysitting and does not think the child choked. Which of the following would the nurse do *first*?
○ 1. Perform the abdominal thrust maneuver.
○ 2. Call an ambulance to take the toddler to the emergency room.
○ 3. Determine the child's oxygen saturation level.
○ 4. Carry the child next door for a chest radiograph.

159. The nurse is assessing a child's skeletal traction and notices that the weights are on the floor. Which of the following would the nurse do *next*?
○ 1. Raise the weights so that the child can move up in bed.
○ 2. Notify the physician immediately.
○ 3. Put the foot of the bed on blocks.
○ 4. Move the child up in bed.

160. Some parents ask about food requirements for school-aged children. The nurse explains that compared with the food requirements of preschoolers and adolescents, the food requirements of school-aged children are not as great because they have a lower
○ 1. growth rate.
○ 2. metabolic rate.
○ 3. level of activity.
○ 4. hormonal secretion rate.

161. When assessing a 17-year-old client with depression for suicide risk, which of the following questions would be *best*?
○ 1. "What movies about death have you watched lately?"
○ 2. "Can you tell me what you think about suicide."
○ 3. "Has anyone in your family ever committed suicide?"
○ 4. "Are you thinking about killing yourself?"

162. Which of the following is a major risk factor for having a low-birth-weight baby?
○ 1. Heredity.
○ 2. Smoking.
○ 3. Drug use during pregnancy.
○ 4. Poor nutrition.

163. Which of the following techniques is best for the nurse to use in evaluating the parents' ability to administer ear drops correctly?
○ 1. Observe the parents instilling the drops in the child's ear.
○ 2. Listen to the parents as they describe the procedure.

○ 3. Ask the parents to list the steps in the procedure.

○ 4. Ask the parents whether they have read the handout on the procedure.

164. Ibuprofen (Motrin) is prescribed for a client with osteoarthritis. Which of the following instructions about ibuprofen should the nurse include in the client's teaching plan?

○ 1. Report the development of tinnitus.

○ 2. Increase vitamin B_{12} intake.

○ 3. Take with food or antacids.

○ 4. Have the complete blood count monitored monthly.

165. When a client has had surgery for a ruptured appendix, the nurse should document the wound as

○ 1. clean.

○ 2. clean-contaminated.

○ 3. contaminated.

○ 4. infected.

166. A staff member states, "I don't know why Mary is so depressed. She lives in an exclusive part of town and has gorgeous clothes. Her husband seems to care about her very much. She really has it all." Which of the following would the nurse conclude from the staff member's statement?

○ 1. An accurate assessment of the client has been made.

○ 2. The staff member is jealous of the client.

○ 3. There is no reason for the client to be depressed.

○ 4. The staff member needs teaching about major depression.

167. The mother tells the nurse that she does not understand why her child had another attack. He was not around any of the things that trigger his asthma. The nurse explains to the mother that asthma attacks may be triggered by various mechanisms, including certain food allergies, and states that which of the following foods would most likely be responsible for such an allergic reaction?

○ 1. Whitefish.

○ 2. Tossed salad.

○ 3. Hamburger patty.

○ 4. Fudge brownies.

168. When preparing to administer a tapwater enema, in which position should the nurse place the client?

○ 1. Supine.

○ 2. Semi-Fowler's.

○ 3. Right lateral.

○ 4. Left Sims'.

169. Which of the following is a risk factor for the development of pressure ulcers?

○ 1. Ambulating less than twice a day.

○ 2. An indwelling urinary catheter.

○ 3. Decreased serum albumin.

○ 4. Elevated white blood cell count.

170. A 42-year-old woman was admitted to hospital with a hemoglobin of 6.5 g/dL. She is experiencing symptoms of cerebral tissue hypoxia. Which of the following nursing interventions would be *most* important?

○ 1. Plan frequent rest periods throughout the day.

○ 2. Assist the client in ambulating to the bathroom.

○ 3. Check the temperature of the water before the client showers.

○ 4. Refer the client to occupational therapy for energy conservation interventions.

171. A client has been diagnosed with multiple myeloma. Which of the following laboratory values should the nurse expect to find in a client with multiple myeloma?

○ 1. Polycythemia vera.

○ 2. Decreased serum protein.

○ 3. Hypocalcemia.

○ 4. Bence Jones protein.

172. The nurse is caring for a multigravid client in active labor who has contractions occurring 2 to 3 minutes apart and lasting 45 seconds. After the administration of an epidural anesthetic, the client's blood pressure drops from 124/80 to 84/60 mm Hg. Which of the following would the nurse expect the physician to order *next*?

○ 1. Atropine sulfate.

○ 2. Ephedrine.

○ 3. Methylergonovine.

○ 4. Oxytocin.

173. A major intervention for the prevention of lung cancer is

○ 1. to encourage the public to install high-efficiency particulate air filters (HEPA filters) in their homes.

○ 2. to encourage cigarette smokers to have yearly chest radiographs.

○ 3. to offer strategies for smoking cessation.

○ 4. to recommend that homes and apartments be checked for asbestos leakage.

174. A client diagnosed with tuberculosis (TB) is taking medication for the treatment of TB. The nurse should instruct the client that he will be safe from infecting others approximately how long after initiation of the chemotherapy regimen?

○ 1. Within 48 hours after initiating chemotherapy.

○ 2. Two to 3 weeks after initiation of chemotherapy.

○ 3. Results vary with each client, so it is difficult to predict.

○ 4. After completion of 6 months of chemotherapy.

175. Which of the following client statements indicates that a client with major depression and suicidal ideation is improving?

○ 1. "I'll go to group when I have more energy."

○ 2. "I only think about killing myself at night."

○ 3. "My kids need me to be around."

○ 4. "I want everyone to leave me alone."

176. A nulligravid client at 34 weeks' gestation visits the clinic complaining of flu-like symptoms and a bull's eye–like rash. She reports that she went camping last weekend and may have gotten a tick bite. The client is diagnosed with Lyme disease. Which of the following medications would the nurse expect the physician to order?

○ 1. Tetracycline (Panmycin).

○ 2. Doxycycline (Vibramycin).

○ 3. Penicillin. (Pen-Vee K).

○ 4. Gentamicin (Garamycin).

177. The physician orders an amnioinfusion for a multigravid client in active labor. When preparing the client's teaching plan, the nurse would include which of the following as a likely reason for using this procedure?

○ 1. Early decelerations.

○ 2. Meconium-stained fluid.

○ 3. Very short umbilical cord.

○ 4. Multifetal pregnancy.

178. A client is scheduled for a surgical procedure. When planning the client's care, the nurse would consider that which of the following conditions will increase the client's risk for complications after surgery?

○ 1. A history of diabetes.

○ 2. A history of sensitivity to aspirin.

○ 3. A history of osteoarthritis.

○ 4. A history of chronic low back pain.

179. A 36-year-old man is receiving three different chemotherapeutic agents for Hodgkin's disease. The nurse explains to the client that the three drugs are given over an extended period because

○ 1. the three drugs can be given at lower doses.

○ 2. the second and third drugs increase the effectiveness of the first drug.

○ 3. the first two drugs are toxic to cancer cells, and the third drug promotes cell growth.

○ 4. the three drugs have a synergistic effect and act on the cancer cells with different mechanisms.

180. Which of the following should the nurse write on the parents' care plan as an expected client outcome for the nursing diagnosis of Anticipatory Grieving related to their child's death? The parents will

○ 1. keep to themselves until 3 months after the baby's death.

○ 2. be able to discuss their feelings with each other.

○ 3. immerse themselves in work and outside activities.

○ 4. act as if nothing has happened.

Correct Answers and Rationale

The letters in parentheses following the rationale identify the step of the nursing process (A, D, P, I, E), client needs (1, 2, 3, 4, 5, 6, 7, 8, 9, 10), and nursing care area (O, Y, M, X). See the inside front cover for the key.

1. 1. The colleague needs to provide the nurse with information about spouse abuse. Giving information about reasons for staying is useful for decreasing the nurse's frustration. Although expressing empathy is appropriate, it does not help the nurse understand the client's needs and behaviors. Telling the nurse that there will be another chance is not helpful and fails to educate the other nurse about the dynamics of abuse. Although dependence is a problem, women who are abused can overcome this and leave if they have support, not criticism. Saying that abused women almost never leave does not help the nurse understand the client's needs and behaviors. (I, 1, X)

2. 3. First, convert micrograms to milligrams: 200 μg = 0.2 mg. Then, 0.2 mg / x mL = 0.2 mg / 1 mL, so x = 1.0 mL. (I, 8, M)

3. 3. Viral gastroenteritis may be communicable, and all of the other children are already at risk for infection. The infant should be placed in a private room.

4. 4. The neonate would be considered large for gestational age (LGA) because the neonate weighs more than 4000 g (90th percentile). Therefore, the nurse needs to assess for the possibility of complications. Common complications for an LGA neonate include hyperbilirubinemia from the bruising and polycythemia, cephalohematoma, caput succedaneum, molding, phrenic nerve paralysis, and fractured clavicle. Hypoglycemia, not hyperglycemia, is a problem for the LGA neonate, because glycogen stores are quickly used to maintain the weight. Hypercalcemia is not usually found in LGA neonates. Hypocalcemia is common in infants of diabetic mothers. Hypermagnesemia may occur in neonates whose mothers received large doses of magnesium sulfate to treat severe preeclampsia. (A, 9, O)

5. 2. Ovarian enlargement, hyperstimulation syndrome, febrile reaction, and multiple pregnancies are considered adverse effects of menotropins. If ovarian enlargement occurs, the drug should be discontinued to prevent damage to the ovary. Pulmonary edema is not associated with menotropin use. Visual disturbances and breast tenderness are associated with the use of clomiphene citrate (Clomid), another drug prescribed for infertility treatment. (E, 8, O)

6. 1. Organ Procurement Organizations are responsible for organ recovery in the United States. These organizations have offices in major cities, and provide services on a local, state, and regional basis. The agency is the repository for information about tissues and organs and their distribution. The American Transplant Association coordinates recipients of transplants. The American Hospice Foundation is involved with hospice care. The American Association of Critical Care Nurses is involved with professional critical care nurses. (P, 1, M)

7. 3. Fluid accumulates in the base of the pleura postoperatively. The lower chest tube, called the posterior or lower tube, will drain serous and serosanguineous fluid that accumulates as a result of the surgical procedure. A larger-diameter tube is usually used for the lower tube to ensure drainage of clots. Air rises, and the anterior or upper tube is used to remove air from the pleural space. The practice of "milking" the tubes to prevent clots is becoming less common; the surgeon's orders must be followed regarding this procedure. (A, 10, M)

8. 1. Elderly clients are a high-risk group for depression. The classic symptoms of depression frequently are masked, and depression present differently in the aging population. Depression in late life is underdiagnosed because the symptoms are incorrectly attributed to aging or medical problems. Impairment of cognition in a previously well elderly client or psychosomatic complaints may be the presenting symptom of depression. Traditional therapies are usually effective. (A, 3, M)

9. 4. Fears of the adolescent include body changes and loss of control. The young adolescent is typically concerned about the inability to control body changes and feelings and about embarrassment. The typical adolescent is more concerned about being separated from the peer group than from the family and schoolwork and is realistically worried about experiencing pain and loss of control. (A, 3, Y)

10. 2. The mother's statements reveal that she is having problems with parenting. Therefore, a referral to a parenting education program is the most appropriate measure at this time. (P, 1, X)

11. 2. The nurse acts in a reasonable and prudent manner to correctly identify a client by checking the client's armband and asking the client's name. Omitting to do so is an act of negligence. *Res judicata* and *stare decisis* are legal doctrines used to guide the courts in making decisions. Vicarious liability is a concept in which the

employer is held liable for the nurse's act. It was established after precedent-setting cases in the 1960s. (I, 1, M)

12. 2. Morphine can cause respiratory depression, leading to respiratory arrest. The nurse should assess the client's respiratory rate before administration and throughout the course of analgesic treatment. Morphine does not affect blood pressure, pulse rate, or temperature. (I, 8, M)

13. 1. Anger is a natural result of feelings of loss and helplessness in normal, healthy people. It is a natural response to coping with a sick child. Nurses should recognize anger in clients and families. Parents are usually able to control their anger in a socially acceptable manner. Nurses can assist clients and families to overcome helplessness and anger in an acceptable manner. (I, 1, Y)

14. 3. Supervised activities that promote walking are behavioral management strategies that help a client such as this. The client's cognitive and memory impairment would not be conducive to playing bingo. Allowing the behavior at selected intervals would further encourage the client to wander. The client should not be restrained in a chair. (I, 1, M)

15. 3. With a new complaint of numbness in the fingers, the nurse needs to first assess the circulation to evaluate color, evidence of swelling, and presence of pulses to determine whether there is any circulatory compromise. Once the nurse had evaluated the child's circulatory status, the next action would be to verify the arm's position above the level of the heart. Notifying the physician would not be done until the child's neurovascular status and position are checked. Cutting the cast would be done only with a physician's order. (I, 9, Y)

16. 4. The second-generation antihistamines do not cross the blood–brain barrier and therefore do not cause sedation or psychomotor dysfunction. They are much more expensive than first-generation antihistamines. The effectiveness is similar. The medications are rapidly absorbed in 1 to 2 hours after oral administration on an empty stomach. (I, 8, M)

17. 3. LBP is commonly associated with overuse or an injury to the soft tissue structures. It is estimated that 50% to 70% of people will experience musculoskeletal back pain at some time. Although the other causes of pain must be excluded, the initial treatment of LBP is usually aimed at decreasing the inflammatory response to the tissue injury. (D, 4, M)

18. 2. At the time of a major crisis, the client suffering a great loss is best helped by being encouraged to talk about his experience and describe his feelings. Crisis interventions focus on re-establishing emotional equilibrium and preventing decompensation. Telling the client that everything will be fine is a cliché and inappropriate. Asking the client to stop talking so that the nurse can write notes places more emphasis on the nurse's needs than on the client's needs. Telling the client to think more about what happened for further discussion the next day is not helping him with the crisis. (I, 5, X)

19. 2. Beclomethasone is an inhaled steroid used for the maintenance treatment of asthma. The steroid can precipitate overgrowth of fungus, such as oral *Candida albicans*. Rinsing the mouth well after each use decreases the incidence of oral fungal infections. (I, 8, M)

20. 1. The incident report should be given to the nurse manager. The incident report should not be placed on the chart because it is considered a confidential communication and cannot be subpoenaed by a client or used as evidence in lawsuits. It is appropriate, ethical, and legally required that the fall be documented in the chart. Unless there is a change in the client's condition reflecting an injury from the fall, there is no need to notify the family. If the family does need to be notified, the nurse manager or the physician should place the call. (I, 1, M)

21. 2. General wound care is appropriate initially. This includes washing the bite area with lots of water, because infections occur frequently with animal bites, especially those on the arms or hands. Next, the mother should be advised to determine the extent of the injury and then to follow-up with the child's physician if needed. A trip to the local care center would be warranted if the bite injury was extensive or there was severe bleeding. Although knowledge of when the child last had a tetanus vaccination is important, the child's wound takes priority. For rabies injections, there needs to be a history of rabies or unusual behavior in the pet. (I, 9, Y)

22. 4. The biophysical profile uses a sonogram to assess five parameters, including fetal breathing movements, fetal movements, fetal tone, amniotic fluid volume, and fetal heart rate activity. A nonstress test is used to evaluate fetal heart rate activity. (I, 3, O)

23. 2. Chemoprophylaxis should be given to household contacts and close contacts only. To prevent community outbreaks, chemoprophylaxis with rifampin 600 mg twice a day for 2 days or a single dose of Cipro 500 mg is indicated for household and close contacts of clients with *H. influenzae* meningitis. (I, 8, Y)

24. 2. Infants and toddlers younger than 2 years of age should not be placed on a fat-restricted diet, because cholesterol and other fatty acids are required for continued neural growth. After the age of 2 years it is believed that no harm is done by encouraging a child to eat a variety of foods, maintain a desirable body

weight, limit saturated fat and cholesterol, and increase fiber. (D, 4, M)

25. 1. The petroleum jelly is thought to smother the lice. Pediculicide should not be applied to the face or close to the eyes. Bacitracin ointment will not kill the lice. (I, 8, M)

26. 1. A major goal of safety and accident prevention focuses on having all cleaning supplies and medications locked up. Toddlers are great climbers and can very quickly get into what they should not. The child should not play in the bathroom even if the parent is present, because the child will think that it is okay to play with these items when the parent is not present. Playing with cords could lead to possible strangulation. The child-protective cabinets locks should work unless they were installed incorrectly or are defective. (E, 2, Y)

27. 4. Steroid therapy can mask the signs of infection, making an atypical presentation. (A, 8, M)

28. 4. Fever is generally not thought to be a sign of impaired renal function related to long-term use of gentamycin. The client should report signs of decreasing urinary function such as decreased output, unusual appearance of the urine, or edema. (A, 8, M)

29. 4. Plastic blocks are the most appropriate toy for a toddler in a croup tent. Because the blocks are plastic, they can be washed. For the pull toy to be used, the child would need to leave the mist tent, which is not advisable at this time. Although crayons may be appropriate for a mist tent, any paper, including story books, would become damp, crumble, and provide an environment for the growth of microorganisms. (I, 3, Y)

30. 2. Febrile seizures commonly occur as the fever rises. The exact cause of febrile convulsions is not known. Infants and young toddlers are the age groups primarily affected. Febrile seizures typically do not follow immunization administration. (I, 9, Y)

31. 4. Oral contraceptive use, pregnancy, and lactation are situations that increase demand for folic acid. With supplementation, a response should cause the reticulocyte count to increase within 2 to 3 days after therapy has begun. It is not necessary to take folic acid on an empty stomach. A client may safely take both iron and folic acid supplementation. (I, 8, M)

32. 4. Although acrocyanosis may be present for 24 to 48 hours after birth, central cyanosis of the trunk indicates decreased oxygenation from respiratory distress or another disease state (eg, cardiac anomalies). This should be reported to the physician and evaluated further. Maternal lochia serosa in scant amount is a normal finding 1 week postpartum, as is a nonpalpable maternal fundus. Presence of a neonatal tonic neck reflex is a normal finding in a 1-week-old neonate. (A, 9, O)

33. 4. Severe inflammatory acne is often treated with tetracycline or erythromycin. Isoretinoin is a retinoic acid derivative. Cephalexin and azithromycin are not used to treat acne. (A, 8, M)

34. 4. People with hip fractures have been found to have low vitamin K intakes; vitamin K plays an important role in production of at least one bone protein. Heavy alcohol use is a risk factor because it causes fluid excretion resulting in heavy losses of calcium in urine. If the antacid contains aluminum or magnesium, a net loss of calcium can occur. High-fiber diets bind up some of the dietary calcium. (D, 4, M)

35. 1. The postrape examination is important for detecting the possibility of venereal disease, which can be spread through rape. Additionally, if the victim or the rapist was not using a contraceptive, postcoital contraceptive methods should be discussed. The information provided does not indicate anxiety or physical injury, such as periurethral tears, as an issue, and these are not the primary reason for the examination. Menstrual difficulties are not a common result of rape unless pregnancy has resulted. (I, 6, X)

36. 3. The nurse should question the use of any local anesthetic agent with epinephrine on the hands or feet, because the epinephrine is a vasoconstrictor and can cause ischemia and gangrene of extremities. The nurse should suggest that the intern use bupivacaine (Marcaine) without epinephrine for the local anesthetic agent. An intern should be trained in suturing small superficial incisions, and the cosmetic effect should be acceptable. The client's room should be a sufficiently aseptic environment because there is no other client in the room. (D, 1, M)

37. 2. Chills are a normal response of the body's immune system to infection and are not a response of the sympathetic nervous system to pain. Tachycardia, increased respiratory rate, and dilated pupils are sympathetic effects. (A, 10, Y)

38. 3. In dark-skinned clients, cyanosis can best be detected by examining the conjunctiva, lips, and oral mucous membranes. Examining the retinas, nail beds, or inner aspects of the wrists is not an appropriate assessment for determining cyanosis in any client. (A, 4, M)

39. 3. 0.9 mg $/ x$ mL $= 0.6$ mg $/ 5$ mL; $x = 7.5$ mL. (I, 8, M)

40. 1. A biophysical profile includes a nonstress test; evaluation of fetal breathing movements, gross body movements, and fetal tone; and amniotic fluid volume measurement. Because an ultrasound analysis is used during the test, the client should plan to drink 1 to 2 L of fluid before the test to ensure a full bladder, which provides better visualization of the fetus. The client does not need to be NPO before the test. The client does not need to

remain in the clinic for 4 hours after the test. However, if the client were scheduled for a contraction stress test, she would be observed as an outpatient for 1 to 4 hours after the test to make certain that the contractions had stopped. The client does not need to eat a high-fiber meal after the test. A high-fiber meal typically is indicated after certain radiographic procedures, such as an upper gastrointestinal series. (I, 9, O)

41. 3. The physician will most likely order packed red blood cells to alleviate the anemia of sickle cell disease. During pregnancy, sickle cell crises are more common and produce excruciating pain due to ischemia and infarction of various organs. Infections and pulmonary complications are also more common. Morphine or meperidine may be used to treat the client's pain. A transfusion of platelets may be ordered for clients exhibiting symptoms of the HELLP syndrome (hemolysis, elevated liver enzymes, and low platelets). An infusion of granulocytes may be ordered for a pregnant client diagnosed with aplastic anemia who develops an infection. Red cell transfusions and platelet transfusions also may be ordered for these clients to treat anemia or to control hemorrhage. Whole blood typically is used for a client who is hemorrhaging (eg, postpartum hemorrhage). The whole blood not only treats the anemia but also replaces blood volume. (P, 8, O)

42. 2. About 25% of the teenager's diet can come from snacks. This is a way for teenagers to obtain protein, thiamine, riboflavin, vitamin B_6, magnesium, and zinc. Although not all snacks are low in fat or contain these nutrients, the nurse should encourage the mother to provide snacks with these nutrients. (P, 4, M)

43. 3. Applying a water-soluble lubricant to the nares helps alleviate sore nares when a nasogastric tube is in place. (I, 9, M)

44. 1. Hindus do not eat beef. Sufficient protein can be obtained from lentils and fish. (A, 8, M)

45. 3. Although monitoring vital signs frequently is important, for the first few days the primary concern in burn care is fluid and electrolyte balance, with the goal being to replace fluid and electrolytes lost. With burns, fluid and electrolytes move from the interstitial spaces to the burn injury and are lost. These must be replaced. Once the child's fluid and electrolyte status has been addressed and fluid resuscitation has begun, preventing wound infection is a priority and efforts to control the child's pain can be initiated. (I, 10, Y)

46. 1. Sabin's polio vaccine is given by oral route. Salk's vaccine is given by deep injection into the largest muscle available if a killed viral vaccine is needed. A killed virus is given to immunocompromised children. (I, 4, Y)

47. 4. The nurse does not administer naloxone (Narcan), because naloxone is the antidote for morphine, not mida-

zolam (Versed). The benzodiazepine-receptor antagonist for midazolam is flumazenil (Romazicon). (D, 8, M)

48. 3. The client should be seated upright with arms raised and crossed in front and supported by the overbed table. The client's head should rest on the arms. This position allows for outward expansion of the chest wall and promotes collection of the pleural fluid at the base of the thorax. (P, 9, M)

49. 3. Three or more servings of dairy products meets the calcium requirement. This can be obtained through milk, cheese, yogurt, and foods such as tofu. Spinach contains oxalates, which decrease the availability of calcium. Six to eleven servings of whole grains are recommended. Vitamin A supplements are not necessary in vegetarian diets, because most vegetarian diets are rich in vitamin A. Vitamin A supplements can lead to anorexia, irritability, hair loss, and damage to the fetus. (P, 7, O)

50. 1. Intracellular microorganisms such as viruses and parasites invade the myocardium to survive. These microorganisms damage the vital organelles and cause cell death in the myocardium. The myocardium becomes weak, leading to heart failure; then T lymphocytes invade the myocardium in response to the viral infection. The T lymphocytes respond to the viral infection by secreting cytokines to kill the virus, but they also kill the virus-infected myocardium. Myocardial infarction, renal failure, and liver failure are not direct consequences of a viral or parasitic infection. (E, 2, M)

51. 2. The compensatory mechanism for respiratory acidosis is the renal system. In respiratory acidosis the kidneys will conserve bicarbonate (HCO_3^-) in an attempt to correct the acidosis. Excretion of HCO_3^- would exacerbate the body's acidosis. The lungs cannot compensate for a problem that arises in the respiratory system. (A, 10, M)

52. 2. Amiodarone is metabolized in the liver and excreted in the bile and feces. Liver toxicity has been reported, so the nurse will want to monitor the client's liver enzymes. Amiodarone does not affect the hemoglobin, CPK, or urinary function. (I, 10, M)

53. 2. Antibiotics are the drug of choice in treating otitis media. Antihistamines, ear drops, and cotton in the ears are not helpful and are not recommended. (I, 9, Y)

54. 2. Yogurt is high in protein because it is made from milk. The other choices are much higher in carbohydrates than protein except for bacon, which is higher in fat. (I, 7, Y)

55. 2. The extracellular fluid compartment consists of two divisions, interstitial and intravascular. Prominent neck veins, hypertension, and bounding pulse are indicative of fluid excess in the intravascular (plasma) compartment. Fluid excess occurring in the interstitial compartment would lead to clinical findings related to tissue edema. Extra fluid in the intracellular compartment would lead to central nervous system changes, such as confusion. (D, 10, M)

56. 3. Ciprofloxacin (Cipro) does not affect the aPTT level. It increases the theophylline level by 15% to 30% and may increase the PT level. Iron decreases the absorption of ciprofloxacin. (I, 8, M)

57. 3. Pediculosis capitis or head lice can be spread by close contact or sharing of head gear or combs and brushes with other children. Sharing craft supplies, swimming, or showering usually does not provide close enough contact to permit transmission. (D, 10, Y)

58. 1. In the first trimester, ultrasound scanning typically is ordered to determine the gestational age. This is especially important for a client with a history of irregular menstrual cycles to establish an accurate delivery date. There is no reason at this point in pregnancy to determine whether twins are present. This might be indicated if the fundal height were larger than the gestational age may indicate. Identifying the gender of the fetus is not a reason for an ultrasound examination unless there is a history of sex-linked genetic disorders. Pelvic adequacy can be determined by physical examination. If the client has a borderline pelvis, an ultrasound scan cannot confirm this. Pelvimetry can be done, but it is not performed as frequently anymore. (I, 3, O)

59. 2. The nurse should prepare to insert a nasogastric tube. The data collected provide evidence that the client is experiencing an upper gastrointestinal bleed secondary to a peptic ulcer. The client will be placed on NPO status and a nasogastric tube will be inserted to provide gastric decompression and alleviate vomiting. Administering antiemetics is not a priority action for a client who is hypotensive and vomiting coffee-ground emesis. Assessment of client stressors is appropriate after emergency care has been provided and the client stabilized. A modified Trendelenburg position is inappropriate for clients who are vomiting. (I, 10, M)

60. 3. If the client is symptomatic, suggesting decreased cardiac output, he will need to be treated, because maintaining circulation is the key goal. A temporary pacemaker can be inserted until the client is stable and the underlying etiology is determined. Cardiac catheterization with an electrophysiology study would follow insertion of the pacemaker. Bypass surgery is done when the arteries are occluded by plaque. An aortic balloon pump is used when pump failure is the problem. (P, 10, M)

61. 4. Refined grains are fortified with folic acid. Folic acid fortification is expected to prevent more than half of all neural tube defects. Vitamin C, which has multiple functions, is already added to many beverages and is widely available in many foods. Niacin maintains the normal functioning of the digestive tract and aids in energy metabolism. It is already added to enriched bread prod-

ucts and is widely available from many food sources. Vitamin B_{12} is involved in many metabolic processes. It is essential for the development of normal red blood cells. Many cereals, juices, soy, and bread products are fortified with vitamin B_{12}. (P, 7, M)

62. 3. The sudden onset of bright red drainage of this magnitude needs to be further assessed. Assessing vital signs is an important nursing action to determine whether there have been any changes in the client's status. Additional steps would include reinforcing the dressing and notifying the physician. Increasing the intravenous flow rate does not address the bleeding. Changing the dressing would be done only if the physician ordered it. (I, 9, M)

63. 2. Acute renal failure can occur secondary to a decrease in circulating fluid volume because of renal hypoperfusion. Paralytic ileus, adrenal insufficiency, and inappropriate antidiuretic hormone release can result in fluid volume alterations but do not occur secondary to a decrease in circulating fluid volume, (A, 10, Y)

64. 4. The goal that has the highest priority when a client has a massive bleed from esophageal varices is to maintain a patent airway. (I, 10, M)

65. 4. A client who is taking phenelzine (Nardil), a monoamine oxidase inhibitor (MAOI), needs to avoid foods that are rich in tyramine, because this food–drug combination can cause a hypertensive crisis. The client should be given a list of foods to avoid and should report headaches, palpitations, and a stiff neck to the physician immediately. Drinking 10 to 12 glasses of water each day is important to teach the client who is receiving lithium therapy. (P, 8, X)

66. 3. Clients with open fractures are particularly susceptible to infections. If not treated promptly, these infections can lead to the development of osteomyelitis. Localized symptoms of osteomyelitis include tenderness, swelling, and warmth at the site of infection, as well as unrelieved severe bone pain. Systemic symptoms include fever, chills, night sweats, and malaise. Avascular necrosis occurs when the blood supply to a bone is interrupted, most commonly in intracapsular hip fractures. Compartment syndrome is most commonly associated with fractures of the distal humerus and proximal tibia; it results from an increase in pressure on the nerves and blood supply within a closed tissue compartment. Fat embolism syndrome is associated most frequently with fractures of the long bones, ribs, and pelvis, which may or may not be open fractures. (E, 9, M)

67. 4. Impaired Verbal Communication is a priority nursing diagnosis for the client after a total laryngectomy because the client will have a tracheostomy. These clients frequently require teaching on methods of communication after surgery. Risk for Impaired Skin Integrity, Excess

Fluid Volume, and Ineffective Thermoregulation are not priority nursing diagnoses associated with laryngectomy surgery. (D, 10, M)

68. 3. The retina is especially susceptible to damage in a client with chronic hypertension. The arterioles supplying the retina are damaged. Such damage can lead to vision loss. (P, 9, M)

69. 3. Milia are white papules resulting from plugged sebaceous ducts that disappear by 2 to 4 weeks of age. Parents should be instructed to avoid scratching them to prevent secondary infection. Term neonates generally have many creases on the soles of their feet. Preterm neonates may have only a few creases due to their immaturity. Strawberry hemangiomas are elevated areas formed by immature capillaries which will disappear over time. Port wine stains are deep, dark red discolorations that require laser therapy for removal. Erythema toxicum is a newborn rash or "flea bite" rash that requires no treatment and disappears over time. (P, 3, O)

70. 4. Clients with fractures of the long bones, such as the femur, are particularly susceptible to fat embolism syndrome (FES). Signs and symptoms include chest pain, dyspnea, tachycardia, and cyanosis. Changes in mental status are caused by hypoxemia and can be the first symptoms noted in FES. The client can also be restless and febrile and can develop petechiae. Osteomyelitis is infection of the bone; signs and symptoms of osteomyelitis do not include respiratory symptoms. Compartment syndrome causes signs of localized neurovascular impairment, not systemic symptoms. Venous thrombosis occurs in the lower extremities and is caused by venous stasis. (D, 9, M)

71. 2. A small tuft of hair and an indentation at the base of the neonate's spine is termed spina bifida occulta. This condition usually occurs between the L5 and S1 vertebrae with failure of the vertebrae to completely fuse. There are usually no sensory or motor deficits with this condition. Spina bifida cystica includes meningocele, myelomeningocele, and lipomeningocele. Meningocele is characterized by a sac-like protrusion filled with spinal fluid and meninges. Usually, this condition is associated with sensory and motor deficits. Myelomeningocele is characterized by a sac-like protrusion filled with spinal fluid, meninges, nerve roots, and spinal cord. With myelomeningocele, there are usually sensory and motor deficits. (A, 3, O)

72. 1. The primary purpose of instilling 5 mL of normal saline before suctioning a tracheostomy tube is to thin the secretions to be suctioned. (I, 9, M)

73. 3. The client with emphysema has a chronically elevated carbon dioxide level. As a result, the normal stimulus for breathing in the medulla becomes ineffective. Instead, peripheral pressoreceptors in the aortic arch and carotid arteries, which are sensitive to oxygen blood levels, stimulate respirations. This is in response to low oxygen levels that have developed over time. If the client receives high concentrations of oxygen, the blood level of oxygen will rise excessively, the stimulus for respiration will decrease, and respiratory failure may result. Oxygen is not cooled. Humidification or administration of the oxygen through nasal cannula will not prevent depressed ventilation if the flow rate of the oxygen is too high. (I, 10, M)

74. 1. Protein intake is a concern in all vegetarian diets. Combining two incomplete proteins to make a complete protein (with all of the essential amino acids) can improve the client's protein intake. Rice with beans or tofu provides a complete protein. Soy milk would provide vitamin D and calcium, not protein. Yogurt provides vitamin D and calcium, not sufficient protein. Corn and rice do not make up a complete protein. However, corn and beans would be a complete protein. (I, 7, O)

75. 3. The client should be encouraged to join the community arthritis support group so that she can share her feelings with others who are facing similar experiences with this chronic illness and can identify with her concerns. A hobby will not help her resolve her feelings of being alone. Seeking counseling or discussing her feelings with a minister may be helpful, but these activities will not necessarily help the client to understand that there are many individuals who must adjust their lifestyles because of arthritis and that she is not alone. (I, 5, M)

76. 2. For the client who is unable to sit through meals to maintain adequate nutrition, the nurse would offer the client nutritious finger foods and fluids that he can consume while "on the run." Foods high in protein and carbohydrate, such as half of a peanut butter sandwich, will help to maintain nutritional needs. Adequate fluid intake is necessary, especially if the client has been started on lithium therapy. Directing the client to his room to eat is not helpful because the client will not stay in his room long enough to eat. Asking the client's family to bring his favorite foods or asking the client about his food preferences is not helpful in ensuring adequate nutrition for the hyperactive client who is unable to sit and eat. (P, 6, X)

77. 4. Telling the client to get her laundry and then showing her how to use the machine helps keep the client from becoming overly dependent on the nurse, establishes boundaries between the client and the nurse, and promotes positive self-worth. The statement, "Sure, I have time; I'll do it for you," is not therapeutic because it increases the client's dependency. Telling the client that she will have to wait because the nurse doesn't have time dismisses the client and insinuates that the nurse will do the laundry later, thus fostering dependency. Asking, "Can your family do it for you?" is not appropriate because the client is capable of doing her own laundry.

This statement places responsibility on the family instead of the client. (I, 6, X)

78. 2. Early signs and symptoms of hypermagnesemia include drowsiness, lethargy, nausea, and vomiting. Flushed skin is one sign of hypernatremia. Severe thirst is associated with hyperglycemia. Tremors are associated with hypomagnesemia. (E, 9, M)

79. 3. When blood glucose drops, the pancreas secretes the hormone glucagon. The glucagon travels to the liver, where it stimulates the liver to release glucose. The muscle does not release glucose into the bloodstream. Glucagon does not stimulate intestinal absorption of glucose. Glucagon works only at the liver. (D, 10, M)

80. 3. This statement is critical in nature and judgmental on the nurse's part. It is inappropriate for the nurse to make a comment like this at shift report or at any time. (I, 1, M)

81. 1. The nurse would teach personnel to communicate with clients in a calm, matter-of-fact manner, using short sentences and a moderate tone of voice. This approach promotes orientation, reinforces cognitive–perceptual functions, and decreases anxiety. A cheerful tone and humor are inappropriate, possibly leading to misperceptions by the client with cognitive–perceptual impairment. Using abstract terms and a loud tone of voice increases anxiety and may lead to misunderstanding. Lengthy explanations delivered with a quiet voice tone will lead to frustration and increased anxiety. (I, 1, X)

82. 1. During the emergent phase of burn care, one of the most significant problems is hypovolemic shock. The development of hypovolemic shock can lead to impaired blood flow through the heart and kidneys, resulting in decreased cardiac output and renal ischemia. Efforts are directed toward replacing lost fluids and preventing hypovolemic shock. Preventing infection and controlling pain are important goals, but preventing circulatory collapse is a higher priority. It is too early in the stage of burn injury to promote wound healing. (P, 10, M)

83. 2. A client with multiple sclerosis may have a sense of optimism and euphoria, particularly during remissions. Euphoria is characterized by mood elevation with an exaggerated sense of well-being. Inappropriate laughter, slurring of words, and visual hallucinations are uncharacteristic of euphoria. (A, 10, M)

84. 1. The "rule of nines" is used to determine the percentage of the client's body surface area that was burned. Medical treatment, including fluid volume replacement therapy, is based on the percentage of body surface area burned. (A, 10, M)

85. 2. The "click" the nurse feels when abducting the femur is made by the head of the femur as it slips into the acetabulum. This is Ortolani's sign and indicates a dislocated hip. This is not a normal finding for a 2-month-old. The nurse needs to gather additional information by checking for unequal leg lengths and asymmetry of the gluteal and thigh folds. Once the nurse has obtained additional assessment information, then the nurse would notify the physician. Usual medical treatment involves keeping the hip joint in an abducted position through triple diapering or a Pavlik harness. The goal of treatment is to keep the head of the femur centered in the acetabulum. Treatment needs to begin as soon as possible. Usually, the earlier treatment is started, then the better the outcome is. (I, 4, Y)

86. 4. Warfarin sodium (Coumadin) interferes with clotting factors II—prothrombin, VII, IX, and X. The nurse should monitor the PT and evaluate for the therapeutic effects of Coumadin. A therapeutic PT range is between 1.5 and 2.5 times the control value. It may also be reported as an International Normalized Ratio (INR), a standardized system that provides a common basis for communicating and interpreting PT results. The PTT is monitored in clients who are receiving heparin therapy. Serum potassium levels and arterial blood gas values are not affected by Coumadin. (E, 8, M)

87. 4. The lower abdominal pain is most likely caused by bladder spasms. A common cause of bladder spasms after TURP is blood clots obstructing the catheter; therefore, the nurse's first action should be to assess the patency of the catheter. Auscultating the abdomen for bowel sounds would be appropriate after patency of the catheter has been established. The nurse should assess for bladder spasms before administering an analgesic. A sitz bath would not relieve bladder spasms that are caused by an obstructed catheter. (I, 10, M)

88. 2. The parents of an infant with a congenital defect are frequently in a state of shock when the child is first born. The parents go through a period of grieving for the normal child they did not have. There are no data yet to support the other nursing diagnoses. (D, 5, Y)

89. 1. The nurse should not automatically discard the partial fill of imipenem–cilastatin (Primaxin) found at the client's bedside until further investigation is done. The nurse should recognize the cost of medications such as imipenem–cilastatin and consult with the pharmacist after identifying information on the partial fill that was found. The nurse should also ascertain whether the client received the last dose of imipenem–cilastatin. If the client did not receive the last dose, the nurse should notify the physician that the client did not receive the dose, receive orders, document, implement the orders, and complete an incident report. The nurse should administer the new partial fill of imipenem–cilastatin (Primaxin) so that the client can receive the antibiotic on time. (D, 2, M)

90. 2. For a client with moderate anxiety, the nurse would initially lead the client to a less stimulating environment and help him discuss his feelings. Doing so helps the client to gain control over anxiety that could be over-

whelming. Telling the client that it would be best to lie down until he is calmer is not appropriate because the client is too anxious to benefit from this intervention. Suggesting that the client try relaxation exercises could be helpful after the nurse takes the client to a less stimulating environment and allows the client to vent and discuss his feelings. Getting some medication to help the client relax is an intervention that the nurse would carry out later after trying to help the client decrease anxiety through ventilation and relaxation exercises. (I, 6, X)

91. 1. Clients who are receiving anticoagulant therapy should consult the physician before undergoing any dental work. The dentist should also be aware that the client is taking anticoagulants. A soft toothbrush is desirable for oral hygiene if the client is receiving anticoagulant therapy. It helps prevent the gums from bleeding. Rectal suppositories are contraindicated during anticoagulant therapy, because insertion of them may cause bleeding. Stool softeners may be used instead to prevent straining, which also may promote bleeding. Green leafy vegetables should not be eaten in excess because of their vitamin K content, which may alter the effectiveness of the anticoagulant therapy. (P, 8, M)

92. 3. Increasing the client's fluid intake to 3000 mL/day, unless contraindicated, is the most appropriate action. Typically, clients who are immobilized by skeletal traction are given stool softeners. Treating constipation with diet, increased fluids, and stool softeners is preferred to the administration of an enema. Placing the client on the bedpan will not encourage a bowel movement. Range-of-motion movements maintain joint mobility but do not stimulate peristalsis. (I, 7, M)

93. 4. Risk factors for postoperative pulmonary complications include malnourishment, which is indicated by the client's height and weight. Although keeping feelings inside can be problematic, it would not be considered a postoperative risk risk for pulmonary complications. The absence of dyspnea on exertion is not indicative of postoperative complications. The client's age does not necessarily place her at increased risk. (A, 3, M)

94. 2. Administering an antiemetic before beginning chemotherapy and then routinely around the clock helps prevent nausea and vomiting. Waiting until the client requests it may be too late because nausea is already present. (P, 8, Y)

95. 1. Greenish-colored amniotic fluid is caused by the passage of meconium, usually secondary to a fetal insult during labor. Meconium passage also may be related to an intact gastrointestinal system of the neonate, especially those neonates who are full term or of postdate gestational age. Amnioinfusion may be used to treat the condition and dilute the fluid. Cloudy-colored amniotic fluid is associated with an infection caused by bacteria or a sex-

ually transmitted disease. Severe yellow-colored fluid is associated with Rh incompatibility or erythroblastosis fetalis. (D, 3, O)

96. 1. The pH of 7.24 indicates that the client is acidotic. The carbon dioxide level is normal, but the HCO_3 level is decreased. These findings, in addition to the Kussmaul respirations, indicate that the client is in metabolic acidosis. (D, 10, M)

97. 3. Black, tarry stools indicate the presence of a slow upper gastrointestinal (GI) bleed. The longer the blood is in the system, the darker it becomes as the hemoglobin is broken down and iron is released. Vital sign changes, such as an increased pulse, are not evident with slow GI bleeds. Nausea and abdominal cramps can occur but are not definitive signs of GI bleeding. (E, 10, M)

98. 1. Most adolescents with Osgood-Schlatter disease are able to continue to exercise and use ice afterward. Ibuprofen also may be ordered. Because Osgood-Schlatter disease is self-limited, crutches or physical therapy is unnecessary, and the adolescent usually does not need to stop playing football. Only in severe cases would the adolescent have to stop playing sports. (I, 10, Y)

99. 3. Iron supplements will darken the stools. Iron supplements should not be taken on an empty stomach because they can cause gastric irritation. Iron is constipating, and a daily bulk-forming laxative should be started prophylactically. A straw should be used when taking liquid iron to avoid discoloring the teeth. (I, 8, M)

100. 1. A client with generalized anxiety disorder needs to learn cognitive and behavioral strategies to cope with anxiety appropriately. In doing so, the client's anxiety decreases and becomes more manageable. The client may need assertiveness training, reframing, and relaxation exercises to adaptively deal with anxiety. (I, 6, X)

101. 4. Deep-breathing helps prevent microatelectasis and pneumonitis and also helps force air and fluid out of the pleural space into the chest tubes. It does not decrease blood flow to the lungs or control the rate of air flow. The diaphragm is the major muscle of respiration; deep-breathing causes it to descend, thereby increasing the ventilating surface. (D, 9, M)

102. 2. When applying an Ace bandage to a leg, start at the distal end and move toward the trunk in order to support venous return. Tension should be kept even and not increased with each turn to prevent circulatory impairment. Overlapping each layer twice when wrapping can also impair circulation. The clips securing the bandage should be placed on the outer aspect of the leg to avoid creating a pressure point on the other leg. (E, 7, M)

103. 1. Spermicidal agents work by destroying the spermatozoa before they enter the cervix. In addition, some spermicides alter the vaginal pH to a strong acidic environment, which is not conducive to survival of spermatozoa. Spermicides do not prevent the spermatozoa from entering the uterus, but the diaphragm or condom is a barrier. (I, 3, O)

104. 4. A low dose of haloperidol (Haldol) is helpful in controlling dementia-induced paranoia and hallucinations. Methylphenidate (Ritalin) would be indicated if the primary symptoms were apathy and social withdrawal. Lorazepam (Ativan) would be ordered if the client were anxious and agitated. Nefazodone (Serzone) would be used if depression were prominent. (P, 8, X)

105. 1. Increased fremitus can be present in bacterial pneumonia, indicating the presence of pulmonary consolidation. Additional findings would include crackles, bronchial breath sounds, and dullness on percussion. Bilateral expiratory wheezing and resonance on percussion are not present in bacterial pneumonia. Vesicular breath sounds are normal and would not be an expected finding in bacterial pneumonia. (A, 10, M)

106. 3. Acute pancreatitis is very painful; management involves interventions for pain management. Although alcohol abuse is often implicated in pancreatitis, drug and alcohol counseling will be an individual consideration. Risk for injury and ineffective airway clearance are not typically associated with acute pancreatitis. (A, 9, M)

107. 3. Increased intracranial pressure can cause vomiting, particularly in children whose fontanels are closed. An infant with an open anterior fontanel may have less vomiting because the cranium can respond, expanding with increased intracranial pressure. The best course of action is to wait a few minutes and then refeed the child. Making the child NPO may not be helpful because this is not a gastrointestinal problem. Because this is an expected event, notifying the physician is not necessary. Antiemetic medications frequently make a client sleepy, making neurologic checks difficult to interpret. (I, 9, Y)

108. 1. The air is injected into the long-acting insulin first. Air is then injected into the short-acting insulin and the short-acting insulin is withdrawn. Then the long-acting insulin is withdrawn. It does matter which insulin is drawn up first, because the nurse does not want to contaminate the short-acting insulin with the long-acting insulin. A low-dose insulin syringe is used because a total of 5 units of insulin is needed. (P, 1, M)

109. 2. Solids should be introduced at about age 5 to 6 months. Full-term infants use up their prenatal iron stores within 4 to 6 months after birth. Cow's milk contains insufficient iron. (I, 3, Y)

110. 3. Diminished breath sounds during an acute asthma attack are a serious sign of airway obstruction, fatigue, and impending respiratory failure. Wheezing, coughing, and the production of sputum indicate the presence of airflow through the lungs and are less ominous symptoms. (A, 9, M)

111. 1. Cardiomyopathies can be treated medically for a period of time. The only other treatment for the disease is a heart transplant. (E, 9, M)

112. 1. Clients should use an electric razor, instead of a straight-edge razor, on any skin areas that are receiving radiation. The skin should be cleansed daily with a mild soap, not harsh antibacterials. Lotion should be removed from the skin before any treatment and then reapplied after the treatment. The radiated skin area needs to be kept clean, dry and open to air. (I, 7, M)

113. 3. A moderate amount of bloody drainage could indicate active bleeding. The priority action would be to apply pressure to the area and call for help. Assessing the airway or pulse or administering oxygen does not address the bleeding. (A, 9, M)

114. 4. Because valproic acid is associated with thrombocytopenia and hypofibrinogenemia, routine follow-up blood work would consist of monitoring platelet and fibrinogen levels for decreases. A complete blood count and serum electrolyte level are not necessary. Aspartate transaminase (AST), not alkaline phosphatase, is routinely monitored to evaluate for hepatic toxicity, a possible but rare effect of valproic acid. Valproic acid has no effect on cholesterol levels. (I, 8, Y)

115. 3. Bacterial conjunctivitis is very contagious. Attention should be paid to thorough handwashing, a major means of stopping the transmission of the disease. Closing the day care center for 1 week is not necessary because thorough handwashing will stop the spread of the infection. Keeping the children out for 48 hours is not necessary. A child may return to day care after being treated for 24 hours. Although the parents of each child should be told about the outbreak, doing so will not help to curtail or prevent the spread of the infection. (I, 2, Y)

116. 3. The client's mobility status is the best indicator of risk for development of a pressure sore. Nutritional and circulatory status are other factors that can contribute to pressure sore development, but immobility, even in the presence of adequate nutrition and circulation, is the leading cause of pressure sores. Disorientation can cause a client to neglect making needed position changes, but the underlying factor will be immobility. (E, 9, M)

117. 1. Ketosis is an adaptation to prolonged fasting or carbohydrate deprivation. The body takes partially broken-down fat fragments and combines them into ketone bodies, which the brain can then use for energy. Hypoglycemia is more likely to occur than hyperglycemia, although glucagon assists in preventing this from happening. Metabolic syndrome refers to syndrome X, which includes an abnormal lipid profile and a tendency to gain weight in the abdomen. Lactic acidosis is

a metabolic reaction that occurs when oxygen is reduced or not present. (D, 10, M)

118. 1. The nurse should stop and assess the client further. Encouraging the client to continue to move his lower extremities to avoid orthostatic hypotension is also appropriate. A chair should be available for the client to sit down. Obtaining the client's blood pressure and heart rate are important when exercising. These values can be used to predict when the oxygen demand becomes greater than the oxygen supply. Calling for help is not necessary for the complaint of midsternal burning. If the doctor has ordered nitroglycerin, the nurse can administer it; however, stopping the activity may restore the balance. (I, 10, M)

119. 2. The statement, "If I forget a dose, it's no big deal, I'll just take it when I remember it," indicates a knowledge deficit. The nurse should reinforce that the client should take dexamethasone (Decadron) as prescribed and at the same time each day. The drug has to be tapered off and cannot be stopped abruptly. The physician should be notified when the client is under additional stress (eg, infection, surgery, illness). The client can have an allergic reaction to inactive ingredients contained in dexamethasone. (E, 8, M)

120. 1. A child with moderate dehydration, described as a loss of 50 to 90 mL/kg of body fluid, would have oliguria, gray skin color, increased pulse rate, and poor skin elasticity. A child with severe dehydration, described as a loss of more than 100 mL/kg of body fluid, would have a rapid and thready pulse, very poor skin elasticity, and mottled skin color. A child with mild dehydration, described as a loss of less than 50 mL/kg of body fluid, would have pale skin color, decreased skin elasticity, decreased urine output, and normal or increased pulse rate. (A, 9, Y)

121. 1. Oropharyngeal candidiasis, or thrush, is the most common infection associated with the early symptomatic stages of HIV infection. Thrush is characterized by whitish-yellow patches in the mouth. Various other opportunistic diseases can occur in clients with HIV infection, but they tend to occur later, after the diagnosis of AIDS has been made. Dyspnea can be indicative of pneumonia, which is caused by a variety of infective organisms. Bloody diarrhea is indicative of cytomegalovirus infection. Hyperpigmented lesions are indicators of Kaposi's sarcoma. (A, 10, M)

122. 2. Postpartum infection is a leading cause of maternal mortality in the United States. Typical treatment for the condition is intravenous antibiotic therapy with drugs such as clindamycin or gentamicin, or both. Cultures of the lochia will also be obtained. The neonate can continue to breast-feed as long as the mother desires. A switch to bottle-feeding is not necessary. The uterus tends to be firm, with increased cramping to rid the uterus of the infection. The client should be encouraged to remain in bed in a Fowler's position to allow for drainage of the lochia. (I, 9, O)

123. 1. The mother needs further instructions when she says, "I should position the baby the same way for each feeding." This can contribute to sore nipples. The position should vary for each feeding to prevent repeated pressure on the same area each time. Grasping the entire areola and nipple will help to decrease the nipple soreness. Air drying the breasts and not using a hand pump will help to decrease the nipple soreness. (E, 9, O)

124. 1. During an acute attack of vertigo, it is best for the client to lie down in a darkened, quiet room and to avoid sudden position changes. A low-sodium diet may be helpful in decreasing the number of attacks, but it is not recommended during the attack. Headaches are not a component of the vertigo attack. Because vertigo is frequently accompanied by nausea and vomiting, the client will not want to eat or drink. Fluids are usually administered parenterally to maintain hydration and administer medications. (P, 10, M)

125. 3. The American Academy of Pediatrics recommends that all neonates should receive only formula or breast milk for the first 4 to 6 months of life. Cereal will not help the neonate sleep through the night and may result in allergies and other digestive disorders. (I, 3, O)

126. 2. Once the client has stated that he is allergic to a substance, the nurse would be negligent to ignore the client's statement and administer the substance. The nurse should check the chart for allergies and call the physician for an alternative antibiotic prescription. (D, 1, M)

127. 1. Jaundice that persists past the third or fourth day of life and pale, light-colored stools are associated with biliary atresia. Alkaline phosphatase levels will also be elevated. Surgical intervention is necessary to remove the blockage. Rh isoimmunization and ABO incompatibility are associated with neonatal anemia as the red blood cells are hemolyzed by the antibodies. Jaundice is seen within 24 hours after birth. Esophageal varices are associated with cirrhosis of the liver and large amounts of bleeding when the vessels rupture. The child will exhibit manifestations of anemia, such as pallor, and may experience hemorrhage and shock. (D, 9, O)

128. 1. Most parents find it especially difficult to allow a child who was unable to be normally active before corrective heart surgery to lead a normal and active life after surgery. These parents are less likely to be apprehensive about persuading the child of the need for rest, about postoperative complications, or about the child's siblings treating the child as a handicapped person. (P, 7, Y)

129. 3. After abdominal surgery, the reason for inserting a nasogastric tube is to *decompress* the gastrointestinal tract until peristaltic action returns. *Compression* may be used to control bleeding esophageal varices. *Lavage* is used to remove substances from the stomach or control bleeding. *Gavage* is used to provide enteral feedings. (A, 10, M)

130. 3. The most common long-term problem experienced by children with cleft palate repair is speech problems. These children frequently need speech therapy for a period of time. Hearing problems may occur as a result of chronic ear infections and the placement of myringotomy tubes. A poor self-concept may develop in any child. However, if a child with a cleft palate receives adequate parenting and support, this should not occur. Chronic sinus infections are more commonly associated with asthma, not with this defect. (I, 9, Y)

131. 2. Feeding solutions that have not been infused after hanging for 8 hours should be discarded because of the increased risk for bacterial growth. Sitting the client upright during the feeding helps prevent aspiration of the feeding. A gastric residual of 25 mL is considered acceptable. A gastric residual of 100 to 150 mL, or a residual greater than 100% of the previous hour's intake, indicates delayed emptying. The feeding solution should be at room or body temperature. (E, 9, M)

132. 3. Furosemide (Lasix) is a loop diuretic and inhibits the reabsorption of sodium and chloride from the proximal and distal renal tubules and the loop of Henle. Lasix promotes a sodium diuresis, resulting in a loss of potassium and serious electrolyte imbalances. Furosemide does not effect the BUN. (D, 10, M)

133. 3. Suctioning the respiratory tract for prolonged periods depletes the client's oxygen supply and causes hypoxia. It is recommended that each suctioning pass not exceed 15 seconds. (I, 7, M)

134. 2. The most appropriate action is to encourage the daughter to talk to her mother about the end-of-life issues first to reach a consensus or agreement. This is a family decision. Immediately informing the physician or preparing to remove the client from life support would be premature if the family is not in agreement. Although a copy of the living will should be on the client's chart, it is up to the daughter to show it to her mother. (I, 2, X)

135. 4. Contraindications for t-PA or alteplase recombinant (Activase) therapy include current active internal bleeding, 3 hours or longer since the onset of symptoms of a stroke, and severe hypertension. Age greater than 65 years is not a contraindication of the therapy. (I, 9, M)

136. 1. Extreme muscle weakness is present in both cholinergic crisis and myasthenic crisis. In cholinergic crisis, intravenous edrophonium chloride (Tensilon), a cholinergic agent, does not improve muscle weakness; in myasthenic crisis, it does. (E, 10, M)

137. 3. For a complete breech, the buttocks present, the feet and legs are flexed on the thighs, and the thighs are flexed on the abdomen. For a frank breech, the buttocks present with the hips flexed and the legs extended against the abdomen and chest. This is the most common type of breech presentation. For a compound breech, the buttocks present together with another part, such as a hand. This is a rare occurrence. For an incomplete breech, one or both feet or the knees extend below the buttocks. This can also be termed a single footling or double footling breech. (D, 10, O)

138. 1. It is important that the client understand that alcohol should be avoided for at least 1 year after an episode of hepatitis. Sexual intercourse does not need to be avoided, but the client should be instructed to use condoms until the HbsAG antigen measurement is negative. The client will need to restrict activity until liver function tests are normal; this will not occur within 1 to 2 weeks. Jaundice will subside as the client recovers; it is not a permanent condition. (E, 9, M)

139. 4. The individual who is bulimic is most commonly college-aged and female. She uses bingeing and purging to control her weight. Sometimes excessive exercise is also used. Use of regular exercise, calorie-counting, and occasional use of diet medication to maintain normal weight is not considered dysfunctional in our society. (I, 6, X)

140. 2. Swollen cervical lymph nodes are characteristic of early Hodgkin's disease. Difficulty breathing and swallowing are not early signs. The disease originates in the lymphatic system, not the liver. (A, 4, M)

141. 1. Parents are typically quick to notice changes in their infant's physical appearance. The removal of the infant's hair may be upsetting to them if they have not been told why it is being done. Hair is removed on the scalp at the site of needle insertion for intravenous therapy to provide better visualization and a smooth surface on which to attach tape to secure the needle. Sedatives are not ordinarily prescribed before intravenous fluid administration. Holding the infant is encouraged to provide comfort. (P, 8, Y)

142. 1. Abdominal pain can be a significant problem in acute pancreatitis. An expected outcome is to decrease or eliminate the pain the client is experiencing. Patterns of bowel elimination and liver function are not typically affected by the pancreatitis. The client should avoid all alcohol. (E, 10, M)

143. 3. The most appropriate initial response by the nurse would be to test the child's blood glucose level. These symptoms are consistent with hypoglycemia but could

also be used by the child to avoid participation in planned activities. Administering milk or fruit juice during a mild reaction may also be appropriate if testing cannot be done. Notifying the physician may be appropriate after the child's glucose level has been obtained and emergency treatment has been initiated if the child is experiencing hypoglycemia. Returning the child to previous activities is not appropriate until either testing or administering treatment has been done. (P, 9, Y)

144. 3. Normally, breasts are about the same size. They can vary in size before menstruation due to breast engorgement caused by hormonal changes. It is not necessary for a physician to check this slight change in breast size. The changes in breast size this client described are most likely caused by hormonal changes, not a benign cyst or normal growth and development. (I, 3, M)

145. 2. Traditional Chinese medicine describes health as the balance of yin and yang. It describes health as harmony between the mind, body, and soul. (E, 5, M)

146. 2. Before an IVP, the client should be assessed for allergies to iodine. Shellfish is a source of iodine, so people who are allergic to shellfish should not receive an IVP. Asking the client whether he or she has ever had an IVP before can help determine the degree of teaching needed before the procedure, but that is not the most important question. Neither the client's last bowel movement nor urinary incontinence has any relationship to an IVP. (P, 9, M)

147. 3. Progestin alone has no effect on breast milk or breast-feeding. Estrogen suppresses milk output. Testosterone is not given as an oral contraceptive. (A, 9, M)

148. 2. In this situation, the client has indicated that she is not willing to leave the abusive boyfriend because of potential economic concerns and other children in the household. The nurse should explain the cycle of abuse (ie, tension-building phase, battering incident, and honeymoon phase). The priority intervention is to assist the client to make concrete plans for the safety of herself and her children. The client should identify the safest, quickest routes out of the house and be able to identify where she will go once the cycle of violence escalates. Contacting a social worker at this time is not appropriate because the client is not ready to leave the abusive situation. The nurse can tell the client that these services are available, but it is up to the client to determine whether a referral is necessary. Telling the client that she shouldn't allow anyone to hit her or her children does not assist the client to make plans for her safety and the children's safety should the violence escalate. The client may have a flat affect or feel extreme humiliation from the abuse. The client may also be feeling that the abuse is her fault. When the

client is ready to leave the abusive situation and receive continuous counseling, efforts can be taken to increase her self-esteem and prevent additional violence. The client should be made aware of the available services in the community for women who are involved in abusive relationships. The location and phone numbers for available shelters should be provided to the client. Giving her a brochure related to the statistics about violence against women is not helpful and, if found by the abuser, may lead to further violence. (I, 6, O)

149. 2. The client who is taking sulfadiazine should be instructed to drink at least 8 glasses of water a day to prevent the development of crystalluria. Sulfadiazine should be taken on an empty stomach with a full glass of water. It does not affect the color of the urine and does not require that the client's urinary output be measured. (I, 8, M)

150. 3. The client is demonstrating loose associations. Therefore, the nurse needs to clarify the meaning of and the connection between ideas. The nurse's statement about Halloween makes the assumption that the client is talking about Halloween from the mention of black cats and black hats. Asking if the client has a black cat reinforces the client's loose association. The statement about time going faster ignores the client's statement entirely. (I, 6, X)

151. 1. MID results from multiple small blood clots in the brain. Therefore, the most critical factor is using anticoagulants to reduce the risk of more infarcts. Administering benzodiazepines such as lorazepam to decrease choreiform movements is associated with Huntington's disease. Although depression is common with MID, managing depression-related symptoms will not slow the progression of MID. Managing symptoms by increasing dopamine availability is appropriate for clients with Parkinson's disease. (P, 6, X)

152. 2. Checking the carotid artery pulse in a child during CPR provides information about perfusion of the brain. The brachial pulse is checked in an infant because the infant's short and often fat neck makes it difficult to palpate the carotid pulse. The femoral and radial arteries might indicate perfusion to the peripheral body sites, but the critical need is for adequate circulation to the brain. (I, 10, Y)

153. 2. Nephrotic syndrome is characterized by massive proteinuria caused by increased glomerular membrane permeability. Other symptoms include peripheral edema, hyperlipidemia, and hypoalbuminemia. Because of the edema, clients retain fluid and may gain weight. Hematuria is not a symptom related to the nephrotic syndrome. (A, 10, M)

154. 2. Because the child has a history of severe hypoxic episodes, having oxygen readily available at the bedside is most important. Should the child experience another hypoxic episode, oxygen could be administered easily and quickly. Although morphine causes peripheral dilation, which causes the blood to remain in the periphery, decreasing system volume, oxygen administration is the priority. Typically a child with tetralogy of Fallot with episodes of hypoxia does not require suctioning. (P, 9, Y)

155. 1. Although individuals differ, the most likely attitude of a Mexican American client is to bear pain stoically, to endure pain as a part of God's will, and to delay seeking treatment. (A, 5, M)

156. 1. When a client voids frequent, small amounts, the nurse should suspect that the client is retaining urine. Palpating for a distended bladder is the first assessment that the nurse should perform to verify this suspicion. Obtaining an order to catheterize for a residual urine may be appropriate as a follow-up activity. Obtaining a urine specimen for culture is not a first priority. The nurse would not encourage an increased fluid intake until further assessment of the situation is completed. (I, 10, M)

157. 3. It is appropriate for the client to be on a low-sodium diet to help decrease fluid retention. Dry skin and pruritus are common in renal failure. Lotions are used to relieve the dry skin, and antihistamines may be used to control itching; corticosteroids are not used. Pain is not a major problem in chronic renal failure, but any analgesics that are excreted by the kidneys must be avoided. It is not necessary to measure abdominal girth daily, because ascites is not a clinical problem in renal failure. (E, 10, M)

158. 1. The most frequent cause of respiratory distress in a toddler with no history of an illness is foreign body aspiration. The nurse should immediately begin abdominal thrusts. The nurse cannot wait for the ambulance or chest radiography report. Someone other than the nurse can check the oxygen saturation level. (I, 2, Y)

159. 4. The traction weights should be hanging freely to maintain pull. The child needs to be moved up in bed with the weights left untouched to continue countertraction. Then the nurse can determine whether blocks are necessary to maintain the child in the correct position. Raising the weights is inappropriate, because doing so interferes with countertraction. The physician does not need to be notified. The nurse can easily correct the problem by moving the child up in bed. (I, 9, Y)

160. 1. Children between ages 6 and 12 years have a slower growth rate than do younger children and adolescents. As a result, their food requirements are comparatively less. (I, 3, Y)

161. 4. Asking whether the client is thinking about killing herself is the most direct and therefore the best way to

assess suicidal risk. Knowing whether the client has recently watched movies on suicide and death, what the client thinks about suicide, or about previous suicides of family members will not tell the nurse whether the client herself is thinking about committing suicide right now. (A, 6, X)

162. 4. Proper nutrition before and during pregnancy helps to ensure that the uterus will be able to support the growth of a healthy placenta. If the placenta never develops properly, the fetus will fail to thrive and the infant may have a low birth weight. (A, 9, M)

163. 1. Return demonstrations are the best way to evaluate a person's ability to perform a skill. This technique enables the teacher to observe not only the learner's sequencing of steps of the procedure but also the learner's ability to perform the skill. (E, 8, Y)

164. 3. Ibuprofen (Motrin) should be taken with food or antacids to avoid the development of gastrointestinal distress. Tinnitus is not a side effect of ibuprofen; it is a sign of salicylate toxicity. There is no need to increase vitamin B_{12} intake. The complete blood count is not typically monitored monthly, although clients should be told to report signs of unusual bleeding, because ibuprofen can prolong bleeding time. (P, 8, M)

165. 4. When the client has a ruptured appendix, the nurse should document the surgical wound as an infected wound, because bacterial organisms are present in the wound and there are signs of infection (eg, inflammation, skin separation, purulent drainage). A clean wound is documented when no cavities have been entered and there is a low risk of infection. A clean-contaminated wound is recorded when a cavity such as the gastrointestinal, genitourinary, or respiratory tract has been entered under controlled conditions and there is greater risk for an infection than with a clean wound. A contaminated wound is when a traumatic, open, accidental wound has occurred or when a break in sterile technique occurred in a surgical wound and there is a high risk for infection. (A, 2, M)

166. 4. The nurse concludes that the staff member needs teaching about depression, specifically the biologic basis of major depression, when the staff member states the client has no reason to be depressed because "she really has it all." Major depression or endogenous depression is caused by alterations of neurotransmitters, primarily serotonin and norepinephrine. Genetics and hereditary also predispose an individual to develop depression. Therefore, there may not be an external cause or a reason for depression to develop. Depression that occurs from an external cause is known as reactive depression; it could be caused by a loss or a life stress. (D, 6, X)

167. 4. In asthma, the airways react to certain external and internal stimuli, including allergens, infections, exer-

cise, and emotions. Food allergens commonly associated with asthma include wheat, egg white, dairy products, citrus fruits, corn, and chocolate. (I, 7, Y)

168. 4. When administering an enema, the nurse should position the client in a left Sims' position. Placing the client in this position facilitates the flow of fluid into the rectum and colon. It also allows the client to flex the right leg forward, adequately exposing the rectal area. (I, 7, M)

169. 3. Risk factors for the development of pressure ulcers include poor nutrition, indicated by a decreased serum albumin level. According to the *Guidelines for Pressure Ulcers* published by the Agency for Healthcare Research and Quality, other risk factors include immobility, incontinence, and decreased sensation. A client who does not ambulate often can be repositioned frequently to prevent pressure ulcers. Having an indwelling Foley catheter does not normally increase the risk for development of a pressure ulcer unless pressure from the tubing impinges on urethral or other tissue. An elevated white blood cell count does not place a client at risk for pressure ulcers. (A, 9, M)

170. 2. Cerebral hypoxia is commonly associated with dizziness. The greatest risk of injury to a client with dizziness is a fall. Frequent rests and energy conservation measures should be included in the client's plan of care, but safety from falls is the greatest need. Checking the shower water temperature is not critical for this client, who will not be showering because of her fall risk. (P, 1, M)

171. 4. A characteristic finding in multiple myeloma is that of Bence Jones protein in the urine. Other laboratory findings include increased serum protein, hypercalcemia, anemia, thrombocytopenia, and hyperuricemia. Polycythemia vera is not found in multiple myeloma. (A, 10, M)

172. 2. Ephedrine is the drug of choice when the client's blood pressure falls after administration of an epidural anesthesia. Atropine sulfate is used with general anesthesia to dry the secretions and prevent aspiration. It is the antidote for poisoning by several species of mushrooms. It is also used to treat cardiovascular collapse from cholinergic drugs. Methylergonovine is used for severe postpartum hemorrhage. It does exert an antihypotensive effect. Oxytocin, a vasoconstrictor, is used to stimulate uterine contractions. It is not as effective as ephedrine to raise the client's blood pressure, and the client does not need additional uterine stimulation. (P, 8, O)

173. 3. Epidermoid cancer involving the larger bronchi is almost entirely associated with heavy cigarette smoking. The American Cancer Society reports that smoking is implicated in more than 80% of lung cancers in men and women. The prevalence of lung cancer is related to the duration and intensity of the smoking. The best intervention for nurses is to encourage smoking cessation. HEPA filters can reduce allergens, but they do not prevent lung cancer. Chest radiographs aid in detection of lung cancer but do not prevent it. Exposure to asbestos has been implicated as a risk factor, but cigarette smoking is the major risk factor. (I, 3, M)

174. 2. The client needs to take the prescribed medications for approximately 2 to 3 weeks before discontinuing precautions against infecting others. Effectiveness of the drug therapy is determined by negative sputum spears obtained on three consecutive days. Although results can vary among clients, the majority respond to therapy within 2 to 3 weeks. (I, 8, M)

175. 3. The statement, "My kids need me," indicates an improvement in the client's condition because the client is stating a reason for wanting to live rather than hopelessness and worthlessness. Stating that he will go to group when he has more energy conveys the presence of fatigue and withdrawal, key features of depression. Saying that he only thinks about killing himself at night indicates the presence of suicidal ideation and recurrent thoughts of death, and thus continued depression. Stating, "I want everyone to leave me alone," indicates the presence of withdrawal, depressed mood, and a lack of focus on present activities. (E, 6, X)

176. 3. Penicillin is the drug of choice to treat Lyme disease in pregnant women. Tetracycline and doxycycline are contraindicated during pregnancy because they have been associated with fetal defects. Gentamicin is not used for Lyme disease but is useful for treating gram-negative bacterial infections. It may be teratogenic to the fetus and is not used during pregnancy. (P, 8, O)

177. 2. Amnioinfusion is the addition of sterile fluid into the uterus to supplement or dilute amniotic fluid that is meconium stained. Amnioinfusion may be used when there is evidence of variable decelerations caused by cord compression, not early decelerations. Amnioinfusion is not used for short umbilical cords. There is no treatment for an abnormally short umbilical cord. Electronic fetal monitoring, not amnioinfusion, is used for multi-fetal pregnancies. (P, 9, O)

178. 1. As a chronic condition that affects many body systems, diabetes is a risk factor for surgery. The client's blood glucose levels and insulin requirements need to be closely monitored before and after surgery. Being sensitive to aspirin does not pose a risk for the client in surgery. Osteoarthritis is not a systemic condition and does not place the client at risk during surgery. Chronic low back pain is not a systemic condition that places the client at risk for surgery; however,

it can be exacerbated by positioning on the operating room table. (P, 9, M)

179. 4. Multiple drug regimens are used because the drugs have a synergistic effect. The drugs have different cell cycle lysis effects, different mechanisms of action, and different toxic side effects. They are usually given in combination to enhance therapy. Dosage is not affected by giving the drugs in combination. The second and third drugs do not increase the effectiveness of the first. It is not true that the first two drugs are toxic to cancer cells while the third drug promotes cell growth. (I, 10, M)

180. 2. The parents need to discuss their feelings with each other to begin the healing process. Avoiding discussing their feelings causes each one to become isolated and to grieve without support. Working long hours is detrimental to the grieving process; there is no time to come to terms with what has occurred. Acting as if nothing has happened is avoiding the issue. (D, 5, Y)

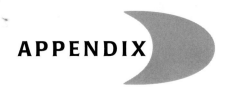

State and Territorial Boards of Nursing

For information about the dates, requirements, and specifics of writing the examination in your state, contact the appropriate state board of nursing. The address, telephone and fax numbers, and Website address (if available) are provided below.

(*Note*: This contact information is current as of April 2001)

Alabama Board of Nursing
RSA Plaza, Suite 250
770 Washington Avenue
Montgomery, Alabama 36130-3900

Phone: (334) 242-4060
FAX: (334) 242-4360
http://www.abn.state.al.us

Alaska Board of Nursing
Department of Commerce and
    Economic Development
Division of Occupational Licensing
3601 C Street, Suite 722
Anchorage, Alaska 99503

Phone: (907) 269-8161
FAX: (907)-269-8196
http://www.dced.state.ak.us/occ/pnur/htm

American Samoa Health Services
Regulatory Board
LBJ Tropical Medical Center
Pago Pago, American Samoa 96799

Phone: 011 (684) 633-1222
FAX: 011 (684) 633-1869
(No Web address as of April 2001)

Arizona State Board of Nursing
1651 East Morten Avenue, Suite 150
Phoenix, Arizona 85020

Phone: (602) 331-8111
FAX: (602) 906-9365
http://www.azboardofnursing.org

Arkansas State Board of Nursing
University Tower Building, Suite 800
1123 South University
Little Rock, Arkansas 72204

Phone: (501) 686-2700
FAX: (501) 686-2714
http://www.state.ar.us/nurse

California Board of Registered Nursing
400 R Street, Suite 4030
Sacramento, California 95814-6239

Phone: (916) 322-3350
FAX: (916) 327-4402
http://www.rn.ca.gov

California Board of Vocational Nurse
and Psychiatric Technician Examiners
2535 Capitol Oaks Drive, Suite 205
Sacramento, California 95833

Phone: (916) 263-7800
FAX: (916) 263-7859
http://www.bvnpt.ca.gov

Colorado Board of Nursing
1560 Broadway, Suite 880
Denver, Colorado 80202

Phone: (303) 894-2430
FAX: (303) 894-2821
http://www.dora.state.co.us/nursing

Connecticut Board of Examiners for
    Nursing
Division of Health Systems
    Regulations
410 Capitol Avenue, MS#12HSR
PO Box 340308
Hartford, Connecticut 06134-0328

Phone: (860) 509-7624
Fax: (860) 509-7553
http://www.state.ct.us/dph

Delaware Board of Nursing
Cannon Building, Suite 203
861 Silver Lake Boulevard
Dover, Delaware 19904

Phone: (302) 739-4522
FAX: (302) 739-2711
(No Web address as of April 2001)

District of Columbia Board of
    Nursing
Department of Health
825 North Capitol Street,
    NE—2nd Floor
Washington, DC 20002

Phone: (202) 442-4778
FAX: (202) 442-9431
(No Web address as of April 2001)

Florida Board of Nursing
4080 Woodcock Drive, Suite 202
Jacksonville, Florida 32207

Phone: (904) 858-6940
FAX: (904) 858-6964
*http://www.doh.state.fl.us/mqa/nursing/
rnhome.htm*

Georgia Board of Nursing
237 Coliseum Drive
Macon, Georgia 31217-3858

Phone: (912) 207-1640
FAX: (912) 207-1363
http://www.sos.state.ga.us/ebd-rn

Georgia State Board of Licensed
    Practical Nurses
327 Coliseum Drive
Macon, Georgia 31217-1640

Phone: (912) 207-1300
FAX: (912) 207-1363
http://www.sos.state.ga.us/ebd-lpn

Guam Board of Nurse Examiners
1304 East Sunset Boulevard
Barrgada, Guam 96913

Phone: 011 (671) 475-0251
FAX: 011 (671) 477-4733
(No Web address as of April 2001)

Hawaii Board of Nursing
PO Box 3469
Honolulu, Hawaii 96801

Phone: (808) 586-3000
FAX: (808) 586-2689
http://www.state.hi.us/dcca/pvoffline

Idaho Board of Nursing
PO Box 83720
280 North 8th Street, Suite 210
Boise, Idaho 83720-0061

Phone: (208) 334-3110
FAX: (208) 334-3262
http://www.id.us/ibn/ibnhome/htm

Illinois Department of Professional
    Regulation
James R. Thompson Center
100 West Randolph, Suite 9-300
Chicago, Illinois 60601

Phone: (312) 814-2715
FAX: (312) 814-3145
http://www.dpr.state.il.us

Indiana State Board of Nursing
Health Professions Bureau
402 West Washington Street,
    Room #041
Indianapolis, Indiana 46204

Phone: (317) 232-2960
FAX: (317) 232-4236
*http://www.state.in.us/hpb/boards/
    isbn*

Iowa Board of Nursing
River Point Business Park
400 SW 8th Street, Suite B
Des Moines, Iowa 50309-4685

Phone: (515) 281-3255
FAX: (515) 281-4825
*http://www.state.ic.us/government/
    nursing*

Kansas State Board of Nursing
Landon State Office Building
900 SW Jackson, Suite 551-S
Topeka, Kansas 66612-1230

Phone: (785) 296-4929
FAX: (785) 296-3929
http://www.ksbn.org

Kentucky Board of Nursing
312 Wittington Parkway,
    Suite 300
Louisville, Kentucky 40222-5172

Phone: (502) 329-7000
FAX: (502) 329-7011
http://www.kbn.state.ky.us

Louisiana State Board of Nursing
3510 North Causeway Boulevard,
    Suite 501
Metairie, Louisiana 70002

Phone: (504) 838-5332
FAX: (504) 838-5349
http://www.lsbn.state.la.us

Maine State Board of Nursing
158 State House Station
Augusta, Maine 04333-0158

Phone: (207) 287-1133
FAX: (207) 287-1149
http://www.state.me.us/nursingbd

Maryland Board of Nursing
4140 Patterson Avenue
Baltimore, Maryland 21215-2299

Phone: (410) 585-1900
FAX: (410) 358-3530
http://www.dhmh.state.md.us/mbn/

Massachusetts Board of Registration
    in Nursing
Commonwealth of Massachusetts
239 Causeway Street, Suite 500
Boston, Massachusetts 02114

Phone: (617) 727-9961
FAX: (617) 727-1630
http://www.state.ma.us/reg/boards/rn

Michigan CIS/Office of Health Services
Ottawa Towers North—4th Floor
611 West Ottawa
Lansing, Michigan 48933

Phone: (517) 373-9102
FAX: (517) 373-2179
http://www.cis.state.mi.us/bhser/genover.htm

Minnesota Board of Nursing
2829 University Avenue, SE, Suite 500
Minneapolis, Minnesota 55414

Phone: (612) 617-2270
FAX: (612) 617-2190
http://www.nursingboard.state.mn.us

Mississippi Board of Nursing
1935 Lakeland Drive, Suite B
Jackson, Mississippi 39216

Phone: (601) 987-4188
FAX: (601) 364-2352
http://www.msbn.state.ms.us/licenapps.htm

Missouri State Board of Nursing
3605 Missouri Boulevard
Jefferson City, Missouri 65102

Phone: (573) 751-0681
FAX: (573) 751-0075
http://www.ecodev.state.mo.us/pr/nursing

Montana State Board of Nursing
301 South Park
Helena, Montana 59620-0513

Phone: (406) 444-2071
FAX: (406) 444-7759
*http://www.com.state.mt.us/license/pol/
    index.htm*

Nebraska Health and Human
    Services System
Department of Regulation and
    Licensure
Nursing Section
301 Centennial Mall Square
Lincoln, Nebraska 68509-4986

Phone: (402) 471-4376
FAX: (402) 471-3577
http://www.hhs.state.ne.us/crl/nns.htm

Nevada State Board of Nursing
1755 East Plumb Lane, Suite 260
Reno, Nevada 89502

Phone: (775) 688-2620
FAX: (775) 688-2628
http://www.nursingboard.state.nv.us

New Hampshire Board of Nursing
78 Regional Drive - Building B
Concord, New Hampshire 03302-6527

Phone: (603) 271-2323
FAX: (603) 271-6605
http://www.state.nh.us/nursing

New Jersey Board of Nursing
PO Box 45010
Newark, New Jersey 07101

Phone: (973) 504-6586
FAX: (973) 648-3481
http://www.state.nj.us/lps/ca/medical.htm

New Mexico Board of Nursing
4206 Louisiana Boulevard, NE
Suite A
Albuquerque, New Mexico 87109

Phone: (505) 841-8340
FAX: (505) 841-8347
http://www.state.nm.us/clients/nursing

New York State Board of Nursing
Education Building
89 Washington Avenue
2nd Floor, West Wing
Albany, New York 12234

Phone: (518) 473-6999
FAX: (518) 474-3706
http://www.op.nysed.gov/nurse/htm

North Carolina Board of Nursing
3724 National Drive, Suite 201
Raleigh, North Carolina 27612

Phone: (919) 782-3211
FAX: (919) 781-9461
http://www.ncbon.com

North Dakota Board of Nursing
919 South 7th Street, Suite 504
Bismarck, North Dakota 58504-5881

Phone: (701) 328-9777
FAX: (701) 328-9785
http://www.ndbon.org

Northern Mariana Islands
Commonwealth Board of Nurse
    Examiners
Public Health Center
PO Box 1458
Saipan, MP 96950

Phone: 011 (670) 234-8950
FAX: 011 (670) 234-8930
(No Web address as of April 2001)

Ohio Board of Nursing
17 South High Street, Suite 400
Columbus, Ohio 43215-3413

Phone: (614) 466-3947
FAX: (614) 466-0388
http://www.state.oh.us/nur

Oklahoma Board of Nursing
2915 North Classen Boulevard,
    Suite 524
Oklahoma City, Oklahoma 73106

Phone: (405) 962-1800
FAX: (405) 962-1821
(No Web address as of April 2001)

Oregon State Board of Nursing
800 NE Oregon Street, Suite 465
Portland, Oregon 97232

Phone: (503) 731-4745
FAX: (503) 731-4755
http://www.osbn.state.or.us

Pennsylvania State Board of
    Nursing
124 Pine Street
Harrisburg, Pennsylvania 17101

Phone: (717) 783-7142
FAX: (717) 787-0822
*http://www.dos.state.pa.us/bpoa/nurbd/m
    ainpage.htm*

Commonwealth of Puerto Rico
Board of Nurse Examiners
Room 202, Stop 18
800 Roberto H. Todd Avenue
Santurce, Puerto Rico 00908

Phone: (787) 725-8161
FAX: (787) 725-7903
(No Web address as of April 2001)

Rhode Island Board of Nurse Regis-
    tration
and Nursing Education
105 Cannon Health Building
3 Capitol Hill, Room 104
Providence, Rhode Island 02908-5097

Phone: (401) 222-3855
Fax: (401) 222-2158
http://www.health.state.ri.us

South Carolina State Board of Nurs-
    ing
110 Centerview Drive, Suite 202
Columbia, South Carolina 29210

Phone: (803) 896-4550
FAX: (803) 896-4525
http://www.llr.state.sc.us/pol/nursing

South Dakota Board of Nursing
4300 South Louise Avenue, Suite C-1
Sioux Falls, South Dakota 57106-3124

Phone: (605) 362-2760
FAX: (605) 362-2768
http://www.state.sd.us/dcr/nursing

Tennessee State Board of Nursing
Cordell Hull Building, 1st Floor
426 Fifth Avenue North
Nashville, Tennessee 37247

Phone: (615) 532-5166
FAX: (615) 741-7899
*http://170.142.76.180/bmf-bin/bmf-
    proflist.pl*

Texas Board of Nurse Examiners
333 Guadalupe, Suite 3-460
Austin, Texas 78701

Phone: (512) 305-7400
FAX: (512) 305-7401
http://www.bne.state.tx.us

Texas Board of Vocational Nurse
    Examiners
William P. Hobby Building, Tower 3
333 Guadalupe, Suite 3-400
Austin, Texas 78701

Phone: (512) 305-8100
FAX: (512) 305-8101
http://www.bvne.state.tx.us

Utah State Board of Nursing
Heber M. Wells Building, 4th Floor
160 East 300 South
Salt Lake City, Utah 84111

Phone: (801) 530-6628
FAX: (801) 530-6511
http://www.commerce.state.ut.us

Vermont State Board of Nursing
109 State Street
Montpelier, Vermont 05609-1106

Phone: (802) 828-2396
FAX: (802) 828-2484
http://vtprofessionals.org/nurses

Virgin Islands Board of Nurse Licen-
    sure
PO Box 4247, Veterans Drive Station
St. Thomas, US Virgin Islands 00803

Phone: (340) 776-7397
FAX: (340) 777-4003
(No Web address as of April 2001)

Virginia Board of nursing
6606 West Broad Street, 4th Floor
Richmond, Virginia 23230-1717

Phone: (804) 662-9909
FAX: (804) 662-9512
http://www.dhp.state.va.us

Washington State Nursing Care
Quality Assurance Commission
Department of Health
1300 Quince Street, SE
Olympia, Washington 98504-7864

Phone: (360) 236-4740
FAX: (360) 236-4738
http://www.doh.wa.gov/nursing

West Virginia Board of Examiners
for Registered Professional Nurses
101 Dee Drive
Charleston, West Virginia 25311-1620

Phone: (304) 558-3596
FAX: (304) 558-3666
http://www.state.wv.us/nurses/rn

West Virginia State Board of Examiners
for Licensed Practical Nurses
101 Dee Drive
Charleston, West Virginia 25311-1620

Phone: (304) 558-3572
FAX: (304) 558-4367
http://www.lpnboard.state.wv.us

Wisconsin Department of Regulation and Licensing
1400 Washington Avenue
PO Box 8935
Madison, Wisconsin 53708-8935

Phone: (608) 266-0145
FAX: (608) 261-7083
http://www.drl.state.wi.us

Wyoming State Board of Nursing
2020 Carey Avenue, Suite 110
Cheyenne, Wyoming 82002

Phone: (307) 777-7601
FAX: (307) 777-3519
http://nursing.state.wy.us

Lippincott's Review Series
makes study time
SWING!

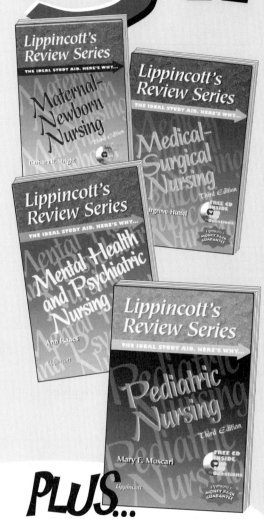

Lippincott's Review Series combines a comprehensive outline format and extensive self-testing to make learning complex concepts easy and fun! Whether you're preparing for the NCLEX or just looking for a review of nursing essentials, **Lippincott's Review Series** is a sure hit.

- **Nursing Alert and Key Concept icons** highlight critical information.
- **Categorized Questions** tie each question to the NCLEX exam.
- **Chapter study questions** offer fun ways to apply your knowledge.
- **Comprehensive examination** evaluates competency for each subject area.
- **Rationale for responses** reveals the how and why behind every answer.

THE NEW EDITIONS INCLUDE NEW LEARNING FEATURES:
- Nursing Process Overview
- Drug Charts
- Client and Family Teaching Boxes
- Development Boxes in the Pediatric review
- FREE CD-ROM with hundreds of NCLEX-style questions

PLUS...

Lippincott's Review Series is GUARANTEED TO WORK!

MONEY-BACK GUARANTEE
We're so confident that **Lippincott's Review Series** will enhance your study skills and test performance, we will refund your money if you fail to pass the NCLEX exam.

Check out the other Lippincott's Review Series chart-toppers...
Community and Home Health Nursing
Critical Care Nursing
Fluids and Electrolytes, 2/E
Pharmacology
Pathophysiology, 2/E

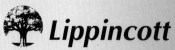

Lippincott
The Roots of Nursing Knowledge

CO/CP G243-01

Available at your bookstore or call TOLL-FREE
800•638•3030
or visit our Websites at www.LWW.com or www.nursingcenter.com

INSTALLATION INSTRUCTIONS

CD-ROM for Lippincott s Review for NCLEX-RN
7th edition

SYSTEM REQUIREMENTS

Windows 95 or higher

486/66 Processor or higher

16 MB RAM

6 MB Free Hard Disk Space

CD-ROM Drive

640 x 480 Color Monitor or higher

256 Colors or higher

INSTALLATION

Insert the CD-ROM into your CD-ROM drive.

Click on the **Start** button, and then click **Run**.

At the command line, type **D:\setup.exe.** (*Note*: The letter D represents the CD-ROM drive. If your
drive is designated by a different letter, use your drive letter instead.)

Click **OK**.

Follow the online instructions.

TECHNICAL SUPPORT

If you experience difficulty viewing the text, it may be the result of the color settings on your system.
Should you need assistance or have any questions regarding the use or content of this CD-ROM, please
contact our Technical Support department by telephone at 800-638-3030 or 410-528-4010, by fax at
410-528-4422, or by e-mail at *techsupp@LWW.com*. Technical support is available from 8:30 AM to
5:00 PM (EST), Monday through Friday.